SEDATION
A Guide to Patient Management

STANLEY F. MALAMED, D.D.S.
Professor and Chair
Section of Anesthesia and Medicine
University of Southern California School of Dentistry
Los Angeles, California

CHRISTINE L. QUINN, D.D.S.
University of California
Los Angeles, California

Health Sciences Center
School of Dentistry
Los Angeles, California

Author of *Chapter 37, The Geriatric Patient,* and
Chapter 39, The Physically Compromised Patient

THIRD EDITION
with **266** *illustrations*

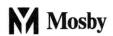 Mosby

A Harcourt Health Sciences Company
St. Louis   Philadelphia   London   Sydney   Toronto

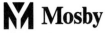

Executive Editor: Linda L. Duncan
Developmental Editor: Melba Steube
Project Manager: Carol Sullivan Weis
Senior Production Editor: Pat Joiner
Designer: Sheilah Barrett
Manufacturing Supervisor: Karen Lewis
Cover art: Celia Johnson

THIRD EDITION

Printed in the United States of America

Mosby, Inc.
11830 Westline Industrial Drive
St. Louis, Missouri 63146

Library of Congress Cataloging-in-Publication Data
Malamed, Stanley F.
      Sedation : a guide to patient management / Stanley F. Malamed : chapter 37, the geriatric patient and chapter 39, The physically compromised patient by Christine L. Quinn.—3rd ed.
      p. cm.
      Includes bibliographical references and index.
      ISBN 0-8151-5736-3
      1. Sedatives.   2. Anesthesia in dentistry.   I. Quinn, Christine L.
II. Title.
      [DNLM: 1. Anesthesia, Dental.   2. Anxiety—prevention & control.   3. Pain—prevention & control.   WO 460 M236 1994]
RK512.S44M35 1994
617.9′676—dc20
DNLM/DLC   94-32507

01 02 03 04 / 9 8 7 6

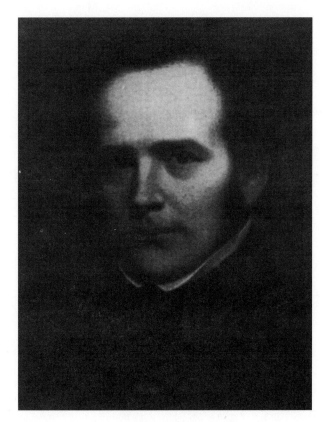

Horace Wells (1815-1848)

To **Francis Foldes, M.D.** for having instilled in me an everlasting fascination in the art and science of anesthesiology, and to **Norman Trieger, D.M.D., M.D.,** and **Thomas Pallasch, D.D.S., M.S.** for having made possible a career that has provided me with continual challenge, interest, and enjoyment, one that I would change for no other, and to **Horace Wells, D.D.S.** who 150 years ago discovered anesthesia

Preface

Hartford Connecticut, December 10, 1844 ... One hundred and fifty years ago Samuel Cooley, a clerk in a retail store, ran around a stage in an intoxicated state, little realizing the major role he was playing in forever altering the degree of pain and suffering that patients throughout the world would experience during surgery. Cooley had come to attend a popular science lecture in which advances in science were demonstrated. One demonstration was of the intoxicating effects of "laughing gas," which Cooley volunteered to inhale. Also in attendance on that fateful evening was Horace Wells, a local dentist who, on seeing Cooley injure his leg but continue to run about as though nothing had happened, considered there might be a clinical application for this "laughing gas." On the following day, December 11, 1844, nitrous oxide ("laughing gas") was administered to Dr. Horace Wells, rendering him unconscious and able to have a wisdom tooth extracted without any awareness of pain.

The world had forever been changed.

In this year of the sesquicentennial celebration of the discovery of anesthesia so much is taken for granted. Local anesthetics are administered to patients when a surgical procedure might be ever so slightly painful. *Yet in 1844 these drugs did not exist.* When fearful patients require treatment a variety of techniques are available—intravenous conscious sedation; intramuscular sedation; oral, rectal, transmucosal, and intranasal sedation; and general anesthesia. These techniques of drug administration were not available in 1844. Drugs are available that are able to provide relief from extreme anxiety and fear while the patient retains consciousness; yet these drugs provide amnesia (a lack of memory) of the entire procedure. These drugs did not exist in 1844.

No longer does a patient about to undergo dental or surgical procedures face that prospect with utter hopelessness and despair. Dentistry has long recognized that many persons are frightened of the dental experience and to its credit has taken steps to prepare the dental professional to recognize and manage these patients. In its approach to the management of pain and anxiety, the dental profession has remained in the forefront of all the health professions.

Publication of the *Guidelines for the Teaching of Pain and Anxiety Control and the Management of Related Complications* (ADA, 1979) put forth a cohesive document aimed at providing well-constructed standards for teaching the future generations of dental students and dentists safe and effective techniques of managing pain and anxiety. A dentist graduating from a dental school in the United States in the past 20 years has received training (albeit to varying degrees of clinical proficiency) in these important areas. For phobic patients seeking dentists able to manage their dental fears, the search is usually short. More and more dentists promote their ability and desire to "cater to cowards." The public has been the ultimate beneficiary of that chance encounter between Mr. Samuel Cooley and Dr. Horace Wells in December 1844.

This third edition of *Sedation: A Guide to Patient Management* is, as were its predecessors, designed for the student of medicine or dentistry on a doctoral, postdoctoral, or continuing education level. It is meant to be comprehensive, providing basic concepts needed to fully understand the drugs and techniques and how they work, step-by-step descriptions of the various techniques, and a look at potential complications and emergencies that might arise. More than anything else, this edition of *Sedation* is designed to be used with a course in sedation that provides for the clinical management of patients in a controlled (supervised) environment. Only through this type of program can the techniques described in this book be used in a dental or medical practice in a safe and effective manner.

Changes have occurred in several areas in this third edition. A new chapter (Chapter 10) has been added; this chapter introduces alternative routes of drug administration that have received considerable scrutiny over the past several years. These routes—sublingual, transdermal, and intranasal—may have a place in the dental armamentarium for patient management. Monitoring continues to be an area of ever-increasing importance. The pulse oximeter was introduced in the second edition (1989) as a valuable addition to patient safety during general anesthesia, deep sedation, and parenteral conscious sedation. Its importance continues to grow. In addition, the next generation of monitoring has appeared—capnography. Although not yet considered as essential during conscious sedation, capnography has made significant inroads into monitoring during deep sedation and general anesthesia. And drugs—midazolam has become a part of the everyday armamentarium for IV and IM sedation just 8 years after its clinical introduction in the United States; flumazenil, a benzodiazepine antagonist, joins naloxone in providing an "umbrella of safety" as a means of reversing the clinical actions of previously administered drugs; and propofol, the most recent addition to the armamentarium of IV drugs, adds an entirely new dimension to outpatient anesthesia. Rapid-acting, short-acting propofol appears to be the most nearly ideal drug for short surgical procedures on ambulatory dental and medical patients.

As stated in the previous editions of *Sedation,* the ultimate aim of this book remains the same: to help dental patients, to enable them to receive the quality of care they truly deserve, and to enable them to do receive care in an atmosphere of relaxation, mental ease, and safety.

In November 1994, the American Dental Association recognized dental anesthesiology as a dental specialty.

How times have changed in 150 years!

STANLEY F. MALAMED

Acknowledgments

I would like to thank many persons for their assistance, encouragement, and in many cases, patience during the time it has taken to produce not only the original manuscript for *Sedation,* but also this third edition. I would especially like to thank Norman Goldberg for the excellent photography, and Jerry Drucker and Dr. Diane Conly for their assistance as models. Thanks are also due to John Glueckert, research librarian at the University of Southern California School of Dentistry, for his assistance in locating many obscure references.

Dr. Christine L. Quinn has again co-authored two chapters in this edition: the geriatric patient (Chapter 37) and the physically compromised patient (Chapter 39). Her knowledge and expertise in these areas adds much to these chapters.

In addition, I must thank my friends at Mosby–Year Book: Linda Duncan and Melba Steube. Their not-so-gentle reminders provided me on occasion with a much-needed stimulus.

Finally, I thank my computer, for having made this job somewhat more enjoyable and at times more challenging (where did Chapters 15 to 21 go?) to complete and for making life more bearable for the entire Malamed family.

Note

The treatment modalities and the indications and dosages of all drugs in *Sedation: A Guide to Patient Management* have been recommended in the medical literature. Unless specifically indicated, drug dosages are those recommended for adult patients.

The package insert for each drug should be consulted for use and dosages as approved by the FDA. Because standards of usage change, it is advisable to keep abreast of revised recommendations, particularly those concerning new drugs.

Contents

SECTION ONE

Introduction

CHAPTER 1

Introduction

The words "fear," "anxiety," and "pain" have long been associated with dentistry. Throughout the years the public has thought, and has been taught, that dentistry hurts. The public's image of the dentist has borne this out. Surveys have consistently shown that although dentistry as a profession is highly respected by the public,[1] the image of the dentist as one who enjoys hurting people is still retained by a majority of persons. In a recent survey of the most common fears of adults, fear of going to the dentist ranked second only to the fear of public speaking (Table 1-1).[2]

Is the image of the dentist justified? Of course not; indeed, it never truly was. Unfortunately, however, our predecessors in dentistry did not have at their disposal the array of equipment and medications for the management of pain and anxiety that are available today. Yet history has recorded that members of the dental profession have consistently been in the forefront in the research and development of new techniques and medications for the management of pain and anxiety. Horace Wells (a dentist) and William T.G. Morton (dentist and physician), in the 1840s, were the founders of anesthesia and the first to employ nitrous oxide (N_2O) (Wells) and ether (Morton) for the management of pain during surgical procedures.[3] Prior to this time dental care consisted to a great degree of the removal of root tips without any form of anesthetic, except for alcohol, which was frequently used preoperatively (and perhaps still is).[4] Surgery prior to the introduction of anesthesia consisted almost exclusively of the amputation of limbs that had become infected and gangrenous.[3] As in dentistry, these procedures were of necessity performed without the aid of any form of anesthesia.

In the area of intravenous (IV) medications and outpatient general anesthesia the dental profession again led the way. With the introduction of the IV barbiturates in the late 1930s, Victor Goldman and Stanley Drummond-Jackson in England and Adrian Hubbell in the United States pioneered the techniques of IV general anesthesia for ambulatory oral surgery patients.[5,6] It was not until the 1970s that the medical profession, realizing the merits of short-stay surgery, began to use these same techniques.[7]

Dentistry has indeed been at the forefront in the fight against pain. In the 1990s virtually all dental procedures may be successfully completed in the absence of any patient discomfort through the administration of local anesthetics and/or the use of other techniques (such as electronic dental anesthesia). However, the dental consumers, our patients, may not be aware of this, or they may consider that the injection of a local anesthetic is the most traumatic part of the entire dental procedure. How then are we to manage these patients?

As dentistry developed, dentists gained the reputation of being "tooth doctors." Dental education was for many years predicated on the fact that the dentist was responsible for the oral cavity of the patient, and dental school curricula illustrated this. Early dentists were trained to manage their patients' dental requirements only. The possible interaction

Table 1-1. Our most common fears

Fear	Percentage
Public speaking	27
Going to dentist	21
Heights	20
Mice	12
Flying	9
Other/no fears	11

From *Dental Health Advisor,* Spring 1987 (survey of 1000 adults).

between dental treatment and the overall health of the patient was either unknown or was ignored.

As medicine became more sophisticated, it became very apparent that dental care could and indeed did have a significant impact on the overall health of patients. Dental schools amended their curricula, adding courses in medicine and physical evaluation.[8] The dentist became even more alert to the fact that treatment in the oral cavity could profoundly influence a patient's well-being and conversely that the patient's health could significantly affect the type of dental treatment offered. The use of the patient-completed medical history questionnaire became a standard in the 1950s, followed by the routine recording of vital signs (1970s). The direction today, in the 1990s, is toward more in-depth training in physical evaluation, including heart and lung auscultation.

Unfortunately, until the late 1960s and early 1970s few dental schools in the United States (the University of Pittsburgh and Loma Linda University being notable exceptions) provided the graduate dentist with a thorough background in the recognition and management of fear and anxiety. Until recently, the dentist could only treat the teeth of a patient who was known to be healthy enough (physically) to withstand the stresses of dental therapy. The "mind" of the patient (their psychological attitude toward dentistry) was almost entirely ignored. The absence, at all levels of education, of training programs in the recognition and management of anxiety implied that anxiety did not exist or that it was of little or no importance. The doctor would treat the patient as well as he or she could, given the clinical circumstances, and quite often the quality of the dentistry demonstrated the difficulty in patient management. General anesthesia was always available for those few patients who were absolutely unable to tolerate treatment; however, the most common type of dentistry performed under general anesthesia was extractions. For conservative dental care little or no thought was given to the patient's state of mind during treatment.

Under the sponsorship of three organizations—the American Dental Association (ADA), the American Dental Society of Anesthesiology (ADSA), and the American Association of Dental Schools (AADS)—four "Workshops on Pain Control" were held (1964, 1965, 1971, and 1977). From these workshops came the "Guidelines for Teaching the Comprehensive Control of Pain and Anxiety in Dentistry," which established the outline for three levels of training in various techniques of pain and anxiety control: the undergraduate dental program, the graduate (residency) program, and a continuing education program.[9]

The 1970s saw the establishment by dental schools of viable programs in the area of sedation. Although the level of training still varies considerably from school to school, the dental student today receives, at a minimum, a solid background in the subject of anxiety and fear of dentistry and the techniques available in their management. Dentists today are aware that many patients are somewhat afraid of receiving dental treatment. This awareness is the first step required for the effective treatment of the patient's fears and anxieties. Add to this the almost universal availability of one or more techniques of sedation (usually iatrosedation, oral sedation, and inhalation sedation) and it becomes possible for the dentist to effectively and safely manage virtually all patients seeking dental care.

In the past few years, however, it has also become quite obvious that many dentists (and physicians) who had not received training in the use of these techniques prior to graduation from school have begun to use these techniques in their private practices without the benefit of appropriate postgraduate training programs. In too many cases this has resulted in death or serious injury to patients.[10] Lawmakers in many states have taken action to halt this trend, either by prohibiting dentists from using certain techniques of sedation or anesthesia or by requiring a special permit or license if the doctor is to use the techniques.[11] The Dentists Insurance Company (TDIC) in California published a retrospective study of deaths related to drug administration in dental practice.[12] Three major areas of fault were found:

1. Inadequate preoperative evaluation of the patient
2. Inadequate monitoring during the procedure
3. Lack of knowledge of the pharmacology of the drug(s) being administered

Whenever medications are administered to a patient, it is imperative that the doctor be fully cognizant of these three areas, as well as of any others that are involved in the ultimate safety of a drug technique. Failure to adequately prepare ourselves to administer medications to patients safely can only result in these techniques being taken forcibly away from us.

One of my goals in preparing this book was to provide the doctor with appropriate background information concerning the various techniques of sedation that are most frequently employed in the typical outpatient setting. As was previously stated in the Preface, this book is not intended to be used as a sole source of knowledge concerning these techniques. Only when used in conjunction with a course of study that involves using these procedures in the actual management of patients can a doctor become truly capable of safely administering the medications discussed in this book. Of greater importance perhaps is the level of training required for each of these techniques. At the end of the chapter or section on each technique, recommendations are presented that outline the level of training deemed appropriate for the doctor to be able to employ the technique in a safe and effective manner.

• • •

This book is divided into eight sections. Section One is introductory, presenting an outline of the "problem" that all members of the dental profession face: the problem of fear and anxiety, which is confronted by dental practitioners throughout the world on a daily basis.

Section Two introduces the concept of sedation and of the spectrum of pain and anxiety control. The dental and medical professions have at their disposal a wide array of techniques that can be employed in patient management. The availability of these to the dentist will increase the possibility of a successful outcome of treatment. Also included in Section Two are chapters on preoperative physical evaluation of the patient and monitoring of the patient during the various sedative procedures. The section ends with an introduction to two nondrug techniques of sedation: iatrosedation and hypnosis. These techniques are extremely valuable in the management of virtually all patients.

Sections Three, Four, and Five present an in-depth look at the subject of pharmacosedation. Section Three presents discussions of three techniques of sedation: oral, rectal, and intramuscular (IM). Considerable attention is devoted to the clinical pharmacology of the drugs discussed in an effort to discourage the use of agents that might be deemed inappropriate for certain procedures and to encourage the use of other medications that have proved to be safe and effective.

Sections Four and Five are each devoted to one technique: Section Four to inhalation sedation, and Section Five to intravenous (IV) sedation. Because I believe that these are the two most effective and, when used properly, the safest of all sedative procedures, I have presented a complete and up-to-date discussion of these valuable techniques. It cannot be overemphasized that in the absence of considerable supervised clinical experience the reading of these sections does not constitute preparation adequate to permit anyone to safely use these techniques of drug administration.

Section Six provides the reader with an introduction to general anesthesia, another important method of pain and anxiety control. Training in this subject requires a considerably greater length of time: a minimum of 1 year (and preferably 2 years) of full-time training.

Section Seven addresses the subject of emergencies in the dental office. Preparation for and management of emergencies are reviewed in this section. The most important aspect of training for emergencies—prevention—has been the subject of all of the chapters that precede this section. Although it may appear to some that the subject of emergencies and complications takes up an inappropriately large part of this book, it is my belief that this subject can never be discussed too often or too thoroughly. When the techniques discussed in this book are used properly, the number of emergencies and complications that do occur will be minimal. Although a lack of complications is the goal, success at this goal does have inherent risks: the doctor may become complacent with a technique that works "all the time" and thereby become a little less vigilant. It is at times like this that problems do occur. If the doctor is aware of the possible complications associated with a procedure, then these may be recognized and managed more effectively when and if they do develop.

Finally, Section Eight discusses four groups of "special" patients. Management of the pediatric, geriatric, medically compromised, and disabled patient requires a degree of knowledge and training on the part of the doctor and dental staff beyond that needed for the typical patient. These four groups of patients are not uncommon in the dental office and, unfortunately, present all too many doctors with significant problems in management. It is important for the doctor to be aware of the subtle changes in treatment protocol that may be required in the management of these patients. A doctor knowledgeable in the management of these patients will have available a greatly expanded pool of potential patients.

• • •

As will be mentioned throughout this textbook, no single technique of sedation can ever be considered a panacea. Failures are to be expected on occasion with every technique of sedation. Though failures are frustrating for the doctor, they must be considered an unavoidable aspect of any sedation procedure, for as long as some patients retain even the slightest degree of consciousness, they will respond inappropriately to stimulation. It is only with the loss of consciousness (general anesthesia) that a significantly greater success rate can be expected; however, most doctors (both dentists and physicians) do not have the training necessary to employ techniques in which unconsciousness is produced purposefully. As the doctor becomes more experienced with the techniques of sedation, failure rates will decrease. Patients will sense a doctor's unease and unfamiliarity with a "new" technique, and this uncertainty is transferred to the patient, thereby decreasing the chance of a successful result. With increased experience, the doctor will become increasingly comfortable with the procedure and so too will the patient, thereby increasing the rate of success.

The greater the number of different sedation techniques that the doctor has available for patient management, the greater the probability of a successful result. The only way to become successful with these techniques is to receive appropriate supervised training. Acceptable courses are listed semiannually in the *Journal of the American Dental Association*[13] and bimonthly in *Anesthesia Progress.*

REFERENCES

1. Professions with prestige (National Opinion Research Center report on job status), *Washington Post* 115:p WH5, March 31, 1991.
2. *Dental Health Advisor,* Spring, 1987.
3. Bankoff G: *The conquest of pain: the story of anesthesia.* London, 1946, MacDonald.
4. Sykes WS: *Essays on the first hundred years of anaesthesia.* Edinburgh, 1960, E & S Livingstone.
5. Drummond-Jackson SL: Evipal anesthesia in dentistry, *Dental Cosmos* 77:130, 1935.
6. Hubbell AO, Adams RC: Intravenous anesthesia for dental surgery with sodium ethyl (1-methylbutyl) thiobarbituric acid, *JADA* 27:1186, 1940.
7. White PF: Outpatient anesthesia—an overview. In White PF, ed: *Outpatient anesthesia.* New York, 1990, Churchill Livingstone.
8. Curricular guide for physical evaluation, *J Dent Educ* 48:219, 1984.
9. Council on Dental Education: American Dental Association, Guidelines for teaching the comprehensive control of pain and anxiety in dentistry, *J Dent Educ* 36:62, 1972.
10. Newcomer K: "Dentist waited outside while patient died," *Rocky Mountain News,* August 4, 1992.
11. Department of State Government Affairs, American Dental Association, 1992.
12. de Julien LF: Causes of severe morbidity/mortality cases, *J Calif Dent Assoc* 11:45, 1983.
13. Council on Dental Education, Continuing education course list for January–June, 1994, Chicago, American Dental Association.

CHAPTER 2

Pain and anxiety in dentistry

August 14, 1984

Dear Dr. Malamed: I am writing to you in hope that you can give me some information on dentists who use conscious sedation in their practice. In reading the Los Angeles Times article June 4, 1984 . . . I finally found the right course I could take to get my teeth worked on.

For the last 5 years I have been trying to find a solution to my problem. I have an overwhelming fear of dentists and a very sensitive mouth. When I read the article and found out about various types of anesthesia that are available to dentists, I found light at the end of the tunnel. I do not, however, know how to find these dentists who are trained in the field. . . . I would appreciate any help you can give me.

Thank you

The writer of the preceding letter is unusual, not because she is afraid of dentistry, but because she was able to write this letter in an effort to seek help for herself.

In the United States it is estimated that somewhere between 6% and 14% of the population (14,000,000 to 34,000,000 people) voluntarily avoid seeking dental care because of their fear of dentistry.[1] These individuals will put off treatment until they are in such pain that home remedies are no longer effective. They are categorized as severe anxiety patients and represent a dual problem in management, for the doctor will have to treat both the patients' acute dental problem and their psychological emergency. I once gave a talk entitled "The Pain of Fear."[2] This title aptly describes the dilemma faced by the acutely fearful dental patient: fear of pain keeps the patient from seeking needed dental care until the pain, which is exacerbated by this fear, ultimately forces the patient to the dental office. Such patients present the doctor with a significant problem. Attempts to treat these patients without acknowledging their fear usually lead to great frustration and increased stress

for the doctor as well as an increased level of fear for the patient.[3] Kahn et al.[4] surveyed a group of dentists and reported that 57% of those responding stated that the most stressful factor in their dental practices was the "difficult patient."

Much more typically seen than the person with severe anxiety—the vast majority of those seen in the dental office—is the patient who does not harbor any irrational fears* of dental treatment. However, this patient does experience a degree of heightened anxiety as the scheduled dental appointment nears. This apprehension over dental treatment does not prevent the patient from appearing in the office, for this patient is genuinely concerned about maintaining oral hygiene and does not want to experience the pain of a toothache. This patient will be categorized

---

*The terms *fear* and *anxiety* are often used interchangeably, as is the case in this text. However, there is a distinction to be made between them.

Fear tends to be a short-lived phenomenon, disappearing when the external danger or threat passes. It includes a feeling that something terrible is going to happen; physiologic changes including tachycardia, profuse perspiration, and hyperventilation; and overt behavioral movements such as becoming jittery or shaking. These clinical manifestations comprise what is called the "fight or flight" response.[1,5]

Anxiety, in contrast, is not likely to be dispelled as quickly. The emotional response is usually an internal one and is not readily recognized. Weiss and English[6] define anxiety as "a specific unpleasurable state of tension which indicates the presence of some danger to the organism." Anxiety tends to be a learned response, acquired from personal experience or secondarily through the experiences of others. Anxiety arises from anticipation of an event, the outcome of which is unknown.[7]

Milgrom[1] states that a major difference between fear and anxiety is the immediacy of the threat to the person. A response to an immediate threat is fear. Properly employed in the dental situation the term *anxiety* is used to connote reactions that develop in anticipation of or at the thought of dentistry, while *fear* refers to the reaction occurring at the dental office.

as having low to moderate anxiety and will appear on a regular basis for scheduled dental care because such a patient knows that avoiding needed dental treatment will only lead to more significant (and painful) problems later. However, while in the dental office this patient has somewhat sweaty palms and a more rapid heartbeat, and would admittedly much rather be somewhere else.

In 1972 the Ad Hoc Committee on Research and Faculty Training in Pain Control in Dentistry[8] reported that "the threat and fear of pain constitutes one of the great obstacles to the acceptance of dental services in the United States, considered by some to be greater than the financial barrier." With the arrival of prepaid dental care and health insurance coverage for many millions of Americans, it has become quite obvious that it is not only the financial aspect of dental care that prevents patients from seeking treatment.

If this is so, then we in the dental profession have been neglecting a very important aspect of the management of our patients. With the great technical advances that have been achieved in dentistry in recent years, almost all areas of dental treatment can be undertaken with greater skill, a greater degree of accuracy, and less trauma, and they can be completed in less time. Yet despite these advances, the problems of fear and anxiety persist.

A large part of the problem can be assumed to be a carry-over from the recent past, when many dental patients were severely traumatized both physically and psychologically in the process of receiving routine dental care. Because of the lesser degree of scientific knowledge available at the time, a certain level of discomfort (pain) was to be expected. "Grin and bear it" was a commonly heard cliché.

The children of that era are the adults of today, and because they carry with them many psychological scars and bitter memories of "going to the dentist," today's dental professional is faced with a multiplicity of management problems when these patients appear for treatment.

Anxious patients present a problem to the dentist not only when they appear for treatment but also when their children require treatment. Anxiety is contagious, and even though the apprehensive adult will usually make every attempt to mask their true feelings about "the dentist" (for it is "childish" to be afraid of the dentist), their feelings usually manage to make themselves evident to the child. Every dentist is familiar with the child who appears at the first dental appointment already "knowing" that the drill is going to hurt. The problem of anxiety and its management in the pediatric patient are discussed more fully in Chapter 36.

This is our problem.

BASIC FEARS

What are the causes of our patients' fear of dentistry? Most persons harbor five universal fears:
1. Fear of pain
2. Fear of the unknown
3. Fear of helplessness and dependency
4. Fear of bodily change and mutilation
5. Fear of death

When the stress of the dental situation is superimposed onto these fears, many patients find themselves unable to successfully cope and they exhibit "dental phobia"—an irrational fear of dentistry and all that it represents.

Each of the above fears may easily be transferred into the dental situation. As will be demonstrated, the *fear of pain* is easily the most significant fear harbored by the typical dental patient. How often does one hear the plaintive question "Is it going to hurt?" from a patient just before a procedure is to start? In fact, how do most patients select their dentist? Because of the superior quality of dental care or because the doctor has a reputation for being "painless" and caring? Each of us has heard a patient say, "It's nothing personal, Doctor, but I don't like dentists." In a recent survey it was found that patients who were not experiencing dental pain when they appeared for routine treatment fully expected that at some time during their treatment they would experience pain, and the person most likely to inflict this pain on them was the dentist.[1]

Fear of the unknown is present in varying degrees whenever a person is confronted with a new situation, be it attempting to cross a furnished room for the first time in the dark or facing a new and threatening dental procedure. Fortunately, this fear can be effectively eliminated or at least modulated through a technique of iatrosedation (Chapter 7) called preparatory communications. The doctor need merely discuss the planned procedure with the patient, describing in nontechnical and nonthreatening terms the nature of the planned procedure.

The *fear of helplessness and dependency* is, unfortunately, more difficult to eliminate in dentistry. Because of the nature of dental care, the patient is both unable to observe the treatment and is usually placed in a very vulnerable position—the supine position. Most persons will experience a feeling of unease at this time, especially when they are receiving treatment from a stranger—a doctor or hygienist with whom they are not well acquainted. As the patient becomes more familiar with the doctor or hygienist, this feeling of helplessness should resolve.

In the area of pharmacosedation the fear of helplessness and dependency also appears. Consider that we are asking already apprehensive patients to lie back in the dental chair (a vulnerable position) and to permit virtual strangers to administer medications that will alter their level of consciousness and decrease even further the degree of control they possess over their body. Examples will be presented throughout the book of ways in which a patient's active participation may be enlisted during certain procedures. Such activities will increase the patient's sense of being in control, thereby allaying the feeling of helplessness.

One personality type—the authoritarian—will prove very difficult to manage with the use of pharmacosedation. This individual, the "executive type," is a "take-charge" person who likes to be in complete control of the situation at all times. Where anxiety exists and pharmacosedation is indicated, this patient will prove somewhat more difficult to sedate successfully. The success of pharmacosedation is based, in part, on a patient's desire to simply "let go" and relax. Authoritarian patients will often prove unwilling or unable to release control of their mind to the drug(s) being employed. The doctor will label this patient as "resistant" or say that the patient "fought the medication."

The *fear of bodily change or mutilation* is common in all aspects of medicine but is especially evident in dentistry. The oral cavity is both a richly innervated and a psychologically important region of the body. All aspects of dental care have potentially great psychological overtones. Though at times these may seem illogical to the doctor, they must be dealt with for treatment to succeed. Changes in the size and shape or configuration of the body may have a profound effect on the patient's overall outlook and attitude. The loss of teeth, for example, in today's society may represent the process of growing old, a situation that could prove to be extremely disturbing psychologically to the patient.

The *fear of death* is also ever present. Placed in a vulnerable position in the dental chair, patients next have a multitude of hands and instruments placed into their mouth. Drugs are injected that remove the patient's ability to feel, and then a high-speed handpiece is placed in the mouth, with a bur rotating several hundred thousand times per minute. Many sensations and feelings race through the typical patient's mind at this time: Can I breathe with all this equipment and these hands in my mouth? Will I move my tongue too close to the drill and have it injured? Will the doctor slip and injure me? Add to this the feelings of a patient when the use of sedation is recommended, in light of the many media reports of death and injury related to the use of drugs in dental offices.[9,10]

The fear of death in the dental office has probably been accentuated because of the seeming popularity of this subject in the mass media. Several nationwide television programs (for example, *20/20*) have presented exposés on the dangers of anesthesia and sedation in dentistry.[9] Reaction from patients has been as expected: an increased reluctance to permit the doctor to administer any drugs, even local anesthetics and N_2O-O_2 sedation, for their treatment.

DENTAL FEARS

Table 2-1 presents the results of a survey of dental patients in which they were asked to list, in order of fearfulness, a number of situations that commonly occur in the dental office. As can be seen from this list virtually every procedure that is performed in the dental office is capable of being viewed as frightening by the patient.[11]

Most of these fear-producing situations are easily understood, for example, extractions and drilling. However, several situations might easily be overlooked by the doctor. Being told that "you have bad teeth" (No. 3), "holding a syringe and needle in front of you" (No. 4), and "dentist laughs as he looks in your mouth" (No. 7) are situations that are almost entirely avoidable if the dentist is made aware of them. We all develop habits during our professional careers, most of them good, with but a few of them negative. The manner in which we present ourselves to our patients may be the most important of all the habits we develop. Through the use of proper treatment protocols combined with an appropriate professional attitude and demeanor, these three fear-producing situations may be eliminated or diminished.

Our profession has taken great strides toward the elimination of dental pain. With the many excellent local anesthetics available to us today, pain is not usually a problem during dental treatment. In fact, with the disposable equipment available today and the use of recommended injection technique, the injection of local anesthetic solution can become virtually

Table 2-1. Ranking of dental situations from the most fearful to the least fearful

Situation	Total group	Low fear group	High fear group
Dentist is pulling your tooth	1	1	2
Dentist is drilling your tooth	2	2	1
Dentist tells you you have bad teeth	3	3	3
Dentist holds syringe and needle in front of you	4	4	6
Dentist is giving you a shot	5	5	4
Having a probe placed in a cavity	6	6	5
Dentist laughs as he looks in your mouth	7	7	10
Dentist squirts air into a cavity	8	8	7
Sitting in the dentist's waiting room	9	9	8
Dentist laying out his instruments	10	10	13
Nurse tells you it's your turn	11	12	9
Getting in the dentist's chair	12	11	11
Dentist is putting in the filling	13	13	14
Thinking about going to the dentist	14	15	12
Dentist cleans your teeth with a steel probe	15	14	16
Getting in your car to go to the dentist	16	16	15
Dentist looks at your chart	17	17	17
Dentist places cotton in your mouth	18	18	18
Calling dentist to make an appointment	19	19	19
Dental assistant places bib on you	20	20	20
Dentist squirts water in your mouth	21	21	21
Making another appointment with the nurse	22	22	22
Dentist is cleaning your teeth	23	23	23
Dentist asks you to rinse your mouth	24	24	24
Dentist tells you he is through	25	25	25

From Gale E: *J Dent Res* 51:964, 1972

100% painless and atraumatic. Of interest therefore is the finding in Table 2-1 that the statement "dentist holds syringe in front of you" was considered to be more fear provoking than "dentist giving you a shot." The anticipation of the injection produces more fear then the actual injection!

Dental fear does exist. The first step in the management of a patient's fear of dentistry must be the recognition that it is present. All members of the dental and medical office staff must be ever alert to clues that might signify the presence of heightened anxiety in a patient. The methods of recognizing the presence of anxiety and fear will be discussed in Chapters 5 and 7.

Ignoring the presence of dental fears provokes many negative responses from the patient. One of the most common is the response of the pain reaction threshold to heightened anxiety. Murray[12,13] demonstrated that of the many variables that influence the pain reaction threshold of a patient, anticipation and anxiety appear to be the most important. Apprehensive patients do in fact have a lowered pain

reaction threshold. The patient will respond adversely to stimulation (e.g., pressure) that in the more relaxed patient would not be interpreted as painful. When anxiety is reduced or eliminated through psychosedation, the patient's subjective experience of pain declines significantly.[14]

Pain and anxiety are related circularly. According to Schottstraedt,[15] "Pain is a source of anxiety, anxiety is a factor that increases pain, and increased pain incites further anxiety." Ignoring fears and anxieties increases the frustration and stress of the doctor and staff and increases the likelihood of stress-related emergency situations developing in the patient.

Ignoring a patient's fear of dentistry will not make the fears go away. Ignoring a patient's fears of dentistry may, however, make the patient go away. The following is a transcript of an interview with an apprehensive dental patient that illustrates this point:

I remember when I was in high school, I had a bad experience with a guy who I had to go to like every week for a couple of months and I hated going to this guy because he wasn't very . . . he didn't have very much empathy for

. . . at least me. . . . I don't know about the rest of his patients. And he kept saying, "Oh, that doesn't hurt. . . . Come on, you're just a sissy," which wasn't cool. . . . He wasn't just hurting my mouth, but he was hurting my ego . . . and when I was in high school, I just couldn't handle both.

But what he was doing was like he'd give me a prescription of a bunch of sedative pills to take before I went. So I'd take about a double dose, and I'd have to have somebody drive me to the dentist and there I was. . . . I don't know if they were like reds (secobarbital) or whatever, but I remember I felt out of it, but I felt uncomfortable. It wasn't a good experience. Going to him really, really, really touched off my fear of going back again because I didn't go back to the dentist for a long time after that.[16]

The rest of this book is devoted to the various methods involved in the recognition of anxiety and in its management. The dental and medical practitioners of today have at their disposal a plethora of techniques that are quite effective in the management of a patient's fears and anxieties. Many of the techniques to be discussed involve the administration of drugs to the patient to achieve the desired goal, whereas other techniques may prove effective in the absence of drug administration. It is one of the goals of this book to help the doctor to be able to select the appropriate psychosedative technique for a given patient so that fears of the dental situation may be managed in the least traumatic but still clinically effective manner.

REFERENCES

1. Milgrom P, Weinstein B, Kleinknecht R et al: *Treating fearful dental patients.* Reston, Va, 1985, Reston Publishing.
2. Malamed SF: "The pain of fear." Lecture to the California Dental Society of Anesthesiology, October, 1975, San Francisco, Calif.
3. Friedman N: Iatrosedation. In McCarthy FM, ed: *Emergencies in dental practice,* ed 3. Philadelphia, 1979, Saunders.
4. Kahn RL, Cooper C, Mallenger M: Dentistry: what causes it to be a stressful profession? *Int Rev Appl Psych* (in press).
5. Cannon WB: *Bodily changes in pain, hunger, fear and rage,* ed 2. New York, Appleton-Century-Crofts, 1929.
6. Weiss E, English OS: *Psychosomatic medicine.* Philadelphia, 1957, Saunders.
7. Pearson RE: Anxiety in the dental office. In Bennett CR: *Conscious-sedation in dental practice,* ed 2. St Louis, 1978, Mosby.
8. National Institute of Health: Report of the Ad Hoc Committee II on research and faculty training in pain control in dentistry, Feb 9-10, 1972.
9. Diamond J, producer: ABC News Show #335, In the dentist's chair, Sept 29, 1983.
10. Newcomer K: "Dentist waited outside while patient died," *Rocky Mountain News,* August 4, 1992.
11. Gale E: Fears of the dental situation, *J Dent Res* 51:964, 1972.
12. Murray JB: Psychology of the pain experience. In Weisenberg M, ed: *Pain: clinical and experimental perspectives.* St Louis, 1975, Mosby.
13. Murray JB: The puzzle of pain, *Percep Mot Skills* 28:887, 1969.
14. Jones A, Bentler PM, Petry G: The reaction of uncertainty concerning future pain, *J Abnorm Psychol* 71:87, 1966.
15. Schottstraedt WW: *Psychophysiologic approach in medical practice.* Chicago, 1960, Year Book Medical.
16. Interview, Department of Human Behavior, University of Southern California School of Dentistry, Los Angeles, Calif, 1975.

SECTION TWO

Spectrum of pain and anxiety control

Sections Two through Six present what might be called the answer to the problem that was initially presented in Section One (the problem of fear and anxiety in dentistry). The answer includes all of the techniques that can be termed sedation *as well as those termed* general anesthesia; *this terminology will be defined in this section.*

In Chapter 3 the reader will be introduced to the concept of sedation. The term will be defined and then discussed in relation to general anesthesia, a state that many persons readily confuse with sedation. The various stages of anesthesia, of which sedation is one, will be described.

Chapter 4, The Spectrum of Pain and Anxiety Control, illustrates the wide variety of patient management techniques that are available to the dentist and physician. Advantages and disadvantages of these techniques will be discussed and the techniques compared.

Prior to the administration of any drug to a patient, or for that matter prior to treatment of any sort, it is imperative that the doctor fully evaluate the patient to determine his or her ability to withstand the stresses involved in the planned treatment. This evaluation must be even more comprehensive whenever a drug is to be administered to the patient during treatment. In addition, all patients receiving sedative medications or general anesthesia must be monitored to varying degrees throughout the entire procedure. Chapters 5 and 6 present extremely important guidelines that should be employed every time drug administration is considered. Failure to properly evaluate a patient prior to treatment (Chapter 5) and failure to monitor the patient during treatment (Chapter 6) have been responsible for many cases of morbidity and mortality.[1] The importance of these two chapters to the safety of the techniques that follow cannot be overstated.

In Chapter 7 the reader is introduced to the first of the two major categories of psychosedation—nondrug techniques. Although several nondrug techniques are available, two, iatrosedation and hypnosis, are used to a greater degree than the others. Iatrosedation, known by various names, represents the building block on which the success or failure of all pharmacosedative procedures (involving the administration of drugs) will be based. Whether we are aware of it or not, all doctors employ iatrosedation in their office on all of their patients. Hypnosis, on the other hand, is a technique that must be learned in a more formal setting. When employed appropriately, its success rate in management of both pain and fear is quite acceptable.

REFERENCE

1. de Julien LF: Causes of severe morbidity/mortality cases, *J Calif Dent Assoc* 11:45, 1983.

CHAPTER 3

Introduction to sedation

The primary aim of this book is to aid the doctor in the management of pain and anxiety in the dental patient, for it is these two items that either singly or in combination produce most of the difficulties associated with patient management today.

How may pain and anxiety be managed successfully and safely in the dental office? Pain associated with dental treatment is managed effectively through the administration of local anesthetic drugs prior to the start of treatment. These chemicals prevent passage of the nerve impulse beyond the site at which they are deposited. Although the tooth or soft tissues have received a noxious stimulus (e.g., drill, currette), the propagated nerve impulse will travel only as far as the site at which the local anesthetic drug was deposited. The rapid influx of sodium ions into the interior of the nerve (the process responsible for continued propagation of the nerve impulse) is prevented, the impulse is terminated, and the patient feels no discomfort.

As was noted in Chapter 2, however, the *fear* of pain is a major deterrent to the receipt of dental care today. Patients who are not in pain fear the visit to the dental office because they feel that at some time during their dental treatment they will be hurt.[1] The fear of pain produces a heightened anxiety in these patients, a factor that occasionally leads to the avoidance of dental care until they are truly in pain.

How can dentistry alter its image of being painful? It is a fact today that virtually all dental care can be completed without discomfort to the patient. With the availability of a wide variety of excellent local anesthetics it is possible to achieve clinically adequate pain control in almost all situations. The most difficult pain management problems usually occur in endodontically involved teeth, and only rarely in this situation is effective pain control unattainable.

The administration of a local anesthetic is also considered to be a traumatic procedure by most patients and, indeed, by many doctors (Table 2-1).[2,3] Yet even this aspect of dental care need not be traumatic. Local anesthetic injections may be administered atraumatically anywhere in the oral cavity, including the palate. The technique of the atraumatic injection of local anesthetics is presented in various textbooks of local anesthesia.*

Yet the possibility of pain and the administration of local anesthetics are not the only things about dentistry that produce fear in patients. Doctors with extensive clinical experience have probably heard patients express fear of almost every possible procedure that we are called on to carry out.

How then can we manage these overly fearful patients? The answer is to induce a state of consciousness (or, more precisely, altered consciousness) in which a person is more relaxed and carefree than previously. Over the years many names have been given to this state. Names such as chemamnesia,[4] sedamnesia,[5] twilight sleep,[6] relative analgesia,[7] and comedication[8] have been used to describe the state of consciousness that is now called sedation.

Many definitions of this important term have been given over the years; however, in 1971, following the Third Pain Control Conference sponsored by the ADA, American Dental Society of Anesthesiology, and American Association of Dental Schools, the "Guidelines for Teaching the Comprehensive Control of Pain and Anxiety in Dentistry," were published.[9] These guidelines established a standard for training all dental personnel in this important area of patient management. Included in these guidelines

---

*The reader is referred to the *Handbook of Local Anesthesia,* by S.F. Malamed (St. Louis, ed 3, 1991, Mosby-Yearbook), for an in-depth discussion of this technique.

are definitions of terms that were adopted to describe the various techniques and levels of consciousness and awareness discussed in the document. The following definitions, extracted from the 1992 revision of this document, will be used throughout this book.[10]

general anesthesia   The elimination of all sensation, accompanied by the loss of consciousness.

analgesia   The diminution or elimination of pain in the conscious patient.

local anesthesia   The elimination of sensations, especially pain, in one part of the body by the topical application or regional injection of a drug.

conscious sedation   A minimally depressed level of consciousness that retains the patient's ability to independently and continuously maintain an airway and respond appropriately to physical stimulation and verbal command and that is produced by a pharmacological or nonpharmacologic method or combination thereof.

The Academy of Pediatric Dentistry, in its "Guidelines for the Elective Use of Conscious Sedation, Deep Sedation, and General Anesthesia in Pediatric Patients" added another term describing a level of consciousness that lies between sedation and general anesthesia. It is termed deep sedation.[10]

deep sedation   A controlled state of depressed consciousness accompanied by partial loss of protective reflexes, including the inability to continually maintain an airway independently and/or respond purposefully to verbal command, and is produced by a pharmacologic or nonpharmacologic method or a combination thereof.

One of the most frequent misunderstandings between the doctor and the patient relates to the patient's misinterpretation of the term *sedation*. In the minds of many of our patients sedation is synonymous with general anesthesia, unconsciousness, and sleep. In addition, I have encountered more than a few health professionals, including physicians and dentists, who also misapply or misuse these terms.

Sedation is one of the stages of anesthesia. It is that stage of anesthesia in which the patient is still conscious but is under the influence of a CNS depressant drug. The definition of "conscious" is extremely important because it provides a baseline description of all the techniques of sedation to be discussed in this book.

conscious   Capable of a rational response to command, with protective reflexes intact, including the ability to independently and continuously maintain a patient airway.

The definition of "conscious" has been altered slightly in recent years in that the word "rational" has been replaced by "appropriate." This was considered necessary because some patients who receive sedation within the dental or medical office will be unable to respond rationally to command. Such persons might include the very young patient, or the physically or mentally disabled. Deaf patients will be unable to respond rationally to the spoken word, but will be able to respond appropriately, given their handicaps.

Pain-relieving and anxiety-relieving techniques in which the patient retains consciousness may be termed *sedative techniques*. Procedures producing the loss of consciousness, even for the shortest of times, must be considered general anesthesia. These latter procedures will be discussed in Chapters 31 and 32.

THE STAGES OF GENERAL ANESTHESIA

In the mid-1840s Francis Plomely described three stages of general anesthesia.[11] In 1847 John Snow added a fourth, overdose.[12] It was not, however, until World War I that Guedel[13] more clearly described the signs and symptoms of the various stages of anesthesia. Guedel's classification of the stages of anesthesia has been accepted throughout the world and is considered to be one of the important contributions to the science of anesthesiology. Four stages of anesthesia were described:

I. Stage of analgesia
II. Stage of delirium
III. Stage of surgical anesthesia
IV. Stage of respiratory paralysis

Guedel based his observations on the following parameters:

1. Character of the respirations
2. Eyeball activity
3. Pupillary changes
4. Eyelid reflex (presence or absence)
5. Swallowing or vomiting

Guedel's observations were based primarily on the effects of the gaseous anesthetic ether. As the nature of the practice of anesthesiology evolved over the years, it became obvious that the signs and symptoms described for ether were not always observed with many of the newer agents being developed. In 1943 Gillespie added several new factors to Guedel's criteria.[14]

6. Respiratory response to skin incision
7. Secretion of tears
8. Assessment of pharyngeal and laryngeal reflexes

An overview of the basic pattern of action of general anesthetics (and other CNS depressant drugs) may provide a better understanding of the stages and planes of anesthesia. The basic pattern of action consists of a descending depression of the central nervous system. CNS depressants (general anesthetics, antianxiety drugs, sedative-hypnotics, narcotics, alcohol) first depress the cerebral cortex, producing a loss of sensory function, followed by a loss of motor function. Then the basal ganglia and cerebellum are depressed, followed by the spinal cord and finally the medulla. Medullary depression leads to depression of the respiratory and cardiovascular systems and is the usual cause of death from drug overdose. Guedel's four stages of anesthesia are based on this progressive depression of the central nervous system: stage I, analgesia or altered consciousness, corresponds to the action of drugs on higher cortical centers (sensory). The various techniques of psychosedation lie within this stage. Stage II, delirium or excitement, corresponds to the depressant action of drugs on higher motor centers. The patient is unconscious at this stage. Stages I and II comprise what

is termed the induction stage of general anesthesia. In stage III, surgical anesthesia, spinal reflexes are depressed, producing skeletal muscle relaxation. Stage IV, medullary paralysis, corresponds to depression of respiratory and cardiovascular centers of the medulla, producing first respiratory arrest and then cardiovascular collapse.

The stages of general anesthesia, as defined by Guedel and modified by Gillespie, will now be described in greater detail. They are illustrated in Fig. 3-1.

Stage I: analgesia (Fig. 3-1)

The first stage of anesthesia starts with the initial administration of the CNS depressant drug and continues until the patient loses consciousness. The patient is conscious throughout this stage and is capable of response to command and may therefore provide the administrator with information (con-

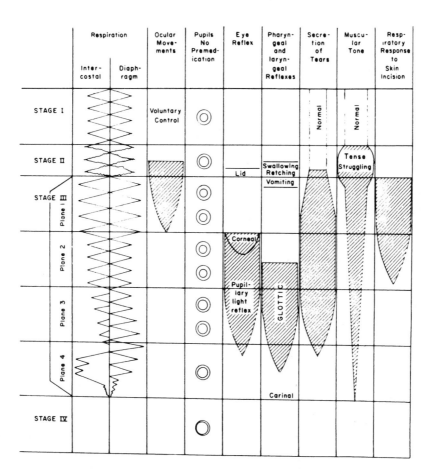

Fig. 3-1. Classic signs of unpremedicated diethyl ether anesthesia as described by Guedel and modified by Gillespie. (From Allen GD: *Dental anesthesia and analgesia: local and general,* ed 2. Baltimore, 1979, Williams & Wilkins.)

cerning, for example, the presence or absence of pain). The portions of the brain that are of most recent phylogenetic development are depressed earliest, primarily the cerebral cortex. Depression of the cerebral cortex results in diminished intellect, memory, integrative functions, and perception of time and space.

Though this phase is called the stage of analgesia, pain may in fact be present and the pain reaction threshold may be unaltered. However, because of the degree of CNS depression, especially depression of the cerebral cortex, the patient's response to noxious stimulation may prove to be diminished.

The techniques of sedation to be described throughout this textbook provide the doctor with a patient who is in stage I of anesthesia. These techniques include oral, rectal, IM, submucosal, intranasal, inhalation, and IV sedation. The patient is relaxed and cooperative, with a decreased awareness of the surroundings, and may exhibit a diminished response to stimulation.

The patient in stage I is under the influence of the drug but is technically awake. Any person who has ever received nitrous oxide-oxygen (N_2O-O_2) or taken a "sleeping pill" or antianxiety drug such as diazepam or even alcohol has technically been in stage I of anesthesia.

1. Respiration is normal.
2. Eye movements are normal, with voluntary movement possible (e.g., the patient is able to follow the examiner's finger from left to right).
3. Protective reflexes are intact.
4. Amnesia (the lack of recall) may or may not be present. Some techniques (e.g., intravenous sedation) will provide a degree of amnesia, although most will provide little or no amnesia. In some techniques, such as N_2O-O_2 inhalation sedation, amnesia is extremely variable; however, patients will usually exhibit a diminished sense of time. A 2-hour appointment may seem to have been only 15 minutes.

CNS depression that places a patient into the lighter levels of stage I is entirely appropriate for use in the dental or medical office for outpatient procedures. Training is required for the safe and effective use of these procedures; however, the length and degree of training are not as extensive or intensive as that required for the administration of general anesthesia. As the depth of CNS depression (sedation) deepens, as may be seen in IM, submucosal, and IV sedation, the patient's ability to respond appropriately, as well as the function of the protective reflexes, diminishes.

Additional training for the doctor and staff becomes critical, as does an increase in the level of monitoring of the patient. However, the patient in stage I is able to maintain a patent airway ("independently and continuously") and to clear the airway should foreign material enter the region of the larynx or pharynx.

Once the patient becomes unable to respond appropriately to command or the protective reflexes are depressed, the patient is technically unconscious; stage I ends and stage II begins.

Unfortunately there is no objective sign that reliably indicates the point of transition from stage I to stage II. A commonly used sign of this transition is the eyelid reflex. Gentle stroking of the eyelashes provokes lid closure in the conscious patient. Lack of response to this stimulus is commonly used to indicate entry of the patient into stage II of anesthesia. However, some patients in light stage I do not maintain their eyelid reflex.

Stage II: delirium

Stage II of anesthesia is called the stage of delirium or excitement. When employed in outpatient general anesthesia, this stage is called ultralight general anesthesia.

In stage II the level of CNS depression is greater than in stage I, and the patient loses consciousness. Stage II starts with the loss of consciousness and progresses until entry into the stage of surgical anesthesia.

Early in stage II the respiratory pattern of the patient may be somewhat irregular. As CNS depression deepens, the character of breathing becomes regular once again, marking the end of stage II and entry into stage III. The patient's reflexes may be exaggerated in the earlier part of stage II. The patient will overreact to stimulation. Restraints are recommended whenever procedures are carried out in this stage. In response to stimulation, especially noxious stimulation, patients may cry out and attempt to move their extremities. Indeed, observers of patients undergoing the extraction of third molars while receiving ultralight general anesthesia with intravenously administered barbiturates will often state that they thought the patients were suffering because of their reactions to the stimulation produced during the removal of the teeth. However, the first response of these patients upon regaining consciousness is often the question, "When are you going to start?"

Because reflexes are hyperactive in this stage, extreme care must be taken to prevent blood, saliva, or foreign materials from reaching the level of the patient's larynx, where laryngospasm may be provoked (Chapters 27 and 31). Only procedures of short duration should be contemplated in stage II and then only by persons who have received thorough training in general anesthesia. Well-trained assistants (doctors or auxiliaries) are responsible for protection of the patient's airway via suctioning and screening off with gauze packing while another person is responsible for continued maintenance of a patent airway. Although the patient continues to breathe spontaneously, in the absence of a patent airway the exchange of O_2 and CO_2 will not occur.

1. Respirations are irregular early in stage II but become more regular as stage II progresses.
2. Eyeballs oscillate involuntarily, a movement termed *lateral nystagmus*.
3. Pupils react to light normally.
4. Skeletal muscle tonus is increased with muscular rigidity present in some patients early in stage II. Muscle tonus decreases as stage II deepens.
5. The laryngeal and pharyngeal reflexes (swallowing and laryngeal closure) are still quite active early in stage II but become progressively more obtunded as stage II deepens.

Entry into stage II is undesirable when attempting to employ sedative techniques. Entry into it is an indication that oversedation has occurred. If the doctor has not received adequate training in the recognition and management of the unconscious patient, significant morbidity and even mortality can occur. When stage III is the goal, it is usual to induce anesthesia relatively rapidly so as to pass the patient through stage II as quickly as possible, thereby minimizing the possibility of overreaction to stimulation.

Treatment for a patient who has inadvertently entered into stage II is either to increase the level of CNS depression (administer additional drug) to bring the patient into stage III of anesthesia or to simply maintain the patient in stage II and permit a slow return to stage I as the cerebral blood level of drug decreases through redistribution.

Stage III: surgical anesthesia

Further CNS depression brings the patient to a level at which respiratory regularity once again occurs. This heralds the onset of stage III of anesthesia, a stage that lasts until breathing ceases (onset of stage IV). Most surgical procedures in medicine are performed at this level of CNS depression.

Entry into stage III is marked by several signs:

1. The respiratory irregularity observed in stage II disappears. Respiration is automatic and involuntary, responding to the level of CO_2 within the blood.
2. Muscular tonus is lost, unlike the increased muscular tonus seen in stage II. The patient's head may now be moved from side to side, and the mouth may be opened with ease.
3. Swallowing and reflex respiratory arrest will not occur if the anesthesiologist suddenly increases the concentration of an inhalational anesthetic. Both of these responses will occur in stage II.

For a more accurate determination of the depth of anesthesia, stage III is divided into four planes. The major differences in physical signs in these planes relates to the character of respiration, the character of eyeball movements, the presence or absence of certain reflexes, and the size of the pupils. The planes of anesthesia were introduced by Gillespie in 1943.[14]

Plane 1 of stage III

Plane 1 is entered once respiratory regularity is regained. Respirations become full, regular, and automatic, and are equally thoracic and abdominal in character.

Eyeballs oscillate slowly during this plane, and the pupils respond to light normally. Pharyngeal reflexes that induce vomiting when an oral airway is inserted are gradually diminished as plane 1 continues. The swallowing, retching, and vomiting reflexes disappear in that order during the induction of general anesthesia and reappear in reverse order on recovery from anesthesia.

Tears are secreted throughout plane 1. The tendency of the patient to breathe deeply and more rapidly as the skin incision is made decreases as plane 1 deepens. Peripheral vasodilation develops in plane 1.

Plane 2 of stage III

Plane 2 begins when the eyeballs cease to oscillate and become eccentrically fixed. Plane 2 ends when the intercostal muscles weaken and thoracic respiration becomes decreased.

Respiration remains regular, but because the depth of breathing is diminished, tidal volume is decreased.

If patients have not received premedication, pupillary size increases in plane 2 (dilation). However because of the almost routine administration of preoperative medications, pupillary signs are rather inconsistent and are no longer used as reliable indicators of the level of general anesthesia. Narcotics produce pupillary constriction, while belladonnas such as atropine produce dilation of the pupils.

The protective reflexes, such as laryngeal closure (laryngospasm), begin to disappear in plane 2. Secretion of tears diminishes in this plane, and the respiratory response (increased rate and depth) to skin incision disappears.

Plane 3 of stage III

Plane 3 is entered as thoracic respiration decreases and the abdominal component of respiration increases. This is produced either by the beginning paralysis of the intercostal muscles or by a weakening of the diaphragm. As plane 3 deepens, intercostal paralysis becomes complete and respiration is produced entirely by the diaphragm. Tidal volume is decreased and inspiration is now of shorter duration than exhalation.

The diaphragm may exhibit excessive or jerking movements during plane 3. During abdominal operations this may interfere with the surgical procedure, leading the surgeon to request a deeper plane of anesthesia. In fact, lightening of the anesthetic level to plane 2 is all that is required for diaphragmatic movements to become more rhythmical and smooth. Another means of providing the surgeon with a more ideal surgical field is to keep the patient in plane 3 of anesthesia but to assist or control the patient's ventilation.

It is not recommended that plane 3 be used during surgery for extended periods of time. The upper portions of plane 2 and lower plane 1 are suitable for most procedures once the surgeon has explored the abdomen, exposed the surgical site, and mobilized the organs.

In mid to lower plane 3, the pupillary reaction to light is gradually lost. Tear secretion continues to diminish in plane 3.

Plane 4 of stage III

From the onset of paralysis of the intercostal muscles until respiratory arrest occurs, the patient is in plane 4. Activity of the diaphragm progressively decreases as plane 4 deepens until spontaneous breathing ceases entirely. Pupils dilate and little or no muscle tonus is to be found.

A response known as tracheal tug is often encountered in plane 4. Dripps et al.[15] state that although there is no single satisfactory explanation for tracheal tug, it may be the result of an attempt by accessory muscles of respiration to augment respiratory exchange.

Stage IV: medullary paralysis

Stage IV begins with the onset of respiratory arrest and ends with the cessation of effective circulation (cardiac arrest). Essentially, stage IV is a stage of reversible clinical death. By definition clinical death occurs with the cessation of effective respiration and circulation. With the application of controlled ventilation and the lightening of the depth of CNS depression, the patient may recover from this overly deep level of anesthesia. Stage IV of anesthesia is rarely sought intentionally. If respiration needs to be terminated temporarily during surgery (as in abdominal surgery in which skeletal muscle relaxation is necessary to enter the abdomen), the patient is maintained in stage III and a muscle relaxant drug such as d-tubocurarine, pancuronium, or atricurium is administered.

Stage IV of anesthesia will be encountered in the emergency room of the hospital when cases of drug overdose are treated. Management of the patient in stage IV involves the application of basic and advanced life support, primarily effective ventilation with O_2, until redistribution and biotransformation of the offending agent(s) produce a lower plasma level.

SUMMARY

The reader should be aware of the four classic stages of anesthesia because whenever a technique of sedation involving the administration of a drug is to be used, the patient will enter one or more of these stages. Stage I of anesthesia is the stage that is called the stage of analgesia or the stage of sedation. This is the stage in which all of the techniques presented in Sections Three, Four, and Five may be placed.

The patient in stage I is conscious, but is under the influence of the drug(s). The patient is relaxed and cooperative, and may be amnesic. Vital signs are minimally altered, protective reflexes are intact, and the patient is able to maintain a patent airway.

In order for a doctor to be able to safely manage a patient in stages II or III of anesthesia a minimum of 1 full year, and preferably 2 or more years, of training in anesthesiology is necessary. The ability to safely manage the unconscious patient requires a significantly greater period of time to learn well.

Within the practice of dentistry there are indications for the use of stages II and III. Stage II is indicated primarily with outpatient oral surgery procedures, and stage III may be indicated for longer or more traumatic procedures of any type.

The next chapter will introduce the many techniques of sedation and general anesthesia that are presently available for use by the dental and medical professions for the management of both pain and anxiety. In subsequent sections of this book each of these techniques will be reviewed in considerable depth so as to impart to the reader a degree of knowledge that will, when combined with adequate clinical and didactic training, permit the employment of these techniques in a safe and effective manner.

REFERENCES

1. Milgrom P, Weinstein P, Kleinknecht T et al: *Treating fearful dental patients.* Reston, Va, 1985, Reston Publishing, p 23.
2. Gale E: Fears of the dental situation, *J Dent Res* 51:964, 1972.
3. Fiset L, Milgrom P, Weinstein P et al: Psychophysiological responses to dental injections, *JADA* 111(4):578, 1985.
4. Monheim LJ: *General anesthesia in dental practice,* ed 3. St Louis, 1968, Mosby.
5. Carnow R, Schaffer AB: Application of the concept of augmenter-moderator-reducer to dental patient management. In Spiro SR: *Amnesia-analgesia techniques in dentistry.* Springfield, Ill, 1972, Charles C Thomas.
6. Berns J: Twilight sedation—a substitute for lengthy office intravenous anesthesia, *J Conn State Dent Assoc* 37:4, 1963.
7. Langa H: *Relative analgesia in dental practice: inhalation analgesia with nitrous oxide.* Philadelphia, 1968, Saunders.
8. Hamburg HL: *The joy of sedation: a beginner's manual to newer sedative techniques for the dentist and dental student.* Hamburg, NY 1978, Hamburg.
9. Council on Dental Education: American Dental Association, Guidelines for teaching the comprehensive control of pain and anxiety in dentistry, *J Dent Educ* 36:62, 1972.
10. American Academy of Pediatric Dentistry, Guidelines for the elective use of conscious sedation, deep sedation, and general anesthesia in pediatric patients, *1992-1993 Reference Manual,* Chicago, 1993, American Academy of Pediatric Dentistry.
11. Lee JAA, Atkinson RS: *A synopsis of anesthesia,* ed 5. Baltimore, 1964, Williams & Wilkins.
12. Snow J: *The inhalation of the vapour of ether in surgical operations.* London, 1847, Churchill.
13. Guedel AF: *Inhalation anesthesia: a fundamental guide,* New York, 1937, Macmillan.
14. Gillespie NA: The signs and reflex reactions of the stages of anesthesia, *Anesth Analg* 22:275, 1943.
15. Dripps RD, Eckenhoff JE, Vandam LD: *Introduction to anesthesia,* ed 8. Philadelphia, 1992, Saunders.

CHAPTER 4

The spectrum of pain and anxiety control

A number of techniques are available to the dental and medical professional to aid in the management of a patient's fears and anxieties regarding dental care and surgery. To some this statement may be self-evident; however, to others the availability of a variety of techniques may come as something of a surprise. The aim of this chapter is to introduce the concept of the *spectrum of pain and anxiety control.* This spectrum, which is presented graphically in Fig. 4-1, demonstrates that there are indeed quite a number of techniques available to manage patients' fears and anxieties. This chapter introduces the various techniques included in this spectrum, and subsequent chapters discuss them in depth.

In Fig. 4-1 the vertical bar about three quarters of the way across the spectrum indicates a very significant barrier: the point at which consciousness is lost. All techniques found to the right of the bar fall under the heading of general anesthesia, and all techniques to the left of the bar may correctly be termed psychosedation, sedation, or (less correctly) conscious sedation.

The techniques of sedation may further be divided into those that require the administration of drugs to achieve a desirable clinical effect and those that do not. The former may be termed *pharmacosedation* techniques; the latter may be called *iatrosedative (iatrosedation)* techniques. These terms will be further defined at other points in this book.

The bar representing the point at which consciousness is lost is significant in that it identifies a level of training that must be achieved by the doctor before various techniques can even be considered. Without elaborating at this point (educational requirements for specific techniques will be discussed in appropriate sections of the book), it may be stated that the absolute minimum of training recommended for the use of general anesthesia is not less than 1 year (full time), with 2 full years preferred. These guidelines for general anesthesia, as well as those for techniques of sedation, have been accepted by the American Dental Association, the American Dental Society of Anesthesiology, and the American Association of Dental Schools.[1]

The duration of time necessary to adequately prepare the doctor to employ the various techniques of sedation safely and effectively will vary from technique to technique and from doctor to doctor. Many dentists and dental hygienists will be fully prepared on graduation from dental school to enter into private practice knowledgeable in the safe and effective use of some of these techniques. Many others, however, will not have this ability, and for these persons continuing education courses are available.[2] For inhalation sedation with nitrous oxide (N_2O) and oxygen (O_2), a minimum course of 2 to 3 days, including patient management, is recommended; for IV sedation, a much more extensive program, including patient management, is required.[3]

In recent years outpatient surgery in the practice of medicine has greatly increased in popularity. Minor surgical procedures on the limbs, trunk, and face are easily completed with the administration of local anesthetics by general surgeons, dermatologists, and plastic and reconstructive surgeons.[4] Other health professionals, such as podiatrists, are also extensively involved in outpatient surgery.[5] Until recently, however, there was little consideration given to the degree of patient anxiety toward this type of surgical procedure. The patient faces these nondental surgical procedures with the same dread as may be noted in dental patients. The techniques and concepts dis-

22

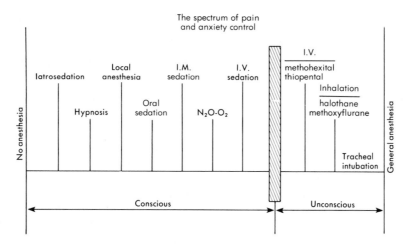

Fig. 4-1. Spectrum of pain and anxiety control. Illustration of many of the techniques available in medicine and dentistry for patient management. Vertical bar represents the loss of consciousness.

cussed in this textbook are as appropriate for non-dental surgery as they are in dentistry.

Many techniques of pain and anxiety control are available to the health professional. Which ones if any are used is a very personal choice. Some doctors will feel comfortable using a technique with which others may be quite uncomfortable. Having several techniques available at his or her disposal will enable the doctor to tailor the appropriate sedation technique to a given patient. There is no panacea, nor is any one technique always indicated or always effective. To rely solely on one technique for sedation is to invite failure.

NO ANESTHESIA

The extreme left-hand portion of the spectrum of pain and anxiety control (Fig. 4-1) comprises that small group of patients who will require absolutely no sedation or local anesthesia during their dental treatment. Although these patients are quite rare, it is probable that a dentist or hygienist will be called upon to treat one or more of these persons at some time. For whatever reason—anatomical, physiological, psychological, cultural, or religious—these patients either do not feel pain or do not react to it, and they are able to tolerate any form of dental treatment without the need for drug intervention of any sort.

Although such patients may not feel any pain during their dental treatment, such may not be the case with the dentist or hygienist called on to treat them. The following incident actually took place: The pa-

tient, a pleasant 26-year-old woman requiring periodontal surgery (soft tissue), requested that the doctor not use any medications at all during her treatment because she did not require them. After a futile attempt to dissuade the patient from what was assumed to be a foolhardy course, the doctor agreed to begin the surgical procedure without local anesthesia only if the patient would consent to receive it if at any time during the surgery pain was present. The surgical procedure required approximately 45 minutes to complete, during which time the patient displayed absolutely no evidence of discomfort, to the complete amazement of the dental personnel who had gathered around to watch. Vital signs (blood pressure, heart rate, and rhythm) monitored during the procedure demonstrated essentially no deviation from baseline values. Not so with the doctor and assistant. Following the procedure, which proceeded smoothly, they were bathed in perspiration. The doctor said that he felt quite uncomfortable throughout the procedure because he knew that the patient *should* be in pain. Indeed, he stopped many times to ask the patient how she was feeling. He also said that he could almost feel the pain for the patient. "I was uncomfortable for the patient," he said. At the next surgical appointment the doctor and assistant were quite pleased when the patient consented to their request to give her local anesthesia for the surgery. When asked why she had changed her mind, the patient stated that she did it for the sake of the doctor and the assistant. She had noticed *their* discomfort at the prior visit and, although she still did not require the pain-controlling medication, felt it prudent to receive it to allow the doctor to be more relaxed during her treatment.

It is important to separate this small group of patients who truly do not require anesthetics from those patients who similarly request that they not receive local anesthesia because they are quite fearful of injections. It is somewhat easier to recognize such a patient prior to starting the planned procedure. But if the doctor is unable to recognize the anxiety and proceeds to dental treatment, it usually becomes painfully obvious, to both the doctor and the patient, to which group the patient truly belongs.

IATROSEDATION

Iatrosedation, defined as the relief of anxiety through the doctor's behavior, stands as the building block for all other forms of psychosedation. The term and the technique of iatrosedation were created many years ago by Dr. Nathan Friedman, chairman and founder of the Department of Human Behavior, University of Southern California School of Dentistry.[6] Discussed in greater detail in Chapter 7, iatrosedation may briefly be described as a process involving a number of steps: recognition by the doctor of the patient's anxieties toward dentistry, management of the information gathered by the doctor from the patient, and a commitment by the doctor to aid the patient in dental treatment.

Simply stated, iatrosedation is a technique of communication between the doctor and the patient that creates a bond of trust and confidence. A patient possessing trust and confidence in the doctor (physician, dentist, or other health professional) is well on the way to being more relaxed and cooperative, without the need for supplemental pharmacosedation.[7]

Another important benefit of the use of iatrosedation in the practice of medicine and dentistry is the prevention of possible medicolegal complications. Lack of effective communication between the health professional and the patient is one of the leading causes of suits brought against medical and dental professionals. In some estimates up to 37% of all malpractice actions are a result of a lack of communication and trust between the doctor and patient.[8]

Iatrosedation alone may in some situations remove all of a patient's fears and anxieties about the upcoming treatment, permitting us to then proceed in a normal manner, without the need for pharmacosedation. More often, however, iatrosedation alone will produce a decrease in the patient's level of anxiety to the point that the use of supplemental pharmacosedation will enable the patient to more readily accept and tolerate the planned treatment.

OTHER NONDRUG PSYCHOSEDATIVE TECHNIQUES

In addition to the technique of iatrosedation, there are other methods available in order to decrease a patient's fear and anxiety about dentistry without the administration of drugs.

Hypnosis has been used for many years for the management of both pain and anxiety. When employed by a trained hypnotherapist, in the proper clinical environment, and on the appropriate patient, hypnosis has proved to be a highly effective method of achieving both a relaxed and a pain-free treatment environment.

Other nondrug techniques for achieving pain and anxiety control are available. Some are not new, having been introduced to the medical and dental professions years ago. Interest in these techniques has waxed and waned over the years. They may prove to be effective in the hands of some medical and dental practitioners. Textbooks that provide in-depth coverage of these potentially valuable procedures are available and recommended.

Nondrug techniques are mentioned here for the sake of completeness. Developments in this field are occurring so rapidly that it is virtually impossible to include all of them in our compendium of available techniques. Nondrug techniques for the management of either pain or anxiety or both include acupuncture,[9] acupressure, audioanalgesia,[10] biofeedback,[11] electroanesthesia (TENS, EA, EDA),[12] and electrosedation.

ROUTES OF DRUG ADMINISTRATION

To this point in discussing the management of patient anxiety, we have not yet employed any technique that required administration of a drug. Sedation produced without the administration of drugs is termed iatrosedation. The use of drugs to control anxiety is termed pharmacosedation. The three methods we have introduced thus far will permit us to manage but a small percentage of our fearful patients. One advantage that these iatrosedative techniques possess is their ability to increase the effectiveness of any drugs that might need to be administered for the definitive management of the patient's dental fears. Even though we may have to turn to pharmacosedation, the great majority of patients in whom iatrosedation has been employed will require a smaller dose of the drug(s) to bring about a comparable degree of sedation.[13]

Table 4-1. Comparison of routes of drug administration

Route	Cooperation*	First-pass effect	Used for sedation†	Children/adults	Titration	Maximum sedation level recommended‡
Topical	2	–	0	na	–	na
Sublingual	2	–	1	–/+	–	1
Intranasal	1	–	2	+/?	–	1
Oral	2	+	1	+/+	–	1
Rectal	1	+	1	+/+	–	1
Transdermal	1	–	1	–/+	–	1
Subcutaneous	1	–	1	+/+	–	1
IM/SM	0	–	2	+/+	–	1
Inhalation	2	–	2	+/+	+	1
Intravenous	2	–	2	+/+	+	2
Intraarterial	2	–	0	na	–	na
Intrathecal (spinal)	2	–	0	na	+	na
Intramedullary	1	–	0	na	+	na
Intraperitoneal	0	–	0	na	–	na

Key: *Cooperation required, 2; cooperation not critical, 1; cooperation not necessary, 0.
†Strongly recommended, 2; somewhat recommended, 1; not recommended, 0.
‡Moderate to deep, 2; light to moderate, 1.
na, not applicable.

Drugs may be administered through 14 routes. (See Table 4-1.) The first 13 of these routes are used within the practice of medicine, and the first 10 can be used within the practice of dentistry and are covered here. The intraperitoneal route is used in veterinary medicine. These routes are

1. Topical
2. Sublingual
3. Intranasal (IN)
4. Oral
5. Rectal
6. Transdermal
7. Subcutaneous (SC)
8. Intramuscular (IM)
9. Inhalation (pulmonary)
10. Intravenous (IV)
11. Intraarterial (IA)
12. Intrathecal (within the spinal cord)
13. Intramedullary
14. Intraperitoneal

Topical

The absorption of drugs through intact skin is quite poor; however, topically applied local anesthetics can be used to produce anesthesia of tissues where skin is absent, such as the mucous membranes of the mouth, nose, throat, trachea, bronchi, esophagus, stomach, urethra, bladder, vagina, and rectum.[14] Topical anesthesia, as used in dentistry, is a highly effective method of relieving some of the fear and pain potentially involved in the administration of local anesthetics via injection.[15] Topical application of drugs other than local anesthetics is not common.

Sublingual

Certain drugs can be administered sublingually, that is, they can be absorbed into the blood through the mucous membranes of the oral cavity. Examples of the clinical use of sublingual drug administration include nitroglycerin and nifedipine for management of anginal pain[16] and triazolam for sedation in pediatrics.[17]

An advantage of sublingual drug administration is that the drug enters directly into the central circulation, bypassing the enterohepatic circulation. In this way the drug does not encounter the hepatic first-pass effect in which a percentage of the drug is biotransformed before ever having the opportunity to enter the general circulation and to reach its target organ (e.g., brain).[18]

Intranasal

A more recent addition to the drug administration armamentarium has been the intranasal (IN) route. Intranasal drugs have been employed primarily in pediatric patients as a means of circumventing the need for injection or oral drug administration in unwilling patients.[19] Absorption of IN drugs occurs directly into the central circulation, bypassing the enterohepatic circulation. Clinical trials have demonstrated that the absorption and bioavailability of intranasally administered drugs were close to those of IV administration, with peak plasma levels of the agent occurring 10 minutes following administration.[20,21]

Midazolam, a water-soluble benzodiazepine[19-22] and sufentanil,[22] an opioid analgesic, have received the most attention for the IN route of administration.

Oral

The oral route is the most commonly employed route of drug administration. It possesses advantages over parenteral routes of administration that make it quite useful in various situations involving the management of pain and anxiety. This route, however, possesses several significant disadvantages that must also be considered.

Advantages include an almost universal acceptance by patients, ease of administration, and relative safety. Patients today are accustomed to taking medications by mouth, so it is quite rare for the doctor to encounter an adult patient objecting to the oral route of administration. The younger child, however, may often be an unwilling recipient of orally administered drugs. Unwanted drug effects, such as overdosage, idiosyncrasy, allergy, and drug side effects may occur whenever a drug is administered by any route, but such reactions are less likely to develop when a drug is administered orally, and when they do develop, they are normally less intense than those reactions that develop following parenteral administration. This is not meant to imply that life-threatening situations do not arise following oral drug administration. Indeed, cardiac arrest and anaphylaxis after oral drug administration have been reported.[23,24]

Disadvantages of oral drug administration include a long latent period, unreliable drug absorption, an inability to easily achieve a desired drug effect (titration), and a prolonged duration of action. These are significant disadvantages that serve to limit the clinical use of the oral route in the management of pain and anxiety.

Orally administered drugs must reach the stomach and small intestine, where most absorption into the circulatory system occurs. For most drugs the onset of clinical effectiveness is not noted for approximately 30 minutes, the latent period. Drug absorption continues, and a peak plasma concentration equivalent to the greatest degree of clinical effectiveness (pain or anxiety relief) is reached. With most orally administered drugs this maximal clinical effect develops approximately 60 minutes after administration. Because of this slow onset of action and the delay in reaching maximal effect, it is impossible to titrate via the oral route. Titration is defined as the administration of small incremental doses of a drug until the desired clinical action is observed. The ability to titrate a drug allows the administrator control over the drug's actions and its ultimate effect. Titration eliminates the need to make an educated "guesstimate" of the appropriate dose of a drug for a patient. The lack of ability to titrate via the oral route of administration is a considerable handicap to the effective use of this technique when central nervous system (CNS) depressant drugs are administered. The clinician must administer a predetermined dose to the patient. This dose will be determined after consideration of a number of factors (discussed fully in Chapter 8). However, once the drug is administered, it becomes virtually impossible to enhance quickly its actions should the initial dose prove inadequate or to reverse its effects rapidly should an undesirable reaction develop.

The duration of action of most orally administered pain- and anxiety- controlling drugs is prolonged, approximately 3 to 4 hours. This duration is unacceptable for most dental procedures (for sedative drugs especially) because the patient will remain under the influence of the drug well into the posttreatment period and be unable to leave the doctor's office unescorted. Patients receiving CNS depressant drugs via the oral route must be advised against operating potentially dangerous machinery or driving a car (see drug package insert for all oral CNS depressants).

Orally administered drugs may be safely and effectively employed for the management of pain in the postoperative period and for the management of anxiety in the preoperative period. Because of the significant disadvantages associated with it, the oral route of drug administration is not recommended for routine use in the management of intraoperative pain and anxiety. The oral route of drug administration will be more fully discussed in Chapter 8.

Rectal

The rectal route of drug administration is only occasionally employed in the practice of dentistry. Its major use occurs within the practice of pediatric dentistry, where it is more common to encounter patients who are either unwilling or unable to take drugs by mouth.[25,26]

Advantages and disadvantages of the rectal route are similar to those of the oral route of administration. This route of administration will be discussed more fully in Chapter 9.

* * *

The techniques of drug administration that follow are techniques in which the drug is absorbed directly from the site of its administration into the cardiovascular system, effectively bypassing the gastrointestinal (GI) tract. Such techniques are given the name *parenteral,* in contradistinction with the oral and rectal routes of administration, in which drugs are absorbed from the GI tract into the cardiovascular compartment. These routes are termed *enteral* routes of administration. Common usage of the term parenteral usually denotes drug administration by injection with a syringe (e.g., IM, SC, IV). Intranasal and sublingual administration might properly be termed parenteral as drug absorption is directly into the central circulation.

Transdermal

The transdermal route is a means of administering medication, bypassing the GI tract, without the need for injection.[27] The drugs most frequently administered by the transdermal route are scopolamine (primarily for the prevention of motion sickness and postsurgical nausea and vomiting),[28,29] nitroglycerin (for angina pectoris),[30] and nicotine (for smoking cessation).[31] Opioids, such as fentanyl, have also been employed via the transdermal route of administration for postsurgical analgesia.[32]

Transdermal administration of drugs is considered when a long-term course of drug is necessary. Though rarely necessary in dentistry, there are situations (e.g., postsurgery) where transdermally administered analgesics might prove advantageous. Potential drawbacks to transdermal drug administration include the development of decreased responsiveness to the drug[33] and adverse skin reactions at the site of application.[34]

Subcutaneous

The SC route of administration involves the injection of a drug beneath the skin into the subcutaneous tissues. It is useful for the administration of nonvolatile, water- or fat-soluble hypnotic and narcotic drugs. Drugs capable of producing irritation, such as diazepam, should not be administered subcutaneously.

The rate of drug absorption into the cardiovascular system will vary with the blood supply to the tissue. As subcutaneous tissues have a relatively limited blood supply, absorption of drugs following subcutaneous administration is usually delayed.

This slow rate of absorption following SC injection limits the effectiveness of this route in dentistry. Other, more rapidly effective and controllable techniques are preferred and available.

Intramuscular

Intramuscular administration is a parenteral technique that maintains several advantages over the enteral techniques discussed, making it potentially useful in the management of pain and anxiety. However, the IM route pales in comparison to other parenteral methods of administration, especially the inhalation and IV routes. Of the four major techniques employed in dentistry (oral, IM, inhalation, and IV), IM is the least commonly used.

Submucosal (SM) drug administration is similar to IM administration and is most often employed in pediatric dentistry. Its advantages and disadvantages are similar to those discussed for IM administration, except that the absorption of the drug is somewhat more rapid via the SM than the IM route.[35] Clinical consequences of this are significant, including a somewhat more rapid onset of drug effect. Because of this more rapid onset, it is also possible for undesirable drug actions to be noted more rapidly and to be somewhat more intense than those following IM administration. Problems associated with the SM technique will be reviewed in Chapter 10.

Advantages of IM administration over enteral routes include its more rapid onset of action (shorter latent period)—approximately 10 minutes—and a more rapid onset of a maximal clinical action—approximately 30 minutes. Another advantage is the usually more reliable absorption of a drug into the cardiovascular system following IM than oral administration. In other words, 50 mg of a drug administered intramuscularly will produce a more pronounced clinical effect than the same dose of the same drug given by mouth or rectally. Patient cooperation is not as essential as it is with most other techniques. This advantage is of particular importance in pediatric patients who are commonly unwilling to cooperate in the administration of a drug. The child need only be restrained momentarily while the drug is administered.

Disadvantages of IM administration include its 10-minute latent period, a time factor that makes titration impossible. In addition, it is impossible to retrieve the drug should overdose develop; patients may not be willing to accept the injection necessary to administer the medication; the prolonged duration of action (about 2 to 4 hours or more) requires that the patient be accompanied from the doctor's office by a responsible companion; and there is a possibility of injury to the tissues at the site of the injection caused by either the drug or the needle.

Several sites are available for IM injections. Whatever the site selected by the doctor, it is important to become familiar with the anatomy of the area before administering any medication via the IM route.

As with the oral route, the IM route possesses several significant disadvantages. It is in fact not commonly used in dental practice; however, there are many situations in which this route is valuable. The inability to titrate medications accurately makes it unwise to attempt to reach deeper levels of sedation or pain control with this route, unless the drug administrator is well trained in general anesthesia and maintains continual access to the patient (i.e., does not send the patient home). In adult patients there are limited indications for the administration of pain- and anxiety-controlling drugs via the IM route because the IV route is more effective, reliable, and controllable. One indication is when a longer duration of drug action is desirable, as in postsurgical pain relief or when naloxone or flumazenil are employed following IV drug administration. In the disabled patient and in the recalcitrant child, however, all techniques that require a degree of patient cooperation (oral, inhalation, IV) may prove impossible to employ effectively, and the IM route may be the only means of sedation available. General anesthesia may prove to be the only alternative treatment available to this patient. IM and SM administration of medications for pain and anxiety control is discussed further in Chapter 10.

Inhalation (Pulmonary)

A variety of gaseous agents may be administered by inhalation to produce either sedation or general anesthesia. In dental practice, however, the inhalation route is virtually synonymous with the use of nitrous oxide (N_2O) and oxygen (O_2). Nitrous oxide, the first general anesthetic, has been in use since 1844 in both medicine and dentistry. It is estimated that more than 35% of dentists practicing in the United States use this agent as an aid in patient management.[36] In addition, 13 states (1993 data) have enacted legislation permitting dental hygienists to administer N_2O-O_2.[37]

The advantages and disadvantages discussed relate to inhalation sedation in general and to the use of

N_2O-O_2 in particular. The latent period observed in the inhalation route is usually quite short. Arguably, the inhalation route provides the most rapid onset of clinical action. The drug enters the cardiovascular system after a rapid passage through the mouth or nose, the trachea, and the lungs. With some inhalation agents, such as N_2O, clinical effects may become noticeable as quickly as 15 to 30 seconds after inhalation. This extremely short latent period is used to advantage to permit the administrator to titrate the agent to the patient. The ability to titrate is a major reason why N_2O-O_2 inhalation sedation is considered by many to be the most ideal sedative technique currently available. In addition, the administrator of the gases also possesses the ability to reverse the actions of the drug rapidly should this become necessary. Indeed, the inhalation route is the only one in which drug actions can be quickly adjusted to either increase or to decrease the depth of sedation. With IV sedation, drug action may easily be enhanced; however, it is not possible to lessen the level of sedation unless a specific pharmacological antagonist is available.

Recovery from inhalation sedation is also quite rapid. In an outpatient medical or dental practice rapid recovery is important because it permits the doctor to discharge most patients receiving N_2O-O_2 from the office unaccompanied by a responsible adult companion. Most patients may return to their work, drive a motor vehicle, or operate machinery without undue concern for their well-being.

There are a few disadvantages associated with the use of the inhalation route. Nitrous oxide is not a very potent anesthetic, and when employed with at least 20% O_2 (as it always should be) there will be a certain percentage of patients in whom this technique will fail to produce its desired actions. Patient cooperation is required for the successful use of inhalation sedation, the lack of such cooperation being a significant disadvantage. This will most often be observed in the management of disruptive children and disabled children and adults. In the dental setting, patients must be capable of breathing through their noses. As used in the operating room setting, as a component of a general anesthetic, inhalation agents may be administered through both the mouth and nose; this is of course not possible in dentistry. Patients unable to breath comfortably through their nose will find the use of inhalation sedation in dentistry quite uncomfortable. Physicians and other health professionals employing N_2O-O_2 while treating patients at sites other than the oral cavity (i.e., leg, foot) will be able to use either the nose or mouth as a portal of entry for the gaseous agents, an advantage over their dental colleagues.

Two minor disadvantages of the inhalation route include the size and cost of the equipment and the additional training and expense required for the safe administration of N_2O-O_2. It is especially important that all health personnel employing this technique be well trained in all aspects of its clinical application.

Nitrous oxide-oxygen inhalation sedation is the technique of choice for most dental procedures and many minor surgical procedures that require intraoperative anxiety control. Pain, however, is not consistently controlled when N_2O-O_2 is employed, and its use as an analgesic in lieu of local anesthesia is not recommended primarily because of the high level of effectiveness of local anesthetics and because of the increased incidence of unwanted side effects that may accompany the increased concentration of N_2O that is required to produce profound analgesia. Inhalation sedation is described in depth in Section Four, Chapters 11 through 20.

Intravenous

The IV route of drug administration represents the most effective method of ensuring predictable and adequate sedation in virtually all patients. Effective blood levels of medications are achieved quite rapidly.

Advantages of IV drug administration include its short latent period of about 20 to 25 seconds (permitting medications to be titrated) and the ability to rapidly enhance the action of a drug, if necessary. In clinical practice a drug used intravenously for sedation will require approximately 2 to 8 minutes to reach its desired clinical effect. An additional advantage possessed by many intravenously administered drugs used for the reduction of anxiety is that they are capable of providing amnesic periods of varying duration. Dental or surgical procedures that are feared by the patient, such as the administration of local anesthetics, may be carried out during the amnesic period.

Disadvantages of intravenously administered medications include an inability to reverse the actions of the drugs after they have been injected. Although it is possible to reverse the actions of some medications (e.g., narcotics, anticholinergics, and benzodiazepines) through the use of specific antagonists, this is not the case with all IV agents. The rapid onset of action of intravenously injected drugs, as well as their

accentuated clinical actions, will lead to more exaggerated problems with overdosage, side effects, and allergic manifestations than are seen with other less effective modes of drug administration. The entire office staff must, therefore, be well trained in the use of these drugs, as well as in the recognition and management of associated adverse reactions and emergencies.

Cooperation from the patient is a requirement if a successful venipuncture is to be accomplished. Many children do not permit venipuncture to be performed; therefore IV sedation is rarely attempted in these disruptive patients. Conversely, a cooperative child, willing to permit a venipuncture, probably does not require as profound a technique as IV sedation for his or her dental care. Intraoral injections of local anesthetics might possibly be carried out with a little more patience on the part of the doctor, and perhaps with another technique of sedation, such as inhalation sedation. However, disabled patients (both physically and mentally) are usually good candidates for IV sedation. These patients may be incapable of cooperation during dental therapy, but once sedated, they frequently become readily manageable.

Intravenous sedation may not be suitable for all dentists and physicians. Many doctors are uncomfortable with the technique during their early exposure to it; however, they gradually become more comfortable and relaxed as they gain experience. A small percentage, however, will remain uneasy with the technique and will be unable to provide dental or surgical care up to their usual standards. It is important to remember that regardless of the route of drug administration employed, the quality of care should not be compromised.

Intravenous sedation is not a panacea. Indeed, no technique of sedation is a panacea. Although IV sedation is the most effective technique of sedation currently available, an occasional patient will be encountered in whom IV drugs will prove ineffective. A concern of many involved with the teaching of IV sedation is that intravenously administered drugs will always prove to be effective if a large enough dose is administered. In many cases, however, this course of action will result in the loss of consciousness (general anesthesia, not sedation), and unless the doctor and staff are well versed in managing the unconscious patient, grave complications may develop.

The IV route of administration is most often reserved for the management of the more fearful patient. Drugs and techniques are available that permit the effective management of fear for varying lengths of time. Intravenous drug administration is occasionally used for patients in whom it is difficult to achieve adequate pain control with local anesthetic administration alone. Small doses of narcotic analgesics administered intravenously in conjunction with intra-oral local anesthesia may produce adequate pain control without increased risk to the patient. Intravenous sedation is discussed in detail in Section Five, Chapters 21 through 30.

Thus far we have been able to manage successfully approximately 99% of our dental patients using one or more of the techniques discussed. In the remaining 1% various factors, such as intense fear or biological variability, act to produce management failures. General anesthesia will usually be required for these patients.

We now approach a very important barrier in the spectrum of pain and anxiety control (see Fig. 4-1). When we cross this barrier, we are dealing with the unconscious patient and general anesthesia. The patient can no longer respond to commands, and his protective reflexes are no longer operative.

GENERAL ANESTHESIA

The importance of general anesthesia in dentistry is illustrated by the fact that in excess of 5 million persons annually receive general anesthesia on an ambulatory basis in the United States, the overwhelming majority of these in outpatient dental settings (private practice, surgi-centers).[38] About 16% of all general anesthetics administered in the United States annually are administered in conjunction with dental care.[39]

General anesthesia was the first technique of pain and anxiety control introduced into medical and dental practice. Though still used extensively in the practice of medicine (although the use of sedation is growing rapidly), its use in dentistry has declined since the introduction of the techniques of sedation. There are several advantages to the use of general anesthesia: a rapid onset of action, high effectiveness, and reliability. However, its disadvantages frequently outweigh its advantages. These include an increased risk to the patient and the requirement of an intensive training program in general anesthesia to prepare the doctor to manage the unconscious patient safely. Most general anesthetics employed in dentistry are used for oral surgery; however, there are many indications for their use in other procedures, such as restorations and hygiene, especially in the disruptive child or in the disabled patient.[40]

The step from management of the conscious patient (sedation) to management of the unconscious patient (general anesthesia) is a big one, requiring an absolute minimum of 1 full year of training in the principles and techniques of general anesthesia.[41] General anesthesia will be further discussed in Section Six, Chapters 31 and 32.

REFERENCES

1. American Dental Association, Council on Dental Education: Guidelines for teaching the comprehensive control of pain and anxiety in dentistry, *J Dent Educ* 36:62, 1972.
2. American Dental Association: Continuing education directory, Chicago, 1993, The Association.
3. American Dental Association, Council on Dental Education: Guidelines for teaching the comprehensive control of pain and anxiety in dentistry, Part III, Chicago, 1993, The Association.
4. Bernal-Sprekelsen M, Schmelzer A: Local anesthesia of the head and neck, *Anesth Pain Control* 1(2):81, 1992.
5. Davis JE: Ambulatory surgery . . . how far can we go? *Med Clin North Am* 77(2):365, 1993.
6. Friedman N: Iatrosedation. In McCarthy FM, ed: *Emergencies in dental practice*, ed 3. Philadelphia, 1979, Saunders.
7. Milgrom P: Treatment of the distrustful patient. In Milgrom P et al: *Treating fearful dental patients*. Reston, Va, 1985, Reston Publishing.
8. Shapiro RS, Simpson DE, Lawrence SL et al: A survey of sued and nonsued physicians and suing patients, *Arch Intern Med* 149(10):2190, 1989.
9. Santamaria LB: Non-pharmacologic techniques for treatment of post-operative pain, *Minerva Anestesiol* 56(7-8):359, 1990.
10. Mayer R: Dental treatment measurements in children using audioanalgesia, *Zahnarztliche Mitteilungen* 81(14):1370, 1991.
11. Friis-Hasche E, Hutchings B: Psychology of phobias in relation to dental anxiety, *Tandlaegebladet* 94:(2):42, 1990.
12. Status report: transcutaneous electrical nerve stimulation (TENS) units in pain control, Council on Dental Materials, Instruments, and Equipment, *JADA* 116(4):540, 1988.
13. Malamed SF: A most powerful drug, *J Calif Acad Gen Dent* 4:17, 1979.
14. Norris RL Jr: Local anesthetics, *Emerg Med Clin North Am* 10(4):707, 1992.
15. Daublaender M, Roth W, Kleeman PP: Clinical investigation of potency and onset of different lidocaine sprays for topical anaesthesia in dentistry, *Anesth Pain Control Dent* 1(1):25, 1992.
16. Diker E, Ertuerk A, Akguen G: Is sublingual nifedipine administration superior to oral administration in the active treatment of hypertension? *Angiology* 43(6):477, 1992.
17. Garzone PD, Kroboth PD: Pharmacokinetics of the newer benzodiazepines, *Clin Pharmacokinet* 16(6):337, 1989.
18. Motwani JG, Lipworth BJ: Clinical pharmacokinetics of drug administered bucally and sublingually, *Clin Pharmacokinet* 21(2):83, 1991.
19. Saint-Maurice C, Landais A, Delleur MM et al: The use of midazolam in diagnostic and short surgical procedures in children, *Acta Anaesthesiol Scand Suppl* 92:39, 1990.
20. Rey E, Delaunay L, Pons G et al: Pharmacokinetics of midazolam in children: comparative study of intranasal and intravenous administration, *Eur J Clin Pharmacol* 41(4):355, 1991.

21. Walbergh EJ, Wills RJ, Eckhert J: Plasma concentrations of midazolam in children following intranasal administration, *Anesthesiology* 74(2):233, 1991.

22. Karl HW, Keifer AT, Rosenberger JL et al: Comparison of the safety and efficacy of intranasal midazolam and sufentanil for preinduction of anesthesia in pediatric patients, *Anesthesiology* 76(2):209, 1992.

23. Safranek DJ, Eisenberg MS, Larsen MP: The epidemiology of cardiac arrest in young adults, *Ann Emerg Med* 21(9):1102, 1992.

24. Gill CJ, Michaelides PL: Dental drugs and anaphylactic reactions: report of a case, *Oral Surg* 50:30, 1980.

25. Flaitz CM, Nowak AJ, Hicks MJ: Evaluation of anterograde amnesic effect of rectally administered diazepam in the sedated pedodontic patient, *J Dent Child* 53:17, 1986.

26. Mattila MA, Ruoppi MK, Ahlstron-Bengg E et al: Diazepam in rectal solution as premedication in children, with special reference to serum concentrations, *Br J Anaesth* 53:1269, 1981.

27. Asmussen B: Transdermal therapeutic systems—actual state and future developments, *Methods and Findings in Exper Clin Pharmacol* 13(5):343, 1991.

28. Scopderm: transdermal hyoscine for motion sickness, *Drug Ther Bull* 27(23):91, 1989.

29. Santamaria LB, Fodale V, Mandolfino T et al: Transdermal scopolamine reduces nausea, vomiting and sialorrhea in the postoperative period in teeth and mouth surgery, *Minerva Anesthesiol* 57(9):686, 1991.

30. Todd PA, Goa KL, Langtry HD: Transdermal nitroglycerin (glyceryl trinitrate). A review of its pharmacology and therapeutic use, *Drugs* 40(6):880, 1990.

31. McKenna JP, Cox JL: Transdermal nicotine replacement and smoking cessation, *Am Fam Physician* 45(6):2595, 1992.

32. Calis KA, Kohler DR, Corso DM: Transdermally administered fentanyl for pain management, *Clin Pharm* 11(1):22, 1992.

33. Parker JO: Nitrate tolerance. A problem during continuous nitrate administration, *Eur J Clin Pharmacol* 38(suppl 1):21, 1990.

34. Hogan DJ, Maibach HI: Adverse dermatologic reactions to transdermal drug delivery systems, *J Am Acad Dermatol* 22(5), pt. 1):811, 1990.

35. Roberts SM, Wilson CF, Seale NS et al: Evolution of morphine as compared to meperidine when administered to moderately anxious pediatric dental patients, *Pediatr Dent* 14(5):306, 1992.

36. Jastak JT, Donaldson D: Nitrous oxide, *Anesth Prog* 38(4-5):172, 1991.

37. Department of Educational Surveys: Legal provisions for delegating functions to dental assistants and dental hygienists, Chicago, 1993, American Dental Association.

38. Rosenberg M, Weaver J: General anesthesia, *Anesth Prog* 38(4-5):172, 1991.

39. Craig DC, Ponte J: General anaesthesia for dental surgery, *Dent Update* 111:37, 1988.

40. Cichon P, Bader J: Dental care of the handicapped in intubation anesthesia. The outpatient dental care of handicapped patients in intubation anesthesia at a rehabilitation center, *Schweiz Monatsschr Zahnmed* 100(6):741, 1990.

41. American Dental Association Council on Dental Education. Guidelines for teaching the comprehensive control of pain and anxiety in dentistry, Part II, Chicago, 1992, The Association.

CHAPTER 5

Physical and psychological evaluation

Prior to starting any treatment on a new patient, it is important for the doctor and staff to become aware of that patient's medical history. This is true in all situations, regardless of whether or not the patient is to receive drugs for pain or anxiety control. Because dental care can have a profound effect on both the physical and psychological well-being of the patient, it is extremely important for the person treating the patient to know beforehand the most likely problems to be encountered. It has been stated that "when you prepare for an emergency, the emergency ceases to exist."[1] Prior knowledge of a patient's physical status will enable the doctor to modify the proposed treatment plan to meet the patient's limit of tolerance better. This is of special importance whenever the administration of a drug for the management of pain or anxiety is planned. The administration of certain drugs used in dentistry is specifically contraindicated in some disease states. Knowledge of these contraindications is critical if potentially serious complications are to be avoided.

GOALS OF PHYSICAL AND PSYCHOLOGICAL EVALUATION

In the following discussion a comprehensive but easy-to-use program of physical evaluation will be described.[2] Used as recommended it will allow the doctor to assess accurately the potential risk presented by any patient prior to the start of treatment. The following are the goals that are sought in the use of this system:

1. To determine the patient's ability to tolerate physically the stresses involved in the planned dental treatment
2. To determine the patient's ability to tolerate psychologically the stresses involved in the planned dental treatment
3. To determine if treatment modifications are indicated to enable the patient to better tolerate the stresses of dental treatment
4. To determine whether the use of psychosedation is indicated
5. To determine which technique of sedation is most appropriate for the patient
6. To determine whether contraindications exist to any of the medications to be employed

The first two goals involve the patient's ability to tolerate the stress involved in the planned dental care. Stress may be of either a physiologic or psychological nature. Patients with underlying medical problems are usually less able to tolerate the usual levels of stress associated with various types of dental care. These patients will be more likely to undergo an acute exacerbation of their medical problems during these periods of stress. Such disease processes include angina pectoris, epilepsy, asthma, and sickle cell disease. Although most of these patients will be able to tolerate the planned dental care in relative safety, it is the obligation of the doctor and staff to determine, first, whether this problem does exist, and second, the severity of the problem.

Excessive stress can also prove detrimental to the nonmedically compromised (e.g., "healthy") patient. Fear, anxiety, and pain produce acute changes in the normal homeostasis of the body that may prove to be detrimental. Many patients suffer from fear-related emergencies, including hyperventilation and vasodepressor syncope (fainting).

The third goal is to determine whether or not the usual treatment regimen for a patient requires modification in order to enable the patient to tolerate the stress of treatment better. In many cases a healthy patient will be psychologically unable to tolerate the planned treatment. Treatment may be modified to minimize the stress faced by this patient. The medically compromised patient will also benefit from treatment modification aimed at minimizing stress. The Stress Reduction Protocols that will be introduced in this chapter are designed to aid the doctor in minimizing treatment-related stress in both the healthy and medically compromised patient.

In those instances in which it is believed that the patient will require some assistance in coping with his or her dental treatment, the use of psychosedation should be considered. The last three goals involve the determination of the need for use of these techniques, selection of the most appropriate technique, and selection of the most appropriate drug(s) for patient management.

PHYSICAL EVALUATION

The term *physical evaluation* will be employed to discuss the steps involved in fulfilling the mentioned goals. Physical evaluation in dentistry consists of the following three components:

1. Medical history questionnaire
2. Physical examination
3. Dialogue history

With the information (data base) collected from these three steps the doctor will be better able to (1) determine the physical and psychological status of the patient (establish a risk factor classification for the patient), (2) seek medical consultation, if indicated, and (3) institute appropriate modifications in the dental treatment plan, if indicated. Each of the three steps in the evaluation process will be discussed in general terms, with specific emphasis placed on their importance in the evaluation of the patient for whom the use of pharmacosedative techniques is being considered.

Medical history questionnaire

The use of a written, patient-completed medical history questionnaire is a moral and legal necessity in the practice of both medicine and dentistry. In addition, these questionnaires provide the doctor with valuable information about the physical, and in some cases the psychological, condition of the prospective patient.

Many types of medical history questionnaire are available; however, most are simply modifications of two basic types: the "short" form and the "long"

form. The short-form medical history questionnaire provides basic information concerning a patient's medical history and is best suited for use by a doctor with considerable clinical experience in physical evaluation. When using the short-form history the doctor must have a firm grasp of the appropriate dialogue history required to aid in a determination of the relative risk presented by the patient. The doctor should also be experienced in the use of the techniques of physical evaluation and their interpretation. Unfortunately, most doctors employ the short form or a modification of it in their office primarily because of convenience to the patient. The long form, on the other hand, provides a more detailed data base concerning the physical condition of the prospective patient. It is used most often in teaching situations and represents a more ideal instrument for teaching physical evaluation.

In recent years computer-generated medical history questionnaires have been developed. These permit the patient to enter their responses to questions on a keyboard. Whenever a positive response is given, the computer will bring up additional questions related to the positive response. In essence the computer asks the questions called for in the dialogue history.

Either form of medical history questionnaire may be used to determine the physical status of the patient accurately. Either form of medical history questionnaire can also prove to be entirely worthless. The ultimate value of a medical history questionnaire will rest on the ability of the doctor to interpret its meaning and then to elicit additional information through physical examination and dialogue history. The medical history questionnaire used at the University of Southern California (USC) School of Dentistry (Fig. 5-1) has combined the best of both short and long forms.[3]

Although both forms of medical history questionnaire are valuable in the determination of a patient's physical risk during treatment, a decided failing of most available health history questionnaires is the absence of questions relating to the patient's attitude toward dentistry. It is recommended therefore that one or more questions be added to the questionnaire that relate to this all-important subject. The following questions are included in the USC School of Dentistry adult health history questionnaire:

1. Have you ever had a bad experience in the dentistry office?
2. Do you feel very nervous about having dentistry treatment?

MEDICAL HISTORY

CIRCLE

1. Are you having pain or discomfort at this time? . . . . YES   NO
2. Do you feel very nervous about having dentistry treatment? . . . . YES   NO
3. Have you ever had a bad experience in the dentistry office? . . . . YES   NO
4. Have you been a patient in the hospital during the past two years? . . . . YES   NO
5. Have you been under the care of a medical doctor during the past two years? . . . . YES   NO
6. Have you taken any medicine or drugs during the past two years? . . . . YES   NO
7. Are you allergic to (i.e., itching, rash, swelling of hands, feet or eyes) or made sick by
   penicillin, aspirin, codeine, or any drugs or medications? . . . . YES   NO
8. Have you ever had any excessive bleeding requiring special treatment? . . . . YES   NO
9. Circle any of the following which you have had or have at present:

Heart Failure	Emphysema	AIDS
Heart Disease or Attack	Cough	Hepatitis A (infectious)
Angina Pectoris	Tuberculosis (TB)	Hepatitis B (serum)
High Blood Pressure	Asthma	Liver Disease
Heart Murmur	Hay Fever	Yellow Jaundice
Rheumatic Fever	Sinus Trouble	Blood Transfusion
Congenital Heart Lesions	Allergies or Hives	Drug Addiction
Scarlet Fever	Diabetes	Hemophilia
Artificial Heart Valve	Thyroid Disease	Venereal Disease (Syphilis, Gonorrhea)
Heart Pacemaker	X-ray or Cobalt Treatment	Cold Sores
Heart Surgery	Chemotherapy (Cancer, Leukemia)	Genital Herpes
Artificial Joint	Arthritis	Epilepsy or Seizures
Anemia	Rheumatism	Fainting or Dizzy Spells
Stroke	Cortisone Medicine	Nervousness
Kidney Trouble	Glaucoma	Psychiatric Treatment
Ulcers	Pain in Jaw Joints	Sickle Cell Disease
		Bruise Easily

10. When you walk up stairs or take a walk, do you ever have to stop because of pain in your chest,
    or shortness of breath, or because you are very tired? . . . . YES   NO
11. Do your ankles swell during the day? . . . . YES   NO
12. Do you use more than 2 pillows to sleep? . . . . YES   NO
13. Have you lost or gained more than 10 pounds in the past year? . . . . YES   NO
14. Do you ever wake up from sleep short of breath? . . . . YES   NO
15. Are you on a special diet? . . . . YES   NO
16. Has your medical doctor ever said you have a cancer or tumor? . . . . YES   NO
17. Do you have any disease, condition, or problem not listed? . . . . YES   NO
18. WOMEN: Are you pregnant now? . . . . YES   NO
    Are you practicing birth control? . . . . YES   NO
    Do you anticipate becoming pregnant? . . . . YES   NO

*To the best of my knowledge, all of the preceding answers are true and correct. If I ever have any change
in my health, or if my medicines change, I will inform the doctor of dentistry at the next appointment
without fail.*

_____   _____   _____
Date   *Faculty Signature*   *Signature of Patient, Parent or Guardian*

MEDICAL HISTORY / PHYSICAL EVALUATION UPDATE

Date   *Addition*   *Student/Faculty Signatures*

_____   _____   _____   _____

_____   _____   _____   _____

_____   _____   _____   _____

Fig. 5-1. University of Southern California medical history questionnaire. Room is provided
on the bottom of the form for periodic updates of the patient's medical condition.

It has been my experience that many adult patients are reluctant to express their fears about the proposed treatment to the doctor, hygienist, or assistant for fear of being labeled a "baby." This is especially true of young men, usually under 35 years of age. These persons, rather than expressing their fears, will attempt to "take it like a man" or "grin and bear it." Unfortunately, all too often the outcome of such "manly" behavior is an episode of syncope. In situations in which an open admission of their fears prior to treatment is usually nonexistent, my experience has been that these same patients will volunteer this information in writing if questions are included in the medical history questionnaire. Other means of identifying dental fear and anxiety will be discussed later in this chapter.

The USC questionnaire will be reviewed, providing the basic significance of each of the questions as well as their relevance to the possible use of sedation. More detailed discussion of the use of the various techniques of sedation in the presence of specific medical problems is presented in Chapters 38 and 39.

QUESTION 1. Are you having pain or discomfort at this time?

Comment: The primary thrust of this question is related to dentistry. The question is asked to try to determine what it was that actually brought the patient to seek dental care at this time. Should pain or discomfort be present, it may be necessary for the doctor to treat the patient at this first visit; in a more normal (nonemergent) situation, treatment would not begin until future visits.

QUESTION 2. Do you feel very nervous about having dentistry treatment?

QUESTION 3. Have you ever had a bad experience in the dentistry office?

Comment: The inclusion of questions relating to a patient's attitude toward dentistry is a significant addition to the medical history questionnaire. Most questionnaires, unfortunately, ignore questioning along this important line. It has been my experience that many adult patients, who would never verbally admit to being fearful, willingly indicate their fears or prior negative experiences on the written questionnaire. In-depth dialogue history must seek to determine the reasons for these positive responses.

QUESTION 4. Have you been a patient in the hospital during the past 2 years?

Comment: Knowledge of the reason(s) for hospitalization of the patient greatly increases the doctor's ability to evaluate the patient's ability to tolerate the stresses involved in dental treatment adequately.

QUESTION 5. Have you been under the care of a medical doctor during the past 2 years?

Comment: As with the previous question, knowledge of any medical problems for which the patient required medical intervention can greatly increase the ability to evaluate more fully the patient prior to the start of treatment.

QUESTION 6. Have you taken any medicine or drugs during the past 2 years?

Comment: Awareness of any drugs or medications taken by a patient for the control or treatment of a medical disorder is vitally important. It is not uncommon for patients to take medications but be unaware of the medical condition for which it has been prescribed. In addition, many (most) patients do not even know the name of the medication they are taking. For these two reasons, it is essential that the doctor have available one or more means of identifying these medications, which patients may have with them. Several sources are available, including the *Physician's Desk Reference* (*PDR*), *Facts and Comparisons*, and *Clinical Management of Prescription Drugs* (Long, 1984).[4] The *PDR*, although primarily a compilation of drug package inserts, is a valuable resource, containing a picture section that allows the identification of a drug should the patient not be aware of its name.

Knowledge of the drugs and medications being taken by a patient is essential because (1) it permits identification of the medical disorder being treated, (2) there are potential side effects to most drugs, some of which may be of significance in dentistry (such as postural hypotension), and (3) drug–drug interactions can develop between a patient's medication and drugs administered during dental treatment. Table 5-1 lists drug–drug interactions involving sedative and anesthetic drugs that are used in dentistry.

QUESTION 7. Are you allergic to (i.e., itching, rash, or swelling of hands, feet, or eyes) or made sick by penicillin, aspirin, codeine, or any drugs or medications?

Comment: Question 7 seeks to determine if adverse drug reactions (ADRs) have occurred in the patient. Adverse drug reactions are not uncommon; the most frequently reported reactions being labeled "allergy." However, true allergic drug reactions are relatively uncommon in spite of their great frequency in reporting. The doctor must evaluate all ADRs quite thoroughly, especially in those situations in which closely related drugs are to be administered to or prescribed for the patient. Evaluation of alleged allergy and other adverse drug reactions is discussed further in Chapter 35.

QUESTION 8. Have you ever had any excessive bleeding requiring special treatment?

Comment: Bleeding disorders, such as hemophilia, can lead to modification in certain forms of dental treatment (e.g., surgery, local anesthetic administration, venipunc-

Table 5-1. Drug–drug interactions involving sedative/anesthetic drugs

Drug	Interacting agent	Resulting action
Anesthetics, general	Antidepressants	Hypotension
	Antihypertensives	Hypotension
Barbiturates	Alcohol	Enhanced sedation: ↑ respiratory depression
	Anticoagulants, oral	↓ Anticoagulant effect
	Antidepressants	↓ Antidepressant effect
	β-adrenergic blockers	↓ β-blocker effect
	Corticosteroids	↓ Steroid effect
	Digitalis	↓ Digitalis effect
	Doxycycline	↓ Doxycycline effect
	Griseofulvin	↓ Griseofulvin effect
	Phenothiazines	↓ Phenothiazine effect
	Quinidine	↓ Quinidine effect
	Rifampin	↓ Barbiturate effect
	Valproic acid	↓ Phenobarbital effect
Benzodiazepines	Alcohol	Enhanced sedation
	Barbiturates	Enhanced sedation; ↑ respiratory depression
Meperidine	Barbiturates	↑ CNS depression
	Curariform drugs	↑ Respiratory depression
	Monoamine oxidase inhibitors (MAOIs)	Hypertension
Phenothiazines	Alcohol	↑ Sedation
	Guanethidine	↓ Phenothiazine effect
	Levodopa	↓ Levodopa effect
	Lithium	↓ Phenothiazine effect
Sympathomimetic amines (epinephrine)	Antidepressants	↑ Sedation
	Antihypertensives	↓ Phenothiazine effect
	β-adrenergic blockers	↓ Levodopa effect
	Halogenated anesthetics	↓ Phenothiazine effect
	Digitalis drugs	Hypertension, hypertensive crisis
	Indomethacin	↓ Antihypertensive effect
	MAOIs	Hypertension with epinephrine
		Cardiac dysrhythmias with epinephrine
		↑ Cardiac dysrhythmias
		Severe hypertension
		Hypertensive crisis

Modified from Council on Dental Therapeutics: Clinical products in dentistry, *JADA* 107:885, 1983.

ture) and must therefore be made known to the doctor prior to the start of treatment.

QUESTION 9. Circle any of the following that you have had or have at the present time:

Comment: This question presents a list of the more common illnesses and disorders afflicting the adult population in the United States.

Heart failure

Comment: The severity of heart failure must be determined through the dialogue history. If more serious congestive heart failure (CHF) is present (e.g., dyspnea at rest), the patient will require strict modifications in the planned dental treatment and possibly the administration of supplemental oxygen throughout treatment. Sedation is not contraindicated but should be restricted (if possible) to a "light" level in patients with more severe heart failure (ASA III or IV).

Heart disease or attack

Comment: Heart attack is the lay term for myocardial infarction. Knowledge of the severity, residual damage, and time elapsed since its occurrence is essential, as treatment modifications may be warranted for this patient. Stress reduction is usually indicated.

Angina pectoris

Comment: A history of angina usually indicates the presence of a significant degree of coronary artery atherosclerosis. The risk factor for the typical anginal patient is an ASA III. Stress reduction is strongly recommended in these patients.

High blood pressure

Comment: Elevated baseline or preoperative blood pressure measurements are not uncommonly obtained in the dental or surgical environment primarily because of the added stresses associated with dental treatment or surgery. Whenever patients report a history of high blood pressure, the doctor should determine the antihypertensive drug(s) they are taking as well as their side effects and potential drug interactions. Postural (orthostatic) hypotension is a side effect of many antihypertensive drugs. Guidelines for clinical evaluation of risk based on blood pressure determinations are presented later in this chapter (Table 5-4). The use of stress-reduction techniques is strongly recommended in patients with histories of high blood pressure.

Heart murmur

Comment: Heart murmurs are not uncommon; however, not all murmurs are clinically significant. The doctor should seek to determine whether a murmur is functional (nonpathologic), if clinical signs and symptoms of either valvular stenosis or regurgitation are present, and if antibiotic prophylaxis is warranted. The major clinical symptom associated with a significant murmur is undue fatigue. Current regimens for antibiotic prophylaxis are presented in Table 5-2. Sedation may be employed with these patients as deemed necessary.

Rheumatic fever

Comment: A history of rheumatic fever should lead the doctor to an in-depth dialogue history seeking the presence of rheumatic heart disease (RHD). If RHD is present, antibiotic prophylaxis is indicated to minimize the risk of subacute bacterial endocarditis (SBE). Additional treatment modification may be desirable to further minimize risk to the patient depending on the degree of cardiac involvement. The use of the stress-reduction protocols, including sedation, may be necessary in these patients.

Congenital heart lesions

Comment: An in-depth dialogue history is called for to determine the nature of the lesion and, of greater significance, the degree of disability (if any) it produces. Medical consultation may be required, especially if the patient is a child and/or if the defect is uncorrected. Prophylactic antibiotics may be required prior to treatment. The use of stress-reduction protocols, including sedation, may be necessary in these patients.

Scarlet fever

Comment: Produced by group A β-hemolytic streptococci, scarlet fever rarely produces cardiovascular sequelae such as valvular damage. However, dialogue history should seek to determine the presence of any cardiovascular damage secondary to scarlet fever. The use of the stress-reduction protocols, including sedation, may be necessary in these patients.

Artificial heart valve

Comment: With thousands of artificial valves being placed annually in the United States,[5] it is not uncommon to be called upon to provide dental care for these patients. The primary concern of the doctor is to determine which antibiotic regimen for prophylaxis is appropriate for the patient during dental treatment. Medical consultation prior to the start of therapy is usually recommended in these patients. The use of stress-reduction protocols, including sedation, may be necessary in these patients.

Heart pacemaker

Comment: Pacemakers are implanted beneath the skin of the upper chest or the abdomen, with pacing wires extending into the myocardium. The most frequent indication for the use of a pacemaker is the presence of a clinically significant dysrhythmia. Fixed-rate pacemakers provide the heart with a regular, continuous rate of firing regardless of the inherent rhythm of the heart, whereas the more commonly employed demand pacemakers remain inactive while the rhythm of the heart is normal but take over pacing when the inherent rhythm of the heart becomes abnormal. Although there is little indication for the administration of antibiotics in these patients, medical consultation is recommended prior to the start of the initial treatment to obtain the recommendations of the patient's physician. The effect of stress on the patients cardiac rhythm should be ascertained during this consultation, as well as a discussion of the possible use of sedation, if needed, during the patient's dental care.

Heart surgery

Comment: This very general term may include any procedure from the implantation of a pacemaker to a valve replacement to coronary artery bypass surgery to a heart transplant. A "yes" response to this question should elicit a vigorous dialogue history. Medical consultation should be considered if there is any uncertainty remaining about the patient's physical condition or about the requirement for sedation during dental care.

Artificial joint

Comment: The replacement of hips, knees, and elbows with prosthetic devices has become quite common. It is uncertain, however, whether the bacteremia produced during many dental procedures significantly increases the risk of joint infection. For this reason it is recommended that consultation with the patient's surgeon be obtained prior to the start of any dental procedure. There are no contraindications specifically related to the artificial joint to the use of sedation in these patients.

Table 5-2, A. Recommended standard and alternate prophylactic regimens for dental, oral, or upper respiratory tract procedures*

---

*For patients able to take amoxicillin/penicillin**

Amoxicillin 3.0 g orally 1 hour before procedure, then 1.5 g 6 hours after initial dose.

For patients allergic to amoxicillin/penicillin†

Erythromycin ethylsuccinate 800 mg or erythromycin stearate 1.0 g orally 2 hours before procedure, then one-half the dose 6 hours after initial dose.
Or:
Clindamycin 300 mg 1 hour before procedure, then 150 mg 6 hours after initial dose.

For standard risk patients unable to take oral medications

Ampicillin 2.0 g IV or IM 30 minutes before procedure, then 1.0 g ampicillin IV or IM (or 1.5 g amoxicillin orally)* 6 hours after initial dose.
For ampicillin/amoxicillin/penicillin-allergic patients unable to take oral medications:
Clindamycin 300 mg IV 30 minutes before a procedure and 150 mg IV (or orally)‡ 6 hours after initial dose.

For high-risk patients for whom the practitioner desires to use a parenteral regimen

Ampicillin 2.0 g IV or IM plus gentamicin 1.5 mg/kg IV or IM (not to exceed 80 mg) one-half hour before procedure, followed by 1.5 g oral amoxicillin 6 hours after the initial dose. Alternatively, the parenteral regimen may be repeated 8 hours after the initial dose.
For amoxicillin/ampicillin/penicillin-allergic patients considered to be at high risk:
Vancomycin 1.0 g IV administered over one hour, starting 1 hour before the procedure. No repeat dose is necessary.

From Committee on Rheumatic Fever, Endocarditis, and Kawasaki Disease of the Council on Cardiovascular Disease in the Young of the American Heart Association: Prevention of bacterial endocarditis—recommendations by the American Heart Association, *JAMA* 264:2219, 1990.
NOTE: Initial pediatric doses are listed below. Follow-up doses should be one-half the initial dose. Total pediatric dose should not exceed total adult dose.
   Amoxicillin: 50 mg/kg
   Erythromycin ethylsuccinate or stearate: 20 mg/kg
   Clindamycin: 30 mg/kg
*Includes those with prosthetic heart valves and other high risk patients.
†The following weight ranges may also be used for the initial pediatric dose of amoxicillin.
   <15 kg (33 lbs), 750 mg amoxicillin.
   15-30 kg (33-66 lbs), 1500 mg amoxicillin
   >30 kg (66 lbs), 3,000 mg amoxicillin (full adult dose)
NOTE: Initial pediatric dosages are listed below. Follow-up oral doses should be one-half the initial dose. Total pediatric dose should not exceed total adult dose.
   Ampicillin: 50 mg/kg
   Clindamycin: 10 mg/kg
   Gentamicin: 2.0 mg/kg
   Vancomycin: 20 mg/kg
   Amoxicillin: No initial dose recommended in this table. 25 mg/kg is the follow-up dose.
‡Some patients unable to take oral medications prior to a procedure may be able to take them after the procedure.

Anemia

Comment: Determine the nature of the anemia. *Iron deficiency anemia* is relatively common in the adult population, especially among younger women. The concern with anemic patients is the decreased ability of their blood to carry oxygen. This may be of special significance during procedures in which hypoxia is more likely to develop. Although this should never occur during dental care, the use of deeper levels of IM or IV sedation, without supplemental oxygen administration, is more likely to produce hypoxia, which would be of greater clinical consequence in anemic patients.

Sickle cell anemia (see Sickle cell disease)

Comment: Sickle cell anemia will be seen in some black patients. A differentiation between sickle cell disease and sickle cell trait must be made. The avoidance of hypoxia is of great importance in these patients.

Methemoglobinemia

Comment: Methemoglobinemia can develop when patients receive large doses of certain drugs, such as the local anesthetics prilocaine and articaine.[6] Other drugs, including analgesics such as acetanilid and acetaminophen, can

Table 5-2, B. Cardiac conditions*

Endocarditis prophylaxis recommended

†Prosthetic cardiac valves, including bioprosthetic and homograft valves

†Previous bacterial endocarditis, even in the absense of heart disease

†Surgically constructed systemic-pulmonary shunts

Most congenital cardiac malformations

Rheumatic and other acquired valvular dysfunction, even after valve surgery

Hypertrophic cardiomyopathy

Mitral valve prolapse with valvular regurgitation

Endocarditis prophylaxis not recommended

Isolated secundum atrial septal defect

Surgical repair without residua beyond 6 months of:

    Secundum atrial septal defect

    Ventricular septal defect

    Patent ductus arteriosus

Previous coronary artery bypass graft surgery

Mitral valve prolapse without valvular regurgitation‡

Physiologic, functional, or innocent heart murmurs

Previous Kawasaki disease without valvular dysfunction

Previous rheumatic fever without valvular dysfunction

Cardiac pacemakers and implanted defibrillators

From Council on Dental Therapeutics and American Heart Association: Preventing bacterial endocarditis: a statement for the dental profession, *JAMA* 122:87, 1991.

*This chart lists selected conditions but is not meant to be all-inclusive.

†These patients are at high risk for developing bacterial endocarditis.

‡Individuals with mitral valve prolapse associated with thickening and/or redundancy of the valve leaflets may be at increased risk for bacterial endocarditis, particularly men over the age of 45 years.

Table 5-2, C. Dental or oral surgical procedures

Endocarditis prophylaxis recommended

Dental procedures likely to induce gingival or mucosal bleeding, including professional cleaning

Surgical operations involving respiratory mucosa (maxillary sinus)

Incision and drainage of infected tissue

Intraligamentary injections

Endocarditis prophylaxis not recommended

Dental procedures not likely to induce gingival or mucosal bleeding such as simple adjustment of orthodontic appliances or fillings above the gum line.

Injection of local intraoral anesthetic (except intraligamentary injections)

Shedding of primary teeth

New denture insertion

From Council on Dental Therapeutics and American Heart Association: Preventing bacterial endocarditis: a statement for the dental profession, *JAMA* 122:87, 1991.

This chart lists selected procedures but is not meant to be all-inclusive.

produce elevated blood levels of methemoglobin. Patients with congenital methemoglobinemia should avoid receiving any drugs that can elevate methemoglobin blood levels. Sedation can be employed in patients with any of these forms of anemia, but the avoidance of hypoxia should be a cardinal concern throughout the procedure.

Stroke

Comment: Stroke or cerebral vascular accident (CVA) must be evaluated carefully, for patients with a history of CVA are also at greater risk when exposed to hypoxic levels of oxygen. When sedation is necessary, only lighter levels, such as those provided by inhalation sedation, are recommended. Transient cerebral ischemia (TCI) (see Fainting or Dizzy Spells) is a prodromal syndrome of CVA and must be evaluated carefully. Medical consultation for both CVA and TIA is suggested.

Kidney trouble

Comment: The nature of the kidney problem should be determined. Treatment modifications, including antibiotic prophylaxis, may be in order for several chronic forms of kidney disease. The use of CNS depressants and local anesthetics in patients with renal disease is discussed in Chapter 38.

Ulcers

Comment: The presence of stomach (peptic) or intestinal (duodenal) ulcers may indicate the presence of acute or chronic anxiety and of the possible use by the patient of medications such as tranquilizers, H_1 antagonists, and antacids. Knowledge of which drugs are being taken is important before additional medications are administered during treatment. Sedation may be required for the management of a more fearful patient.

Emphysema

Comment: Emphysema is a form of chronic obstructive pulmonary disease (COPD). The emphysematous patient has a decreased respiratory reserve to draw on in the event that the cells of the body require additional oxygen. Oxygen therapy during dental treatment is strongly recommended in more severe emphysema. Only lighter levels of sedation should be employed.

Cough

Comment: The presence of a chronic cough may be indicative of active tuberculosis or other chronic respiratory disorder such as chronic bronchitis. The administration of

CNS depressants, especially those with greater respiratory depressant properties (e.g., barbiturates, narcotics) must be carefully evaluated in these patients with diminished respiratory reserve.

Tuberculosis

Comment: The status of the disease (active or arrested) should be determined prior to the start of any dental treatment. Medical consultation is recommended if any doubt persists, with possible modification of dental therapy. Inhalation sedation is not recommended for use in patients with active tuberculosis because of the likelihood of contamination of the rubber goods (mask, tubing, reservoir bag) and the difficulty in sterilizing them. If the doctor treats many patients with tuberculosis, disposable rubber goods for inhalation sedation units are available. Patients can be issued their own set of rubber goods for inhalation sedation.

Asthma

Comment: Asthma represents a partial obstruction of the lower airway. The doctor must determine the nature of the asthma (allergic vs. nonallergic), its frequency of occurrence, the causative factors in its onset (e.g., stress), how the patient manages an acute episode, any drugs that the patient may be taking on a regular basis to minimize the risk of an acute episode developing, drugs being used to terminate an acute episode of bronchospasm, and whether hospitalization has been necessary for the patient's asthma.

Sedation is not contraindicated in asthmatics. However, certain drugs, such as barbiturates and narcotics (especially meperidine) should be avoided, if possible, as their use in asthmatics is associated with a greater occurrence of acute bronchospasm. The use of inhalation anesthetics that irritate the respiratory mucosa is contraindicated in asthmatics.

Hay fever

Comment: Hay fever indicates the presence of allergy to a foreign protein material (e.g., pollen, cat dander, dust, dirt). Dental treatment with sedation should be avoided, if possible, during periods in which acute exacerbations are more frequent.

Sinus trouble

Comment: Sinus trouble may indicate the presence of allergy (to be pursued via dialogue history) or of an upper respiratory infection (e.g., cold). Although sedation is not contraindicated, supplemental oxygen administration may be desirable throughout the procedure. Inhalation sedation may be ineffective if the patient has difficulty breathing through his or her nose.

Allergies or hives

Comment: Any allergy must be thoroughly evaluated prior to the start of any dental care and drug administration.

Diabetes

Comment: A positive response requires further inquiry to determine the type of diabetes, its severity, and the level of control of the diabetes. The patient with diabetes does not usually represent a significant risk during dental therapy or during the administration of drugs for the management of pain or anxiety. The greatest concern relating to the management of this patient relates to the possible effect of dental care on the patient's posttreatment eating habits. Dosages of insulin may require modification in situations in which the patient cannot maintain a normal food intake.

Thyroid disease

Comment: The presence of clinically evident hyperthyroidism or hypothyroidism should lead the doctor to be more cautious in the administration of certain drug groups (vasopressors [hyperthyroid], CNS depressants [hypothyroid]) to these patients. On most occasions, however, the patient seen will have been hyperthyroid or hypothyroid at one time, but at the present, because of either surgical intervention, radiation, or drug therapy, the patient will be functioning at a normal level of thyroid hormone activity (euthyroid). The euthyroid patient does not represent an unusual risk to the administration of anesthetic or sedative drugs.

X-ray or cobalt treatment
Chemotherapy (cancer, leukemia)

Comment: The presence or prior existence of cancer of the head or neck may require specific modifications in dental therapy. Irradiated tissues may have a decreased resistance to infection and a diminished vascularity with reduced healing capacity. There is no specific contraindication to the administration of any drug for pain or anxiety control. Many patients with cancer may also be receiving long-term therapy with CNS depressants such as antianxiety drugs, hypnotics, or narcotics. Consultation with the patient's physician may be in order before treatment is begun.

Arthritis
Rheumatism
Cortisone medicine

Comment: A history of arthritis may be associated with chronic use of salicylates (aspirin) or other nonsteroidal antiinflammatory drugs (NSAIDs), some of which may alter blood clotting. Arthritic patients may also be receiving long-term corticosteroid therapy with the possible risk of acute adrenal insufficiency. Such patients may require modification in the dosage of corticosteroids during the period of dental therapy to enable them to respond more appropriately to any additional stress associated with their treatment. An additional consideration relates to the possible difficulty the doctor may have in attempting to place the patient in the recommended position (supine with feet elevated slightly) for sedation. Modification in this position may be necessary to accommodate the patient's physical disability.

Glaucoma

Comment: Glaucoma will be of concern for those patients in whom an anticholinergic is to be administered to diminish salivary gland secretions or for their vagolytic actions. Atropine, scopolamine, and glycopyrrolate are contraindicated in these patients.

Pain in the jaw joints

Comment: Chronic temporomandibular joint (TMJ) pain is seen with increasing frequency today. Evaluation as to the cause(s) should be sought. In the event that the mandibular range of motion is decreased extreme care must be taken when considering the use of deeper levels of sedation or of general anesthesia to ensure that airway patency can be maintained throughout the procedure.

Aids
Hepatitis A (infectious)
Hepatitis B (serum)
Liver disease
Yellow jaundice
Blood transfusion
Drug addiction

Comment: The preceding diseases are either highly transmissable (HIV and AIDS, hepatitis A and B) or are possible indicators of a state of hepatic dysfunction. When any of these disorders is encountered, the doctor should seek to determine the status of the disease process and of the patient via consultation with the patient's physician.

Most of the drugs that will be discussed in this text undergo biotransformation in the liver. The presence of significant liver dysfunction will lead to a decreased rate of drug inactivation and to an increased risk of prolonged clinical duration of action and possibly overdose.

In patients who have undergone blood transfusion or who are admitted (past or present) intravenous drug abusers there is a higher than normal incidence of liver dysfunction and HIV infection. In addition, intravenous drug abusers also have a significantly greater risk of valvular damage in the heart and may require antibiotic prophylaxis. The routine use of universal precautions (gloves, masks, glasses) by health care providers minimizes cross-infection during parenteral sedation and general anesthesia.

Hemophilia

Comment: Hemophilia and other bleeding disorders must be fully evaluated prior to the start of any procedure, especially one in which bleeding may occur. It is prudent to avoid (where possible) the administration of regional nerve blocks in which the risk of positive aspiration of blood is great (inferior alveolar, posterior superior alveolar). In most instances alternative techniques of pain control are available.

The use of parenteral sedation techniques, especially the intravenous route, is not contraindicated if in the doctor's opinion the benefits associated with this procedure outweigh the possible risk of postoperative bleeding.

Veneral disease (syphilis, gonorrhea)
Cold sores
Genital herpes

Comment: The possibility of infection of the doctor is increased in these patients. Where oral lesions are present, dental treatment should be postponed, if possible. The use of universal precautions provides the operator with a degree of protection but not absolute protection.

Epilepsy or seizures

Comment: The type(s) of seizure, its frequency, and the drug(s) used to prevent its occurrence should be determined prior to the start of dental treatment. Stress reduction and other treatment modifications are frequently in order during treatment of these patients, as stress is a major precipitating factor of seizures.

The use of sedation is indicated wherever fear or anxiety is noted. Many of the parenteral drugs used for sedation possess anticonvulsant actions. Diazepam, midazolam, or pentobarbital may be administered intravenously to terminate seizures. Their use as sedatives decreases the likelihood of a seizure developing during dental treatment.

Inhalation sedation with N_2O-O_2 may also be used in epileptic patients who exhibit dental fear or anxiety.

Fainting or dizzy spells

Comment: The presence of chronic postural (orthostatic) hypotension or of symptomatic hypotension or anemia may be detected by this question. Transient ischemic attacks, a form of "prestroke," may also be detected by this question. Further evaluation, including consultation with the patient's physician, is recommended prior to dental treatment or the use of pharmacosedative techniques.

Nervousness
Psychiatric treatment

Comment: The presence of undue nervousness (in general or specifically related to the planned treatment) and the need for psychiatric care should alert the doctor prior to the start of dental therapy. These patients may be receiving any number of drugs for the management of their disorders, drugs that in many instances may interact with other CNS depressants used in dentistry for the control of anxiety (Table 5-1). Medical consultation is usually desirable in these cases.

Sickle cell disease

Comment: Sickle cell disease is seen exclusively in the black patient. A sickle cell crisis can be precipitated during periods of unusual stress or when the patient does not receive an adequate supply of oxygen (hypoxia). When sickle cell disease is present, oxygenation of the patient during dental treatment is strongly recommended and is deemed essential during parenteral sedation techniques.

Bruise easily

Comment: A positive response to this statement may indicate the presence of a bleeding disorder, which should be evaluated prior to the start of dental or surgical treatment. Parenteral sedation techniques as well as regional nerve blocks involving a greater risk of bleeding (e.g., inferior alveolar and posterior superior alveolar nerve blocks) should be avoided until the bleeding problem is corrected.

QUESTION 10. When you walk up the stairs or take a walk, do you ever have to stop because of pain in your chest, shortness of breath, or because you are very tired?

Comment: Although the patient may have indicated in question 9 that he does not have angina or heart failure, clinical signs and symptoms usually associated with these (and other) problems may be present. A positive response to this question should lead the doctor to consider deferring the planned procedure until the patient's physician can be contacted for further evaluation of the patient's status.

QUESTION 11. Do your ankles swell during the day?

Comment: Congestive heart failure immediately comes to mind when one thinks of swelling of ankles (pitting edema or dependent edema); however, there are several other conditions in which this is observed. These include varicose veins, pregnancy (during the latter stages), and renal dysfunction. In addition, healthy persons who spend much of their time standing on their feet (e.g., letter carriers) may also exhibit edematous ankles.

QUESTION 12. Do you use more than two pillows to sleep?

Comment: Persons with more severe CHF exhibit orthopnea, which is the inability to breathe comfortably when lying down. These patients may require additional pillows under their back, in effect propping them up in bed, so that they may breathe more comfortably.

The use of more than two pillows (3+ pillow orthopnea) should be considered significant, prompting medical consultation prior to the start of dental care. Modifications in dental treatment may include altering the position of the dental chair to avoid the supine position. Additionally, the use in parenteral sedation of drugs that are known to significantly depress respiration (such as narcotic agonists and barbiturates) should be avoided, if possible.

QUESTION 13. Have you lost or gained more than 10 pounds in the past year?

Comment: The question refers primarily to any unexpected gain or loss of weight (as opposed to dieting). Such weight changes may be observed in patients with heart failure (increased weight) or with widespread carcinoma (weight loss), among other disorders (hyperthyroidism [loss], hypothyroidism [increase], anorexia nervosa [decrease]). Medical consultation should be considered prior to any dental care to determine the cause of the change in weight and the significance to the overall physical status of the patient.

QUESTION 14. Do you ever wake up from sleep short of breath?

Comment: Paroxysmal nocturnal dyspnea is a clinical manifestation of more severe left heart failure. Medical consultation is recommended. Treatment modifications include positional changes and the possible use of supplemental oxygen.

QUESTION 15. Are you on a special diet?

Comment: This question will elicit dietary modifications resulting from certain medical disorders such as diabetes, high blood pressure, elevated cholesterol levels, heart failure, and also diets that the patient may be on (either through a physician's consultation or a personal dieting plan) in an attempt to lose or gain weight.

In most situations in which a patient is on a carefully planned and monitored dietary plan there are no contraindications to the use of any technique of sedation.

QUESTION 16. Has your medical doctor ever said you have a cancer or tumor?

Comment: This question refers to comments made previously concerning x-ray or cobalt treatment, as well as chemotherapy.

QUESTION 17. Do you have any disease, condition, or problem not listed?

Comment: The patient is permitted to comment on specific matters not previously discussed. Examples of disorders that might be mentioned at this time that will affect the administration of many common drugs used in dentistry include porphyria, atypical plasma cholinesterase, and malignant hyperthermia (hyperpyrexia).

QUESTION 18. Women: are you pregnant now? Are you practicing birth control? Do you anticipate becoming pregnant?

Comment: Pregnancy represents a relative contraindication to extensive elective dental care, particularly during the first trimester. Consultation with the patient's physician is recommended. The use of pharmacosedative techniques should receive careful consideration, weighing the risks versus the benefits to be gained in their use. Of the available techniques, inhalation sedation with N_2O-O_2 is the most highly recommended. Table 5-3 lists many commonly used drugs and their possible fetal effects.

Table 5-3. Known fetal effects of drugs

Drug	Effect
Amobarbital	No adverse effects reported
Anesthetics, local	No adverse effects in dentistry
Atropine	Sympathomimetic effects
Barbiturates	Concentration is greater in fetus than mother because fetal kidneys are unable to eliminate barbiturate
Bupivacaine	Does not cross placenta readily; no adverse effects in dentistry
Chlordiazepoxide	In initial 42 days of pregnancy, congenital abnormalities more frequent
Diazepam	In first trimester, cleft lip and palate increased fourfold
Epinephrine	No adverse effects reported for dental use
Halothane	May be hazardous to pregnant operating room personnel
Hydroxyzine	Hypotonia reported
Lidocaine	No adverse effects reported in dentistry
Meperidine	Decreased neonatal respiration
Mepivacaine	No adverse effects reported in dentistry
Meprobamate	Possible increased congenital abnormalities during first 42 days of pregnancy
Morphine	With chronic usage, smaller newborns; withdrawal symptoms noted
N_2O	With few exposures, no adverse effects reported when a 30% oxygen level is maintained and employed as an anesthetic for dental procedures; evidence suggests an increase in spontaneous abortion among wives of heavily exposed (>9 hours/week) dentists and female chariside assistants; increase in congenital anomalies in offspring of heavily exposed (>9 hours week) dental chairside assistants
Pentazocine	Fetal addiction and withdrawl symptoms of hypertonia, tremors, hyperactivity, and inability to feed
Promethazine	Congenital hip dislocation
Prilocaine	No adverse effect reported in dentisty
Scopolamine	No adverse effects reported

Modified from Council on Dental Therapeutics, *JADA* 107:887, 1983.

After completing the medical history questionnaire (in ink), the patient should sign it. In addition, the doctor should also sign the questionnaire after reviewing it. After any prolonged absence from the office (6 or more months) the questionnaire should be updated. The entire history need not be redone, although this would represent the ideal. The following questions need only be asked:

1. Has there been any change in your general health since your last visit?
2. Are you now under the care of a physician? If so, what is the condition being treated?
3. Are you taking any drug or medicine?

If a positive response is obtained, a detailed dialogue history with the patient should follow. The responses to these questions are recorded on the patient's chart (in the section for progress notes). Where significant changes are present, the entire questionnaire should be redone.

Physical examination

The medical history questionnaire is quite important to the overall assessment of a patient's physical and psychological status. However, there are limitations to the questionnaire. For the questionnaire to be valuable the patient must (1) be aware of the presence of any medical condition, and (2) be willing to share this information with the doctor.

Most patients will not knowingly deceive the doctor by omitting important information from the medical history questionnaire, although cases in which such deception has been attempted are on record. A patient seeking treatment for an acutely inflamed tooth decides to withhold from the doctor the fact that he had a myocardial infarction 2½ months earlier because he knows that to tell the doctor would mean that he would not receive treatment. Another example is that of an HIV-positive individual withholding this information from the doctor for fear of being refused treatment.

The other factor, a patient's knowledge of his physical condition, is a much more likely cause of misinformation on the questionnaire. Most "healthy" persons do not visit their physician regularly for routine checkups. In fact, recent information has suggested that annual physical examination be discontinued in the younger healthy patient because annual physical examination has not proven to be as valuable an aid in preventive medicine as was once thought.[7] In addition, most patients simply do not visit their physicians on a regular basis, doing so instead whenever they become ill. From this premise it therefore stands to reason that the true state of the patient's physical condition may be unknown to the patient. Feeling well, though usually a good indicator of health, is not a guarantee of good health.[8] Many disease entities may be present for a considerable length of time without exhibiting any overt signs or symptoms that warn the patient of their presence (e.g., high blood pressure, diabetes mellitus). When signs and symptoms are present, they are frequently mistaken for other, more benign problems. Although they may answer questions on the medical history questionnaire to the best of their knowledge, patients cannot give a positive response to a question unless they are aware that they do, in fact, have the condition. The first few questions on most histories refer to the length of time since the patient's last physical examination. The value of the remaining answers, dealing with specific disease processes, can be gauged from the patient's responses to these initial questions.

Because of these problems, which are inherent in the use of a patient-completed medical history questionnaire, the doctor must look for additional sources of information about the physical status of the patient. Physical examination of the patient provides much of this information. This consists of

1. Monitoring of vital signs
2. Visual inspection of the patient
3. Function tests, as indicated
4. Auscultation of heart and lungs and laboratory tests, as indicated.

Minimal physical evaluation for all potential patients should consist of (1) measurement of vital signs and (2) visual inspection of the patient.

The primary value of the physical examination is that it provides the doctor with important information concerning the physical condition of the patient immediately prior to the start of treatment, as contrasted with the questionnaire, which provides historical information. The patient should undergo this minimal physical evaluation at an initial visit to the office, prior to the start of any dental treatment. Readings obtained at this time, called baseline vital signs, are recorded on the patient's chart.

Vital signs

There are six vital signs:
1. Blood pressure
2. Heart rate (pulse) and rhythm
3. Respiratory rate
4. Temperature
5. Height
6. Weight

The techniques of recording vital signs as well as guidelines for their interpretation follow.

Blood pressure

Technique. The following technique is recommended for the accurate manual determination of blood pressure.[9] A stethoscope and sphygmomanometer (blood pressure cuff) are the required equipment. The most accurate and reliable of these devices is the mercury-gravity manometer. The aneroid manometer, probably the most frequently employed, is calibrated to be read in millimeters of mercury (mm Hg or torr) and is also quite accurate, if well maintained. Rough handling of the aneroid manometer may lead to erroneous readings. It is recommended that the aneroid manometer be recalibrated at least annually by checking it against a mercury manometer. Many automatic blood pressure monitoring devices are now available, their cost ranging from under $100 to several thousand dollars. Likewise, their accuracy varies widely.[10] The use of automatic monitors simplifies the monitoring of vital signs, but doctors should be advised to check the accuracy of these devices periodically (comparing values with those of a mercury manometer).

For routine preoperative monitoring of blood pressure the patient should be seated in the upright position. The arm should be at the level of the heart—relaxed, slightly flexed, and supported on a firm surface (e.g., the arm rest of the dental chair). The patient should be permitted to sit for at least 5 minutes before the blood pressure is recorded. This will permit the patient to relax somewhat so that the recorded blood pressure will be closer to the patient's normal baseline reading. During this time other nonthreatening procedures may be carried out, such as review of the medical history questionnaire.

The blood pressure cuff should be deflated before being placed on the arm. The cuff should be wrapped evenly and firmly around the arm, with the center of the inflatable portion over the brachial artery with the rubber tubing lying along the medial aspect of the arm. The lower margin of the cuff should be placed approximately 1 inch (2 to 3 cm) above the antecubital fossa (the patient should still be able to flex the elbow). A blood pressure cuff is too tight if two fingers cannot be placed under the lower edge of the cuff. Too tight a cuff will decrease venous return from the arm, leading to erroneous measurements. A cuff is too loose (a much more common problem) if it may be easily pulled off of the arm with gentle tugging. A slight resistance should be present when a cuff is properly applied.

The radial pulse in the wrist should be palpated and then the pressure in the cuff increased rapidly to a point approximately 30 mm Hg above the point at which the pulse disappears. The cuff should then be slowly deflated at a rate of 2 to 3 mm Hg per second until the radial pulse returns. This is termed the *palpatory systolic pressure*. Remaining pressure in the cuff should be released to permit venous drainage.

Determination of blood pressure by the more accurate auscultatory method requires palpation of the brachial artery, located on the medial aspect of the antecubital fossa. The earpieces of the stethoscope should be placed facing forward, firmly in the recorder's ears. The diaphragm of the stethoscope must be placed firmly on the medial aspect of the antecubital fossa, over the brachial artery. To reduce extraneous noise, the stethoscope should not touch the blood pressure cuff or rubber tubing.

The blood pressure cuff should be rapidly inflated to a level 30 mm Hg above the previously determined palpatory systolic pressure. Pressure in the cuff should be gradually released (2 to 3 mm per second) until the first sound is heard through the stethoscope. This is referred to as the systolic blood pressure.

As the cuff deflates further, the sounds undergo changes in quality and intensity. As the cuff pressure approaches the diastolic pressure, sounds become dull and muffled and then cease. The diastolic blood pressure is best indicated as the point of complete cessation of sounds. In some instances, however, complete cessation of sound does not occur. In these instances the point at which the sounds became muffled will be the diastolic pressure. The cuff should be slowly deflated to a point 10 mm Hg beyond the point of disappearance, and then totally deflated.

Should additional recordings be necessary, a wait of at least 15 seconds is required before reinflating the blood pressure cuff. This permits blood trapped in the arm to leave, providing more accurate readings.

Blood pressure is recorded on the patient's chart or sedation/anesthesia record as a fraction: 130/90 R or L (arm on which recorded).

Common errors in technique. There are some relatively common errors associated with the recording of blood pressure, leading to obtaining inaccurate readings (too high or too low). Lack of awareness of these may lead to unnecessary referral for medical consultation, added financial burden to the patient, and a loss of faith in the doctor.

1. Applying the blood pressure cuff too loosely produces falsely elevated readings. This probably represents the most common error in recording blood pressure.

2. Use of the wrong cuff size can result in erroneous readings. A "normal adult" blood pressure cuff placed on an obese arm will produce falsely elevated readings. This same cuff applied to the very thin arm of a child or adult will produce false low readings. Sphygmomanometers are available in a variety of sizes. The width of the compression cuff should be approximately 20% greater than the diameter of the extremity on which the blood pressure is being recorded (Fig. 5-2).

3. An auscultatory gap may be present (Fig. 5-3) representing a loss of sound (a period of silence) between systolic and diastolic pressures, the sound reappearing at a lower level. For example, systolic sounds are noticed at 230 mm Hg; however, the sound then disappears at 198 mm Hg, reappearing at approximately 160 mm Hg. All sound is lost at 90 mm Hg. The ausculatory gap occurred between 160 and 198 mm Hg. In this situation, if the person recording the blood pressure has not palpated (estimated) the systolic blood pressure prior to auscultation, the cuff might be inflated to some arbitrary pressure, say 165 mm Hg. At this level the recorder would pick up no sound because this lies within the auscultatory gap. Sounds would first be noted at 160 mm Hg, with their disappearance at 90 mm Hg, levels well within therapy limits (see guidelines for blood pressure, next subsection). In reality, however, this patient has a blood pressure of 230/90, a significantly elevated blood pressure that represents a greater risk to the patient during dental treatment (in fact, this patient is not considered to be a candidate for elective dental care). Although the auscultatory gap occurs only infrequently, the possibility of error may be eliminated by first using the palpatory technique. The pulse will be present throughout the gap (disappearing, in our example, at 230 mm Hg), although the sound will not be present. Although there is no pathologic significance to its presence, the auscultatory gap is found most often in patients with high blood pressure.

4. The patient may be anxious. Having one's blood pressure recorded may produce anxiety, causing transient elevations in blood pressure, primarily the systolic. This is even more likely

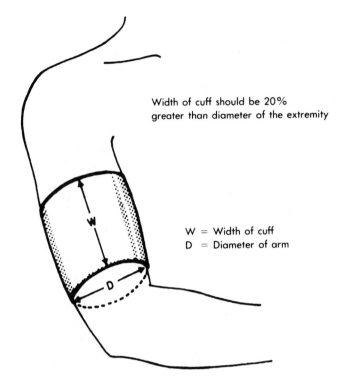

Width of cuff should be 20%
greater than diameter of the extremity

W = Width of cuff
D = Diameter of arm

Fig. 5-2. Determination of proper size of blood pressure cuff. (From Burch GE, DePasquale NP: *Primer of clinical measurement of blood pressure,* St Louis, 1962, Mosby.)

to be noted in a patient who is to receive sedation for management of their dental fear. For this reason it is recommended that baseline measurements of vital signs be obtained at a visit prior to the actual start of treatment, perhaps the first office visit, when the patient will only be completing various forms. Measurements are more likely to be the norm for the particular patient at this time.

5. Blood pressure is based on the Korotkoff sounds (Fig. 5-4) produced by the passage of blood through occluded, partially occluded, or unoccluded arteries. Watching a mercury column or needle on an aneroid manometer for "pulsations" will lead to the recording of falsely elevated systolic pressures. Pulsations of the dial are noted approximately 10 to 15 mm Hg before the first Korotkoff sounds are heard.

6. Use of the left or right arm will produce differences in recorded blood pressure. A difference of 5 to 10 mm Hg exists normally between arms, the left arm being slightly higher.

Guidelines for clinical evaluation. The USC physical evaluation system is based on the American Society of Anesthesiologists (ASA) Physical Status Classifica-

tion System.[11] It provides four risk categories based on a patient's medical history and physical evaluation. The ASA categories for blood pressure recordings in adults are presented in Table 5-4.[12]

For the adult patient with a baseline blood pressure in the ASA I range (<140/<90 mm Hg) it is suggested that the blood pressure be recorded every 6 months, unless specific dental treatment demands more frequent monitoring. The parenteral administration of any drug (local anesthesia, intramuscular, intravenous, inhalation sedation, or general anesthesia) mandates the more frequent recording of vital signs (see Chapter 6).

Patients with blood pressures in the ASA II, III, or IV categories should be monitored more frequently (e.g., at every appointment), as outlined in the guidelines. Patients with known high blood pressure should also have their blood pressure monitored at each visit to determine if their blood pressure is adequately controlled. It is not possible to gauge a blood pressure by "looking" at a person or by asking "how they feel." The routine monitoring of blood pressure in all patients according to the treatment guidelines will effectively minimize the occurrence of acute complications of high blood

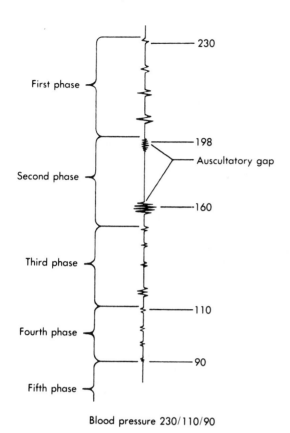

Blood pressure 230/110/90

Fig. 5-3. Korotkoff sounds illustrating auscultatory gap. Sound is heard at 230 torr, disappears at 198 torr, and reappears at 160 torr. Sound disappears (fifth phase) at 90 torr. (From Burch GE, DePasquale NP: *Primer of clinical measurement of blood pressure,* St Louis, 1962, Mosby.)

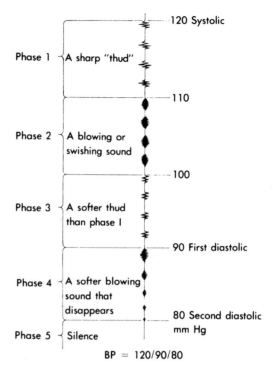

BP = 120/90/80

Fig. 5-4. Korotkoff sounds. Systolic blood pressure is recorded at the first phase, diastolic blood pressure at the point of disappearance of sound (fifth phase). (From Burch GE, DePasquale NP: *Primer of clinical measurement of blood pressure,* St Louis, 1962, Mosby.)

pressure (e.g., hemorrhagic cerebrovascular accident).

When parenteral or inhalation sedation techniques or general anesthesia is to be employed, there is a greater need for obtaining baseline vital signs. One factor that will be used to evaluate a patient's recovery from sedation and ability to be discharged from the office will be a comparison of the posttreatment vital signs with the baseline values.

Still another reason for routine monitoring of blood pressure relates to the management of medical emergencies. After the basic steps of management in each emergency, certain specific steps are necessary for definitive treatment. Primary among these is the monitoring of vital signs, particularly blood pressure. Blood pressure recorded during an emergency situation provides an important indicator of the status of the cardiovascular system. However, unless a baseline or nonemergency blood pressure had been re-

corded earlier, the measurement obtained during the emergency is less significant. A recording of 80/50 mm Hg is less ominous in a patient with a preoperative reading of 110/70 mm Hg than if the pretreatment recording were 190/110 mm Hg. The absence of blood pressure is an indication for beginning cardiopulmonary resuscitation.

The normal range for blood pressure in younger patients is somewhat lower than that in adults. Table 5-5 presents a normal range of blood pressure in infants and children.

Heart rate and rhythm

Technique. Heart rate (pulse) and rhythm may be measured at any readily accessible artery (Fig. 5-5). Most commonly employed for routine measurement are the *brachial artery,* located on the medial aspect of the antecubital fossa, and the *radial artery,* on the radial and ventral aspects of the wrist.

When palpating an artery, the fleshy portions of the first two fingers (index and middle) should be used. Gentle pressure must be applied in order to feel the pulsation, but do not press so firmly that the artery is occluded and no pulsation is felt. The

Table 5-4. Guidelines for blood pressure (adult)

Blood pressure (mm Hg or torr)	ASA classification	Dental therapy consideration
<140 and <90	I	1. Routine dental management 2. Recheck in 6 months, unlesss specific treatment dictates more frequent monitoring
140 to 160 and/or 90 to 94	II	1. Recheck blood pressure prior to dental treatment for 3 consecutive appointments; if all exceed these guidelines, medical consultation is indicated 2. Routine dental management 3. Stress-reduction protocol as indicated
160 to 200 and/or 95 to 115	III	1. Recheck blood pressure in 5 minutes 2. If blood pressure is still elevated, a medical consultation prior to dental therapy is warranted 3. Routine dental therapy 4. Stress-reduction protocol
>200 and/or >115	IV	1. Recheck blood pressure in 5 minutes 2. Immediate medical consultation if still elevated 3. No dental therapy, routine or emergency,* until elevated blood pressure is corrected 5. Refer to hospital if immediate dental therapy indicated

*When the blood pressure of the patient is slightly above the cut-off for category IV and where anxiety is present, the use of inhalation sedation may be employed in an effort to diminish the blood pressure (via the elimination of stress) below the 200/115 level. The patient should be advised that if the N_2O-O_2 succeeds in decreasing the blood pressure below this level, the planned treatment will proceed. However, should the blood pressure remain elevated, the planned procedure will be postponed until the elevated blood pressure has been lowered to a more acceptable range.

Table 5-5. Normal blood pressure for various ages (figures have been rounded off to nearest decimal place)

Ages	Mean systolic ±2 S.D.	Mean diastolic ±2 S.D.
Newborn	80 ± 16	46 ± 16
6 mo-1 year	89 ± 29	60 ± 10*
1 yr	96 ± 30	66 ± 25*
2 yr	99 ± 25	64 ± 25*
3 yr	100 ± 25	67 ± 23*
4 yr	99 ± 20	65 ± 20*
5-6 yr	94 ± 14	55 ± 9
6-7 yr	100 ± 15	56 ± 8
7-8 yr	102 ± 15	56 ± 8
8-9	105 ± 16	57 ± 9
9-10 yr	107 ± 16	57 ± 9
10-11 yr	111 ± 17	58 ± 10
11-12 yr	113 ± 18	59 ± 10
12-13 yr	115 ± 19	59 ± 10
13-14 yr	118 ± 19	60 ± 10

From Nadas AS, Fyler DC: *Pediatric cardiology,* ed 3. Philadelphia, 1972, Saunders
*In this study the point of muffling was taken as the diastolic pressure

thumb ought not to be used to monitor pulse because it contains a fair-size artery.

Guidelines for clinical evaluation. Three factors should be evaluated while the pulse is monitored:

1. The heart rate (recorded as beats per minute)
2. The rhythm of the heart (regular or irregular)
3. The quality of the pulse (thready, weak, bounding, full)

The heart rate should be evaluated for a minimum of 30 seconds, and ideally for 1 minute. The normal resting heart rate for an adult ranges from 60 to 110 beats per minute. It is frequently lower in a well-conditioned athlete and elevated in the fearful individual. However, clinically significant pathology may also produce slow (bradycardia [<60 per minute]) or rapid (tachycardia [>110 per minute]) heart rates. It is suggested that any heart rate under 60 or above 110 beats per minute (adult) be evaluated (initially via dialogue history). Where no obvious cause is present (endurance sports, anxiety), medical consultation should be considered.

The normal heart maintains a relatively regular rhythm. Irregularities in rhythm should be confirmed and evaluated via dialogue history and/or medical consultation prior to the start of treatment.

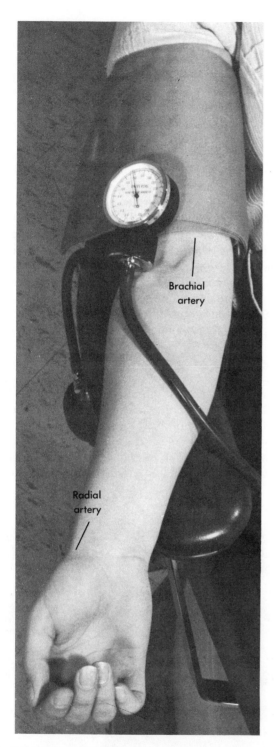

Brachial
artery

Radial
artery

Fig. 5-5. Location of brachial artery and radial artery. Brachial artery is located in the medial half of the antecubital fossa; the radial artery is located in the lateral volar aspect of the wrist.

The occasional *premature ventricular contraction (PVC)* is so common that it is not necessarily considered to be abnormal. Premature ventricular contractions may be produced by smoking, fatigue, stress, various medications (e.g., epinephrine), and alcohol. More frequent PVCs are usually associated with a damaged or an ischemic myocardium. However, where PVCs are present at a frequency of five or more per minute, especially if they appear at irregular intervals, medical consultation should definitely be sought. Patients with five or more PVCs per minute are considered to be at greater risk for sudden cardiac death (ventricular fibrillation)[13] and are more and more likely to have automatic defibrillators implanted into their abdomen.[14] Clinically, PVCs are detected by palpation, as a break in a generally regular rhythm in which a longer-than-normal pause (a skipped beat) is noted, followed by the resumption of a regular rhythm.

A second disturbance in the pulse is termed *pulsus alternans.* It is not truly a dysrhythmia but a regular heart rate that is characterized by a pulse in which strong and weak beats alternate. It is produced by the alternating contractile force of a diseased left ventricle. Pulsus alternans is observed frequently in severe left ventricular failure, severe arterial high blood pressure, and coronary artery disease. Medical consultation is indicated.

Many other dysrhythmias may be noted by palpation of the pulse. The "irregular irregularity" of *atrial fibrillation* is noted in hyperthyroid patients and warrants pretreatment consultation. *Sinus arrhythmia* is detected frequently in healthy adolescent patients. It is noted as an increase in heart rate followed by a decrease in rate that is correlated with the breathing cycle (the heart rate increases during inspiration, decreases with expiration). Sinus arrhythmia is not indicative of any cardiac abnormality and therefore does not require pretreatment consultation.

The quality of the pulse is commonly described as full, bounding, thready, or weak. These adjectives relate to the subjective "feel" of the pulse and are used to describe situations such as a "full bounding" pulse (as noted in severe arterial high blood pressure) or a "weak thready" pulse often noted in patients with hypotension and signs of shock. Table 5-6 presents the range of normal heart rates in children of various ages.

Respiratory rate

Technique. Determination of the respiratory rate must be made surreptitiously. Patients aware that their breathing is being observed do not breathe normally. Therefore, it is recommended that respiration be monitored immediately after the heart rate. The fingers are left on the patient's radial or brachial pulse after the heart rate has been determined; however, the doctor counts respirations (by observing the rise and fall of the chest) instead, for a minimum of 30 seconds, ideally for 1 minute.

Guidelines for clinical evaluation. Normal respiratory rate for an adult is 14 to 18 breaths per minute. Bradypnea (abnormally slow rate) may be produced by, among other causes, narcotic administration, and tachypnea (abnormally rapid rate) is seen in fever and alkalosis. The most common change in ventilation in dentistry will be hyperventilation, an abnormal increase in the rate and depth of respiration. It is also seen, but much less frequently, in diabetic acidosis. The most common cause of hyperventilation in dental and surgical settings is extreme psychological stress.

Any significant variation in respiratory rate should be evaluated prior to treatment. The absence of spontaneous ventilation is always an indication for artificial ventilation. Table 5-7 presents the normal range of respiratory rate at different ages.

Table 5-6. Average pulse rate at different ages

Age	Lower limits of normal	Average	Upper limits of normal
Newborn	70	120	170
1–11 mo	80	120	160
2 yr	80	110	130
4 yr	80	100	120
6 yr	75	100	115
8 yr	70	90	110
10 yr	70	90	110

From Behrman RE, Vaughn VC III: *Nelson textbook of pediatrics,* ed 12. Philadelphia, 1983, Saunders. Reprinted by permission.

Table 5-7. Respiratory rate by age

Age	Rate/minute
Neonate	40
1 wk	30
1 yr	24
3 yr	22
5 yr	20
8 yr	18
12 yr	16
21 yr	12

Blood pressure, heart rate and rhythm, and respiratory rate are the vital signs that provide information about the functioning of the cardiorespiratory system. It is suggested that they be recorded as a part of the routine physical evaluation for all potential patients. Recording of the remaining vital signs—temperature, height, and weight—although desirable, may be considered as optional. However, in cases in which parenteral medications are to be administered, especially in lighter weight, younger, or older patients, recording of a patient's weight becomes considerably more important.

Temperature

Technique. Temperature should be monitored orally. The thermometer, sterilized and shaken down, is placed under the tongue of the patient, who has not eaten, smoked, or had anything to drink in the previous 10 minutes. The thermometer remains in the closed mouth for 2 minutes before removal. Disposable thermometers (Fig. 5-6) as well as digital thermometers are equally accurate and easy to use (Fig. 5-7). Forehead thermometers are effective in situations in which the patient's behavior will not permit use of an oral thermometer (Fig. 5-8)

Guidelines for clinical evaluation. The "normal" oral temperature of 98.6° F (37.0° C) is only an average. The true range of normal is considered to be from 97° F to 99.6° F (36.11° C to 37.56° C). Temperatures vary (from 0.5° F to 2.0° F) during the day,

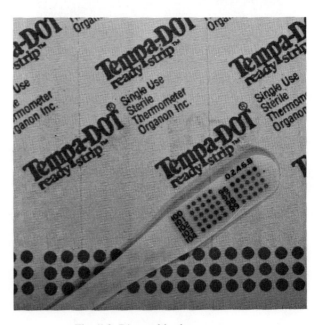

Fig. 5-6. Disposable thermometer.

being lowest in the early morning and highest in the late afternoon.

Fever represents an increase in temperature beyond 99.6° F. Temperatures in excess of 101° F (38.33° C) usually indicate the presence of an active disease process. Evaluation of the cause of the fever is necessary prior to treatment. When dental or periodontal infection is considered to be a probable cause of elevated temperature, immediate treatment (e.g., incision and drainage, pulpal extirpation, or extraction) and antibiotic and antipyretic therapy are indicated. If the patient's temperature is 104° F (40.00° C) or higher, pretreatment medical consultation is indicated.

The planned treatment, especially any treatment involving the administration of CNS depressants, should be postponed, if possible, until the cause of the elevated temperature is determined and treated.

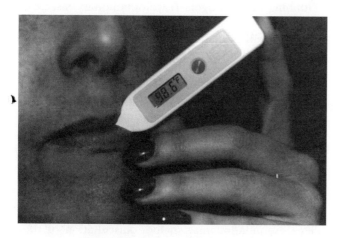

Fig. 5-7. Digital thermometer.

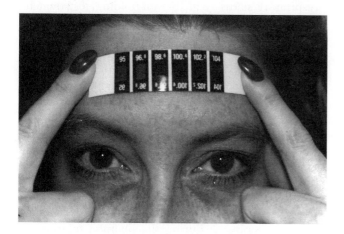

Fig. 5-8. Forehead thermometer.

Height and weight

Technique. Patients should be asked to state their height and weight. The range of normal height and weight is quite variable and is indicated on charts developed by various insurance companies. New guidelines of range of normal height and weight have been published (Table 5-8).

Guidelines for clinical evaluation. Gross obesity or underweight may be an indication of an active disease process. Obesity will be noted in various endocrine disorders such as Cushing's syndrome, whereas extreme underweight may be noted in pulmonary tuberculosis, malignancy, and hyperthyroidism. Anorexia nervosa should also be considered where an extremely underweight individual is encountered. In all instances of gross obesity or extreme underweight, pretreatment medical consultation is recommended.

Excessively tall persons are referred to as giants, whereas persons who are decidedly shorter than normal are called dwarfs. In both instances endocrine gland dysfunction may be present. Medical consultation is usually not necessary for these patients.

Whenever a pharmacosedative technique is to be employed in which titration is not possible (intramuscular [IM] or submucosal [SM]) the approxi-

Table 5-8. Acceptable weights (in pounds) for men and women.[1,2]

Height	Age	
	19-34 Years	*35 years and older*
5'0"	97-128	108-138
5'1"	101-132	111-143
5'2"	104-137	115-148
5'3"	107-141	119-152
5'4"	111-146	122-157
5'5"	114-150	126-162
5'6"	118-156	130-167
5'7"	121-160	134-172
5'8"	125-164	138-178
5'9"	129-169	142-183
5'10"	132-174	146-188
5'11"	136-179	151-194
6'0"	140-184	155-199
6'1"	144-189	159-205
6'2"	148-195	164-210

[1]Weights based on weighing in without shoes or clothes.
[2]Source: United States Department of Agriculture and United States Department of Health and Human Resources, 1990.

mate weight of the patient must be obtained. One method used to determine the appropriate dose of drug for the patient is the patient's lean body weight (Chapters 10 and 36). It is suggested that the patient be weighed on a scale in the doctor's office rather than relying on the patient to tell you his or her weight.

Visual inspection of the patient. Visual observation of the patient will provide the doctor with valuable information concerning the medical status and the patient's level of apprehension toward the planned treatment. Observation of the patient's posture, body movements, speech, and skin can assist in a diagnosis of possibly significant disorders that may previously have gone undetected. Management of many of these patients will be discussed in Chapters 38 and 39.

Patients with CHF and other chronic pulmonary disorders may be forced to sit in a more upright position in the chair because of significant orthopnea. The arthritic patient with a rigid neck may need to rotate his entire trunk when turning toward the doctor to view an object from the side. Recognition of these factors will better enable the doctor to determine necessary treatment modifications.

Involuntary body movements occurring in conscious patients may connote significant disorders. Tremor is noted in disorders such as fatigue, multiple sclerosis, parkinsonism, hyperthyroidism, and of great importance to dentistry, hysteria and nervous tension.

The character of a patient's speech may also be significant. For example, CVA may cause muscle paralysis leading to speech difficulties. Anxiety over impending treatment may also be noted by listening to a patient's speech. Rapid response to questions or a nervous quiver to the voice may indicate the presence of increased anxiety and the possible need for sedation during treatment.

Other disorders may be uncovered by the detection of odor on the patient's breath. A sweet, fruity odor of acetone is present in diabetic acidosis and ketosis. The smell of ammonia is noted in uremia. Probably the most likely odor to be on the breath of a patient is that of alcohol. Detection of alcohol on a patient's breath should lead the doctor to consider the possibility of heightened anxiety or of drug abuse. The planned pharmacosedative procedure should be canceled in a patient who is "self-medicated."

The skin is a vast source of information about the patient. It is my belief that the doctor should shake hands on greeting the patient as a matter of routine. Much information can be gathered from the feel of a patient's skin. For example, the skin of a very apprehensive person will feel cold and wet, a patient with a hyperthyroid condition will be warm and wet, and the skin of a patient with diabetic acidosis will be warm but dry.

Looking at skin is also valuable. The color of the skin is significant. Pallor may indicate anemia or heightened anxiety. Cyanosis, indicating heart failure, chronic pulmonary disease, or polycythemia will be most notable in the nail beds and gingiva. Flushed skin may point to apprehension, hyperthyroidism, or elevated temperature, and jaundice may indicate past or present hepatic disease.

Additional factors revealed through a visual examination of the patient include the presence of prominent jugular veins (in a patient seated upright), an indication of possible right heart failure; clubbing of the fingers (cardiopulmonary disease); swelling of the ankles (seen in right heart failure, varicose veins, renal disease, and in the latter stages of pregnancy); and exophthalmos (hyperthyroidism).

For a more complete discussion of the art of observation and its importance in medical diagnosis the reader is referred to a truly excellent textbook, *Mosby's Guide to Physical Examination*.[15]

Additional evaluation procedures. Following completion of these three steps (medical history questionnaire, vital signs, and physical examination), it may, on occasion, be necessary to follow up with additional evaluation for specific medical disorders. This examination may include auscultation of the heart and lungs, testing for urinary or blood glucose levels, retinal examination, function tests for cardiorespiratory status (e.g., breath-holding test, match test), electrocardiographic examination, and blood chemistries. At present many of these tests are used in dental offices but do not represent a standard of care in dentistry. However, when general anesthesia or certain sedation techniques are to be employed, the level of routine pretreatment evaluation may require some or all of these evaluations.

Dialogue history

After patient information has been collected, the doctor next reviews with the patient all positive responses on the questionnaire, seeking to determine the severity of these disorder(s) and the potential risk they represent during the planned treatment. This process is termed the dialogue history, and it forms an integral part of patient evaluation. The doctor must put to use all available knowledge of the disease to assess accurately the degree of risk to the patient.

Several examples of dialogue history are presented below. For a more in-depth description of dialogue history for specific disease states, the reader is referred to the *Handbook of Medical Emergencies in the Dental Office*.[16]

In response to a positive reply to the question "Are you diabetic?" the dialogue history that follows includes these questions:

1. What type of diabetic are you (insulin-dependent [type-I] or non–insulin-dependent [type-II])?
2. How do you control your diabetes (oral medication or injectable insulin)?
3. How often do you check your blood or urine for sugar, and what are the measurements (monitoring the degree of control of the disease)?
4. Have you ever required hospitalization for your diabetic condition?

The following is a dialogue history to be initiated with a positive reply to angina pectoris:

1. What precipitates your angina?
2. How frequently do you suffer anginal episodes?
3. How long do your anginal episodes last?
4. Describe a typical anginal episode.
5. How does nitroglycerin affect the anginal episode?
6. How many tablets or sprays do you normally need to terminate the episode?
7. Are your anginal episodes stable (similar in nature), or has there been a recent change in their frequency, intensity, radiation pattern of pain, or response to nitroglycerin (seeking unstable or preinfarction angina)?

Dialogue history should be completed for every positive response noted on the medical history. A written note should be included on the questionnaire that summarizes the patient's response to the questions. For example, "heart attack" is circled. Written, by the doctor, next to this on the questionnaire is the statement "June 1990," implying that the patient stated they suffered their heart attack in June 1990.

RECOGNITION OF ANXIETY

Thus far the primary thrust of our evaluation of the patient has been the medical history. Few, if any, questions have been directed at the patient's feelings toward the upcoming treatment. The typical medical history questionnaire (long form) has questions that ask "Do you have fainting spells or seizures?" and "Have you had any serious trouble associated with any previous dental treatment?" The short-form history contains no questions that relate to this important area. Heightened anxiety and fear of dentistry or surgery are stresses that can lead to the exacerbation of medical problems such as angina, seizures, or asthma or to other stress-related problems, such as hyperventilation or vasodepressor syncope. One of the goals of patient evaluation is to determine if the patient is psychologically able to tolerate the stresses that are associated with the planned dental treatment. Two methods are available to recognize the presence of anxiety. First is the medical history questionnaire, and second is the art of observation.

Earlier in this chapter it was recommended that one or more questions that relate to a patient's attitudes toward dentistry be included in the medical history questionnaire. It has been our experience at the USC School of Dentistry that patients who will not verbally admit their fears to their doctor will in fact record on the chart that they are apprehensive. A positive response to any of these questions should alert the doctor to begin a more in-depth interview with the patient, seeking to determine the cause of their fear of dentistry.

In the absence of such questions or in the absence of a positive response to such questions, careful observation of the patient will enable the doctor and staff members to recognize the presence of unusual degrees of anxiety. Some adult patients will volunteer to the doctor and staff that they are quite apprehensive; however, the vast majority of apprehensive adult patients (both male and female) will do everything within their power to attempt to conceal their anxiety. The usual feeling of patients is that their fear is irrational and probably even a bit childish and that they are the only persons who feel this way. They do not wish to tell the doctor of their fear because they are afraid of being labeled "childish." Because this attitude exists in many adults, all members of the dental and medical office staff should be trained to recognize clinical signs and symptoms of heightened anxiety.

Although there are a number of levels into which anxiety may be subdivided, for the purposes of this discussion two will be discussed: moderate anxiety and severe (neurotic) anxiety.

Patients with severe anxiety will usually not attempt to hide this fact from the doctor. In fact, these persons usually do everything within their power to avoid having to become dental patients. It is estimated that between 14 and 34 million adults in the United States avoid regular dental care because of their intense fears.[17] These persons constitute the severe anxiety group. When in the dental or medical office, they may be recognized by the following:

1. Increased blood pressure and heart rate
2. Trembling
3. Excessive sweating
4. Dilated pupils

Severely apprehensive and fearful patients will most often appear in the dental office when they are suffering from a severe toothache or infection. On questioning, they state that they have had this problem for quite some time, not just a few days, and have exhausted every available means of home remedy (e.g., toothache drops and alcohol), which apparently worked for some time. The reason that they are finally in the dental office is that for the past few nights they have been unable to sleep because of the intense pain that none of their home remedies could alleviate. These patients are driven by their pain to the dental office where their usual expectation is to have the offending tooth removed. These patients represent quite a management problem for the dentist. Although they desire to have their problem treated, when the time arrives for treatment to begin, their underlying fear of dentistry comes to the forefront, and it often becomes impossible for them to tolerate the procedure. In addition, and by no means of secondary importance, the doctor is often faced with the unpleasant prospect of either having to extract an acutely inflamed tooth or to extirpate the pulp of an acutely sensitive tooth—two situations in which achieving clinically adequate pain control can be difficult, even in the best of circumstances.

Because of these factors, severely anxious patients will very often be candidates for the use of either IV sedation or general anesthesia. Other techniques, such as oral, IM, or inhalation sedation, used as suggested, will have little likelihood of success primarily because of their limited effectiveness or the constraints that are properly placed on their use. Younger children with severe anxiety and fear levels are candidates for either IM or IV sedation or for general anesthesia.

It is much more common to see patients with moderate degrees of dental anxiety. Many of these adult patients will try to hide their fears from the doctor because they believe that, being adults, they should not admit to being afraid of the dentist. Children, on the other hand, being less inhibited than the typical adult, will immediately let the office staff know their feelings toward dentistry. Assuming then that adult patients may attempt to hide their fears, the doctor and staff should remain observant both prior to and during the planned treatment.

"Front-office" staff (such as the receptionist) will be able to overhear patients conversations in the waiting room, or patients might ask important questions of the receptionist, such as "Is the doctor gentle?" or "Does the doctor use gas?" The receptionist should be trained to inform the doctor or chairside staff immediately whenever a patient makes statements that might indicate an increased degree of concern about the upcoming treatment. This is also true for chairside personnel.

Shaking hands with the patient may lead to a presumption of anxiety when the patient's palms are cold and sweaty, especially when the office is not especially cool. Discussing a patient's prior dental experiences may give an indication of the dental anxiety status. The patient who has a history of emergency care only (e.g., extractions or incision and drainage [I & D]) but who cancels or does not appear for subsequent (more routine) treatment may be a fearful individual. A patient with a history of multiple canceled appointments may also be a fearful patient. This history should be discussed with the patient in an attempt to determine the reasons behind this pattern of treatment (or nontreatment).

The patient, once seated in the chair, should be watched and listened to. Apprehensive patients remain alert and on guard at all times. They sit at the edge of the chair, eyes roaming around the room viewing everything. Their posture appears to be unnaturally stiff, their arms and legs tense. They may nervously play with a handkerchief or tissue, occasionally being unaware that they are doing so. The "white-knuckle" syndrome may be observed, in which the patient clutches the arm rest of the dental chair tightly enough that their knuckles turn white. Profuse diaphoresis (sweating) of the palms and forehead may be noted, explained by the patient as "Gee, it's hot in here!" The moderately apprehensive patient will be overly willing to aid the doctor. Actions are carried out quickly, usually without thinking. Questions to this patient are answered very quickly, usually too quickly.

Once anxiety is recognized, be it through the questionnaire or by observation, the patient must be confronted with it. The straightforward approach is surprisingly successful, "Mr. Smith, I see from your medical history that you have had several unpleasant experiences in a dental office. Tell me about them." Or when the anxiety was determined visually, "Mrs. Smith, you appear to be somewhat nervous today. Is something bothering you?" I have been truly astonished at how rapidly patients will drop all pretense at being calm once it is known that the doctor is aware of their fears. They usually will say, "Doctor, I didn't think you could tell" or "I thought I could handle it." Then, seek to determine the exact source of the patient's fears, such as injections or the drill. Once fears are made known, steps may be instituted to minimize the development of adverse situations related to them.

The patient with moderate anxiety will usually be manageable. In most cases psychosedation will prove to be effective in patient management. This may involve the administration of a drug (pharmacosedation) and/or a nondrug form of sedation (iatrosedation). General anesthesia will be needed only rarely for effective management of these patients.

With the information that has now been gathered concerning the patient's past and present medical and dental histories, vital signs, and physical examination, the basic goals of evaluation can now be completed.

DETERMINATION OF MEDICAL RISK

Having completed all of the components of the physical evaluation and a thorough dental examination, the doctor next takes all of this information and answers the following questions:

1. Is the patient capable, physically and psychologically, of tolerating in relative safety the stresses involved in the proposed treatment?
2. Does the patient represent a greater risk (of morbidity or mortality) than normal during this treatment?
3. If the patient does represent an increased risk, what modifications will be necessary in the planned treatment to minimize this risk?
4. Is the risk too great for the patient to be managed safely as an outpatient in the medical or dental office?

In an effort to answer these questions the USC School of Dentistry developed a physical evaluation system that attempts to assist the doctor in categorizing patients from the standpoint of risk factor orientation.[18,19] Its function is to place each patient in an appropriate risk category so that dental care can be provided to the patient in comfort and with greater safety. The system is based on the ASA Physical Status Classification System, which will now be described.

PHYSICAL STATUS CLASSIFICATION SYSTEM

In 1962 the American Society of Anesthesiologists adopted what is now referred to as the ASA Physical Status Classification System.[11] It represents a method of estimating the medical risk presented by a patient undergoing a surgical procedure. The system was designed primarily for patients about to receive a general anesthetic, but since its introduction the classification system has been used for all surgical patients regardless of anesthetic technique (e.g., general anesthesia, regional anesthesia, sedation). The system has been in continual use since 1962 virtually without change and has proved to be a valuable method of determining surgical and anesthetic risk prior to the actual procedure.[20] The classification system follows:

ASA I: A patient without systemic disease; a normal, healthy patient

ASA II: A patient with mild systemic disease

ASA III: A patient with severe systemic disease that limits activity but is not incapacitating

ASA IV: A patient with incapacitating systemic disease that is a constant threat to life

ASA V: A moribund patient not expected to survive 24 hours with or without operation

ASA E: Emergency operation of any variety; E precedes the number indicating the patient's physical status (e.g., ASA E-III)

When this system was adapted for use in a typical outpatient dental or medical setting, ASA V was eliminated, and an attempt made to correlate the remaining four classifications with possible treatment modifications for dental treatment. Fig. 5-9 illustrates the USC physical evaluation form on which a summary of the patient's physical and psychological status is presented, along with planned treatment modifications.

In the discussion of the ASA categories to follow the terms *normal,* or *usual,* activity is used, along with the term *distress.* Definitions of these terms follow: *normal,* or *usual,* activity is defined as the ability to climb one flight of stairs or to walk two level city blocks, and *distress* is defined as undue fatigue, shortness of breath, or chest pain. Fig. 5-10 illustrates the ASA classification system based on the ability to climb one flight of stairs. Each of the ASA classifications are reviewed, with specific examples listed.

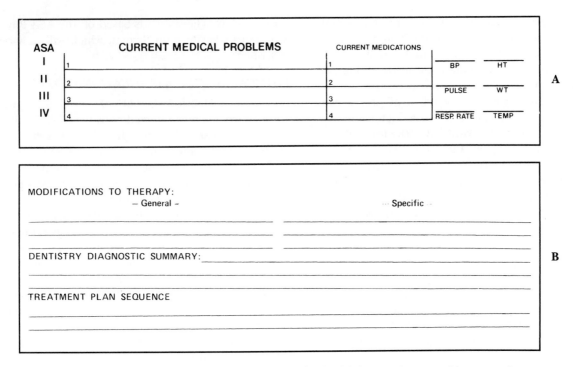

ASA	CURRENT MEDICAL PROBLEMS	CURRENT MEDICATIONS			
I	1	1	BP	HT	A
II	2	2	PULSE	WT	
III	3	3			
IV	4	4	RESP. RATE	TEMP	

MODIFICATIONS TO THERAPY:
— General —   ··· Specific ··

DENTISTRY DIAGNOSTIC SUMMARY: B

TREATMENT PLAN SEQUENCE

Fig. 5-9. A, The physical evaluation section on the health history form provides room for summary of medical problems, vital signs, and ASA classification. **B**, Possible treatment modifications are listed on the patient's chart.

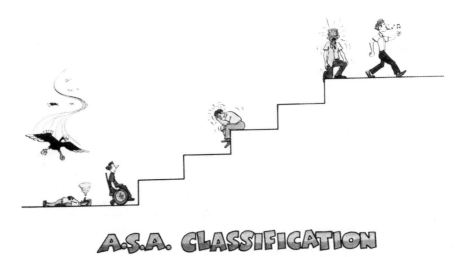

Fig. 5-10. ASA classification for CHF. (Courtesy Dr. Lawrence Day.)

ASA I

ASA I patients are considered to be normal and healthy. They are able to carry out normal activity without distress. They are able to walk up a flight of stairs or walk two level city blocks without distress.

Review of this patient's medical history, physical evaluation, and any other parameters that have been evaluated indicates no abnormalities. Physiologically, this patient should be able to tolerate the stresses involved in the planned treatment with no added risk of serious complications. Psychologically this patient should represent little or no difficulty in handling the proposed treatment. Healthy patients with little or no anxiety are classified as ASA I. Therapy modifications are usually not warranted in this patient group. The ASA I patient is a candidate for any sedation technique or for outpatient general anesthesia. The ASA I patient represents a green light (Go!) for treatment.

ASA II

ASA II patients have a mild systemic disease, are healthy but present with extreme anxiety and fear toward dentistry, or are older (>60 years) or pregnant. ASA IIs are able to complete normal activities but must rest on completion because of distress. The ASA II can walk up one flight of stairs or walk two level city blocks but must rest at the completion of the task because of distress (chest pain, undue fatigue, or shortness of breath).

ASA II patients are generally somewhat less stress tolerant than ASA I patients. However, they still represent a minimal risk during treatment. Routine treatment is in order with the consideration for treatment modifications or special considerations as warranted by the particular condition. Examples of such modifications include the use of prophylactic antibiotics or sedative techniques, limiting the duration of treatment, and possible medical consultation. There are no general limitations on the use of pharmacosedative procedures for the ASA II patient. Outpatient general anesthesia may be employed in ASA II patients. The ASA II patient represents a yellow light for treatment (proceed with caution!).

Examples of ASA II patients are (1) the healthy, pregnant female; (2) any healthy patient over 60 years of age; (3) a healthy but extremely phobic patient; (4) patients with drug allergy or atopic patients (multiple allergies present); (5) adult blood pressure between 140-159 mm Hg and/or 90-94 mm Hg; (6) patients with non–insulin-dependent diabetes (NIDDM, or type-II, diabetes); (7) patients with well-controlled epilepsy (no seizures within past year); (8) patients with well-controlled asthma; and (9) patients with a history of hyperthyroid or hypothyroid conditions who are under care and presently in a euthyroid condition.

ASA III

ASA III patients have severe systemic disease that limits activity but is not incapacitating. An ASA III is able to walk up a flight of stairs or walk two level city blocks but must stop (at least once) before reaching their goal, because of distress.

The ASA III patient does not exhibit signs or symptoms of distress while at rest (e.g., in the waiting room), however in stressful situations (e.g., dental chair), signs and symptoms develop.

ASA III patients are less able to tolerate stress than those classified as ASA II. Elective dental care is still appropriate. However, the need for stress-reduction techniques and other treatment modifications is increased. Serious consideration should be given to treatment modifications in the ASA III. Outpatient general anesthesia is not usually recommended in this group; however, many of the pharmacosedation techniques may be employed, although with some potential modification as to the length of procedure and the depth of sedation. The ASA III represents a yellow light for treatment (proceed with caution!).

Examples of ASA III patients include: (1) the well-controlled insulin-dependent diabetic (IDDM, type I, diabetes); (2) the patient with symptomatic thyroid disease (hypo- or hyperthyroid); (3) status postmyocardial infarction more than 6 months with no residual complications; (4) status postcerebrovascular accident more than 6 months with no residual complications; (5) adult blood pressure between 160-199 mm Hg and/or 95-114 mm Hg; (6) epilepsy, but less well controlled (several seizures or more per year); (7) asthma, less well controlled, stress- or exercise-induced, and/or a history of hospitalization because of the asthma; (8) angina pectoris (stable angina); (9) congestive heart failure, with orthopnea (> 2 pillow) and/or ankle edema; (10) COPD—emphysema or chronic bronchitis).

ASA IV

ASA IV patients have an incapacitating disease that is a constant threat to life. The ASA IV patient is unable either to walk up a flight of stairs or to walk two level city blocks.

ASA IV patients exhibit signs and symptoms of their medical problem(s) at rest. Seated in the waiting room of the dental or medical office such patients exhibit undue fatigue, shortness of breath, or chest pain. Patients in this category have a medical problem that is of greater significance than the planned dental treatment. Elective care should be postponed until the patient's medical condition has improved to at least an ASA III. The ASA IV patient represents a significant risk during treatment.

The management of dental emergencies, such as infection and pain, in the ASA IV patient should be treated as conservatively as possible until the patient's physical condition improves. When possible, emergency care should be noninvasive, consisting of the prescription of medications such as analgesics for pain and antibiotics for infection. In situations in which it is felt that immediate intervention is required (I & D, extraction, pulpal extirpation), it is recommended that, wherever possible, the patient receive such care within the confines of an acute care facility (e.g., hospital). Although the risk to the patient is still significant, the chance of survival should an acute medical emergency arise will be increased.

The ASA IV patient represents a red light for treatment (stop; do not proceed!).

Examples of ASA IV patients include: (1) unstable angina pectoris (preinfarction angina); (2) status postmyocardial infarction within the past 6 months: (3) status postcerebrovascular accident within the past 6 months; (4) adult blood pressure greater than 200 mm Hg and/or 115 mm Hg; (5) uncontrolled dysrhythmias (require medical consultation); (6) severe CHF or COPD confining the patient to wheelchair and/or requiring that the patient receive supplemental oxygen therapy; (7) uncontrolled epilepsy; (8) uncontrolled IDDM.

ASA V

ASA V: A moribund patient not expected to survive 24 hours with or without operation. The ASA V is almost always a hospitalized patient with an end-stage disease. The ASA V is not a candidate for elective dental care. However, dental care is frequently required for the management of any intraoral and dental problems that arise. The nature of the dental care rendered is palliative—the relief of any pain and infection that is noted. The physical condition of the ASA V patient is fragile at best. The use of local anesthetics and other CNS depressants should be undertaken with as much care as possible. Patients should be monitored throughout the procedure.

The ASA V represents a red light for elective treatment (stop: do not proceed!).

Examples of ASA V patients include: (1) end-stage cancer; (2) end-stage heart and/or lung disease; (3) end-stage renal disease; (4) end-stage hepatic disease; (5) end-stage infectious disease (e.g., AIDS).

This system is quite easy to employ when a patient has an isolated medical problem. However, many patients are seen with histories of several significant diseases. On these occasions the doctor must weigh the significance of each disease and make a judgment as to the appropriate ASA category. The system is not meant to be inflexible but, rather, to function as a relative value system based on the doctor's clinical judgment. When the doctor is unable to determine the clinical significance of one or more disease processes, consultation with the patient's physician or other medical or dental colleagues is recommended. In all cases, however, the ultimate decision on whether to treat or to postpone treatment must be made by the treating doctor. Liability rests solely in the hands of the doctor who treats or does not treat the patient.

STRESS REDUCTION PROTOCOLS

At this point in our pretreatment evaluation of the patient we have reviewed all of the history and physical evaluation data and assigned a physical status classification. Most patients will be assigned an ASA I or ASA II status (85% in most private dental practices), with fewer still being categorized as ASA III (about 14%), and IV.[21]

As has been discussed, every dental or surgical procedure is potentially stress-inducing. Such stress may be of a physiologic nature (pain, strenuous exercise) or of a psychological nature (anxiety, fear). In both types, however, one of the responses of the body involves an increased release of catecholamines (epinephrine and norepinephrine) from the adrenal medulla into the cardiovascular system. This results in an increased workload on the cardiovascular system (increased rate and strength of myocardial contraction and an increased myocardial oxygen requirement). Although the ASA I patient may be quite able to tolerate such changes in cardiovascular activity, ASA II, III, and IV patients will be increasingly less able to safely tolerate these changes. The patient with stable angina (ASA III) may respond with an episode of chest discomfort, and various dysrhythmias may develop. Patients with CHF may develop pulmonary edema. Patients with noncardiovascular disorders may also respond adversely when faced with increased levels of stress. For example, the patient with asthma may develop an acute episode of breathing distress, whereas the epileptic patient may suffer a seizure.

Unusual degrees of stress in the ASA I patient may be responsible for several psychogenically induced emergency situations, such as hyperventilation or vasodepressor syncope.

Interviews with fearful dental patients have demonstrated that many will begin to worry about their upcoming dental or surgical appointment 1 or more days before the appointment. These persons may be unable to sleep well at night prior to the appointment, thus arriving for the procedure fatigued and even more stress intolerant. The risk presented by this patient during actual treatment is increased even further.

The Stress Reduction Protocols are two series of procedures that, when used either individually or collectively, act to minimize stress during treatment and thereby decrease the risk presented by the patient.[2,22] These protocols are predicated on the belief that the prevention or reduction of stress ought to begin prior to the start of treatment and continue throughout the treatment period and, if indicated, into the postoperative period.

Stress-reduction protocol: Normal, healthy, but anxious patient

1. Recognition of anxiety
2. Premedication the night prior to scheduled appointment, as needed
3. Premedication immediately prior to scheduled appointment, as needed
4. Appointment scheduled in morning
5. Minimize office waiting time
6. Psychosedation during therapy, as needed
7. Adequate pain control during therapy
8. Length of appointment variable
9. Postoperative pain/anxiety control

Stress reduction protocol: Medical risk patient (ASA II, III, and IV)

1. Recognition of medical risk
2. Medical consultation prior to treatment, as needed
3. Appointment scheduled in morning
4. Preoperative and postoperative vital signs monitored and recorded
5. Psychosedation during therapy, as needed
6. Adequate pain control during therapy
7. Length of appointment variable—not to exceed patient's limits of tolerance
8. Postoperative pain/anxiety control

Recognition of medical risk and anxiety

Recognition of these factors represents the starting point for the management of stress in the dental or surgical patient. Medical risk assessment will be accurately determined by strict adherence to the measures previously described in this chapter. The recognition of anxiety is often a more difficult task. As has been described, visual observation of the patient as well as verbal communication can provide the doctor with clues to the presence of anxiety.

Medical consultation

Medical consultation should be considered in those situations in which the doctor is uncertain about the degree of risk represented by the patient. Medical consultation is neither required nor recommended for all patients with medical problems. In all cases it must be remembered that a consultation is but a request for additional information concerning a specific patient or disease process. The doctor is seeking information that will aid in determining the degree of risk and therapy modifications that may be needed. The final responsibility for the care and safety of the patient rests solely with the person who treats him.

Premedication

Many apprehensive patients state that their fear of dentistry or surgery is so great that they are unable to sleep well the night before their scheduled appointment. Fatigued the next day, these patients are less able to tolerate any additional stresses placed on them by their treatment. Should the patient be medically compromised, the risk of an acute exacerbation of the patient's medical problem is greatly increased. In the ASA I patient such additional stress may provoke a psychogenically induced response. A clinical manifestation of increased fatigue includes a lowered pain reaction threshold, in which the patient is more likely to respond to any given stimulus as being painful than is a well-rested patient.

Whenever it has been determined that heightened anxiety exists, it should also be determined whether this anxiety interferes with the patient's sleep. Restful sleep the night prior to a scheduled appointment is desirable. Oral sedation is one method of achieving this goal. An antianxiety or sedative-hypnotic drug such as diazepam, triazolam, or flurazepam may be prescribed to be taken 1 hour before sleep. Appropriate dosages of these and other agents are discussed in Chapter 8.

As the scheduled appointment approaches, the anxiety level of the patient will heighten. In many cases the administration of an antianxiety or sedative-hypnotic drug approximately 1 hour prior to the scheduled appointment will decrease the patient's anxiety level to a degree such that the thought of dental or surgical treatment is no longer as frightening. Oral medications should be administered approximately 1 hour prior to the scheduled start of treatment to permit a therapeutic blood level of the agent to develop. Oral agents may be taken by the patient while at home or at the dental office. Wherever a CNS depressant drug has been prescribed to be taken by the patient at home, the doctor must advise the patient against driving a car or operating other potentially hazardous machinery. The appropriate use of oral antianxiety or sedative-hypnotic drugs is an excellent means of diminishing preoperative stress. Premedication might also include the need for preoperative antibiotic prophylaxis. Indications and protocols are found in Table 5-2.

Appointment scheduling

Apprehensive or medically compromised patients are best able to tolerate stress when well rested. For most persons the most ideal time to schedule their dental treatment will be early in the day. This is also the case for apprehensive or medically compromised children.

If treatment is scheduled for the afternoon the apprehensive patient must contend for many hours with the ominous specter of the dental or surgical appointment, casting a pall over everything the patient does prior to it, allowing him or her more time to think and to worry about it. The patient becomes more anxious, thereby increasing the likelihood of adverse psychogenic reactions. The morning appointment permits this patient to "get it over with" and to then continue with usual activities unburdened by anxiety.

For the medically compromised patient the situation is somewhat similar. As fatigue sets in, the patient becomes less and less able to manage any increase in stress. An appointment scheduled later in the day following many hours at work and driving through traffic will present the doctor with a medically compromised patient with little or no ability to handle the additional stress of dental care adequately. An earlier appointment provides the doctor and the patient with a degree of flexibility in patient management.

Minimized waiting time

Once in the dental or medical office setting, the fearful patient should not be made to remain in the waiting room or dental chair for extended periods before treatment begins. It is well-known that anticipation of a procedure can induce more fear than the actual procedure.[23] Sitting and waiting allow the patient to smell dental odors and hear dental sounds and to fantasize about the "horrible things" that are going to happen. Cases of serious morbidity and of death have occurred in the waiting room in dental offices prior to treatment beginning.[24] This factor is of greater significance in the apprehensive patient.

Vital signs (preoperative and postoperative)

Prior to the start of treatment on the medically compromised patient it is recommended that the doctor measure and record the patient's vital signs. (Vital signs may be recorded by a trained auxiliary.) Those signs monitored should include blood pressure, heart rate and rhythm, and respiratory rate. Comparison of these preoperative signs to the baseline values recorded at an earlier visit can serve as an indicator of the patient's physical and emotional status on the day of treatment. Although especially relevant to patients with cardiovascular disease, it is recommended that vital signs be recorded on all medically compromised (all ASA IV, III, and appropriate ASA II) patients. Postoperative vital signs should also be measured and recorded in the dental chart for these same patients.

Psychosedation during therapy

Should additional stress reduction be considered appropriate during treatment, any of the techniques of sedation or general anesthesia may be considered. The means of selecting the appropriate technique for a given patient will be discussed in subsequent sections of this book. Nondrug techniques include iatrosedation and hypnosis, whereas the more commonly used pharmacosedation procedures include oral, inhalation, IM, and IV sedation. The primary goal of all these techniques is the same: the decrease or elimination of stress in a conscious patient. When used as described in this book, this goal may readily be achieved without additional risk to the patient.

Adequate pain control during therapy

For stress reduction to be successful it is essential that adequate pain control be obtained. The successful management of pain is probably of greater importance in the medically compromised patient than in the ASA I individual. The potentially adverse actions of endogenously released catecholamines on cardiovascular function in the patient with clinically significant heart or blood vessel disease warrant the inclusion of vasoconstrictors in the local anesthetic solution.[25] Without adequate control of pain, sedation and stress reduction are impossible to achieve.

Duration of treatment

The duration of treatment is of significance to both medically compromised and fearful patients. In the absence of any medical factors indicating the need for shorter appointments, the length of the appointment should be decided on by the doctor after consideration of the patient's desires. In many instances a healthy but apprehensive patient (ASA I) may prefer to have as few dental appointments as possible, regardless of their length. Appointments 3 hours or longer may constitute the preferred management for this otherwise healthy patient (assuming of course, that the doctor, too, is an ASA I or II). However, attempting to satisfy the patient's (or parents' or guardians') desires for longer appointments is inadvisable when the doctor believes that there are appropriate reasons for shorter appointments. Cases of serious morbidity and of death have occurred when the doctor complied with parents' wishes to complete the dental treatment of their child in one long appointment.

Unlike the fearful ASA I patient, the medically compromised patient should not be permitted to undergo longer appointments. In a dental chair 1 hour of treatment is stressful for many persons. Even an ASA I patient may have difficulty tolerating 2- or 3-hour appointments. To permit the higher risk patient to undergo extended treatments may unnecessarily increase risk. Dental appointments in the medically compromised patient should be shorter and not exceed the limit of the patient's tolerance. Signs that this limit has been reached include evidence of fatigue, restlessness, sweating, and evident discomfort by the patient. The most prudent means of managing the patient at this time is to terminate the procedure as expeditiously as possible and to reschedule the treatment.

Postoperative control of pain and anxiety

Of equal importance to preoperative and intraoperative pain and anxiety control is the management of pain and anxiety in the posttreatment period. This is especially relevant for the patient who has undergone a potentially traumatic procedure (i.e., endodontics, periodontal or oral surgery, extensive oral reconstruction, or restorative procedures). The doctor must carefully consider the possible complications that could arise during the 24 hours immediately following treatment, discuss these with the patient, and then take steps to assist the patient in managing them. These steps include any or all of the following, when indicated:

1. Availability of the doctor via telephone around the clock
2. Pain control: prescription for analgesic medications, as needed
3. Antibiotics: prescription for antibiotics, if the possibility of infection exists
4. Antianxiety agents, if in the doctor's opinion the patient may require them

5. Muscle relaxant agents after prolonged therapy or multiple injections into one area (i.e., inferior alveolar nerve block)

The availability of the doctor by telephone around the clock has become a standard of care in the health professions. With answering services, beepers, and telephone answering machines readily available, the patient should be able to contact the doctor whenever necessary.

Several studies have demonstrated that unexpected pain is rated as being more uncomfortable than expected pain.[23] Should the possibility of discomfort (pain) exist following a procedure, the patient should be forewarned, and an analgesic medication made available. Where the possibility of posttreatment pain has not been discussed and it does develop, the patient immediately thinks that something has gone wrong. Such pain is recorded as being more intense and anxiety provoking than pain that is expected (e.g., the patient has been advised of its likelihood) because of the emotional component of unexpected pain, which is not found in pain that is expected.[17] Should the posttreatment pain, which has been discussed, fail to materialize, the patient will be all the more relaxed and confident in the doctor's abilities.

Through the use of the steps included in the stress-reduction protocol, patient management has been enlarged to include the preoperative and postoperative periods as well as the intraoperative period. These protocols have made it possible to manage the dental health needs of a broad spectrum of fearful and medically compromised patients with a minimal complication rate. Specific procedures included in the protocols will be expanded throughout this textbook.

REFERENCES

1. Goldberger E: *Treatment of cardiac emergencies,* ed 5. St Louis, 1990, Mosby.
2. McCarthy FM: Stress reduction and therapy modifications, *J Calif Dent Assoc* 9:41, 1981.
3. McCarthy FM: A new, patient-administered medical history developed for dentistry, *JADA* 111:595, 1985.
4. Skidmore-Roth L: *Mosby's 1990 nursing drug reference.* St Louis, 1990, Mosby.
5. Little JW: Prosthetic implants: risk of infection from transient dental bacteremias, *Compendium* 12(3):160, 1991.
6. Bardoczky GI, Wathieu M, D-Hollander A: Prilocaine-induced methemoglobinemia evidenced by pulse oximetry, *Acta Anaesthesiol Scand* 34(2):162, 1990.
7. Smith DM, Lombardo JA, Robinson JB: The preparticipation evaluation, primary care, *Clinics in Office Practice* 18(4):777, 1991.

8. Brady WF, Martinoff JT: Validity of health history data collected from dental patients and patient perception of health status, *JADA* 101:642, 1980.

9. American Heart Association: Recommendations for human blood pressure determination by sphygmomanometry, Dallas, 1967, The Association.

10. Zachariah PK, Sheps SG, Smith RL: Clinical use of home and ambulatory blood pressure monitoring, *Mayo Clin Proc* 64(II): 1436, 1989.

11. American Society of Anesthesiologists: New classification of physical status, *Anesthesiology* 24:111, 1963.

12. Malamed SF: Blood pressure evaluation and the prevention of medical emergencies in dental practice, *J Prev Dent* 6:183, 1980.

13. Adgey AAJ et al: Acute phase of myocardial infarction: prehospital management of the coronary patient, *Minnesota Med* 59:347, 1976.

14. Damiano RJ Jr: Implantable cardioverter defibrillators: current status and future directions, *J Cardiovasc Surg* 7(I):36, 1992.

15. Seidel HM, Ball JW, Dains JE et al: *Mosby's guide to physical examination*, ed 2. St Louis, 1991, Mosby.

16. Malamed SF: *Medical emergencies in the dental office*, ed 4. St Louis, 1993, Mosby.

17. Milgrom P, Weinstein B, Kleinknecht R et al: *Treating fearful dental patients*. Reston, VA, 1985, Reston Publishing.

18. McCarthy FM, Malamed SF: *Physical evaluation manual*. Los Angeles, 1975, University of Southern California School of Dentistry.

19. McCarthy FM, Malamed SF: Physical evaluation system to determine medical risk and indicated dental therapy modifications, *JADA* 99:181, 1979.

20. Owens WD, Felts JA, Spitznagel EL Jr: ASA physical status classifications: a study of consistency of ratings, *Anesthesiology* 49: 239, 1978.

21. Malamed SF: ASA physical status, unpublished data, 1992.

22. Malamed SF: The stress reduction protocols: a method of minimizing risk in dental practice. Paper presented at the fifth annual Continuing Education Seminar in Practical Considerations in IV and IM Dental Sedation, Mt. Sinai Medical Center, Miami, 1979.

23. Corah NL, Gale EN, Illig SJ: Assessment of a dental anxiety scale, *JADA* 97:816, 1981.

24. Matsuura H: Analysis of systemic complications and deaths during dental treatment in Japan, *Anesth Prog* 36:219, 1989.

25. Glover J: Vasoconstrictors in dental anaesthetics contrainidication—fact or fallacy, *Aust Dent J* 13:65, 1968.

CHAPTER 6

Monitoring

The word *monitor* comes from the Latin *monere*, "to remind, admonish." One definition of monitor is "to observe and evaluate a function of the body closely and constantly."[1] A second definition is "an apparatus which automatically records such physiological signs as respiration, pulse (heart rate and/or rhythm), and blood pressure in an anesthetized patient or one undergoing surgical or other procedures."[2]

Monitoring of appropriate physiologic functions of a patient, during both sedative procedures and general anesthesia, permits the early detection of adverse side effects that may be produced by drugs or by clinical actions, including, for example, hemorrhage or underventilation.[3] Early detection of these problems permits corrective measures to be instituted at a time when they will effectively prevent serious complications from developing.

Since the first edition of this textbook in 1985, there has been an increased emphasis placed on monitoring of patients during sedation and general anesthesia. The first specific, detailed mandatory standards for minimal patient monitoring during anesthesia in medicine were developed by the Risk Management Committee of the Department of Anesthesia, Harvard Medical School, in Boston, Massachusetts, in 1985.[4] Although some of this emphasis stems from the normal elevation of the standard of care, a major impetus came from studies that evaluated critical accidents occurring during anesthesia. It was demonstrated that up to 80% of these critical events were preventable and could be attributed to human error and a lack of vigilance.[5,6] It was felt that the routine application of minimal monitoring devices would enable the detection of subtle physiologic changes, allowing proper measures to be taken before the situation deteriorated into a catastrophe.[7]

In 1986 the American Society of Anesthesiologists (ASA) Committee on Standards of Care[8] developed the ASA Standards for Basic Intraoperative Monitoring as a national standard. Prior to the Harvard and ASA standards, formal guidelines for monitoring during sedation in dentistry were limited to but a few states that had previously instituted regulations defining the practice of anesthesia (general anesthesia and sedation) in dentistry, in essence providing guidelines for treatment. There was a considerable increase in implementation of guidelines in the years immediately following their publication. By July 1987 30 states had enacted regulations governing the use of general anesthesia in dentistry, and 27 were regulating parenteral sedation.[9] As of June 1994 these figures had become 48 for general anesthesia and 46 for parenteral sedation.[10] Specific requirements for monitoring during parenteral sedation or general anesthesia are usually described in these regulations. In addition, specialty organizations within dentistry have produced sedation/anesthesia guidelines for use within their specialty. Guidelines have been forthcoming from the American Association of Oral and Maxillofacial Surgeons,[11] the American Academy of Pediatric Dentistry,[12] and the American Academy of Periodontology.[13] The national governing bodies of dentistry in several countries have also produced guidelines for the use of parenteral sedation and general anesthesia.[14,15]

The Subcommittee on Standards of Care of the American Dental Society of Anesthesiology[16] has created monitoring guidelines that take into account the unique aspects of sedative and anesthetic care delivery in the dental office setting. These guidelines represent an amalgamation of the Harvard and ASA standards and continue to stress the triad of oxygenation, ventilation, and circulation (the Airway,

Breathing, and **C**irculation of basic life support). The ADSA monitoring guidelines are presented as an appendix at the end of this chapter.

In a report comparing 43 cases of morbidity or mortality (M & M) from pharmacosedation and general anesthesia in the dental office, the M & M was characterized as occurring in a young, healthy patient in whom multiple pharmacological agents were used with limited monitoring and resuscitative efforts. Heart rate was *not* monitored in 68%, respiration in 77%, blood pressure in 77%, tissue oxygen saturation in 92%, and heart rhythm in 96%.[17] The authors concluded, and other experts agreed, that lack of adequate monitoring is a key factor in the majority of morbid and mortal events.[17,18] If, as Jastak[18] has stated, subtle *trends* in vital signs are not detected because appropriate monitoring is not used, the morbid event eventually recognized by the practitioner is often the last in a series of physiologic distress signals, and, of course, results in the clinician's response being too little and too late.

The implementation of monitoring guidelines has been associated with improved anesthesia care and a downward adjustment of anesthesia malpractice insurance premiums.[19,20]

An apparatus that measures a physiologic function may correctly be termed a monitor only if it delivers an audible or visual warning when the function being measured falls outside of predetermined parameters (e.g., blood pressure <90 mm Hg or >200 mm Hg). In the absence of a warning system the device is more truly a measuring instrument than a monitor. The effectiveness of the monitor usually rests with the person administering the sedation or general anesthesia.

Because the terms *monitoring* and *measurement* are so frequently used interchangeably, the term *monitoring* will be used throughout this chapter. Many techniques and devices are available to assist in monitoring the sedated or anesthetized patient. In general these devices are designed to measure the functioning of the following:

Central nervous system (CNS)
Respiratory system
Cardiovascular system
Temperature

Devices are termed *invasive* and *noninvasive.* Whenever possible, monitors should be noninvasive. Indeed, for routine monitoring noninvasive monitoring is essential. Invasive devices hurt, their placement is time-consuming, they are costly, and their use has unacceptable risks in many instances.[3] Invasive monitors include arterial lines for measurement of blood gases and central venous pressure. Although they provide highly accurate measurements of important physiologic parameters, there is an increased risk associated with their use, in that complications are more likely to develop because of the very nature of the techniques. In addition, invasive monitors are often quite time-consuming to prepare for use. In the outpatient dental or surgical environment, where only sedation techniques are employed, the use of invasive monitors is rarely justified. However, in cases in which inpatient general anesthesia is to be used, particularly when the patient is categorized as ASA IV, III, or II (see Chapter 5), the use of additional, highly accurate monitoring procedures is warranted. Noninvasive monitors are easier to employ and are not associated with a greater risk. Some may suffer from a diminished level of accuracy (when compared with invasive monitoring of the same physiologic parameter). However, recent devices, such as pulse oximeters and capnographs (end-tidal CO_2 monitors), have been shown, by and large, to be quite accurate. For outpatient sedation techniques employed in dentistry and medicine, noninvasive devices prove to be quite acceptable for monitoring of patients during and after treatment. The requirements of the ideal monitoring device are as follows[21]:

1. Safe
2. Reliable
3. Noninvasive
4. Easily interpreted display
5. Easy to calibrate
6. Stable
7. Portable
8. Easily integrated with other monitoring equipment
9. No technical aid required
10. Inexpensive

In the pages that follow monitoring equipment ranging in price from but a few dollars to several thousand dollars will be described. Our goal in monitoring the sedated or anesthetized patient is to increase patient safety during the procedure. As will be evident as we procede, it is not necessary to employ sophisticated and expensive equipment to achieve this goal.

ROUTINE PREOPERATIVE MONITORING

Prior to treatment of any dental or medical patient vital signs should be recorded as a part of routine

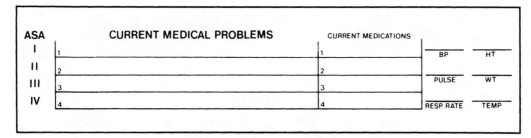

Fig. 6-1. Baseline vital signs are recorded on the right side of the patient's chart.

pretreatment patient evaluation (see Chapter 5). Vital signs recorded at this pretreatment visit include blood pressure, heart rate and rhythm, and respiratory rate. Additional vital signs to be monitored as indicated include temperature, height, and weight.

These values should be recorded on the patient's chart (Fig. 6-1) and serve as baseline values, to which values obtained during treatment will be compared. Baseline vital signs should be recorded during a non-threatening period when they are likely to be more nearly normal for that patient. A patient's first visit to a dental office, when no invasive dental procedure is planned, is likely to provide reliable baseline values.

Pulse (heart rate and rhythm)

Monitoring of the pulse, and heart rate and rhythm, are reviewed in Chapter 5. Pulse monitoring is recommended for all patients as a part of the routine preoperative evaluation. Values below 60 or greater than 110 beats per minute (in the adult) should be evaluated prior to treatment.

Preoperative recording of the heart rate and rhythm should be made whenever any drug (including local anesthetic) is to be administered. Monitoring of the heart rate and rhythm at *regular intervals* is desirable during parenteral sedation techniques, such as intramuscular (IM), submucosal (SM), and intravenous (IV) sedation. Monitoring of these vital signs on an every-15-minute (q 15 m) or every-5-minute (q 5 m) basis is suggested. Specific time frames will be discussed later in this chapter, but a very basic rule of thumb is that the greater the degree of CNS depression and the less able a patient is to respond appropriately to command, the more frequently vital signs must be evaluated.

In techniques of sedation in which a more profound level of CNS depression is sought (IM, submucosal) *continuous monitoring* of the pulse is consid-

Table 6-1. Arteries employed for pulse determination

Artery	Location
Radial	Ventrolateral wrist
Brachial	Medial antecubital fossa
Carotid	Groove between trachea and sternocleidomastoid muscle in neck
Labial	Upper lip
Facial	Cheek
Superficial temporal	Anterior to tragus of ear

ered mandatory. Continuous pulse monitoring is also mandatory for all forms of general anesthesia.

The heart rate and rhythm may be measured either manually or by electronic methods. When recording the heart rate manually, the fleshly portions of one or two fingers are gently placed over a superficial artery for at least 30 seconds (preoperative recording). When monitoring during sedation or general anesthesia, a period of 10 to 15 seconds is usually employed, although 30 seconds is still suggested. Arteries that are accessible for monitoring of the pulse are listed in Table 6-1. The radial and brachial arteries are most often employed in routine situations. The superficial temporal artery is frequently used during general anesthesia. The facial or labial arteries are accessible when working in or around the oral cavity. Palpation of the carotid artery is usually reserved for emergency situations.

It is suggested that the doctor palpate a large artery on the patient at the start of a procedure so that he or she will know its precise location at a later time when, perhaps, conditions have deteriorated and the pulse may be weak or absent. The feel of a strong, regular pulse beneath one's fingers during a deep sedation or general anesthesia case is greatly reassuring to the doctor!

Fig. 6-2. A, Pulse monitor provides a continuous measurement of heart rate with either a visual or auditory signal or both. **B,** Pulse is detected through probe placed on finger or earlobe.

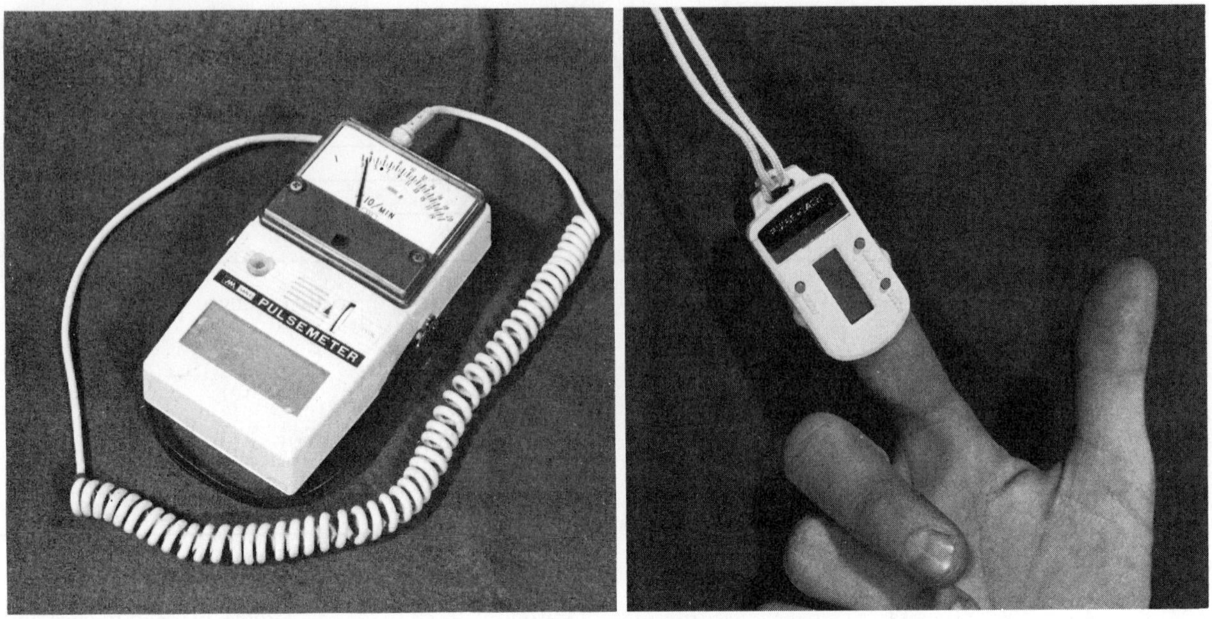

A rough but consistent estimate of systolic blood pressure may be obtained via palpation of three of the aforementioned arteries. Where the radial artery pulse is palpable, the systolic blood pressure is at least 80 mm Hg. A brachial artery pulse will be palpable at a systolic pressure of 70 mm Hg, and a carotid artery pulse is present at a systolic reading of 60 mm Hg. Therefore, if both the carotid and brachial pulses are noted but the radial pulse is absent, it can be stated that (barring anatomic anomalies) the systolic blood pressure is greater than 70 mm Hg (brachial) but less than 80 mm Hg (appearance of radial). This technique is used almost exclusively in emergency situations in which blood pressure monitoring apparatus is not immediately available or in which it is impossible to hear the sounds produced.

Pulse monitors (Fig. 6-2, *A* and *B*) provide a continuous measurement of the heart rate. These devices usually involve a simple electromechanical or optical transducer that is placed on a patient's fingertip or earlobe. A photoelectric beam is interrupted by the flow of blood through the finger following each contraction of the heart. This interruption produces a visual and/or audio signal.

In addition to their primary function(s), many monitoring devices such as the pulse oximeter, automatic vital signs monitor, and the electrocardio-graph (ECG) also provide the heart rate. Either a digital display or a graph on the oscilloscope is provided. Recommendations for heart rate monitoring are found in Tables 6-2 and 6-3.

Blood pressure

The technique of recording blood pressure is presented in Chapter 5. Monitoring blood pressure is the second method, along with the heart rate and rhythm, of determining the status of the patient's cardiovascular system. Blood pressure levels should be determined on a routine basis for all potential patients as a part of their pretreatment physical evaluation. For adult patients a blood pressure in excess of 200 mm Hg systolic or 115 mm Hg diastolic represents an ASA IV risk, requiring medical consultation and management prior to the start of elective dental or surgical care. Blood pressure values for younger patients will vary, being somewhat lower than usual adult values. Table 5-5 presents representative blood pressures for children.

Patients with an ASA I blood pressure determination at their first office visit will have their blood pressure rechecked every 6 months, when their medical history is updated or on those occasions when the planned treatment necessitates the administration of drugs such as sedatives and/or local anesthetics.

Table 6-2. Recommended monitoring for adult patients

Monitor	Local anesthesia			Oral			IM/SM			Inhalation			IV			General anesthesia Outpatient			Inpatient		
	Pr	In	Po	Pr	In	Po	Pr	In	Po	Pr	In	Po	Pr	In	Po	Pr	In	Po	Pr	In	Po
Heart rate	**	0	*	**	0	*	**	**	**	**	**	**	**	**	**	**	**	**	**	**	**
								q 15 m			q 15 m			Cont.			Cont.			Cont.	
Blood pressure	**	*	*	**	*	*	**	**	**	**	*	**	**	**	**	**	**	**	**	**	**
								q 15 m			q 15 m			q 5 m			q 5 m			q 5 min	
ECG	0	0	0	0	0	0	*	*	0	0	0	0	*	*	*	**	**	**	**	**	**
Respiration	**	0	0	**	0	0	**	**	**	**	*	**	**	**	**	**	**	**	**	**	**
	V			V			V	PT	V	V	V	V	V	PT	V	V	PT	V	V	PT/E	V
Oximetry	0	0	0	0	0	0	*	**	**	0	0	0	*	**	**	**	**	**	**	**	**
Temperature	*	0	0	*	0	0	*	0	0	*	0	0	*	0	0	**	*	*	**	**	*

Legends: 0, not essential; *, optional; **, recommended; Pr, preoperative; In, intraoperative; Po, postoperative; Cont., continuous; V, visual; PT, pretracheal stethoscope; E, esophageal stethoscope; q____ m, every____ minutes.

HEART RATE: Heart rate may be monitored by palpation in both the preoperative and postoperative periods; however, it is suggested that when the heart rate is monitored intraoperatively an electrical monitor providing a continuous reading be used. Devices such as the pulse meter, pulse oximeter, and ECG provide continuous heart rate monitoring.

BLOOD PRESSURE (BP): When the recommendation for monitoring BP is **, I suggest the BP cuff be kept on the patient's arm throughout the entire procedure.

ELECTROCARDIOGRAPH (ECG): The ECG provides continuous monitoring of the electrical activity of the heart and the heart rate.

RESPIRATION: Visual monitoring implies a casual observation of the movements of the patient's chest for 30 to 60 seconds to obtain sounds as well). E, the esophageal stethoscope, is inserted into the esophagus during general anesthesia, providing excellent sound quality for both heart and lung sounds.

OXIMETRY: Oximetry provides continuous monitoring of arterial oxygen saturation.

TEMPERATURE: Preoperative temperature monitoring may be done manually, but if intraoperative monitoring of body temperature is required, it is more readily achieved continuously via a rectal or esophageal probe.

Table 6-3. Recommended monitoring for pediatric patients

Monitor	Local anesthesia			Oral			IM/SM			Inhalation			IV			General anesthesia Outpatient			Inpatient		
	Pr	In	Po	Pr	In	Po	Pr	In	Po	Pr	In	Po	Pr	In	Po	Pr	In	Po	Pr	In	Po
Heart rate	**	0	*	**	**	**	**	**	**	**	**	**	**	**	**	**	**	**	**	**	**
					Cont.			Cont.			Cont.			Cont.			Cont.			Cont.	
Blood pressure	**	*	*	**	**	**	**	**	**	**	**	**	**	**	**	**	**	**	**	**	**
					q 15 m			q 15 m			q 15 m			q 5 m			q 5 m			q 5 m	
ECG	0	0	0	0	0	0	*	*	0	0	0	0	*	*	*	**	**	**	**	**	**
Respiration	**	0	0	**	**	**	**	**	**	**	**	**	**	**	**	**	**	**	**	**	**
	V			V	PT		V	PT	V	V	V/PT	V	V	PT	V	V	PT	V	V	PT/E	V
Oximetry	0	0	0	0	0	0	*	**	**	0	0	0	*	**	**	**	**	**	**	**	**
Temperature	*	0	0	*	0	0	*	*	*	*	0	0	*	*	*	**	**	**	**	**	**

Refer to footnotes to Table 6-2.

Blood pressure should be monitored and recorded before, and in some cases after, drug administration.

Whenever sedation techniques are used, particularly those in which more profound levels of sedation are obtainable, such as the parenteral techniques (IM, SM, IV), blood pressure must be monitored more frequently. Specifically, it is recommended that blood pressure be recorded immediately following the administration of any drug and then at least every 15 minutes for the duration of the procedure. The deeper the level of sedation and the less able the patient is to respond appropriately to command, the greater the requirement for the monitoring of blood pressure. During deep sedation and general anesthesia blood pressure is monitored every 5 minutes.

There are several methods of monitoring blood pressure. The preferred method involves auscultation through the use of a stethoscope and sphygmomanometer (blood pressure cuff). The blood pressure cuff is applied to the patient's upper arm and left in place throughout the procedure. It should be placed on the arm closest to the person assigned to monitor the blood pressure (assistant or doctor). However, where an IV infusion is in place, the blood pressure cuff should, if possible, be placed on the opposite arm to prevent a temporary occlusion of the IV line when the cuff is inflated. The same is true where a pulse oximeter is being used. Inflation of the blood pressure cuff will temporarily occlude blood flow through the finger, and the pulse oximeter alarm will be activated.

In some situations, particularly with markedly obese individuals, it may be extremely difficult, if not impossible, to determine blood pressure accurately by auscultation. If this is the case, a palpation blood pressure may be used. After locating the radial artery in the wrist, the examiner should rapidly inflate the blood pressure cuff until the pulse disappears, continuing to inflate for an additional 20 mm Hg to 30 mm Hg. While keeping his or her fingers over the radial artery, the examiner slowly decreases the pressure in the cuff until a pulse is felt. A relatively accurate systolic blood pressure may be obtained in this manner; however, no diastolic pressure is obtainable. When this technique is employed, a note should be entered in the anesthesia record, such as BP:130 mm Hg (palpation).

Blood pressure may also be monitored by automatic devices that eliminate the need for a stethoscope. Some devices simply require the inflation of the blood pressure cuff, after which the deflation is automatic. Pressure is released slowly, and auditory (beeping) and visual (flashing light) monitors announce the systolic and diastolic pressure (and in many cases the heart rate too). Digital readouts are available on most of these devices, and many also provide a printed record. Until recently the accuracy of many of these devices was suspect. For these devices to provide accurate readings the sensor (equivalent to a stethoscope head) had to be placed precisely over the brachial artery and the patient had to sit quite still. Any extraneous movement produced erroneous measurements. The most accurate automatic blood pressure equipment costs several thousand dollars. In recent years second-generation devices have appeared that are significantly more reliable than the earlier models. In addition, the cost of these instruments has become somewhat more reasonable. Two automatic blood pressure devices are shown in Fig. 6-3. Most of the newer blood pressure monitors can be programmed to record blood pressure at regular intervals (every 30 seconds, every 2 minutes, every 4 minutes, etc.). Some devices combine several functions. The device shown in Fig. 6-4 integrates blood pressure, heart rate, electrocardiograph ECG, oxygen saturation, and temperature into one unit.

Yet another means of monitoring blood pressure is through the direct cannulation of an artery. The level of accuracy obtained with this method is unsurpassed by any of the noninvasive techniques previously discussed. The need for this degree of accuracy in blood pressure monitoring during outpatient sedation and general anesthetic procedures is not great considering the limitations we impart on the type of patients treated as outpatients. Indirect techniques of blood pressure monitoring prove quite adequate for the ASA I, II, and III patients. Direct monitoring of arterial blood pressure is indicated both in general anesthetic procedures involving a greater degree of risk (neurosurgery, cardiac surgery) and when the degree of risk presented by the patient (ASA IV or V) is significant. Recommendations for monitoring blood pressure during various techniques of sedation and general anesthesia are found in Tables 6-2 and 6-3.

Electrocardiography

The electrocardiograph (ECG) (Fig. 6-5) monitors both the heart rate and rhythm, warning of the development of possibly significant changes in the electrical activity of the myocardium. Although 12 leads may be employed, standard lead I (right arm → left

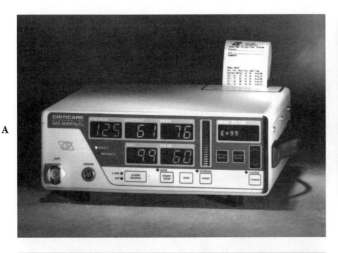

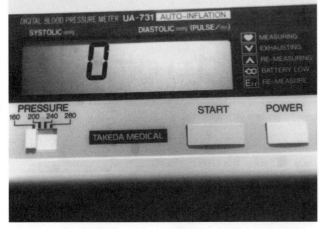

Fig. 6-3. A, Automatic blood pressure monitor provides measurements of systolic, diastolic, and mean arterial pressures as well as of the heart rate. Unit may be programmed to cycle automatically at regular intervals. **B,** Less expensive models are also available.

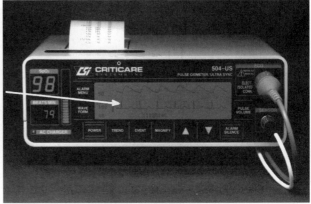

Fig. 6-5. ECG. This model provides both a display screen *(right)* and a permanent written record *(left),* and contains defibrillation paddles (front tray).

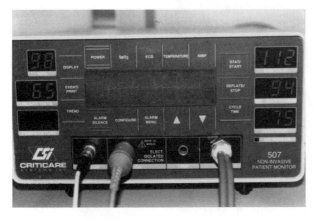

Fig. 6-4. Criticare 507 monitor.

arm) or lead II (right arm → left leg) are most commonly used during anesthesia because they permit excellent detection of dysrhythmias.

The use of the ECG as a tool for monitoring during dental, surgical, and anesthetic procedures has increased dramatically since the 1970s. With the availability of clip-on wrist leads (Fig. 6-6) the ease with which the ECG may be employed has greatly increased its value in many procedures. A number of textbooks on basic electrocardiography are available that enable the reader to become proficient at interpreting ECG tracings.[22] The normal sinus rhythm is illustrated in Fig. 6-7.

Although not recommended for use in all procedures, the ECG does increase one's ability to detect possibly significant changes in the functioning of the myocardium at a time when corrective treatment may usually restore a normal rhythm.

During general anesthesia the appearance of dysrhythmias is more common. Two common causes of dysrhythmias are (1) hypoxia, leading to myocardial ischemia, and (2) endogenous catecholamine release, produced by inadequate pain control or too light a level of anesthesia. Management of dysrhythmias secondary to these causes are usually readily correctable through (1) airway management and ventilation, and (2) providing adequate pain control (e.g., local anesthesia). Recommendations for the use of the ECG during sedation and anesthesia are found in Tables 6-2 and 6-3.

Respiration

Of at least equal if not greater importance than monitoring of cardiovascular function during seda-

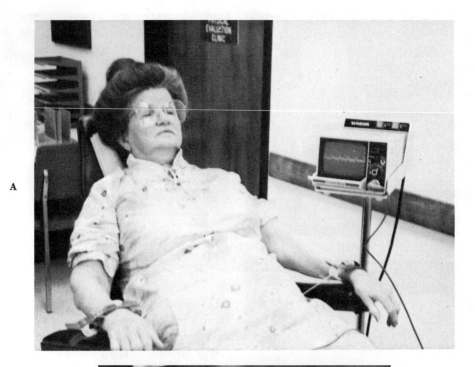

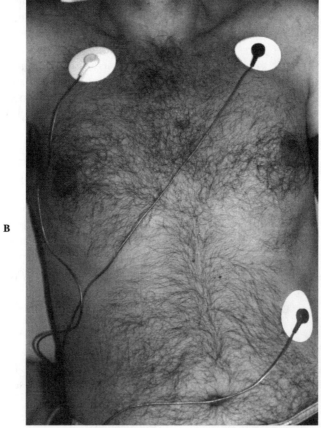

Fig. 6-6. A, ECG using clip-on wrist leads. **B**, ECG electrodes.

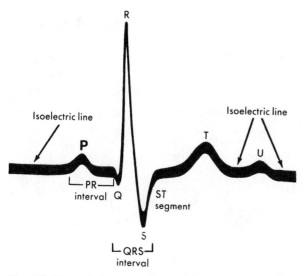

Fig. 6-7. Normal electrocardiographic components of cardiac cycle. (From Phillips RE, Feeney MK: *The cardiac rhythms,* Philadelphia, 1973, Saunders.)

tive and general anesthetic procedures is monitoring of the respiratory status of the patient. Because the drugs used to provide sedation or general anesthesia are CNS and respiratory depressants to a greater degree than they are cardiovascular depressants, changes in breathing will usually be observed well before cardiovascular changes are noted. Alterations in cardiac rhythm (dysrhythmias) observed on the ECG in the ASA I or II patient are likely to be produced by myocardial ischemia, which is most often secondary to respiratory depression or inadequate ventilation produced by the drug(s) that have been administered.

Over the years I have become adamant in my advocacy of respiratory monitoring as an imperative during parenteral sedation and general anesthetic techniques. Morbidities and mortalities have occurred because of respiratory depression (or arrest) that went unrecognized for too long.[23,24] Casual monitoring of respiratory adequacy by observation of the rise and fall of the patient's chest or by observation of the color of the oral mucous membranes is unreliable and not recommended as the sole method of monitoring in those techniques in which more profound levels of sedation or the loss of consciousness are possible.[16]

Respiratory adequacy may be crudely monitored by (1) determining the respiratory rate, (2) observing the rise and fall of the chest wall, (3) observing the color of the mucous membranes (oral and finger nails), and (4) observing the inflation and deflation of the reservoir bag if inhalation sedation or oxygen is being administered (and if the patient is breathing through his or her nose, not mouth breathing).

It must always be remembered that movement of the chest wall is not an absolute guarantee of air exchange between the lungs and the external environment. Chest wall movement indicates that an effort is being made to exchange air and that respiratory arrest has not occurred. The airway may be obstructed (e.g., tongue, foreign body) with no air exchange in the presence of spontaneous efforts at respiration. In addition, respiratory efforts usually indicate that cardiac arrest has not yet occurred because the primary cause of cardiac arrest during sedation and general anesthesia is the occurrence of acute dysrhythmias resulting from ischemia of the myocardium secondary to either respiratory arrest or airway obstruction.

Observing the color of mucous membranes is also unreliable, because cyanosis will not be observed until sometime after the patient has become hypoxic. In addition, placement of a rubber dam is indicated during many dental procedures, especially in patients receiving parenteral sedation or general anesthesia. Rubber dams cover the lips and intraoral soft tissues, obviating this as a means of monitoring.

Visualization of the reservoir bag on an inhalation sedation unit or anesthesia machine is a valid method of determining air exchange if an airtight seal of the mask is maintained. The bag partially deflates during inhalation and reinflates during exhalation. However, if leakage occurs around the sides of the nasal hood or if the patient begins to mouth breathe, the reservoir bag will cease to inflate and deflate during breathing.

While operating in the patient's oral cavity, the doctor, hygienist, or assistant is able to determine if air is being exchanged by the patient. A mirror held in the patient's mouth or in front of his or her nose will fog if air is being exchanged (Fig. 6-8). More effective is holding an ungloved hand in front of the patient's mouth and nose so that air is felt on the palm of the hand if exchange of air is occurring (Fig. 6-9).

Several excellent and inexpensive devices are available for use in monitoring respiratory function. Two such devices are the precordial/pretracheal stethoscope and the esophageal stethoscope. In addition, these devices provide a means of monitoring heart sounds and rate.

The *precordial/pretracheal stethoscope* is extremely valuable as a monitoring device during both general

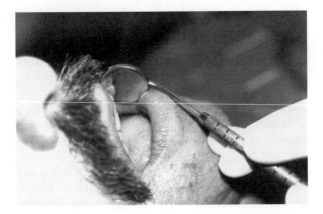

Fig. 6-8. Fogging of mirror indicates exchange of air.

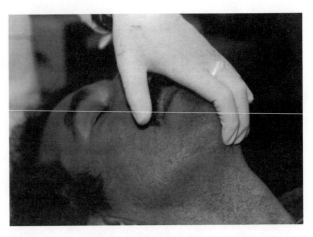

Fig. 6-9. Hand held in front of mouth and nose so air may be felt if air exchange is occurring.

anesthesia and sedation. A weighted stethoscope head is secured with tape (Fig. 6-10) to either the precordial (Fig. 6-11) or pretracheal region (Fig. 6-12) on the patient's chest. Used as a pretracheal stethoscope the weighted head is placed on the neck over the trachea just above the sternal notch. Here it lies above the lower end of the trachea, at or just slightly above its bifurcation into the right and left mainstem bronchi. Tubing connects this stethoscope to a binaural or monaural (Fig. 6-13) earpiece. The custom monaural earpiece is preferred because of its comfort and because it permits the user to carry on normal conversation while continually listening for the sounds associated with the exchange of air. A length of rubber tubing inserted into the listener's ear may also be employed for this purpose. Custom earpieces can usually be obtained from companies that manufacture hearing aids.*

Heart sounds are more easily heard when the weighted stethoscope head is placed in the precordial region, but in some cases heart sounds may overwhelm the more subtle sounds of respiration. Placement in the pretracheal region allows easier recognition of respiratory sounds, but the intensity of heart sounds is diminished. My preference is to place the stethoscope head in the pretracheal region, as my primary goal with this device is to monitor respiration. The weighted stethoscope head is available in adult and pediatric sizes (Fig. 6-14). When placed in the pretracheal region the pediatric head is adequate for both children and adults. The heavier adult stethoscope head is often uncomfortable for the both the child and adult patient.

---

*For example, Miracle Ear—1-800/228-2200 (United States).

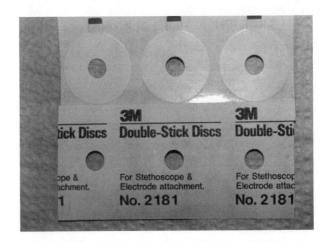

Fig. 6-10. Double-sided tape for pretracheal stethoscope.

The *esophageal stethoscope* is designed for placement into the patient's esophagus through his or her nose or mouth. Heart as well as breath sounds will be heard quite well because of the proximity of the stethoscope to the lungs and heart (see Fig. 32-13). Obviously, the esophageal stethoscope cannot be employed during sedative procedures because the conscious patient is unable to tolerate placement of this tube. The esophageal stethoscope is an extremely valuable monitoring device during general anesthesia. In dental procedures in which a general anesthetic is used, the well-lubricated esophageal stethoscope is inserted through the patient's nose so that it will not interfere with the operative procedure. As with the precordial/pretracheal stethoscope, the esophageal stethoscope may be attached

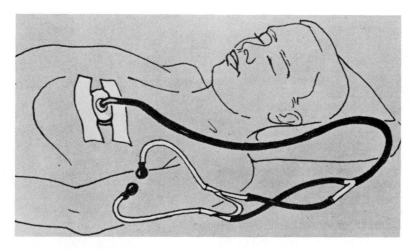

Fig. 6-11. Precordial stethoscope provides an excellent monitor of both heart and respiratory sounds. (From Dripps RD, Eckenhoff JE, Vandam LD: *Introduction to anesthesia,* ed 3. Philadelphia, 1967, Saunders.)

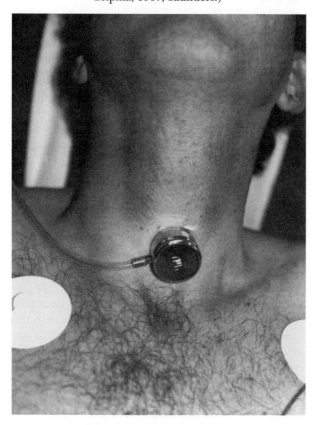

Fig. 6-12. Pretracheal stethoscope on patient's trachea.

to a monaural custom earpiece or a binaural stethoscope. When listening to breathing there are two elements being considered: (1) the rate of breathing, and (2) the presence of abnormal sounds.

The rate in breaths per minute is obtained by counting breaths for 15 or 30 seconds and multiplying by 4 or 2. The most frequent disturbances in rate of breathing are an overly rapid rate (tachypnea) and an unusually slow rate (bradypnea). Tachypnea may indicate the presence of anxiety (e.g., hyperventilation), pathology (e.g., diabetic acidosis and ketosis), or elevated CO_2 levels, whereas bradypnea is observed following the administration of larger doses of the narcotic agonist analgesics (see Chapter 26).

The recognition of abnormal sounds is of vital importance. Normal, unobstructed airflow is relatively quiet, a smooth ''whooshing'' sound being heard in the earpiece. The presence of this sound is indicative of an airway that is patent and should serve as a comforting influence on the doctor. Silence in the earpiece on the other hand is ominous and should trigger a rapid response. Respiratory obstruction (in the presence of exaggerated ventilatory movements) or respiratory arrest (no chest movements and possibly no heart sounds) may have developed and must be corrected immediately. Or it may merely be that the stethoscope has become disconnected from the patient! The presence of the pretracheal, precordial, or esophageal stethoscope decreases the time required for recognition of this potentially serious problem, allowing corrective measures to start more quickly.

Wheezing indicates partial obstruction in the lower airways (i.e., bronchioles) and is termed *bronchospasm* (Chapter 35). Management is required, but bronchospasm is not the immediate, acute, life-threatening situation that total airway obstruction represents. Snoring or the sound of fluid (a gurgling sound) indicates the presence of partial obstruction

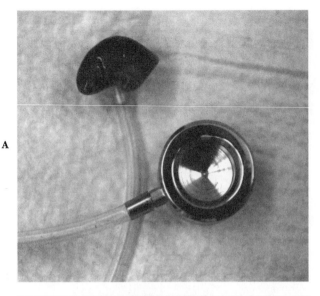

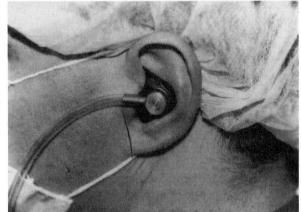

Fig. 6-13. A, Custom-molded earpiece and pretracheal stethoscope. **B,** Molded earpiece in use.

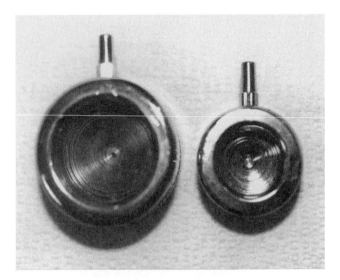

Fig. 6-14. Adult (*left*) and pediatric (*right*) weighted stethoscope heads.

of the upper airway. Snoring most often results when the base of the tongue falls against the posterior wall of the pharynx, whereas the bubbling, gurgling, or crackling sound of fluid indicates the presence of a liquid—blood, saliva, water, or vomitus in the airway. Management of snoring requires elevation of the mandible (head-tilt/chin-lift), which lifts the base of the tongue off of the pharyngeal wall. Where foreign matter is present in the airway of a sedated or unconscious patient three problems may develop: (1) aspiration of foreign matter into the trachea or bronchi with possible development of infection, (2) obstruction of the airway, and (3) laryngospasm.

When the presence of fluid (or other foreign matter) is suspected, immediate management requires suctioning of the posterior pharynx. With removal of

this material, normal breath sounds should return. Table 6-4 describes breath sounds and their management Recommendations for monitoring of respiration during sedative and general anesthetic procedures are found in Tables 6-2 and 6-3.

Pulse oximetry

Monitoring breath sounds and the rate of respiration, although important to patient care during sedation and anesthesia, does not provide an absolutely accurate assessment of the adequacy of ventilatory efforts. Clinically unsuspected hypoxemia occurs considerably more frequently than was thought prior to introduction of oximetry.[24-26] In one study 53% of 296 adult anesthetics demonstrated hypoxia (SpO_2 86% to 90%) during routine surgical procedures.[24] Severe hypoxemia (SpO_2 <81%) was detected in 20% of the patients, yet 70% of these episodes were not detected visually by the anesthetist. McKay and Noble[25] found that 6% of a series of 5000 anesthetics involved critical incidents in which 29 involved SpO_2 readings under 75%. Cote et al,[26] in a single-blind study of 402 pediatric anesthetics, examined the effect of withholding the oximeter and/or capnograph data from the anesthesia team. They identified 59 major desaturation events (SpO_2 <85% for >30 seconds) in 43 patients and 130 minor desaturations (<95% for >60 seconds). Of the 43 major events 41% were first diagnosed by the oximeter (70%), 13 by the anesthesiologist, and 5 by the cap-

Table 6-4. Causes of partial airway obstruction

Sound heard	Probable cause	Management
Snoring	Hypopharyngeal obstruction by the tongue	Repeat head tilt, then proceed to triple airway maneuver, if necessary
Gurgling	Foreign matter (blood, water, vomitus) in airway	Suction airway
Wheezing	Bronchospasm (asthma)	Administer bronchodilator (via inhalation, only if conscious; IM or IV if unconscious)
Crowing	Laryngospasm (partial)	Suction airway; positive pressure O_2

nograph. The authors concluded that "the pulse oximeter is far superior to either the capnograph or clinical judgement in providing the earliest warning of desaturation events."[26] It is thus apparent that monitoring of arterial blood gases (oxygen [O_2] and carbon dioxide [CO_2]) provides more accurate analysis of the effectiveness of ventilation during anesthesia and sedation.

Until recently determination of arterial O_2 and CO_2 levels required invasive techniques that were potentially uncomfortable for the patient, required technical skill, the availability of expensive equipment, and the expenditure of considerable time. Such techniques were, and are, used during major surgical procedures or on high-risk patients, but their use during outpatient procedures was essentially unknown.

In outpatient procedures involving parenteral sedation a knowledge of the oxygen saturation of arterial blood is adequate for clinical purposes, especially in situations in which alveolar ventilation is apt to be constant, as in ASA I, II, and most ASA III patients. A simple noninvasive assessment of arterial oxygenation is clearly advantageous in these situations. The pulse oximeter provides this level of monitoring (Figs. 6-4 and 6-15).

A function of the pulse oximeter—indeed its primary function during sedation and general anesthesia—is the detection and quantification of hypoxemia. Pulse oximeters measure the oxygen saturation of arterial blood. Oxygen saturation refers to the amount of oxygen carried by hemoglobin. Expressed as a percentage, oxygen saturation is the amount of oxygen carried compared with the total oxygen-carrying capacity of hemoglobin. Breathing ambient air at sea level normal arterial O_2 saturation (SpO_2) is 95%; at an altitude of 5000 feet (e.g., Denver, Colorado), 92%; and at 10,000 feet (e.g., Mexico City, Mexico), approximately 88%.

The pulse oximeter is designed to operate on the assumption that hemoglobin exists in two principal

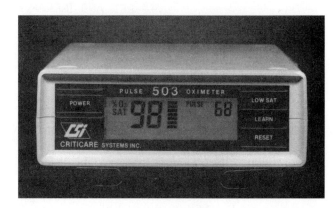

Fig. 6-15. Pulse oximeter.

forms in the blood: (1) oxygenated (with O_2 molecules loosely bound) = HbO_2, and (2) reduced (with no O_2 molecules bound) = Hb. Arterial oxygen saturation (SpO_2) is defined as the ratio of oxygenated hemoglobin (HbO_2) to total hemoglobin (HbO_2 + Hb):

$$SpO_2 = \frac{HbO_2}{HbO_2 + Hb}$$

The pulse oximeter measures the absorption of selected wavelengths of light (660 nm and 910 nm or 940 nm) as they pass through living tissue, such as the fingertip, toe, or earlobe) (Fig. 6-16). HbO_2 and Hb absorb these wavelengths of light to differing degrees. The relative percentages of these two hemoglobins are calculated within the oximeter, and the SpO_2 is displayed on the screen.[27]

The pulse oximeter allows parameters to be determined for all monitored functions (SpO_2, heart rate) above and below which both an audible and visual alarm is triggered (e.g., <90% SpO_2, <50 or >120 beats per minute heart rate). The accuracy of pulse oximeters varies from unit to unit,[28,29] but in general the statement by manufacturers of oximeters that the devices are accurate within ±3% at SpO_2 values

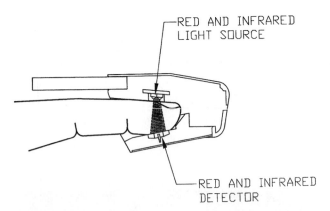

Fig. 6-16. Diagram of pulse oximeter that measures wavelengths of light passing through finger.

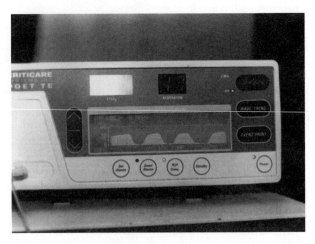

Fig. 6-17. End-tidal CO_2 monitor.

>70% has been confirmed.[30-33] Various other factors, such as the presence of ambient light reaching the sensor,[34] skin pigments,[35] the presence of nail polish or acrylic nails,[36] cold vasoconstriction of the skin,[37] and motion artifact,[38] induce error into the observed reading. In 63 dental visits, 87% to 90% of the 235 desaturation episodes recorded were due to patient movement.[38] In addition, although the response of the oximeter to changes in arterial oxygen saturation is ever more rapid than direct visualization of mucous membranes, there is a time lag between change in respiratory function (e.g., the onset of acute airway obstruction) and its detection by the oximeter. Time lag will vary with the site of placement of the probe (finger, toe) and from oximeter to oximeter[39] and with the temperature of the extremity on which the probe is located.[40] It is estimated that the time lag averages between 20 and 60 seconds on a typical pulse oximeter, using the finger as the site of monitoring.[41]

The use of pulse oximetry has become a standard of care during general anesthesia, whether for inpatients or outpatients.[4,8,16] Pulse oximetry is also considered standard of care during ultralight general anesthesia[11] and deep sedation.[12] Although pulse oximetry is highly recommended for conscious sedation, its use is not at the present time considered a standard of care.[16] The author, in his own practice, considers the pulse oximeter to be an essential part of the armamentarium for all parenteral sedation cases. Used in conjunction with the pretracheal stethoscope, the pulse oximeter permits respiratory function of the sedated or anesthetized patient to be accurately and continuously evaluated, adding a level of increased safety to the procedure.

Does pulse oximetry increase patient safety during anesthesia? Severinghaus[27] concludes that "pulse ox-imetry *probably* did contribute to the increasing safety of anesthesia. In one sense, however, this change may have come through the device's educational role in promoting vigilance and awareness of inadequacies in technique."

Carbon dioxide monitoring

In recent years noninvasive devices for monitoring of carbon dioxide (CO_2) have been developed and gained increasing popularity.[42] Using the principle of infrared absorption, these devices monitor the levels of inspired and end tidal CO_2, providing visual displays as percentage (%) or millimeters of mercury (mm Hg) (Fig. 6-17). Response of the CO_2 monitor is virtually instantaneous, assessing every breath taken by the patient. Arterial oxygen saturation and respiratory rate are also provided. Audible and visual alarms warn the operator if end tidal CO_2 values are less or greater than the selected parameters (<23 mm Hg, or 3%) (>51 mm Hg, or 6.5%) or if apnea occurs. When nitrous oxide (N_2O) is administered concurrently, the percentage of N_2O is also displayed (Fig. 6-18). Although not yet in common use in outpatient anesthesia and sedation, CO_2 monitoring provides another noninvasive means of increasing the safety of sedated or anesthetized patients. With the development of future generations of CO_2 monitors, their use during deep sedation and general anesthesia in outpatients is likely to increase.

Temperature

Monitoring of the patient's body temperature during parenteral sedation is not usually as critical as are the cardiovascular and respiratory parameters discussed. However, it is quite important to determine if a patient has elevated temperature prior to the

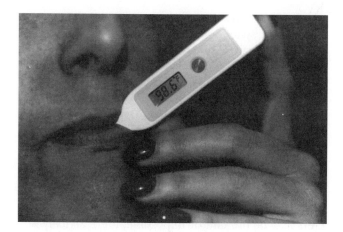

Fig. 6-18. Digital thermometer.

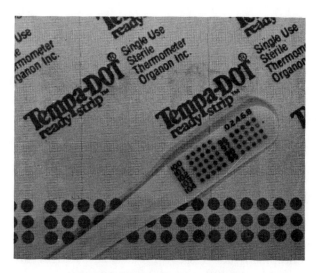

Fig. 6-19. Disposable thermometer.

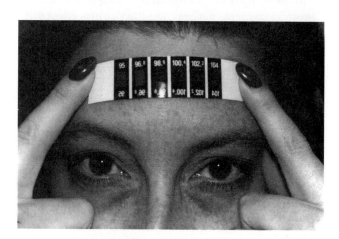

Fig. 6-20. Forehead thermometer.

start of the planned treatment. Fever increases the workload of the cardiovascular and respiratory systems. Heart rate increases with increased temperature as does the rate of respiration. The patient's ability to tolerate stress decreases.

Temperature is most often monitored orally or rectally. In the dental office the most practical method of routinely monitoring temperature is the oral route. Nondisposable thermometers may be used, as may disposable units. When a nondisposable thermometer is employed, it is placed in the sublingual area for 3 to 5 minutes prior to reading the temperature. Digital, nondisposable thermometers are also available, providing a rapid assessment of body temperature (Fig. 6-18). Disposable thermometers utilizing a system of chemicals that melt and recrystallize at specific temperatures have made the monitoring of temperature extremely simple and sanitary. When the unit is placed sublingually, the dots change color according to the patient's temperature within approximately 30 seconds (Fig. 6-19). Where patient compliance is lacking and it is desirable to record the temperature preoperatively, a forehead thermometer may be used, being held firmly against the dry forehead for about 15 seconds. Color changes in the strips occur indicating the patient's temperature. As forehead temperatures are lower than oral temperatures, the forehead thermometer has been adjusted to accommodate this difference (of about 4.5° F or 2.5° C) (Fig. 6-20).

Devices for monitoring body temperature during general anesthesia are available. Temperature probes that monitor rectal or esophageal temperature are most often employed. The esophageal temperature probe is frequently included as a part of the esophageal stethoscope.

The importance of monitoring temperature intraoperatively during general anesthesia is based on the need to prevent severe hypothermia, which develops as body heat is dissipated during abdominal and thoracic surgery, and to monitor for the possible development of malignant hyperthermia (hyperpyrexia), an extremely serious complication during general anesthesia. Monitoring of the body temperature is a standard of care in pediatric general anesthesia.[4,8] Tables 6-2 and 6-3 present my recommendations for monitoring of body temperature during sedation and general anesthesia.

Other monitoring devices and techniques

Other monitoring devices and techniques are available. However, the necessity of using them during the typical outpatient procedure on an

ASA I or II patient in the dental or medical office environment is questionable.

These additional procedures include monitoring of central venous pressure (CVP) as a means of assessing the degree of hydration or fluid requirement occurring during surgery. Monitoring CVP necessitates the passage of a catheter from either the subclavian or the internal jugular vein approximately 10 cm to 15 cm to the junction of the great veins and the right atrium. Central venous pressure monitoring is not recommended for use in the ASA I or II patient undergoing "routine" treatment under general anesthesia.

The level of depression of the CNS may be monitored through the use of the (noninvasive) electroencephalogram (EEG). Predictable changes are noted in the EEG with different anesthetic agents. The need for EEG monitoring during sedative and most outpatient general anesthetic procedures is minimal, and it is not recommended.

Before reviewing the various techniques of sedation and general anesthesia with recommendations for monitoring for each, it must be emphasized that the most important technique of patient monitoring during any sedation technique remains direct communication between the patient and the doctor. The ability of the sedated patient to respond *appropriately* to command is an integral part of the definition of the conscious patient presented in chapter 3. Lack of such an appropriate response is a call for immediate action to determine (and correct) the cause of the lack of response. Direct communication with the patient is a means of determining the level of functioning of the CNS. As virtually all drugs employed in sedation and/or general anesthesia act primarily by depressing the CNS (this is in fact their raison d'être), it is appropriate that the importance of monitoring the CNS be recognized. Monitoring of the respiratory and cardiovascular systems, though important, is considered to be secondary to CNS monitoring during light sedation (e.g., oral benzodiazepine or nitrous oxide-oxygen inhalation sedation). As the depth of CNS depression increases in moderate to deep sedation, the patient's ability to respond appropriately is increasingly diminished warranting intensified monitoring of "other systems." Generalizing to a slight degree, most drugs used during sedation and general anesthesia (CNS depressants) depress the respiratory system to a greater extent than they depress the cardiovascular system—at sedative doses—thus, my emphasis on more intense

monitoring of respiratory function than of the cardiovascular system during sedation. Once unconsciousness occurs, however, effective communication is lost, and the doctor must rely solely on respiratory and cardiovascular monitoring to assess the patient's clinical status.

Monitoring in the pediatric patient proves to be somewhat more difficult if the patient presents a significant management problem. Where oral, SM, or IM sedation is to be employed, the patient may be combative, crying, or screaming, making it virtually impossible for the recommended baseline vital signs to be obtained. Although determining these parameters may be difficult or impossible, there actually is little necessity to monitor the vital signs of the patient during the immediate preoperative period when he or she is extremely active, as the patient's baseline vital signs have been previously recorded at the preoperative visit to the office. Monitoring of the patient, pediatric as well as adult, becomes increasingly more important when the patient, under the influence of the administered CNS depressant drugs, becomes quiet and cooperative. Once this condition is achieved (where dental care can commence), the doctor must be ever more vigilant in monitoring the parameters recommended (CNS, respiratory, cardiovascular). As with the sedated adult patient, monitoring of respiration becomes critical as sedation deepens. Some pediatric sedation techniques include the administration of narcotic agonists, often in combination with other CNS depressants. Respiratory depression is a significant concern in these patients. The probability that the unmanageable pediatric patient has been placed into a physical restraint, such as the Pedi-Wrap or papoose board, increases the possibility of respiratory depression while decreasing the ability to monitor respiration. A rubber dam used to isolate the oral cavity may also be in place, restricting mouth breathing as well as hindering visualization of oral mucous membranes. The use of a pretracheal or precordial stethoscope is therefore considered essential whenever parenteral pediatric sedation or more profound oral sedation is employed, while use of the pulse oximeter is strongly recommended.

RECORDKEEPING

A written record must be prepared for each patient during the administration of sedative or anesthetic drugs. Such records serve several purposes:
1. As a trend plot of vital values
2. As an aid to the clinician's memory

3. As documentation of a patient's response to the administration of drugs and the operative procedure

4. Nonclinically, as a legal document

Although there are similarities in the records maintained for sedative and general anesthetic procedures, a basic difference in the two will be the frequency and level of monitoring. Figs. 6-21 and 6-22 illustrate two types of records available for use in sedation, and Fig. 6-23 also shows a general anesthesia record.

Sedation record

In the sedation form (Fig. 6-21) patient identification is presented on the top of the record. The upper left portion of the record is a summary of the preoperative evaluation (medical history and baseline vital signs) (Fig. 6-23). Intraoperative monitoring and drug administration data are found at the bottom portion of the chart (Fig. 6-24). Time is noted on the top column while directly below are spaces for recording vital signs and dosages of drugs administered. The names of *all* medications administered, including local anesthetics, are listed, and the milligram dose or flow rate (liters per minute) of gases is placed in the appropriate column. At the conclusion of the procedure the right side of the chart is completed (Fig. 6-25), summarizing the drugs administered and discarded, site of needle puncture, fluids administered, treatment rendered, and additional comments.

We recommend as a minimum that *vital signs* be recorded on the chart:

1. Preoperatively
2. Intraoperatively: Following the administration of any drug; every 15 minutes during treatment
3. Postoperatively
4. Prior to discharge

Immediately below the operative record the monitors used during the procedure are identified (Fig. 6-24). Specific monitoring recommendations will be presented in the chapters on specific sedation and general anesthesia techniques. Recommendations for monitoring from the American Dental Society of Anesthesiology are found in the appendix to this chapter.

A summary of the procedure (needles used, IV/IM site, type of IV infusion, and volume administered) and drugs administered is located on the upper right side, immediately below which is a list of total drug doses administered and the amount of medication discarded (Fig. 6-25). The lower right side lists the treatment completed, start and finish times, name of the person to whom the patient is discharged (if appropriate), and comments of interest concerning the procedure. The purpose of the comment section is to provide helpful hints that may improve the quality of subsequent sedation procedures on the same patient. For example, it might be noted that the only readily apparent site for venipuncture was the right antecubital fossa; or that midazolam was somewhat ineffective in producing sedation but changing to diazepam markedly improved the procedure. The doctor then signs the form, which is placed into the patient's dental or medical chart.

General anesthesia record

Because of the nature of general anesthesia, primarily the fact that the unconscious patient is unable to respond to verbal or physical stimulation, the need for intensified monitoring is more important. As described in the preceding section, the frequency and intensity of monitoring are increased as CNS depression increases. Several vital functions (e.g., heart rate and rhythm, respiration, SaO_2, temperature [and increasingly, CO_2]) are monitored continuously, whereas others, including blood pressure, are monitored at regular intervals of approximately 5 minutes. A typical record used in general anesthesia is illustrated in Fig. 6-22. Each of the small, thin vertical lines is an interval of 5 minutes, the thicker, darker lines representing 15 minutes. Drug administration is listed chronologically, as is the performance of specific procedures, such as the start of anesthesia, the start of surgery (i.e., incision made), specific intraoperative procedures, the termination of surgery, and the termination of anesthesia.

Examples of completed sedation and general anesthesia records are presented in Figs. 6-26 and 6-27. The anesthesia record also provides room for monitoring of the patient during the postoperative period in the anesthesia recovery room.

Recordkeeping is an important aid to the doctor in reconstructing events that occurred during a sedative or general anesthetic procedure. Review of records can provide the doctor with information regarding a patient's prior response to certain medications or procedures, possibly alerting the doctor to modify treatment or drug therapy at a subsequent appointment. In addition, well-kept written documentation will greatly assist in a doctor's defense, should a claim be made against the doctor or facility.

Patient's Name: _____ S.S.#: _____ Age: _____ Date: _____ / _____ / _____

Medical Hx:		Current Medications: _____		IV started at _____ a.m./p.m.
	CVS _____	_____		Venipuncture Site _____
	Respiratory System _____	_____		Type of Needle _____
	CNS _____	_____		IV d/c'd at _____ a.m./p.m.
	Liver _____	Allergy: _____		IV Solution & Volume _____ ML
	Kidneys _____	_____		
	Other _____	_____		

Base Line Vital Signs:

ASA: I,   II,   III,   IV

DRUGS ADMINISTERED
– SUMMARY –

Date of V.S.: _____
B.P.: _____ P.R.: _____
R.: _____ T.: _____
Ht.: _____ Wt.: _____
Age: _____

Reason for Sedation: _____
Evaluator: _____
Name of Driver: _____

PREOPERATIVE	INTRAOPERATIVE					POST-OP	DISCHARGE
time	time	time	time	time	time	time	time
Blood Pressure							
Heart Rate							
Respirations							
O$_2$ LPM							
N$_2$O LPM							
___ (mg)							
___ (mg)							
___ (mg)							
___ (mg)							
___ (mg)							
___ (mg)							
___ (mg)							

List all drugs and route of administration (IV, IM)

DRUGS DISCARDED
– SUMMARY –

DENTISTRY TREATMENT

Start _____   Finish _____

Name of person discharged to: _____

Post-Op Medications (if any): _____

Additional Monitoring: precordial stethescope _____   pulse oximeter _____
(check as appropriate)   ECG _____   automatic blood pressure _____

COMMENTS

Student Doctor: _____   AMED Faculty: _____   ☐ Informed Consent
IV Student: _____   Assistants: _____   ☐ Post-Operative Instructions

SAM/USC/SOD
02/85

Fig. 6-21. Sedation record.

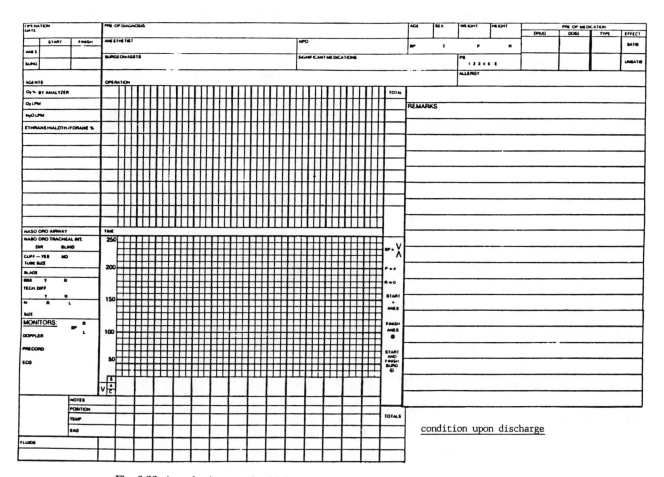

Fig. 6-22. Anesthesia record, which may be used for sedation or general anesthesia.

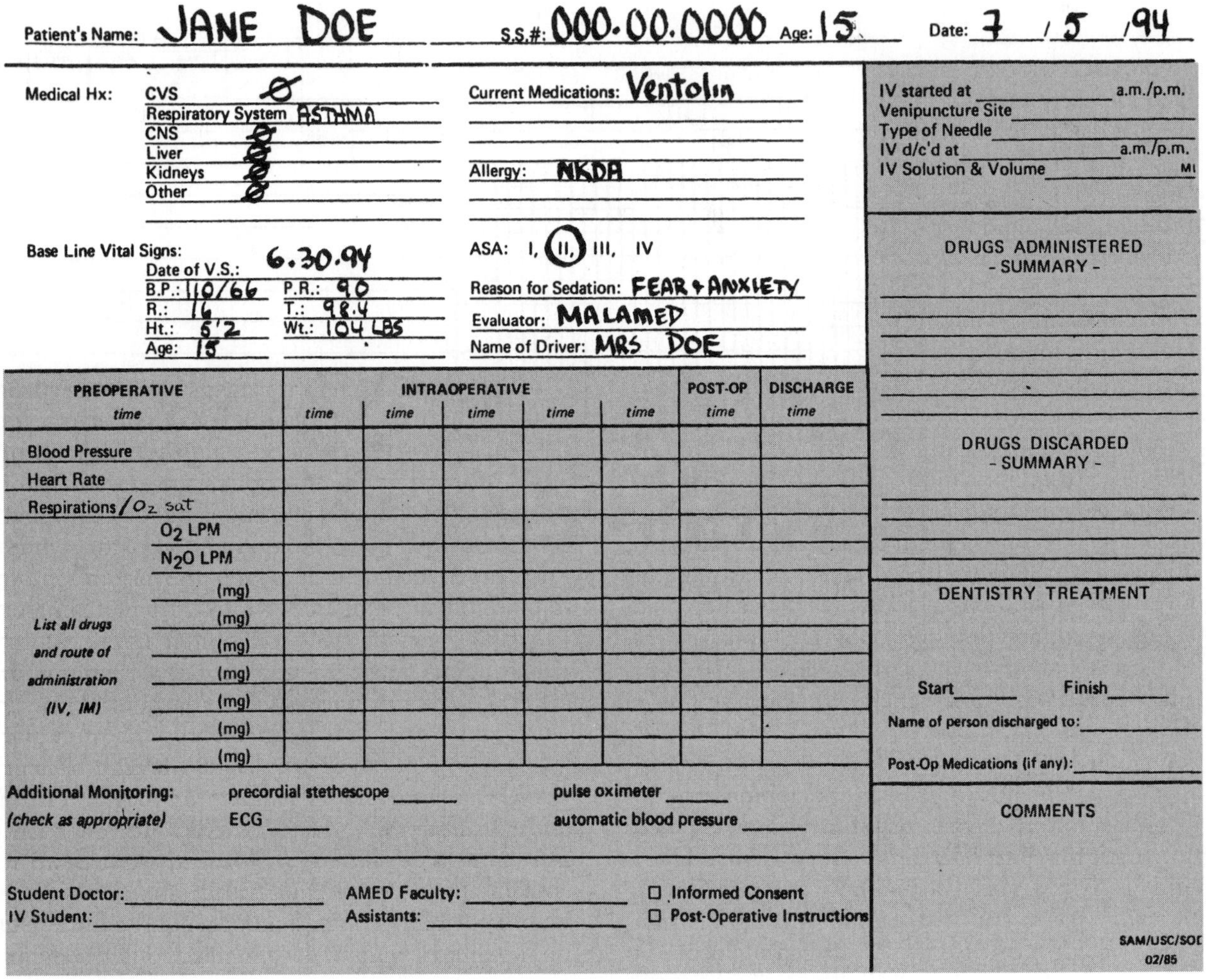

Patient's Name: **JANE DOE**　　S.S.#: **000.00.0000**　Age: **15**　　Date: **7 / 5 /94**

Medical Hx:	CVS ⊘
	Respiratory System **ASTHMA**
	CNS ⊘
	Liver ⊘
	Kidneys ⊘
	Other ⊘

Current Medications: **Ventolin**

Allergy: **NKDA**

Base Line Vital Signs:
Date of V.S.: **6.30.94**
B.P.: **110/66**　P.R.: **90**
R.: **16**　T.: **98.4**
Ht.: **5'2**　Wt.: **104 LBS**
Age: **15**

ASA:　I, (II), III, IV
Reason for Sedation: **FEAR + ANXIETY**
Evaluator: **MALAMED**
Name of Driver: **MRS DOE**

IV started at _____ a.m./p.m.
Venipuncture Site _____
Type of Needle _____
IV d/c'd at _____ a.m./p.m.
IV Solution & Volume _____ ML

DRUGS ADMINISTERED – SUMMARY –

DRUGS DISCARDED – SUMMARY –

DENTISTRY TREATMENT

Start _____　Finish _____

Name of person discharged to: _____

Post-Op Medications (if any): _____

COMMENTS

PREOPERATIVE time	INTRAOPERATIVE					POST-OP time	DISCHARGE time
	time	time	time	time	time		
Blood Pressure							
Heart Rate							
Respirations / O₂ sat							
O₂ LPM							
N₂O LPM							
List all drugs _____ (mg)							
_____ (mg)							
and route of _____ (mg)							
_____ (mg)							
administration _____ (mg)							
(IV, IM) _____ (mg)							
_____ (mg)							

Additional Monitoring:　precordial stethescope _____　　pulse oximeter _____
(check as appropriate)　ECG _____　　automatic blood pressure _____

Student Doctor: _____　AMED Faculty: _____　☐ Informed Consent
IV Student: _____　Assistants: _____　☐ Post-Operative Instructions

SAM/USC/SOD
02/85

Fig. 6-23. Preoperative records for sedation.

Patient's Name: _____ S.S.#: _____ Age: _____ Date: _____ / _____ / _____

Medical Hx:	CVS _____	Current Medications: _____	IV started at _____ a.m./p.m.
	Respiratory System _____	_____	Venipuncture Site _____
	CNS _____	_____	Type of Needle _____
	Liver _____		IV d/c'd at _____ a.m./p.m.
	Kidneys _____	Allergy: _____	IV Solution & Volume _____ ML
	Other _____		

Base Line Vital Signs:		ASA: I, II, III, IV	DRUGS ADMINISTERED – SUMMARY –
Date of V.S.: _____			
B.P.: _____	P.R.: _____	Reason for Sedation: _____	
R.: _____	T.: _____		
Ht.: _____	Wt.: _____	Evaluator: _____	
Age: _____		Name of Driver: _____	

	PREOPERATIVE	INTRAOPERATIVE					POST-OP	DISCHARGE
time	0930	0935	0950	1005	1020	time	1025	1100
Blood Pressure	110/64	116/68	110/60	106/58	104/58		108/60	106/58
Heart Rate	88	96	82	84	84		88	84
Respirations / O₂ sat	98	99	98	98	99		98	98
O₂ LPM		4			6			
N₂O LPM		2			0			
MIDAZOLAM (mg) IV		3						
MEPERIDINE (mg) IV		25						
LIDOCAINE (mg) IM			72					
(mg)								
(mg)								
(mg)								
(mg)								

List all drugs and route of administration (IV, IM)

DRUGS DISCARDED – SUMMARY –

DENTISTRY TREATMENT

Start _____ Finish _____

Name of person discharged to: _____

Post-Op Medications (if any): _____

Additional Monitoring: precordial stethescope __X__ pulse oximeter __X__
(check as appropriate) ECG _____ automatic blood pressure __X__

COMMENTS

Student Doctor: _____ AMED Faculty: _____ ☐ Informed Consent
IV Student: _____ Assistants: _____ ☐ Post-Operative Instructions

SAM/USC/SO?
02/85

Fig. 6-24. Intraoperative records for sedation.

Patient's Name: _____ S.S.#: _____ Age: _____ Date: ____/____/____

Medical Hx:	CVS _____	Current Medications: _____
	Respiratory System _____	
	CNS _____	
	Liver _____	Allergy: _____
	Kidneys _____	
	Other _____	

IV started at **0935** (a.m)/p.m.
Venipuncture Site (R) ANTECUBITAL F.
Type of Needle 21g CATHETER
IV d/c'd at 1025 (a.m)/p.m.
IV Solution & Volume D5W 130 MI

Base Line Vital Signs:
Date of V.S.: _____
B.P.: _____ P.R.: _____
R.: _____ T.: _____
Ht.: _____ Wt.: _____
Age: _____

ASA: I, II, III, IV
Reason for Sedation: _____
Evaluator: _____
Name of Driver: _____

DRUGS ADMINISTERED
- SUMMARY -

MIDAZOLAM 3mg IV
MEPERIDINE 25mg IV
LIDOCAINE 72mg IM(oral)

PREOPERATIVE	INTRAOPERATIVE					POST-OP	DISCHARGE
time	time	time	time	time	time	time	time
Blood Pressure							
Heart Rate							
Respirations / O₂ sat							
O₂ LPM							
N₂O LPM							
(mg)							
List all drugs (mg)							
and route of (mg)							
administration (mg)							
(IV, IM) (mg)							
(mg)							
(mg)							

DRUGS DISCARDED
- SUMMARY -

MIDAZOLAM 2mg
MEPERIDINE 25mg

DENTISTRY TREATMENT
Restorative

Start 0955   Finish 1020

Name of person discharged to: Mrs DOE

Post-Op Medications (if any): n/a

Additional Monitoring: precordial stethescope _____   pulse oximeter _____
(check as appropriate)   ECG _____   automatic blood pressure _____

Student Doctor: Jones   AMED Faculty: Malamed   ☒ Informed Consent
IV Student: SMITH   Assistants: LOPEZ   ☒ Post-Operative Instructions

COMMENTS
Good reins –
Responds well to
midazolam +
meperidine

SAM/USC/SOD
02/85

Fig. 6-25. Postoperative summary.

Patient's Name: _John Smith_   S.S.#: _000-00-0000_   Age: _27_   Date: _06 / 06 / 88_

Medical Hx:		
CVS	Ø	
Respiratory System	Ø	
CNS	Ø	
Liver	Ø	
Kidneys	Ø	
Other	Ø	

Current Medications: _Ø_

Allergy: _Penicillin_

Base Line Vital Signs:
Date of V.S.: _05/27/88_
B.P.: _108/72_   P.R.: _64_
R.: _18_   T.: _98.6_
Ht.: _5'8_   Wt.: _165_
Age: _27_

ASA: (Ⓘ) II, III, IV
Reason for Sedation: _dental fear_
Evaluator: _Jones_
Name of Driver: _Mrs. S. Smith_

IV started at _11:10_   (a.m)/p.m.
Venipuncture Site _Ⓡ AC fossa_
Type of Needle _21g catheter_
IV d/c'd at _11:55_   (a.m)/p.m.
IV Solution & Volume _D5+W 110_ ML

DRUGS ADMINISTERED - SUMMARY -
midazolam 3mg
meperidine 20mg
prilocaine 144mg

DRUGS DISCARDED - SUMMARY -
midazolam 2mg
meperidine 30mg

	PREOPERATIVE time 1100	INTRAOPERATIVE 1115 time	1130 time	1145 time	1200 time	time	POST-OP time	DISCHARGE time
Blood Pressure	114/70	116/70	110/66	108/62			108/60	114/66
Heart Rate	70	68	66	66			68	72
Respirations	16	16	14	16			16	16
O₂ LPM		5						
N₂O LPM								
midazolam (mg)		3						
meperidine (mg)		20						
prilocaine (mg)		144						
(mg)								
(mg)								
(mg)								
(mg)								

List all drugs and route of administration (IV, IM)

DENTISTRY TREATMENT
_Cl II [MO] #14_   _DO #2_
MOD #15

Start _11:25_   Finish _11:50_
Name of person discharged to: _Mrs S Smith_
Post-Op Medications (if any): _Ø_

Additional Monitoring: (check as appropriate)
precordial stethescope _X_   pulse oximeter _x_
ECG _____   automatic blood pressure _x_

COMMENTS
Good veins
Smooth sedation, excellent recovery
Amnesia of injections (intraoral)

Student Doctor: _X_
IV Student: _Y_
AMED Faculty: _SFM_
Assistants: _Z_
☒ Informed Consent
☒ Post-Operative Instructions

SAM/USC/SOD
02/85

Fig. 6-26. Completed sedation record.

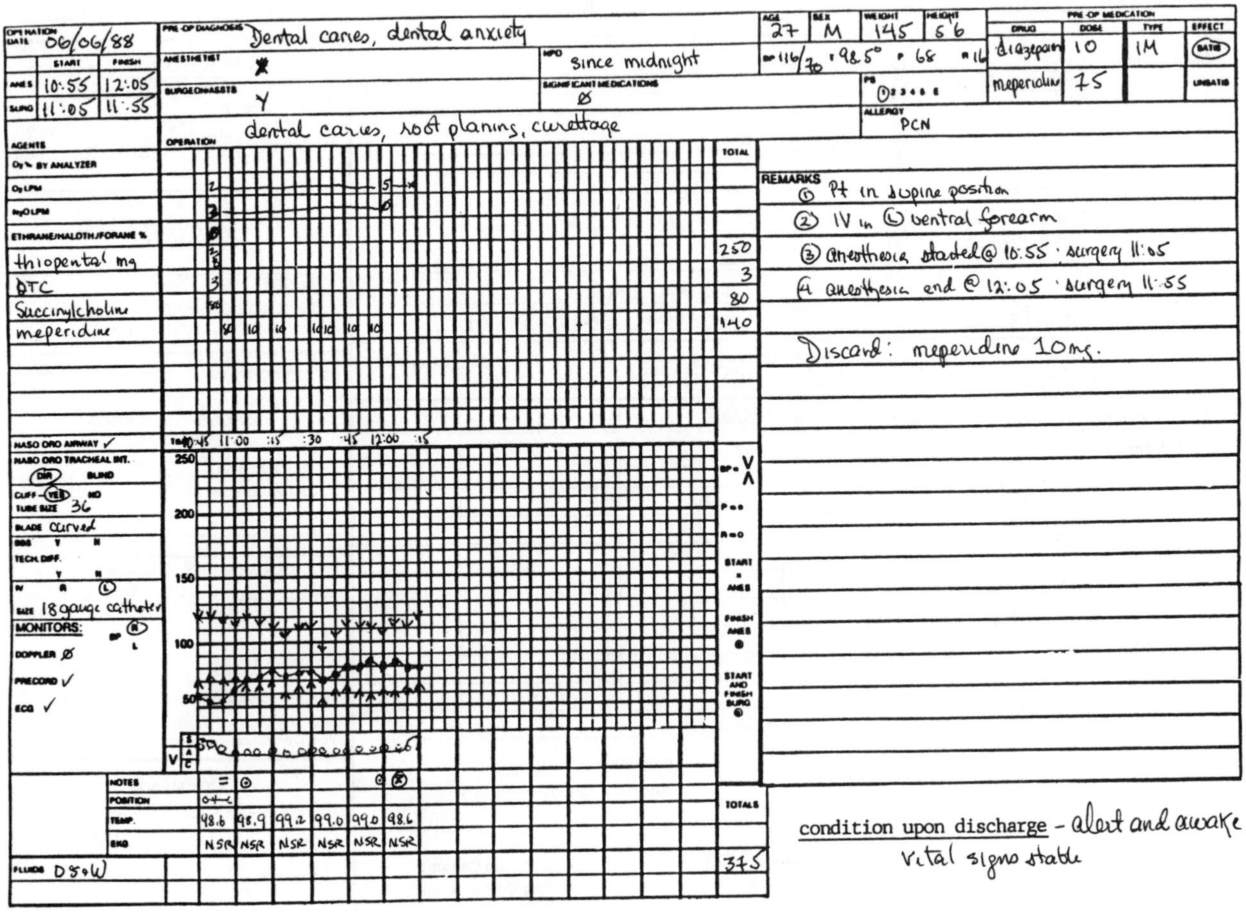

OPERATION DATE	06/06/88		PRE-OP DIAGNOSIS	Dental caries, dental anxiety			AGE 27	SEX M	WEIGHT 145	HEIGHT 5'6		PRE-OP MEDICATION			
	START	FINISH	ANESTHETIST								DRUG	DOSE	TYPE	EFFECT	
ANES	10:55	12:05	X		NPO since midnight		BP 116/70	T 98.5°	P 68	R 16	diazepam	10	1M	SATIS	
SURG	11:05	11:55	SURGEON&ASSTS Y		SIGNIFICANT MEDICATIONS Ø		PS (I) 2 3 4 5 6				meperidine	75		UNSATIS	
					dental caries, root planing, curettage		ALLERGY PCN								

AGENTS	OPERATION																			TOTAL	REMARKS
O₂ % BY ANALYZER																					① Pt in supine position
O₂ LPM			2					5	x												② IV in ⓁL ventral forearm
N₂O LPM			2																		③ anesthesia started @ 10:55; surgery 11:05
ETHRANE/HALOTH./FORANE %			Ø																		④ anesthesia end @ 12:05; surgery 11:55
thiopental mg																				250	
DTC			3																	3	Discard: meperidine 10mg.
Succinylcholine			80																	80	
meperidine			50	10	10	10	10	10	10											140	

NASO ORO AIRWAY ✓	TIME 10:45	11:00	:15	:30	:45	12:00	:15													
NASO ORO TRACHEAL INT.	250																			BP V Λ
DIR (circled) BLIND																				P = •
CUFF YES (circled) NO	200																			R = O
TUBE SIZE 36																				
BLADE curved																				START ANES =
BBS Y N	150																			
TECH. DIFF.																				
Y R (L)																				FINISH ANES ⊕
IV	SIZE 18 gauge catheter																			
MONITORS: BP R (circled)	100																			START AND FINISH SURG ⊗
	L																			
DOPPLER Ø																				
PRECORD ✓	50																			
ECG ✓																				

NOTES		=	⊕		⊗ ⊗										TOTALS	condition upon discharge – *alert and awake*
POSITION	0+←															*vital signs stable*
TEMP.	98.6	98.9	99.2	99.0	99.0	98.6										
EKG	NSR	NSR	NSR	NSR	NSR	NSR										
FLUIDS D5W															375	

Fig. 6-27. Completed anesthesia record.

Because of the potential value of the written sedation or anesthesia record, it is important that these records not be altered after the fact. In addition, it is recommended that these records be kept in pen, not pencil. Should an error or omission be noted after the fact, and it becomes necessary to add, change, or delete something from the written record, a single line should be drawn through the error (without obscuring it, which would increase suspicions), and the correction should be entered and initialed. If this is done at a later date, include both the time and date of the correction. The record should remain with the patient's medical or dental chart as a part of the permanent record.

REFERENCES

1. Urdang L: *Mosby's medical and nursing dictionary.* St Louis, 1983, Mosby.
2. *Dorland's illustrated medical dictionary,* ed 27. Philadelphia, 1988, Saunders.
3. Gravenstein JS, Paulus DA: *Monitoring practice in clinical anesthesia.* Philadelphia, 1982, Lippincott.
4. Eichhorn JH, Cooper JB, Cullen DJ et al: Standards for patient monitoring during anesthesia: Harvard Medical School, *JAMA* 256:1017, 1985.
5. Cooper JB, Newbower RS, Long CD: Preventable anesthesia mishaps: a study of human factors, *Anesthesiology* 49:399, 1978.
6. Keenan R, Bozan CP: Cardiac arrest due to anesthesia, *JAMA* 253:2373, 1985.
7. Emergency Care Research Institute: Death during general anesthesia, *J Health Care Technol* 1:155, 1985.
8. Standards for basic intra-operative monitoring, *ASA Newsletter* 50:13, 1986.
9. American Dental Association: Department of State Government Affairs, Chicago, 1987, The Association.
10. American Dental Association: Department of State Government Affairs, Chicago, 1992, The Association.
11. American Association of Oral and Maxillofacial Surgeons, Committee on Anesthesia: *Office Anesthesia Evaluation Manual,* ed 4. Rosemont, Ill, 1991, The Association.
12. Guidelines for the elective use of conscious sedation, deep sedation, and general anesthesia in pediatric patients, *Pediatr Dent* 7:334, 1985.
13. American Academy of Periodontology: Subcommittee on Anxiety and Pain Control of the Pharmacotherapeutics Committee: *Guidelines for the use of conscious sedation in periodontics.* Chicago, 1990, The Academy.
14. General anaesthesia, sedation and resuscitation in dentistry. Report of an Expert Working Party, prepared for the Dental Advisory Council. London, March 1990.
15. Thompson I: Emergency treatment in Australia, *J Anesth Pain Contr Dent* 1(3):167, 1992.
16. Rosenberg MB, Campbell RL: Guidelines for intraoperative monitoring of dental patients undergoing conscious sedation, deep sedation, and general anesthesia, *Oral Surg* 71:2, 1991.
17. Krippaehne JA, Montgomery MT: Morbidity and mortality from pharmacosedation and general anesthesia in the dental office, *J Oral Maxillofac Surg* 50:691, 1992.
18. Jastak JT: Discussion: Morbidity and mortality from pharmacosedation and general anesthesia in the dental office, *J Oral Maxillofac Surg* 50:698, 1992.
19. Eichhorn JH, Cooper JB, Cullen DJ et al: Anesthesia practice standards at Harvard: a review, *J Clin Anesth* 1:55, 1988.
20. Holzer JF: Liability insurance issues in anesthesiology, *Int Anesthesiol Clin* 27:205, 1989.
21. Lawler PG: Monitoring during general anesthesia. In Gray TC, Nunn JF, Utting JE, eds: *General anesthesia.* London, 1971, Butterworth.
22. Dubin DB: *Rapid interpretation of EKG's,* ed 4. Tampa, Fla, 1989, Cover Publishing.
23. Tiret L, Nivoche Y, Hatton F et al: Complications related to anaesthesia in infants and children. A prospective survey of 40240 anaesthetics, *Brit J Anaesth* 61(3):263, 1988.
24. Moller JT, Johannessen NW, Berg H et al: Hypoxaemia during anaesthesia: an observer study, *Br J Anaesth* 66:437, 1991.
25. McKay WPS, Noble WH: Critical incidents detected by pulse oximetry during anesthesia, *Can J Anaesth* 35:265, 1988.
26. Cote CJ, Rolf N, Liu LM et al: A single-blind study of combined pulse oximetry and capnography in children, *Anesthesiology* 74:980, 1991.
27. Severinghaus JW, Kelleher JF: Recent developments in pulse oximetry, *Anesthesiology* 76:101, 1992.
28. Severinghaus JW: History and recent developments in pulse oximetry, *Scand J Clin Lab Invest Suppl* 214:105, 1993.
29. Kelleher JF: Pulse oximetry, *J Clin Monit* 5:37, 1989.
30. Ralston AC, Webb RK, Runciman WB: Potential errors in pulse oximetry: I. Pulse oximeter evaluation, *Anaesthesia* 46:202, 1992.
31. Webb RK, Ralston RC, Runciman WB: Potential errors in pulse oximetry: II. Effects of changes in saturation and signal quality, *Anaesthesia* 46:207, 1991.
32. Severinghaus JW, Naifeh KH, Koh SO: Errors during profound hypoxia in 14 pulse oximeters, *J Clin Monit* 5:72, 1989.
33. Taylor MB, Whitwam JG: The accuracy of pulse oximeters. A comparative clinical evaluation of five pulse oximeters, *Anaesthesia* 43:229, 1988.
34. Costarino AT, Davis DA, Keon TP: Falsely normal saturation reading with the pulse oximeter, *Anesthesiology* 67:830, 1987.
35. Ries AL, Prewitt LM, Johnson JJ: Skin color and ear oximetry, *Chest* 96:287, 1989.
36. Cote CJ, Goldstein EA, Fuchsman WH et al: The effect of nail polish on pulse oximetry, *Anesth Analg* 67:683, 1988.
37. Langston JA, Lassey D, Hanning CD: Comparison of four pulse oximeters: effects of venous occlusion and cold-induced peripheral vasoconstriction, *Br J Anaesth* 65:245, 1990.
38. Wilson S: Conscious sedation and pulse oximetry: false alarms? *Pediatr Dent* 12:228, 1990.
39. Mendelson Y: Pulse oximetry: theory and applications for noninvasive monitoring, *Clin Chem* 38(9):1601, 1992.
40. Severinghaus JW, Spellman MJ Jr: Pulse oximeter failure thresholds in hypotension and ischemia, *Anesthesiology* 73:532, 1990.
41. Severinghaus JW, Kelleher JF: Recent developments in pulse oximetry, *Anesthesiology* 76(6):1018, 1992.
42. Gudipati CV, Weil MH, Bisera J et al: Expired carbon dioxide: a noninvasive monitor of cardiopulmonary resuscitation, *Circulation* 77(1):234, 1988.

APPENDIX: AMERICAN DENTAL SOCIETY OF ANESTHESIOLOGY GUIDELINES FOR INTRAOPERATIVE MONITORING OF PATIENTS UNDERGOING CONSCIOUS SEDATION, DEEP SEDATION, OR GENERAL ANESTHESIA

The terminology recognized by the American Dental Association for various methods of delivery of nonregional anesthetics and sedatives and the anticipated clinical effect has been previously approved by the House of Delegates in 1985. These include, but are not limited to, the following: enteral, parenteral, conscious sedation, deep sedation, and general anesthesia. The standards endorsed by the ADSA in these guidelines apply to all nonregional dental anesthesia care. They are designed to encourage a high level of quality care in the dental office setting. It should be recognized that emergency situations may require that these standards may be modified on the basis of the judgment of the clinician(s) responsible for the delivery of anesthesia care services. Changing technology; individual states' rules, regulations, or laws; and regulations developed by the parent organization, the American Dental Association, may also supersede the standards listed herein. It should also be recognized that there may be certain situations whereby the standards may be clinically impractical* (e.g., combative patient, emergency surgery) and that adherence to the standards is no guarantee of successful outcome.

When the intention of the practitioner responsible for delivery of anesthesia care is to maintain a state of conscious sedation in a patient, it is that practitioner's responsibility to assess continually that level of sedation. If a change is observed, the type of intraoperative monitoring and the number of personnel present must be consistent with the level of anesthesia.

STANDARD I: QUALIFIED PERSONNEL

Qualified personnel shall be present in the operating room during the anesthesia period.

Objectives

1. During conscious sedation, a minimum of two qualified persons (e.g., doctor and assistant trained to monitor appropriate physiologic parameters) should be present.

2. Because deep sedation and general anesthesia are often indistinguishable entities with regard to the levels of consciousness or unconsciousness, a minimum of three qualified persons must be present during deep sedation and general anesthesia. There should be one person whose sole responsibility is monitoring and recording vital signs continually. This person may be classified as an anesthesia assistant, anesthesia technician, nurse, physician, or dentist.

3. In the event of special circumstances (e.g., an emergency in another location, radiation exposure to personnel), a modification in the number of personnel present may be made according to the best judgment of the clinician responsible for the patient under anesthesia. However, at no time should the monitoring of the patient be interrupted.

STANDARD II: OXYGENATION

During the anesthesia period, the oxygenation of the patient shall be continually evaluated and assured.

Objective

Adequate oxygen concentration must be delivered through inspired gases to be delivered to the body tissues.

Methods

Inspired gas. Fail-safe mechanisms (e.g., automatic nitrous oxide turnoff) must be used on delivery systems before the entry of the gas mixture to the patient's respiratory system. If an anesthesia machine that is capable of delivering more than 80% nitrous oxide (i.e., <20% oxygen) is used, then low-oxygen alarms and oxygen analyzers should be used.

Blood oxygenation. The color of mucosa, skin, or blood should be evaluated on a continual basis. In certain circumstances (e.g., deep sedation, general anesthesia) mechanical monitors should be used to supplement clinical signs. Pulse oximetry is strongly encouraged during deep sedation and general anesthesia, especially in pediatric patients.

STANDARD III: VENTILATION

During the anesthesia period, the ventilation of the patient shall be continually evaluated. When inhalation agents other than nitrous oxide are used, continuous observation of the patient is required.

---

*In certain circumstances the clinician in charge of the delivery of monitored anesthesia care may waive the requirements. Documentation in the patient's chart or anesthesia record is recommended.

Objective

The exchange of oxygen and carbon dioxide from the lungs must be adequately maintained.

Methods

1. During conscious sedation, clinical signs including chest excursion, auscultation of breath sounds, and movement of the reservoir bag on the gas machine (except when a nasal cannula is being used) should be continually monitored. Auscultation of breath sounds can be performed by a precordial or suprasternal stethoscope.
2. During deep sedation and general anesthesia, clinical signs including chest excursion, auscultation of breath sounds, and movement of the reservoir bag on the gas machine must be continuously monitored.
3. During endotracheal anesthesia, breath sounds and chest excursion must be verified after intubation and monitored continually. The use of a capnograph to measure carbon dioxide levels is encouraged.*

STANDARD IV: CIRCULATION

During the anesthesia period, the circulation and its related organ (e.g., heart) should be evaluated.

Objectives

Adequate perfusion of blood must be maintained to permit the exchange of oxygen from the blood to the tissues and carbon dioxide from the tissues to the blood.

Methods

1. When conscious sedation is being used, a blood pressure reading should be made before its use and after its use before discharge.
2. A blood pressure device must be used to continually monitor systolic and diastolic pressure during deep sedation and general anesthesia. The pulse rate should be measured by either peripheral palpation or by mechanical devices. Both the pulse and blood pressure should be properly recorded at regular intervals during deep sedation and general anesthesia.
3. The electrocardiogram should be used to continuously display cardiac rhythm during deep seda-

---

*In certain circumstances the clinician in charge of the delivery of monitored anesthesia care may waive the requirements. Documentation in the patient's chart or anesthesia record is recommended.

tion* and must be used during general anesthesia throughout the anesthesia period.

STANDARD V: BODY TEMPERATURE

During the anesthesia period, the patient's body temperature may need to be evaluated.

Objective

Body temperature should be maintained at or as near to normal as possible. Certain types of anesthetic agents are more commonly associated with excessive body temperature changes. Low body temperatures, although generally less likely to develop during dental or office-type anesthesia, may cause a delay in drug metabolism and patient recovery. High body temperatures may cause a hypermetabolic state and increase oxygen consumption.

Methods

1. An enteral or transcutaneous device should be readily available to monitor body temperature during or after general anesthesia.
2. During general anesthesia, when anesthetic agents that are frequently implicated in malignant hyperthermia (e.g., depolarizing muscle relaxants and volatile gaseous agents) are used, monitoring body temperature continually is encouraged.

TERMINOLOGY

Anesthesia period: Period of time beginning with placement of a needle, mask, or solution into or onto the body until patient has regained sufficient reflexes to be transferred to the recovery area

Conscious sedation: A minimally depressed level of consciousness that retains the patient's ability to maintain the airway independently and continuously and to respond appropriately to physical stimulation and verbal command; produced by pharmacologic and nonpharmacologic methods, alone or in combination

Continual: Repeated regularly and frequently in steady succession

Continuous: Prolonged without any interruption at any time

Deep sedation: A controlled state of depressed consciousness, accompanied by partial loss of protective reflexes, including inability to respond purposefully to verbal command; produced by a pharmacologic or nonpharmacologic methods, alone or in combination

Enteral: A route of drug administration in which the drug is placed directly into the gastrointestinal tract, from which absorption occurs across the entire membrane; includes oral and rectal administration

General anesthesia: A controlled state of unconsciousness accompanied by partial or complete loss of protective reflexes, including inability to maintain an airway independently and to respond purposefully to physical stimulation or verbal command; produced by a pharmacologic or nonpharmacologic method, alone or in combination

May or could: Indicates freedom or liberty to follow a suggested alternative

Parenteral: A route of administration of a drug in which the agent passes by the gastrointestinal tract; includes injections, inhalation, and topical routes

Qualified personnel: Persons with training and credentials to perform specific tasks

Regional anesthesia: Elimination of sensations, especially pain, in one part of the body by topical application or local injection of a drug

Shall or must: Indicates imperative need and/or duty: an indispensable item; mandatory

Should: Indicates the recommended manner to obtain the standard; highly desirable

CHAPTER 7

Nondrug techniques: iatrosedation and hypnosis

In Chapter 4 the overall concept of sedation was described, employing the terms *psychosedation, iatrosedation,* and *pharmacosedation.* Definitions of these terms will be presented at this time to provide groundwork for the remaining sections of this book.

The overall concept of *sedation* was originally defined as "the calming of a nervous, apprehensive individual, through the use of systemic drugs, without inducing the loss of consciousness."[1] Though this definition is essentially an accurate one, it is necessary to further clarify and define it. This is so because clinical techniques exist that act to diminish a patient's fears and anxieties toward dentistry and surgery without using drugs. In addition, the term *sedation,* implying relaxation of the mind, is too broad a term, because it is possible to specifically "relax" or "sedate" the function of other organs, for example, the heart (through the use of beta-blocking drugs, for example). Therefore the more specific term *psychosedation* is suggested when discussing the overall concept of management of fear and anxiety. The term *psychosedative* describes a drug that is capable of producing relaxation of the patient's mind (e.g., CNS depression). There are two major categories of psychosedative techniques: these are *iatrosedative* techniques and *pharmacosedative* techniques.

Iatrosedation will be defined in both a general and a more specific manner. The general definition of *iatrosedation* is those techniques of psychosedation not involving the administration of drugs. This chapter presents an introduction to these extremely valuable patient management techniques. Included in these techniques will be

Acupressure
Acupuncture
Audioanalgesia
Biofeedback
Electronic dental anesthesia (EDA)
Electrosedation
Hypnosis

Iatrosedation and hypnosis will be discussed in some depth in this chapter as they are both important components of the doctor's armamentarium against pain and anxiety. The reader interested in the other techniques listed above is referred to specific references cited for each: acupressure,[2] acupuncture,[3] audioanalgesia,[4] biofeedback,[5] electronic dental anesthesia (EDA),[6] and electrosedation.[7]

IATROSEDATION

Iatrosedation was defined in general terms as any technique of anxiety reduction in which no drug administration was required. At this point a more specific definition of this same term must be presented.

iatrosedation: The relief of anxiety through the doctor's behavior.

This definition of the term *iatrosedation* was formulated by Dr. Nathan Friedman, for many years the chairman of the Section of Human Behavior at the University of Southern California School of Dentistry. The word is derived from the Greek prefix *iatro,* "pertaining to the doctor," and *sedation,* "the relief of anxiety."[8]

The basic concept on which the technique of iatrosedation is based is rather simple: that the behavior of the doctor and staff can have a profound influence on a patient's behavior.

Other names have been applied to this concept by other writers. These include "suggestion," "chairside/bedside manner," and "the laying on of hands." The underlying premise of all these techniques is similar: that one can use himself or herself to aid in relaxing the patient.

How important is iatrosedation in the overall concept of psychosedation? The author of this text has received extensive training in the administration of drugs for pharmacosedation and general anesthesia, yet has received no formal training in any aspect of psychology or human behavior. It might therefore appear that I would have a strong bias toward the use of techniques that require drug administration to achieve sedation. When I first started my training in anesthesiology in 1969, this was indeed true. However, in the ensuing years I have become acutely aware that iatrosedation is an integral part of the success (or possible failure) of every procedure that we in medicine and dentistry attempt. The success or failure of every pharmacosedative procedure also hinges on the use of iatrosedation.

Two classic studies illustrate the importance of human behavior in the control of pain and anxiety. In the first, Egbert et al.[9] demonstrated the value of the preoperative visit by the anesthesiologist to patients about to undergo surgery the next day. Patients were placed in one of three groups.

Group one received a preoperative visit from the anesthesiologist, but no preoperative medication for sedation prior to surgery. The purpose of the preoperative visit was to discuss the upcoming events with the patients and to answer any questions they might pose so as to allay their fears. The second group received a sedative—pentobarbital—1 hour preoperatively, but no preoperative visit from the anesthesiologist. A third group received both the visit from the anesthesiologist and the preoperative pentobarbital.

Results of the study demonstrated that patients in the first group were alert on arrival in the operating room but were quite calm. They did not appear apprehensive. Patients in the second group were drowsy (the effect of the pentobarbital) but did not appear to be calm. In fact, they appeared quite concerned with the activities occurring around them. The third group, receiving both the visit and medication, were both drowsy and calm.

In a second study Egbert[10] once again demonstrated the value of iatrosedative techniques on patients undergoing surgery. Patients scheduled for abdominal surgery were placed in one of two groups.

Group 1 patients were not told about postoperative discomfort (pain) following abdominal surgery.

Patients were told that analgesics would be available if they were required. Group 2 patients ("special care") were told that postoperative discomfort following abdominal surgery was quite usual and normal. The type of discomfort was described as well as its probable location. These patients were also told that analgesics would be available if they should be required.

During the postoperative recovery period, patients in group 1 required twice the number of doses of analgesics for their discomfort as the patients who had been prepared for the discomfort. It appears that when pain is expected and is considered to be normal, the patient is better able to tolerate it. Put another way, it might be stated that pain that is expected by a patient simply doesn't hurt as much as pain that is unexpected. A significant anxiety component is noted with unexpected pain, a reaction that is not present with pain that is expected (is normal). It is this anxiety (the fear that the presence of pain means that something is wrong) that makes the patient experience even more and greater discomfort. A second interesting finding in this study was that patients in the "special care" group recovered from their surgical procedure more rapidly and were discharged from the hospital an average of 2.7 days earlier than the group 1 patients. This may be due to the diminished requirement for analgesic medications in the second group, leading to a reduction in drug-related side effects and complications that might impede recovery and discharge from the hospital.

These two studies by Egbert demonstrate the power of communication. I have been witness to many such demonstrations during the use of sedative drugs in dental practice. Unfortunately not all communication works to the benefit of the doctor. This next case illustrates this point.

A patient received inhalation sedation with N_2O and O_2 for root planing and curettage. The doctor performing the procedure was working with a dental assistant. The patient was receiving approximately 35% N_2O, was quite well sedated, and had a degree of soft tissue analgesia. Treatment was proceeding quite well despite the patient's earlier anxiety and the sensitivity of the tissues. Approximately 20 minutes into the procedure the doctor, who had been conversing casually with the assistant throughout the procedure, made the comment, "Gee, I haven't done one of these (root planing) in about 15 years." Almost immediately, the patient grabbed the nasal hood, pulled it off his nose, sat up, and said to the doctor that he wanted to go home. The patient did not want to be treated by anyone in whom he did not have confidence (even a doctor who was quite capable of doing the procedure well). An offhand remark, meant for the ears of the dental assistant, had destroyed the patient's confidence in the doctor. Another example of the power (albeit negative) of communication.

Yet another example of the power of communication, or the lack of communication, is that of a young man, age 26, who admits to being quite uncomfortable with dental treatment. He stated that his previous doctor would walk into the treatment room, tell the patient to open his mouth, and immediately start treatment, without ever saying hello. The patient was very aware of this and became uncomfortable with his overall care. This doctor suggested that perhaps the patient would be more comfortable if he took a sedative prior to his next appointment. The patient told us that his treatment was even more uncomfortable than it had been previously because, under the influence of the medication, he was even more aware of the doctor's lack of concern for him as a person. Following this treatment the patient changed doctors.

Communication is a powerful ally to the health professional. As these last cases illustrate, even where pharmacosedation is used, communication must never be ignored. Effective communication will make the drugs administered even more effective.

In a recent motion picture, *The Doctor,*[11] a successful surgeon falls ill and enters into the contemporary health care system as a patient experiencing, as never before, the trials and tribulations that befall patients every day in the great hospitals and medical clinics of America. Through his negative experiences the physician learns the value of communication and the importance of empathy in dealing with patients. This award-winning and highly successful film was based on a true story. Incoming residents in family practice medicine at the Long Beach (California) Veterans Administration Hospital begin their hospital career as patients being admitted to the hospital, undergoing the routines all patients face (hospital gowns, blood tests, impersonal attitudes by hospital staff).[12] Much of the commercial success of *The Doctor* was thought to be the fact that audiences (potential patients all) felt that the message of the film struck home. The medical profession, to its credit, has recognized that the great emphasis placed in medical education upon the "scientific process" leads to the isolation of the physician from the patient and has

begun to take steps to right the perceived wrongs. In a recent paper Spiro[13] states that "medical students lose some of their empathy as they learn science and detachment, and hospital residents lose the remainder in the weariness of overwork and in the isolation of the intensive care units that modern hospitals have become." Medical schools have begun to modify their curricula, including in them new programs on communication and human behavior, designed to prevent the impersonalization of the physician.[14]

Similar programs have been in place for years in many dental schools throughout the United States and other countries throughout the world. Yet in the highly competitive world that is dentistry today, it is often the patient who gets lost in the shuffle. The importance of effective communications among the doctor and staff and patient can never be overemphasized. Interestingly, in the venue of continung dental education, among the most popular programs offered are those in practice management—how to have a successful dental practice.[15] The theme of communication is paramount in all of these programs.

Preparatory communication

In the two studies by Egbert[9,10] examples were presented of preparatory communication. Preparatory communication is aimed at minimizing or eliminating a patient's fear of the unknown, one of the most potent fears people harbor. Within the realm of dentistry patients possess many fears that are based on hearsay. Patients faced with the prospect of endodontic therapy become hysterical because of their concept of what a "root canal" is. The thought of the "nerve" being removed from a tooth is an unpleasant one to most persons. However, if the doctor spends but a few moments prior to the start of endodontic therapy describing the treatment or if educational pamphlets are made available to the patient, such fears may be allayed. What is endodontic therapy? In this author's words it may be described as the removal of tissue from the tooth, followed by shaping and filling of the tooth (or canal) with an inert material. When root canal therapy is described in this manner, it appears much less traumatic to the patient.

A few moments spent with a patient describing the planned procedure, prior to the start of a new mode of treatment, serves to allay most of the patient's anxieties. Terms used to describe the treatment should be nonthreatening if preparatory communication is to be effective in decreasing fear. Explaining an endodontic procedure by stating that "we will give you a shot of anesthetic and then remove the nerve from the tooth" will only succeed in increasing a patient's fears. The art of semantics will therefore play an important role in communication between the doctor and patient. Friedman discusses the use of euphemistic language, which is the substitution of mild or inoffensive words for those that may offend or suggest something unpleasant.[8] The word *euphemism* is derived from the Greek *eu* (well) and *phanai* (to speak).

Euphemistic language

The dental vocabulary is replete with threatening words, examples of which are presented below:

Hurt, pain
Needle, shot, injection
Cut
Cauterize
Extract
Drill
Scalpel
Operatory
Nerve

Most health professionals, especially dentists, are acutely aware of the need to avoid using these words. However, occasions do arise when their use seems inescapable. For example, during the administration of a nasopalatine nerve block (perhaps the most difficult intraoral injection to administer atraumatically on a consistent basis) the patient might feel some pain (a negative term). Should the doctor tell the patient prior to the injection, "You will probably feel some pain during this injection" or "This shot will probably hurt a little"? The answer is no, at least not in the manner described. When it is expected that there will be pain, a nonthreatening term, such as *discomfort,* can be substituted. The statement "I will be doing this slowly; if there should be some discomfort please raise your hand and I will stop immediately" relays the same information but does not traumatize the patient psychologically as does the preceding statement.

Examples of other terms that may be used in place of more traumatic ones are *discomfort* or *feel,* in place of *hurt* or *pain,* as in, "I don't expect you to feel this" instead of "This won't hurt." The only word heard by the patient is "hurt." *Novocain* or *local anesthetic,* in place of *needle, shot,* or *injection,* as in "We're going to give you a local anesthetic now," is preferable to "We're going to give you a shot (or injection) now." Canadian dentists have used the word *freeze* in this

situation ("I am going to freeze you now") with great success. In essence the message delivered to the patient who is about to receive an injection of a local anesthetic is nonthreatening.

In pediatric dentistry euphemistic language has always been an important means of describing to the younger patient the instruments and procedures that are to be used. The injection (administration) of a local anesthetic is described as "spraying sleepy water on a tooth," a saliva ejector is called a "vacuum cleaner," and preparation of a tooth with a drill is described as "tickling the tooth." Though the words used for adults may be different, the concept is the same. Describe the procedure in a way that lessens, not heightens, the patient's anxiety. *Remove* may be substituted for *extract* or *extirpate.* That is, "Tissue will be removed from the tooth" instead of "We will have to extirpate the nerve." *Handpiece* is used in place of *drill,* and *treatment room* may be substituted for *operatory.*

Euphemistic language in sedation

Throughout this book examples of euphemistic language will be offered as they relate to the use of pharmacosedation. In describing the feelings a patient will experience during a sedative procedure, or the equipment that is used to deliver the medications to the patient, less threatening words or phrases will be substituted for potentially traumatic ones. An excellent example deals with the administration of diazepam, a drug very commonly used to obtain light levels of sedation via the intravenous route. Because diazepam is not water-soluble, propylene glycol is used as a solvent. Propylene glycol can produce irritation of vein walls as the drug is injected. This irritation may be experienced only slightly or not at all by some patients, whereas it may be considered quite uncomfortable by others. It is suggested that the person administering IV diazepam caution the patient prior to its administration that there is a possibility of discomfort. Should the doctor fail to tell the patient about this possibility and a painful sensation does occur, the patient will probably become quite apprehensive, fearing that something is wrong. This possibility can be eliminated by forewarning the patient. The manner in which this potential "feeling" is described is important. Stating that the patient will experience a painful sensation or that there will be a burning sensation as the drug is injected is likely to put the patient on the alert, increasing an already heightened anxiety level. The patient might well ask, "Why, if this drug is going to hurt when it is being injected, is the doctor using it at all?'' I have found it best to tell the patient receiving diazepam IV that "You may experience a slight warmth in your arm as the medication is administered. This is entirely normal and will pass within a few seconds." In this manner the patient is prepared but not frightened.

Inhalation sedation with N_2O-O_2 is commonly called *gas, laughing gas, sweet air,* or *medicated air* by doctors who feel that the chemical names may be too threatening to their patients.[16]

Yet another euphemistic term relating to sedation comes to mind: with the recent media avalanche of headlines concerning the illicit use of drugs, such as cocaine and narcotics, the very word *drug* has taken on a negative connotation. Use of the word *medication* relays the desired message in a more professional and less intimidating manner.

Iatrosedation: staff and office

The entire dental staff must be alert to the appropriate use of language, for much of a patient's contact in the office will be with persons other than the doctor. In addition, the demeanor of the receptionist, chairside personnel, and all others will add to or detract from the environment in the office. Sedation does not just magically happen when a patient sits down in the dental chair. As was demonstrated in the stress reduction protocols (Chapter 5), the recognition and management of anxiety must start prior to the actual treatment. A receptionist is just as important in the management of anxiety as are chairside personnel. The receptionist is trained to answer the telephone "with a smile," to help reassure the apprehensive patient, and to relay such information to the doctor and other chairside personnel. The apprehensive patient is on the alert for clues on entering the dental office. A positive attitude on the part of the staff, as well as a relaxed environment within the office, will help to allay the patient's fears. A busy, high-pressure office where staff members are constantly running about in a frenzy is not conducive to relaxation. The use of striking colors and loud rock music will also detract from a sedative environment (although patients' musical tastes will vary considerably). Conversely, a low-pressure, relaxed office staff, combined with a toned-down color scheme (earth colors) and a more moderate type of music, provides a warm, cheerful environment that will add to the sedative effect of any medications that may subsequently be employed.[17]

Once the patient arrives in the dental office, his presence should be acknowledged within a minute or two. Even when the doctor may be somewhat delayed in scheduling, the patient should be informed of this and not kept waiting for no apparent reason. The patient should be escorted to the (dental) treatment room (the term *operatory* or *surgery* is threatening to many patients) and seated in the dental chair. At this point the dental assistant can aid the patient's level of comfort by simply adjusting the chair and headrest as may be desired by the patient or by offering the patient a facial tissue. An attitude of concern or empathy should be relayed by the assistant to the patient in order to help establish lines of communication. On entering the treatment room the doctor should always greet the patient, shake hands (personal touches like this are greatly appreciated by the patient, as well as being an aid in recognition of anxiety [cold, sweaty palms]), and spend a moment or two talking before treatment is started. I have been astounded by the number of fearful patients who have stated that the major reason they left a doctor was because "the doctor didn't care about me as a person." A few words spoken to the patient prior to and during treatment help to establish a better working relationship between the treatment team and the patient.

I was present when a dental student was interviewing an apprehensive patient whom he was seeing for the first time. The student had reviewed the patient's medical history questionnaire and was seeking to determine the causes of the patient's fears of dentistry. The audio portion of the tape of this interview demonstrated that the student was quite adept at obtaining the necessary information and at transmitting his desire to work with the patient to help him to diminish his dental fears. However, when seen on video the entire interview was considered a failure. The student doctor, asking all of the appropriate questions and expressing his concern for the patient, was standing with his back toward the patient and reading from a prepared list of questions. At no point during this 20-minute interview did the patient ever see the doctor's face for more than a few seconds at a time!

Clinical demeanor

Why does a patient select one dentist over another? Most patients select a dentist after discussion with friends and relatives. Commonly expressed reasons for selection include the comments that this doctor "is good" or "is painless." It appears therefore that one of the primary considerations used in the selection process is a doctor's clinical demeanor.[18] This does not always mean that the technical quality of the dentistry is superior; it does, however, mean that the doctor "cares about his patients" and makes an effort to be gentle and to provide painless treatment. Many business cards used by dentists include the phrase, "We cater to cowards."

Friedman[19] has stated that "the more threatening an instrument, the more significant your manner of wielding it" becomes to the patient. A gentle touch is appreciated over a rough appearance. Expressions of concern, either verbal or nonverbal, during treatment aid in allaying a patient's fears. A simple statement such as "If for any reason you would like me to stop, simply raise your hand and I will stop immediately" tells the patient of the doctor's concern. A new patient may test this system several times to be certain the doctor was honest, but once convinced will relax and permit treatment to continue.

The goal of iatrosedation

The ultimate goal of iatrosedation is to minimize the patient's requirement for pharmacosedation. Another goal is to open lines of communication so that the patient will not be inhibited from expressing true feelings or desires to the doctor or staff members. When patients are able to express their fears to the doctor prior to treatment, it becomes that much more simple to manage them once treatment starts.

Iatrosedation is an effective technique; however, it may not be adequate by itself to remove the fears of dentistry harbored by all patients. The use of supplemental pharmacosedation may be necessary in the initial phases of patient management. Iatrosedation will effectively minimize the depth of pharmacosedation required to reach a desired clinical level of relaxation or it will maximize the effectiveness of the pharmacosedative technique used.

By communicating with our patients we can begin the process of fear reduction during our initial contact. Through the establishment of rapport with the patient we are able to determine the level of pharmacosedation (if any) required to manage the patient's dental fears and make more effective use of any drugs we might employ. The following case history serves to point up the objectives of iatrosedation.[20]

The patient, a 24-year-old college student, had purposely avoided dental treatment in the past until forced by pain to seek help. His anxieties were related to the sound of the dental handpiece and originated in childhood, when the patient was treated by a dentist who did not use local anesthesia. The patient associated the sound of the handpiece with the pain of tooth preparation. The patient arrived at the University of Southern California School of Dentistry Emergency Clinic with acute pulpitis of the mandibular right first molar.

The patient admitted to an extreme fear of dentistry and stated that in spite of his pain he could not tolerate dental treatment. At the first treatment visit intravenous diazepam, 19 mg, was administered (via titration) to sedate the patient, and after mandibular anesthesia was obtained, the pulp was extirpated without incident. The patient later stated that he had "enjoyed" the dental appointment and wished to become a regular clinic patient.

At subsequent appointments the patient did require the use of pharmacosedative techniques. However, at the end of eight dental visits, spanning a period of 3 months, the patient no longer required the use of pharmacosedation for his dental care. This is the goal to be sought. Through the combined use of iatrosedation and pharmacosedation it is possible to achieve this goal by reeducating the fearful patient, in a majority of cases. This goal may easily be accomplished in those practices in which patients remain for many years, such as in general dental practice, pediatric dentistry, and periodontics. Because of the shorter treatment periods needed in oral surgery and endodontics, this same goal is somewhat more difficult to achieve, though it is still achievable.

As stated in Chapter 3, the goal in initially using pharmacosedation as an aid in patient management is to eventually eliminate its need. The technique of iatrosedation will, of course, be used with each and every patient who appears in the office seeking treatment at each and every appointment.

HYPNOSIS

Hypnosis has been defined as a "special trancelike state in which the subject's attention is focused intensely on the hypnotist, while attention to other stimuli is markedly diminished."[21] Barber[22] defines hypnosis as "an altered state of consciousness characterized by narrowed, heightened attention, and the capacity for producing alterations in memory and perception."

Franz Anton Mesmer (1734-1815), a graduate of the University of Vienna School of Medicine, did much work on the subject of animal magnetism. His work became the subject of controversy throughout Europe and his Magnetic Institute in Paris attracted many influential and rich persons. Banned from Paris, Mesmer moved his institute, along with its ardent followers, to Switzerland. Animal magnetism, or mesmerism, as it came to be known, was an early form of hypnotism and as such was instrumental in the development of a new awareness of the possibilities of making people insensitive to pain. James Esdaile in India performed 73 painless surgical operations using mesmerism; however, the medical communities of the day remained unconvinced of its value and mesmerism remained a controversial topic within the medical community and among the public for many years to come.[23]

In 1837 the first reported case of a tooth extraction using mesmerism was published.[24] It was not until 1843 that the term *hypnotism* was introduced by James Braid.

At the end of the nineteenth century and the beginning of the twentieth century, the foundations of hypnosis were elucidated by Jean-Martin Charcot (1825-1893) and others. Freud initiated the use of hypnosis as a therapeutic tool in psychoanalysis, a role that it still maintains today.[23]

Hypnosis in dentistry

As with iatrosedation, hypnosis serves as a means of providing relaxation without the requirement of drug administration. In addition, hypnosis serves as a means of providing clinically acceptable pain control in many patients, making it a potentially valuable technique in dentistry.

Barber[25] lists the following possible uses of hypnosis in dentistry:

Patient relaxation

Anxiety reduction

Orthodontics (aid in overcoming fear of orthodontics)

Maintenance of comfort during prolonged treatments

Modification of noxious dental habits (e.g., thumb sucking)

Reduction of the need for anesthesia or analgesia

Postoperative analgesia

Substitution for premedication in general anesthesia

Control of reflexes and autonomic processes (i.e., gagging, nausea, salivary flow, bleeding)

Management of difficult patients

Hypnosis is an effective technique as an aid in helping patients to overcome their fears of various procedures. Hypnotic suggestion has proven valuable in eliminating the fear of injections (both intraoral and IV/IM), and the claustrophobic feeling some patients experience when the N_2O-O_2 inhalation sedation nasal hood is placed over their nose.[26] When venipuncture is difficult to achieve because of a patient's fear of needles, hypnosis may prove effective in eliminating or minimizing the fear.[27]

In many cases hypnosis can be employed in place of other, more conventional techniques of pain and anxiety control.[28] When hypnosis is successful, even local anesthetics for pain control may not be required.

Postoperative complications and discomfort can be minimized through the effective use of posthypnotic suggestion, thereby decreasing a patient's requirement for analgesics and other medications with their potential side effects.[22]

The success of hypnosis

Although folklore acknowledges that only 25% of the population is "susceptible" to hypnosis, reports on the success of hypnosis in clinical practice are more positive. Beecher[29] reported that hypnosis is an effective substitute for anesthesia in all but approximately 20% of the surgical population tested. Barber and Mayer,[22] using a technique of hypnotic induction called "rapid induction analgesia," reported that test subjects were able to "dramatically alter their awareness of experimental dental pain, irrespective of hypnotic susceptibility. . . . Ninety-nine percent of unscreened dental patients were able to undergo normally painful dental procedures using only hypnosis, as induced by rapid induction analgesia."

Education in hypnosis

Although many dental schools include training in hypnosis as a part of their curriculum, most practicing dentists are untrained in the effective use of this potentially valuable technique. Two professional groups offer clinical workshops in hypnosis throughout the United States. The reader is referred to them for additional information and training in hypnosis.*

In conclusion, I must restate to the reader the vital importance of iatrosedation in the everyday practice of medicine and dentistry. Iatrosedation must be employed by each of us whenever we are in contact with other human beings, be they are our patients, staff, or simply other persons we come into contact with. Our behavior and our appearance provide these per-

---

*American Society of Clinical Hypnosis, 2250 E. Devon Ave., Suite 336, Des Plaines, IL 60018. Society of Clinical and Experimental Hypnosis, 1294 Kings Park Drive, Liverpool, NY, 13088.

sons with a sense of "like" or "dislike" toward us. For a practice of dentistry or medicine to be successful, an attitude of caring must become an integral part of office philosophy. In the absence of this caring attitude, patients will feel isolated and alienated, increasing their own anxiety levels and producing additional management difficulties for the staff. The successful use of iatrosedation will enhance the effectiveness of the pharmacosedative techniques that will be discussed in the chapters to follow.

REFERENCES

1. Council on Dental Education: *Guidelines for teaching the comprehensive control of pain and anxiety in dentistry*, 1993, ADA.
2. Smith LS: Evaluation and management of the muscle contraction headache, *Nurs Pract* 13(1):20, 1988.
3. Wong T: Use of electrostimulation of acupuncture points in general dental practice, *Anesth Prog* 36(4,5):243, 1989.
4. Mayer R: Stress, anxiety and audio-analgesia in dental treatment measured with the aid of biosignals, *Deutsche Zahnarztliche Zeitschrift* 44(9):692, 1989.
5. Elmore AM: Biofeedback therapy in the treatment of dental anxiety and dental phobia, *Dent Clin North Am* 32(4):735, 1988.
6. teDuits E, Geopferd S, Donly K et al: The effectiveness of electronic dental anesthesia in children, *Pediatr Dent* 15(3):191, 1993.
7. Treschinskii AI, Aznaurian SK, Trotsevich VA: Changes in autonomic homeostasis during anesthesia induction in patients operated on for congenital cleft palate, *Stomatologiia* 70(3):59, 1991.
8. Friedman N: Iatrosedation. In McCarthy FM, ed: *Emergencies in dental practice,* ed 3. Philadelphia, 1979, Saunders.
9. Egbert L, Battit G, Turndoff H et al: Value of the preoperative visit by an anesthetist, *JAMA* 195:553, 1963.
10. Egbert LD: Reduction of post-operative pain by encouragement and instruction of patients: a study of doctor-patient rapport, *N Engl J Med* 270:825, 1964.
11. Ziskin L, producer: *The Doctor,* Hollywood, 1991, Touchstone Films (film).
12. LBVA hospital program, Long Beach, Calif.
13. Spiro H: What is empathy and can it be taught? *Ann Intern Med* 116:843, 1992.
14. Matthews DA, Feinstein AR: A review of systems for the personal aspects of patient care, *Am J Med Sci* 295(3):159, 1988.
15. *Continuing education directory,* Chicago, 1993, ADA.
16. Shedlin M, Wallechinsky D: *Laughing gas, nitrous oxide.* Berkeley, Calif, 1973, And/Or Press.
17. Schmierer A: Use of relaxation sound tracks in the dental office, *Zahnarztliche Praxis* 42(8):286, 1991.
18. Friedman H: The doctor-patient relationship in an intravenous-sedation practice, *Anesth Prog* 23:48, 1976.
19. Friedman N: Iatrosedation. In McCarthy FM, editor: *Emergencies in dental practice,* ed 3. Philadelphia, 1979, Saunders.
20. Malamed SF: A most powerful drug, *J Calif Acad Gen Dent* 4:17, 1979.
21. Seltzer S: *Pain control in dentistry, diagnosis and management.* Philadelphia, 1978, Lippincott.
22. Barber J, Mayer D: Evaluation of the efficacy and neural mechanism of a hypnotic analgesia procedure in experimental and clinical dental pain, *Pain* 4:41, 1977.
23. Lyons AS, Petrucelli RJ: *Medicine: an illustrated history.* New York, 1978, Harry N Abrams.
24. Ring ME: *Dentistry: an illustrated history.* New York and St Louis, 1985, Harry N Abrams and Mosby.
25. Barber J: Acupuncture and hypnosis in dentistry. In Allen GD, editor: *Dental anesthesia and analgesia (local and general),* ed 2. Baltimore, 1979, Williams & Wilkins.
26. DiBona MC: Nitrous oxide and hypnosis: a combined technique, *Anesth Prog* 26:17, 1979.
27. Morse DR, Cohen BB: Desensitization using meditation-hypnosis to control "needle" phobia in two dental patients, *Anesth Prog* 30:83, 1983.
28. Hilgard ER: Pain: its reduction and production under hypnosis, *Proc Amer Philosoph Soc* 115:470, 1971.
29. Beecher HK: *Measurement of subjective responses.* New York, 1959, Oxford University Press.

SECTION THREE

Oral, rectal, and intramuscular sedation

In this and in subsequent sections the techniques of pharmacosedation will be described in detail. Major sections are devoted to inhalation and intravenous (IV) sedation, two of the most useful pharmacosedative techniques. In this section three routes of drug administration are discussed in depth: the oral, rectal, and intramuscular (IM) routes, each of which can prove to be quite effective within the practice of dentistry for the management of pain, fear, and anxiety, while three relatively new and potentially valuable routes of drug administration, sublingual, transdermal, and intranasal, are introduced in Chapter 10.

The oral, rectal, and IM techniques are frequently referred to as premedication, *whereas the term* sedation *is commonly applied to inhalation and IV techniques.* Premedication *is defined as "any sedative, tranquilizer, hypnotic, or anticholinergic medication administered prior to anesthesia."[1] A deciding factor as to whether a technique will be considered premedication or sedation is the latent period of the technique. The latent period is that period of time that elapses between the administration of a drug and its onset of clinical activity.*

In both inhalation and IV drug administration the latent period is quite short, well under 60 seconds. However, in oral, rectal, and IM drug administration, the latent period may range from 15 minutes to more than 30 minutes.

Each of these routes of drug administration may be employed to provide sedation, and will be addressed as such throughout this text, because they all accomplish the stated goal of sedation: "relaxation of an apprehensive person without inducing the loss of consciousness." It is in their clinical application that the distinction between premedication and sedation has developed. The term sedation *is used to describe techniques in which clinical actions develop more rapidly, and the term* premedication *is used to describe those techniques with a more gradual onset of action. The term* sedation *will be used throughout this text in our discussion of all techniques of patient relaxation.*

REFERENCE

1. Urdang L, ed: *Mosby's medical and nursing dictionary*, St Louis, 1983, Mosby.

CHAPTER 8

Oral sedation

The oral route is the oldest of all routes of drug administration and is still the most commonly used route for the administration of drugs. It is also the safest, most convenient, and most economical method of drug administration. The oral route may be used quite effectively in dentistry for the reduction of stress prior to or during dental treatment and as a means of managing preoperative and postoperative pain. Although other techniques of administration may be more reliable and more effective in producing a desired clinical effect, the oral route still maintains a valued place in dentistry's armamentarium against pain and anxiety.

ADVANTAGES

The oral route does possess several advantages over other routes of drug administration:
1. Almost universal acceptability
2. Ease of administration
3. Low cost
4. Decreased incidence of adverse reactions
5. Decreased severity of adverse reactions
6. No needles, syringes, equipment
7. No specialized training

Most adults do not object to taking medications by mouth. For better or for worse, we have become a "pill-popping" society, a fact that makes the prescription of an anxiety-reducing drug prior to dental treatment all the more palatable to the patient. An important exception to this is the young child, who may prove unwilling to accept any medications by mouth.

Oral medications are exceptionally easy for the doctor to administer. In most cases the drug prescribed for premedication will be taken by the patient at home. In other situations the doctor may elect to administer an oral drug to the patient personally on the patient's arrival in the dental office,

in order to ensure proper dosage and time of administration. In either case the administration of drugs via the oral route requires only that the doctor have knowledge of the pharmacologic action of the drug being administered, its side effects and potential drug-drug interactions, and any contraindications to its administration. No special equipment, personnel, or advanced training is required for the safe use of the oral route.

The cost of most medications for oral administration is normally quite low, especially when considering the minimal number of doses employed in dentistry. Although there is significant variation in the cost of drugs, the cost of the oral form of a drug is usually significantly below that of its parenteral counterpart.

Complications are possible whenever drugs are administered, regardless of their route of administration. Drug idiosyncrasy, allergy, and overdose, as well as other adverse actions, can and do occur. Drug-related side effects are less likely to develop following enteral drug administration (i.e., oral, rectal) than they are following parenteral drug administration. In addition, adverse reactions developing following oral administration are often much less intense than those noted following parenteral administration of the same drug. This is not to imply that serious complications do not occur following oral drug administration. Berger et al.[1] reported a cardiac arrest following oral diazepam intoxication, and Gill and Michaelides[2,3] described an anaphylactic response to oral penicillin.

The convenience of the oral route of drug administration is a primary reason for its popularity. This technique can be employed with minimal risk providing that the doctor prescribing the drug(s) is knowledgeable of (1) the pharmacologic actions of the drug being administered; (2) its indications, contraindications, precautions, side effects, and dosage; and (3) the medical history of the patient, especially as it relates to prior drug use, specific contraindications to the use of particular drugs, and prior reactions to the drug to be employed. No special equipment (e.g., needles, syringes), no additional personnel, and no advanced educational training are required when oral medications are used.

The advantages listed above appear to make the use of orally administered drugs quite compelling. However, there are, as with all routes of drug administration, some distinct disadvantages that effectively limit the clinical use of this route of drug administration.

DISADVANTAGES

Disadvantages associated with the oral administration of drugs include the following:

1. Reliance on patient compliance
2. Prolonged latent period
3. Erratic and incomplete absorption of drugs from the GI tract
4. Inability to titrate
5. Inability to readily lighten or deepen the level of sedation
6. Prolonged duration of action

When prescribing drugs for oral administration, the doctor must rely on the patient to take the drug as prescribed (the proper dose at the proper time). Although in many instances patients may in fact medicate themselves properly, oftentimes they will not. This potential problem, termed *noncompliance*, is a significant one in medicine, especially in relation to long-term drug administration (e.g., antihypertensive medications). The Council on Patient Information and Education estimates that 35% to 50% of all prescriptions dispensed by doctors are taken incorrectly by patients and that one in five patients never even bothers to have the prescription filled. One in seven stops taking the medication too soon. Noncompliance rates among patients over 65 years of age are more than 55%.[4] Although noncompliance is not as critical a problem in the dental situation, the administration of too small or too large a dose, too soon or too late, can significantly alter the effectiveness of the drug during dental treatment. One of the more common forms of noncompliance is the taking of a dose larger than that prescribed, the rationale being that "if one (tablet or capsule) is good, then two or more will be better." This type of thinking leads to oversedation, overdose, and other unwanted and unpleasant complications. Fortunately (in this situa-

tion, at least), the erratic and incomplete absorption of orally administered drugs minimizes the development of serious problems from drug overadministration.

On many occasions I have observed this phenomenon in pediatric dental practice: a parent or guardian administers either a tablespoon instead of a teaspoon, or a larger dose than desired, because the child did not take all of the first dose. Significant overdose, with attendant respiratory depression, can develop in this manner if the administered drug is a CNS depressant. The consequences of these actions are formidable, with potential morbidity or mortality the result. The doctor prescribing oral drugs for anxiety reduction must always remember that these drugs are CNS depressants and that excessive CNS depression (e.g., oversedation, general anesthesia) is always a potential problem. To minimize concern over patient noncompliance, the doctor should (1) tell the patient, or the parent or guardian, exactly how much of the drug to take and at what time to take it; (2) write these instructions down and give them to the patient; (3) make sure the prescription is clearly marked with these same instructions; (4) prescribe only the dose the patient is to take (this is warranted even though prescriptions for larger numbers of tablets or capsules are less expensive per item than are single doses); and (5) record the instructions given to the patient, as well as the drug and its dose, in the patient's chart. In those cases in which a patient is known to be unreliable, the patient can be asked to appear in the dental office 1 hour prior to the scheduled treatment, and the drug given to the patient by a member of the office staff.

Another disadvantage of the oral route is its relatively long latent period. Most orally administered drugs have a latent period of approximately 30 minutes. At this time the blood (plasma) level of the drug is at the minimal (therapeutic) level required for clinical activity to be evident. Most absorption of oral drugs occurs from the small intestine with lesser absorption from the stomach. Drug absorption into the cardiovascular system continues and the blood level of the drug increases until a maximal level is reached. With most oral drugs peak blood levels occur approximately 60 minutes following drug ingestion, or 30 minutes following the onset of clinical activity. Peak blood level is equated clinically with maximal drug action (i.e., most intense analgesia or sedation).

In addition to the long latent period, most oral drugs are absorbed erratically and incompletely from the GI tract, which makes consistent clinical results very difficult to achieve. There are a number of factors that act to influence the absorption of drugs from the GI tract:

1. Lipid solubility
2. pH of the gastric tissues
3. Mucosal surface area
4. Gastric emptying time
5. Dosage form of the drug
6. Drug inactivation
7. Presence of food in the stomach
8. Bioavailability of the drug
9. Hepatic "first pass" effect

Absorption

Both the lipid solubility of the drug and the pH of the gastric tissues will affect drug absorption from the GI tract. Lipid-soluble drugs will be absorbed more rapidly than non–lipid-soluble drugs. The pH of the gastric juice is approximately 1.4. Drugs that are organic acids, such as aspirin, freely diffuse across the gastric mucosa into the circulatory system. Drugs that are bases, codeine for example, are poorly absorbed from the highly acid environment of the stomach. As gastric fluid leaves the stomach to enter the small intestine, its pH changes significantly, owing to the addition of biliary, intestinal, and pancreatic secretions. In the intestinal environment, with its pH of approximately 4.0 to 6.0, the absorption of aspirin will be slowed, whereas that of the more basic codeine will be accelerated.

Primary absorption of most drugs occurs from the small intestine rather than from the stomach. This is true even for drugs such as aspirin because the lower gastric pH favors its absorption, yet over 90% of the absorption of aspirin occurs in the small intestine. The primary factor for this is the architecture of the small intestine. It is designed for the process of absorption, containing a considerable surface area, consisting of microvilli, villi, and the folds of Kerckring. The stomach, by contrast, is a relatively smooth organ that is poorly designed for absorption.

Because the small intestine is the primary site for drug absorption, it becomes important to get the drug through the mouth, esophagus, and stomach and into the small intestine as rapidly as possible. The removal of foods and other substances from the stomach occurs by contraction of the antrum of the stomach. The time required for a substance to be expelled from the stomach is termed the *gastric emptying time.* Liquids, when taken alone, require approximately 90 minutes to be removed, and a mixed

meal of food and liquids requires about 4 hours to reach the duodenum. Liquids are discharged from the stomach into the duodenum at a rate of 10 ml per minute. The presence of fat in the stomach will significantly retard gastric emptying time. It is therefore recommended, as a general rule, that oral medications be taken with a glass of water (approximately 8 oz) in the absence of food. In this manner the drug's delivery to the duodenum will be maximal, permitting more reliable absorption. Yet another factor that delays gastric emptying is anxiety. It is estimated that gastric emptying time can be delayed by as much as two times in the fearful patient,[5] thereby retarding the onset of action of antianxiety drugs. Thus a negative cycle is established. Oral antianxiety agents are administered 1 hour prior to treatment to lessen the patient's fear of impending dental or surgical care, yet the very fear that we are seeking to manage inhibits the absorption of the drug into the cardiovascular system. This helps to explain why very apprehensive patients may be poorly sedated when they arrive for treatment in spite of having taken their oral medication as directed by the doctor.

Drugs administered in aqueous solution are more rapidly absorbed than those given as an oily solution or in tablet or capsule form. The tablet or capsule must first dissolve in the gastric fluid before absorption can occur. Once dissolved, the size of the resulting particles of drug is important. The smaller the particle, the greater the rate of drug absorption.[6] There is in fact significant variation in the clinical effectiveness of different forms (i.e., liquid, capsule, tablet) of the same drug (see the next section, Bioavailability).

Some drugs, such as morphine, cannot be administered orally because a significant degree of drug inactivation occurs before they reach the cardiovascular system. Although the acidity of the stomach is the major cause of this, intestinal contents can also affect the actions of oral drugs. The hepatic first pass effect may also be involved. Drugs absorbed from the GI tract (stomach, intestine, colon) are first delivered to the liver via the hepatic portal system before entering into the general circulation. The liver is rich in enzymes that biotransform certain drugs into pharmacologically inactive byproducts. A prime example of this is the antidysrhythmic drug lidocaine. Lidocaine is so completely transformed via hepatic first pass that the drug is essentially useless when administered orally.[7] By modifying the chemical structure of lidocaine a chemical analog was developed, tocainide, which is clinically effective as an oral antidysrhythmic agent.[8] In the area of drugs used for anxiety reduction, there is a subtle (but not clinically significant) hepatic first pass effect noted with the narcotic analgesics.

The presence of food in the stomach will decrease the absorption of drugs into the cardiovascular system by increasing gastric emptying time, and if the drug is bound to food it will not be available for absorption.[9] As mentioned previously, it is recommended that oral drugs be ingested with a full glass of water and in the absence of food (unless the drug specifically requires that it be administered along with food as a means of minimizing gastric upset).

Bioavailability

Two tablets from different manufacturers of the same dosage of the same drug are said to be *chemically* equivalent. If the ensuing blood levels of the drugs are equivalent, they are said to be *biologically* equivalent. They are *therapeutically* equivalent if they are equally effective therapeutically. Drugs that are chemically equivalent are not necessarily biologically or therapeutically equivalent. These differences are termed *bioavailability*. Differences in bioavailability of drugs are most often seen with oral preparations. The differences in absorption of chemically equivalent drugs are related to differences in size of particles or shape of crystals, and the rates of disintegration and dissolution of the drugs.

The slow onset of clinical activity of oral drugs prevents their titration. The ability to titrate a drug permits individualization of drug dosages for all patients. Undersedation or oversedation need not occur when titration is possible. The ability to titrate a drug to clinical effect is one of the greatest safety factors in drug administration. Unfortunately, the 30-minute latent period and 60-minute delay for the drug to reach peak blood level (for most oral drugs) precludes titration. Care must be exacted to avoid underadministration or overadministration of orally administered sedative drugs.

Another disadvantage of orally administered drugs is the inability to either lighten or deepen the level of sedation promptly. Should the effect of the drug prove inadequate, a second dose may be given; however, the same time factors (30 and 60 minutes) will be required to achieve full benefit of the drug, making this an unattractive option. If, on the other hand, the effect of the initial dose proves too intense, there is no effective means of reversing it. This lack of control over the actions of the drug seriously impairs the usefulness of this technique in a typical outpatient dental environment.

The duration of clinical action of most oral drugs is approximately 3 to 4 hours. For the typical 1-hour dental appointment this duration of action is entirely too long. Unfortunately however there is no method of reversing the clinical action of the drug. The patient will most likely remain under the influence of the drug well into the postoperative period and will be unable to leave the dental office unescorted. Patients receiving oral sedation for stress reduction must always be cautioned against driving or operating potentially hazardous machinery. If patients receive oral drugs at home an hour prior to their dental appointment, they should be similarly cautioned.

RATIONALE FOR USE

When the advantages and disadvantages of the oral route are compared, it becomes obvious that there are a number of significant disadvantages associated with the use of this technique. These combine to produce a route of drug administration in which the administrator has little control over the ultimate clinical action of the drug.

This lack of control over drug action is a potential source of danger every time an oral drug is administered. This is particularly so when the drug is a CNS depressant, as are those used in stress reduction. The potential for oversedation, respiratory depression, and loss of consciousness must always be considered when administration of an oral drug for anxiety relief is contemplated.

In spite of the negative factors associated with oral sedation, there is considerable need for orally administered drugs for stress reduction in dentistry. The primary use of the oral route will be in the management of anxiety prior to the dental procedure. However, because of the lack of control over the ultimate drug action, it is strongly suggested that only lighter levels of sedation be sought via this route. Light levels of sedation may prove adequate to reduce anxieties occurring prior to the dental appointment but may prove inadequate in diminishing the fears developing once the patient reaches the dental office and treatment begins. It is possible to achieve deeper levels of sedation with the oral route. The clinician must always keep in mind however the lack of control over drug action and the wide range of individual response to a given drug dose. The possibility of overdose, respiratory depression, impaired consciousness, or unconsciousness is increased as the degree of CNS depression increases. Persons untrained in the management of the unconscious airway ought not attempt to achieve more profound sedation by the oral route. Additionally, the doctor prescribing or administering oral drugs should possess a thorough knowledge of the drug's actions, contraindications, side effects, and precautions. The doctor must also be capable of prompt recognition and management of any adverse reaction that might develop. If deeper levels of sedation are required, a more controllable technique of sedation (i.e., inhalation or IV) should be considered.

What then represents a rational use of the oral route in a typical dental practice? From the standpoint of safety it is important that the clinician never seek to achieve a level of sedation beyond which he or she is comfortable (has been trained to use) and is capable of recognizing and managing any undesirable side effects that might develop. For these reasons the rational use of oral sedation includes only lighter levels of sedation. Deeper levels of sedation should be restricted to more controllable techniques or, when indicated via the oral route, should only be employed by a clinician with prior experience or training in the technique of deep oral sedation and who is fully prepared to manage any adverse reactions that might develop.

The most common use of oral sedation is for the reduction of anxiety in the hours immediately preceding a dental appointment. An antianxiety or sedative-hypnotic drug should be used to reduce anxiety so that the patient will appear in the dental office for the scheduled appointment. More controllable techniques can be used at this time for intraoperative sedation. When using oral drugs for this purpose, the clinician must remember to caution the patient against driving or operating hazardous machinery. If the patient has taken the drug at home, he or she should be advised against driving a car and should be accompanied to the office (driven) by an adult. For medicolegal purposes this should also be noted in the patient's chart.

A second use for oral sedation is one that is often overlooked by the busy clinician. As noted earlier (Chapter 5), not only do patients with fears of dentistry or surgery become apprehensive immediately before the appointment, but often their anxieties begin to build the day before the scheduled appointment. These persons might be unable to sleep the night before the appointment as they anticipate their upcoming "ordeal." These patients will be fatigued when they appear in the dental office the next day, a factor that leads to a decrease in the pain reaction threshold. An antianxiety or hypnotic drug taken 1 hour before sleep the night before the appointment helps to ensure a restful night's sleep and a more fit patient during treatment.

USE OF ORAL SEDATION

1. Sedation the night before treatment to ensure restful sleep.
2. Light levels of sedation for preoperative anxiety reduction.

Other uses of the oral route in dentistry include the administration of drugs to inhibit salivary secretions (antisialagogues), agents to prevent or to manage nausea (antiemetics), and antibiotics.

DRUGS

A large number of drugs are commonly administered via the oral route in the management of anxiety. The overwhelming majority of these are classified as either sedative-hypnotics or antianxiety drugs. Other drug groups that may be used for this purpose are antihistamines and narcotics.

Prior to a discussion of these drugs, a word is in order regarding the appropriate dosages to be used. The clinician must use as much information as is available to make an informed decision regarding the appropriate dose to employ, particularly when using the oral route. Information available to the clinician includes the patient's medical history, age, weight, and previous drug reactions. In addition, the clinician must determine the degree of anxiety present and the level of sedation sought. After consideration of these factors, a drug dose is determined.

A source of information regarding recommended dosages of drugs is the drug package insert. A common problem associated with the use of recommended doses is that they often lead to inadequate anxiety reduction in the dental or surgical setting. There is a reasonable explanation for this; the package insert recommends a certain dose of a drug to induce sedation or sleep in a nonstress situation, such as the home environment. The dose of a drug that would effectively relax an apprehensive individual in the home will probably prove ineffective when the stress of the dental office environment is added to it. For this reason the doses recommended for oral sedation in this chapter and in many textbooks of pediatric dentistry[10,11] may be somewhat higher than those in the package inserts.

Many antianxiety and sedative-hypnotic drugs for oral administration are produced in three dosage forms. When selecting a dosage for stress reduction in dental practice, these three dosage forms of the

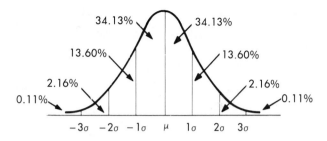

Fig. 8-1. Normal distribution curve ("bell-shaped" curve). Persons will respond to drug dosages in dissimilar ways. Approximately 2.5% of persons will be extremely resistant to a "usual dose," and 2.5% will be quite sensitive to the same dose. (From Bennett CR: *Anesth Prog* 30:106, 1983.)

drug should correlate with the "bell-shaped" curve (Fig. 8-1). The middle dosage form is the average dose, producing clinically effective results (in nonstress situations) in approximately 70% of persons receiving it. The larger dosage form is for persons in whom the smaller dose proves to be ineffective or who have a greater degree of anxiety. The smaller dosage form is for persons in whom the average dose provides too intense a clinical effect, for persons with lesser degrees of anxiety, for the elderly, or for debilitated patients. It must be remembered that the added stresses associated with dental or surgical treatment will increase the percentage of patients requiring larger than "usual" doses for adequate management of their treatment-related fears.

Although titration (individualization of drug dosages) is not possible with orally administered drugs—a significant impediment to their safe use—it is possible, in situations in which oral medications are to be used over multiple appointments, to *titrate by appointment*. This concept was introduced to me by Dr. Ronald Johnson, chairman of the Department of Pediatric Dentistry at the University of Southern California.[12] Quite simply put, titration by appointment means that the doctor will assess the efficacy of sedation achieved at the first appointment with a given drug dosage and if necessary will increase or decrease the dosage or drug(s) administered at subsequent appointments. Therefore, over a period of two to three visits the appropriate dosage for that patient will be achieved (titrated). Titration by appointment is discussed more fully in the chapter on pediatric sedation (Chapter 36).

In the remainder of this chapter the drugs that are administered via the oral route to provide sedation will be reviewed. Drugs will be discussed by their therapeutic category.

1. Sedative-hypnotics
   a. Ethyl alcohol
   b. Barbiturates
   c. Nonbarbiturates
2. Antianxiety drugs
3. Antihistamines
4. Opioid analgesics

SEDATIVE-HYPNOTICS

Sedative-hypnotics are drugs that produce either sedation or hypnosis depending on the dosage of the drug that is administered and the patient's response to it. Lower dosages of these drugs produce a calming effect (sedation), usually associated with a degree of drowsiness and motor incoordination (ataxia), while higher dosages produce hypnosis (a state resembling physiologic sleep).

Sedative-hypnotics are commonly divided into two groups: the barbiturates and the nonbarbiturate sedative-hypnotics. Alcohol, probably the most frequently employed sedative-hypnotic, will be discussed first.

Ethyl alcohol

Alcohol has long been used by apprehensive patients as a means of medicating themselves prior to dental care. Each and every one of us in dentistry has had occasion to manage a patient who was quite well premedicated with alcohol (which was NOT prescribed by the doctor!). The very fact that patients feel that they require some form of sedation in order to "handle" their dental treatment should alert the dental office staff to the probable presence of anxiety (or of a drug abuse problem). The doctor should seek to determine the underlying dental fears harbored by such patients and take the steps necessary to correct or alleviate them.

As common a drug as alcohol may be, its use as a sedative in dentistry has never been popular. In 1923 Niels Bjorn Jorgensen, considered by many to be the "father of sedation in dentistry," first used medicinal alcohol in the management of the fearful adult patient. Jorgensen administered 4 oz of medicinal alcohol, with excellent results. Jorgensen later prescribed aromatic elixir USP in a flavored base, which became known as "Jorgensen's elixir."[13]

McCarthy and Hayden[14] have reviewed the history of alcohol and present a protocol for its use as a sedative in dentistry. McCarthy[15] has stated that many doctors have employed alcohol in their offices, virtually all with resounding success. The following is a review of their recommendations.[14]

The use of alcohol is not contraindicated in pediatric dentistry; however, special precautions and care are necessary to prevent alcohol-induced hypoglycemic reactions. The dosage forms described by the authors refer to the adult patient—one who is legally able to drink alcohol.

The authors recommend use of the term *medicinal alcohol* when discussing the advantages and disadvantages of the drug with respect to informed consent. Eighty proof (40%) distilled neutral spirits are used, flavored if desired or administered in a pleasant vehicle such as fruit or vegetable juice. In order to minimize the possibility of gastritis, the dose of alcohol should be diluted twice, for example, 2 oz of vehicle (juice) to 1 oz of alcohol. The patient should not have consumed any alcohol within the preceding 12 hours, with a maximum consumption of 6 oz of distilled spirits within the past 24 hours. Other CNS depressant drugs ought not be employed along with the alcohol in order to avoid possibly undesirable drug interactions, unless the doctor is thoroughly experienced in sedation and general anesthesia and in basic life support.

The patient is advised to eat a light carbohydrate-rich meal (cereal and milk) 3 hours prior to the dental appointment. This usually provides an empty stomach by treatment time. Approximately 20 minutes before the start of treatment, the alcohol is administered to the patient in the dental office. Maximal blood levels are reached within 20 to 30 minutes following ingestion of a single dose on an empty stomach. The average duration of clinical sedation is 60 minutes, although a degree of sedation will persist for an additional 10 to 20 minutes. In most cases the patient may be dismissed about 80 minutes after the alcohol is administered. The patient may be permitted to drive a car, if in the doctor's opinion the patient is fully recovered from the drug's effects. This represents a significant advantage over other oral and parenteral medications.

Dosage forms are presented in Table 8-1. The higher dosage levels are used at subsequent visits only if the initial doses proved ineffective (an example of titration by appointment). When higher doses are used, the authors recommend that the patient be retained in the dental office for 140 minutes from the time of administration.

The patient is advised to abstain from further alcohol or other CNS depressants for a minimum of 3 hours after discharge. A light carbohydrate-rich meal is recommended after dismissal.

Alcohol-induced hypoglycemia. Alcohol may induce serious hypoglycemia in children and in malnourished adults by reducing the process of gluco-

Table 8-1. Recommended doses of ethyl alcohol

Weight in pounds	First appointment	Subsequent appointments*
100	30 ml (1 oz)	45 ml (1.5 oz)
140	30 ml (1 oz)	60 ml (2 oz)
180	60 ml (2 oz)	90 ml (3 oz)
220	60 ml (2 oz)	90 ml (3 oz)

From McCarthy FM, ed: *Emergencies in dental practice,* ed 3. Philadelphia, 1979, Saunders.
*Increased dosage forms should be used only if first appointment dose proves inadequate.

neogenesis from amino acids. This response is not likely to be observed in a healthy adult receiving the doses suggested for sedation.

Prevention of alcohol-induced hypoglycemia depends on an estimate of the patient's past experience with alcohol, an estimate of the sedative dose, and the patient's ingestion of a light carbohydrate-rich meal 3 hours before sedation.

Contraindications. The use of alcohol as a sedative is contraindicated in patients who have had no social experience with it, are intolerant of it, have an aversion to alcohol for personal or religious reasons, have a history of alcohol-induced hypoglycemia or hypoglycemia caused by diabetes mellitus or malnutrition, have liver disease, or have a prior or present history of alcohol abuse. In addition, the use of alcohol should be avoided in persons taking other CNS depressants, such as barbiturates, antianxiety agents, narcotics, and antidepressants.

The pharmacokinetics of alcohol are reviewed in the paper by McCarthy and Hayden,[14] providing an understanding of why it is possible to administer a CNS depressant drug to a patient preoperatively and then to permit the patient to leave the dental office unescorted and to operate a motor vehicle.

Alcohol is an effective sedative for the relief of mild anxiety. When administered with adequate instructions and in the proper dosage, there are virtually no side effects. The drug is metabolized rapidly and most patients may be permitted to leave the dental office unescorted. Alcohol is as effective an antianxiety agent as oral diazepam or pentobarbital; however, side effects of these other agents, such as depression and headache, are seldom encountered.

Barbiturates

The barbiturates represented the first truly effective drugs for the management of anxiety that were, and still are, widely prescribed. The barbiturates are generalized CNS depressants, depressing the cerebral cortex, the limbic system, and the reticular activating system at therapeutic blood levels. These actions produce a reduction in the anxiety level, decreased mental acuity, and a state of drowsiness. At higher dosage levels depression of the medulla occurs, leading to respiratory depression and possible cardiovascular depression. Barbiturates are capable of producing any level of CNS depression ranging from light sedation through hypnosis, general anesthesia, coma, and death.[16,17]

Pharmacology

Central nervous system. The barbiturates produce a reversible depression of all excitable tissues, the central nervous system being remarkably sensitive. As mentioned previously, barbiturates produce a dose-related depression of the central nervous system, ranging from mild sedation to death. The reticular formation—a complex network of neurons, nuclei, and neural pathways extending through the brainstem from the medulla to the thalamus—is especially sensitive to depression by the barbiturates. The reticular formation is sometimes called the ''ascending reticular activating system'' (ARAS). The ARAS is important in the maintenance of sleep and wakefulness. It appears that the major action of the barbiturates is on the ARAS.

Barbiturates commonly exert a clinical effect that exceeds the expected clinical duration of the drug. For example, an oral dose of secobarbital may produce a sedative effect for only 3 to 4 hours, but there may be a subtle hangover effect, consisting of mood alteration (irritability), drowsiness, and impaired judgment, which may persist for many hours.

Barbiturates lack the ability to obtund the sense of pain; in other words they do not possess any analgesic properties. Patients who receive noxious stimuli after having received barbiturates for sedation will often hyperreact to the stimulus. Patients in pain who receive barbiturates may become aroused, agitated, and even dysphoric. Fortunately, this property of hyperalgesia is not shared by the nonbarbiturate sedative hypnotics. This increased response to pain in patients receiving barbiturates should concern dentists and physicians who are considering the use of these agents for sedation. Effective pain control must be provided whenever barbiturates are used, and if this is not possible, other sedative drugs should be used in their place.

Barbiturates are capable of preventing or terminating convulsive episodes, such as those occurring in grand mal epilepsy or local anesthetic overdose.[18]

In most instances however the barbiturate, to be effective, must be administered intravenously. A notable exception is phenobarbital, an agent that has been administered orally for many years in the preventive management of grand mal epilepsy.

Respiratory system. Barbiturates are respiratory depressants. At sedative doses there is little noticeable effect on respiration; however, at hypnotic levels or higher there is a progressive depression of respiration. These actions of the barbiturates will be reviewed in the section on IV sedation.

Cardiovascular system. At doses normally employed orally for sedation or hypnosis the barbiturates do not exhibit significant cardiovascular effects. Barbiturate-induced depression of the cardiovascular system is not usually seen until a significant degree of CNS and respiratory depression has developed.

Liver. In the therapeutic dosage range barbiturates do not impair normal hepatic function; however, in patients who are hypersensitive to the barbiturates, severe liver damage can develop from therapeutic dosages.

Prolonged use of barbiturates produces a nonspecific increase in the activity of the hepatic microsomal enzyme system. The resultant rise in levels of this enzyme causes an increase in the rate at which many drugs (e.g., barbiturates) are metabolized. The induction of hepatic microsomal enzymes can give rise to drug-drug interactions. For example, barbiturates shorten the prothrombin time of patients receiving anticoagulants[19]; and the potency of digitoxin may be decreased by accelerating its conversion to digoxin.[20] One of the more dangerous side effects produced by the actions of barbiturates on the liver is their ability to increase the synthesis of porphyrins. In patients suffering from acute intermittent porphyria, barbiturates may precipitate an episode of acute abdominal pain, nerve demyelinization, paralysis, and death. Barbiturates are absolutely contraindicated in patients with acute intermittent porphyria.[21]

Termination of clinical activity. The processes responsible for termination of the clinical activity of barbiturates are redistribution of the drug, biotransformation, and renal excretion. All three processes decrease the plasma level of the drug and result in its removal from its primary site of action in the central nervous system.

Redistribution is responsible in large part for the short duration of clinical action noted with the intravenously administered barbiturates thiopental, methohexital, and thiamylal. The drug undergoes redistribution from the brain to other tissue compartments, where it is stored and slowly rereleased into the cardiovascular system, undergoing metabolic transformation when it reaches the liver. The slow release of the barbiturate from its storage site (liver or fat) may be responsible for the hangover effect seen with many barbiturates.

Barbiturates that do not undergo metabolic transformation in the liver are excreted from the body unchanged in the urine. The long-acting barbiturate barbital has approximately 65% to 90% of its total dose removed from the body in this manner, whereas about 50% of a hypnotic dose of phenobarbital or aprobarbital is handled in this manner.

Most barbiturates are eliminated from the body through biotransformation into inactive metabolites. The liver is the primary site for this process. Thiobarbiturates may undergo a small portion of their metabolism in the kidney and brain. The presence of hepatic microsomal enzymes affects the rate of metabolic degradation of barbiturates. Although these enzymes may be present at normal levels in patients with some hepatic diseases, cirrhotic patients may demonstrate an increased sensitivity to the barbiturates. Barbiturates must be administered with caution to patients with hepatic damage. Initial dosages should be decreased. The plasma half-lives (the time required for blood levels of the drug to fall by half) of the barbiturates vary significantly (Table 8-2).

Table 8-2. Classification of barbiturates

Generic	Proprietary	Half-life
Ultrashort-acting		
Hexobarbital	Sombulex	5 hours
Methohexital sodium*	Brevital, Brietal	3.5 to 6 hours
Thiamylal sodium*	Surital	—
Thiopental sodium*	Pentothal	3 to 8 hours
Short-acting		
Pentobarbital sodium	Nembutal	21 to 42 hours
Secobarbital sodium	Seconal	20 to 28 hours
Intermediate-acting		
Amobarbital	Amytal	14 to 42 hours
Butabarbital	Butisol	—
Long-acting		
Phenobarbital	—	24 to 96 hours

*Intravenous agents.

Tolerance. Tolerance develops to the barbiturates, especially when administered on a long-term basis, a situation of minimal significance in dentistry. Persons addicted to barbiturates are often resistant (they hyporespond to the dose administered) to the hypnotic effects of the barbiturates and other depressants; however, tolerance to the hypnotic effects does not increase the lethal dose of the drugs. A hypnotic dose of a barbiturate taken daily for a period of 2 weeks or longer will, at the end of this period, be ineffective in producing or maintaining sleep. Larger doses of the drug will be required to produce the same clinical effect observed with a smaller dose 2 weeks earlier. Of all the sedative-hypnotics (both barbiturate and nonbarbiturate) to be discussed in this chapter, only the benzodiazepines flurazepam and triazolam do not produce this tolerance.[22]

Dependence. The barbiturates are capable of producing both psychological and physical dependence (addiction). Methods of minimizing this problem include prescribing no more than the recommended dose of the drug and terminating the use of the drug at the earliest possible time. Within the realm of dental practice this is not very difficult to achieve.

Oral barbiturates in dentistry

The barbiturates are classified as sedative-hypnotic drugs, which at different dosage levels produce differing levels of CNS depression manifested as relaxation (sedation) or drowsiness (hypnosis). Barbiturates are normally categorized by their duration of clinical action following an average oral dose (where possible). The *long-acting* (16 to 24 hours of clinical CNS depression) and the *intermediate-acting* (6 to 8 hours) *barbiturates* produce clinical levels of sedation for too long a period of time for the usual dental or surgical appointment. The long-acting barbiturates, such as phenobarbital, are commonly employed as anticonvulsants or when long-term sedation is necessary; the intermediate-acting barbiturates are used as "sleeping pills" in specific types of insomnia (where a person has no difficulty in falling asleep but does encounter difficulty in remaining asleep).

Short-acting barbiturates (3 to 4 hours' duration of action), most notably pentobarbital and secobarbital, are better suited for dental situations. They are also used in insomnia where the patient has difficulty in falling asleep but once asleep has no difficulty remaining asleep. Most of the *ultrashort-acting barbiturates* are used intravenously for the rapid induction of general anesthesia. The most frequently employed ultrashort-acting barbiturates are thiopental (Pentothal), thiamylal (Surital), and methohexital (Brevital, Brietal). Hexobarbital, another ultrashort-acting barbiturate, is available in oral preparations. Its clinical applications will be discussed shortly.

The disadvantages of the barbiturates are numerous. In the past 20 years, since the introduction of more effective and pharmacologically specific antianxiety agents, the use of barbiturates has declined.[23] This laudable trend should continue as evidence accumulates regarding the adverse properties of these drugs, including dose-related respiratory depression, the potential for habituation and addiction, the development of tolerance, and drug-drug interactions. In addition, the barbiturates are the drugs most often implicated in suicide attempts.[24]

Another important consideration in the use of barbiturates in dentistry is their inability to obtund pain without inducing a concurrent decrease in the level of consciousness. In sedative doses the barbiturates actually increase a patient's response to noxious stimuli. Barbiturates ought not be administered to patients who are in pain or in whom pain is expected to occur (e.g., postoperatively).[25]

Of the dozen or so barbiturates used clinically, only three (the short- and ultra-short-acting drugs) are of any value in dentistry, and even then only in isolated instances. The IV barbiturates, the intermediate-acting, and the long-acting barbiturates are of little value in contemporary dentistry for preoperative anxiety reduction. The three agents of potential value when administered orally in dentistry and surgery are pentobarbital, secobarbital, and hexobarbital.

Contraindications

Barbiturates are contraindicated in cases of hypersensitivity (allergy), uncontrolled pain, known addiction to sedative-hypnotics, latent or manifest porphyria or familial history of intermittent porphyria, and in respiratory disease when dyspnea or obstruction is present. Barbiturates should be avoided in patients with severe hepatic dysfunction.

Pregnancy and lactation

Barbiturates readily cross the placenta and if administered during pregnancy may have a depressant effect on the fetus. In addition, barbiturates are found in the milk of nursing mothers; therefore their use should be avoided during lactation.

Drug-drug interactions

Barbiturates may decrease the potency of the coumarin anticoagulants. Patients receiving both groups of drugs should undergo more frequent prothrombin determinations. The systemic actions of exogenous hydrocortisone and endogenous cortisol may also be diminished.

Care must be exercised when administering barbiturates to patients receiving other CNS depressant drugs because of the possibility of additive respiratory depression. These drugs include analgesics, other sedatives or hypnotics, alcohol, and antianxiety drugs.

Pentobarbital. Pentobarbital sodium is classified as a short-acting barbiturate. Its onset of action following oral administration is approximately 15 to 30 minutes, with a duration of action of 3 to 6 hours. The half-life of pentobarbital is 21 to 42 hours. The therapeutic index (the ratio of the median lethal dose to median effective dose) of pentobarbital is relatively high, which is unusual for barbiturates. For this reason, as well as for its shorter duration of action, pentobarbital is preferred over most other barbiturates for sedation prior to dental or surgical care. Pentobarbital is available in dosage forms of 50- and 100-mg capsules. The average dose recommended for adult preoperative sedation is 100 mg taken 1 hour before the scheduled appointment. Pentobarbital is packaged in white and yellow capsules. The name "yellow jackets" is frequently applied to this drug in the illicit drug market.

Availability. Pentobarbital sodium (generic): 50- and 100-mg capsules. Nembutal sodium (Abbott): 50- and 100-mg capsules. Pentobarbital is a controlled substance in Schedule II.

Secobarbital. Secobarbital is a short-acting barbiturate, with a half-life of 20 to 28 hours. Its onset of action develops within 15 to 30 minutes, with a duration of action of 3 to 6 hours. The therapeutic index of secobarbital is lower than that of pentobarbital, increasing the risk of unwanted side effects. The recommended dose for preoperative sedation is 100 to 200 mg taken 1 hour before the scheduled treatment. Secobarbital comes in distinctive red capsules from which is derived its street name of "reds."

Availability. Secobarbital sodium (generic): 50- and 100-mg capsules. Seconal sodium (Lilly): 30-, 50-, and 100-mg capsules. Seconal elixir (Lilly): 440 mg secobarbital per 100 ml. Secobarbital is a controlled substance in Schedule II.

Hexobarbital. Hexobarbital, an ultrashort-acting barbiturate, is available in an oral dosage form. Its clinical onset develops rapidly, between 15 and 30 minutes. Hexobarbital is metabolized rapidly and removed from the cardiovascular system within 4 to 5 hours. The usual duration of clinical effectiveness of hexobarbital is 60 to 90 minutes. It is administered approximately 30 minutes prior to treatment in a dose of 250 to 500 mg. Because of its more rapid onset of clinical activity, it is my practice to administer hexobarbital after the patient arrives at the dental office rather than having the patient take it at home.

Availability. Sombulex (Riker): 250-mg tablets.

Summary

The short-acting barbiturates secobarbital and pentobarbital are appropriate for preoperative anxiety control and on rare occasions for more profound intraoperative sedation when more controllable techniques are not available or are contraindicated. The latter use of these drugs cannot be recommended unless the doctor is capable of recognizing and managing any adverse actions that might develop following administration of these drugs. Oversedation, noted as decreased cooperativeness and/or respiratory depression, is the most frequently observed clinical sign. Barbiturates should be used for sedation only when other more effective antianxiety agents (e.g., benzodiazepines) have proved to be ineffective or are unavailable.

Effective sedation with the barbiturates results in drowsiness. The patient *must* be accompanied by an adult and must be warned against operating a motor vehicle or dangerous machinery for the balance of the day.

The ultrashort-acting barbiturate hexobarbital is commonly administered to the patient within the office to achieve a rapid onset of sedation when other techniques of sedation are not available. The drug is administered 30 minutes prior to treatment. The same precautions regarding companion, driving, and dangerous machinery apply.

Nonbarbiturate sedative-hypnotics

Many other drugs share with barbiturates the ability to produce a state of hypnosis. These *nonbarbiturate sedative-hypnotics* share many of the same disadvantages as barbiturates. There are only two ways in which these drugs differ from barbiturates: (1) they are less potent than barbiturates and (2) they are not cross-allergenic with barbiturates. Drugs included in this category are listed below by their major classification:

1. Benzodiazepines
   a. Flurazepam
   b. Temazepam
   c. Triazolam
   d. Lorazepam
   e. Nitrazepam
   f. Midazolam
2. Carbamates
   a. Ethinamate
   b. Meprobamate
3. Chloral derivatives
   a. Chloral hydrate
4. Ethchlorvynol
5. Paraldehyde
6. Glutethimide
7. Methyprylon

Benzodiazepines

The benzodiazepines include some drugs that are categorized as sedative-hypnotics and others that are categorized as antianxiety agents. All benzodiazepines have hypnotic effects to a degree; however, the incidence of side effects and the duration of action of some of these drugs preclude their use in this area. The pharmacology of this important group of drugs will be reviewed in depth in the section on oral antianxiety drugs.

One of the primary benefits gained from using benzodiazepines as sedative-hypnotics instead of barbiturates is the decreased occurrence of the hangover effect so often noted when barbiturates are administered. Additional benefits include a minimal effect on the hepatic microsomal enzyme system and the fact that pharmacologically the benzodiazepines present less of a risk to the patient than do the barbiturates.

Five benzodiazepines have received significant attention as sedative-hypnotics: flurazepam, temazepam, triazolam, lorazepam, and nitrazepam.

Flurazepam. Flurazepam, like most other benzodiazepines, has been demonstrated to produce its clinical action on the hypothalamus and the amygdala. Because of the lack of hepatic microsomal enzyme induction, the dose of flurazepam required to induce sleep does not increase with prolonged administration. Following oral administration flurazepam is rapidly absorbed and distributed; peak plasma levels develop within 30 to 60 minutes. As flurazepam is biotransformed in the liver, the drug should be employed with caution in patients with hepatic dysfunction. The half-life of flurazepam is 47 to 100 hours.

The incidence of side effects occurring with flurazepam administration is approximately 7%. The most often reported side effects include dizziness, drowsiness, lightheadedness, staggering, and ataxia. The hangover effect so often seen with the barbiturates is infrequent with flurazepam.

The clinical effectiveness of a 15- to 30-mg dose of flurazepam has been demonstrated in controlled trials to be equivalent to 100 mg of secobarbital, 100 mg of pentobarbital, 50 mg of amobarbital, 500 mg of glutethimide, and 500 and 1000 mg of chloral hydrate.[26]

Contraindications. The use of flurazepam is contraindicated in hypersensitivity (allergy) to benzodiazepines, and in pregnant females.

Warnings. Patients should be cautioned against operating motor vehicles or hazardous machinery and combining other CNS depressant drugs, such as alcohol, with flurazepam.

Drug interactions. Additive CNS depressant actions may develop when flurazepam is administered to patients receiving other CNS depressants such as alcohol, barbiturates, or narcotics.

Dosage. The usual dose of flurazepam is 30 mg taken 1 hour prior to bedtime. In the elderly or debilitated the 15-mg dose is recommended.

Availability. Dalmane (Roche): 15- and 30-mg capsules. Flurazepam is a controlled substance in Schedule IV.

Temazepam. Temazepam is absorbed slowly after oral administration. Onset occurs within 20 to 30 minutes; however, peak plasma levels require 2 to 3 hours (whereas flurazepam reaches peak levels at 30 minutes to 1 hour). The mean plasma half-life is 10 hours, and there are no significant active metabolites. The primary clinical use of temazepam is for patients having difficulty remaining asleep once falling asleep. Because of its slow onset of action temazepam is not effective in patients having difficulty falling asleep.

Contraindications, warnings, and drug interactions are similar to those for flurazepam (discussed previously).

Dosage. The usual dose is 30 mg 1 hour before bedtime. The 15-mg dosage form should be used initially in the elderly and debilitated.

Availability. Restoril (Sandoz): 15- and 30-mg capsules. Temazepam is a controlled substance in Schedule IV.

Triazolam. Triazolam is another benzodiazepine derivative. It was approved for marketing as a hypnotic in 1982 and has become the most prescribed psychoactive drug in the United States.[27] Triazolam is valuable in dentistry because of its short half-life of 1.5 to 5.5 hours and the fact that it has no active metabolites.[28] Peak plasma levels develop at 1.3 hours (orally). Very little residual drowsiness (hangover) is noted with triazolam.

Triazolam has been used in dentistry as an effective oral drug in the management of pretreatment anxiety.[29,30] Several recent trials have evaluated its effectiveness in pediatric populations.[31,32] The use of oral triazolam in pediatric anxiety control will be discussed more fully in Chapter 36.

Contraindications. Triazolam is contraindicated in pregnant patients.

Warnings. Overdosage of triazolam may develop at four times the recommended therapeutic dosage. Patients receiving triazolam must be cautioned against operating machinery or driving a motor vehicle and against the simultaneous ingestion of alcohol and other CNS depressant drugs.

Anterograde amnesia, of varying severity, and paradoxical reactions have been reported following therapeutic doses of triazolam.[33] Cases of "traveler's amnesia" have been reported by persons taking triazolam to induce sleep while traveling, such as during an airplane flight.[34] In some of these cases insufficient time was allowed for the sleep period prior to awakening and before beginning activity. Halcion has received some extremely negative press during the past few years.[35,36] Great Britain, following reports of several serious complications, including suicide, banned the prescription of triazolam.[37] Following significant discussion of the safety and potential hazard of triazolam, the Food and Drug Administration decided against issuing any prohibitions on the prescription of this drug in the United States.[38]

Drug interactions. Additive CNS depressant actions may develop when triazolam is administered to patients receiving other CNS depressants such as alcohol, barbiturates, or narcotics.

Adverse reactions. The most common adverse side effects noted following triazolam administration are drowsiness (14.0%), headache (9.7%), dizziness (7.8%), and nervousness (5.2%).[39]

Dosage. A hypnotic dose of 0.25 mg 1 hour before bedtime or 1 hour prior to dental treatment will be adequate in most patients, while a dose of 0.125 may be sufficient for selected patients. A dose of 0.5 mg should be reserved for those patients who do not respond adequately to a lower dose since the risk of several adverse reactions increases with the size of the dose administered.

In geriatric or debilitated patients the recommended dosage range is 0.125 to 0.25 mg. Initial dosage in this group should be 0.125 mg.

Availability. Halcion (Upjohn): 0.125- and 0.25-mg tablets. Triazolam is a controlled substance in Schedule IV.

Lorazepam. Lorazepam is absorbed slowly following oral administration, attaining peak plasma levels in 2 hours, with a mean half-life of 12 hours. The drug was marketed in 1977 under the trade name of Ativan. Lorazepam is also available for parenteral administration. Orally the drug is effective as an antianxiety and a hypnotic drug. It is one of the few benzodiazepines that does not possess active metabolites. Hepatic dysfunction (hepatitis, cirrhosis) does not alter the manner in which lorazepam is handled by the liver.

Contraindications. Lorazepam is contraindicated in patients with known sensitivity to benzodiazepines and with narrow-angle glaucoma.

Warnings. Lorazepam is not recommended for patients with a primary depressive disorder or psychosis. Patients receiving lorazepam must be cautioned against operating machinery or driving a motor vehicle and against the simultaneous ingestion of alcohol and other CNS depressant drugs.

Drug interactions. Additive CNS depressant effects develop with the concurrent administration of other CNS depressant drugs, such as narcotics, barbiturates, and alcohol.

Adverse reactions. The most frequently observed side effects of lorazepam are sedation (15.9%), dizziness (6.9%), weakness (4.2%), and ataxia (3.4%).[40]

Because of the greater possibility of unwanted sedation with lorazepam than with other benzodiazepines, its use in the immediate preoperative period should be discouraged unless the doctor desires this effect and if arrangements have been made for the patient to be escorted from the office by an adult companion. The use of lorazepam the evening prior to treatment to ensure a restful night's sleep appears more sensible.

Dosage. The usual adult dosage of lorazepam is from 2 to 6 mg in two or three divided doses. The largest dose should be taken 1 hour before bedtime. For anxiety the initial dose is from 2 to 3 mg per day in two to three doses. Elderly or debilitated patients should receive an initial dose of 1 to 2 mg per day in divided dosages. The safety and effectiveness of lorazepam in patients under 12 years of age has not been established (as is true for most drugs). For preoperative anxiety control or as an aid to sleep prior to dental or surgical treatment, a single dose of 2 to 4 mg may be given 1 hour prior to sleep or to the appointment.

Availability. Ativan (Wyeth): 0.5-, 1-, and 2-mg tablets. Ativan is a controlled substance in Schedule IV.

Nitrazepam. Nitrazepam has been available in the United Kingdom and in Europe for several years. It is not available in the United States (July 1994). Clinically, nitrazepam has the same indications as flurazepam.[41]

The *contraindications, warnings, drug interactions,* and *precautions* to be noted with nitrazepam are similar to those previously noted for flurazepam.[42]

Dosage. The usual dose of nitrazepam for sedation is 5 to 10 mg taken 1 hour prior to bedtime. The 10-mg dose produces considerably more drowsiness than the 5-mg dose.

Availability. Mogadon (Hoffmann-LaRoche): 5-mg tablets and capsules. Also available as 10-mg tablets from other manufacturers.

COMMENT: The benzodiazepines are the preferred drugs for the management of preoperative anxiety in the dental setting. This is also the case in situations where nighttime sedation is desirable. The primary advantage of the benzodiazepines over other sedative-hypnotics, especially the barbiturates, is their relative safety. The benzodiazepines are relatively innocuous when taken alone in intentional or accidental overdosage.[43] In addition, the benzodiazepines do not produce clinically significant hepatic microsomal enzyme induction, nor do they interact with other drugs, such as the coumarin anticoagulants, as do the barbiturates.

Midazolam. Midazolam is available in an oral dosage form as a sedative-hypnotic in several countries. As of July 1994 midazolam was not available in oral preparation in the United States.

The absorption and onset of clinical action of midazolam are more rapid than those of benzodiazepines with which it has been compared.[44,45] Peak action after oral administration occurred within 30 minutes.[46] Monti et al.[47] concluded that a 15-mg oral dose of midazolam was appropriate for patients demonstrating difficulty in falling asleep and that a 30-mg dose was appropriate in patients having difficulties in staying asleep. The actions of midazolam are less apparent after 8 hours than those of other benzodiazepines.[44] Hildebrand et al.[48] concluded that absorption of midazolam is better with oral than intramuscular administration.

The clinical pharmacology of midazolam is discussed in more detail in Chapters 11 and 26.

Midazolam has been employed orally as premedication prior to surgical procedures in medicine[49] as well as in dentistry for adults[50,51] and dentistry for children.[52-55] In areas where the drug is available in an oral form a single dose of 7.5 mg administered 1 hour prior to surgery is usually effective.[50,51] The parenteral form of midazolam has been used with good clinical effect in several studies in the United States where an oral formulation is not available.[49,54,56]

Dosage. The usual dosage of midazolam when used to help induce sleep is 15 mg taken 1 hour before bedtime. Wahlmann et al.[50] administered a dose of 7.5 mg preoperatively for anxiety control in adults prior to oral surgery with little success whereas Luyk,[51] using the same dose, demonstrated significant anxiolysis, amnesia, and patient preference. Using a 10-mg dose of the parenteral form of midazolam orally, Turner and Paech[49] found the drug to be equal to a 20-mg dose of oral temazepam in anxiolysis and sedation prior to day case gynecological surgery.

In pediatrics oral doses of midazolam have proven effective in dosages ranging from 0.2 mg/kg,[54] to 0.4 mg/kg,[57,58] to 0.5 mg/kg,[52,55,56] to 0.75 mg/kg.[55]

Availability. As Dormicum in 7.5-mg tablets. Midazolam is not available in an oral dosage form in the United States as of July 1994.

• • •

The benzodiazepines that I most often prescribe and recommend for their hypnotic effects either for sleep the evening prior to treatment or for preoperative sedation are flurazepam (30 or 15 mg) and triazolam (0.125 and 0.25 mg). Midazolam, though not yet available worldwide in an oral form, is becoming an attractive drug for preoperative sedation in both adults and children.

Carbamates

Two agents, ethinamate and meprobamate, are relatively nonselective CNS depressants that are classified as carbamates. Ethinamate was categorized as a sedative-hypnotic, whereas meprobamate is usually considered an antianxiety drug, although studies have demonstrated that it might more appropriately be considered as a sedative-hypnotic.[59] Meprobamate will be considered with the other antianxiety agents. Ethinamate (Valmid) is rarely employed today for sedation in either dentistry or medicine and an indepth discussion of the drug has been dropped from this edition of *Sedation*. The reader is referred to prior editions (1989 and 1985) for a review of the clinical pharmacology and uses of ethinamate.[60,61]

Meprobamate. Meprobamate is discussed along with other antianxiety agents later in this chapter.

Chloral derivatives

Chloral hydrate. Several drugs classified as chloral derivatives may be used for hypnosis or sedation. Within the practice of dentistry one of these drugs, chloral hydrate, is a popular agent for the management of anxiety, particularly in pediatric dentistry. Chloral betaine and triclofos sodium are other less frequently employed members of this group.

Chloral hydrate, first synthesized in 1832, was the first member of the hypnotic group of drugs. With the introduction of the barbiturates interest in chloral hydrate waned; however, there has been a renewal of interest in it since the 1950s.

Chloral hydrate is available for oral administration in both capsule and liquid formulations.

Chloral hydrate is quite irritating to skin and to mucous membranes. The drug does produce Gl irritation in a high percentage of patients.[62] The incidence of gastric upset may be minimized by diluting the drug or by following the drug immediately with a full glass (8 oz) of water or milk. Although chloral hydrate is available in several preparations, because of the potential for gastric upset the capsule and rectal suppository are frequently the desirable dosage forms. In pediatric dentistry, however, because of the dislike of many children for solid forms of medication, chloral hydrate is administered as an elixir. Unfortunately the elixir has an unpleasant taste, which may be masked by mixing the drug with a suitable liquid such as ginger ale or fruit juice.

Like the barbiturates, chloral hydrate does not possess any analgesic properties; therefore the drug should not be administered to patients in pain as their response may be quite exaggerated. The effect of a therapeutic dose of chloral hydrate on blood pressure and respiration is negligible, similar to those occurring in normal sleep.[63]

Chloral hydrate is rapidly absorbed through the Gl tract into the cardiovascular system and undergoes metabolic degradation in the liver and kidneys into its active form, trichloroethanol. The other chloral derivatives, chloral betaine and triclofos sodium, undergo metabolic degradation into chloral hydrate and then into trichloroethanol. Trichloroethanol is thought to be the active metabolite responsible for the CNS depressant effects of these three agents. The chloral derivatives may be administered safely to patients with hepatic and renal dysfunction. The half-life of chloral hydrate is 7 to 9.5 hours.

Among the untoward effects produced by the irritating properties of chloral hydrate are an unpleasant taste, gastric upset, nausea, vomiting, and flatulence. Other CNS effects considered uncomfortable are lightheadedness, ataxia, and nightmares.[64] The hangover effect is a much less common occurrence than with the barbiturates. Chloral hydrate, though not metabolized by the hepatic microsomal enzyme system, does accelerate the metabolism of drugs such as the coumarin anticoagulants. The toxic oral dose reported for chloral hydrate is 10 g, although death has been reported with as little as 4000 mg (4 g). More important in clinical situations is the dose of chloral hydrate based on patient body weight. The usual oral dose is 50 mg/kg (or about 25 mg/lb) of body weight, with a suggested range of 40 to 60 mg/kg.[62,65,66] In a survey of pediatric residency programs it was determined that chloral hydrate in doses between 25 and 100 mg/kg is the most common drug used for sedation.[67]

Reports of overdose reactions following chloral hydrate administration in pediatric dentistry have been few. However, cases of life-threatening hypotension and respiratory arrest following estimated doses of 86 mg/kg and 118 mg/kg have been reported.[63,68] The GI upset produced by chloral hydrate proves to be advantageous when accidental overdosage occurs. With doses greater than 60 mg/kg, vomiting is frequently noted, thus diminishing the absorption of chloral hydrate from the GI tract and limiting the degree of overdose observed.[62]

Following oral administration the onset of action of chloral hydrate is rapid, drowsiness or a rousable sleep usually developing within 30 to 45 minutes. The duration of action is 2 to 5 hours.

Chloral hydrate is useful as a sedative prior to dental care and as an agent to assist the patient in achieving a restful night's sleep prior to the scheduled treatment. It is an especially useful agent in debilitated, elderly, and younger patients. Chloral hydrate appears to be less effective when given in lower doses or when used for dental care in older handicapped patients.[69-71]

Contraindications. Allergy to the drug or to other chloral derivatives, severe hepatic or renal dysfunction, severe heart disease, and gastritis are contraindications. Chloral hydrate should not be prescribed to nursing mothers as the drug will appear in breast milk.

Warnings. Prolonged use of chloral hydrate may prove to be habit forming. This is unlikely to develop in dental situations because of the manner in which the agent is prescribed.

Drug interactions. As with the barbiturates, chloral hydrate must be used with caution in patients who are concurrently receiving the coumarin anticoagulants. Prothrombin times should be monitored on a more frequent basis. Doses of chloral hydrate should be decreased when administered to patients receiving other CNS depressant drugs, such as alcohol, narcotics, and barbiturates, as additive CNS depression will develop.

Precautions. Chloral hydrate should be used with caution in patients with severe cardiovascular disease, as large doses (significantly greater than therapeutic) may further depress the myocardium. In therapeutic dosages there is no contraindication to the administration of this agent in cardiac risk patients.

Adverse reactions. The most frequently reported adverse effect of chloral hydrate is gastric irritability. The only other adverse reaction, reported on occasion, is the occurrence of a skin rash.

Dosage. The dosages presented here are for the adult patient. Pediatric dosages and use of this drug will be presented in Chapter 36.

The hypnotic dose of chloral hydrate is 500 to 1000 mg taken 15 to 30 minutes prior to bedtime. The usual dose for sedation in a nondental setting is 250 mg; however, when chloral hydrate is administered for surgery or dental procedures, doses of 500 to 1500 mg may be required.

When the capsule form of chloral hydrate is prescribed, the drug should be taken with a full (8-oz) glass of water. If administered as an elixir or syrup, chloral hydrate should be mixed in one half glass of water, ginger ale, or fruit juice.

Availability. Chloral hydrate (generic): 250- and 500-mg capsules; 500 mg/5 ml (tsp) syrup; 500 mg/5 ml (tsp) elixir.

Chloral hydrate is also available in many proprietary forms. The brand names and manufacturers are Aquachloral (Webcon) and Noctec (Squibb).

Ethchlorvynol. Ethchlorvynol is a sedative-hypnotic with a rapid onset (15 minutes to 1 hour) and short duration of action (5 hours). The drug also possesses anticonvulsant and skeletal muscle relaxant properties. Its primary use is for the induction of sleep in a person who has difficulty falling asleep, but once asleep has no difficulty in remaining asleep. In this sense the clinical application of this drug is similar to the short-acting barbiturates secobarbital and pentobarbital. Ethchlorvynol is a bitter-tasting liquid that has a disagreeable odor. Its availability in capsule form overcomes these disadvantages. Its primary advantage over chloral hydrate is the fact that ethchlorvynol is less irritating to the gastric mucosa.

Following oral administration of a hypnotic dose, the clinical onset of signs and symptoms of drowsiness usually develop within 15 to 30 minutes. Peak blood levels occur within 1 to 1½ hours. Ethchlorvynol has a plasma half-life of 10 to 20 hours. The duration of effective hypnosis or sedation is quite short (about 5 hours); therefore it is effective as a sleep-inducing agent in insomniacs and in patients fearful of upcoming treatment. Although the liver is the primary site of metabolic degradation, approximately 10% of the dose is excreted unchanged in the urine. As with chloral hydrate and the barbiturates, ethchlorvynol should be administered with caution to patients taking anticoagulants. In addition, ethchlorvynol should not be administered to patients with porphyria. The hypnotic actions of the drug may be potentiated if a patient takes alcohol concurrently.

The most common side effects of ethchlorvynol are an unpleasant aftertaste, dizziness, nausea and vomiting, hypotension, and facial numbness. A mild hangover effect is frequently reported from the drug in spite of its short duration of action. Patients receiving antidepressants (Table 8-3) should not be administered ethchlorvynol, as delirium may result. Physical dependence may develop to ethchlorvynol with long-term administration of high dosages.

Contraindications. Hypersensitivity (allergy) and porphyria are absolute contraindications to the administration of ethchlorvynol.

Warnings. Patients must be advised not to operate a motor vehicle or other potentially hazardous machinery. Because the drug has the potential for physical and psychological dependence, large doses should not be administered on a long-term basis. This should not be a significant problem within the dental setting.

Drug interactions. Ethchlorvynol may exhibit potentially significant interactions with other CNS depressants, such as alcohol, barbiturates, antianxiety drugs, and narcotics, because these may produce exaggerated depressant effects. Patients receiving oral anticoagulants should have their prothrombin times monitored on a more frequent schedule because hepatic microsomal induction may alter their response to the anticoagulant. Patients receiving monoamine oxidase inhibitors (MAOI) or antidepressants may be more likely to exhibit transient delirium when receiving ethchlorvynol. This is especially likely to develop with amitryptyline.

Precautions. Peripheral neuropathy (facial numbness) has been observed with the administration of excessive dosages.[72] Discontinuance of the drug leads to reversal of the signs and symptoms. When pain is present, ethchlorvynol should be administered only if an analgesic is given concurrently. Care must be observed because a narcotic analgesic combined with ethchlorvynol may produce an exaggerated CNS depression.

Dosage. The usual hypnotic dose is 500 to 750 mg given 30 minutes to 1 hour prior to bedtime the evening before dental treatment. A dose of 1000 mg may be administered at bedtime if insomnia is severe. The drug may also be used effectively for preoperative sedation, administered in the same dosage about 1 hour before the scheduled appointment.

Elderly and debilitated patients should receive smaller dosages.

Availability. Placidyl (Abbott): 200-, 500-, and 750-mg capsules. Ethchlorvynol is a controlled substance in Schedule IV.

Table 8-3. Antidepressants

Tricyclics	*Phenothiazines*	*MAO inhibitors*
Amitriptyline (Elavil)	Acetophenazine (Tindal)	Isocarboxazid (Marplan)
Desipramine (Norpramin)	Chlorpromazine (Thorazine)	Pargyline (Eutonyl)
Imipramine (Tofranil)	Fluphenazine (Permitil, Prolixin)	Phenelzine (Nardil)
Nortriptyline (Aventyl)	Perphenazine (Trilafon)	Tranylcypromine (Parnate)
Protriptyline (Vivactil)	Piperacetazine (Quide)	Pargyline with methyclothiazide (Eutron)
Perphenazine with amitriptyline (Etrafon, Triavil)	Thioridazine (Mellaril)	
	Triflupromazine (Vesprin)	
	Perphenazine with amitriptyline (Etrafon, Triavil)	

Reprinted with permission from Cooke-Waite Laboratories, Inc., New York, NY 10016.

Methaqualone. Methaqualone is a sedative-hypnotic that also possesses anticonvulsant, antispasmodic, local anesthetic, antihistaminic, and antitussive properties.[73] Popular in the "drug culture," methaqualone was reported to have aphrodisiac effects. Clinical studies have failed to confirm this action of the drug.[74] Many persons abusing this drug describe its effects as being similar to those of heroin and claim that the drug produces a dissociative high without the drowsiness produced by the barbiturates. Because of its significant potential for abuse, methaqualone is no longer being produced.

Paraldehyde. Paraldehyde was first introduced into medicine in 1882. The oral form of the medication has a very strong (disagreeable) odor and a disagreeable taste. Rarely used in dentistry, paraldehyde is mentioned here for the sake of completeness. It is categorized as a nonbarbiturate sedative-hypnotic. The main disadvantage to its use is its disagreeable odor. The agent is metabolized in the liver (70% to 80%) and exhaled through the lungs (11% to 28%), and about 1% is excreted in the urine. In patients with hepatic dysfunction, the amount of drug exhaled in the lungs is increased. Following oral administration, sleep usually develops within 10 to 15 minutes.

The primary use of paraldehyde today is in the management of drug abstinence (withdrawal) and other psychiatric states associated with excitement.

Glutethimide. Glutethimide is a piperidine derivative introduced in 1954. Within 1 year it became the sixth most prescribed hypnotic drug because it was thought to be devoid of addiction potential. It does possess a very high therapeutic index. It is now known to have addiction liability and sometimes severe withdrawal symptoms. The use of this agent in medicine has decreased significantly in the past 10 to 15 years, and its use is rare in dentistry.

Pharmacologically, glutethimide is similar to barbiturates in that it produces hypnosis without any analgesic effect. It does not possess anticonvulsant, analgesic, or antitussive properties.

Glutethimide is absorbed quite erratically from the GI tract following oral administration. Onset of action is rapid, usually within 30 minutes. The duration of action of the drug is 4 to 8 hours. Glutethimide is quite lipid-soluble, but poorly soluble in water. Blood levels following equal doses of the drug may vary twofold, although the time required to reach maximal blood levels may vary sixfold. The average plasma half-life is 10 hours. Glutethimide is metabolized primarily in the liver, with approximately 2% of a dose excreted in the urine. Because the agent stimulates the hepatic microsomal enzyme system, patients receiving anticoagulants should be monitored carefully, and the drug is contraindicated in patients with porphyria.

The major side effect is a skin rash (after discontinuation, the rash disappears within a few days). Other, much less frequent side effects include nausea and hangover.

Contraindications. Allergy and porphyria are the only contraindications.

Warnings. Patients receiving glutethimide should be warned against driving a motor vehicle or operating potentially dangerous machinery.

Drug interactions. Other CNS depressants used concurrently with glutethimide may produce exaggerated clinical effects. Patients receiving coumarin anticoagulants should be monitored frequently and their anticoagulant dosages altered as appropriate.

Precautions. In the presence of pain glutethimide should not be prescribed without an analgesic.

Dosage. For induction of sleep the night prior to surgery or dental treatment a dose of 250 to 500 mg is indicated 1 hour before bedtime. For sedation during dental treatment a dose of 500 to 1000 mg is suggested (1 hour before treatment).

Availability. Glutethimide (generic): 500-mg capsules; 250- and 500-mg tablets. Doriden (USV): 500-mg capsules.

Methyprylon. Methyprylon, another piperidine derivative, was introduced in 1955. A dosage of 300 mg is equivalent to 200 mg of secobarbital. Methyprylon is more water-soluble than glutethimide. Approximately 97% of the drug is metabolized in the liver, with 3% excreted unchanged in the urine. The hepatic microsomal enzyme system is stimulated by this drug; therefore the agent should be avoided in patients with porphyria, and those taking anticoagulants should be monitored more closely. The plasma half-life of methyprylon is 4 hours.

Following oral administration clinical hypnosis develops within 45 minutes. The duration of action is 5 to 8 hours.

Side effects are not common after methyprylon administration. Those most frequently observed are hangover, nausea, vomiting, epigastric distress, headache, and rash. The drug can produce habituation, tolerance, physical dependence, and addiction.

Contraindications. Allergy is the only contraindication.

Warnings. Patients should be cautioned against operating a motor vehicle or potentially hazardous machinery. Long-term administration may produce both physical and psychological dependence. This is unlikely to develop within the typical dental situation.

Drug interactions. Patients receiving methyprylon should be cautioned about the additive effects of other CNS depressants, including alcohol.

Precautions. The total daily dose of methyprylon should not exceed 400 mg. Dosages above this level do not provide greater clinical effectiveness but are more likely to produce hypnotic effects and increase the risk of dependence. The usual precautions should be observed in patients with hepatic or renal dysfunction.

Dosage. The usual dosage is 300 mg or one or two tablets of 200 mg (200 or 400 mg) 1 hour either before bedtime the evening prior to dental treatment or 1 hour prior to the scheduled appointment. The patient must be driven to the office by an adult companion.

Availability. Noludar (Roche): 200-mg tablets; 300-mg capsules. Methyprylon is a controlled substance in Schedule III.

ANTIANXIETY DRUGS

Antianxiety drugs are used to manage moderate-to-severe daytime anxiety and tension. Drugs in this group share a similar CNS depressant action: at therapeutic dosages they produce a mild degree of sedation without impairing the patient's mental alertness or psychomotor performance. Groups of medications that are commonly categorized as antianxiety drugs are as follows:

1. Benzodiazepines
   a. Chlordiazepoxide
   b. Diazepam
   c. Oxazepam
   d. Clorazepate
   e. Prazepam
   f. Halazepam
   g. Alprazolam
2. Carbamates
   a. Meprobamate
   b. Tybamate

For the management of anxiety the use of antianxiety drugs is much preferred to the barbiturates, the latter group much more commonly producing the undesirable side effect of loss of alertness. Intentional and unintentional overdosage occurs much more readily with barbiturates, and undesirable actions are noted at dosages just slightly above the usual therapeutic levels. Antianxiety drugs have a wider dosage range of therapeutic activity and thus are less likely to produce unwanted side effects.

Although termed "antianxiety drugs," a more appropriate name for these drugs might be "sedative-antianxiety drugs," for all agents in this group have sedative properties as well as antianxiety actions.

The antianxiety drugs have, in the past, been known by other names, such as "minor tranquilizers," "anxiolytics," "ataratics," "anxiolytic sedatives," and "psychosedatives." The general category "antianxiety drugs" has become the accepted label for this group of medications.

Benzodiazepines

The benzodiazepines are the most effective drugs currently available for the management of anxiety. They also possess skeletal muscle relaxant properties and are anticonvulsants. Over 2000 benzodiazepines have been synthesized since 1933. Clordiazepoxide was the first benzodiazepine introduced (1960). In 1994, in the United States, 11 benzodiazepines are available, seven of which are categorized as antianxiety drugs. These include alprazolam, chlordiazepoxide, clorazepate, diazepam, halazepam, oxazepam, and prazepam. Flurazepam, lorazepam, temazepam, and triazolam are classified as sedative-hypnotics, and clonazepam is approved for use only as an anticonvulsant. Nitrazepam, a sedative-hypnotic, and medazepam, an antianxiety drug, are available only in Europe.

The benzodiazepines are one of the most popular classes of drugs available today. Diazepam has been one of the most prescribed drugs in the United States since 1977. Approximately 30% of all psychotropic drug prescriptions are for benzodiazepines (100 million prescriptions annually). Furthermore, it is estimated that between 5% to 15% of adults in the United States take some form of antianxiety medication. Over one third of hospital inpatients receive a benzodiazepine during their hospitalization. The overuse and possible misuse of the benzodiazepines have come under scrutiny in the last few years. However, in the dental or surgical situation, rational drug prescribing habits will minimize potential misuse of this very important class of antianxiety drugs.

Pharmacology
Mode of action

The benzodiazepines have depressant effects on subcortical levels of the central nervous system. The specific anxiolytic effect of the benzodiazepines is a result of their actions on the limbic system and the thalamus, those areas of the brain that are involved with our emotions and behavior. The benzodiazepines have been called "limbic system sedatives," as they impair neuronal discharge in the amygdala and amygdala-hippocampus nerve transmission. The benzodiazepines depress the limbic system at lower doses than those that depress the reticular activating system and the cerebral cortex. The barbiturates and other sedative-hypnotics, on the other hand, do not exhibit this selective depression, but rather produce a generalized depression of the central nervous system.

Specific receptors for benzodiazepines have been isolated within the spinal cord and the brain. The location of these receptors parallels that of gamma-aminobutyric acid (GABA), the major inhibitory neurotransmitter in the brain, and of glycine, the major inhibitory neurotransmitter in the spinal cord.[62] Benzodiazepines act by intensifying the physiologic inhibitory effects of GABA by interfering with GABA reuptake.[75-77]

One of the most significant features of the benzodiazepines as a group is the very wide margin of safety between therapeutic and toxic doses. Ataxia and sedation develop only at doses beyond those required for antianxiety effects.

Central nervous system

The principal behavioral effects of the benzodiazepines are the following:
1. Reduction of hostile and aggressive behavior (frequently termed "taming").
2. Attenuation of the behavioral consequences of frustration, fear, and punishment (termed "disinhibition," this is the most consistently observed behavioral action of the benzodiazepine antianxiety drugs).

It is interesting that when aggression and hostility are held in check by fear and anxiety, the ingestion of a benzodiazepine or other antianxiety drug may produce a "paradoxical" increase in aggression. Other CNS depressants, such as the barbiturates, can produce these same effects; however, they do so only at doses that produce drowsiness and motor incoordination, and the benzodiazepines commonly achieve this action without these side effects.[78]

Other CNS actions of the benzodiazepines include skeletal muscle relaxant properties and anticonvulsant effects.[79,80] The site of action of the muscle relaxant properties of the benzodiazepines is as yet uncertain; however, it is thought that the effect is central rather than peripheral. Skeletal muscle relaxation appears to be caused by a combination of central depression of the brainstem reticular formation

and depression of polysynaptic spinal reflexes.[79,81] The anticonvulsant action of the benzodiazepines is produced by a depression of epileptiform discharge in the cerebral cortex and an enhancement of electrical activity of Purkinje cells. For effective anticonvulsant activity the benzodiazepines must be administered intravenously (although intramuscularly administered midazolam has terminated seizures).[82] Diazepam and clonazepam are the two benzodiazepines currently approved for anticonvulsant therapy.

Respiratory system

All sedative-hypnotics and antianxiety drugs (including benzodiazepines) are potential respiratory depressants. In the usual therapeutic dosages required for oral use in healthy patients, the benzodiazepines when administered alone do not produce clinically significant respiratory depression and do not potentiate the depressant effects of opiates. Cases of significant respiratory depression and respiratory arrest following oral benzodiazepine ingestion have been reported.[83,84]

Cardiovascular system

Following oral administration to a healthy patient (ASA I), benzodiazepines produce virtually no changes in cardiovascular function. Indeed, the benzodiazepines are employed quite frequently in the management of anxiety and depression associated with cardiac disease. They are preferred to the barbiturates and other sedative-hypnotics in this situation primarily because they do not produce unwanted degrees of CNS depression or restlessness and because they do not produce cardiovascular depression at therapeutic levels.[85]

Liver

The benzodiazepines undergo biotransformation in the liver (see following section); however, they do not stimulate the induction of hepatic microsomal enzymes. Potentially hazardous drug interactions, such as those observed between the barbiturates and the coumarin anticoagulants, do not develop with benzodiazepines. In addition, patients with hepatic dysfunction may receive the benzodiazepines without increased risk of side effect, regardless of the cause of the hepatic dysfunction.

Absorption, metabolism, excretion

Following oral administration, all benzodiazepines are absorbed relatively rapidly and reliably from the GI tract. The rate at which maximum plasma levels

Table 8-4. Onset of peak plasma levels following oral administration of benzodiazepines

Drug	Peak plasma level (hours)
Flurazepam	0.5-1
Midazolam	0.5
Triazolam	1.3
Medazepam	1-2
Alprozolam	1-2
Oxazepam	1-4
Nitrazepam	2
Diazepam	2
Lorazepam	2
Halazepam	2
Temazepam	2-3
Chlordiazepoxide	4
Prazepam	4-6

Table 8-5. Properties of benzodiazepines

	Peak plasma level (hours)	Half-life (hours)	Active metabolites
Alprazolam	1-2	12-15	No
Chlordiazepoxide	4	24-48	Yes
Clorazepate	1	48	Yes
Clonazepam	1-2	18-50	Yes
Diazepam	2	20-70	Yes
Flunitrazepam	—	13.5-36	Yes
Flurazepam	0.5-1	2.3	Yes
Halazepam	2	14	Yes
Lorazepam	2	12	No
Medazepam	1-2	—	—
Midazolam	0.5	1.2-12.3	No
Nitrazepam	2	18-28	No
Oxazepam	1-4	5.7-10.9	No
Prazepam	4-6	63-70	Yes
Temazepam	2-3	10	No
Triazolam	1.3	1.5-5.5	No

develop exhibits significant variation among the different benzodiazepines and among individuals. Approximate time for peak plasma levels following oral administration of several benzodiazepines is shown in Table 8-4.

The benzodiazepines undergo biotransformation in the liver. There is considerable variation in the half-lives of these drugs: diazepam's elimination half-life is 20 to 70 hours, while triazolam's is 1.5 to 5.5 hours. In addition, many of the benzodiazepines have biotransformation products that are pharmacologically as active as the parent drug (Table 8-5).

Chlordiazepoxide has a plasma half-life of between 24 and 48 hours and has as intermediate metabolites two pharmacologically active chemicals, desmethylchlordiazepoxide and demoxepam. The half-life of diazepam ranges between 20 and 70 hours. Pharmacologically active metabolites of diazepam include desmethyldiazepam (half-life of 96 hours), temazepam, and oxazepam. Flurazepam, with a plasma half-life of 2.3 hours, has an active metabolite with a half-life of 47 to 100 hours. Medazepam has three active metabolites: diazepam, desmethyldiazepam, and desmethylmedazepam; and prazepam (half-life 63 to 70 hours) has among its metabolites desmethyldiazepam and oxazepam. Desmethyldiazepam is a metabolite of clorazepate.

Nitrazepam, oxazepam, lorazepam, triazolam, temazepam, and alprazolam are biotransformed into pharmacologically inactive metabolites. The combination of rapid absorption from the GI tract (1 to 4 hours), short elimination half-life (5.7 to 9 hours), and inactive metabolites make oxazepam an attractive agent for the management of anxiety within the dental or surgical environment. Lorazepam, on the other hand, with a slow rate of absorption (2 hours) and a half-life of 12 hours (range 9 to 24 hours), is less appealing. Nitrazepam is employed as a sedative-hypnotic but is not yet available in the United States. Triazolam, with a rapid onset of action and short half-life (1.5 to 5.5 hours), is ideally suited as a hypnotic in dentistry.[29,30,32]

All benzodiazepines are excreted in the feces and urine. The percentage of urinary excretion varies from 80% for flurazepam and oxazepam to 22% for prazepam.

Dependence

Psychological and physiological dependence may develop to benzodiazepines.[86] The incidence of physiological dependence is considerably less than that of psychological dependence. It is not likely to develop unless the patient takes doses much greater than therapeutic over long periods of time. As employed within the dental setting there is little likelihood of this occurring.

Oral benzodiazepines in dentistry

The benzodiazepines represent the most nearly ideal agents for the management of anxiety. In the dental and surgical setting the benzodiazepines are the drugs of choice via the oral route for the management of mild-to-moderate pretreatment anxiety and apprehension. Many benzodiazepines are currently available and many more will surely become available in the future. As there are significant differences in the onset of action and the duration of action among these drugs, the choice of a specific agent should be made only after consideration of the needs of both the patient and the doctor.

Although there are indications for the use of other agents in specific instances, the agents most ideally suited for pretreatment anxiety control via oral administration in the dental and surgical setting are oxazepam and diazepam. For patients requiring anxiety reduction to sleep restfully the evening before their treatment, nitrazepam, flurazepam, and triazolam are preferred.

Contraindications

Allergy, psychoses, and acute narrow-angle glaucoma are contraindications. Benzodiazepines may be administered to patients with open-angle glaucoma if they are receiving appropriate therapy.

Warnings

Patients must be advised against driving a motor vehicle or operating hazardous machinery. Other CNS depressants, such as alcohol, narcotics, and barbiturates, should be avoided while benzodiazepines are being administered. There is some evidence that the use of benzodiazepines (particularly chlordiazepoxide and diazepam) during the first trimester of pregnancy increases the risk of congenital malformations (e.g., cleft palate).[87] Benzodiazepines do cross the placental barrier and are excreted in breast milk.

Benzodiazepines in children

Use of oral diazepam tablets in children under 6 months of age is not recommended. Oral diazepam has been employed successfully in pediatric dentistry. Recommended pediatric dosages are from 0.15 to 0.3 mg/kg.[88,89] Oral forms of chlordiazepoxide and oxazepam are not recommended under the age of 6 years. Clorazepate is not recommended in patients under the age of 18 years. This is a commonly observed statement in the drug package insert of many drugs and is a reflection of an inadequate volume of research data on these age groups.

Drug interactions

Patients should be advised against the concurrent use of benzodiazepines and other CNS depressants. These include alcohol, other psychotropic agents such as phenothiazines, narcotics, barbiturates, and MAO inhibitors, and other antidepressants.

Precautions

Drug dosages should be decreased in elderly or debilitated patients. Initial dosages should be small, with subsequent increases if warranted, as judged by the patient's response (titration by appointment). In this way, the adverse effects of drowsiness and ataxia may be minimized.

Adverse reactions

The most frequently reported adverse reactions following the oral administration of benzodiazepines for anxiety reduction include transient drowsiness (especially in the elderly or debilitated), fatigue, and ataxia.

Paradoxical reactions, though rare, may occur and consist of excitement, hallucinations, insomnia, and rage.[78] Discontinuance of drug administration leads to termination of these effects.

Chlordiazepoxide. Chlordiazepoxide was synthesized by Leo Sternbach in 1955. When tested in 1957, it was demonstrated to possess hypnotic and sedative properties, as well as skeletal muscle relaxant and anticonvulsant actions. The chemical is inactivated when exposed to ultraviolet light, thereby explaining its marketing in capsule form. Chlordiazepoxide may also be used parenterally; however, because of its instability it must be prepared immediately prior to injection. Other benzodiazepines, such as diazepam, midazolam, and lorazepam, being more stable, are preferred to chlordiazepoxide when parenteral administration is required.

On February 24, 1960, the Food and Drug Administration (FDA) approved the marketing of the first benzodiazepine, chlordiazepoxide, under the brand name Librium.

When administered orally, chlordiazepoxide is absorbed well from the GI tract; however, peak plasma levels of the agent do not develop for up to 4 hours. Although adequate anxiety reduction may develop within 1 to 2 hours, the slow onset of an antianxiety effect makes chlordiazepoxide less attractive than other benzodiazepines in the management of anxiety in the pretreatment period in surgery and dentistry.

Hypotension and syncope have been observed following large oral doses of chlordiazepoxide, and there have been reports of usual oral doses exacerbating ventilatory failure in patients with chronic bronchitis.[90] Long-term use of larger than usual dosages may produce physical or psychological dependence or both.

Dosage. The adult dosage of chlordiazepoxide for relief of mild-to-moderate anxiety is 5 or 10 mg 3 to 4 times daily. For relief of severe anxiety and tension the dosage is 20 or 25 mg 3 to 4 times daily. The dosage for geriatric patients or patients with debilitating disease is 5 mg 2 to 4 times daily. The recommended dosage for preoperative apprehension and anxiety is 5 to 10 mg 3 to 4 times daily the day prior to treatment or surgery.

Chlordiazepoxide is not recommended in children under 6 years of age. For older children, treatment should be initiated with the smallest possible dose and increased as required: 5 mg 2 to 4 times daily to start, increased to 10 mg 2 to 3 times daily, if needed.

Availability. Chlordiazepoxide (generic), Librium (Roche), SK-Lygen (Smith Kline and French): 5-, 10-, and 25-mg capsules. Chlordiazepoxide is a controlled substance in Schedule IV.

Diazepam. Diazepam was synthesized in 1959 and was found to be equitoxic to chlordiazepoxide, yet had greater antianxiety, skeletal-muscle-relaxing, and anticonvulsant properties. Diazepam was marketed in December 1963 as Valium and quickly became one of the most prescribed drugs in the United States. By 1966 diazepam was one of the 50 most prescribed drugs, and by the 1970s it was the leader among prescription medications, a position it retained until recently.

Following oral administration, diazepam is rapidly absorbed from the GI tract, achieving peak plasma levels within 2 hours. The drug may be administered 1 hour before contemplated treatment because approximately 90% of the maximal clinical action develops within this time. Because of the prolonged plasma half-life (20 to 70 hours) and the presence of active metabolites, cumulation of effect may develop with prolonged administration of diazepam. However, in the typical dental or surgical situation in which not more than one or two doses are prescribed, this effect is unlikely to develop. Diazepam is highly effective in the preoperative management of apprehension and anxiety. Its rapid onset of action makes it an appropriate agent for use in dental or surgical situations.

Patients receiving the drug at home must be advised against operating a motor vehicle. They should be driven to the medical or dental facility by a responsible adult companion, who can later drive them home. Failure to warn a patient about this potential hazard may lead to legal action should a problem develop before or after treatment. That such problems do occur is seen in a study by Murray, in which 68 automobile drivers taking oral diazepam were monitored for a 3-month period. During this time, 16 of them were involved in accidents, an incidence 10 times greater than that expected.[91] Impaired motor function produced by the benzodiazepine was presumed to be the basis for the increase.

Dosage. The adult dosage for tension and anxiety states is 2 to 10 mg 2 to 4 times daily. For geriatric patients or those with debilitating disease (ASA III or IV), recommended dosages are 2 to 2.5 mg 1 to 2 times daily to start, increasing the dose if needed. The suggested dosage for premedication is 5 to 10 mg 1 hour prior to bedtime or treatment.

Diazepam is not recommended for children under 6 months of age. For older children the recommendation is 1 to 2.5 mg 3 to 4 times daily, increasing the dose if needed. Recommended pediatric dosages range from 0.15 to 0.3 mg/kg.[88,89]

Availability. Valium (Roche): 2-mg, 5-mg, and 10-mg tablets, and as Valrelease in 15-mg capsules. Diazepam is also available generically. Diazepam is a controlled substance in Schedule IV.

Oxazepam. Oxazepam, synthesized in 1961, was marketed in 1965 under the proprietary name Serax. It possesses a short elimination half-life (5.7 to 10.9 hours) and no active metabolites. Oxazepam is therefore quite attractive in situations where short-term anxiety control is required, such as in surgery or dentistry. The incidence of drowsiness is low, usually developing in persons receiving doses of 60 mg daily or greater. Other side effects are similar to those for other members of this drug group.

Oxazepam is rapidly and reliably absorbed following oral administration, peak plasma levels developing within 1 to 4 hours. This, in combination with the lack of active metabolites and a short half-life, make oxazepam a preferred benzodiazepine for use as an antianxiety agent in dentistry.

Dosage. The adult dosage for mild to moderate anxiety and tension is 10 to 15 mg 3 to 4 times daily. For geriatric patients the initial dose is 10 mg 3 times daily, increased if needed to 15 mg 3 to 4 times daily.

An absolute dosage has not been established for children under 12 years of age. Oxazepam should not be taken by patients under 6 years of age.

Availability. Serax (Wyeth): 10-, 15-, and 30-mg capsules; 15-mg tablets. Oxazepam is a controlled substance in Schedule IV.

Clorazepate. Clorazepate (also spelled chlorazepate) is available in the form of two salts: monopotassium and dipotassium salts. The dipotassium salt was marketed in 1972 as Tranxene, and clorazepate monopotassium was marketed in 1972 as Azene. The monopotassium salt reaches peak plasma levels following oral administration in approximately 1 hour, and the dipotassium salt requires 1 to 2 hours. The plasma half-life of both agents is approximately 48 hours.

Clorazepate itself cannot be absorbed from the GI tract. The chemical is hydrolyzed in the stomach to its active form desmethyldiazepam, which is then absorbed, producing the clinical actions of the drug. The rate and extent of absorption of clorazepate from the GI tract is dependent on gastric pH. Antacid therapy will significantly decrease the absorption of clorazepate. Clorazepate is useful in dental and surgical situations; however, oxazepam, because it possesses a shorter half-life, is preferred.

Dosage. For adults the usual daily dosage of monopotassium salt is 13 to 52 mg, divided into 3 or 4 doses or in one dose (13 mg) taken 1 hour before bedtime. The usual adult dosage of dipotassium salt is 15 to 60 mg daily, divided into 2 to 4 doses or in one dose (15 mg) 1 hour before bedtime. The dose for preoperative anxiety control is 13 mg of monopotassium, or 15 mg of dipotassium salt, 1 hour prior to treatment.

For geriatric or debilitated patients the initial dose of monopotassium salt is 6.5 to 13 mg, and of dipotassium salt is 7.5 to 15 mg. Adequate information is not available to establish a dosage in patients under 18 years of age.

Availability. Clorazepate monopotassium—Azene (Endo): 3.25-, 6.5-, and 13-mg capsules. Clorazepate dipotassium—Tranxene (Abbott): 3.75-, 7.5-, and 15-mg tablets. Tranxene-SD (Abbott): 11.25- and 22.5-mg tablets. Clorazepate is a controlled substance in Schedule IV.

Prazepam. Prazepam is a benzodiazepine derivative with a slow rate of absorption following oral administration (peak plasma level in 6 hours) and a relatively long half-life (63 to 70 hours). A major active metabolite is oxazepam. Prazepam was marketed originally in 1977 with the name Verstran, which was later changed to the current name Centrax. Clinical actions and side effects are similar to those of other benzodiazepines. Its slow onset and prolonged duration of action hinder the effective use of this drug for pretreatment anxiety reduction in dentistry and surgery.

Dosage. The usual daily dosage for adults is 30 mg with a range from 20 to 60 mg in 3 to 4 doses. For sleep a dose of 20 mg 1 hour prior to bedtime is usually effective. Elderly or debilitated patients should receive a divided daily dosage of 10 to 15 mg. Safety and effectiveness in patients below the age of 18 years has not been established.

Availability. Centrax (Parke-Davis): 5-, 10-, and 20-mg capsules; 10-mg tablets. Prazepam is a controlled substance in Schedule IV.

Halazepam. Halazepam is rapidly and well absorbed following oral administration; peak plasma levels are reached within 2 hours. Halazepam has a half-life of 14 hours. Its major metabolite, desmethyldiazepam, is quite active.

Dosage. The adult dosage for anxiety reduction is 20 to 40 mg 2 or 3 times daily. The dosage for elderly patients is 20 mg 1 or 2 times daily.

Availability. Paxipam (Schering-Plough): 20- and 40-mg tablets. Halazepam is a controlled substance in Schedule IV.

Alprazolam. Alprazolam is another benzodiazepine derivative being marketed as an antianxiety agent. It reaches peak plasma levels within 1 to 2 hours (orally) and has a half-life of 12 to 15 hours, with no active metabolites.

Dosage. The adult dosage for anxiety reduction is 0.25 to 0.5 mg 3 times a day. The dosage for the elderly or debilitated is 0.25 mg 2 or 3 times daily. Modification in dosage is appropriate based upon patient response.

Availability. Xanax (Upjohn): 0.25-, 0.5-, and 1.0-mg tablets. Alprazolam is a controlled substance in Schedule IV.

• • •

Several other oral benzodiazepines have been mentioned, but because they are unavailable at this time in the United States or their primary indication is not for antianxiety purposes, they are not reviewed in this section. These agents include

Nitrazepam (Mogadon), discussed under sedative-hypnotics

Flurazepam (Dalmane, Roche), discussed under sedative-hypnotics

Midazolam (Hynovel, Dormicum, Versed), discussed under sedative-hypnotics

Medazepam (Nobrium), an antianxiety drug not available in the United States

Flunitrazepam (Rohypnol), a hypnotic not available in the United States

Clonazepam (Clonopin, Roche), an anticonvulsant drug

Lorazepam (Ativan, Wyeth), discussed under sedative-hypnotics

Triazolam (Halcion, Upjohn), discussed under sedative-hypnotics

Temazepam (Restoril, Sandoz), discussed under sedative-hypnotics

For the management of milder degrees of anxiety arising in the dental and surgical environment, there is probably no more effective group of drugs than the benzodiazepines. Pharmacologically they offer significantly greater safety compared to the sedative-hypnotics, especially the barbiturates. Although respiratory and cardiovascular depression may occur following oral administration of benzodiazepines, these are unlikely to develop. The most frequently observed side effect is a degree of sedation.

As safe and as frequently administered as the benzodiazepines may be, it must be remembered that the patient must always be warned against driving a car when these drugs have been administered. Motor coordination may be subtly depressed, a condition that could have serious consequences for both the patient and the doctor.

Although any of the benzodiazepines may be employed therapeutically in dentistry, it is my opinion that for the management of preoperative anxiety on the day of the dental or surgical treatment, diazepam (in a dose of 5 to 10 mg) or oxazepam (15 to 30 mg) is the most practical. When employed to aid in the induction of sleep in a fearful patient the night before the appointment, flurazepam (in a dose of 30 mg) or triazolam (0.25 to 0.5 mg) is suggested. Table 8-6 summarizes the availability of the benzodiazepines.

Carbamates

Meprobamate and tybamate belong to the class of drugs called "propanediol carbamates." Another member of this class, ethinamate, was discussed in the section on nonbarbiturate sedative-hypnotics. Meprobamate and tybamate are commonly classified as antianxiety drugs.

Meprobamate. Meprobamate is somewhat less effective than the benzodiazepines in the management of anxiety. Although the drug is rapidly absorbed from the GI tract, maximal effectiveness develops approximately 3 hours following oral administration. With a half-life of approximately 11 hours, the use of meprobamate in the typical dental situation is rarely justified.

Meprobamate appears to have multiple sites of action within the CNS, including the thalamus and limbic system. Respiratory depression is rare at therapeutic dosages, but has occurred following massive overdoses.[90] Hypotension, though unlikely to occur, has also developed following therapeutic dosages. Metabolized in the liver, meprobamate does induce the production of hepatic microsomal enzymes, and tolerance and physical dependence do develop following prolonged administration. With the introduc-

Table 8-6. Availability of benzodiazepines (oral)

Generic	*Proprietary*	*Class**	*Availability (mg)*	*Dose† (mg)*
Alprazolam	Xanax	AA	0.25, 0.5, 1	0.25-0.5
Chlorazepate with monopotassium	Azene	AA	3.25, 6.5, 13	13
Chlorazepate with dipotassium	Tranxene	AA	3.75, 7.5, 15	15
Chlordiazepoxide	Librium, SK-Lygen, Libritabs	AA	5, 10, 25	10
Clonazepam	Clonopin	AC	0.5, 1, 2	n/a
Diazepam	Valium	AA	2, 5, 10	10
Flunitrazepam	Rohypnol	SH	2	0.25-2
Flurazepam	Dalmane	SH	15, 30	30
Halazepam	Paxipam	AA	20, 40	20-40
Lorazepam	Ativan	SH, AA	0.5, 1, 2	2-4
Medazepam	Nobrium	AA	5, 10	5-10
Midazolam	Dormicum	SH	15	15-30
Nitrazepam	Mogadon	SH	5	2.5-10
Oxazepam	Serax	AA	10, 15, 30	15-30
Prazepam	Centrax	AA	5, 10	10-20
Temazepam	Restoril	SH	15, 30	30
Triazolam	Halcion	SH	0.25, 0.5	0.25-0.5

**AA*, Antianxiety; *AC*, anticonvulsant; *SH*, sedative-hypnotic; *n/a*, not applicable.
†For nighttime sedation or preoperative anxiety control.

tion of the benzodiazepines, the usefulness of meprobamate in dentistry has declined.

Contraindications. Contraindications include acute intermittent porphyria and allergy. Since meprobamate may cause seizures in epileptics, its administration is contraindicated in seizure-prone individuals.

Warnings. Drug dependence has developed following prolonged administration. Though unlikely to develop in surgical and dental situations, careful monitoring of dosages and length of time administered, and avoidance of use in alcoholics or other addiction-prone persons, will minimize risk. Patients receiving meprobamate must be cautioned against driving a motor vehicle or operating hazardous machinery. Meprobamate passes the placental barrier and is also found in breast milk; therefore, it must be used with caution in the pregnant patient and in the lactating woman.

Drug interactions. Additive effects may be observed between meprobamate and other CNS depressants, such as alcohol, sedative-hypnotics, and antianxiety drugs.

Precautions. Elderly and debilitated patients should receive the lowest effective dose of meprobamate. Meprobamate should be used with caution in patients with serious liver or kidney dysfunction. Meprobamate may precipitate seizures in epileptics.

Adverse reactions. The most frequently occurring adverse reactions to meprobamate administration include drowsiness and ataxia, which are more common with daily doses in excess of 1200 mg. Nausea and vomiting, dizziness, headache, and slurred speech also have been reported.

Dosage. The usual adult dosage is 1200 to 1600 mg daily in 3 to 4 divided doses. For use as an oral premedicant in dental or surgical situations a dose of 600 mg 1 hour before treatment is recommended. The usual dosage for children ages 6 to 12 years is 100 to 200 mg 2 or 3 times a day. Meprobamate is not recommended for children under 6 years of age.

Availability. Meprobamate (generic): 200-, 400-, and 600-mg tablets. Equagesic (Wyeth): 200- and 400-mg tablets; 400-mg capsules. Miltown (Wallace): 200-, 400-, and 600-mg tablets. Neuramate (Halsey): 400-mg tablets. Meprobamate is a controlled substance in Schedule IV.

Tybamate. Tybamate, like meprobamate, acts subcortically, producing a depression of the hippocampal and limbic structures of the brain. The actions of tybamate are similar to those of meprobamate, with the notable exception that the half-life of tybamate is only 3 hours. Hepatic microsomal enzyme induction does not occur, nor do the coincident effects of tolerance, accelerated drug metabolism, and interactions with other drugs. The shorter duration of clinical activity of tybamate makes it more suitable than meprobamate for use in dentistry. Metabolized in the liver, approximately 10% of the total dose is excreted unchanged in the urine.

Contraindications. Acute intermittent porphyria and allergy are contraindications.

Warnings. Patients receiving tybamate must be cautioned against operating a motor vehicle or hazardous machinery. Though neither psychological nor physiological dependence has been reported with tybamate, care should be exerted in its administration because dependence has developed with related compounds (meprobamate). The safety of tybamate in pregnant patients has not been established, nor has the safety of tybamate in patients under the age of 6 years.

Drug interactions. In patients receiving tybamate along with other CNS depressants, particularly the phenothiazines, instances of grand mal or petit mal seizures have been reported. In addition, the simultaneous administration of tybamate with CNS depressants may produce potentiation of depressant actions.

Precautions. Elderly and debilitated patients should receive the lowest effective dose, in order to minimize the risk of oversedation. Because tybamate is metabolized in the liver and excreted in the urine, its use should be carefully evaluated in patients with liver or renal dysfunction.

Dosage. The adult dosage is 250 to 500 mg 3 to 4 times daily. The dose for preoperative sedation is 700 mg 1 hour prior to bedtime or the scheduled appointment. The dosage for children ages 6 to 12 years is 20 to 35 mg/kg daily in 3 to 4 equal doses.

Availability. Tybamate is no longer marketed in the United States (1994). However, it is available in many countries as Tybatran (Robins) 125-, 250-, and 350-mg capsules. Tybamate is a controlled substance in Schedule IV.

ANTIHISTAMINES (Histamine blockers)

Sedation and hypnosis are known side effects of some drugs used primarily for other purposes. Such effects occur with many of the antihistamines, drugs used primarily in the management of allergy and motion sickness and as antiparkinsonism agents. Several antihistamines demonstrate this property and in fact are marketed throughout the world primarily as sedative-hypnotics. These agents include methapyrilene, pyrilamine, diphenhydramine, promethazine, and hydroxyzine.

Methapyrilene and pyrilamine are available as nonprescription sedative-hypnotics, usually in combination with scopolamine. Recently, diphenhydramine in 25-mg capsules has been approved by the Food and Drug Administration (USA) as an over-the-counter preparation.

The two antihistamines most frequently employed for sedative-antianxiety properties are promethazine and hydroxyzine. In dentistry these drugs have proved to be quite useful, primarily in pediatric dentistry.

Promethazine. Promethazine is a phenothiazine derivative that is commonly used as an antiemetic for management of nausea and vomiting, for preoperative sedation, for sedation and the relief of apprehension and anxiety, to produce a light sleep from which the patient is easily aroused, and in the management of various forms of allergic reaction.

Promethazine was marketed in 1951 under the brand name Phenergan. Its first reported use in dentistry was in 1959 when it was used in conjunction with meperidine and chlorpromazine in the lytic cocktail (DPT—Demerol, Phenergan, Thorazine). Its primary function in this cocktail was to serve as an antiemetic to control the nausea and vomiting associated with narcotics.

In dentistry, promethazine is frequently used in pediatric sedation. In a 1973 survey of drug use in pediatric dentistry, promethazine was the fourth most frequently employed solo premedicant and the most commonly employed combination drug (with meperidine).[92] More recent surveys find the use of promethazine to remain high, ranking third as a solo premedicant and remaining first (with meperidine) as a combination drug.[93]

Promethazine is a member of a group of drugs termed "phenothiazines," a group of drugs classified as antipsychotics (formerly termed "major tranquilizers"). The primary use of these agents (Table 8-7) is to decrease agitation, hostility, combativeness, and hyperactivity. They are also quite useful in the management of nausea and vomiting, and some members have potent antihistaminic actions. Promethazine differs structurally from the antipsychotic phenothiazines by the presence of a branched sidechain and no ring substitution. It is felt that this structural difference is responsible for the lack of antipsychotic action. Promethazine is an H_1 receptor blocking agent, providing antihistaminic and antiemetic as well as sedative effects.

Table 8-7. Phenothiazines

Generic	Proprietary	Sedative action
Chlorpromazine	Thorazine	High
Promethazine	Phenergan	High
Thioridazine	Mellaril	High
Prochlorperazine	Compazine	Moderate
Promazine	Sparine	Moderate
Trifluoperazine	Stelazine	Moderate
Perphenazine	Trilafon	Low to moderate

All phenothiazines produce some degree of sedation (CNS depression). The action of these drugs is quite different from the barbiturates and other sedative-hypnotics. Two major differences are that (1) phenothiazines, in large doses, do not produce unconsciousness or depress respiration or the cardiovascular system, and (2) the phenothiazines are not addictive.[94,95]

On the negative side all phenothiazines are capable of producing extrapyramidal reactions. They usually develop early in phenothiazine therapy and usually prove quite benign; however, they may require treatment. The incidence of extrapyramidal reactions is greatest with perphenazine, prochlorperazine, and trifluoperazine and lowest with promethazine and thioridazine.[96]

Four types of extrapyramidal reaction may be observed. *Akathisia* (motor restlessness) refers to the compelling need of the patient to be in constant motion. The patient feels he must get up and walk or continuously move about. *Acute dystonias* include perioral spasms (protrusion of the tongue), mandibular tics, facial grimacing, hyperextension of the neck and trunk, and clonic convulsions. These reactions may be accompanied by hyperhidrosis, pallor, fever, and an increase in anxiety. *Parkinsonism,* which consists of tremors, rigidity, shuffling gait, postural abnormalities, masklike facies, and hypersalivation, may also occur. *Tardive dyskinesia* represents a late-appearing neurological syndrome associated with antipsychotic drug use. It is more frequent in older patients and is characterized by choreiform movements of the face, trunk, and extremities.

Management of extrapyramidal reactions in dental situations involves the discontinuance of the offending drug and the possible administration of antiparkinsonism medication, such as diphenhydramine (Benadryl, 50-mg IM or IV in adults) or trihexyphenidyl (Artane, 5 to 15 mg daily, orally).[97]

Many phenothiazines act on the cardiovascular system to produce postural (orthostatic) hypotension and a reflex tachycardia. This is most common with chlorpromazine. The phenothiazines undergo metabolic degradation in the liver and are excreted in the urine and feces.

Contraindications. Known allergy to phenothiazines is a contraindication to the use of promethazine and other phenothiazines.

Warnings. Patients receiving other CNS depressants should be aware of the additive effects of the phenothiazines. These drugs should either be eliminated or their dosages reduced.

Precautions. Patients must be advised against operating a motor vehicle or potentially hazardous machinery. Phenothiazines must be used with caution in patients with a history of convulsive disorders. Phenothiazines may lower the seizure threshold.

Children with acute disease, such as chicken pox, measles, and gastroenteritis, appear much more susceptible to extrapyramidal reactions, especially dystonias, than do adults.

Adverse reactions. The most frequently reported adverse reactions to phenothiazines include dryness of the mouth, blurring of vision, and less commonly dizziness.

Oversedation is the most frequently observed side effect from promethazine. In general, the phenothiazines have a high therapeutic index and are remarkably safe drugs. Extrapyramidal reactions are the most significant side effect of these agents.

Dosage. The adult dose for sedation is 25 to 50 mg 1 hour before treatment; for preoperative sedation, 50 mg 1 hour before bedtime. In children the dose for sedation is 12.5 to 25 mg 1 hour before treatment.

For preoperative sedation in pediatric dentistry the traditional dosage recommendation for promethazine used alone is 2.2 mg/kg, and 1.1 mg/kg when used in combination with other CNS depressants.[98]

Availability. Promethazine (generic): 12.5-, 25-, and 50-mg tablets. Phenergan (Wyeth): 12.5-, 25-, and 50-mg tablets; 6.25 mg/5 ml (1.5% alcohol) syrup; 25 mg/5 ml (1.5% alcohol) syrup fortis.

Hydroxyzine. Hydroxyzine is derived from a group of drugs called "diphenylethanes." Although classified as an antihistaminic, hydroxyzine also possesses sedative, antiemetic, antispasmodic, and anticholinergic properties. Two forms of the agent are available: hydroxyzine hydrochloride (Atarax) and hydroxyzine pamoate (Vistaril). Hydroxyzine is the most popular oral sedative in the practice of pediatric dentistry, with 50% of the responding pedodontists using one or both drugs.[92,93]

The sedative actions of hydroxyzine are not produced by cortical depression. It is thought to suppress some hypothalamic nuclei and to extend its actions peripherally into the sympathetic portion of the autonomic nervous system.

Following oral administration, hydroxyzine is rapidly absorbed from the GI tract, with clinical actions observed within 15 to 30 minutes. Maximal clinical actions develop in 2 hours, with an approximate duration of action of 3 to 4 hours.

The oral liquid form of hydroxyzine hydrochloride (Atarax) is more pleasant-tasting to most patients than the liquid form of hydroxyzine pamoate (Vistaril). This fact is of particular importance in pediatric dentistry.

When administered in combination with narcotics or barbiturates, the dosage of these drugs should be decreased by 50%, because the depressant actions of narcotics and barbiturates are potentiated by hydroxyzine.

Indications for the use of hydroxyzine include total management of long-term anxiety and tension; management of anxiety and tension in which the causative stress is temporary (e.g., dental or other surgical procedures); preoperative medication; allaying of apprehension and anxiety in the cardiac-risk patient; and management of nausea and vomiting. Hydroxyzine is metabolized in the liver and is excreted in the urine.

In dental practice the use of hydroxyzine as a sole agent is limited to the management of children with mild-to-moderate fear. It is often used in combination with either meperidine or chloral hydrate for management of more fearful pediatric patients.

The incidence of side effects is quite low; the most commonly observed is transient drowsiness. Fatal overdosage with hydroxyzine is extremely uncommon and withdrawal reactions following long-term therapy have never been reported.

Contraindications. Previous hypersensitivity to hydroxyzine.

Drug interactions. Hydroxyzine will potentiate the CNS depressant actions of drugs such as barbiturates, narcotics, alcohol, sedative-hypnotics, and antianxiety drugs. Dosages of these drugs should be decreased by 50% when administered concurrently with hydroxyzine.

Precautions. Patients receiving hydroxyzine must be warned against operating a motor vehicle or hazardous machinery. Children receiving hydroxyzine should be kept under observation by their parent or guardian for the remainder of the day.

Dosage. The adult dosage ranges from 25 mg 3 times a day to 100 mg 4 times a day. The dosage for children under the age of 6 years is 50 mg daily in divided doses. The dosage for children over the age of 6 years is 50 to 100 mg daily in divided doses. The dose for preoperative medication in adults is 50 to 100 mg 1 hour preoperatively.

In pediatric dentistry the oral dose of hydroxyzine is 1.1 to 2.2 mg/kg when used as a sole agent for anxiety control. When administered in conjunction with other CNS depressants, such as meperidine or chloral hydrate, the dose of hydroxyzine should be reduced by 50%.[98]

Availability. Hydroxyzine hydrochloride—Atarax (Roerig): 10-, 25-, 50-, and 100-mg tablets; 10 mg/5 ml (0.5% alcohol) syrup.

Hydroxyzine pamoate—Vistaril (Pfizer): 25-, 50-, and 100-mg capsules; 25 mg/5 ml oral suspension.

OPIOIDS (Narcotics)

Opioids are classified as strong analgesics. Their primary indication for use is the relief of moderate-to-severe pain. Beneficially, opioids do alter a patient's psychological response to pain and will suppress anxiety and apprehension. Many of these drugs are used parenterally as preanesthetic medications because of their sedative, antianxiety, and analgesic properties. On the other hand, many anesthesiologists prefer to employ sedative-hypnotics or antianxiety agents preoperatively unless pain is present. In the absence of pain, opioids administered alone frequently produce dysphoria instead of the desired sedation. To achieve antianxiety and sedative effects, narcotics ought not be administered via the oral route. Absorption following oral administration is not as consistent as with parenteral administration, and the incidence of unwanted side effects (postural hypotension, nausea and vomiting) is considerably greater. The resulting sedative effect varies significantly from patient to patient. Respiratory and cardiovascular depression may be noted that can result in airway obstruction, hypoventilation, and hypotension. Oral narcotic administration should be reserved for the management of *pain* when milder analgesics have proved ineffectual.

CONCLUSIONS

The oral route of drug administration may be used successfully for the relief of milder degrees of apprehension and anxiety. Because of the inherent difficulties attendant in achieving precise levels of sedation, it is recommended that only light levels of sedation be sought by the oral route.

A great number of drugs are presently available for the relief of anxiety via oral administration. This chapter has only described the most commonly used drugs in dentistry and surgery and those that appear most applicable to the outpatient environment. In general, these drugs belong to a small number of drug groups: the antianxiety agents, the sedative-hypnotics, and the antihistamines. Ethyl alcohol is also an effective agent for milder anxiety in dentistry.

Although all drugs may be employed by the knowledgeable, well-trained doctor, the more prudent will restrict their prescribing habits to a limited number of drugs with which they are familiar. From the practical point of view, the benzodiazepines have virtually supplanted the barbiturates as the drugs of choice for preoperative anxiety reduction in dentistry and surgery. Although many benzodiazepines are available, oxazepam and diazepam are the most frequently employed and are highly recommended for management of milder levels of anxiety in dentistry. Flurazepam and triazolam, classified as sedative-hypnotics, are useful for mild-to-moderate anxiety and may be administered the evening prior to treatment and occasionally on the day of treatment.

Other drug groups should be considered for use where the benzodiazepines are contraindicated or have proved ineffective and when other more controllable techniques of pharmacosedation are unavailable.

Ease of drug prescription is a minor factor in selection of a suitable agent for premedication, but one that must be considered. The following agents discussed in this chapter are placed in Schedule IV on the Controlled Substances Schedule: the benzodiazepines, chloral hydrate, ethchlorvynol, ethinamate, and meprobamate. Schedule III drugs include butabarbital and glutethimide. Schedule II drugs include amobarbital, pentobarbital, and secobarbital.

REFERENCES

1. Berger R, Green G, Melnick A: Cardiac arrest caused by oral diazepam intoxication, *Clin Pediatr* 14:842, 1975.
2. Gill CJ, Michaelides PL: Dental drugs and anaphylactic reactions: report of a case, *Oral Surg* 50:30, 1980.
3. Johnson AG, Seideman P, Day RO: Adverse drug interactions with nonsteroidal anti-inflammatory drugs (NSAIDs): recognition, management and avoidance, *Drug Safety* 8(2):99, 1993.
4. Brody JE: Personal Health: Ignoring the doctor's orders has become a costly and deadly epidemic, *New York Times* cxli:B-6, Sept. 16, 1992.
5. Magni G, Cadamuro M, Borgherini G et al: Psychological stress and gastric emptying time in normal subjects, *Psychol Rep* 68(3):739, 1991.
6. Sugito K, Ogata H, Goto H et al: Gastric emptying rate of drug preparations. III. Effects of size of enteric micro-capsules with

mean diameters ranging from 0.1 to 1.1 mm in man, *Chem Pharm Bull* 40(12):3343, 1992.

7. Wedlund PJ, Wilkinson GR: Hepatic tissue binding and the oral first-pass effect, *J Pharm Sci* 73(3):422, 1984.

8. Lucas WJ, Maccioli GA, Mueller RA: Advances in oral anti-arrhythmic therapy: implications for the anaesthetist, *Can J Anaesth* 37(1):94, 1990.

9. Zimmermann T, Leitold M: The influence of food intake on gastrointestinal pH and gastric emptying time. Experience with two radiotelemetring methods: (Heidelberg pH capsule system and Flexilog 1010), *Int J Clin Pharmacol Ther Toxicol* 30(11):477, 1992.

10. Wright GZ: Pharmacotherapeutic approaches to behavior management. In Wright GZ, ed: *Behavior management in dentistry for children*, Philadelphia, 1975, Saunders.

11. Anderson JA, Vamm WF Jr, Dilley DC: Pain and anxiety control, part II: pain reaction control—conscious sedation. In Pinkham JR, ed: *Pediatric dentistry: infancy through adolescence*, ed 2. Philadelphia, 1994, Saunders.

12. Johnson R: Personal communications, 1992.

13. Jorgensen NB, Hayden J Jr: *Premedication, local and general anesthesia in dentistry*. Philadelphia, 1967, Lea & Febiger.

14. McCarthy FM, Hayden J Jr: Ethyl alcohol by the oral route as a sedative in dentistry, *JADA* 96:282, 1978.

15. McCarthy M: Personal communication, 1978.

16. Harvey SC: Hypnotics and sedatives: the barbiturates. In Goodman IS, Gilman A, eds: *Pharmacological basis of therapeutics*, ed 5. New York, 1990, Macmillan.

17. Felpel LP: Sedative-hypnotics and central nervous system stimulants. In Neidle EA, Yagiela JA, eds: *Pharmacology and therapeutics for dentistry*, ed 3. St Louis, 1989, Mosby.

18. Bleck TP: Convulsive disorders: status epilepticus, *Clin Neuropharm* 14(3):191, 1991.

19. Rehse K, Kapp WD: Structure activity relationships in oral anticoagulants: barbituric acids and quinolones, *Arch Pharm* 315(6):502, 1982.

20. Leslie SW: Sedative-hypnotic drugs: interaction with calcium channels, *Alcohol Drug Res* 6(6):371, 1985-1986.

21. Pimstone NR: Hematologic and hepatic manifestations of the cutaneous porphyrias, *Clin Dermatol* 3(2):83, 1985.

22. DeTullio P, Kirking DM, Zacardelli DK et al: Evaluation of long-term triazolam use in ambulatory Veterans Administration Medical Center population, *DICP* 23(4):290, 1989.

23. Warneke LB: Benzodiazepines: abuse and new use, *Can J Psychiatry* 36(3):194, 1991.

24. Melander A et al: Anxiolytic-hypnotic drugs: relationships between prescribing, abuse and suicide, *Eur J Clin Pharmacol* 41(6):525, 1991.

25. Nembutal sodium, drug information sheet, Abbott Laboratory, 1993.

26. Loeffler PM: Oral benzodiazepines and conscious sedation: a review, *J Oral Maxillofac Surg* 50(9):989, 1992.

27. Greenblatt DJ: Pharmacology of benzodiazepine hypnotics, *J Clin Psychiatry* 53(suppl):7, 1992.

28. Garzone PD, Kroboth PD: Pharmacokinetics of the newer benzodiazepines, *Clin Pharmacokinet* 16(6):337, 1989.

29. Young ER, Mason D: Triazolam: an oral sedative for the dental practitioner, *Can Dent Assoc J* 54:511, 1988.

30. Lieblich SE, Horswell B: Attenuation of anxiety in ambulatory oral surgery patients with oral triazolam, *J Oral Maxillofac Surg* 49:792, 1991.

31. Meyer ML, Mourino AP, Farrington FH: Comparison of triazolam to a chloral hydrate/hydroxyzine combination in the sedation of pediatric dental patients, *Pediatr Dent* 12(5):283, 1990.

32. Quarnstrom FC, Milgrom P, Moore PA: Experience with triazolam in preschool children, *J Anesth Pain Control Dent* 1(3): 157, 1992.

33. Greenfield DP: What about Halcion? *N J Medicine* 88(12):889, 1991 (editorial).

34. Bixler EO, Kales A, Manfredi RL et al: Next-day memory impairment with triazolam, *Lancet* 337(8745):827, 1991.

35. Medawar C, Rassaby E: Triazolam overdose, alcohol, and manslaughter, *Lancet* 338(8781):1515, 1991.

36. Schneider PJ, Perry PJ: Triazolam—an "abused drug" by the lay press? *DICP* 24(4):389, 1990.

37. Myrhed M: Background and current status. Halcion (triazolam) banned in England—Sweden investigates, *Lakartidningen* 88(47):4035, 1991.

38. Wysowski DK, Barash D: Adverse behavioral reactions attributed to triazolam in the Food and Drug Administration's Spontaneous Reporting System, *Arch Intern Med* 151(10):2003, 1991.

39. Halcion, drug package insert, The Upjohn Company, 1990.

40. Ativan, drug package insert, Wyeth-Ayerst Laboratories, 1992.

41. Christensen P, Lolk A, Gram LF et al: Benzodiazepine-induced sedation and cortisol suppression: a placebo-controlled comparison of oxazepam and nitrazepam in healthy male volunteers, *Psychopharmacology* 106(4):511, 1992.

42. Greenblatt DJ, Harmatz JS, Shader RI: Clinical pharmacokinetics of anxiolytics and hypnotics in the elderly: therapeutic considerations (part I), *Clin Pharmacokinet* 21(3):165, 1991.

43. Miller NS, Gold MS: Benzodiazepines: a major problem; introduction, *J Subst Abuse Treat* 8(1-2):3, 1991.

44. Castleden CM, Allen JG, Altman J et al: A comparison of oral midazolam, nitrazepam, and placebo in young and elderly subjects, *Eur J Clin Pharmacol* 32:253, 1987.

45. Jochemsen R, van Rijn PA, Hazelzet TG et al: Comparative pharmacokinetics of midazolam and loprazolam in healthy subjects after oral administration, *Biopharm Drug Dispos* 7:53, 1986.

46. Langlois S, Kneeft, JH, Chouinard G et al: Midazolam: kinetics and effects on memory, sensorium, and haemodynamics, *Br J Clin Pharmacol* 23:273, 1987.

47. Monti JM, Alterwain P, Debellis J et al: Short-term sleep laboratory evaluation of midazolam in chronic insomniacs: preliminary results, *Arzneimittelforschung* 37:54, 1987.

48. Hildebrand PJ, Elwood RJ, McClean E et al: Intramuscular and oral midazolam: some factors influencing uptake, *Anaesthesia* 38:1220, 1983.

49. Turner GA, Paech M: A comparison of oral midazolam solution with temazepam as a day case premedicant, *Anaesth Intensive Care* 19(3):365, 1991.

50. Wahlmann UW, Dietrich U, Fischer W: The question of oral sedation using midazolam in outpatient dental surgery, *Deutsche Zahnarztliche Zeitschrift* 47(1):66, 1992.

51. Luyk NH, Whitley BD: Efficacy of oral midazolam prior to intravenous sedation for the removal of third molars, *Int J Oral Maxillofac Surg* 20(5):264, 1991.

52. Parnis SJ, Foate JA, vander Walt JH et al: Oral midazolam is an effective premedicant for children having day-care anaesthesia, *Anaesth Intensive Care* 20(1):9, 1992.

53. Payne KA, Coetzee AR, Mattheyse FJ: Midazolam and amnesia in pediatric premedication, *Acta Anaesthesiol Belg* 42(2):101, 1991.

54. Hennes HM, Wagner V, Bonadio WA et al: The effect of oral midazolam on anxiety of preschool children during laceration repair, *Ann Emerg Med* 19(9):1006, 1990.

55. Feld LH, Negus JB, White PF: Oral midazolam preanesthetic medication in pediatric outpatients, *Anesthesiology* 73(5):831, 1990.

56. Weldon BC, Watcha MF, White PF: Oral midazolam in children: effect of time and adjunctive therapy, *Anesth Analg* 75(1):51, 1992.

57. Tolksdorf W, Eick C: Rectal, oral and nasal premedication using midazolam in children aged 1-6 years: a comparative clinical study, *Anaesthetist* 40(12):661, 1991.

58. Molter G, Altmayer P, Castor G, Buech U. Oral premedication with midazolam in children, *Anaesthesiol Reanim* 16(2):75, 1991.

59. Greenblatt DJ, Shader RI: Meprobamate: a study of irrational drug use, *Am J Psychiatry* 127:1297, 1971.

60. Malamed SF: *Sedation, a guide to patient management*, ed 2. St Louis, 1989, Mosby.

61. Malamed SF: *Sedation, a guide to patient management*. St Louis, 1985, Mosby.

62. Moore P, Haupt M: Sedative drug therapy in pediatric dentistry. In Dionne RA, Phero JC, eds: *Management of pain and anxiety in dental practice*. New York, 1992, Elsevier.

63. Nordenberg A, Dalisle G, Izukawa T: Cardiac arrhythmias in a child due to chloral hydrate ingestion, *Pediatrics* 47:134, 1971.

64. Greenberg SB, Faerber EN, Aspinall CL et al: High-dose chloral hydrate sedation for children undergoing MR imaging: safety and efficacy in relation to age, *Am J Roentgenol* 161(3):639, 1993.

65. Judish GF, Andreasen S, Bell EB: Chloral hydrate sedation as a substitute for examination under anesthesia in pediatric ophthalmology, *Am J Ophthalmol* 89:560, 1982.

66. Thompson JR, Schneider S, Ashwal S et al: The choice of sedation for computed tomography in children: a prospective evaluation, *Neuroradiology* 143:475, 1982.

67. Cook BA, Bass JW, Nomizu S et al: Sedation of children for technical procedures: current standard of practice, *Clin Pediatr* 31(3):137, 1992.

68. Troutman KC: Misuse of chloral hydrate in sedating a pediatric patient, ADSA Mortality and Morbidity Conference, ADSA Annual Meeting, Boston, 1984.

69. Moore PA: Therapeutic assessment of chloral hydrate premedication for pediatric dentistry, *Anesth Prog* 31:191, 1984.

70. Smith RC: Chloral hydrate sedation for handicapped children: a double-blind study, *Anesth Prog* 24:159, 1977.

71. Barr ES: Oral premedication in children, *Anesth Analg* 41:201, 1962.

72. Kolpek JH, Parr MD, Marshall ML et al: Ethchlorvynol pharmacokinetics during long-term administration in a patient with hyperlipidemia and hypothyroidism, *Pharmacotherapy* 6(6):323, 1986.

73. Ionescu-Pioggia M, Bird M, Cole JO: Subjective effects of methaqualone, NIDA Research Monograph 95:455, 1989.

74. Ionescu-Pioggia M et al: Methaqualone, *Int Clin Psychopharmacol* 3(2):97, 1988.

75. Richter JJ: Current theories about the mechansms of benzodiazepines and neuroleptic drugs, *Anesthesiology* 54:66, 1981.

76. Study RE, Barker JC: Cellular mechanisms of benzodiazepine action, *JAMA* 247:2147, 1982.

77. Tallman JF, Paul SM, Skolnick P et al: Receptors for the age of anxiety: pharmacology of the benzodiazepines, *Science* 207:274, 1980.

78. Greenblatt DJ, Miller LG, Shader RI: Benzodiazepine discontinuation syndromes, *J Psychiatr Res* 24(suppl 3):73, 1990.

79. Oreland L: The benzodiazepines: a pharmacological overview, *Acta Anaesthes Scand* 88(suppl):13, 1988.

80. Lacey DJ: Status epilepticus in children and adults, *J Clin Psychiatry* 49(suppl):33, 1988.

81. Simiand J, Keane PE, Biziere K et al: Comparative study in mice of tetrazepam and other centrally active skeletal muscle relaxants, *Arch Int Pharmacodyn Ther* 297:272, 1989.

82. Mayhue FE: IM midazolam for status epilepticus in the emergency department, *Ann Emerg Med* 17(6):643, 1988.

83. Classen DC, Pestotnik SL, Evans RS et al: Intensive surveillance of midazolam use in hospitalized patients and the occurrence of cardiorespiratory arrest, *Pharmacotherapy* 12(3):213, 1992.

84. Daneshmend TK, Bell GD, Logan RF: Sedation for upper gastrointestinal endoscopy: results of a nationwide survey, *GUT* 32(1):12, 1991.

85. Greenblatt DJ, Shader RI: *Benzodiazepines in clinical practice.* New York, 1974, Raven Press.

86. Edwards JG, Cantopher T, Olivieri S: Benzodiazepine dependence and the problems of withdrawal, *Postgrad Med* 66(suppl 2):27, 1990.

87. Laegreid L et al: Congenital malformations and maternal consumption of benzodiazepines, *Develop Med Child Neurol* 32(5):432, 1990.

88. Badalaty MM, Houpt MI, Koenigsberg SR et al: A comparison of chloral hydrate and diazepam sedation in young children, *Pediatr Dent* 12(1):33, 1990.

89. Palma-Aguirre JA, Rodriguez-Palomares C: Indications and contraindications for analgesics and antibiotics in pediatric dentistry, *Practica Odontol* 10(1):11, 1989.

90. Jacobsen D, Frederichsen PS, Knutsen KM et al: Clinical course in acute self-poisonings: a prospective study of 1125 consecutive hospitalized patients, *Hum Toxicol* 3(2):107, 1984.

91. Murray JB: Effects of valium and librium on human psychomotor and cognitive functions, *Genet Psychol Monogr* 109(20):167, 1984.

92. Wright GZ, McAulay DJ: Current premedicating trends in pedodontics, *J Dent Child* 40:185, 1973.

93. Wright GZ, Chiasson RC: The use of sedation agents by Canadian pediatric dentists, *Pediatr Dent* 9(4):308, 1987.

94. Jones KF: Preoperative medications in operative dentistry for children, *J Dent Child* 36:93, 1969.

95. Pautola A, Elomaa M: The use of promethazine and diazepam in dental treatment of apprehensive children, *Suom Hammaslaak Toim* 67:226, 1971.

96. Skorin L Jr, Onofrey BE, DeWitt JD: Phenothiazine-induced oculogyric crisis, *J Am Optometr Assoc* 58(4):316, 1987.

97. Lopez-Rois F et al: Drug-induced extrapyramidal syndrome: apropos of 22 cases, *Anales Espanoles de Pediatria* 26(2):91, 1987.

98. Council on Dental Therapeutics: *Accepted dental therapeutics*, ed 39, Chicago, 1982, ADA.

CHAPTER 9

Rectal sedation

The rectal route of drug administration has seen a resurgence of interest in anesthesiology and, to a lesser extent, dentistry in recent years.[1] Historically the rectal route of drug administration was employed for the administration of smoke ("fumigation") for resuscitation[2] and the administration of anesthetics. An ether boiler for rectal application was developed in 1847 by Pirogoff.[3] With the advent of more reliable routes of drug administration (e.g., IV and inhalation), the rectal route became less commonly used.

There remain certain situations in which rectal drug administration may prove to be valuable. These include the administration of a drug to a patient who is unwilling or unable to take drugs orally. In most instances this patient is a child or a handicapped adult requiring sedation either to permit treatment to proceed[4-6] or as a preliminary to the induction of general anesthesia.[7-9] Another situation in which rectally administered drugs are warranted is the administration of antiemetics to patients with nausea and vomiting. Although parenteral administration is preferred (if the patient is present in the office where the drug may be injected), rectal administration can be used if the patient objects to the injection or if the patient is at home. Another indication for rectal administration of drugs is analgesics for postoperative control of pain.[10]

Advantages of the rectal route include a rapid onset of clinical activity; a decreased incidence and intensity of drug-related side effects; the lack of a needle, syringe, or other equipment; the avoidance of an injection; ease of administration (many children who vehemently object to oral medications will not object to this route); and its low cost.

In the past it was thought that rectally administered drugs were absorbed directly into the systemic circulation via the vena cava, circumventing the enterohepatic circulation, thereby negating the hepatic first-pass effect, which so influences the clinical activity of most drugs administered enterally.[11] The superior rectal vein empties into the inferior mesenteric vein and thence into the portal system. The middle and inferior rectal veins empty into the internal iliac vein and the inferior vena cava.[12,13] However, it has been demonstrated that hepatic clearance is *the* main factor affecting bioavailability of rectally administered drugs.[1] This may be due to the fact that blood flow occurs through anastomoses that interconnect the superior, middle, and inferior rectal venous systems, thereby producing a hepatic first-pass effect with rectally administered drugs. Other potential factors, such as adsorption by feces, intraluminal degradation by microorganisms, metabolism within the mucosal cell, and lymphatic drainage do not significantly affect the fate of rectally administered drugs.

Comparing the oral, nasal, and rectal administration of the water-soluble benzodiazepine midazolam, Tolksdorf[7] found that children aged 1 to 6 years accepted the oral drug better than rectal or nasal, but that the rectally administered midazolam had the most rapid onset of action and fewer side effects in the postoperative period. In several studies peak levels of clinical action were noted rapidly following rectal administration. Roelofse et al,[4] noted good anxiolysis, sedation, and cooperation 30 minutes after rectal administration of midazolam, while Kraus et al,[14] noted peak plasma levels of midazolam at 7.5 minutes.

Disadvantages of the rectal route include the inconvenience to the administrator and patient, variable absorption of some drugs from the large intestine, possible irritation of the intestines by some drugs, inability to reverse the action of the drug easily, prolonged recovery with some drugs, and the inability to titrate precise individual dosages.

The primary use of rectal drug administration in both medicine and dentistry is the management of uncooperative patients, whether children or adults. The drug may be administered by the parent at home 1 hour prior to the appointment; however it is strongly suggested that rectally administered sedatives be administered in the medical or dental office by the doctor or a staff person. Signs and symptoms of sedation develop rapidly with many rectal drugs, clinical sedation being evident at 15 to 30 minutes.[4,14] The possibility of oversedation exists, and it would therefore be beneficial for the patient to be in a situation in which oversedation could be easily managed. An automobile en route to the doctor's office is not a desirable location.

Because of the lack of control maintained over the clinical actions of the drug, rectal administration ought not to be used in an effort to achieve deeper levels of sedation unless the doctor is well versed in anesthesiology and in management of the airway of the unconscious patient. The recommended use of rectal sedation is for the induction of light to moderate sedation where other, more controllable methods of anxiety control (IV, inhalation) may be employed if needed during treatment. Rectally administered drugs may provide a level of patient management adequate for many procedures, such as root planing and curettage,[5] and restoration or extraction of primary teeth,[6] but it may prove inadequate for procedures such as radiographs that require a patient to remain still for a period of time.[15]

The administration of rectal drugs is often considered to be difficult for the administrator and uncomfortable for the patient. Of 80 patient children receiving rectal premedication, deWaal et al[16] reported that 66 (82.5%) accepted rectal instillation well, 12 (15%) moderately well, and 2 (2.5%) poorly.

The patient receiving rectal drugs for sedation should receive supplemental oxygen as well as monitoring via pulse oximetry and pretracheal stethoscope. Personnel and equipment for resuscitation must always be available.

DRUGS

Many drugs are administered rectally. Ideally a drug for rectal administration will be available as a suppository, although in several cases (e.g., midazolam) drug formulations designed for parenteral administration have been employed successfully. Historically the two major drug groups that have been employed rectally are the barbiturates and narcotics.

Barbiturates
    Phenobarbital
    Secobarbital
    Pentobarbital
    Thiopental
    Methohexital
Narcotics
    Hydromorphone
    Oxymorphone
Promethazine
Chloral hydrate
Benzodiazepines
    Diazepam
    Midazolam
Ketamine

Phenobarbital

Phenobarbital is classified as a long-acting barbiturate. It is a rather safe medication for sedation of infants and younger children. It is also indicated for use in prolonged vomiting, in convulsive states, and in general when oral sedatives cannot be administered. The prolonged duration of action of this agent restricts its use in surgery and in dentistry.

Dosage. The usual dose for children is 1 mg/kg to 6 mg/kg body weight daily in three divided doses.

Availability. Phenobarbital sodium (generic): 8-, 16-, 32-, 65-, 100-, and 130-mg suppositories. Hypnette (Fleming); 8- and 16-mg suppositories. Phenobarbital is classified as a Schedule II drug.

Secobarbital

Secobarbital sodium is a short-acting barbiturate sedative-hypnotic. It is recommended for preoperative sedation or for helping a patient obtain a restful night's sleep prior to a dental appointment. It may be used in both children and adults.

Dosage. For adults the usual dose is 120 to 200 mg 1 hour before bedtime or prior to the scheduled dental appointment. The usual pediatric dose is 15 to 60 mg for infants up to 6 months of age, 60 mg for children 6 months to 3 years old, and 60 to 120 mg for older children.

Availability. Secobarbital sodium (generic): 8-, 50-, 65-, 100-, 130-, and 195-mg suppositories. Seconal sodium (Lilly): 30-, 60-, 120-, and 200-mg suppositories. Secobarbital is classified as a Schedule II drug.

Pentobarbital

Pentobarbital sodium is another short-acting barbiturate sedative-hypnotic that is available in suppository form. Its applications are similar to those of secobarbital sodium. Because of its relatively short duration of action (3 to 4 hours), pentobarbital is an excellent choice for sedation via the rectal route.

Dosage[17]

Age (weight)	Usual dose
Adults (average to above average weight)	120-200 mg
Children	
2 months-1 year (10-20 lbs)	30 mg
1-4 years (20-40 lbs)	30-60 mg
5-12 years (40-80 lbs)	60 mg
12-14 years (80-110 lbs)	60-120 mg

Availability. Pentobarbital sodium (generic): 16-, 32-, 65-, 130-, and 195-mg suppositories. Nembutal sodium (Abbott): 30-, 60-, 120-, and 200-mg suppositories. Pentobarbital is classified as a Schedule II drug.

Thiopental

Thiopental sodium is an ultrashort-acting CNS depressant commonly employed for the induction of general anesthesia via the IV route. It is also available as a rectal suspension for use in achieving deep sedation. Its primary use is in the uncooperative patient in whom other techniques of sedation are unavailable and where the duration of the planned procedure is short (not more than 15 minutes). The effective dose of thiopental for deep sedation is 44 mg/kg, which is approximately 10 times the intravenous dose for general anesthesia.[11] Giovannitti and Trapp[11] recommended that once sedation has been achieved rectally, an IV infusion be established and maintained throughout treatment. Where the planned treatment cannot be completed in 15 minutes, other sedative drugs should be administered IV before the patient becomes uncooperative.

Because of the pharmacology of the barbiturates in general and the uncertainty of drug response following rectal administration, thiopental is not recommended for use by doctors who have not had thorough training in general anesthesia and in maintenance of the unconscious airway. Larsson et al[18] reported elevated P_{CO_2} levels after rectal induction of anesthesia with either thiopentone (thiopental [30 mg/kg]) or methohexitone (methohexital [20 or 30 mg/kg]). The authors concluded that the use of rectal induction of anesthesia with barbiturates carries an increased risk of hypoventilation in infants under the age of 2 years.

Dosage.[19] For preoperative sedation the average dose is 1 g/75 lb body weight (1 g/34 kg). This is equivalent to 13.5 mg/lb or 29.4 mg/kg. The total dose should not exceed 1000 mg to 1500 mg in children weighing 75 lb or more and 3000 mg to 4000 mg in adults over 200 lb. A cleansing enema is rarely required prior to administration of this agent. The volume administered rarely induces defecation. The effective dose for deep sedation is 44 mg/kg.[11]

Availability. Pentothal (Abbott) rectal suspension: 400 mg/g of suspension. Thiopental is classified as a Schedule IV drug.

Methohexital

Methohexital (Brevital, Brietal), like thiopental, is classified as an ultrashort-acting barbiturate. Used intravenously methohexital produced ultralight general anesthesia of a somewhat shorter duration than thiopental. Methohexital has also been used via rectal instillation for premedication prior to the induction of general anesthesia in children.[1,20-23] As mentioned in the discussion of rectal thiopental, the use of rectal barbiturates for sedation or induction of anesthesia carries an increased risk of hypoventilation.[18]

Dosage. A dose of 20 mg/kg of methohexital is the usually recommended rectal dose for premedication as a sole agent. A dose of 10 mg/kg of methohexital following IM atropine and meperidine produces equal results.[23]

Availability. Methohexital is classified as a Schedule IV drug.

Hydromorphone

Hydromorphone is an opioid analgesic whose primary indication is for the relief of pain. One of the advantages of this agent is that the incidence of nausea and vomiting from hydromorphone is quite low. Sleep that occurs following its administration is produced by the relief of pain, not hypnosis.

Hydromorphone is administered rectally to provide long-lasting pain relief. The onset of action of the drug occurs within 30 minutes, and it has a duration of action of 4 to 5 hours.

Dosage.[24] The usual dose is 3 mg 1 hour prior to bedtime.

Availability. Dilaudid (Knoll): 3-mg suppositories. Dilaudid is classified as a Schedule II drug.

Oxymorphone

Oxymorphone is a rapid-acting opioid analgesic used primarily for the management of pain. It also produces sedation and is therefore indicated for use in preoperative sedation. Following oral or rectal administration the onset of action occurs within 30 minutes; the duration of action is approximately 6 hours.

Dosage.[25] The usual adult dosage is 5 mg every 4 to 6 hours. The safe use of oxymorphone in children under age 12 years has not been established.

Availability. Numorphan (DuPont): 5-mg suppositories. Oxymorphone is classified as a Schedule II drug.

Promethazine

The pharmacology of promethazine, a phenothiazine derivative, has been discussed in the section on oral sedation (Chapter 8). Promethazine may also be administered rectally for preoperative sedation and in the management of nausea and vomiting.

Dosage. The usual adult dose is 25 to 50 mg 1 hour before bedtime. For preoperative sedation of adults the dose is 50 mg 1 hour before treatment. For sedation of children the usual dose is 12.5 to 25 mg 1 hour before treatment.

Availability. Phenergan (Wyeth): 12.5-, 25-, and 50-mg suppositories.

Chloral hydrate

Chloral hydrate, a nonbarbiturate sedative-hypnotic, has been reviewed in Chapter 8. Chloral hydrate is also used rectally for preoperative sedation.

Dosage. For adults for preoperative sedation or to aid in falling asleep the night prior to dental treatment the usual dose is 650 mg to 1300 mg 1 hour before treatment or bedtime. The dosage for children is discussed in Chapter 35.

Availability. Rectules (Fellows): 650- and 1300-mg suppositories. Chloral hydrate is classified as a Schedule IV drug.

Diazepam

Diazepam has been used rectally for two specific purposes in medicine: management of epilepsy,[26] and management of anxiety in a variety of clinical settings, including terminal cancer patients[27] and adults for sedation during oral surgery.[28] The pediatric use of rectal diazepam has been well received.[29] Mattila et al[30] stated that the rectal solution of diazepam is a faster and more effective and reliable alternative to either tablets or suppositories and to the uncertain intramuscular (IM) injection of diazepam. Diazepam is not available at this time in the United States in a rectal formulation. However, it is available in this form in many countries, where its administration rectally has been well accepted.

Flaitz et al[31] reported on the effective use of rectally administered diazepam for pediatric sedation in dentistry. Using the intravenous (IV) formulation of diazepam, a dosage of 0.6 mg/kg was administered rectally. Effective levels of both sedation and anterograde amnesia were found in most patients. A potential complication of the rectal administration of diazepam is intestinal irritation, the incidence of which is thought to be quite low.[32]

Midazolam

Midazolam, a recently introduced water-soluble benzodiazepine, has received considerable attention as a rectally administered drug for premedication or sedation.*

Various doses of rectal midazolam have been used, ranging from 0.2 mg/kg to 5.0 mg/kg. It appears that a rectal dose of approximately 0.35 mg/kg[4,14,37] to 0.5 mg/kg[7,16] provides a rapid onset of action, a high level of successful sedation, with minimal intra- or postoperative complications. Roelofse et al[4] observed that 23% of the 60 patients receiving rectal midazolam exhibited disinhibition reactions, particularly those receiving a dose of 0.45 mg/kg. Reactions observed included agitation/excitement, restlessness/irritation, disorientation/confusion, and emotional/crying responses.

Midazolam is not available in a rectal formulation. The parenteral formulation of midazolam has been used, diluting 2 ml of midazolam with 8 ml of distilled water.[16] This volume is then instilled behind the anal sphincter using a suitable plastic applicator. Midazolam has not been observed to produce irritation of the rectal mucosa.

Studies in which response of vital signs and other physiologic parameters were monitored following rectal midazolam administration show no clinically significant changes in arterial blood pressure, heart rate, oxyhemoglobin saturation, or end-tidal carbon dioxide concentrations.[9,33]

Availability. Midazolam is not available as a rectal formulation, nor is it recommended for rectal administration in the United States. As of the writing of this text (July 1994), only France and Switzerland have approved the pediatric use of midazolam via rectal administration.[41] Midazolam is classified as a Schedule IV drug.

---

*References 4, 6-7, 9, 14-16, 33-40

Ketamine

Ketamine, a cyclohexane derivative, is classified as a dissociative anesthetic. First reported in 1969, ketamine produces a surgical depth anesthesia by interrupting afferent impulses reaching the cerebral cortex.[42] During dissociative anesthesia the patients appear to be awake—their eyes may be open, their mouth moving—yet they are incapable of purposefully reacting to environmental stimulation with appropriate motor responses.[43] The pharmacology of ketamine will be discussed in greater detail in Chapter 32. Although used primarily via the IM and IV routes, ketamine has also been administered rectally for premedication or sedation.[1,36,40] Holm-Knudsen et al[36] used 10 mg/kg ketamine and 0.2 mg/kg midazolam for induction of general anesthesia in healthy 2- to 10-year-olds, reporting that no cases of rectal irritation or unpleasant dreams occurred and that postoperative analgesia was good. vander Bijl et al. also administered rectal ketamine (5 mg/kg) and midazolam (0.3 mg/kg) to patients 2 to 9 years old. They reported that 30 minutes after administration of the two drugs good anxiolysis, sedation, and cooperation were obtained in most patients. The group receiving midazolam alone appeared to be more efficacious and had fewer adverse effects than the group receiving ketamine alone (but no statistical difference was noted).[40]

An often reported side effect of ketamine, via any route of administration, is vivid dreams or hallucinations.[44] Such adverse events are rarely noted in pediatric patients, who generally tolerate ketamine anesthesia quite well. Ketamine should not be used by doctors who have not been trained in general anesthesia and in the management of the airway of the unconscious patient.

Lytic cocktail

The lytic cocktail is a combination of meperidine (Demerol), promethazine (Phenergan), and chlorpromazine (Thorazine), also known as DPT. Used intramuscularly, DPT is commonly used in hospitals (especially in the emergency department) during painful procedures. The efficacy of this mixture is poor, especially when compared with alternative approaches, and it has been associated with a high frequency of adverse effects.[45,46] It has been used rectally in pediatrics. A dose of 0.07 ml/kg was administered to patients ranging in age from 1 to 12 years.[47] One milliliter of lytic cocktail contains 28 mg meperidine, 7 mg promethazine, and 7 mg chlorpromazine. Satisfactory sedation was achieved before operation in most patients, but following the operation rectally premedicated patients were less sedated than a control group receiving IM DPT.

That the lytic cocktail has fallen into disfavor is noted by the statement in a U.S. Department of Health and Human Services' *Clinical Practice Guideline on Acute Pain Management*.[48] Their conclusion is that the lytic cocktail "is not recommended for general use and should be used only in exceptional circumstances."

COMPLICATIONS OF RECTAL ADMINISTRATION

There are several complications associated with the rectal administration of drugs. Primary among these is the initiation of a bowel movement by instillation of a large volume of fluid into the rectum.[11] The incidence of this complication is not documented, but it is estimated to occur in 5% to 10% of patients.[11]

Irritation of rectal mucosa, even to the extent of ulceration, is possible with certain drugs and with prolonged rectal administration.[49] Long-term rectal administration of acetylsalicylic acid has produced rectal ulceration. However, even single-dose rectal instillation has produced rectal irritation.

The potential for oversedation or the production of general anesthesia, both with attendant risk of airway obstruction produced by the tongue, must be considered whenever rectally administered drugs are intended to provide deep sedation. This risk is increased where barbiturates, opioid agonists, and ketamine are used. The occurrence of oversedation, inadvertent general anesthesia, or airway obstruction is decreased where rectal benzodiazepines are employed.

SUMMARY

The use of rectally administered drugs has increased in popularity in many countries, especially since the introduction of midazolam in the 1980s. Clinical trials have demonstrated that rectally administered drugs are usually well accepted and well tolerated and provide a rapid onset of action with a minimum of adverse effects or complications. Rectally administered drugs provide an alternative to the oral and parenteral routes, which might prove difficult to employ or be contraindicated in certain populations such as pediatric and handicapped patients.

Rectal sedation should be considered only by doctors who are well versed in the pharmacology of the drug(s) to be employed, in the potential side effects and complications of the technique and drug(s), and who are proficient in the management of the unconscious patient and airway. In addition, I strongly recommend that supplemental oxygen be administered to all patients receiving deep sedation via rectal drugs, that an IV infusion be maintained throughout the procedure, and that monitoring of the patient be continuous, including pulse oximetry and a pretracheal stethoscope.

Where rectal sedation is to be employed I suggest the drug be administered in the office to ensure proper dosing and monitoring following administration. Whenever possible, the use of benzodiazepines, midazolam or diazepam, should be considered. Opioids, barbiturates, ketamine, and the lytic cocktail ought not be employed rectally unless specific indications for their administration exist and adequately trained personnel are available to manage the patient during and after the sedation.

REFERENCES

1. Jantzen JP, Diehl P: Rectal administration of drugs. Fundamentals and applications in anesthesia, *Anaesthesist* 40(5):251, 1991.
2. American Heart Association: National Academy of Sciences and National Research Council standards for cardiopulmonary resuscitation (CPR) and emergency cardiac care (ECC), *JAMA* 227(suppl):833, 1974.
3. Sykes WS: *Essays on the first hundred years of anaesthesia,* Edinburgh, 1960, ES Livingstone.
4. Roelofse JA, vander Bilj P, Stegmann DH et al: Preanesthetic medication with rectal midazolam in children undergoing dental extractions, *J Oral Maxillofac Surg* 48(8):791, 1990.
5. Diner MH, Fortin RC, Marcoux P: Behavioral influences of rectal diazepam in solution on dental patients with mentally and physically handicapping conditions, *Spec Care Dent* 8(1): 19, 1988.
6. Kraemer N, Krafft T, Kinzelmann KH: Treatment of deciduous teeth under rectal Midazolam sedation, *Deutsche Zahnarztliche Zeitschrift* 46(9):609, 1991.
7. Tolksdorf W, Eicj C: Rectal, oral and nasal premedication using midazolam in children aged 1-6 years. A comparative clinical study, *Anaesthesist* 40(12):661, 1991.
8. Kasaba T, Nonoue T, Yanagidani T et al: Effects of rectal premedication and the mother's presence on induction of pediatric anesthesia, *Masui Jpn J Anesthes* 40(4):552, 1991.
9. Spear RM, Yaster M, Berkowitz ID et al. Preinduction of anesthesia in children with rectally administered midazolam, *Anesthesiology* 74(4):670, 1991.
10. Maunuksela EL, Ryhaenen P, Janhunen L: Efficacy of rectal ibuprofen in controlling postoperative pain in children, *Can J Anaesth* 39(3):226, 1992.
11. Giovannitti JA, Trapp LD: Adult sedation: oral, rectal, IM, IV. In Dionne RA, Phero JC, eds. *Management of pain and anxiety in dental practice.* New York, 1991, Elsevier.
12. De Boer A, De Leede L, Breimer D: Drug absorption by sublingual and rectal routes, *Br J Anaesth* 56:69, 1984.
13. De Boer A, Moolenaar F, Leede L et al: Rectal drug administration: clinical pharmacokinetic considerations, *Clin Pharmacokinet* 7:285, 1982.
14. Kraus GB, Gruber RG, Knoll R et al. Pharmacokinetic studies following intravenous and rectal administration of midazolam in children, *Anaesthesist* 38(12):658, 1989.
15. Coventry DM, Martin CS, Burke AM: Sedation for paediatric computerized tomography—double-blind assessment of rectal midazolam, *Eur J Anaesthesiol* 8(1):29, 1991.
16. deWaal FC, Huisman J, Veerman AJ: Rectal premedication with midazolam in children. A comparative clinical study, *Tijdschr Kindergeneesk* 56(2):82, 1988.
17. Pentobarbital package insert, Chicago, 1992, Abbott Laboratories.
18. Larsson LE, Nilsson K, Andreasson S et al: Effects of rectal thiopentone and methohexitone on carbon dioxide tension in infant anesthesia with spontaneous ventilation, *Acta Anaesthesiol Scand* 31(3):227, 1987.
19. Pentothal rectal syringe package insert, Chicago, 1992, Abbott Laboratories.
20. Bjorkman S, Gabrielsson J, Quaynor H et al: Pharmacokinetics of IV and rectal methohexitone in children, *Br J Anaesth* 59: 1541, 1987.
21. Quaynor H, Corbey M, Bjorkman S: Rectal induction of anaesthesia in children with methohexitone, *Br J Anaesth* 57:573, 1984.
22. Liu L, Gaudreault P, Friedman P et al: Methohexital plasma concentrations in children following rectal administration, *Anesthesiology* 62:567, 1985.
23. Karhunen U: Sleep effect of rectal methohexital (10 mg/kg) in children premedicated for anaesthesia, *Devel Pharmacol Ther* 11(2):92, 1988.
24. Dilaudid drug package insert, Whippany, NJ, 1989, Knoll Pharmaceuticals.
25. Numorphan drug package insert, Garden City, NY, 1985, DuPont Multi-Source.
26. Dhillon S, Ngwane E, Richens A: Rectal absorption of diazepam in epileptic children, *Arch Dis Child* 57:264, 1982.
27. Ehsanullah RS, Galloway DB, Gusterson FR et al: A double-blind crossover study of diazepam rectal suppositories, 5 mg and 10 mg, for sedation with advanced malignant disease, *Pharmatherapeutica* 3:215, 1982.
28. Lundgren S: Serum concentration and drug effect after intravenous and rectal administration of diazepam, *Anesth Prog* 34: 128, 1987.
29. Knudsen F: Plasma-diazepam in infants after rectal administration in solution and by suppository, *Acta Paediatr Scand* 66: 563, 1977.
30. Mattila MA, Ruoppi MK, Ahlstrom-Bengg E et al: Diazepam in rectal solution as premedication in children, with special reference to serum concentrations, *Br J Anaesth* 53:1269, 1981.
31. Flaitz CM, Nowak AJ, Hicks MJ: Evaluation of anterograde amnesic effect of rectally administered diazepam in the sedated pedodontic patient, *J Dent Child* 53:17, 1986.
32. Lundgren S, Rosenquist J: Comparison of sedation, amnesia, and patient comfort produced by intravenous and rectal diazepam, *J Oral Maxillofac Surg* 42:646, 1984.
33. Roelofse JA, de V Joubert JJ: Arterial oxygen saturation in children receiving rectal midazolam as premedication for oral surgical procedures, *Anesth Prog* 37(6):286, 1990.
34. Piotrowski R, Petrow N: Anesthesia induction in children: propofol in comparison with thiopental following premedication with midazolam, *Anaesthesist* 39(8):398, 1990.

35. Molter G, Castor G, Altmayer P: Psychosomatic, sedative and hemodynamic reactions following preoperative administration of midazolam in children, *Klin Padiatr* 202(5):328, 1990.

36. Holm-Knudsen R, Sjogren P, Laub M: Midazolam and ketamine for rectal premedication and induction of anesthesia in children, *Anaesthesist* 39(5):255, 1990.

37. Roelofse JA, Stegmann DH, Hartshorne J et al: Paradoxical reactions to rectal midazolam as premedication in children, *Int J Oral Maxillofac Surg* 19(1):2, 1990.

38. Tolksdorf W, Bremerich D, Nordmeyer U: Midazolam for premedication of infants. A comparison of the effect between oral and rectal administration, *Anasthesiol, Intensivmed Notfallmed* 24(6):355, 1989.

39. Saint-Maurice C, Esteve C, Holzer J et al: Better acceptance of measures for induction of anesthesia after rectal premedication with midazolam in children. Comparison of results of an open and placebo-controlled study, *Anaesthesist* 36(11):629, 1987.

40. vander Bijl P, Roelofse JA, Stander IA: Rectal ketamine and midazolam for premedication in pediatric dentistry, *J Oral Maxillofac Surg* 49(10):1050, 1991.

41. Moore PA: Pediatric medication with rectal midazolam in children undergoing dental extractions. Discussion, *J Oral Maxillofac Surg* 48:797, 1990.

42. Corssen G, Groves EH, Gomez S et al: Ketamine—its place in anesthesia for neurosurgical diagnostic procedures, *Anesth Analg* 48:181, 1969.

43. Jeffers GE, Dembo JB: Deep sedation. In Dionne RA, Phero JC, eds: *Management of pain and anxiety in dental practice*. New York, 1991, Elsevier.

44. Becsey L, Malamed S, Radnay P et al: Reduction of the psychotomimetic and circulatory side effects of ketamine by droperidol, *Anesthesiology* 37:536, 1972.

45. Benusis KP, Kapaun D, Furnam LJ: Respiratory depression in a child following meperidine, promethazine, and chlorpromazine premedication: report of a case, *J Dent Child* 46:50, 1979.

46. Nahata N, Clotz M, Krogg E: Adverse effects of meperidine, promethazine, and chlorpromazine for sedation in pediatric patients, *Clin Pediatr* 24:558, 1985.

47. Laub M, Sjogren P, Holm-Knudsen R et al: Lytic cocktail in children. Rectal versus intramuscular administration. *Anaesthesia* 45(2):110, 1990.

48. U.S. Department of Health and Human Services: Clinical practice guideline: acute pain management: operative or medical procedures and trauma, publication no. 92-0032, Rockville, Md, 1992, U.S. Department of Health and Human Services, Public Health Service, Agency for Health Care Policy and Research.

49. van Hoogdalem E, de Boer AG, Breimer DD: Pharmacokinetics of rectal drug administration, part I. General considerations and clinical applications of centrally acting drugs, *Clin Pharmacokinet* 21(1):11, 1991.

CHAPTER 10

Sublingual, transdermal, and intranasal sedation

In recent years efforts have been directed at seeking alternative routes of drug administration for use where more traditional routes are not available or where patient cooperation is lacking. Such situations include younger children or infants where cooperation does not exist, older patients requiring long-term drug therapy where noncompliance with administration recommendations is a serious problem, victims of burns or trauma, or life-threatening emergencies where other routes of administration are not present, yet rapid onset of drug action is necessary.

Three routes of drug administration, sublingual (SL), transdermal, and intranasal (IN), will be discussed. As will be noted in the following text, the use of these techniques is becoming increasingly popular in many areas of medicine. One or more may have application in dentistry; only time will tell.

Transdermal administration is most often employed for sustained-action drug administration, for example, scopolamine as an antimotion sickness therapy, whereas *sublingual* and *intranasal* administration provide a considerably more rapid onset of clinical action.

SUBLINGUAL SEDATION

The use of sublingual administration of drugs has a long history. Indeed sublingual administration of nitroglycerin tablets has been the recommended route for management of anginal pain for decades. Sublingual placement of nitroglycerin tablets usually provides relief from anginal discomfort within 2 minutes.

An advantage of sublingual administration is that the drug enters directly into the systemic circulation, almost entirely bypassing the enterohepatic circulation. The drug avoids the hepatic first-pass effect, in which a percentage of the drug is biotransformed before ever having the opportunity to enter the general circulation and to reach its target organ (e.g., brain).[1-3] Harris et al[4] have stated that sublingual delivery of drugs gives rapid absorption and good bioavailability for some drugs, although this site is not well suited to sustained-delivery systems. Patient cooperation is important to the success of the SL route of administration, therefore minimizing the use of this route in many pediatric and other uncooperative patients.[5]

Among the drugs that have been employed sublingually are nitroglycerin in the management of angina pectoris, acute pulmonary edema, and acute myocardial infarction;[6] heparin, in the prophylaxis of atherosclerotic disease;[7] nifedipine, a calcium channel blocker, for the management of acute hypertensive urgencies and emergencies[8-13]; opioids, such as meperidine and buprenorphine, for relief of pain in cancer[14-15] or following abdominal or gynecological surgery;[5,16] and sedatives for premedication and conscious sedation.[17-19]

Nitroglycerin

Nitroglycerin is employed sublingually in the management of anginal discomfort. Rapid SL absorption provides venodilation within 2 minutes. The rapidity of onset and degree of vasodilation observed makes nitroglycerin the drug of choice in managing angina pectoris. Side effects of SL nitroglycerin are few and usually not severe. However, in certain individuals SL nitroglycerin has provoked severe side effects. Brandes et al report on 35 cases of nitroglycerin-induced hypotension, bradycardia, apnea, and unconsciousness, concluding that this is a drug-induced effect of nitroglycerin that is independent of the route of administration and is unpredictable. They recommend close monitoring whenever nitroglycerin is administered.[20]

Therapeutic advantage may be taken of the hypotensive side effect of nitroglycerin in the management of acute hypertensive episodes. Acute hypertensive episodes are classified as either "urgencies" or "emergencies," the level of blood pressure elevation determining the classification. Hypertensive emergencies involve significantly greater blood pressure elevations and require more aggressive and immediate treatment than do hypertensive urgencies.[8] Although nitroglycerin has been employed effectively sublingually, the calcium channel blocker nifedipine has received considerably more attention in management of both hypertensive urgencies and emergencies. Sublingual nifedipine is absorbed rapidly, leading to improved myocardial perfusion, increased coronary blood flow, and decreased coronary vascular resistance.[9] A capsule of nifedipine is punctured several times (in the dental office an explorer or small round bur will be sufficient for this purpose), placed under the tongue, and sucked on by the patient. Nifedipine SL has been employed in the management of clonidine overdose, which produces severe hypertension and altered mental status. Sublingual nifedipine (20 mg) produces a rapid decline in blood pressure and improved mental status.[10] As with nitroglycerin, SL nifedipine used for management of acute hypertensive episodes may produce symptomatic hypotension in some patients.[13] Vital signs should be monitored closely whenever SL nifedipine is used.

Opioids

Four studies have reported on the efficacy of SL administration of opioids. Kortilla et al[16] compared SL buprenorphine to intramuscular (IM) oxycodone as a preanesthetic medication. Preoperatively the SL opioid produced less drowsiness and sedation and alleviated patients' apprehension significantly less than oxycodone. However, in the recovery room moderate to severe pain was more common with oxycodone than with SL buprenorphine. Sublingual buprenorphine was as effective as IM oxycodone for pain relief. However, two patients receiving SL opioid developed severe respiratory depression postoperatively. The authors concluded that SL opioids can provide good postoperative pain relief for gynecological procedures performed under anesthesia, but

that patients must be monitored because of the potential for respiratory depression. In a similar study Carl et al[5] compared SL and IM buprenorphine and IM meperidine for pain control following major abdominal surgery. Patients receiving SL buprenorphine were significantly more conscious in the immediate postoperative period than either IM group, yet all three groups demonstrated equal pain relief. Sedation and nausea were the most common complications in all three groups. Three cases of IM meperidine and one of IM buprenorphine required Intermittent positive pressure ventilation (IPPV) for respiratory depression. They concluded that SL opioids are useful for postoperative pain and exhibited administrative advantages when patients were able to cooperate. Two studies have looked at the use of opioids for the long-term relief of cancer pain, concluding that SL morphine has enabled patients whose cancer pain is refractory to traditional methods of drug delivery to obtain satisfactory control of their symptoms.[14-15]

Fentanyl lollipop (lozenge)

Fentanyl has also been formulated as a lozenge or lollipop that has demonstrated advantages as a preoperative sedative in children. The use of oral transmucosal fentanyl citrate (OTFC) has been studied as an alternative to oral and parenteral medication in younger or older patients who are unwilling or unable to tolerate orally administered drugs.[21-28] Although several dosages have been evaluated, most studies indicated that a dose of 15 μg/kg to 20 μg/kg provides the optimal sedation and anxiolysis preoperatively.[21-22] Acceptance of the lollipop was reported as universal in most studies, a significant advantage over most other forms of drug administration.[21-25] The objective onset of sedation was noted to develop from 10 minutes[23] to 30 minutes[21] following administration of the lollipop. After beginning OTFC, 60% of patients became drowsy or sedated in 12 to 30 minutes.[25] When volunteers were asked to rapidly suck the lollipop (as opposed to permitting it to passively dissolve), a more rapid onset of a pleasant feeling (the first subjective sensation) was observed. However, the onset of subjective sedation or analgesia was no more rapid than with passive dissolution.[22]

The use of fentanyl lollipops is not without the potential for side effects. Significant decreases in respiratory rate and SpO$_2$ have been reported.[2,21,23,27] Management of these episodes of opioid-induced respiratory depression was simple: reminding the patient to breathe.[21] Other side effects noted with some frequency included pruritis[21,24,27] in 80%[21] to 90%[24] of patients preoperatively and 33% to 70% postoperatively;[21] postoperative nausea (30% to 58%[21]); and vomiting (50% to 83%),[21,24,26-27] which was not significantly reduced by the prophylactic administration of the antiemetic droperidol.[26]

The conclusion reached by most authors is that OTFC is a reliable means of inducing rapid, noninvasive, preoperative sedation for pediatric outpatients undergoing short operations[26,28] or in the emergency department.[25] They further observe that OTFC use is associated with potentially significant reductions in respiratory rate and SpO2 and a high incidence of postoperative nausea and vomiting and pruritis.[26] In the absence of controlled clinical trials in dental outpatients it seems prudent, at this time, to withhold recommendation of this method of opioid administration for preoperative sedation in dentistry.

Sedatives

Several studies have reported on the use of the SL route for preoperative sedation. Two have compared the SL administration of a benzodiazepine to oral administration. Gram-Hansen et al,[17] administering 2.5 mg lorazepam either orally or SL prior to gynecological surgery, found a maximal plasma concentration at 40 minutes orally and 60 minutes after SL. Garzone and Kroboth,[18] looking at alprazolam and triazolam, found peak concentrations that occurred earlier and were higher following SL than oral administration. Sublingual lormetazepam (2.5 mg) followed in 35 minutes by IV diazepam (10 mg) was compared to SL placebo followed in 35 minutes by IV diazepam (10 mg) in patients undergoing surgical removal of impacted third molars.[19] A rapid onset of sedation was noted after SL lormetazepam, whereas the course and duration of postoperative sedation, measured using standard psychometric tests, were similar following both treatments. Surgeons' ratings indicated that SL lormetazepam was comparable to IV diazepam, but patients ratings indicated greater satisfaction with and preference for IV diazepam. Significant anterograde amnesia was found following both treatments. The authors indicate that SL lormetazepam may have a role in anesthesia as a premedicant and for conscious sedation.

Conclusions

The SL route of drug administration possesses possible uses in dentistry in two distinct areas. First, for the management of preoperative fears and anxiety the use of certain drugs such as benzodiazepines appears to provide a level of sedation comparable to orally administered drugs. The onset of action also appears comparable to oral drugs. The second possible use for SL administration in dentistry is in management of postoperative pain. Sublingual opioid administration appears to provide adequate pain relief with a lesser degree of sedation than IM opioids. The potential for opioid-induced respiratory depression is still present. Therefore the usual postoperative monitoring practices must be continued when SL opioids are employed. Patient cooperation is essential for SL delivery of drugs to be effective. The use of SL administration in younger children or any uncooperative patient is therefore not recommended.

TRANSDERMAL SEDATION

The administration of drugs through the skin (transdermally) has been in existence for a long time. In the past the most commonly applied systems were topically applied creams and ointments for dermatological disorders. The occurrence of systemic side effects with some of these formulations is indicative of absorption through the skin. In a broad sense the term *transdermal delivery system* includes all topically administered drug formulations intended to deliver the active ingredient into the general circulation.[29] Serious consideration for the transdermal delivery of drugs for systemic therapy began with a number of revolutionary ideas in the early 1970s.[30] It is only since the 1980s, however, that modern transdermal therapeutic systems (TTS) have been successfully marketed.[31] Drugs such as nitroglycerin (angina),[32] scopolamine (antimotion sickness),[33,34] clonidine (high blood pressure),[35] estradiol (postmenopause),[36] and nicotine (smoking cessation)[37] are the current prominent representatives that have met expectations regarding therapeutic benefits based on TTS applications. The use of opioids via TTS for pain management has recently met with considerable clinical success.[38,39]

A major advantage of TTS is the avoidance of the hepatic first-pass effect. Other advantages include simplified dosage regimens, enhanced compliance, reduced side effects, and improved disease therapy.[40]

The intact skin provides an efficient barrier against percutaneous absorption of drugs.[41] This barrier function can be ascribed to the structure of the stratum corneum, which consists of alternating lipoidal and hydrophylic regions, making the skin relatively impermeable. This impermeability of skin is associated with its dual functions as a protective barrier against invasion by microorgamisms and the prevention of the loss of physiologically essential substances such as water. Elucidation of factors that contribute to this impermeability has made the use of skin as a route for controlled systemic drug delivery possible.[29] To deliver drugs for systemic therapy through the skin, skin permeability needs enhancing by either modifying the drug molecules or applying skin permeation enhancers to reduce the barrier property of the skin.[42] Traditionally, the enhancement of skin permeability is considered to be the result of either the improvement of drug lipophilicity and the partition of drugs into the skin or from the direct actions of skin permeation enhancers on the chemical structure and/or composition of lipids and proteins in the stratum corneum.

A number of transdermal delivery systems are currently employed that allow for effective absorption of drugs (of low molecular mass) across the skin.[43] The most widely used system is the membrane-permeation–controlled system. A second system is the microsealed system, a partition-controlled delivery system that contains a drug reservoir with a saturated suspension of the drug in a water-miscible solvent homogeneously dispersed in a silicone elastomer matrix. A third system is the matrix-diffusion–controlled system, and a fourth system, recently made available, is the gradient-charged system. Nitroglycerin TTS is based on a multilayered laminated polymeric structure. A layer of vinyl chloride copolymer or terpolymer containing the drug is sandwiched between two or more layers of polymeric films. The nitroglycerin is released from the device at a controlled rate by a process of diffusion through the reservoir and one of the outer layers, which can function as a rate-controlling membrane.[44] Advanced transdermal systems are being developed, including iontophoretic and sonophoretic systems, thermosetting gels, prodrugs, and liposomes.[29] Penetration enhancers such as Azone may allow the delivery of larger size molecules such as proteins and polypeptides.

Systemic and localized side effects may be noted with the use of transdermal drug delivery systems. These have included skin inflammation and allergy[31,42,45] and drug tolerance.[32,46] Side effects produced by the drug are similar to those noted with other routes of drug delivery.

The onset of clinical activity of TTS administered drugs is slow, thus the primary use of this technique for sustained-release drug therapy. After application of a transdermal fentanyl patch, fentanyl is absorbed into the skin beneath the patch, where a depot forms in the upper skin layers. Plasma fentanyl concentrations are barely detectable for about 2 hours after patch placement. From 8 to 12 hours after patch placement, plasma concentrations approximate those achieved with equivalent IV doses of fentanyl.[39]

Opioids

Interest in the use of transdermal drug delivery systems in dentistry centers on postoperative pain control. Opioids, particularly fentanyl, have received attention in the management of both chronic (cancer) and acute (postoperative) pain.

Mosser[38] describes the unique pharmacokinetics of the transdermal system, including a prolonged time to peak analgesic effect, a long elimination half-life, and the skin depot concept, in recommending fentanyl over parenterally administered opioids in the treatment of cancer pain. Calis et al[39] also recommend fentanyl TTS for management of chronic, cancer-related pain. The use of TTS for acute postoperative pain is not as well accepted. Though Clotz and Nahata[47] state that the transdermal fentanyl patch seems to provide the same degree of analgesia as a continuous IV infusion, Calis et al[39] state that the overall efficacy and safety of the transdermal fentanyl system for the treatment of postoperative pain has not been adequately evaluated.

Antiemetics

A second area in which TTS drug delivery systems have potential utility in dentistry is antiemetic drugs. Swallowed blood is a very potent emetic following oral surgical procedures. In addition, the administration of opioid analgesics during the surgical procedure or postoperatively is associated with a degree of nausea and vomiting.

Scopolamine was among the first drugs employed transdermally for the management of motion sickness.[48] Administered transdermally the duration of effect was 72 hours compared to a 3- to 6-hour duration when administered orally or parenterally. Transdermal administration is associated with a lower incidence of side effects than orally or parenterally administered scopolamine. The most commonly observed side effects following transdermal administration have been dry mouth, drowsiness, and impairment of ocular accommodation, including blurred vision and mydriasis. Systemic side effects, such as adverse CNS effects, difficulty in urinating, rashes, and erythema have been reported only occasionally. The efficacy of transdermal scopolamine in preventing nausea and vomiting in post-surgical patients was evaluated by Schuh et al.[49] Scopolamine has a well-documented postoperative antiemetic effect. One study has demonstrated a 50% reduction of emetic symptoms compared with placebo.[50] In this study of cholecystectomy patients (a procedure with a high incidence of postoperative emesis), the antinausea and antiemetic effect of scopolamine TTS was insufficient and significantly less than that seen with IV droperidol (7.5 mg).[49] In the droperidol group 45% of patients did not have nausea, and vomiting occurred in only 25%, whereas in the scopolamine TTS group only 15% did not become nauseous and 50% vomited. Further study is warranted to determine the efficacy of transdermal scopolamine as an antiemetic following oral surgical procedures.

Conclusions

Transdermal drug delivery systems provide an easy, reliable mechanism of administering drugs in situations in which rapid onset is not important. Transdermal delivery systems bypass the enterohepatic circulation, thereby providing a more reliable clinical action. With many drugs, efficacy of transdermal delivery is equivalent to continuous intravenous infusion, yet in a noninvasive system.

It appears that the transdermal use of opioids might prove advantageous in dental situations in which long-term pain control is required but where patient compliance is suspect. Drug-related side effects following transdermal delivery, though less frequent, are the same as those noted when other administration techniques are employed. Oversedation and respiratory depression must be considered whenever opioids are employed. The use of transdermal scopolamine as an antiemetic following dental surgery requires additional research before its use can be recommended.

INTRANASAL SEDATION

Another recent addition to the drug administration armamentarium has been the intranasal (IN) route. Intranasal drugs have been employed primarily in pediatrics as a means of circumventing the need for injection or oral drug administration in unwilling patients.[51-52] Absorption of IN drugs occurs directly into the central circulation, bypassing the enterohepatic circulation.[53] Clinical trials have demonstrated that absorption and bioavailability of IN administered drugs is close to those of IV administration with peak plasma levels of the agent occurring approximately 10 minutes following administration.[54-60]

Midazolam, a water-soluble benzodiazepine,[51-52,54-61] and sufentanil,[56,62] an opioid analgesic, have received the most attention via the IN route of administration.

Midazolam

Midazolam has been demonstrated to provide a consistent level of CNS activity following IN administration.[52,54-61] A dose of 0.2 mg/kg appears to be the most effective in pediatric patients for premedication prior to general anesthesia,[57-58,61,63] with somewhat larger doses recommended for sedation adequate to permit treatment.[64]

Compared to oral administration the mean IN absorption rates (tmax) of flurazepam, midazolam, and triazolam were 1.7, 2, and 2.6 times faster, respectively, compared with oral dosing.[65] When children accept oral administration at all they appear to accept it better than IN administered drugs.[63] Intranasal drugs are administered by either the parent or the doctor using a 1-ml or 3-ml syringe without a needle with the child seated on the parent's lap. Some children were temporarily distressed at the instillation of the fluid (drug) into the nose, but all rapidly settled down again in the presence of their parents.[51] An undiluted solution of the drug should be used to avoid large volumes of liquid being instilled into the nose and possibly entering the pharynx and producing coughing or sneezing, with attendant expulsion of the drug and decreased absorption. Rose et al[60] found IN midazolam to be slightly more effective than oral diazepam as preanesthetic medication in children, producing anxiolysis and sedation with rapid onset. Buenz and Gossler[57] suggest that with the advent of a more concentrated solution of midazolam (>5 mg/ml) IN application is also conceivable as a premedication in adults.

The IM and IN routes of midazolam administration have been compared. There were no significant differences in the onset of sedation (12.42 ± 4.07 min for IM; 15.26 ± 7.99 min for IN), the degree of sedation, and in the response to venipuncture.[58] Theissen et al[66] compared IM and IN midazolam for sedation in adults prior to endoscopy of the upper GI tract.[66] Sedation was equivalent in both groups with three patients ($n = 10$) in the IM group experiencing retrograde amnesia (0 in the IN group). There were no significant differences in the degrees of anterograde amnesia in either group. Intranasal administration of midazolam was concluded to be a simple, nontraumatic, well-tolerated alternative to the IM route of sedation for bronchoscopy in adults.

Several studies have compared IN midazolam to

IV midazolam. The half-life of midazolam is similar (2.2 hr IN vs. 2.4 hr IV) following IM and IV administration in children ages 1 year to 5 years.[56] At 10 minutes following IN administration the mean plasma concentration of midazolam was 57% of the IV group.[59]

An additional finding noted by one observer was the association of IN instillation of midazolam with a sense of euphoria that occurred almost immediately, which was not observed when midazolam was administered by other routes.[63]

Two studies utilized IN midazolam for procedures akin to dental care. In one, IN midazolam was employed in adults for sedation during upper GI endoscopy, comparing well to IM midazolam.[66] Only two patients ($n = 20$) receiving IM or IN midazolam had a bad opinion of their experience as compared with four of the nine receiving placebo. Intranasal midazolam was employed for sedation prior to ophthalmologic examination in children ranging in age from 3.5 months to 10 years.[64] An IN midazolam dose of 0.35 mg/kg to 0.5 mg/kg provided rapid onset of sedation, which was adequate in all cases to permit ocular examination. In all of the IN midazolam studies reported, oxygen saturation was monitored throughout the procedure, including recovery. No instances of significant desaturation were reported.

Intranasal midazolam in a dose of approximately 0.2 mg/kg appears to be an acceptable alternative to both oral and IM administration of midazolam for premedication prior to additional IV sedation or general anesthesia. A larger dose, 0.35 mg/kg to 0.5 mg/kg, may be necessary where the IN drug is the sole route of sedative administration. It may be of significant value as an alternative in cases in which IM sedation is necessary such as venipuncture in the uncooperative child or adult. Where more profound and more controllable levels of sedation are desired the IV route is recommended. Intranasal midazolam provides the level of sedation adequate to permit separation of the child from the parent and to enable the patient to tolerate venipuncture with minimal distress.

Sufentanil

Sufentanil was one of the first drugs to receive attention via the IN route of administration for preoperative sedation.[62] When compared, both IV and IN sufentanil (IV and IN dose of 15 μg) had rapid onset of action and limited duration.[67] At 10 minutes, all patients ($n = 8$) in the IV group were sedated compared with only two in the IN group. However no significant differences in sedation were observed

in either group at 20 to 60 minutes. These findings are in agreement with measured plasma levels of sufentanil, which are significantly lower following IN than IV at 5 and 10 minutes, being 36% and 56% of those after IV dosing, respectively. From 30 minutes plasma concentrations were virtually identical following both IN and IV sedation. An important finding was a clinically significant decrease in PaO_2 at 5 minutes after IV administration of sufentanil that was not observed following IN administration.[67] In a pediatric trial (ages 6 months to 7 years) for premedication, doses of 0.15, 0.30, and 0.45 μg/kg of sufentanil were administered IN prior to induction of general anesthesia.[68] Patients receiving sufentanil were more likely to separate willingly from their parents and to be judged as calm at or before 10 minutes compared with placebo-treated patients. However, patients receiving 0.45 μg/kg had a higher incidence of vomiting in the recovery room and during the first postoperative day. When compared with IN midazolam, IN sufentanil was accepted more readily by children but produced a significantly greater incidence of decreased PaO_2.[51]

Intranasal sufentanil produces a euphoric effect in addition to anxiolysis and sedation.[68] Its onset of action is similar to that of midazolam. However, the potential decrease in PaO_2 and the increased potential for nausea and vomiting seen following IN sufentanil administration call for intensified monitoring (oximetry and visual observation) during both the perioperative and postoperative periods. The use of IN midazolam does not appear to be associated with either of these two clinical actions.

Conclusions

The IN route of drug administration appears to be of some value in dentistry. The rapid onset of action enables IN drugs to be employed in situations in which speed is of the essence, such as in premedication of the uncooperative child. Although some degree of cooperation is necessary, IN drugs are more readily administered than oral drugs when no patient cooperation is available. As a noninvasive technique, IN administration has none of the potential side effects and complications that are associated with IM drug administration (see Chapters 4 and 11).

The two drugs that have been the most studied to date, sufentanil and midazolam, have been demonstrated to be quite effective intranasally. The IN use of sufentanil is associated with the potential development of significant opioid-related side effects, such as nausea, vomiting, and respiratory depression. The benzodiazepine midazolam provides clinical actions that are similar to sufentanil's, but it is not associated with these side effects. Intensive monitoring should be employed whenever IN drugs are administered.

REFERENCES

1. Aliberti G, D'Erasmo E, Oddo CM et al: Effect of the acute sublingual administration of ketanserin in hypertensive patients, *Cardiovasc Drugs Ther* 5(4):697, 1991.
2. DeBoer A, DeLeede L, Breimer D: Drug absorption by sublingual and rectal routes, *Br J Anaesth* 56:69, 1984.
3. Motwani JG, Lipworth BJ: Clinical pharmacokinetics of drug administered buccally and sublingually, *Clin Pharmacokinet* 21(2):83, 1991.
4. Harris D, Robinson JR: Drug delivery via the mucous membranes of the oral cavity, *J Pharm Sci* 81(1):1, 1992.
5. Carl P, Crawford ME, Masden NB et al: Pain relief after major abdominal surgery: a double-blind controlled comparison of sublingual buprenorphine, intramuscular buprenorphine, and intramuscular meperidine, *Anesth Analg* 66(2):142, 1987.
6. Schneider W, Bussmann WD, Hartmann A et al: Nitrate therapy in heart failure, *Cardiology* 79(suppl 2):5, 1991.
7. Kanabrocki EL, Bremner WF, Sothern RB et al: A quest for the relief of atherosclerosis: potential role of intrapulmonary heparin—a hypothesis, *Q J Med* 83:259, 1992.
8. Gonzalez-Ramallo VJ, Muino-Miguez A: Hypertensive crises and emergencies: the concept and initial management, *An Med Interna* 7(8):422, 1990.
9. Cohn PF: Effects of calcium channel blockers on the coronary circulation, *Am J Hypertension* 3(12, part 2):299, 1990.
10. Dire DJ, Kuhns DW: The use of sublingual nifedipine in a patient with clonidine overdose, *J Emerg Med* 6(2):125, 1988.
11. Garcia JY Jr, Vidt DG: Current management of hypertensive emergencies, *Drugs* 34(2):263, 1978.
12. Bauer JH, Reams GP: The role of calcium entry blockers in hypertensive emergencies, *Circulation* 75(6 pt 2):V174, 1987.
13. Wachter RM: Symptomatic hypotension induced by nifedipine in the acute treatment of severe hypertension, *Arch Intern Med* 147(3):556, 1987.
14. Ripamonti C, Bruera E: Rectal, buccal, and sublingual narcotics for the management of cancer pain, *J Palliative Care* 7(1):30, 1991.
15. Shepard KV, Bakst AW: Alternate delivery methods for morphine sulfate in cancer pain, *Cleve Clin J Med* 57(1):48, 1990.
16. Korttila K, Hovorka J: Buprenorphine as premedication and as analgesic during and after light isoflurane-N$_2$O-O$_2$ anaesthesia. A comparison with oxycodone plus fentanyl, *Acta Anaesthesiol Scand* 31(8):673, 1987.
17. Gram-Hansen P, Schultz A: Plasma concentrations following oral and sublingual administration of lorazepam, *Int J Clin Pharmacol Ther Toxicol* 26(6):323, 1988.
18. Garzone PD, Kroboth PD: Pharmacokinetics of the newer benzodiazepines, *Clin Pharmacokinet* 16(6):337, 1989.
19. O'Boyle CA, Barry H, Fox E et al. Controlled comparison of a new sublingual lormetazepam formulation and IV diazepam in outpatient minor oral surgery, *Br J Anaesth* 60(4):419, 1988.
20. Brandes W, Santiago T, Limacher M: Nitroglycerin-induced hypotension, bradycardia, and asystole: report of a case and review of the literature, *Clin Cardiol* 13(10):741, 1990.

21. Streisand JB, Stanley TH, Hague B et al: Oral transmucosal fentanyl citrate premedication in children, *Anesth Analg* 69(1):28, 1989.
22. Stanley TH, Hague B, Mock DL et al: Oral transmucosal fentanyl citrate (lollipop) premedication in human volunteers, *Anesth Analg* 69(1):21, 1989.
23. Stanley TH, Leiman BC, Rawal N et al: The effects of oral transmucosal fentanyl citrate premedication on preoperative behavioral responses and gastric volumes and acidity in children, *Anesth Analg* 69(3):328, 1989.
24. Nelson PS, Streisand JB, Mulder SM et al: Comparison of oral transmucosal fentanyl citrate and an oral solution of meperidine, diazepam, and atropine for premedication in children, *Anesthesiology* 70(4):616, 1989.
25. Lind GH, Marcus MA, Mears SL et al: Oral transmucosal fentanyl citrate for analgesia and sedation in the emergency department, *Ann Emerg Med* 20(10):1117, 1991.
26. Friesen RH, Lockhart CH: Oral transmucosal fentanyl citrate for preanesthetic medication of pediatric day surgery patients with and without droperidol as a prophylactic anti-emetic, *Anesthesiology* 76(1):46, 1992.
27. Feld LH, Champeau MW, van Steennis CA et al: Preanesthetic medication in children: a comparison of oral transmucosal fentanyl citrate versus placebo, *Anesthesiology* 71(3):374, 1989.
28. Ashburn MA, Streisand JB, Tarver SD et al: Oral transmucosal fentanyl citrate for premedication in paediatric outpatients, *Can J Anaesth* 37(8):857, 1990.
29. Ranade VV: Drug delivery systems. 6. Transdermal drug delivery, *J Clin Pharmacol* 31(5):401, 1991.
30. Merkle HP: Transdermal delivery systems, *Methods Find Exper Clin Pharmacol* 11(3):135, 1989.
31. Asmussen B: Transdermal therapeutic systems—actual state and future developments, *Methods Find Exper Clin Pharmacol* 13(5):343, 1991.
32. Todd PA, Goa KL, Langtry HD: Transdermal nitroglycerin (glyceryl trinitrate). A review of its pharmacology and therapeutic use, *Drugs* 40(6):880, 1990.
33. Scopoderm: transdermal hyoscine for motion sickness, *Drug Therap Bull* 27(23):91, 1989.
34. Parrott AC: Transdermal scopolamine: a review of its effects upon motion sickness, psychological performance, and physiological functioning, *Aviat Space Environ Med* 60(1):1, 1989.
35. Lowenthat DT, Matzek KM, MacGregor TR: Clinical pharmacokinetics of clonidine, *Clin Pharmacokinet* 14(5):287, 1988.
36. Balfour JA, Heel RC: Transdermal estradiol. A review of its pharmacodynamic and pharmacokinetic properties, and therapeutic efficacy in the treatment of menopausal complaints, *Drugs* 40(4):561, 1990.
37. McKenna JP, Cox JL: Transdermal nicotine replacement and smoking cessation, *Am Fam Physician* 45(6):2595, 1992.
38. Mosser KH: Transdermal fentanyl in cancer pain, *Amer Family Physic* 45(5):2289, 1992.
39. Calis KA, Kohler DR, Corso DM: Transdermally administered fentanyl for pain management, *Clin Pharm* 11(1):22, 1992.
40. Geraets D, Burke T: Sustained-release dosage forms, *Iowa Med* 80(3):141, 1990.
41. Wiechers JW: The barrier function of the skin in relation to percutaneous absorption of drugs, *Pharm Weekbl* (scientific edition) 11(6):185, 1989.
42. Xu P, Chien YW: Enhanced skin permeability for transdermal drug delivery: physiopathological and physiochemical considerations, *Crit Rev Ther Drug Carrier Syst* 8(3):211, 1991.

43. Karzel K, Liedtke RK: Mechanisms of transcutaneous absorption. Pharmacologic and biochemical aspects, *Arzneimittelforschung* 39(11A):1487, 1989.

44. Shah KR, Ng S, Zeoli L et al: Hercon technology for transdermal delivery of drugs, *J Biomater App* 1(2):239, 1986.

45. Hogan DJ, Maibach HI: Adverse dermatologic reactions to transdermal drug delivery systems, *J Am Acad Dermatol* 22(5): 811, 1990.

46. Anderson KA: A practical guide to nitrate use, *Postgrad Med* 89(1):67, 1991.

47. Clotz MA, Nahata MC: Clinical uses of fentanyl, sufentanil, and alfentanil, *Clin Pharm* 10(8):581, 1991.

48. Clissold SP, Heel RC: Transdermal hyoscine (scopolamine). A preliminary review of its pharmacodynamic properties and therapeutic efficacy, *Drugs* 29(3):189, 1985.

49. Schuh R, Tolksdorf W, Hucke H: Transdermal scopolamine or droperidol in the prevention of postoperative nausea and vomiting in cholecystectomy patients. *Anasthesiol, Intensivmedapie Notfallmed* 22(6):261, 1987.

50. Palazzo MG, Strunin L: Anaesthesia and emesis. I: Etiology, *Can Anaesthet Soc J* 31(2):1788, 1984.

51. Wilton NCT, Leigh J, Rosen DR et al: Preanesthetic sedation of preschool children using intranasal midazolam, *Anesthesiology* 69:972, 1988.

52. Saint-Maurice C, Landais A, Delleur MM et al: The use of midazolam in diagnostic and short surgical procedures in children, *Acta Anaesthes Scand Suppl* 92:39, 1990.

53. Sarkar MA: Drug metabolism in the nasal mucosa, *Pharmaceutic Res* 9(1):1, 1992.

54. Rey E, Delaunay L, Pons G et al: Pharmacokinetics of midazolam in children: comparative study of intranasal and intravenous administration, *Eur J Clin Pharmacol* 41(4):355, 1991.

55. Walbergh EJ, Wills RJ, Eckhert J: Plasma concentrations of midazolam in children following intranasal administration, *Anesthesiology* 74(2):233, 1991.

56. Rey E, Delaunay L, Pons G et al: Pharmacokinetics of midazolam in children: comparative study of intranasal and intravenous administration, *Europ J Clin Pharmacol* 41(4):355, 1991.

57. Buenz R, Gossler M: Intranasal premedication of young children using midazolam (Dormicum). Clinical experience. *Anaesthesiol Intensivmed Notfallmed Schmerzther* 26(2):76, 1991.

58. de Santos P, Chabas E, Valero R et al. Comparison of intramuscular and intranasal premedication with midazolam in children, *Revista Espanola de Anesthesiol Reanimac* 38(1):12, 1991.

59. Walbergh EJ, Wills RJ, Eckhert J: Plasma concentrations of midazolam in children following intranasal administration, *Anesthesiology* 74(2):233, 1991.

60. Rose E, Simon D, Haberer JP: Premedication with intranasal midazolam in pediatric anesthesia, *Ann Fr Anesth Reanim* 9(4): 326, 1990.

61. Karl HW, Keifer At, Rosenberger JL et al: Comparison of the safety and efficacy of intranasal midazolam and sufentanil for preinduction of anesthesia in pediatric patients, *Anesthesiology* 76(2):209, 1992.

62. Vercauteren M, Boech E, Hanegreefs H et al: Intranasal sufentanil for pre-operative sedation, *Anaesthesia* 43:270, 1988.

63. Tolksdorf W, Eick C: Rectal, oral and nasal premedication using midazolam in children aged 1-6 years. A comparative clinical study, *Anaesthetist* 40(12):661, 1991.

64. Gobeaux D, Sardnal F, Cohn H et al: Intranasal midazolam in pediatric ophthalmology, *Cah Anesthesiol* 39(1):34, 1991.

65. Lui CY, Amidon GL, Goldberg A: Intranasal absorption of flurazepam, midazolam, and triazolam in dogs, *J Pharm Sci* 80(12): 1125, 1129, 1991.

66. Theissen O, Boileau S, Wahl D et al: Sedation with intranasal midazolam for endoscopy of the upper digestive tract, *Ann Fr Anesth Reanim* 10(5):450, 1991.

67. Helmers JH, Noorduin H, van Peer A et al: Comparison of intravenous and intranasal sufentanil absorption and sedation, *Can J Anaesth* 36(5):494, 1989.

68. Henderson JM, Brodsky DA, Fisher DM et al: Pre-induction of anesthesia in pediatric patients with nasally administered sufentanil, *Anesthesiology* 68(5):671, 1988.

CHAPTER 11

Intramuscular sedation

The intramuscular (IM) route of drug administration is a parenteral technique, in which the drug enters directly into the cardiovascular system without first passing through the GI tract. Parenteral techniques possess an advantage over enteral techniques (oral, rectal) in that the drug does not first have to pass through the enterohepatic circulation before entering the systemic circulation. This eliminates several disadvantages of the oral route, including possible hepatic first-pass effect, presence of food in the stomach, and delayed gastric emptying. The advantages and disadvantages of the IM route were discussed in Chapter 4 and are summarized in Table 11-1.

Probably the most significant negative associated with the IM route is the inability to titrate the drug to a desired clinical effect. The doctor is unable to consistently predict the proper dose to administer in any given patient, leading to the use of an "educated guesstimate" based upon several factors to be discussed shortly. Although the dose is frequently appropriate, there are situations in which the calculated dose has proved ineffective, thereby leading to an inability to treat the patient; but more significantly there are occasions when the calculated dose has proved too great for the patient, leading to possibly dire consequences for both the patient and the doctor.[1-4]

The IM route of drug administration is indicated for use in almost any patient; however, several factors must be considered when determining the depth of sedation that can (should) be safely sought via this route. As mentioned, the inability to titrate is a prime negative consideration, as is the inability to rapidly reverse the actions of the drug.

Suggested use of the IM route in the dental office includes the following:

1. The adult patient, when other, more controllable, parenteral routes (IV, inhalation) are unavailable
2. The disruptive pediatric patient, in whom other routes have proved ineffective
3. The disruptive handicapped adult or child patient in whom other routes have proved ineffective
4. The disruptive pediatric or handicapped adult or child patient as premedication prior to the use of IV sedation or general anesthesia
5. The administration of emergency drugs to any patient (where the IV route is unavailable)

The last factor, the administration of emergency drugs, is the reason I believe that all dental personnel should be trained in intramuscular drug administration. Although IV drug administration is more rapidly effective than IM administration, in an emergency situation the IM route may be the only practical route immediately available.

The depth of sedation sought via the IM route will vary considerably, from lighter levels of anxiolysis (in a frightened but otherwise healthy adult) to deeper levels of sedation in the unmanageable or handicapped child or adult in whom the only alternative to IM sedation is general anesthesia. It must be stated here (as it will be over and over again throughout this text) that the doctor administering drugs to a patient must know his or her limitations in drug usage. Important factors in deciding the depth of sedation to which a patient may safely be brought include (1) the physical status of the patient, (2) the training of the doctor and staff, and (3) the availability of trained personnel and equipment for the prompt and effective management of any emergency situation that might conceivably arise as a result of the use of a drug or coincident with its use. Deep

Table 11-1. Advantages and disadvantages of intramuscular premedication

Advantages	Disadvantages
Rapid onset of action (15 minutes)	Inability to titrate (15-minute onset)
Maximal clinical effect (30 minutes)	Inability to reverse drug action
More reliable absorption (than oral, rectal)	Prolonged duration of drug effect
Patient cooperation not as essential	Injection needed
	Possible injury from injection

RECOMMENDED USE OF THE
INTRAMUSCULAR ROUTE

*For sedation in the following types of patients:

1. The adult patient, when IV and inhalation routes are unavailable
2. The disruptive pediatric or adult patient in whom other routes have proved ineffective
3. The disruptive handicapped adult or child in whom other routes have proved ineffective

*Premedication prior to IV sedation or general anesthesia in the disruptive pediatric or handicapped adult or child patient
  *Administration of antiemetics and anticholinergics
  *Administration of emergency drugs where the IV route is unavailable

---

sedation must not be employed by a doctor who is not well versed in the art and science of anesthesiology and in the management of the unconscious airway.

In the normal, healthy adult there are few indications for IM sedation. Most adults, though not "liking it," will tolerate the IM injection of a drug. If the patient can psychologically tolerate this traumatic event (the "sticking of a needle into the skin"), then the IV route of administration is preferred. The IV route is more controllable than is the IM route. If a needle is to be inserted into a patient's body for the purpose of administering a CNS depressant drug, it is much preferred, for reasons of safety and effectiveness, to administer such drugs intravenously. IV administration offers immensely more control over the drug's actions and in many cases unwanted reactions to the drug can be quickly reversed (e.g., with the administration of naloxone or flumazenil). In the absence of superficial veins elective venipuncture and IV sedation is contraindicated; the inability to breathe through the nose, or poor clinical experience in the past with inhalation sedation, contraindicates N_2O-O_2. In these situations IM sedation in an adult patient should receive serious consideration.

In the child the IM technique is much more frequently indicated. Both IV and inhalation sedation do require some patient cooperation for any degree of success to be achieved. The overtly disruptive child will neither permit a venipuncture nor allow a nasal hood to be placed and secured over the nose, thus dooming these two valuable techniques to failure. In such a situation the IM route may be the only sedative route with a likelihood of success. Failure of this technique will most likely mean that the patient will have to receive dental care under general anesthesia.

Some physically or mentally handicapped patients, both pediatric and adult, are unable to tolerate dental care in the usual manner and are therefore candidates for sedative techniques. Though many of these patients are manageable with oral, inhalation, or intravenous sedation, disruptive handicapped patients may require IM drugs as a means of calming them prior to the use of other, more controllable sedative techniques.

Another use of the IM route in dentistry is the administration of nonsedative drugs. These drugs may also be administered orally or rectally; however, because of the increased reliability of absorption and clinical activity noted with the IM route, this technique should be considered when these drugs are used. Drugs frequently employed via this route are the anticholinergics (atropine, scopolamine, glycopyrrolate) and the antiemetics (trimethobenzamide, chlorpromazine). These agents will be discussed later in this chapter.

The suggested uses of IM drug administration in dentistry are presented in the accompanying box.

Submucosal sedation

A variation on intramuscular drug administration called "submucosal (SM) administration" has been developed by pediatric dentistry.[5] In the SM technique the CNS depressant drug is injected into the mucous membrane in either the maxillary or mandibular buccal fold. An advantage of SM administration over IM is a slightly more rapid onset of clinical action.[6,7] However this same rapid onset of action may also be associated with a more rapid appearance of undesirable drug actions, such as respiratory depression. As originally developed, the SM route was used for the administration of opioid agonists such as alphaprodine.[8] The technique has fallen into disfavor because of a significant number of serious adverse reactions that were noted in conjunction with the SM administration of alphaprodine.[1-3,5] The SM route will be discussed in greater detail in the chapter on pediatric sedation (Chapter 36).

SITES OF INTRAMUSCULAR DRUG ADMINISTRATION

Four sites are available for IM drug administration.[9-11] Proper site selection will vary from patient to patient and is an important factor in the safety of this technique. The sites most commonly employed for the administration of IM drugs are the following:

1. Gluteal area
2. Ventrogluteal area
3. Vastus lateralis
4. Deltoid area

Each of these potential sites for IM drug administration has specific advantages and disadvantages that must be considered before final site selection is made.

Gluteal area

The upper outer quadrant of the gluteal region is the most frequently used site for IM drug administration in adults.[12] The gluteus maximus is the muscle most commonly injected.

The gluteal region extends superiorly to the anterior superior iliac spine (Fig. 11-1). With this as a landmark the region is divided into quadrants. The upper outer quadrant is the most anatomically safe since it is at a distance from the sciatic nerve and the superior gluteal artery.[13] The lower inner aspect of the upper outer quadrant is the preferred site within this quadrant.

The gluteal region in the adult can accept between 4 to 8 ml of solution.[10,13] In addition, the skin of this region is relatively thin and is more easily penetrated by the needle.

The upper inner quadrant is unacceptable as an IM injection site because it contains the roots of the sacral plexus. The lower inner quadrant contains the sciatic nerve. Ceravolo et al. report a nerve injury rate of up to 8% following IM injection into the gluteal region.[13]

For injection into the upper outer quadrant the patient should be lying face down on a bed or examining table with the toes in and arms hanging off the table.[14] This permits maximal relaxation. Although this site is also employed with the patient

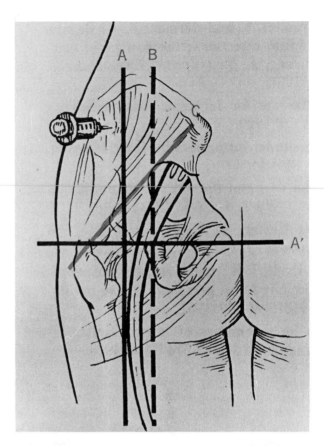

Fig. 11-1. Gluteal region, divided into quadrants. The upper outer quadrant is the recommended site for intramuscular injection. Lines *A* and *A'* represent boundaries in classic IM technique. Line *B* demonstrates ease with which landmark may be displaced, increasing the risk of sciatic nerve injury. (From Grohar ME: *How to give an intramuscular injection.* New York, 1980, Pfizer Laboratories.)

standing, it is not as highly recommended, for the muscles do not relax as well in this position. Muscle tissue that is contracted will not accommodate the injected fluid, forcing it upward into the subcutaneous tissues, where absorption is less reliable and slower and where certain chemicals are more likely to produce tissue irritation and damage. Additionally, the administration of IM drugs into contracted muscle is thought to be more uncomfortable than IM injection into relaxed muscle.[11]

Of the four available IM injection sites, the gluteal region is the least well perfused, having 20% lower perfusion than the deltoid.[15] As the rate-limiting step in the absorption of IM drugs is perfusion, the rate of onset of action of drugs administered in the gluteal region is somewhat slower than that seen elsewhere.[10,13]

The gluteal region requires some degree of patient

disrobing in order for the injection to be properly administered. This may, in some instances, limit the utility of the gluteal region in the adult patient within the dental office; however, with the assistance of the parent/guardian, this site may readily be employed in the pediatric patient with little or no loss of modesty.

Ventrogluteal region

The ventrogluteal region lies in close proximity to the gluteal region. Its primary use is for IM injection in patients who are bedridden and unable to lie face down.[13]

The site is located between three bony landmarks that are usually quite readily palpated. These are the anterior superior iliac spine, the iliac crest, and the greater trochanter of the femur. Anatomically this region lies at some distance from the sciatic nerve and other anatomically important structures.[14]

To properly employ this site the anterior superior iliac spine is located with the tip of the index finger (Fig. 11-2). The left hand is pressed onto the hip with the palm of the hand over the greater trochanter and the fingers pointed toward the patient's head. The index and middle fingers are spread as far as possible, forming a V, the tip of the ventrally placed finger pressed down on the soft tissue over the anterior superior iliac spine, preventing movement of the skin. The needle puncture is made between these fingers and aimed just below the iliac crest.

The ventrogluteal region in an adult is capable of managing between 4 to 8 ml of solution.

This site is rarely employed in the typical dental office situation. Where bedridden patients are treated, this IM site warrants consideration.

Vastus lateralis

The anterior aspect of the thigh is probably the safest region in which to deposit IM drugs. Although not of consequence in the typical dental situation, this muscle mass is capable of receiving considerable volumes of solution, up to 15 ml, whereas the gluteal and ventrogluteal can accommodate approximately 6 to 8 ml each before muscle distortion and dissection occur, leading to increased pain during and after injection.

The site for injection in the vastus lateralis muscle is a narrow rectangular band running along the anterior lateral aspect of the thigh (Fig. 11-3). The region begins approximately one hand breadth above the knee and runs to the same distance below the greater trochanter of the femur.[14]

Anatomically the vastus lateralis site contains no

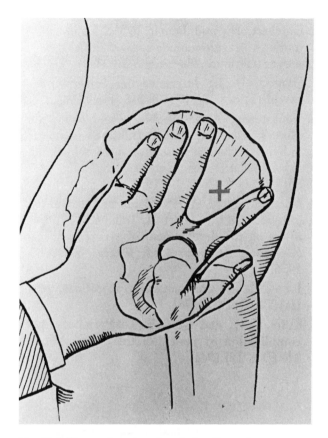

Fig. 11-2. Ventrogluteal region. Index finger locates anterior iliac spine, index and middle fingers spread apart forming a V. Needle puncture occurs between fingers (**X**) and is aimed toward iliac crest. (Courtesy Abbott Laboratories.)

structures of importance (Fig. 11-4). Overly deep penetration of the needle may strike the femur, producing discomfort and possible needle breakage. All significant anatomical structures are located on the medial and posterior aspects of the thigh (the femoral artery and vein and the sciatic nerve).

This site is strongly recommended for use in small children.[10] Injection in the gluteal muscles is contraindicated in children who have not yet begun to walk because of the lack of maturity and development of their gluteal musculature. The gluteal region ought not to be chosen until at least 1 full year after the child has begun to walk.[17]

Some degree of disrobing is required when the vastus lateralis site is used. The site is more readily accessible in the woman wearing a skirt or dress, but it is of absolute importance that a female assistant be present with the doctor in the treatment room throughout the time that the injection is given. In any patient wearing pants or slacks, a greater degree

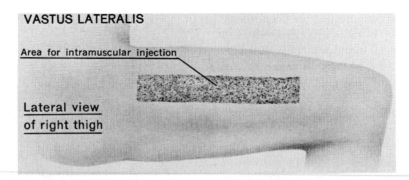

Fig. 11-3. Location of vastus lateralis injection site on anterior lateral aspect of thigh. Preferred site for IM drug administration in infants and children. (From Grohar ME: *How to give an intramuscular injection.* New York, 1980, Pfizer Laboratories.)

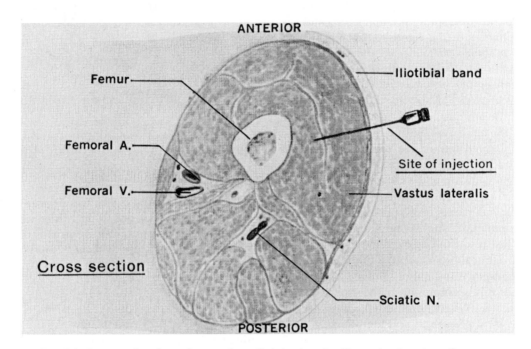

Fig. 11-4. Cross section through vastus lateralis injection site illustrating location of anatomically significant structures. (From Grohar ME: *How to give an intramuscular injection.* New York, 1980, Pfizer Laboratories.)

of disrobing is required, a fact that may discourage use of this site. In the pediatric patient this site may readily be employed, with the assistance of the patient's parent or guardian.

In adult or larger pediatric patients who are unmanageable (e.g., combative) and where IM drug administration is considered mandatory, injection of the drug into the vastus lateralis muscle through the patient's clothing is appropriate. Though sterile technique cannot be maintained in this situation, it is unlikely that complications will be noted. This consideration is of especial importance when a life-threatening situation develops (e.g., anaphylaxis)

and immediate drug therapy is warranted (e.g., epinephrine).

The vastus lateralis muscle is capable of receiving between 8 and 15 ml of injected drug (in adults) without distortion or dissection of muscle fibers. This represents the largest available reservoir for IM drugs in the adult body.

Deltoid

The deltoid muscle is easily accessible in the upper third of the arm. The injection is given between the upper and lower portions of the deltoid muscle (Fig. 11-5), thereby avoiding the radial nerve.

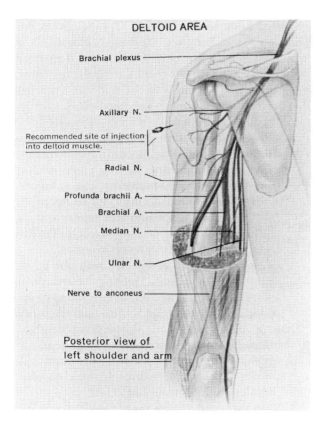

DELTOID AREA

Brachial plexus

Axillary N.

Recommended site of injection into deltoid muscle.

Radial N.

Profunda brachii A.

Brachial A.

Median N.

Ulnar N.

Nerve to anconeus

Posterior view of left shoulder and arm

Fig. 11-5. Mid-deltoid injection site in upper third of arm. (From Grohar ME: *How to give an intramuscular injection.* New York, 1980, Pfizer Laboratories.)

The boundaries of the deltoid region form a rectangle. The superior border is formed by the lower edge of the acromion (the outward extension of the spine of the scapula). The inferior boundary lies opposite the axilla or armpit. The side boundaries are two lines drawn parallel to the arm, about one third to two thirds of the way around the lateral aspect of the upper arm.

Advantages of this site include its easy access in most patients. It is important that the patient not be permitted to simply roll up the shirt sleeve to expose the injection site, for if the sleeve is tight it may not permit visualization of the entire site, in which case the injection might be administered inferior to the desired area and in too close proximity to the radial nerve. The patient should be required to remove his shirt or blouse in order to expose the entire injection site. A female assistant must be with the doctor (male or female) if the patient is female. Another positive factor in the deltoid region is a more rapid absorption of the injected drug into the cardiovascular system than is seen with any of the other IM injection sites. Perfusion is 20% greater in the deltoid region than in the gluteal region.[13]

Table 11-2. Comparison of IM injection sites

IM injection site recommended for:	Perfusion	Maximum volume (ml for adult)	Infant	Child	Adult
Vastus lateralis	2	8-15	+	+	+
Gluteal/ventrogluteal	3	4-8	−	−	−/+
Deltoid	1	4	−	−	−

1 = most vascular
3 = least vascular

The deltoid region is not recommended for use in the infant or child who has not yet begun to walk.[10]

The degree of disrobing required to visualize the injection site is not usually of significance in the deltoid region, making this the most easily employed IM injection site within the practice of dentistry. This site may be used with the patient lying down, sitting, or standing.

Probably the only negative feature of this site, other than the anatomy, is its lack of size; it is only able to accommodate up to 4 ml of solution (adult). However, this is not of significance in dentistry as it is rare to ever administer more than 3 ml IM. Giovannitti and Trapp[18] suggest the deltoid muscle as the preferred site for IM sedation in the dental environment.

Site selection

Selection of the site for IM injection in dentistry is predicated on several factors, including the size (age) of the patient, degree of patient cooperation, and volume of solution to be injected. In the younger (smaller) pediatric patient, the preferred site for IM injection is the vastus lateralis, whereas in older children the vastus lateralis and the deltoid regions are recommended. In the adult, the preferred sites for IM injection are the deltoid region, vastus lateralis, and either gluteal injection sites.

Table 11-2 compares the four IM injection sites.

ARMAMENTARIUM

Very few items are required for the administration of an IM injection. Included in this list are the following:
1. Sterile, disposable syringe (1 to 2 ml) with needle (18-, 20-, or 21-gauge) of appropriate length
2. Alcohol sponges
3. Sterile gauze
4. Band-aid type of bandage
5. Desired medication

There is a very real concern for self-inflicted puncture injuries amongst health professionals with pos-

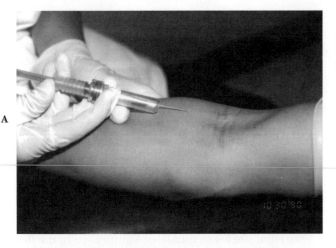

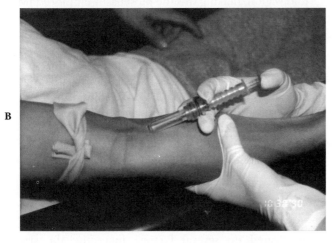

Fig. 11-6. Self-sheathing needle and syringe. **A,** Sheath unit with sheath retracted. **B,** Sheath unit with sheath over needle. (Courtesy Square One Medical, Camarillo, Calif.)

sible infection with either HIV or hepatitis.[19-22] Syringes and other devices (such as the "Sharps" container) have been developed that permit IM drug administration with a minimum risk of needle-stick injury.[23-25] These "safe syringes" prevent accidental needlestick following drug administration through a self-locking sheath that covers the exposed (and contaminated) needle. One such device is illustrated in Fig. 11-6.

TECHNIQUE

The appropriate injection site for the IM injection must be selected. After disrobing the patient if necessary, the doctor must carefully palpate the site on every patient to determine the precise anatomic landmarks. Visual examination alone should never

be relied upon to determine landmarks. From the point of view of propriety (and medicolegally) it is important that the doctor have another staff member present in the treatment room during the injection, especially if the patient is of the opposite sex from the doctor. The following are step-by-step instructions for the administration of an IM injection[10,14]:

1. Cleanse the skin thoroughly using a suitable antiseptic (e.g., isopropyl alcohol). Apply friction while cleansing the area with a circular motion from the injection site outward. The antiseptic should be permitted to dry prior to injection. Injection into a moistened area may introduce antiseptic into the tissues, which will lead to discomfort and possibly to tissue irritation.

2. Grasp the tissue to be injected with one hand, keeping the tissue taut. Holding the syringe in a dartlike grasp, introduce the needle to its appropriate depth (deep within muscle tissue) with one quick motion. Although the depth of insertion will vary from patient to patient, the needle should not be inserted, for safety reasons, more than approximately three quarters of its length into tissue (Fig. 11-7).

3. With the needle at its proper depth, aspirate, pulling the plunger of the syringe back slightly to determine if the needle tip lies within the lumen of a blood vessel. Rotate the syringe a quarter turn and reaspirate, to assure that the needle tip was not lying against the wall of a vessel. If blood appears in the syringe at any time, withdraw the syringe from the tissue and prepare a different injection site. In the uncooperative pediatric or adult patient it may prove difficult or impossible to perform this step as described. Aspiration should be performed whenever possible prior to IM injection.

4. Following negative aspiration, inject the drug slowly. In most IM injections the solution flows quite easily into the tissues. Rapid injection produces increased patient discomfort and should be avoided. Release the pressure that has been maintained on the tissues during needle insertion. Maintaining the pressure during injection of the drug may force solution to backtrack along the path of needle insertion into the subcutaneous tissues, where tissue irritation may occur, or out of the tissue through the injection site. Release of pressure prevents this from occurring.

5. Holding a dry sterile gauze in the other hand

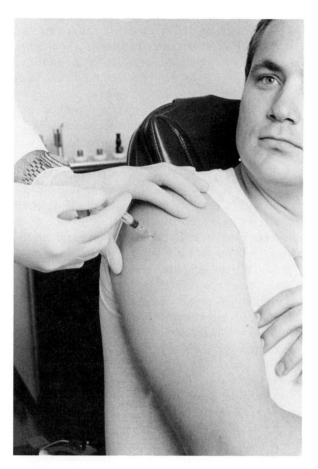

Fig. 11-7. Area to be injected is grasped with one hand, holding tissue taut, while the syringe, held in a dart-like grasp, is inserted to the proper depth.

(non-syringe-holding hand), slowly withdraw the needle from the tissue. Place the dry gauze over the puncture point for approximately 2 minutes, to prevent bleeding. A bandage can be placed over the site at this time.

Care must be taken with the now contaminated needle to prevent accidental percutaneous puncture of the treating staff. The used needle/syringe should be disposed of in a Sharps container.

6. Massage or rub the injection site to increase the blood flow through the area and speed up drug absorption.

7. Record in the patient's chart the date, time of injection, site of injection, drug used, and dose.

8. Observe the patient during the post-IM injection period for the onset of sedation and/or undesirable actions (e.g., syncope, overdose, allergy).

COMPLICATIONS

Though rare, complications can arise following IM drug administration. In most cases the complication appears to be directly related to the site of needle entry and drug deposition.[26]

The needle itself is capable of producing injury to structures through which it passes. Nerve damage, consisting of paralysis (usually of the sciatic nerve in gluteal injection), hyperesthesia, or paresthesia, has been reported following IM injection. In addition, inadvertent IV and intraarterial drug administration have occurred, as well as air embolism, periostitis, and hematoma. Many of these complications have potentially serious consequences and should of course be avoided. Knowledge of anatomy and proper injection technique will minimize these complications.

The drugs that are administered intramuscularly are, in some cases, capable of producing injury to the tissues into which they are deposited. Injuries such as *abscess, cyst and scar formation, and necrosis and sloughing of skin* at the injection site may occur. Although these are potential complications with all drugs, there are a few drugs that, because of their pH or viscosity, are more apt to produce these problems. These drugs include diazepam and hydroxyzine. Improper injection technique, specifically when the drug has not been injected deep into the muscle, or when the tissue is kept taut following the injection of the drug with leakage of the drug into the subcutaneous tissues as the needle is withdrawn, is a common cause of this problem.

Nerve injury of any type is managed conservatively. In many cases the injury may not be noted by the patient for several days following IM injection or in the case of a younger patient or a handicapped patient, possibly for several months, thus emphasizing the importance of precise record keeping. The site of injection should always be recorded when an IM drug is given. When injury is detected, the patient should return to the office so that the nature and extent of the injury may be noted on the chart. Unless the injury is severe the management of choice for most nerve injury is "tincture of time." Most minor traumatic injuries to nerves will resolve with time. In most instances normal function will return within 6 months. The patient should be advised of this time factor at the onset. Some few cases of nerve injury will not resolve completely within 6 months, requiring additional time (an unknown duration), or in fact may never return completely to normal function. Periodic examination of the patient during this time span (e.g., once every month) is recommended, to keep the doctor informed of any progress and to keep the patient aware of the doctor's concern.

Discomfort secondary to the injury should be manageable with milder analgesics, such as aspirin, acetaminophen, or another NSAID. If more potent analgesics are required, consultation with a physician is recommended, as this might indicate a greater degree of injury.

If the injury appears more severe at the onset, the patient should be referred to a physician, preferably a neurologist, for examination. Management in most instances will be consistent with that described. Referral to a physician should also be given serious consideration if the patient appears to be dissatisfied with the progress of his recovery or with the management of the injury by the "dental doctor." Prior to referral of the patient to the physician, a telephone call from the dentist, explaining the circumstances surrounding the case, is appropriate.

Although legal action following nerve injury does occur, the percentage of such cases is extremely small. A patient who is satisfied with the treatment is less likely to initiate a legal action than the patient who believes that the care rendered is below the usual standard.

Inadvertent IV or intraarterial (IA) drug administration ought never occur. Proper IM technique recommends aspiration prior to injection of the drug. The presence of blood in the syringe indicates a positive aspiration. The doctor should remove the syringe from the injection site, apply pressure to the site to prevent hematoma, and reinject the patient at a different site.

Because the drugs being administered for sedation are CNS depressants, the clinical signs and symptoms attending this complication (accidental IV or IA administration) will be related to the degree of CNS depression that develops. This may range from a slightly oversedated patient—one who is conscious but sedated to a degree beyond which the doctor feels comfortable—to the patient who may be unconscious but breathing (requiring airway management), to the unconscious patient whose breathing is quite depressed or who may be apneic. This latter patient will require airway management and artificial ventilation. The pharmacology and the blood levels of the drug(s) injected will determine the severity of the reaction that develops. Some antianxiety drugs, such as benzodiazepines (e.g., midazolam) and hydroxyzine, are less likely to produce (though they are capable of producing) significant CNS depression than are the barbiturates and opioids.

Management of the oversedated patient consists primarily of airway maintenance and, when necessary, assisted or controlled ventilation. In addition, some drugs, such as the opioids and benzodiazepines, have pharmacologic antagonists that may be administered in these circumstances. Their use, and a more detailed discussion of the management of the oversedated patient, will be found in Chapters 28 and 35.

Air embolism has been reported following IM drug administration. With proper technique in loading a syringe with a drug there ought not be any air remaining in its barrel. In addition, avoidance of inadvertent intravascular injection (see previous discussion) will prevent this occurrence.

Periostitis is an inflammation of the periosteum. If acute, it may be associated with severe pain and suppuration and is usually secondary to infection. The condition usually becomes chronic in nature and is characterized by tenderness and swelling of the tissues overlying the bone. It may also be produced by the inadvertent striking of the needle against the periosteum during insertion. Proper technique involves grasping the tissue being injected between the fingers, pulling it off the bone, and inserting the needle to the proper depth (varying from patient to patient and from site to site). This technique will minimize the development of periostitis.

If the patient complains of soreness, tenderness, and swelling at the site of an IM injection 2 or more days following injection, the complaint should be evaluated by bringing the patient to the office, examining the area and, if need be, seeking a medical consultation. Management of milder degrees of periostitis involve "tincture of time" and the maintenance of good relations with the patient. If signs of suppuration and swelling appear, antibiotics are indicated (usually penicillin). Medical consultation should be sought in this latter situation.

Hematoma is, by definition, a tumor consisting of effused blood. It develops following puncture of a blood vessel, either an artery or a vein. Clinically a small but gradually enlarging swelling, bluish in color, will be observed at the site of needle insertion, either during injection or, more commonly, after withdrawal of the syringe from the tissues. Management consists of pressure applied directly to the site of bleeding for a minimum of 2 minutes. If the site subsequently becomes sore, heat can be applied to it (but not less than 4 hours after the bleeding ceases) and mild analgesics may be administered. The effused blood will be gradually resorbed into the cardiovascular system, a process requiring 7 to 10 days.

COMPLICATION OF IM INJECTIONS

Nerve injury
    Paralysis
    Paresthesia
    Hyperesthesia
Intravascular injection
    IV
    Intraarterial
Air embolism
Periostitis
Hematoma
Abcess
Cyst and scar formation
Necrosis and sloughing of skin

Heat should not be applied to the site of a hematoma within the first few hours as heat produces vasodilation, a process that may restart the bleeding.

An *abscess* may occur following IM injection if either the needle or the solution injected was contaminated. Management consists of antibiotics (penicillin) and immediate medical consultation. Prevention consists of sterile technique in handling both drugs and equipment.

Cyst formation, *scarring*, and *necrosis* and *sloughing* of tissues may also occur. Although several factors may be responsible for these, many are produced by the tissues' reaction to the injected drug. Drugs that are irritating to the tissues are more commonly involved in these complications. Injection of drugs into superficial tissues is another cause of this problem. Management should consist of referral to a physician, preferably a dermatologist. Complications of IM injections are listed in the box above.

DETERMINATION OF DOSAGE

The many factors that influence the way in which a drug acts in a given patient were discussed in Chapters 4 and 8. With IM administration of CNS depressants, the influence of these various factors becomes quite important. How then can the informed clinician safely determine the appropriate IM dose of the drug or drugs that are to be administered to a patient for intraoperative sedation?

Most drugs that are administered intramuscularly have their dosages determined, in large part, by the body weight of the patient. Although this is far from an absolute guarantee of proper dosage, in most situations a therapeutically effective result will occur.

Other factors that should be considered in determining the dosage include the degree of anxiety of the patient, the level of sedation desired, the patient's age, the patient's health status, prior response of the patient to CNS depressant drugs, and the education and experience of the drug's administrator.

For the adult patient dosages for the drugs discussed will be based primarily on body weight, expressed in milligrams per pound or milligrams per kilogram. From this dose the doctor will subtract or add additional drug as determined from the other factors mentioned. For example, a patient weighing 150 pounds is to receive a drug, the recommended dose of which is 0.5 mg/lb. The calculated dose of this drug for the patient is therefore 75 mg. If the patient were a normal, healthy individual (ASA I), this dose would be appropriate; however, if this patient is older, has a history of cardiovascular or other serious systemic disease, or has a history of overreaction to average drug dosages, a smaller dose (e.g., 50 mg) might be administered. The level to which the drug dosage is decreased is left to the clinical judgment of the doctor administering it. Conversely, an ASA I patient demonstrating high levels of anxiety, with a history of hyporesponding to drugs of a nature similar to that being administered, might be given a dose somewhat greater than that determined strictly by body weight.

In the pediatric patient the same factors must be considered when determining the dosage of a drug. The patient's age is often considered in determining the dosage of a drug. For example, for a given drug the dose for a 3-year-old patient may be 12.5 mg, while the dose for a 4-year-old is 25 mg. Dosages based solely on the patient's age are apt to lead to inaccuracies, as patients of the same age will vary considerably in physical stature and body weight. The patient's age should not be the primary factor by which the dose of a drug is determined.

Several rules have been used for years in the determination of pediatric drug dosages. Clark's rule takes the weight of the child in pounds and divides it by 150 (the weight of the average adult in pounds). The resultant fraction is multiplied by the adult dosage of the drug.

Clark's rule:

$$\text{Pediatric dose} = \frac{\text{Weight of child (lb)}}{150} \times \text{Adult dose}$$

Young's rule divides the age of the child in years by the age of the child plus 12, multiplying this number by the adult dose.

Table 11-3. Determination of children's doses from adult doses on the basis of body surface area

Weight		Approximate surface area in square meters	Approximate percentage of adult dose*
(kg)	*(lb)*		
2	4.4	0.15	9
4	8.8	0.25	14
6	13.2	0.33	19
8	17.6	0.40	23
10	22.0	0.46	27
15	33.0	0.63	36
20	44.0	0.83	48
25	55.0	0.95	55
30	66.0	1.08	62
35	77.0	1.20	69
40	88.0	1.30	75
45	99.0	1.40	81
50	110.0	1.51	87
55	121.0	1.58	91

Adapted from Done AK: In Modell W, ed: *Drugs of choice 1972-1973*. St Louis, 1972, Mosby.
*Based on average adult surface area of 1.73 square meters.

Young's rule:

$$\text{Pediatric dose} = \frac{\text{Age of child (yr)}}{\text{Age} + 12} \times \text{Adult dose}$$

A factor that has proved to be even more accurate in determining effective pediatric dosages is the body surface area of the patient. Table 11-3 permits a determination of the approximate surface area of the patient. The pediatric dosage will be determined as a percentage of the usual adult dosage, based on the average adult surface area of 1.73 square meters.

Most of the drugs discussed in this chapter will have their dosages presented on a milligram per pound or kilogram of body weight basis. Though not the most accurate method available, this is today the most frequently employed technique of determining IM drug dosage. The reader may employ the surface area method of determining pediatric dosages for any drug listed in this book by simply referring to Table 11-3.

Dosages based upon body weight (e.g., 1 mg/kg or 0.5 mg/lb) are determined by the middle of the "bell-shaped" curve (see Fig. 8-1). Approximately 70% of patients will respond appropriately to this dose with 15% being undersedated. Unfortunately, another 15% will respond in an exaggerated manner—oversedation.

The degree of education and experience of the drug administrator has a significant bearing on the

---

DETERMINANTS OF IM DOSE

Body weight
Degree of anxiety
Level of sedation desired
Age
Health status
Prior response to CNS depressant drugs
Education and experience of drug administrator
Surface area (pediatric patient)

---

level of sedation to which the patient may safely be taken, which will obviously influence the drug dosage to be administered. Doctors who have completed residency training in anesthesiology will be better able to administer larger dosages of drugs to patients in a safe manner than doctors who have merely completed a short postgraduate program. All dental personnel involved in patient management should be adept in monitoring vital signs and in recognizing and managing life-threatening emergencies, including the ability to perform basic life support.

DRUGS

A myriad of drugs is available for the management of anxiety via IM administration. The level of sedation may vary from lighter levels (conscious sedation) to levels approaching unconsciousness (deep sedation). Although certain drugs are more apt to produce more profound sedation than others, any of the drugs listed below can produce overly deep sedation. When determining the dosage of the drug or drugs to be administered intramuscularly, it must always be remembered that the administrator cannot control the drug's action, that titration is not possible, via this route. Care and prudence must be exercised whenever IM drugs are administered to any patient, but especially to pediatric, geriatric, and medically compromised patients. The following outline lists drugs that are frequently employed via IM administration for sedation in dentistry. As will be noted with specific drugs, different levels of training are recommended for the safe use of many of these agents. In some situations the doctor should have received training in general anesthesia and be capable of managing the unconscious airway before ever considering the use of the drug in question.

Antianxiety drugs and sedative-hypnotics
Chlordiazepoxide
Diazepam

Lorazepam
Midazolam
   Antihistamines
Promethazine
Hydroxyzine
   Barbiturates
Secobarbital
Pentobarbital
   Opioid analgesics
Morphine
Meperidine
Fentanyl
   Opioid agonist/antagonists
Pentazocine
Butorphanol
Nalbuphine
   Dissociative anesthetic
Ketamine hydrochloride
   Anticholinergics
Atropine
Scopolamine
Glyocopyrrolate

Antianxiety drugs and sedative-hypnotics

In this grouping of drugs I have included the benzodiazepines, barbiturates, and antihistamines, drugs that are commonly used for light-to-moderate levels of conscious sedation when employed as solo agents. It is not uncommon to combine one of the drugs in this category with an opioid analgesic to provide deeper levels of sedation. When so doing it is necessary for the doctor and all staff members to have been thoroughly trained in general anesthesia and patient monitoring.

Chlordiazepoxide. Chlordiazepoxide (Librium) is one of but a few benzodiazepines that are available for parenteral administration.

Patients receiving chlordiazepoxide parenterally should be cautioned against the operation of a car or other potentially hazardous machinery for the remainder of the day.

Because the parenteral preparation of chlordiazepoxide is not very stable, the agent is prepared for use immediately prior to its administration. Two milliliters of an IM diluent (provided with the drug) is injected into the ampule of chlordiazepoxide powder (100 mg). The solution is agitated slowly and gently until the powder is completely dissolved. This provides a solution of chlordiazepoxide at 50 mg/ml.

Chlordiazepoxide should be administered deep into muscle to minimize discomfort and to optimize absorption. It is recommended that the drug be deposited slowly into the upper outer quadrant of the gluteus muscle.[27] Any unused agent should be discarded. Following parenteral administration deep into muscle, the onset of action will be approximately 15 minutes. Maximal clinical effect arises 30 minutes following injection, with a gradual decrease in clinical action over the next 3 to 5 hours.[28]

Because of the necessity to prepare chlordiazepoxide immediately before injection, the agent is rarely employed within the dental profession for IM sedation. Other benzodiazepines and other classes of drugs are more readily available for parenteral administration.

Dosage. The usual adult dose for preoperative sedation is 50 to 100 mg 1 hour before treatment. The usual dose for elderly or debilitated patients is 25 to 50 mg 1 hour before treatment. Chlordiazepoxide injectable is not recommended in patients below the age of 12 years.

Availability. Librium (Roche): 5-ml dry-filled ampule, containing 100 mg chlordiazepoxide hydrochloride in dry crystalline form; 2-ml ampule of Special Intramuscular Diluent, containing 1.5% benzyl alcohol, 4% polysorbate 80, 20% propylene glycol, 1.6% maleic acid, and sodium hydroxide (to adjust pH to 3.0). When prepared for injection the concentration of the chlordiazepoxide is 50 mg/ml. Chlordiazepoxide is classified as a Schedule IV drug.

Diazepam. Diazepam (Valium) is commonly employed via the IM route in preoperative anxiety control in the hospital setting. It is employed in dentistry via this route, but because of the availability of the IV route, IM administration of diazepam is infrequently used.

Another reason for the infrequent use of diazepam IM were the results of early studies on the absorption of diazepam from IM injection sites. Diazepam injectable is an extremely lipophilic drug and early studies on absorption of IM diazepam were conflicting.[29-32] Peak plasma levels were noted 60 minutes following oral dosing while IM dosing required 90 minutes.[32] Absorption of diazepam from IM injection sites may be slow or incomplete or both because of its lipophilic nature. However, a recent report indicates that IM diazepam absorption appears to be more rapid when the drug is injected into the deltoid rather than the gluteal or vastus lateralis muscle groups.[33] The most likely explanation is the higher blood flow per gram of tissue in the deltoid muscle group.[31] In the gluteal area the depth of injection may be a factor in the completeness of absorption of diazepam. Given equal doses of diazepam via the oral and IM routes, the oral dose will be absorbed more completely than the IM dose, and in many cases the rate of onset will be shorter via the oral route than with the IM route.[32] However, diazepam deposited deeply into muscle (preferably the deltoid) can produce satisfactory sedation in most patients.

Contraindications. Parenteral diazepam should be avoided in patients with known hypersensitivities to it or other benzodiazepines, in patients with acute narrow-angle glaucoma, and in patients with narrow-angle glaucoma unless they are receiving appropriate therapy.

Warnings. When used in combination with other CNS depressants, particularly opioid analgesics, the dosage of the opioid should be decreased by approximately one third to minimize the occurrence of oversedation or of other more serious complications.

Diazepam should not be employed during the first trimester of pregnancy because an increased risk of congenital malformations has been observed. Diazepam crosses the placental barrier, potentially producing depression of the fetus. Its use in pregnancy is not recommended.

Injectable diazepam dosages should be decreased when patients are receiving other CNS depressants, such as barbiturates, phenothiazines, opioids, and alcohol.

Elderly and debilitated patients usually require decreased dosages of diazepam to achieve a desired clinical effect.

Dosage. The usual adult dose for preoperative sedation is 10 mg 30 minutes to 1 hour before treatment. The preferred injection site for diazepam is the deltoid muscle. Regardless of the IM injection site, diazepam should be deposited deep into muscle to avoid discomfort and provide more reliable absorption.[35] The dose for elderly or debilitated patients is 2 to 5 mg 30 minutes to 1 hour prior to treatment. The dose of parenteral diazepam for children should not exceed 0.25 mg/kg of body weight, administered deep into the gluteal or deltoid regions. For example, a child weighing 20 kg (44 lb) will receive a dose of 5 mg IM diazepam. Since the introduction of midazolam the IM use of diazepam has markedly diminished.

Availability. Valium (Roche): 5 mg/ml in 2-ml ampules and 10-ml vials; 5 mg/ml in 2-ml preloaded syringes. Injectable diazepam also contains 40% propylene glycol, 10% ethyl alcohol, 5% sodium benzoate, benzoic acid, and 1.5% benzyl alcohol. Diazepam is classified as a Schedule IV drug.

Lorazepam. Lorazepam (Ativan) is another benzodiazepine available for use parenterally. Its action following parenteral administration is primarily that of sedation rather than anxiolysis. A potential benefit of IM lorazepam is that it frequently provides a degree of amnesia. This lack of recall is maximal within 2 hours of IM injection.

Because the agent is virtually insoluble in water, its onset of action may prove to be prolonged in some patients although, like diazepam, the onset of action will be about 15 minutes in most patients. Peak plasma levels of lorazepam are seen in 60 to 90 minutes.[35] The duration of action of lorazepam following IM administration is approximately 6 to 8 hours. The major side effect is excessive sleepiness and a prolonged amnesic period.

Odugbesan and Magbagbeola[36] recommended that the IV route be preferred to IM for administration of lorazepam, providing a somewhat more rapid onset of activity. Patients receiving lorazepam IM must not be permitted to leave the dental office unescorted and must be advised of the possibly enhanced CNS depressant actions of other agents such as opioids, alcohol, and barbiturates. Because of the prolonged duration of action of lorazepam, this agent is seldom employed in the practice of dentistry.

Warnings. Lorazepam should not be administered to pregnant patients as it may increase the risk of congenital malformation. Patients must be advised against driving a car or operating hazardous machinery for a period of 24 to 48 hours, a period of time that may severely limit the usefulness of this agent in an ambulatory dental patient.

Precautions. Additive CNS depression is observed when lorazepam is administered concurrently with barbiturates, alcohol, opioids, phenothiazines, antidepressants, scopolamine, and MAOIs. When scopolamine is used concurrently with lorazepam, the incidence of hallucinations and irrational behavior is increased. The IM use of lorazepam has resulted in discomfort at the injection site, including a sensation of burning, or observed redness. The overall incidence of burning and pain is about 17% immediately after the injection and 1.4% 24 hours later. Two percent of patients receiving IM lorazepam had redness immediately after the injection, 0.5% after 24 hours.[35]

Dosage. The usual adult dose of lorazepam for preoperative sedation is 0.05 mg/kg (0.025 mg/lb) to a maximum of 4 mg. The agent should be administered undiluted deep into the muscle mass. If dilution is desired (it is not recommended for IM injection), sterile water for injection, sodium chloride injection, and 5% dextrose injection are compatible solutions. The use of lorazepam in patients under the age of 18 years is not recommended because of insufficient data.

Availability. Ativan (Wyeth): 2 mg/ml and 4 mg/ml in 10-ml vials. The drug should be stored in a refrigerator. Lorazepam is classified as a Schedule IV drug.

Midazolam. Midazolam (Versed, Dormicum, Hypnovel) is a water-soluble benzodiazepine recently approved for use in the United States. It is well absorbed following intramuscular administration, and has been employed with increasing frequency as an alternative to the opioid agonists as a means of pretreatment anxiety control. In the author's clinic midazolam IM has been employed with great success as a sole agent or in conjunction with IV midazolam in the management of handicapped patients (adult and pediatric) as well as in the management of behavioral problems in pediatric dentistry.[37,38] These techniques are described in detail in Chapters 36 and 39. IM midazolam provides a degree of retrograde amnesia in many patients following IM administration.[39]

Warnings. Midazolam, like other CNS depressants, can produce respiratory depression. This is especially likely to occur in patients who are receiving other CNS depressants (opioids, barbiturates) concurrently and in patients with preexisting cardiopulmonary disease. Special care must be taken whenever midazolam is administered to these patients.

Dosage. For use in the extremely fearful pediatric or handicapped patient, I have employed an IM dose of 0.15 mg/kg.[37,38] Dosages should be decreased in the presence of cardiorespiratory disease or other indicators of increased responsiveness to benzodiazepines. Continuous monitoring of the patient is essential once the drug is administered.

Availability. Versed (Roche Labs): 1 mg/ml and 5 mg/ml in 2-ml and 5-ml ampules. Midazolam is classified as a Schedule IV drug.

• • •

The benzodiazepines chlordiazepoxide and lorazepam are seldom employed in dentistry via the IM route. The primary dental indication for the use of lorazepam IM might be a patient about to undergo a long dental appointment (over 3 hours) or one in whom a degree of amnesia is desired. Diazepam has received considerable use as an IM agent for preoperative sedation, although primarily in hospital situations rather than in dentistry. When injected deep into muscle, especially the deltoid, it appears to be an effective preoperative sedative. Midazolam, a water-soluble benzodiazepine, has proved to be a very effective IM sedative agent, especially in the pediatric and handicapped population.

Antihistamines (histamine blockers)

Two drugs classified as antihistamines are commonly administered via the IM route for sedation prior to dental treatment. They are used primarily in pediatric dentistry but may also be used effectively in the adult patient.

The pharmacology of these agents, promethazine and hydroxyzine, has been reviewed in Chapter 8, as these drugs are also effective anxiolytics when administered orally. In this section the clinical pharmacology of these agents following IM administration will be presented.

Promethazine. Promethazine hydrochloride, a phenothiazine derivative, is frequently employed via the IM or IV route for the management of anxiety. Other indications for use of this drug include the management of allergic reactions and motion sickness and use as an antiemetic and as a preoperative sedative.[40]

When administered parenterally subcutaneous injection is contraindicated because promethazine produces localized tissue irritation that may possibly lead to necrosis and sloughing. Deep IM administration is preferred to subcutaneous administration. The risk of this complication is considerably diminished with IM administration because of the superior vascularity of muscle. Onset of action following IM administration is rapid (10 to 15 minutes). The duration of action, however, is quite long, the patient usually feeling the effects of the drug for up to 24 hours. If the patient is a child, the parent must be cautioned to watch the child during this time, not permitting bicycle riding or participation in any hazardous activities. The adult patient must also be cautioned and advised not to drive a car or operate hazardous machinery.

As the degree of sedation produced by IM promethazine as a sole IM agent will be mild, it is common for promethazine to be administered in conjunction with an opioid whenever more profound sedation is required. Occasionally promethazine will be administered in combination with a barbiturate and an atropine-like agent. This latter combination is employed commonly as premedication for the hospitalized patient about to undergo surgery and general anesthesia. It is extremely important to remember that when promethazine is combined with an opioid, the dose of the opioid must be decreased by 25% to 50%; if it is combined with a barbiturate the barbiturate dose must be reduced by 50%. Promethazine may produce additive effects with other CNS depressants or the effect may be one of potentiation. In either case the administration of average doses of both CNS depressants is likely to result in excessive degrees of CNS and possible respiratory depression.

In addition to its antihistaminic, sedative, and antiemetic effects, promethazine also possesses anticholinergic properties. For this reason promethazine is not recommended for patients with narrow-angle glaucoma, prostatic hypertrophy, stenosing peptic ulcer, pyloroduodenal obstruction, and bladderneck obstruction. Because these medical disorders are rarely mentioned on the typical medical history questionnaire, the doctor considering use of promethazine must question the patient specifically about these problems.

When used as a sole agent in pediatric dentistry, promethazine is effective in the management of children with lesser degrees of anxiety. It will not, however, be effective in the management of children with extreme apprehension or of the disruptive, unmanageable child. In these situations promethazine will be combined with other CNS depressants, most commonly opioids, such as meperidine. A discussion of the use of these drugs in combinations will be presented in Chapter 36.

Dosage. The usual dose of promethazine for adults for preoperative sedation is 25 to 50 mg 1 hour prior to treatment. The dose as an antiemetic is 12.5 to 25 mg every 4 hours. The dose for children for preoperative sedation is 0.5 mg/lb or 1.0 mg/kg, not to exceed 50 mg.

Availability. Phenergan (Wyeth-Ayerst): 25 and 50 mg per ml.

Hydroxyzine. Hydroxyzine hydrochloride is available for parenteral administration. The drug is not recommended for IV, intraarterial, or subcutaneous administration because of adverse reactions that have occurred following its administration via these routes.[41]

Advantages of hydroxyzine in dentistry include its antiemetic and sedative actions, and the fact that it potentiates the CNS depressant actions of opioids and barbiturates, permitting their dosages to be decreased by as much as 50%.

As with promethazine, hydroxyzine as a sole agent will prove effective in management of lesser degrees of anxiety; however, unless combined with opioids, barbiturates, or inhalation sedation (N_2O-O_2), promethazine will be ineffective in more severe anxiety.

Patients must be cautioned not to drive a car or to operate hazardous machinery for up to 24 hours following administration of IM hydroxyzine hydrochloride.

Because of possible tissue irritation following injection, the preferred IM injection site in adults is the upper outer quadrant of the buttock or the vastus lateralis; in children the vastus lateralis is preferred.[42] The deltoid region should not be employed until it is well developed (adults and teenagers), and the lower and middle third of the upper arm should never be used because of the risk of radial nerve injury.

Dosage. The usual adult dose of hydroxyzine for preoperative sedation is 25 to 100 mg 1 hour prior to treatment. The dose for use as an antiemetic is 25 to 50 mg. The dose for children for preoperative sedation is 0.5 mg/lb (1.0 mg/kg) 1 hour prior to treatment. The antiemetic dose for children is 0.5 mg/lb (1.0 mg/kg).

Availability. Vistaril (Pfizer): 25 and 50 mg/ml in 1-ml ampules and 10-ml multiple-dose vials.

• • •

Promethazine and hydroxyzine are effective agents for IM sedation. Though primarily employed in pediatric dentistry, and then usually in conjunction with opioids, these drugs can be employed in the adult patient with success. Though the dosage range is quite wide, the doctor will select the appropriate dose of the drug after consideration of the factors discussed previously in this section. When used as sole agents, their greatest effect will be in the patient exhibiting milder levels of anxiety or one in whom only a light level of sedation is desired.

Barbiturates

Two barbiturates, secobarbital and pentobarbital, are employed via the IM route for preoperative sedation. The depth of sedation achieved with either of these agents will usually be somewhat more profound than that seen previously with the benzodiazepines or antihistamines. Caution is advised when these agents are employed intramuscularly because of the lack of control maintained over the drug's effect and the respiratory depressant properties of the barbiturates.[43] Use of barbiturates is recommended only to those doctors with the knowledge and ability to adequately monitor, recognize, and manage any adverse actions involved with use of these drugs. The pharmacology of these drugs has previously been discussed (Chapter 8).

Secobarbital. Secobarbital is a short-acting barbiturate that will produce clinical activity within 10 to 15 minutes following IM administration, with a duration of sedative action of approximately 3 to 4 hours.

A potential drawback to the use of secobarbital is that the drug begins to hydrolyze on exposure to moisture in the air or in aqueous solution. For this reason the drug should be administered within 30 minutes of being withdrawn from its container. For IM administration the most practical concentration of secobarbital is 50 mg/ml.

Dosage. The usual dose for adults or children for preoperative sedation is 1.0 mg/lb of body weight. For lighter levels of sedation or anxiety control, the dose may be decreased to 0.5 to 0.75 mg/lb.

Availability. Secobarbital sodium: 50 mg per ml in 1-, 2-, 10-, 20-, and 30-ml vials. Seconal sodium (Lilly): 250-mg ampule dry powder (dilute with 5 ml of sterile water for injection); 50 mg/ml in 20-ml vial or 2-ml disposable syringe. Secobarbital is classified as a Schedule II drug.

Pentobarbital. Pentobarbital, like secobarbital, is a short-acting barbiturate, employed for the production of sedation. This drug will be discussed in much greater depth in the section on IV sedation as a component of the Jorgensen technique. It may also be administered intramuscularly; however, solutions of pentobarbital are quite alkaline and have the ability to injure tissues into which they are deposited. IM pentobarbital must be administered deep into a large muscle mass, such as the upper outer quadrant of the gluteal region. The onset of action will develop within 10 to 15 minutes with a duration of action of 3 to 4 hours.[44]

The parenteral solution is composed of pentobarbital sodium, propylene glycol 40%, alcohol 10%, and water for injection at a pH of 9.5.

Use of pentobarbital is contraindicated in patients with allergy to any barbiturate or those with porphyria.

Though frequently used alone, when administered in conjunction with other CNS depressants (e.g., opioids) the dose of the opioid must be decreased to avoid possible oversedation or respiratory depression. Use of this agent with opioids should be limited to the doctor who has received training in patient monitoring and in recognition and management of the unconscious patient.

Dosage. Dosage should be calculated on the basis of age, weight, and the patient's condition. The usual adult dose is 150 to 200 mg; the child's dose frequently ranges from 25 to 80 mg. In all cases the drug is administered approximately 15 to 30 minutes prior to the scheduled appointment.[44]

Availability. Pentobarbital sodium (generic): 50 mg/ml in 1-, 2-, 5-, 20-, 30-, and 50-ml vials; 120 mg/ml in 10-ml vials; 130 mg/ml in 10-ml vials; 325 mg/ml in 10-ml vials. Nembutal sodium (Abbott): 50 mg/ml in 2-, 5-, 20-, and 50-ml vials. Pentobarbital is classified as a Schedule II drug.

• • •

The short-acting barbiturates secobarbital and pentobarbital are on occasion employed via the IM route for preoperative sedation. Though effective, the doctor must be aware of the potential for respiratory depression and excessive sedation that is inherent in the use of barbiturates. When these drugs are combined with other CNS depressants, the possibility of undesirable actions increases. The entire chairside staff must be fully prepared to recognize and manage any possible complications.

Opioid agonists

The opioid agonists (OAs), though classified as strong analgesics, are frequently used for the management of anxiety in both medicine and dentistry. Though opioids may be employed as solo agents in this regard, this is uncommon; more often they are administered conjointly with nonopioid CNS depressants such as benzodiazepines, barbiturates, or antihistamines to provide a greater depth of sedation than the latter drugs can produce by themselves.

The administration of opioids by any route of administration, but particularly parenterally, must be approached with caution. As will be seen in the discussion of the pharmacology of these potent drugs, a significant number of potentially serious side effects and drug-drug interactions may be observed following opioid administration. Although the incidence of these side effects is dose-related, many serious problems have been encountered following dosages well within the "normal" range. Because these drugs are quite potent, the doctor is cautioned to be absolutely certain, beyond any degree of doubt, that his or her entire staff is fully prepared, both mentally and technically, to recognize and manage any opioid-induced side effect. Without this preparation opioid analgesics should not be used.

There is a need for these drugs in dentistry. Opioid agonists are valuable in the management of postoperative discomfort following surgical procedures. In this regard the most practical route of administration frequently is the oral route, although most OAs possess a significant hepatic first-pass effect and are more effective following parenteral administration. However, it may be more prudent to forgo parenteral administration of OAs when the patient is an ambulatory outpatient. If a drug-related problem develops after the patient is discharged, assistance might not be immediately available. Parenteral administration of OAs for postoperative discomfort in the hospitalized, nonambulatory patient is much more practical and is indeed the more common method of administration.

Another use of OAs in dentistry is in the management of more intense degrees of anxiety and fear. All OAs possess the ability to produce a state of sedation, and advantage may be taken of this to aid in patient management. The use of these opioid agonist analgesics as sole agents for the management of anxiety is not always the most effective approach. Larger doses of the OAs must be administered to achieve a desired level of sedation when administered alone than when opioid agonists are administered concurrently with other nonopioid CNS depressants. As most of the adverse effects of the opioid agonists are potentially more serious than those of nonopioids (though even nonopioids may produce morbidity and mortality) and are dose-related, it simply makes sense (1) to avoid the use of OAs unless there is a definite reason for their use and (2) to employ the smallest clinically effective dose of the OA.

An ever-growing number of OAs have been introduced into clinical practice. However, a small group of these drugs probably represents 99% of all OAs employed by the profession. These agents include meperidine, alphaprodine,* and fentanyl (and its congeners alfentanil and sufentanil). To these must be added the opioid agonist/antagonists exemplified by pentazocine, butorphanol, and nalbuphine.

Pharmacology. Morphine, though not commonly employed in dentistry because of its prolonged duration of action, is recognized as the prototypical opioid agonist. Its pharmacology will be reviewed in some depth as being representative of the entire group. The other OAs employed in dentistry will be discussed later and the differences in their actions from those of morphine will be pointed out.

Mechanism of action. Recent research has provided a significant body of information concerning the mechanisms of action of OAs. Four major stereospecific receptors for OAs and opioid antagonists have been located within the central nervous system, the spinal cord, the trigeminal nucleus, the brainstem solitary nuclei and area postrema of the medulla, the medial thalamus, the limbic system (amygdala), and the periaqueductal gray matter of the mesencephalon (brainstem).[45] The periaqueductal gray matter has been identified as a site important to opioid-induced analgesia, as well as to the perception of pain. In addition to the discovery of these receptors, endogenous opioid-like substances called "enkephalins" and "endorphins" have been isolated.[46] These agents possess potent opioid-like properties and are receiving extensive examination as to their role in the management of pain.

Mu receptors are thought to be responsible for supraspinal analgesia, respiratory depression, euphoria, and physical dependence; *kappa* receptors are associated with alterations in affective behavior; *sigma* receptors are involved in the dysphoria, hallucinations, and vasomotor stimulation associated with some opioids; while *delta* receptors appear to modulate the actions of the mu receptors.[47-49] Table 11-4 summarizes the actions of these four receptors. Opioid agonists (OAs) are drugs that bind with the mu, kappa, and delta fibers. Opioid agonist/antagonists (OAAns) possess either agonist or antagonist actions at the various receptors, and opioid antagonists (OAns) possess antagonist actions at the receptors.

It is likely that the OAs and the endogenous opioids, endorphins, and enkephalins act to alter pain perception and pain reaction by inhibiting neuronal activity at their receptor sites through a decrease in sodium conductance through ion channels in nerve membranes. That opioid receptors are found in certain areas of the CNS in greater abundance than in others lends credence to this theory. Opioid agonists modify both components of the pain experience: the perception of pain and the reaction of the patient to pain. The presence of opioid receptors within the substantia gelatinosa of the spinal cord, the trigeminal nucleus, and the periaqueductal gray matter provides a reasonable explanation of the effect of OAs on pain perception, while the identification of opioid receptors located within the amygdala of the limbic system and the medial thalamus

---

*Alphaprodine was withdrawn from clinical use in the United States in 1986. It is still in clinical use in other countries.

Table 11-4. Classification of opioid receptors

Receptor	Effect	Agonist	Antagonist
mu$_1$	Supraspinal analgesia	b-endorphin	Naloxone
		Morphine	Pentazocine
mu$_2$	Depression of ventilation	Morphine	Naloxone
		Meperidine	
	Indifference or euphoria	Sufentanil	
		Alfentanil	
	Miosis	Fentanyl	
	Bradycardia		
	Hypothermia		
	Physical dependence		
delta	Modulates u	Leuenkephalin	Metenkephalin
kappa	Miosis	Dynorphin	
	Sedation	Pentazocine	
	Analgesia	Butorphanol	
sigma	Dysphoria	Ketamine?	Naloxone
	Tachycardia	Pentazocine	
	Tachypnea		
	Mydiasis		

aids in explaining their effects on the reaction to pain. Patients receiving OAs may still perceive pain, but their reaction to it is usually quite diminished. The side effect of nausea and vomiting is explained by the presence of opioid receptors within the area postrema of the medulla, while their presence within the solitary nuclei explains the antitussive, hypotensive, and GI effects of OAs. The two primary areas influenced by morphine are the central nervous system and the GI tract, the only areas in which opioid receptors have been found.

Central nervous system effects. Morphine produces analgesia, drowsiness, changes in mood, and mental clouding. Of significance is the fact that morphine produces analgesia without producing the loss of consciousness. Following a therapeutic dose of morphine (10 to 15 mg) to patients in pain or feeling anxiety or fear, any or all of these may disappear. Pain may be diminished in intensity or eradicated completely, accompanied frequently by drowsiness. The extremities become quite heavy, the body becomes warm, itching develops on the face (most frequently the nose or upper lip), and the mouth becomes dry. Some patients may become euphoric.

Interestingly, when the same dose of morphine is administered to a pain-free patient, the reaction may not be as pleasant. Many patients report dysphoria rather than euphoria, consisting of increased anxiety or fear and frequently of nausea or vomiting.

With increased doses (15 to 20 mg) the subjective effects of morphine are increased. Drowsiness is increased, euphoria (when present) is accentuated, and patients in severe pain not relieved by smaller doses report relief. The side effects of nausea and vomiting, and respiratory depression are also accentuated.

Morphine and the other OAs appear to be much more effective in the relief of dull, aching, continuous pain than that of a sharp, intermittent nature. Patients frequently report that they still feel the pain but that it no longer bothers them. It appears that the OAs primarily affect those systems responsible for the affective responses to noxious stimuli. Therefore when patients no longer respond to pain in the usual manner, their ability to tolerate the noxious stimulus may be dramatically increased although their ability to perceive the pain is relatively unaltered.

Pupillary responses. Morphine and many other OAs produce a dose-related constriction (miosis) of the pupil. Although the pupil will still respond to changes in light, miosis produced by morphine will be evident even in total darkness. Marked miosis and pinpoint pupils are considered to be pathognomonic of OA overdose. Atropine (and related agents) administered concurrently with OAs counteracts morphine-induced miosis.

Respiratory responses. Morphine and the other OAs produce a dose-related respiratory depression. Respiratory depression is observed even at therapeutic doses of morphine and is the most significant undesirable effect of the opioid agonists. Opioid-induced respiratory depression is a major factor in many instances of morbidity and mortality occurring following IM or IV sedation.[18]

Morphine depresses the responsiveness of the medullary respiratory centers to CO_2, as well as depressing the pontine and medullary centers that regulate respiratory rhythm and rate. Clinically it is observed that the rate, minute volume, and tidal exchange are all depressed by opioid agonists. Normal respiratory rates of 16 to 20 per minute may decrease to as few as 3 to 4 per minute following overdose. Maximal respiratory depression following morphine administration will develop 7 minutes after IV administration, 30 minutes after IM administration, and 90 minutes after subcutaneous administration. Respiratory depression may be present for up to 4 to 5 hours following morphine administration.

All opioid agonists are capable of producing respiratory depression. When equianalgesic doses are administered, the degree of respiratory depression is not significantly different from that produced by morphine.[50]

Nausea and emetic actions. Nausea and vomiting produced by morphine and other OAs are products of the direct stimulation of the chemoreceptor zone for emesis, located in the area postrema of the medulla. This emetic effect is counteracted by opioid antagonists.

It is significant that the incidence of nausea and vomiting is considerably greater in ambulatory patients than in recumbent patients. Nausea occurs in approximately 40% and vomiting in 15% of ambulatory patients receiving 15 mg morphine subcutaneously. It is probable that the emetic effect is produced in part by a peripheral effect on the vestibular apparatus of the ear and by orthostatic hypotension.[51]

As most dental patients are ambulatory the potential for nausea and vomiting following OA administration in dentistry is increased. Reversal of the OA with an antagonist prior to discharge of the patient might be considered as a means of minimizing this occurrence, but it must be remembered that the continued presence of the OA in the blood in the immediate postoperative period will aid in the management of any pain that might develop. Additionally, it has been found that reversal of opioid agonists not only reverses their adverse actions (respiratory depression, nausea, vomiting), but also reverses their analgesic actions as well. Routine reversal of opioid agonists by opioid antagonists prior to patient discharge is not recommended. Use of opioid antagonists should be reserved for those few situations where their administration is essential to the patient's safety. Probably the most effective means of minimizing the occurrence of nausea and vomiting following opioid administration is to minimize the dose administered to the patient, as this complication is dose-related.

Cardiovascular effects. Morphine in therapeutic doses has virtually no effect on blood pressure and heart rate or rhythm when patients are in the supine position.[50] Actions on the cardiovascular system do not develop until doses well into the overdose range are administered, and even then the cardiovascular system is not affected to a great degree. The most significant factor in hypotension developing following OA overdose is hypoxia. In the presence of opioid overdose with adequate oxygenation, the blood pressure will usually be maintained within normal limits.

Postural (orthostatic) hypotension does increase in incidence and severity with increasing doses of morphine and other OAs, a factor to be considered in the usual dental office environment. This is thought to be a result of peripheral vasodilation occurring as a result of histamine release associated with OA administration. Whenever the patient is shifted from the supine to the more upright position, the ability of the cardiovascular system to respond to the actions of gravity will be depressed by the OA. Slower changes in patient positioning are essential to prevent or minimize postural hypotension. Minimizing OA doses will further diminish the incidence of this dose-related situation. Postural hypotension is most likely to be noted with morphine and meperidine (which provoke the greatest release of histamine).

Another result of OA histamine release is the possible development of pruritus at the site of administration. This effect is responsible for the flushed feeling and itching that develop in some patients following IV administration. This will be discussed in detail in the section on IV sedation.

OAs have little or no effect on the myocardium, producing either an increase in heart rate or no change. The cerebral circulation, likewise, is little affected by therapeutic doses of morphine. However, in the presence of respiratory depression and elevated CO_2 levels, cerebral blood vessels dilate and intracranial pressure increases.

Gastrointestinal tract effects. Morphine produces constipation by decreasing motility of the stomach,

Table 11-5. Comparison of opioid agonists and opioid-agonist/antagonists via IM or submucosal injection

	Onset (min)	Peak action (min)	Duration (hours)	Adult dose	Pediatric dose (mg/kg)
Opioid agonists					
Morphine	20	30-90	Up to 7	5 to 15 mg	0.1-0.2
Meperidine	10-15	30-60	2-4	50 to 100 mg	1-2
Alphaprodine	5-10	30	1-2	0.4 to 1.2 mg/kg	0.3-0.6
Fentanyl	5-15	30	1-2	0.05 to 0.1 mg	—
Opioid agonist/antagonists					
Pentazocine	15-20	—	3-5	30 mg	—
Butorphanol	10	30-60	3-4	2 to 4 mg	—
Nalbuphine	15	—	3-6	10 mg/70 kg	—

duodenum, and colon, as well as diminishing both pancreatic and biliary secretions. Because morphine increases biliary tract pressure, its use in patients with biliary colic may produce an increase in pain rather than relief.

Smooth muscle effects. Morphine and other OAs increase smooth muscle tonus throughout the body, such as in the ureters, urinary bladder, uterus, and bronchioles. While therapeutic doses of OAs do not produce significant bronchospasm, their administration to patients with asthma may aggravate their condition, possibly precipitating bronchospasm. OAs ought to be avoided in patients with a history of asthma (a relative contraindication).

Tolerance, physical dependence, and abuse potential. The development of tolerance and physical dependence following repeated use is a characteristic of all opioid agonists. This represents one of the limiting factors in the use of these agents. Within dentistry the potential for producing addiction in a patient through use of OAs for sedation is quite unlikely to develop; however, the presence of opioid agonists within the office does increase the potential for unauthorized use of the drugs by persons unassociated with the dental office (after-hours robbery) or unfortunately by dental personnel themselves. While not as significant a problem in dentistry as within the medical community, opioid abuse by health professionals does occur and must be scrupulously guarded against.

Opioid agonists, as Schedule II drugs, must be stored in a locked cabinet or storage area. Precise records as to the use of these drugs are mandatory, so that anyone can determine the fate of a package of OAs. These records will be reviewed in the section on IV sedation.

Absorption, distribution, biotransformation, and excretion. Opioid agonists are rapidly absorbed following subcutaneous, submucosal (SM), or IM injection (Table 11-5). Owing to a significant hepatic first-pass effect, parenteral doses of OAs are considerably more effective than equal doses administered orally (only 30% of an oral dose of morphine reaches the systemic circulation).

Morphine leaves the blood rapidly and is distributed to the kidney, liver, lungs, and spleen. The major portion of the drug is found in skeletal muscle. Accumulation of the drug in tissues is rare, and within 24 hours the tissue concentration of morphine is quite low.

The OAs undergo biotransformation within the liver and are excreted in the urine. Only a small fraction of the administered dose is found unmetabolized in the urine.

Contraindications. The only absolute contraindication to the use of morphine is the presence of allergy.

Warnings. Opioid agonists should not be administered to patients with head injury or increased intracranial pressure, because of the respiratory depressant actions of these drugs and their ability to increase intracranial pressure. Within the typical dental environment this is an unlikely occurrence.

Morphine and other OAs should be used cautiously if at all in patients with asthma, chronic obstructive pulmonary disease (COPD), or any degree of respiratory depression, hypoxia, or hypercarbia. Even the usual therapeutic doses of OAs in these patients may significantly decrease respiratory drive while simultaneously increasing airway resistance to the point of producing apnea.

Patients receiving OAs must be cautioned against operating motor vehicles or other hazardous machinery. Orthostatic hypotension, nausea, and vomiting are more likely to develop in ambulatory patients receiving OAs.

Opioid agonists cross the placenta and may produce respiratory depression of the fetus. The use of OAs in the pregnant patient should only be considered following consultation with the patient's physician and only if other techniques and drugs are unavailable. The benefit versus the risk of drug administration should always be considered.

Drug interactions. Opioid agonists must be used with caution in patients who are receiving other CNS depressants, such as other OAs, phenothiazines, benzodiazepines, sedative-hypnotics, tricyclic antidepressants, and alcohol. Exaggerated clinical effects, including respiratory depression, hypotension, profound sedation, and unconsciousness may (and have) develop(ed).

The use of meperidine in patients receiving MAOIs is contraindicated because patients have experienced unpredictable, severe, occasionally fatal reactions. Because the therapeutic actions of the MAOIs may continue for 14 days following their discontinuance, meperidine should not be used until at least 2 weeks following the last dose of the MAOI. A list of these drugs is presented in Table 8-3. The reactions are of two types. Some responses involve unconsciousness, severe respiratory depression, cyanosis, and hypotension, resembling acute opioid overdose. Other responses are characterized by hyperexcitability, convulsions, tachycardia, hyperpyrexia, and hypertension. The use of opioid antagonists in the management of these reactions has not always proved effective.

Precautions. Doses of OAs must be decreased in patients who are elderly or debilitated or are known to be sensitive to CNS depressants. Among these are patients with cardiovascular, pulmonary, or hepatic disease. Doses should also be decreased in patients with hypothyroid conditions, alcoholism, convulsive disorders, asthma, Addison's disease, and prostatic hypertrophy or urethral stricture.

Opioid agonists may aggravate preexisting convulsions in patients with seizure disorders. Convulsions may develop in patients without a history of seizures if the OA is administered in a dose considerably above that recommended, because of the development of tolerance.

Adverse reactions. The most significant adverse reaction associated with the administration of opioid agonists is respiratory depression. The degree of respiratory depression is dose-dependent; however, some degree of depression is usually present even with therapeutic doses for most OAs. All aspects of respiration are depressed, but probably the most observable change is the respiratory rate, which will be reduced significantly from the normal adult range of 16 to 20 per minute to as little as 3 to 4 per minute. Respiratory rates below 8 per minute following administration of OAs should be carefully evaluated, and if necessary, treatment instituted to correct the situation.

In addition to respiratory depression, respiratory arrest, cardiovascular depression, and cardiac arrest have been noted following OA administration.

Among the more common side effects of the OAs are light-headedness, dizziness, nausea, vomiting, and diaphoresis (sweating). These appear to be more common in ambulatory patients. Because most of these effects are dose-related, the use of smaller doses, as recommended in this book, should minimize the occurrence of these undesirable effects. If side effects develop despite lower doses, the ambulatory patient should be advised to lie down, avoiding unnecessary positional changes, a maneuver that frequently alleviates the symptoms.

Other adverse reactions associated with opioid agonists include euphoria, dysphoria, headache, insomnia, agitation, tremor, uncoordinated muscular movements, transient hallucinations, disorientation, visual disturbances, dry mouth, constipation, biliary tract spasm, flushing of the face, tachycardia, bradycardia, palpitation, faintness, syncope, urinary retention, reduced libido, pruritus, urticaria, skin rashes, and edema. In other words, the OAs are capable of producing just about any and every side effect that most other drugs (or even nondrugs) may produce.

Overdosage. Overdosage produced by opioids is manifested by respiratory depression, primarily a decrease in the rate and tidal volume of breathing. In more profound overdose the patient may lose consciousness, with pupils becoming constricted (miosis), muscles flaccid, and skin cold and clammy. Bradycardia or hypotension or both may be present. Respiratory arrest may develop.

The primary goal in the management of overdose of any OA is airway maintenance and the delivery of oxygen to the lungs, cardiovascular system, and brain. Ventilation may need to be assisted or indeed controlled by the person managing the patient. Once a patent airway is established and oxygenation assured, the administration of an opioid antagonist may be considered. Naloxone is the drug of choice, administered via the IV route, if available, or IM if necessary. Other drugs and measures that may be considered are oxygen, IV fluids, and vasopressors. More specific details of management of drug-related overdose will be discussed in Chapter 28.

Morphine. The pharmacology of morphine has been discussed at great length in the preceding section. Morphine is used as the sulfate (frequently abbreviated as MS). Following IM or subcutaneous administration, the onset of action develops within 20 minutes, with a peak effect between 30 and 90 minutes. Unfortunately for most dental situations the average duration of clinical effect of morphine sulfate is approximately 7 hours. Approximately 90% of the dose administered is excreted within 24 hours, primarily in the urine.

Morphine is employed primarily as an analgesic, but it is also used commonly as a preoperative sedative prior to surgery and general anesthesia. Morphine is absorbed more reliably following parenteral administration than oral administration primarily because of a significant hepatic first-pass effect.

Dosage. The usual adult dose of morphine for preoperative sedation is 5 to 15 mg 30 minutes preoperatively. The usual dose for children for preoperative sedation is 0.1 to 0.2 mg/kg (0.05 to 0.1 mg/lb).

Availability. Morphine sulfate: 8, 10, and 15 mg/ml in 1-ml ampules; 15 mg/ml in 20-ml vials. Morphine is classified as a Schedule II drug.

Meperidine. Meperidine was first synthesized in 1939 and was studied as an atropine-like agent.[50] Its analgesic properties quickly became recognized, and its atropine-like properties are today listed under side effects of the drug.

Following IM or subcutaneous administration, the onset of action of meperidine is more rapid than that of morphine (10 to 15 minutes), and its duration of action is somewhat shorter (2 to 4 hours). Maximal effectiveness develops between 30 and 60 minutes. Meperidine is probably the most commonly used opioid agonist in dental practice, its clinical onset and duration of action being quite amenable to the typical dental appointment. At a dose of 80 to 100 mg meperidine is equianalgesic with 10 mg morphine sulfate. Meperidine is approximately half as effective orally as parenterally.

Peak respiratory depression following IM administration of meperidine develops in 1 hour with a return toward normal at 2 hours, although respiration may be measurably depressed for up to 4 hours. Opioid antagonists readily reverse opioid-produced respiratory depression. As with morphine sulfate, meperidine produces virtually no untoward effect on the cardiovascular system at therapeutic doses. Ambulatory patients are more likely to experience postural hypotension. Although IV meperidine may produce a tachycardia, IM meperidine seldom does.

Meperidine produces less smooth muscle spasm, less constipation, and less depression of the cough reflex than equianalgesic doses of morphine sulfate.

Dosage. The usual adult dose for preoperative sedation is 50 to 100 mg intramuscularly 30 to 90 minutes prior to treatment. The usual dose for children for preoperative sedation is 0.5 to 1.0 mg/lb (1 to 2 mg/kg) intramuscularly 30 to 90 minutes prior to treatment.

Availability. Meperidine: 25 mg/ml in 1-ml ampules; 50 mg/ml in 1-ml ampules and 30-ml vials; 75 mg/ml in 1- and 1.5-ml ampules; 100 mg/ml in 1-, 2-, 20-, and 30-ml ampules and vials. Demerol (Sanofi Winthrop): 25, 50, 75, and 100 mg/ml ampules and vials. Meperidine is classified as a Schedule II drug.

COMMENT: For IM administration of meperidine and other OAs, it is reasonable to employ one of the more concentrated dosage forms of the medication (e.g., 50 mg/ml), so as to minimize the volume of solution injected. On the other hand, when administered intravenously, more dilute concentrations of these same drugs are recommended, so as to minimize the risk of mistakenly administering too large a dose.

Meperidine with promethazine. Meperidine (Demerol) is combined with the phenothiazine/antihistamine promethazine (Phenergan) to produce a drug combination that is commonly employed in pediatric dentistry. The pharmacology of the individual agents has previously been discussed. This drug combination came into being because several clinical studies demonstrated that promethazine potentiated the analgesic and sedative properties of the opioid agonist meperidine. The dose of meperidine necessary to produce clinically effective sedation or analgesia could be reduced by almost 50% when promethazine was added.[52]

The combination is clinically useful in pediatric dentistry, not because of its analgesic actions, but because the mixture produces more sedation than the use of either drug alone. Available in both oral and injectable forms, its primary effectiveness has been in IM administration.

Following IM administration the combination will produce a clinical effect within 15 to 30 minutes, with a duration of action of 3 to 4 hours.

Dosage. The usual adult dose for preoperative sedation is 25 to 50 mg of each component (1 to 2 ml) 15 to 30 minutes prior to treatment. Although the *Physician's Desk Reference* indicates a recommended dose for children of 0.5 mg/lb of body weight,[53] many pediatric dentistry textbooks indicate a smaller dose: 0.02 mg/kg (0.01 mg/lb) intramuscularly 15 to 30 minutes preoperatively.[54,55]

Availability. Mepergan (Wyeth): 25 mg meperidine and 25 mg promethazine per ml. Mepergan is classified as a Schedule II drug.

Alphaprodine. Alphaprodine is a synthetic opioid analgesic, introduced in 1949 as Nisentil. Its initial primary indications were in obstetrics as an analgesic during labor and delivery, urologic procedures, and surgical procedures. Dentistry became interested in alphaprodine because of its advantages over meperidine: its rapid onset and shorter duration of action. Alphaprodine became quite well accepted in pediatric dentistry, where it was one of the most used drugs in the management of the disruptive child.

Unfortunately, the use of alphaprodine in dentistry was associated with an incidence of morbidity and mortality quite out of proportion to its use. Although most of these cases were the result of the administration of inappropriate doses of the drug, as well as an absence of adequate patient monitoring, the manufacturer of alphaprodine, Roche Laboratories, voluntarily withdrew the agent from the market in September 1980.[56] Following a series of retrospective studies,[5,7,57] alphaprodine was reintroduced. Following its reintroduction, a number of additional serious incidents were reported,[4,58] and alphaprodine was again voluntarily withdrawn from the market in 1986. At this time (1994) alphaprodine is no longer available for clinical use in the United States or Canada. During the period of its brief reappearance there was considerable debate over the appropriateness of its use in outpatient procedures by doctors who had not received training in general anesthesia and in the management of the unconscious airway.

Alphaprodine is an effective opioid agonist that can also produce sedation. The drug may be employed effectively and safely by the doctor who understands its pharmacology, is prepared to adequately monitor the patient, and is able to recognize and manage any adverse reactions associated with its administration. Though this same statement may be made for any of the drugs presented in this textbook, it is especially important when dealing with opioid agonists and particularly significant in relation to alphaprodine, which may have a greater respiratory depressant action than other opioid agonists. The respiratory depressant action of alphaprodine is of longer duration than the drug's clinical effectiveness for analgesia or sedation.

Alphaprodine is a rapid-acting OA that possesses a short duration of action. Except for these properties, alphaprodine is pharmacologically similar to morphine and meperidine.[57] A 50-mg dose of alphaprodine is equianalgesic to 10 mg morphine. Alphaprodine is therefore somewhat more potent than meperidine (10 mg morphine sulfate = 50 mg alphaprodine = 80 mg meperidine).

As with other OAs, alphaprodine exerts its actions primarily on the central nervous system and smooth-muscle-containing organs. Metabolized in the liver, alphaprodine is excreted in the urine and feces. The half-life of alphaprodine is 131 minutes (IV administration).[59]

Following submucosal administration, which has been its primary route of administration in pediatric dentistry, the onset of action is 10 minutes (range 2 to 30 minutes), with a duration of action of from 1 to 2 hours.[60] This is considerably shorter than meperidine (2 to 4 hours). Maximal clinical action develops within 30 minutes.

The manufacturer (Roche) recommends that alphaprodine be administered only via the IV, subcutaneous, and submucosal routes. They state that alphaprodine should never be administered intramuscularly because its absorption is too unpredictable. The only indication for the use of alphaprodine in children is within pediatric dentistry, and then only via submucosal administration.[61]

In submucosal administration, the drug is deposited into the mucobuccal fold adjacent to the mandibular molars or in the maxilla. It is usually deposited into the site of a previously administered local anesthetic. In defense of this technique is the statement that this technique is less painful for the patient. However, even if the local anesthetic did not contain a vasoconstrictor, the absorption of the drug from the buccal mucosa would be only slightly more rapid than from any other extraoral site of subcutaneous administration.[6,7] If a vasoconstrictor is included in the local anesthetic, as it frequently is, the rate of absorption of alphaprodine will be substantially delayed because of the diminished blood flow through the region. Another factor mitigating against this practice is the fact that many of the agents with which alphaprodine is combined prior to submucosal injection (e.g., promethazine) are capable of producing tissue damage and discomfort at the site of administration. An additional reason for not recommending this technique is that it is usually more appropriate to administer sedative drugs prior to the administration of the local anesthetic, so as to diminish any adverse response to this procedure, as opposed to after the local anesthetic has been injected.

Most serious complications resulting from the administration of alphaprodine were attributed to several factors as follows:

1. Inappropriate dosage of alphaprodine
2. Combinations of CNS depressants administered
3. Inadequate monitoring of patient
4. Lack of preparedness in emergency management

The rapid onset of clinical action of alphaprodine requires that the entire treatment staff remain vigilant in their monitoring of the patient from the moment the drug is administered. The degree of patient response to verbal and physical stimuli is observed, and the frequency and depth of respiration are observed continuously by the doctor or the assistant. Where a rubber dam is employed even greater care is required as the dam obscures visibility of the oral cavity (behind the dam) and to a degree may increase the risk of respiratory obstruction. Use of a precordial/pretracheal stethoscope is essential, and the use of pulse oximetry highly recommended. Where available, capnography should also be employed.

In an apparent overresponse to the reported cases of alphaprodine morbidity and mortality, the manufacturers of alphaprodine at one time stated in the package insert that routine opioid reversal with naloxone should be performed following each pediatric procedure when alphaprodine is administered.[62] Fortunately this recommendation was deleted from subsequent inserts. Opioid antagonists need not be administered unless there is a rational therapeutic reason for their being given. As with all CNS depressants, the dose of alphaprodine must be decreased when administered in the presence of other CNS depressants. The use of alphaprodine in pediatric practice will be reviewed in depth in Chapter 36.

Dosage. The usual adult dose for preoperative sedation is 0.4 to 1.2 mg/kg subcutaneously 10 to 30 minutes before treatment. The usual dose for children for preoperative sedation is 0.3 to 0.6 mg/kg (0.136 to 0.27 mg/lb) submucosally 10 to 30 minutes before treatment.

Availability. Nisentil (Roche) is no longer available in the United States or Canada, but remains available elsewhere: 40 mg/ml in 1-ml ampules and 60 mg/ml in 10-ml vial. As an opioid analgesic alphaprodine was classified as a Schedule II drug.

Fentanyl. Fentanyl is a rapid-onset, short-duration opioid agonist with qualitative clinical actions similar to morphine and meperidine. Fentanyl is, however, significantly more potent than these other two agents, a dose of 0.1 mg being equianalgesic to 10 mg morphine and 75 mg meperidine. In other words, 1 mg of fentanyl is equianalgesic with 100 mg morphine or 750 mg meperidine.[62]

As do other OAs, fentanyl produces a dose-related respiratory depression. The respiratory depression produced by fentanyl may however be of longer duration than its analgesic action. Fentanyl appears to produce less nausea and vomiting than do most other OAs. Other OA actions are also observed: miosis, bradycardia, bronchoconstriction, and euphoria. A potentially serious reaction to fentanyl administration is muscular rigidity, which is quite rare, developing primarily after IV administration and involving most muscles, but particularly the muscles of the chest wall and muscles of respiration.[63] This will be discussed in depth in the section on IV sedation.

Fentanyl is used primarily via the IV route, either alone or as the opioid component of Innovar (consisting of fentanyl and droperidol), for the induction and maintenance of neuroleptanesthesia (see Section Six). Additionally, fentanyl is employed to provide sedation preoperatively and is used postoperatively as an analgesic.

The onset of action of fentanyl following IM administration is 5 to 15 minutes; maximal effect develops within 30 minutes, and the duration of action is approximately 1 to 2 hours. These figures demonstrate that fentanyl is an OA whose clinical actions are quite well suited to the typical, short (1-hour) dental or surgical appointment. Fentanyl, in the proper hands, is a useful drug for the management of pain and anxiety, via either the IV or IM route.

Dosage. The usual adult dose for preoperative sedation is 0.05 to 0.1 mg intramuscularly 30 to 60 minutes preoperatively. The dosage must be decreased in the elderly, the debilitated, and patients who have received other CNS depressants. Though recommended for IV administration, there is no recommended dose of fentanyl for children via the IM route.[64]

Availability. Sublimaze (Janssen): 0.05 mg/ml in 2- and 5-ml ampules. Fentanyl is classified as a Schedule II drug.

• • •

Alfentanil and **sufentanil** are congeners of fentanyl that are gaining popularity in short procedures. They are similar to fentanyl in most properties. The primary use of alfentanil and sufentanil is via the intravenous route. They are discussed in greater detail in Chapter 26.

• • •

The opioid agonist analgesics just presented are those most frequently employed intramuscularly in both medicine and dentistry in the management of anxiety in the preoperative period. From the practical point of view the most useful OAs for most dental procedures would be those possessing the shortest duration of action: alphaprodine and fentanyl, sufentanil and alfentanil. With the loss of alphaprodine from our IM armamentarium other short-acting OAs must be evaluated for efficacy and safety. The IM administration of fentanyl and its congeners has not received much attention with dentistry. Their primary use is via IV administration, where their short duration makes them appropriate for many short procedures. Meperidine with its longer history of use as well as its longer duration of action is the most commonly used opioid agonist in dentistry and medicine, being administered either IM or IV. In pediatric dentistry meperidine was used less often than alphaprodine, due primarily to its longer duration of action, but it is much more commonly employed today. Morphine, though an excellent agent, is infrequently used IM in outpatient dentistry and surgery because of its long duration of action.

Opioid agonist/antagonists

Three opioid agonist/antagonists are available for use via the IM and IV routes. These drugs differ from the opioid agonists in that they possess not only opioid-like properties (agonist) but also have opioid antagonist actions as well. The systemic effects described earlier for morphine, as the prototypical opioid, are the agonistic actions. Antagonistic actions include (1) prevention of agonist effects if administered prior to or simultaneously with the OA, (2) reversal of agonist effects if administered after the OA, and (3) precipitation of acute withdrawal syndrome almost immediately in the opioid-dependent individual. One compound, naloxone, is considered to be a pure antagonist and is an important agent in the management of opioid overdose. Its actions and use will be described later (Chapter 25). Pentazocine, butorphanol, and nalbuphine are drugs with mixed agonist and antagonist activities and are discussed next.

Pentazocine. Pentazocine is a product of research aimed at developing an effective analgesic with little or no abuse potential. It possesses agonistic properties as well as very weak antagonistic actions ($\frac{1}{50}$ as potent as nalorphine as an antagonist). Its actions mimic those of morphine, including a sense of euphoria. Since its introduction in the 1960s, many instances of psychological and physical dependence to pentazocine have been documented. Because of its antagonistic properties the administration of pentazocine to opioid-dependent persons may precipitate acute withdrawal syndrome, an action not produced by opioid agonists.[65]

The action of pentazocine on the cardiovascular system differs somewhat from that of morphine. With high doses the blood pressure and heart rate of the patient are seen to rise. Other actions of pentazocine, such as those on uterine smooth muscle and the GI tract, are similar to those of morphine.

Pentazocine is approximately one third as potent as morphine following IM administration, 10 mg of morphine sulfate being equianalgesic to 30 mg pentazocine. It is metabolized in the liver and has a half-life of approximately 12 hours. Following IM administration the onset of action develops within 15 to 20 minutes. Duration of action will be approximately 3 to 5 hours.[66]

Side effects, including respiratory depression, *warnings*, and *contraindications* to the use of pentazocine are similar to those for morphine and the other opioids. Pentazocine-induced respiratory depression may be antagonized by naloxone.

Dosage. The usual adult dose for preoperative sedation is 30 mg intramuscularly or subcutaneously 15 to 30 minutes prior to treatment. IM administration is preferred to subcutaneous administration because of possible tissue irritation and damage associated with subcutaneous administration. The administration of pentazocine in children under the age of 12 years is not recommended.[67]

Availability. Talwin (Sanofi Winthrop): 30 mg/ml in 1-, 1.5-, 2-, and 10-ml ampules. Pentazocine is classified as a Schedule IV drug.

Butorphanol. Butorphanol is a potent analgesic that has an onset of action within 10 minutes following IM administration, reaching a peak level of clinical activity at 30 to 60 minutes, with a duration of analgesia of 3 to 4 hours. An opioid agonist/antagonist, its antagonistic actions are approximately 30 times that of pentazocine and about $\frac{1}{40}$ those of naloxone. In analgesic properties, butorphanol is 3.5 to 7 times more potent than morphine (2 mg = 10 mg).[68]

Side effects of butorphanol are similar to those of

other OAs, including the possibility of respiratory depression. Though 2 mg of butorphanol does produce respiratory depression equivalent to that produced by 10 mg of morphine, increasing the dose of butorphanol to 4 mg does not appreciably add to the degree of respiratory depression. This one factor should make butorphanol (and nalbuphine) an important drug in dentistry's armamentarium against anxiety and pain. Although the magnitude of respiratory depression observed with butorphanol appears not to be dose-related (above the 2-mg dose), the duration of respiratory depression is dose-related. Naloxone rapidly reverses respiratory depression produced by butorphanol.[69]

The cardiovascular effects of butorphanol are similar to pentazocine, including an increased blood pressure and heart rate. In addition, it increases the work of the heart by increasing pulmonary artery pressure, left ventricular end-diastolic pressure, and pulmonary vascular resistance. For these reasons the use of butorphanol is contraindicated in patients with recent myocardial infarction, coronary insufficiency, or ventricular dysfunction.[67]

Butorphanol has received attention in both medicine and dentistry as an agent for preoperative sedation. It may be administered either intravenously or intramuscularly.

Dosage. The usual adult dose for preoperative sedation is 2 mg intramuscularly 15 to 30 minutes prior to treatment. Doses larger than 4 mg are not recommended because of a lack of sufficient information.[67]

Availability. Stadol (Mead Johnson): 1 and 2 mg/ml in 1- and 2-ml vials. Butorphanol is not classified as a Schedule drug.

Nalbuphine. Nalbuphine is another analgesic possessing opioid agonist/antagonist properties. Nalbuphine is equipotent with morphine on a milligram basis. Following IM administration, the onset of action develops within 15 minutes, with a duration of action of from 3 to 6 hours. The plasma half-life of nalbuphine is 5 hours. The opioid antagonistic activity of nalbuphine is one fourth that of nalorphine and 10 times that of pentazocine.[70]

As with butorphanol, the ***actions***, ***side effects***, ***contraindications***, and ***warnings*** are similar to those of the opioid agonists. The one major difference in pharmacology between butorphanol and nalbuphine is the absence of any increased cardiovascular workload with nalbuphine. Its use is not contraindicated in cardiovascular-risk patients.[71]

At the usual IM therapeutic dose of 10 mg (for a 70-kg patient), nalbuphine produces respiratory depression equivalent to 10 mg morphine sulfate. Increasing the dosage of nalbuphine does not appreciably increase the degree of respiratory depression. Naloxone readily reverses respiratory depression produced by nalbuphine.

Dosage. The usual adult dose of nalbuphine for preoperative sedation is 10 mg/70 kg 15 to 30 minutes prior to the procedure. The dose should be adjusted, based on the patient's physical and emotional status, the depth of sedation desired, the patient's age, and the presence of other CNS depressants. Due to a lack of clinical experience, the administration of nalbuphine to patients under the age of 18 years is not recommended.[71]

Availability. Nubain (Du Pont): 10 mg/ml in 1-, 2-, and 10-ml ampules. Nalbuphine is not classified as a Schedule drug.

• • •

The opioid agonist/antagonists offer the significant advantage over the opioid agonists (morphine, meperidine, alphaprodine, fentanyl) of a decrease in dose-related respiratory depression. Although this action will not be of great significance in the doses usually employed for sedation in dentistry (up to 2 mg butorphanol or 10 mg nalbuphine), accidental overadministration of these agents is less likely to lead to serious respiratory depression or respiratory arrest. As with the opioid agonists, the doctor using these drugs must be prepared to both recognize and manage any unwanted side effects produced by these agents. Their presumed safety is not an excuse to forego routine patient monitoring during the procedure. To do so is an invitation to disaster.

Nonsteroidal antiinflammatory drugs

Ketorolac. Ketorolac is a new nonsteroidal antiinflammatory drug (NSAID) possessing appropriate solubility and minimal tissue irritation, making it suitable for intramuscular injection. Ketorolac, the most potent NSAID known, relieves pain through inhibition of arachidonic acid synthesis at the cyclooxygenase level and possesses no central opioid effects.[72] Ketorolac has analgesic potencies comparable to morphine with the following intramuscular equivalence: 30 to 90 mg ketorolac = 6 to 12 mg morphine.[73] Ketorolac is recommended as being effective for moderate to severe pain. It is useful by itself or in combination with opioids, decreasing the required dose of opioid by approximately 45%.[72,74]

is especially useful where opioids are contraindicated, especially to avoid respiratory depression and sedation. Where ketorolac proves to be ineffective in pain management, opioids should be considered.[75]

Following IM administration, peak blood levels are reached in 45 to 50 minutes.[74] It is administered as a 30- to 60-mg IM loading dose followed by 15 or 30 mg IM every 6 hours, with a maximum first-day dose of 150 mg and 120 mg on subsequent days up to a recommended maximum of 5 days. The lower dosage range is recommended for elderly patients, patients weighing less than 50 kg, and patients with impaired renal function.[74]

Availability. Toradol (Syntex): 15 mg/ml Tubex cartridge-needle unit, 1-m syringe; 30 mg/ml 1-ml syringe and 2-ml syringe.

Dissociative anesthesia

Ketamine. Ketamine is a phencyclidine derivative that is administered parenterally to produce a state called "dissociative anesthesia."[76] Following its administration, the patient becomes mentally dissociated from his environment. Phencyclidine is used in veterinary medicine, and has become a popular drug of abuse, known as "angel dust." Ketamine may be used to produce a state of general anesthesia (its primary use) or in subanesthetic doses to produce a state resembling sedation. Within 5 to 8 minutes following IM administration, the patient loses consciousness. Recovery occurs within 10 to 20 minutes, but it is several hours before the patient is fully recovered. Unconsciousness produced by ketamine differs significantly from that produced by the more traditional general anesthetics. Dissociative anesthesia will be described in detail in Chapters 26 and 32.

Pharmacology. Ketamine exerts its dissociative effects by interrupting the cerebral association pathways and by depression of the thalamocortical tracts. The reticular activating system, the limbic system, and the medulla are but little affected.

The cardiovascular system is stimulated following ketamine administration (most general anesthetics depress the cardiovascular system). Increases occur in the mean arterial pressure, heart rate, and cardiac output brought about by direct stimulation by ketamine. The median elevation in blood pressure following IM ketamine is about 20% to 25% above preanesthetic levels. Airway patency is easily maintained following ketamine administration. Muscle tonus is actually increased, in direct contrast to decreased muscle tonus seen with other general anesthetics. Protective reflexes are also maintained, but there is

some degree of diminution of their effectiveness. Administration of overly large doses of ketamine may produce apnea.[77] The administrator of this agent must be ever vigilant during patient treatment with this drug.

Ketamine undergoes biotransformation in the liver into alcohols, which are excreted in the urine.

The use of ketamine is contraindicated in patients with high blood pressure, severe psychiatric disorders, increased intracranial pressure, epilepsy, arteriosclerotic heart disease, and cerebrovascular accident.[78]

Probably the major adverse action observed following ketamine administration is the development of unpleasant dreaming, confused states, and frightening or upsetting hallucinations in the recovery period. These are more likely to occur in adults than in children. When they do occur in children they are usually less intense.[79]

Ketamine must not be employed in either anesthetic or subanesthetic doses by a doctor who is not trained in anesthesiology. The differences between a ketamine-induced state of general anesthesia and the more traditional stage three anesthesia may tempt the unqualified person to believe that they are able to safely employ this drug in their practice. Rest assured that this is not the case! I have had over 1000 case experiences with ketamine and can attest to the fact that this drug can, although it is only on very rare occasion, produce some very severe and frightening situations. Doctors not fully prepared for these reactions will be unable to respond to them effectively, much to their patient's detriment.

The reader is referred to Chapters 26 and 32 for a more complete discussion of this agent, its dosages and availability, and the concept of dissociative anesthesia.

Anticholinergic drugs

The anticholinergics atropine, scopolamine, and glycopyrrolate are also called "cholinergic blocking agents," "belladonna alkaloids," "and antimuscarinic drugs." They are commonly employed in general anesthesia and are frequently of use in dentistry. Their primary use in dentistry is for the reduction of salivary flow. In addition, their vagolytic actions are effective in the prevention or treatment of bradycardia. These drugs may be administered subcutaneously, intramuscularly, or intravenously. The anticholinergics act as competitive antagonists of the postganglionic receptor located at the neuroeffector junction of the parasympathetic nervous system.

Pharmacology[80]

Eye. The anticholinergics block parasympathetic receptors in the sphincter of the iris and the ciliary muscle, producing dilation of the pupil (mydriasis) and an inability of the eye to accommodate (cycloplegia). There is little effect on intraocular pressure, except in patients with narrow-angle glaucoma, where significant increases in intraocular pressure may result. Narrow-angle glaucoma represents a contraindication to use of these agents.

Respiratory system. Administration of the anticholinergics removes the parasympathetic nervous system's control over bronchial smooth muscle, leaving it under sole control of the sympathetic nervous system, which produces bronchodilation. Secretion of all glands within the oral cavity, pharynx, and respiratory tract is inhibited. These drugs are frequently used prior to the induction of general anesthesia to minimize the risk of laryngospasm. This desirable action is a result of the decrease in secretions within the respiratory tract.

Salivary glands. All parasympathetically mediated salivary secretions are completely inhibited by these agents. It is not uncommon for the patient receiving one of these agents to complain to the doctor that his mouth is overly dry, making it difficult to swallow or to speak.

Gastrointestinal tract. The anticholinergic agents inhibit gastrointestinal motility.

Cardiovascular system. The actions of the vagus nerve on the heart are diminished when anticholinergic drugs are administered. This is termed a "vagolytic effect" and is of importance during the induction and maintenance of general anesthesia. There is an increase in heart rate following administration of usual therapeutic doses (0.4 to 0.6 mg) of atropine and scopolamine. Glycopyrrolate does not produce this effect to the same degree.

Urinary tract. Anticholinergic drugs inhibit contractions of the bladder and ureter and produce dilation of the pelvis of the kidney, all of which act to produce urinary retention. In the presence of prostatic hypertrophy, this retention is more likely to develop.

Body temperature. The anticholinergics inhibit sweating through their action on the cholinergic fibers of the sympathetic nervous system that innervate the sweat glands. Body temperature rises following administration of these agents. Elevation in temperature is the most serious and potentially life-threatening result of overdosage of these agents.

Motion sickness. The anticholinergics have been employed for centuries in the management of motion sickness. They appear to act on the vestibular end organs and on the cerebral cortex or on both. Scopolamine is more effective as an anti–motion sickness agent than is atropine. Recently scopolamine has become available for this use in the form of a transdermal patch (Chapter 10).

Absorption, metabolism, and excretion. These drugs are rapidly absorbed following IM administration. The liver is primarily responsible for their biotransformation and the kidney is the main route of excretion. The half-life of atropine is 4 hours.

Contraindications. Anticholinergics are contraindicated in patients with glaucoma (acute narrow-angle), adhesions between the iris and the lens of the eye, and asthma. Their use in patients with prostatic hypertrophy is contraindicated because of the risk of urinary retention.

Drug interactions. Anticholinergics should be used with caution in patients receiving other medications that possess anticholinergic actions. These include tricyclic antidepressants, antipsychotics, antihistamines, and antiparkinsonism drugs.

Adverse reactions. Although there is great potential for individual variation in response to these drugs, the following is the usual pattern of adverse response to atropine:

Dose	Response
0.5 mg	Slight drying of mouth, bradycardia, inhibition of sweating
1.0 mg	Greater dryness of nose and mouth, increased thirst, slowing then acceleration of the heart, slight mydriasis
2.0 mg	Very dry mouth, tachycardia with palpitation, mydriasis, slight blurring of near vision, flushed dry skin
5.0 mg	Increase in above symptoms, disturbance of speech, difficulty in swallowing, headache, hot dry skin, restlessness
10.0 mg and above	Above symptoms to extreme degree, ataxia, excitement, disorientation, hallucinations, delirium, coma

"Red as a beet, dry as a bone, and mad as a hatter" describes the patient during an anticholinergic overdose.

Atropine. Atropine sulfate is a very commonly used drug in general anesthesia, both preoperatively and during the surgical procedure. Its primary functions during this time are (1) the inhibition of secretions within the respiratory tract, thereby minimizing the risk of laryngospasm but not preventing it, and (2) the vagolytic action of the drug on the heart, minimizing the risk of vagally induced bradycardia. Atropine is more effective than scopolamine as a vagolytic agent but does not possess the CNS sedative or amnesic actions of scopolamine; however, these actions will not be observed following IM administration but rather will be seen after IV administration.

The recommended adult parenteral dose of atropine (0.4 to 0.6 mg) does not produce an increase in intraocular pressure and is not contraindicated in patients with glaucoma. If such an increase in pressure does develop, it may be counteracted with topically applied pilocarpine.

Following IM administration atropine produces clinical actions within 10 to 15 minutes, with a duration of action of 90 minutes.

Dosage. The usual adult dose is 0.4 to 0.6 mg intramuscularly, 10 to 20 minutes prior to treatment. For children the following dosage schedule for parenteral atropine is recommended in the drug product insert[81]:

7 to 16 lb—0.1 mg
17 to 24 lb—0.15 mg
24 to 40 lb—0.2 mg
40 to 65 lb—0.3 mg
65 to 90 lb—0.4 mg
Over 90 lb—0.4 to 0.6 mg

Availability. Atropine sulfate: 0.3, 0.4, 0.5, 0.6, 1.0, and 1.3 mg/ml. Atropine is not classified as a Schedule drug.

Scopolamine. Scopolamine hydrobromide possesses the same pharmacologic properties as atropine, but in some cases to differing degrees. The vagolytic action of scopolamine is less than that of atropine, as is its effect in producing mydriasis. In addition, where atropine produces a stimulation of the central nervous system, scopolamine depresses the cerebral cortex. Scopolamine possesses a more intense drying effect than atropine.

Scopolamine is primarily used for its ability to produce sedation and amnesia. Following IM administration the onset of action is 10 to 15 minutes, with a duration of action of approximately 90 minutes.

A possible side effect of scopolamine is the occurrence of excitement, restlessness, disorientation, and delirium during the postoperative recovery period.[82] This action is not observed with atropine or glycopyrrolate. Emergence delirium, as it is known, is more likely to be observed in the very young or older adult patient, and it may be treated effectively with physostigmine (1 to 3 mg IV or IM). This is more common following IV than IM scopolamine administration. Emergence delirium will be discussed more fully in Chapter 28.

Dosage. The usual adult dose is 0.32 to 0.65 mg 10 to 15 minutes prior to the procedure. The dose for children 6 months to 3 years is 0.1 to 0.15 mg; for children 3 to 6 years, 0.15 to 0.2 mg; for children 6 to 12 years, 0.2 to 0.3 mg.[83]

Availability. Scopolamine hydrobromide: 0.3, 0.4, and 0.6 mg/ml. Scopolamine is not classified as a Schedule drug.

Glycopyrrolate. Glycopyrrolate (introduced in 1961) is another anticholinergic, similar in many ways to atropine and scopolamine. Following IM administration, glycopyrrolate acts within 10 to 15 minutes, exerts a maximal effect in 30 to 45 minutes, and has a duration of action of approximately 7 hours, considerably longer than the other anticholinergics.

Because glycopyrrolate is a quaternary ammonium compound, it does not pass through lipid membranes, such as the blood-brain barrier, as do atropine and scopolamine (tertiary amines, which pass easily through lipid membranes). Glycopyrrolate does not produce sedation or emergence delirium, as does scopolamine.

The drying effect of a 0.2-mg dose of glycopyrrolate is equal to that of 0.4-mg atropine. Glycopyrrolate offers the same vagolytic action as atropine and scopolamine; however, and importantly, glycopyrrolate does not produce tachycardias or dysrhythmias as frequently as the other anticholinergics. This action may be significant in the cardiac-risk patient receiving these medications (a beneficial effect), or in situations in which the doctor wishes to increase a too-slow heart rate (glycopyrrolate would not be indicated).

Glycopyrrolate offers an attractive alternative to atropine and scopolamine when long-duration drying action is desired during dental procedures.

Dosage. The usual adult dose is 0.1 to 0.2 mg intramuscularly 30 to 60 minutes prior to treatment. The dose for children is between 0.004 and 0.01 mg/kg 30 to 60 minutes prior to treatment.[84]

Availability. Glycopyrrolate hydrobromide (Robins) 0.2 mg/ml. Glycopyrrolate is not classified as a Schedule drug.

• • •

The anticholinergics are most often used in conjunction with parenterally administered CNS depressants. The primary goal in their use is usually a reduction in salivary flow leading to the production of a dry operating field; a secondary goal during IM sedation is the vagolytic actions of the drug. CNS depression produced by scopolamine via the IM route will usually be insignificant compared to the other drugs being employed. Although all three agents are

Table 11-6. Comparison of anticholinergic actions

	Atropine	*Scopolamine*	*Glycopyrrolate*
Effect on secretions	Effective	Effective	Effective
Vagolytic action	Effective	Less than atropine	Effective
Tachycardia, dysrhythmias	Yes	Yes	Less likely
Effect on eye	Mydriasis	Less than atropine	Mydriasis
Effect on CNS	Stimulates	Depresses cortex	Stimulates

effective and safe when used in therapeutic dosages, scopolamine should not be used if the sole aim in using an anticholinergic is the production of a dry field or its vagolytic actions. Atropine or glycopyrrolate are more appropriate in this regard. Scopolamine is indicated for use when a degree of CNS depression or amnesia is desired, although IV administration produces a much more reliable effect than does IM administration. In addition, scopolamine has the disturbing ability to produce emergence delirium; the other anticholinergics do not. Table 11-6 compares the actions of the anticholinergics.

IM techniques

The drugs discussed in this chapter are those most often used as IM sedative agents. The box classifies these agents into useful therapeutic categories. Group A includes the most effective drugs via the IM route when lesser degrees of anxiety are present.

Used alone, group A drugs provide light-to-moderate levels of conscious sedation in most patients. The benzodiazepines diazepam, lorazepam, and midazolam are preferred to the barbiturates secobarbital and pentobarbital, while promethazine and hydroxyzine are less often used IM.

Lorazepam is long-acting and thus rarely indicated for IM administration in outpatients. Diazepam should be injected deeply into muscle to decrease tissue irritation and to maximize its absorption, which might still be inconsistent. Water-soluble midazolam has provided clinicians with a highly effective, rapid-onset IM agent in the benzodiazepine class. Midazolam is extremely effective in the initial management of both handicapped patients and pediatric patients who are precooperative or uncooperative and will not voluntarily be seated in the dental chair. The use of midazolam in these situations is discussed fully in Chapters 36 and 39.

The IM administration of barbiturates is less enthusiastically recommended because of the greater degree of respiratory depression accompanying therapeutic doses. Pentobarbital may irritate tissues into

---

+---+
| ***DRUGS EMPLOYED IN INTRAMUSCULAR*** |
| ***SEDATION*** |
| |
| *Group A*   *Group B*   *Group C* |
| Diazepam*   Morphine†   Atropine |
| Lorazepam†   Meperidine   Scopolamine |
| Midazolam   Alphaprodine§   Glycopyrrolate† |
| Promethazine   Fentanyl |
| Hydroxy-   Alfentanil |
| zine*   Sufentanil |
| Secobarbital‡ Pentazocine |
| Pentobarbi-   Butorphanol |
| tal*   Nalbuphine |
| |
| *May irritate tissues at injection site unless deposited |
| deep into tissues. |
| †Long duration of action limits outpatient use.|
| ‡Must be prepared immediately prior to administration. |
| §No longer available in United States. |
+---+

which it is deposited and should therefore be injected deep into muscle.

Promethazine is a reliable agent for IM administration, providing slightly longer durations than midazolam or diazepam.

Hydroxyzine must be injected deep into muscle to avoid tissue irritation.

When administered as discussed, group A drugs usually provide a level of conscious sedation adequate to permit treatment of adult patients with milder degrees of anxiety or to place the fearful pediatric or handicapped patient into the dental chair where other, more controllable techniques of drug administration may be employed (i.e., IV and/or inhalation).

Group B drugs are the opioid agonists and agonist/antagonists. Their most rational use is for pain control in the posttreatment period. Though they will also provide a variable degree of sedation, their primary use for this indication cannot be recommended. Group A drugs are more specific and effective in managing anxiety and have the additional benefit of producing fewer adverse effects (specifically, respiratory depression).

Group B drugs are frequently administered in combination with a group A drug in the management of patients with greater degrees of dental or surgical fear. Dosages must be decreased from their "normal" levels when they are administered alone because of the very real possibility of additive or potentiating actions, especially CNS and respiratory depression. Combinations of group A and B drugs are most often used to provide deep sedation in pediatric (Chapter 36) and handicapped (Chapter 39) patients for the management of the overtly disruptive or uncooperative patient. Use of any group B drug for sedation or analgesia requires that the doctor and staff closely monitor the patient and quickly recognize and manage any adverse reactions.

Group C drugs, the anticholinergics, may be administered alone or in combination with group A or B drugs. They function not to provide CNS sedation (although scopolamine, to a minor degree, may do so), but rather to provide a vagolytic action (glycopyrrolate does this to a lesser degree) and to reduce secretions in the oral cavity and respiratory tract. Doses of group C agents need not be reduced when used in combination with group A and/or B drugs.

For decreasing salivary flow only, atropine is most recommended. Glycopyrrolate maintains this action for too long a period of time for most dental procedures. Scopolamine may produce CNS depression and emergence delirium, the latter occurring more commonly in patients under 6 years and over 65 years of age. The IM administration of two drugs from the same therapeutic category (i.e., meperidine and fentanyl or diazepam and midazolam) is only rarely recommended. Table 11-7 summarizes the recommended use of the drug groups listed.

Commonly used IM drug combinations

Diazepam or midazolam and opioid agonist. The combination of benzodiazepine and an opioid is used in both medicine and dentistry for both adult and pediatric patients. As the clinical effect of both diazepam and midazolam lasts 3 to 4 hours following IM administration, the selection of an appropriate opioid is important. IM morphine, with a duration of up to 7 hours, is too long-acting for most medical and dental procedures. Where a patient may be kept under continual observation for several hours immediately posttreatment, and where posttreatment pain is a significant factor, IM morphine may be indicated. Shorter-acting opioids, such as meperidine, fentanyl, sufentanil, and alfentanil, are more appropriate for administration with midazolam or diazepam. Another problem arises where diazepam is to be used. Being lipid-soluble, diazepam cannot be mixed in the same syringe with any of the opioids (which are water-soluble). Two IM injections must therefore be administered. Water-soluble midazolam, on the other hand, which may be combined in the same syringe with the opioids, usually represents the most reasonable choice for an intramuscularly administered benzodiazepine.

Promethazine plus opioid. Because of the moderate duration (2 to 4 hours) of promethazine, it may be combined with meperidine, fentanyl and its congeners, or alphaprodine in the same syringe. Promethazine and meperidine are marketed in a premixed form, Mepergan. This combination is rather popular in pediatric medicine and dentistry for management of the overtly disruptive patient. Promethazine functions both as an antiemetic to counter the effect of the opioid and to provide an added degree of sedation. This injectable drug combination is available as Mepergan. Each milliliter of Mepergan

Table 11-7. Recommended use of drug groups

Drug group	Recommendation	Level of sedation*
A alone (benzodiazepines)	High	Light to moderate
A alone (nonbenzodiazepines)	Low (but better than B alone)	Moderate to deep
B alone	Low	Moderate to deep
C alone	High	For ↓ secretions
A and B	High	Moderate to deep
A and C	High	Light to moderate and ↓ secretions
B and C	Low	Moderate to deep and ↓ secretions
A, B, and C	High	Moderate to deep and ↓ secretions

*Level of sedation may vary considerably with the same mg/kg dose from patient to patient. Level indicated is *usual* level sought. The training and ability of the sedation team to safely manage the patient ultimately determine the level of sedation that should be employed.

contains 25 mg promethazine and 25 mg meperidine. Govannitti[18] considers this combination to be the most ideal choice for intramuscular sedation. Suggested doses are 0.7 mg/kg promethazine and 1.0 mg/kg meperidine. Each drug is drawn up individually into the same syringe and administered IM. If after 45 minutes sedation is inadequate, N_2O-O_2 sedation may be added.[18]

Hydroxyzine plus opioid. Similar to promethazine and opioid in depth and duration, hydroxyzine may be combined with meperidine or fentanyl. Hydroxyzine serves to minimize opioid-induced nausea and vomiting and to provide a degree of sedation. It is used primarily in management of the acutely disruptive or uncooperative child. This technique as well as promethazine plus opioid may also be used in adults.

Barbiturate plus opioid. Providing a slightly longer duration and a slightly greater depth of sedation than the preceding combinations, the combination of either pentobarbital or secobarbital and an opioid is more likely to produce significant respiratory depression. Respiratory monitoring is more essential when this combination is used.

Pentobarbital, meperidine, and scopolamine. Commonly called "twilight sleep," this combination is similar to the preceding one with the added effects of the scopolamine providing for a slightly greater depth of sedation and the production of a degree of amnesia in some patients. This technique was employed for many years as preoperative sedation prior to the induction of general anesthesia. When used intravenously this combination is termed the "Jorgensen technique."

Meperidine, promethazine, and chlorpromazine. This combination is probably more familiar by the name "lytic cocktail" or by its abbreviation, DPT, taken from the proprietary names of the three agents Demerol, Phenergan, and Thorazine. DPT is rarely employed today for sedation, primarily because of the chlorpromazine and its potentially significant side effects (see Phenothiazines). It provides a long duration and a moderately deep level of sedation. Administration of this technique for IM sedation is actively discouraged.[85,86]

Monitoring during IM sedation

A significant change in the use of IM/SM sedation since the initial publication of this book in 1985 has been the increasing importance of monitoring whenever IM/SM agents are used. The more intense the depth of sedation obtained, the greater the level of monitoring required to ensure patient safety.

Where conscious sedation is the goal, direct communication with the sedated patient is the most important monitor (CNS), although respiratory and cardiovascular monitoring is also necessary. However, patient responsiveness is diminished when deep sedation is the goal, and monitoring of other systems must be intensified.

Vital signs (BP, heart rate and rhythm, respiratory rate) must be checked continuously or at regular intervals throughout the period of sedation (which always starts before the actual dental or surgical treatment and extends into the posttreatment period). The use of the pretracheal stethoscope has become a standard of care for IM/SM techniques. In pediatrics, placement of the stethoscope over the precordium is acceptable, although its placement over the trachea, immediately superior to the sternal notch, is preferred. In adults pretracheal placement is preferred.

The use of pulse oximetry should become a standard of care for IM/SM conscious and deep sedation although at present it is not. The combination of a pretracheal stethoscope and pulse oximetry provides the doctor with an immediate and continuous "feel" as to the respiratory status of the sedated patient, which is important since the respiratory system is the system most readily influenced (after the CNS) by the IM/SM agents employed for sedation.

Additional monitoring techniques, such as capnography and electrocardiography, are rarely employed at the present time and are not considered to be essential monitors during IM/SM conscious sedation, although the use of the capnograph during deep sedation is becoming increasingly popular. Monitoring of the electrical activity of the myocardium (ECG) during conscious or deep sedation is not considered by this author to be of as critical importance as respiratory monitoring.

SUMMARY

The IM route of drug administration has some definite advantages over oral administration; however, when compared to the inhalation and IV routes, the IM route fares poorly. In adults the only rationale for the IM route is a lack of success with other, more controllable, routes. In pediatrics or with handicapped patients, however, the IM (or SM) route may prove to be the only effective patient management technique available aside from general anesthesia.

Drugs administered intramuscularly must have their dosages carefully calculated. Once administered IM, it is difficult, if not impossible, to reverse the actions of most drugs. Basic management of overly sedated patients must consist primarily of basic life support: airway maintenance, breathing (spontaneous, assisted, or controlled), and circulation. Doctors employing the IM route must be adept at patient monitoring and be trained in management of the unconscious airway.

REFERENCES

1. Hine CH, Pasi A: Fatality after use of alphaprodine in analgesia for dental surgery: report of a case, *JADA* 84:858, 1972.
2. Okuji DM: Hypoxic encephalopathy after the administration of alphaprodine hydrochloride, *JADA* 103:50, 1981.
3. Goodson JM, Moore PA: Life-threatening reactions following pedodontic sedation: an assessment of narcotic, local anesthetic and antiemetic drug interaction, *JADA* 107:239, 1983.
4. Moore PA, Goodson JM: Risk appraisal of narcotic sedation for children, *Anesth Prog* 32:129, 1985.
5. Alphaprodine, *Pediatr Dent* 4 (special issue 1), 1982.
6. Trapp L, Goodson JM, Price DC: Evaluation of oral submucosal blood flow at dental injection sites by radioactive xenon clearance in beagle dogs, *J Dent Res* 56:889, 1977.
7. Caudill WA et al: Absorption rates of alphaprodine from the buccal and intravenous routes, *Pediatr Dent* 4:168, 1982.
8. Metroka DC, Marchesani JR, Carrel R: A submucous technique utilizing a narcotic and a potentiator, *J Pedod* 4:124, 1980.
9. Jensen ST, Coke JM, Cohen L: Intramuscular injection technique, *JADA* 100:700, 1980.
10. Zelman S: Notes on techniques of intramuscular injection: the avoidance of needless pain and morbidity, *Am J Med Sci* 241:563, 1961.
11. Evans E, Proctor J, Fratkin M et al: Blood flow in muscle groups and drug absorption, *Clin Pharmacol Ther* 17:44, 1975.
12. Ceravolo FJ, Meyers HE, Michael JJ et al: Full dentition periodontal surgery using intravenous conscious sedation: a report of 10,000 cases, *J Periodontol* 57:383, 1986.
13. Greenblatt D, Koch-Weser J: Intramuscular injection of drugs, *N Engl J Med* 295:542, 1976.
14. Grohar ME: How to give an intramuscular injection, New York, 1980, Pfizer Laboratories.
15. Greenblatt D, Shader R, Koch-Weser J: Serum creatinine phosphokinase concentration after intramuscular chlordiazepoxide and its solvent, *J Clin Pharmacol* 16:118, 1976.
16. Reference deleted in proof.
17. Greenblatt DJ, Koch-Weser J: Intramuscular injection of drugs, *N Engl J Med* 295:542, 1976.
18. Giovannitti JA, Trapp LD: Adult sedation: oral, rectal, IM, IV. In Dionne RA, Phero JC, eds: *Management of pain and anxiety in dental practice*. New York, 1991, Elsevier.
19. Siew C, Chang SB, Gruninger SE et al: Self-reported percutaneous injuries in dentists: implications for HBV, HIV, transmission risk, *JADA* 123(7):36, 1992.
20. McCray E, Cooperative Needlestick Surveillance Group: Occupational risk of acquired immunodeficiency syndrome among health care workers, *N Engl J Med* 314(17):1127, 1986.
21. Jagger J, Hunt EH, Brand-Elnaggar J et al: Rates of needlestick injury caused by various devices in a university hospital, *N Engl J Med* 319:284, 1988.
22. Stricof RL, Morse DL: HTLV-III/LAV seroconversion following deep intramuscular needlestick injury, *N Engl J Med* 314:1115, 1986.

23. Kerr D: New product to protect nurses from needlesticks, *Calif Nurs Rev* 39, May/June 1990.
24. Ribner BS, Landry MN, Gholson GL et al: Impact of a rigid, puncture resistant container system upon needlestick injuries, *Infect Control Hosp Epidemiol* 8:63, 1987.
25. Edmond M, Khakoo R, McTaggart B et al: Effect of bedside needle disposal units on needle recapping frequency and needlestick injury, *Infect Control Hosp Epidemiol* 9:114, 1988.
26. Hanson DJ: Intramuscular injection injuries and complications, *Gen Pract* 27:109, 1963.
27. Librium injectable, drug product insert, Roche Laboratory, 1988.
28. Greenblatt DJ, Shader RI, Koch-Weser J: Slow absorption of intramuscular chlordiazepoxide, *N Engl J Med* 291:1116, 1974.
29. McCaughey W, Dundee JW: Comparison of the sedative effects of diazepam given by the oral and intramuscular routes, *Br J Anaesth* 44:901, 1972.
30. Gamble JAS: Plasma levels of diazepam, *Br J Anaesth* 45:1085, 1973.
31. Kortilla K, Linnoila M: Absorption and sedative effects of diazepam after oral administration and intramuscular administration into the vastus lateralis muscle and the deltoid muscle, *Br J Anaesth* 47:857, 1975.
32. Moolenaar F, Bakker S, Visser J et al: Biopharmaceutics of rectal administration of drugs in man. IX: comparative biopharmaceutics of diazepam after single rectal, oral, intramuscular and intravenous administration in man. *Int J Pharmaceutics* 5:127, 1980.
33. Divoll M, Greenblatt DJ, Ochs HR et al: Absolute bioavailability of oral and intramuscular diazepam: effect of age and sex, *Anesth Analg* 62:1, 1983.
34. Reference deleted in proof.
35. Ativan, drug product insert, Wyeth-Ayerst Labs, 1991.
36. Odugbesan CO, Magbagbeola JA: Parenteral premedication with lorazepam—a dose/response study, *Afr J Med Medical Sci* 14(1-2):65, 1985.
37. Malamed SF, Quinn CL, Hatch HG: Pediatric sedation with intramuscular and intravenous midazolam. *Anesth Prog* 36:155, 1989.
38. Malamed SF, Gottschalk HW, Mulligan R et al: Intravenous sedation for conservative dentistry for disabled patients, *Anesth Prog* 36:140, 1989.
39. Theissen O, Boileua S, Wahl D et al: Sedation with intranasal midazolam for endoscopy of the upper digestive tract, *Annals Fr Anesth Reanim* 10(5):450, 1990.
40. Phenergan, drug product insert, Wyeth-Ayerst Labs, 1991.
41. Allen GD: *Dental anesthesia and analgesia*, ed 2. Baltimore, 1979, Williams & Wilkins.
42. Vistaril, drug product insert, Pfizer Inc, 1991.
43. Harvey SC: Hypnotics and sedatives: the barbiturates. In Goodman IS, Gilman A, Rall TW et al, eds: *Pharmacological basis of therapeutics,* ed 7. New York, 1985, Macmillan.
44. Nembutal, drug product insert, Abbott Labs, 1991.
45. Chang KJ, Cuatrecasas P: Heterogeneity and properties of opiate receptors, *Fed Proc* 40:2729, 1981.
46. Gebhart GF: Opioid analgesics and antagonists. In Neidle EA, Yagiela JA, eds: *Pharmacology and therapeutics for dentistry*, ed 2. St Louis, 1984, Mosby.
47. Phillips WJ: Central nervous system pain receptors. In Faust RJ, ed: *Anesthesiology review*. New York, 1991, Churchill Livingstone.

48. Shields SE: Pharmacokinetics of epidural narcotics. In Faust RJ, ed: *Anesthesiology review*. New York, 1991, Churchill Livingstone.

49. Way EL: Sites and mechanisms of basic narcotic function based on current research, *Ann Emerg Med* 15:1021, 1986.

50. Jaffe JH, Martin WR: Opioid analgesics and antagonists. In Gilman AG, Goodman LS, Rall TW et al, eds: *The pharmacological basis of therapeutics*, ed 7. New York, 1985, Macmillan.

51. Manzini JL, Somoza EJ, Fridlender HI: Oral morphine in the treatment of patients with terminal disease, *Medicina* 50(6): 532, 1990.

52. Roberts SM, Wilson CF, Seale NS et al: Evaluation of morphine as compared to meperidine when administered to the moderately anxious pediatric dental patient, *Pediatr Dent* 14(5):306, 1992.

53. Mepergan, drug product insert, Wyeth-Ayerst, 1991.

54. Wright GZ: Pharmacotherapeutic approaches to behavior management. In Wright GZ, ed: *Behavior management in dentistry for children*. Philadelphia, 1975, Saunders.

55. Anderson JA, Vamm WF Jr, Dilley DC: Pain and anxiety control, part II: pain reaction control—conscious sedation. In Pinkham JR, ed: *Pediatric dentistry: infancy through adolescence*, ed 2. Philadelphia, 1994, Saunders.

56. Troutman KC: Use of alphaprodine in pediatric dentistry. Symposium, Los Angeles, December 14 and 15, 1981. *Pediatr Dent* 4(special):156, 1982.

57. Chen DT: Alphaprodine HC1: characteristics, *Pediatr Dent* 4: 158, 1982.

58. Del Vecchio PJ Jr: 20/20, *Am Dent Assoc News* 14:4, 1983 (letter).

59. Caudill WA et al: Absorption rates of alphaprodine from the buccal and intravenous routes, *Pediatr Dent* 4(special):168, 1982.

60. Creedon RL: Alphaprodine. In Wright GZ, ed: *Behavior management in dentistry for children*. Philadelphia, 1975, Saunders.

61. Nisentil, drug product information, Roche Laboratories, 1986.

62. Wiullens JS, Myslinski NR: Pharmacodynamics, pharmacokinetics, and clinical uses of fentanyl, sufentanil, and alfentanil, *Heart Lung* 22(3):239, 1993.

63. Ackerman WE, Phero JC, Theodore GT: Ineffective ventilation during conscious sedation due to chest wall rigidity after intravenous midazolam and fentanyl, *Anesth Prog* 37(1):46, 1990.

64. Sublimaze, drug product information, Janssen Pharmaceutica, 1989.

65. Hsu JY, Lian JD, Shu KH et al: Pentazocine addict nephropathy: a case report, *Chung-hua I Hsueh Tsa Chih (Chinese Medical Journal)*, 49:207, 1992.

66. Houde RW: Analgesic effectiveness of the narcotic agonist-antagonists, *Br J Clin Pharmacol* 7:297S, 1979.

67. Talwin, drug product information, Winthrop Pharmaceuticals, 1992.

68. Vandam LD: Butorphanol, *N Engl J Med* 302:381, 1980.

69. Laffey DA, Kay NH: Premedication with butorphanol: a comparison with morphine, *Br J Anaesth* 56:363, 1984.

70. Pinnock CA, Bell A, Smith G: A comparison of nalbuphine and morphine as premedication agents for minor gynaecological surgery, *Anaesthesia* 40:1078, 1985.

71. Nubain, drug product information, DuPont, 1989.

72. Cataldo PA, Senagore AJ, Kilbride MJ: Ketorolac and patient controlled analgesia in the treatment of postoperative pain, *Surg Gynecol Obstet* 176(5):435, 1993.

73. Buckley MMT, Brogden RN: Ketorolac—a review, *Drugs* 39:86, 1990.

74. Lassen K, Epstein-Stiles M, Olsson GL: Ketorolac: a new parenteral nonsteroidal anti-inflammatory drug for postoperative pain management, *J Post Anesth Nursing* 7(4):238, 1992.

75. Acute Pain Management Guideline Panel. Acute pain management operative or medical procedures and trauma. Clinical Practice Guideline. AHCPR Pub. No. 92-0032, Rockville, Md: Agency for Health Care Policy and Research, Public Health Service, U.S. Department of Health and Human Services, Feb 1992, p 104.

76. Reich DL, Silvay G: Ketamine: an update on the first twenty-five years of clinical experience, *Can J Anesth* 36(2):186, 1989.

77. White PF, Ham J, Way WL et al: Pharmacology of ketamine isomers in surgical patients, *Anesthesiology* 52:231, 1980.

78. Ketalar, drug product information, Parke-Davis, 1990.

79. Roelofse JA, Vander-Bijl P: Adverse reactions to midazolam and ketamine premedication in children, *Anesth Prog* 38(2): 73, 1992.

80. Greenblatt DJ, Shader RI: Anticholinergics, *N Engl J Med* 288: 1215, 1973.

81. Atropine, drug product information, Elkins-Sinn, 1992.

82. Holzgrafe RE, Vondrell JJ, Mintz SM: Reversal of postoperative reactions to scopolamine with physostigmine, *Anesth Analg* 52: 921, 1973.

83. Scopolamine hydrobromide, drug product information, CIBA Pharmaceuticals, 1992.

84. Robinul, drug product information, AH Robins, 1992.

85. US Dept Health Human Resources: Management of postoperative and procedural pain in infants, children and adolescents. In *Clinical practice guideline: acute pain management: operative or medical procedures and trauma*, Rockville, Md, 1992.

86. Nahata M, Clotz M, Krogg E: Adverse effects of meperidine, promethazine, and chlorpromazine for sedation in pediatric patients, *Clin Pediatr* 24:558, 1985.

SECTION FOUR

Inhalation sedation

In the technique of inhalation sedation, gaseous agents are absorbed from the lungs into the cardiovascular system. Although any of a number of inhalation anesthetics may be administered by this route for the production of sedation (see Section Six), only one, nitrous oxide, is used by any appreciable number of health professionals (including, but not limited to, dentists, physicians, and podiatrists). This section will therefore be devoted to a discussion of the use of nitrous oxide and oxygen (N_2O-O_2) inhalation sedation.

Inhalation sedation with nitrous oxide (N_2O) and oxygen (O_2) has significant advantages over other techniques of sedation yet possesses no disadvantages of importance. This technique is an important part of the armamentarium for the management of fear and anxiety; indeed the number of health professionals using N_2O-O_2 has risen steadily during the past decade. In the United States it is estimated that approximately 40% of practicing dentists currently use N_2O-O_2,[1] while virtually all dental graduates today enter into dental practice proficient in its safe and effective use.[2] In addition, a growing number of states have modified their dental practice acts to permit the registered dental hygienist to administer N_2O-O_2.[3] In fields other than dentistry health professionals are beginning to use this valuable technique of sedation to their patients' benefit. In anesthesia N_2O-O_2 has been used for more than 100 years as an important component of most general anesthetics, primarily as a means of permitting other more potent and potentially dangerous general anesthetics to be used effectively in lower doses and consequently in a safer manner. In the past 20 years N_2O-O_2 has been used by emergency

medical personnel, both in the hospital and in mobile coronary care units, to decrease or to eliminate pain in the victim of an acute myocardial infarction.[4] Many dermatologists, plastic and reconstructive surgeons, urologists, radiologists, and ophthalmologists have begun to utilize N_2O-O_2 as an aid in patient management during minor surgical or diagnostic procedures.[5,6] In the practice of podiatric medicine there has been a significant increase in interest in this technique in recent years.[7]

Much of the current interest in inhalation sedation has occurred following a change in the basic concept concerning the goals sought when using N_2O-O_2. Once used solely as a general anesthetic (1800s) and later as an analgesic (1940s to 1950s), N_2O-O_2 is now employed to produce conscious sedation. Safety to the patient is significantly increased because the sedated patient remains conscious (and responsive) throughout the procedure. In addition there have been important changes in the design of the inhalation sedation unit used to deliver these gases. Derived from the operating room general anesthesia machine, today's inhalation sedation unit has incorporated into it safety features that make the technique of inhalation sedation one that is virtually free of significant risk to the patient.

This section consists of a series of smaller chapters than the preceding section. It is hoped that this will enable the reader to more effectively locate material that is of importance to him or her. Subsequent chapters in this section will provide in-depth discussions of the development of inhalation sedation; the advantages, disadvantages, and indications for inhalation sedation; the pharmacology of the gases employed and the mechanisms by which gaseous anesthetics produce their effect; the armamentarium for inhalation sedation; techniques for administration of N_2O-O_2; complications associated with its administration; and current concerns about N_2O, including chronic exposure, recreational abuse, and the occurrence of sexual phenomena. Concluding chapters will discuss practical considerations concerning the use of inhalation sedation and the educational guidelines established that relate to this important technique.

In this year 1994 we are preparing to celebrate the one hundred fiftieth anniversary of the "discovery" of anesthesia. Nitrous oxide was the first drug employed to achieve this magical state that enables surgeons to successfully complete surgical procedures on patients without the dreaded presence of pain.

REFERENCES

1. Jones TW, Greenfield W: Position paper of the ADA ad hoc committee on trace anesthetics as a potential health hazard in dentistry, *JADA* 95:751, 1977.
2. Council on Dental Education Accreditation: *Guidelines for U.S. dental schools.* Chicago, American Dental Association, 1994.
3. Department of Educational Surveys: Legal provisions for delegating functions to dental assistants and dental hygienists, Chicago, 1993.
4. Stern MS et al: Nitrous oxide and oxygen in acute myocardial infarction, *Lancet* 1:397, 1975.
5. Corboy JM: Nitrous oxide analgesia for outpatient surgery, *J Am Intra-ocular Implant Soc* 10(2):232, 1984.
6. Cruickshank JC, Sykes SH: Office sedation, *Adv Dermatol* 7:291, 1992.
7. Harris WC Jr et al: Nitrous oxide and valium use in podiatric surgery for production of conscious sedation, *J Am Podiatr Assoc* 72(10):505, 1982.

CHAPTER *12*

Inhalation sedation: historical perspective

The story of the development of inhalation sedation as used today in medicine and dentistry is a fascinating one, for it is also the story of the development of the art and science of anesthesiology. Nitrous oxide (N_2O), the most commonly used inhalation anesthetic agent in dentistry and indeed in all of medicine, is credited as being the first anesthetic to be employed clinically for the elimination of surgical pain. The story of the discovery of this agent and of its subsequent trials and tribulations, as well as those of the persons involved in its discovery, is presented so that the reader may be better able to appreciate the agent, the equipment, and the technique that we take so much for granted today—more than 200 years since the discovery of N_2O and 150 years since it was first employed as a general anesthetic.

BEGINNINGS (PRE-1844)

As difficult as it is to imagine, the gases oxygen (O_2) and N_2O were once unknown. It was not until 1771 that Karl Scheele and the Englishman Joseph Priestley (1733-1804), working independently, discovered O_2. In 1727 O_2 had been prepared by Stephen Hales; however, he did not recognize that it was an element, and credit for the discovery of O_2 is given to Scheele and Priestley. The year following the discovery of O_2 Priestley discovered N_2O.[1]

During the late 1700s a branch of science known as pneumatic medicine came into being. Thomas Beddoes's Pneumatic Institute in Bristol, England, became one of the major centers of investigation of the newly discovered gaseous "vapors." It was at this time that Sir Humphrey Davy (1778-1829) became interested in the study of these gaseous agents. In 1795, at the age of 17, Davy had become apprentice to the surgeon J. B. Borlase, and during his stay with Borlase had experimented with N_2O and the effects of its inhalation. Davy became the superintendent of the Pneumatic Institute in 1798, and a year later published his book *Researches, Chemical and Philosophical; Chiefly Concerning Nitrous Oxide.* In this book Davy hinted that the inhalation of N_2O might be used to diminish pain during surgical procedures. He also provided the still commonly used nickname "laughing gas." The following is an excerpt from Davy's work on N_2O in which he explains the effects of the agent on himself following self-administration for a toothache and gingival inflammation:

On the day when the inflammation was the most troublesome, I breathed three large doses of nitrous oxide. The pain always diminished after the first four or five inspirations; the thrilling came on as usual, and uneasiness was for a few minutes swallowed up in pleasure. As the former state of mind returned, the state of organ returned with it; and I once imagined that the pain was more severe after the experiment than before. . . . As nitrous oxide in its extensive operation appears capable of destroying physical pain, it may probably be used with advantage during surgical operations in which no great effusion of blood takes place.[2]

Unfortunately, both Davy and the rest of the medical profession failed to take serious notice of N_2O and to employ it for the relief of pain during surgery. One of the reasons for this failure to even try these newer gaseous agents was the fact that during the late 1700s and early 1800s "ether frolics" and "laughing gas demonstrations" were a popular source of entertainment and enjoyment among younger people (Fig.

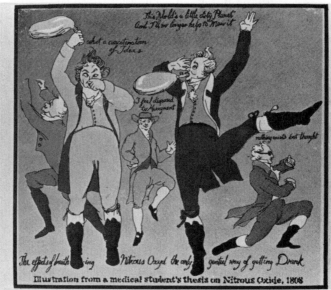

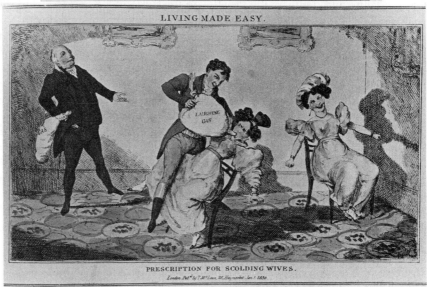

Fig. 12-1. N_2O was used exclusively in a social setting in the early 1800s, as illustrated by these drawings from publications of that era. (From Shedlen M, Wallechinsky D: *Laughing gas, nitrous oxide.* Berkeley, Calif, 1973, And/Or Press.)

12-1). Ether (ethyl ether) had been first described by Valerius Cordus in Germany in 1540, who called it "sweet vitriol."[1] In 1794 Beddoes[3] reported that ether produced a deep sleep. As with N_2O, however, ether had also been used as a source of entertainment in the late eighteenth and early nineteenth centuries. The thought that agents such as ether and N_2O, which were commonly used to produce intoxication, could ever be employed during surgery as a means of abolishing pain was offered serious consideration by very few persons.

One of these persons, Henry Hill Hickman (1800-1830), an English physician, experimented with the use of carbon dioxide (CO_2) for the creation of "suspended animation." Hickman successfully performed surgical procedures on animals utilizing the inhalation of CO_2 to abolish pain during the procedure. In 1824 Hickman's paper, "A Letter on Suspended Animation," was published.[4] Unfortunately, the medical profession did not take notice, and Hickman's potentially important research was ignored and forgotten.

In 1831 yet another volatile agent, chloroform, was discovered. Working independently, Von Liebig (1803-1873) in Germany, Guthrie (1782-1848) in New York, and Soubeiran (1793-1858) in France are credited with its discovery.

In 1842 two other ambitious men took the great step forward and successfully administered ether to a patient during a surgical procedure. In Rochester, New York, Dr. W.E. Clark administered ether to a patient having a tooth extracted by a dentist, Dr. Elijah Pope. In Georgia, Dr. Crawford W. Long administered ether to John Venable for the removal of a tumor from his neck. It is interesting that neither of these persons thought this discovery important enough to write about it in the scientific journals. Dr. Long finally wrote about his use of the agent, stating that he had used it on three occasions in 1842 and on at least one occasion annually since that time.[5] The date of Long's paper was 1849, years after he had originally used ether clinically. The purpose of the paper was to lay claim to the title of the "Founder of General Anesthesia," which was at that time being contested between Morton, Wells, and Jackson—three men who shall be discussed shortly.

Thus for several more years patients requiring surgery were left with the same two options they had faced for centuries: endure the surgical procedure without benefit of any means of abolishing pain or elect not to have the surgery and face probable death.

However, as the 1840s progressed, things were about to change. It is interesting that one of these great changes occurred in a most unusual setting—a popular science lecture during which volunteers from the audience were permitted to experience the effects of N_2O.

THE EARLY DAYS (1844-1862)

On December 10, 1844, in the town of Hartford, Connecticut, Professor Gardner Quincy Colton presented a popular science lecture. Professor Colton was an itinerant, traveling around the countryside presenting his show of new scientific and quasi-scientific discoveries to eager audiences. In his show N_2O gas was discussed and demonstrated, and as a part of the demonstration male volunteers were invited from the audience to partake of the effects of N_2O. Women were also permitted to try N_2O, but not in the presence of the men. A private session was held for the women.

A Hartford dentist, Dr. Horace Wells (1815-1848), was in the audience on this particular evening (Fig.

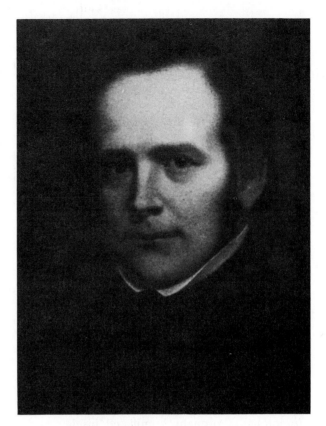

Fig. 12-2. Horace Wells (1815-1848).

12-2). Wells had a productive dental practice, but being an especially sensitive person, had difficulty in dealing with the terrible anguish and suffering of his patients. In the early 1840s in dentistry as in medicine, medications for the prevention and relief of pain were nonexistent. At the demonstration a store clerk by the name of Samuel Cooley volunteered to receive N_2O. Breathing 100% N_2O from a spigot attached to a bladder bag filled with the gas, Cooley quickly became intoxicated, running about the stage. During his running about, Cooley's leg hit the side of a table quite hard, yet Cooley continued to carry on as before, apparently oblivious of his injury. The skin had been broken, the wound bleeding, but there was no indication that Cooley either felt discomfort or was even aware of the injury. Wells spoke with Cooley after the incident and confirmed that he had been unaware of the injury.

Wells discussed this occurrence with Professor Colton and arranged for a demonstration of N_2O at Wells's dental office the next day. At the office, on December 11, 1844, a reluctant Colton served as the anesthesiologist as another dentist, Dr. John Riggs, extracted a wisdom tooth from Dr. Wells. After recovering from the effects of the N_2O, Wells stated that he had been totally unaware of the procedure and that there had been absolutely no pain associated with it.[6]

Wells was taught the process of manufacturing N_2O by Professor Colton, and shortly thereafter began using N_2O in his dental practice with great success.

Through his association with William T.G. Morton, Wells was able to gain permission to demonstrate his newly found technique to the medical students and faculty at the prestigious Harvard Medical School. Morton, a dentist who became a student and later a partner of Dr. Wells in Hartford, eventually left dentistry, becoming a medical student at Harvard. Morton was present in the audience on this fateful day. Using a medical student volunteer as a patient, Dr. Wells administered N_2O to the patient through a newly developed inhaler. As the patient lapsed into unconsciousness, Wells had to remove the inhaler, pick up his instruments, and attempt to extract the volunteer's infected tooth. During the extraction attempt the patient cried out. The audience, assuming that the procedure had failed, proceeded to boo and hiss Wells until he was forced to leave the demonstration hall, thoroughly humiliated, his demonstration a failure.[7]

On awakening, the patient stated that he was unaware that anything had happened, did not remember crying out, and had no memory of the attempted extraction. Unfortunately for Wells, this admission came too late. Wells returned to Hartford and continued his practice of dentistry, as well as the use of N_2O. Over the next year or so, however, ether gradually became the most important of the inhalation anesthetics.

There are several possible explanations for the "failure" of the demonstration given by Horace Wells. The first and most likely reason is that Wells had to function in the dual capacity of both the anesthesiologist and surgeon. Today it is quite apparent that the performance of two such important tasks by one person is not only extremely difficult but also increases risk to the patient during the procedure. However, at the time of Wells's demonstration there was no experience to judge from, for this was the first time such a procedure had been attempted. Though the patient was anesthetized by the N_2O initially, at the point at which Wells began the extraction of the tooth he had to stop the administration of the gas to the patient. Breathing only room air, the patient would naturally begin to recover from the effects of

the N_2O, regaining consciousness. The pharmacokinetics of nitrous oxide are such that the gas maintains a rapid onset of action and an equally rapid termination of action when its administration is discontinued.

A second possible explanation is the concept of biological variability. As is well known today and has been stressed throughout this text, people respond differently when given the same dose of a drug. This concept is illustrated with the so-called "bell-shaped," or normal distribution, curve. Unfortunately for Wells, in 1844 this concept was unknown. The patient may have been what would today be called a hyporesponder, a patient requiring a larger dose of a medication to achieve a desired clinical action.

The third possible explanation for the so-called failure is the lack of knowledge of the various levels of anesthesia. After the patient recovered, he stated that he had been unaware of any discomfort and of his crying out. These responses of Wells's patient are associated with the type of anesthesia commonly known as ultralight general anesthesia. At this level the patient is indeed unconscious, although minimally. He is quite able to react to pain and move about in response to it; however, because of the level of CNS depression he is unable to remember anything occurring at this time.

Unfortunately for Wells, the medical profession, and the many patients requiring surgery at that time, this information was unknown. Surgery continued for a short while longer without the benefit of pain-relieving medications.

Within a year or so of his ill-fated demonstration of N_2O, a discouraged Wells abandoned the practice of dentistry. He ceased to publicize N_2O and to attempt to introduce it into clinical use, although he personally knew that it could be used successfully. He was able to earn a living by partaking in several strange occupations—buying pictures in Paris, France, to sell in the United States and traveling around the countryside with a troupe of singing canaries. Wells continued to experiment with newer inhalation agents and soon became addicted to chloroform. Many of the founders of anesthesia became addicted to the chemicals they discovered, for they had no one to experiment on but themselves. The concept of addiction was unknown at the time and proved to be a terrible personal price to pay for the introduction of newer drugs and chemicals.[8]

In May 1848 Horace Wells was asked by a friend to provide him with a vial of sulfuric acid so that the friend could throw it at a prostitute who earlier had damaged his clothes. The friend then asked Wells if he would like to continue doing this, but Wells declined. Several days later, after Wells had inhaled some chloroform, he returned alone to Broadway in New York and while under the influence of the chloroform threw sulfuric acid at two other prostitutes. Arrested and placed in jail for these acts, Wells took his own life. The following are excerpts from the last letters written by Horace Wells.[9]

Sunday, 7 o'clock P.M.

... I again take up this pen to finish what I have to say. ... Before 12 tonight to pay the debt of Nature; yes, if I were free to go tomorrow I could not live and be called a villain. God knows I am not one. ... Oh, what misery I shall bring on all my near relatives, and what still more distresses me is the fact that my name is familiar to the whole scientific world as being connected with an important discovery. And now, while I am scarcely able to hold my pen, I must to all say farewell! ... Did I live I should become a maniac. The instrument of my destruction was obtained when the officer who had me in charge permitted me to go to my room yesterday.

Horace Wells

To my dear wife

I feel that I am fast becoming a deranged man, or I would desist from this act. I can't live and keep my reason, and on this account God will forgive the deed. I can say no more.

Horace Wells

On May 30, 1848, Horace Wells, later acknowledged as the founder of anesthesia, committed suicide while in jail by cutting the femoral artery in his left thigh with a razor. Prior to this act, Wells had inhaled some chloroform to produce insensibility to the pain.

Interestingly N_2O was reintroduced in 1863 by Professor Colton in New Haven, Connecticut, and became the most commonly used inhalation anesthetic, a position it still maintains today.

William T.G. Morton (1819-1868) is the next major character in the story of the development of anesthesia. Morton learned of the idea of inhalation anesthesia from Wells, under whom he was a student of dentistry and later an associate in dental practice in Hartford. Morton later entered into medical school at Harvard, and it was through Morton's con-

nections that Wells obtained the invitation to his ill-fated demonstration of N_2O anesthesia. Morton was a member of the audience at that demonstration. A more effective anesthetic gas was required, and Morton began to experiment with ether. How Morton came to work with ether became a topic of considerable discussion and controversy as the years passed. It is possible that he learned of ether through "ether parties" that were at the time a frequent entertainment of the medical students or that he was pushed into its use through a professor of his at Harvard, Charles Thomas Jackson (1805-1880), a physician and chemist.

Morton experimented to a small degree on animals (his family dog) and on himself prior to his first use of ether on a patient. That patient, Mr. Eben Frost, received ether for the extraction of a tooth on September 30, 1846. Morton recorded the incident as follows:

Toward evening a man residing in Boston came in, suffering great pain, and wishing to have a tooth extracted. He was afraid of the operation, and asked if he could be mesmerized. I told him I had something better, and saturating my handkerchief, gave it to him to inhale. He became unconscious almost immediately. It was dark, and Dr. Hayden held the lamp while I extracted a firmly-rooted bicuspid tooth. There was not much alteration in the pulse and no relaxing of the muscles. He recovered in a minute and knew nothing of what had been done for him. He remained for some time talking about the experiment. This was the 30th of September 1846.[8]

Morton continued to experiment with ether, both on his own and with Dr. Henry J. Bigelow, for whom Morton administered ether for over 37 operations. All of these cases were done prior to the famous demonstration of ether at the Massachusetts General Hospital in 1846.[10]

On October 16, 1846 (now called Ether Day), Morton administered ether to Gilbert Abbott (Fig. 12-3). The famous surgeon John Collins Warren excised a tumor from the jaw of Mr. Abbott. Though considered to be an absolute success, in fact Morton's demonstration was little more successful than Wells's had been. Abbott later mentioned that when the incision was first made it felt as though his neck had been scratched by a hoe. However, unlike Wells, Morton was not hissed out of the operating theater. The reason for this is twofold: first, Dr. Bigelow had attested to Dr. Warren the success of ether; therefore, Warren was more inclined to believe that this new agent was not a fraud but in fact the real thing. Second, and of considerable importance, is the fact that Morton was

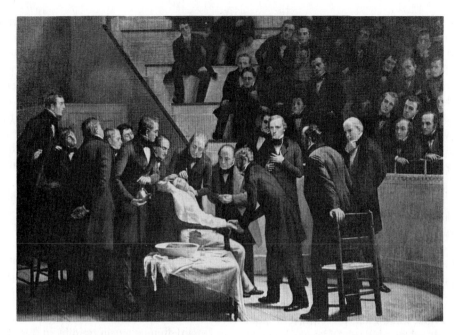

Fig. 12-3. William T.G. Morton administering ether to Gilbert Abbott as John Collins Warren removes tumor from neck of Abbott in the famed Ether Dome at the Massachusetts General Hospital, October 16, 1846. (Boston Medical Library in The Francis A. Countway Library of Medicine.)

a physician and not a dentist. Dentistry at the time was looked down upon by the medical profession as a mere trade. That Wells should have even attempted to demonstrate his new technique to such an august group, including Warren, was, sad to say, quite laughable. His audience was filled with cynics and disbelievers. Morton, on the other hand, being a member of the "club," was more readily accepted. When the endorsement of Bigelow is added, it is readily seen why the less than absolutely successful procedure was proclaimed as the great event it truly was. In the words of John Collins Warren, "Gentlemen, you have witnessed a miracle. This is no humbug!"[10-12]

Ether had been for many years a popular agent for enjoyment. Ether follies were a popular form of entertainment, especially among medical students. Morton, acutely aware that if he were to suggest that this same agent be used for a serious purpose he might also be laughed at, modified the agent. He added a dye to it and called it Letheon, thus gaining acceptance for it among his colleagues.[13] The surgical amphitheater at the Massachusetts General Hospital in which this famed event took place has been preserved and is today known as the Ether Dome.

News of Morton's "etherization" spread rapidly throughout the United States and Europe, creating a degree of celebrity for Morton. On December 21,

1846, Dr. Robert Liston performed the first surgical procedure under "etherization" in England. Almost immediately following the introduction of etherization into surgery by Morton, Dr. Charles T. Jackson came forward to lay claim to its discovery, stating that it was he who had suggested its use to Morton, had advised him about the nature of the agent, and had advised him of the best manner in which to administer it. The controversy was only beginning. Soon Morton, Wells, and Jackson were engaging in bitter accusations and secret deals, each in an effort to prove that it was he in fact who was the sole founder of anesthesia. To complicate the matter still further, Crawford W. Long, who had first administered ether in 1842, came forward in 1849 to lay claim to this title.[14]

The name etherization was used for only a short time, as a more acceptable name for this new technique was being sought. Among the terms offered for this process were the following: aethereal influence, aethereal inhalation, aetherealization, aetherization, anaestheticization, anaesthism, anodyne process, apathisation, ethereal state, etherification, hebetization, lethargic state, letheonization, narcotism, somniferous agent, sopor, soporization, soporized state, and stupefaction.[10]

It was Oliver Wendell Holmes, the physician and

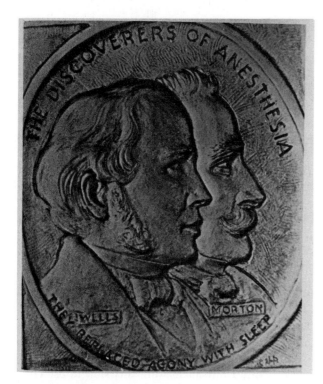

Fig. 12-4. William T.G. Morton and Horace-Wells—the discoverers of anesthesia.

author, who suggested the name anesthesia. At the height of the controversy over the founding of anesthesia, Holmes wrote to Morton:

Everybody wants to have a hand in the great discovery. All I will do is to give you a hint or two as to the names to be applied to the state produced and to the agent. The state should, I think, be called anesthesia. The adjective will be anesthetic. Thus we might say the "state of anesthesia" or the "anesthetic state."[6]

The name *anesthesia,* as suggested by Holmes, had been used by Plato in 400 B.C. to describe the absence of feelings in a philosophical sense. In the first century A.D. Dioscorides also used the term to denote the absence of physical sensation.

Morton shortly gave up the practice of dentistry, devoting his time to the practice of anesthesia. Morton was the first person to specialize full-time in the field of anesthesiology (Fig. 12-4). In addition, he was also involved in the manufacture of anesthetic inhalers and other devices for the administration of anesthetic gases.

Morton fought bitterly seeking to obtain recognition as the founder of anesthesia. Three times he petitioned the Congress of the United States for such recognition, and he spoke personally with President James Knox Polk, but during his lifetime Morton was never granted recognition as the father of ether anesthesia. Morton died of a cerebral hemorrhage in 1868, a discouraged and disappointed man. His tombstone reads: "Inventor and Revealer of Inhalation Anesthesia: Before Whom, in All Time, Surgery was Agony; By Whom, Pain in Surgery was Averted and Annulled; Since Whom, Science has Control of Pain."

As to the matter of who was the discoverer of anesthesia, the question is still debated. However, in 1864 the American Dental Association passed the following resolution:

Therefore Be It Resolved, by the American Dental Association, that to Horace Wells, of Hartford, Connecticut (now deceased), belongs the credit and honor of the introduction of anesthesia in the United States of America, and we do firmly protest against the injustice done to truth and the memory of Dr. Horace Wells, in the effort made during a series of years and especially at the last session of Congress, to award the credit to other persons or person.[14]

In 1870 the American Medical Association followed suit, and a resolution, introduced by Dr. H.R. Storer of Massachusetts, was passed recognizing the discovery of anesthesia by Horace Wells: "Resolved, that the honor of the discovery of practical anesthesia is due to the late Dr. Horace Wells of Connecticut."[15]

Despite the controversy surrounding the discovery of anesthesia, the use of both N_2O and Letheon, as Morton's ether was known, was quite slow in developing. Bitter opposition to these new drugs was found within both the medical and dental professions in the United States in the late 1840s. In 1848 the American Society of Dental Surgeons stated in regard to the use of ether and chloroform: "Hence, in all minor operations in surgery their administration is forbidden; and that their demand in the practice of dental surgery is small."[16] The Dental News Letter of July 1849, which was published in Philadelphia, stated "The Letheon is still used to considerable extent in Boston, for extraction of teeth; while in this city and in most other places, so far as we have been able to learn, it has been generally abandoned."[17] It was claimed that the use of ether encouraged charlatanism.

The development of anesthesia in England will now be discussed. In England in the late 1840s and early 1850s the discoveries of Wells and Morton were well received. In addition, chloroform, which had been introduced in 1831, became widely used.[11] Two names—John Snow and James Young Simpson—must be mentioned. John Snow (1813-1858) became the first physician after Morton to specialize in anesthesia. During his career he designed new inhalers for the delivery of anesthetics, primarily ether, which he used for extractions. In 1847 Snow published his classic textbook *On the Inhalation of Ether* and in 1858 *On Chloroform and other Anaesthetics.*[18,19]

James Young Simpson (1811-1870) was an English obstetrician (Fig. 12-5). On January 19, 1847, Simpson introduced the use of ether into his obstetrical practice. Whereas he liked the drug and the lessening of discomfort it brought his patients, Simpson disliked the disagreeable odor and the potential for nausea and vomiting associated with ether. He began to search for a better agent.

Simpson and his assistants, Keith and Matthew Duncan, began to experiment on themselves by inhaling various chemicals. Although their research was not extensive, it did produce a very valuable clinical agent. In November 1847, at the suggestion of David Waldie, a pharmacist from Liverpool, Simpson and his assistants experimented with perchloride of formyl, or chloroform, as it is known today. They found that chloroform worked quite well, and Simpson almost immediately began to use it as a means of alleviating the pains of childbirth.

Immediately, Simpson found himself embroiled in controversy with the Church of England. The propriety of abolishing pain during childbirth was the major point of contention. The argument used by the anti-Simpson clergy came from the Bible (Genesis III:16):

Unto the woman he said, I will greatly multiply thy sorrow and thy conception; in sorrow thou shalt bring forth children, and thy desire shall be to thy husband, and he shall rule over thee.

Simpson was quite able to cope with the controversy and continued to use chloroform as an analgesic to diminish labor pains. However, because of the controversy other physicians were very slow to use chloroform. However, on April 7, 1853, John Snow administered chloroform analgesia to Queen Victoria at the birth of Prince Leopold, despite the fact that *The Lancet* stated in no uncertain terms that the use of chloroform in normal labor is never justified in any circumstances. Despite this, Queen Victoria received chloroform analgesia for a period of 53 minutes, the chloroform administered by a handkerchief. As mentioned by Snow in his subsequent book on chloroform, the Queen expressed herself as greatly relieved by the administration.[19] Indeed, on April 14, 1857, Snow again administered chloroform analgesia to the Queen at the birth of Princess Beatrice.

The use of chloroform as an analgesic and the administration of anesthetics for the relief of pain during childbirth received a great boost by the actions of Queen Victoria. The field of anesthesia began to grow, as did its problems.

On November 10, 1847, Simpson published an account of his experiences with chloroform. This report was published only 6 days after Simpson first began to use chloroform and contained a glowing account of its anesthetic capabilities. Unfortunately, as is known today, all drugs possess undesirable as well as desirable effects. At the time of publication of Simpson's report the undesirable effects of chloroform were unknown (or unreported). Its ability to produce sudden cardiac arrest remained unknown

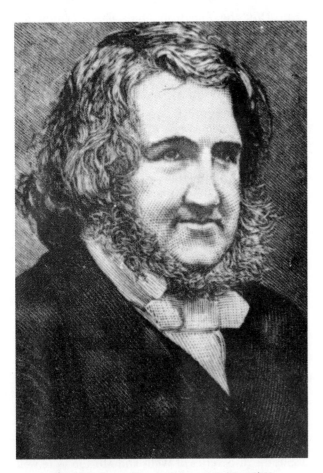

Fig. 12-5. James Young Simpson (1811-1870).

for approximately 11 weeks, until January 28, 1848, when Dr. Meggison, an untrained country doctor, administered chloroform to a 15-year-old patient, Hannah Greener, who "died like a shot rabbit" on receiving chloroform.[20] Today it is known that the effects of epinephrine on the myocardium and heart rhythm are exaggerated by chloroform, producing possibly fatal ventricular fibrillation.[21] Hannah Greener was, in the words of Dr. Meggison, "fretting all the day before 'crying continually and wishing she were dead rather than submit to it'."[22]

Simpson could not believe that chloroform could have been responsible for the death of Hannah Greener. He stated, in defense of chloroform, that the death of Hannah Greener had been caused by the brandy and water that had been poured into her mouth while she was unconscious, in an attempt at resuscitation. He said that Greener had drowned from this fluid. The fact is, we will never know what killed Hannah Greener. Deaths from light chloroform anesthesia continued to be reported, but the older generation of doctors as well as chloroform advocates refused to believe that a very small dose of chloroform could possibly kill a patient. It was not until 1911, when A. Goodman Levy published the results of his experiments on epinephrine and light chloroform anesthesia, that a possible mechanism of Hannah Greener's death was finally and satisfactorily explained—the propensity of chloroform to induce cardiac dysrhythmias, especially in the presence of elevated plasma epinephrine.[21]

During the ensuing 10 years (1850 to 1860) the use of ether and chloroform in dentistry became quite widespread and deaths continued to be reported. Controversy developed over the use of these agents within both medicine and dentistry. Thomas, in his interesting paper, "Some Early Papers on Dental Anaesthesia,"[23] cites two authors, Fowell[24] and Tomes,[25] regarding these agents. Fowell is quoted:

Some persons, I am sorry to say, have become so enamored of chloroform or ether . . . as to refuse to permit the operation (of dental extraction) without its assistance . . . but when it comes to the removal of a tooth, which is an act simple in its execution and quick in its effect, I must confess that I think it is indiscreet."

Tomes stated: "We surely use a great power to overcome a very trifling difficulty, when we give chloroform preparatory to extracting an ordinary tooth." Tomes was also aware of the advantages of analgesia as opposed to general anesthesia: "On many occasions the patient has been perfectly aware of the steps of the operation, has felt the instrument grasp the tooth . . . and yet has felt little or no pain."

At the beginning of the 1860s ether and chloroform were the dominant forms of anesthesia being used in the medical and dental professions. Nitrous oxide was used, but not as extensively, primarily because of the difficulties in its manufacture and storage.

ANESTHESIA DEVELOPS (1863-1898)

In July 1863 Gardner Quincy Colton, the man who had given Horace Wells the idea of using N_2O as an anesthetic in 1844, reintroduced N_2O to the dental profession. Nitrous oxide had not been in very common use since the death of Wells and the introduction of ether and chloroform. Colton established "dental institutes" in cities throughout the United States. These institutes specialized in tooth extractions under N_2O general anesthesia. One hundred percent N_2O was administered, the patient's nose being held closed by the administrator as the patient inhaled through their mouth. Colton soon became the most renowned figure in the world of N_2O. By the year 1881, 18 years after his reintroduction of N_2O, Colton had administered N_2O to 121,709 persons without a death. Each of these cases has subsequently been documented.[26] That Colton was able to obtain such an outstanding record using an anesthetic gas without supplemental O_2 is truly outstanding. Yet Colton would have argued that the use of 100% N_2O was perfectly safe because the oxygen molecule attached to the nitrogen (N_2) would provide the cells of the body with whatever oxygen they required. It is now known that this oxygen is not available for use by the body. Fortunately, the vast majority of cases reported by Colton were of only 1 or 2 minutes in duration (tooth extraction); however, some did last for as long as 16 minutes without adverse effect, according to Colton. In addition, such was the clinical experience and technical excellence of Colton that he was able to administer this drug to more than 120,000 persons without a single death, in spite of the fact that his entire practice was based on an incorrect principle!

Dr. Edmund W. Andrews (1824-1904), a physician born in Vermont, was one of the founders of the Chicago Medical College, the forerunner of the Northwestern School of Medicine. However, Andrews's major claim to fame, and indeed a most significant one in the history of anesthesia, was the addition of 20% O_2 to N_2O. Andrews published his findings in the *Chicago Medical Examiner* in 1868, titled "The Oxygen Mixture; A New Anesthetic Combination."[27] Andrews claimed this combination to be safer and more pleasant than any anesthetic mixture then known. In 1862 Joseph T. Clover (1825-1882) had introduced the mixture of chloroform and air. Clover also sought to make ether anesthesia safer by inducing anesthesia with N_2O and then maintaining anesthesia by adding ether to the N_2O. Indeed, Andrews was right in his thoughts about the combination of 20% O_2 and 80% N_2O. His concept of the use of this agent as well as all other anesthetics still holds true today, 126 years later.

In 1868 Paul Bert, a student of the great Claude Bernard, wrote that the use of 100% N_2O for more than 2 minutes would bring about signs and symptoms of asphyxia. Bert designed an apparatus capable of delivering 25% O_2 and 75% N_2O.[28]

Shortly thereafter, in 1872 in England, liquid N_2O became commercially available to the dental and medical professions, making its use much more practical and considerably safer. No longer did physicians and dentists have to manufacture their own N_2O with the risk of including impurities in the gas.

In 1881 two developments that had profound effects on the use of N_2O occurred in widely separate parts of the world. In St. Petersburg, Russia, an obstetrician, S. Klikovitsch, first used N_2O as an analgesic to relieve the pains of labor. As the years passed, the production of analgesia was to become a primary indication for the use of N_2O.

In the same year in Philadelphia the S. S. White Manufacturing Company began to supply liquified N_2O to the medical and dental professions. It also introduced an apparatus that permitted the delivery of the gas from the cylinder to the patient. This device revolutionized and simplified the administration of N_2O and provided a great boost to its use.

Sir Frederick Hewitt (1857-1916) invented the first practical anesthesia machine for administering N_2O and O_2 in fixed proportions in 1887. By the year 1889 N_2O-O_2 analgesia was being used in dentistry during cavity preparation in Liverpool, England. There were several problems associated with the use of N_2O-O_2 analgesia at that time. The use of very low-speed handpieces, with no local anesthesia (by 1890 cocaine injection into the gums was becoming an accepted method of pain control) or poor local anesthesia, plus the fact that much of the N_2O and O_2 being used was impure, led to a significant number of side effects, such as nausea, vomiting, and excitement. As the 1890s continued, the use of N_2O-O_2 analgesia gradually declined.

THE TWENTIETH CENTURY

By 1898 both Hewitt in England and White in the United States had developed new devices for the administration of N_2O-O_2. In 1902 the Cleveland Dental Manufacturing Company introduced a machine designed by Charles K. Teter, D.D.S. This machine could deliver O_2, N_2O, and other anesthetic gases. Eight years later (1910) two of the major manufacturers of anesthesia equipment entered into the marketplace. J.A. Heidbrink, of Minneapolis, Minnesota, modified the 1902 Teter machine and introduced a new model for the administration of N_2O and O_2. Heidbrink's interest in anesthesia began while he was a dental student. He had suffered such excruciating pain during the extraction of his third molars without the benefit of anesthesia that he decided to correct the situation. Also in 1910 E.I. McKesson, M.D., introduced the first intermittent-flow machine with accurate percentage control for N_2O-O_2. McKesson soon became the undisputed international authority on N_2O anesthesia and a leader in its development.

Teter, Heidbrink, and McKesson, by virtue of the many papers they wrote and lectures and clinical demonstrations they presented, were largely responsible for the increased use of N_2O-O_2 anesthesia for surgical operations throughout the United States.[29,30]

Periods of interest in N_2O were invariably followed by periods of almost total neglect. Two such periods of heightened interest occurred between 1913 and 1918 and between 1932 and 1938. Failures and side effects with the technique were not uncommon, even with the advent of newer machines and the increasing purity of the gases. The technique of N_2O anesthesia was not taught at any dental school or in any postgraduate program during this time; thus it was difficult for a dentist to learn the technique. The manufacturers of the anesthesia machines provided courses for doctors, but the quality of these courses was uniformly poor by modern standards.

A good description of the use of N_2O-O_2 analgesia in dentistry in 1923 is provided by Nevin and Puterbaugh:

For its administration the patient is seated comfortably in the dental chair and the nasal inhaler adjusted carefully in order to avoid leakage about its margin and waste of the anesthetic. Since the patient does not lose consciousness at any time the mouth is left uncovered, no prop between the teeth being required. Before the anesthetic is started it is explained to the patient that he is to administer his own anesthetic. He is directed to breathe through his nose until a sense of numbness and stiffness comes over him which is felt extending to his finger tips, at which time his teeth, when snapped sharply together, will feel like wooden pegs set in wooden jaws. He is told that in this state he will feel no pain; that he need not go to sleep but that when he feels he is about to lose consciousness he is then to breathe through his mouth and by so doing he will remain awake. He is repeatedly reminded that while he will feel the vibration of the bur and be conscious of everything that is going on, the sense of pain will be entirely obtunded; that should he feel the slightest indication of pain he is to breathe entirely through his nose until the pain disappears. Nitrous oxid [sic] and oxygen are then turned on in proportion of twenty per cent oxygen and eighty per cent nitrous oxid. This mixture is administered throughout and, being of the same oxygen percentage as atmospheric air, there are no asphyxial symptoms exhibited at any time during the administration. Patients take quite an interest in this type of anesthesia for they feel that they are a part of its administration and willingly endeavor to cooperate for its success. This method may be safely employed for periods up to one half hour; if continued longer it is occasionally followed by nausea and slight headache, which, of course, should be avoided by arranging for a greater number of sittings of shorter periods each.

The types of operations best suited to analgesia are the excavation of hypersensitive dentin, the preparing of roots for the adaptation of crowns and bridges, the scaling of deep pyorrhea pockets, etc. It will not obtund pain sufficiently to permit of the removal of vital pulps or the extraction of teeth or the lancing of abscesses, all of which require complete anesthesia for their performance.[31]

Throughout the 1930s and into the 1940s most dentists who used N_2O worked with N_2O-O_2 in a ratio of 80%-20% described previously, although many still employed 100% nitrous oxide general anesthesia. The number of dentists using N_2O increased as the 1940s passed, the purity of the gases improved, and the quality of the machines for gas delivery increased, yet the success rate of N_2O-O_2 analgesia still remained low.[32]

During the 1940s fundamental changes in pain control in dentistry occurred. The use of local anesthesia as the primary means of pain control became more accepted. In 1945 lidocaine, the first of the newer, more effective, amide-type local anesthetics was introduced into clinical use. N_2O, which had been introduced in 1844 as a means of eliminating pain, was no longer the "ideal" drug for this task. Over the next few years the manner in which nitrous oxide was used was modified. Rather than seeking the elimination of pain as its primary goal, N_2O could now be used for the management of anxiety and the production of relaxation (sedation). With this change in the goal being sought came

changes in technique, dosage, and the approach to the patient.

In 1947 the third edition of Dr. Harry M. Seldin's classic textbook, *Practical Anesthesia for Dental and Oral Surgery: Local and General,* was published. In Chapter 22, The Administration of Nitrous Oxide and Its Mixtures, Dr. Seldin describes the ways in which the drug was used in the 1940s:

The administration of nitrous oxide is no longer limited to the use of the gas by itself. In order to obviate the haphazard technique of "straight" nitrous oxide anesthesia, to reduce the possibility of unfavorable sequelae, and to extend the operating time, oxygen has been added. . . . Nitrous oxide is given in one of three ways:

1. Pure nitrous oxide, with the exclusion of air or oxygen, usually referred to as "straight nitrous oxide."
2. Nitrous oxide with air.
3. Nitrous oxide with oxygen.

Straight Nitrous Oxide. Pure nitrous oxide without the addition of air or oxygen was the first form in which the gas was employed for the purpose of producing unconsciousness. Today, in spite of the tremendous advances in the art of anesthesia, some practitioners still persist in the use of so-called "straight nitrous oxide."

The technique is simplicity itself. The pure gas is delivered to the patient from . . . the tank. . . . As soon as the patient shows the classical signs of asphyxia (thirty to sixty seconds): dilated pupils, absence of all reflexes, cyanosis, clonic muscular spasms, and jactitation, the inhaler is removed, a gauze pack forced into the posterior part of the mouth, and the operation commenced. The exodontist must work at top speed, usually with little regard for the oral tissues. It is evident that lacerations and sharp bony processes are inevitable when extensive exodontia must be completed in the two minutes or so available before consciousness returns. . . . Many of the pioneers in dental anesthetics developed unusual speed and dexterity, and could accomplish an unbelievable amount of work with a single administration. . . .

There are certain limitations to this method. The period of anesthesia is very short, being frequently less than thirty seconds and rarely longer than one minute. . . . When the operation requires more time, the patient often recovers sufficiently to interfere with the procedure.

However, in light of the present knowledge of anesthetic gases, there is very little justification for the rather crude method described. The addition of oxygen to the nitrous oxide has immeasurably improved operative technique under anesthesia. Speed ceases to be the prime factor.[33]

The term "blue gassing" refers to this technique of administration of pure N_2O. Blue gassing was employed in dentistry for many years, even well into the

1950s and early 1960s. Seldin goes on to describe two other techniques of N_2O anesthesia:

Nitrous Oxide—Air Mixtures. Although narcosis with gas and air has been employed, it can hardly be recommended. This method is extremely trying for the anesthetist, and the end result is not particularly gratifying. In addition to the prevalence of asphyxial symptoms . . . anesthesia is not smooth, and nausea appears almost routinely after anesthesias of more than five minutes' duration; the recovery of the patient is uncomfortably retarded. Most of these deleterious effects may be attributed to the high percentage of nitrogen included in the anesthetic mixture.

Nitrous Oxide—Oxygen Mixtures. Mixtures of nitrous oxide with oxygen have held and still hold a paramount and proved position in dental anesthesia.

Seldin describes two induction techniques—the first is the slow induction technique in which the patient is administered a N_2O-O_2 ratio of 93%-7% for 1 minute. As signs of excitement develop, 100% N_2O is administered until the patient reaches the third stage of anesthesia. Sufficient O_2 is then added to maintain the desired plane of anesthesia. In the rapid induction technique, 100% N_2O is given for 45 to 60 seconds until the patient reaches the third stage of anesthesia, at which point 10% O_2 is added. The percentage of O_2 is changed to meet the needs of the patient:

The anesthetic level is a variable depending upon the type of individual and may differ within the limits of 5 to 80 per cent of oxygen and 20 to 95 per cent of nitrous oxide. Any point within these rather widely-divergent extremes may be required to maintain different subjects at an even keel in the normal plane in the third stage.

Seldin then recommends "setting the dial at 100% oxygen for several inhalations" at the end of the procedure." In discussing analgesia with N_2O, he states:

It is evident that analgesia with nitrous oxide and oxygen is an exceedingly safe procedure, because nitrous oxide is in itself the least harmful anesthetic known to the profession. . . . Analgesia may be maintained without the slightest danger for periods of thirty minutes and longer on any patient, regardless of age. As a matter of fact, elderly patients frequently make the best cases.

The concepts of individual variation and titration are discussed by Seldin:

After the first few inhalations, each subject becomes a law unto himself, and his personal needs in respect to the proper mixture of these gases must be determined by the various symptoms of analgesia manifested by him from one

minute to the next. In fact, considerable variations in the dial settings may be detected for the same person from day to day. This proves the falsity and irrationality of the recommendations made by gas-machine demonstrators that a standard percentage setting, consistently maintained, will induce and sustain perfect analgesia on all patients, irrespective of age or physical condition.

Many of the so-called modern concepts underlying the use of inhalation anesthetics and other parenterally administered drugs were discussed in Seldin's textbook. Much of the impetus for the use of N_2O-O_2 analgesia and sedation stems from the his writings and lectures.

MODERN TIMES (1950-PRESENT)
The development of courses and guidelines

In the 1950s and 1960s N_2O was becoming more frequently used in dentistry. The use of 100% N_2O was decreasing rapidly, and, with the advent of newer local anesthetics for operative pain control, N_2O-O_2 became a very popular agent for the management of the apprehensive dental patient. Interest in the field of anesthesiology in dentistry grew, and in 1953 the American Dental Society of Anesthesiology was formed. In the ensuing years this organization has led the way in advancing the standards and practices in the use of anesthesia (general, local, and sedation) within dentistry in the United States.[34,35]

A few dental schools added courses in inhalation sedation to the dental curriculum as the 1950s gave way to the 1960s. Postgraduate programs in inhalation sedation increased in number; however, with but few exceptions their quality remained low. One man, however, Dr. Harry Langa, presented postgraduate programs of quality throughout these years. Dr. Langa began using N_2O in 1936 and presented his first course in 1949. Between that time and the publication of the second edition of his classic textbook, *Relative Analgesia in Dental Practice: Inhalation Analgesia and Sedation with Nitrous Oxide,* in 1976, he had trained more than 6000 dentists to use this technique safely. Today his book remains the most comprehensive textbook devoted solely to inhalation sedation with N_2O (Fig. 12-6).[36]

As schools and other organizations began to present courses in inhalation sedation, it became obvious that the level of training being offered and its quality varied considerably. It was decided that standards ought to be established for the teaching of the various techniques of pain and anxiety control in dentistry. In 1962 the American Dental Society of Anesthesiology held the first of four workshops, at-

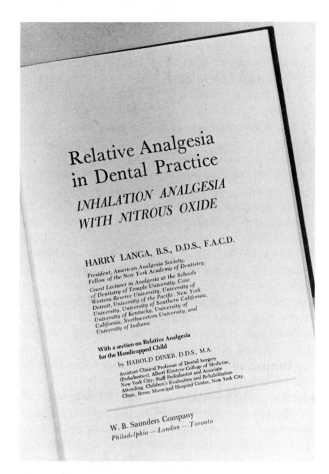

Fig. 12-6. *Relative Analgesia in Dental Practice: Inhalation Analgesia with Nitrous Oxide,* Harry Langa's classic text on N_2O and O_2. (From Langa H: *Relative analgesia in dental practice: inhalation analgesia with nitrous oxide.* Philadelphia, 1968, Saunders.)

tended by representatives of 43 dental schools, out of which came the *Guidelines for Teaching the Comprehensive Control of Pain and Anxiety in Dentistry.* Included within these guidelines is an outline for inhalation sedation courses.[37] The most recent version of these recommendations is presented in Chapter 20.[38] With the adoption of these guidelines the overall quality of training in inhalation sedation was significantly improved. Three primary areas—the undergraduate dental student, the graduate dental student, and continuing education for the postgraduate student—were addressed by the guidelines.

The anesthesia machine

Another area requiring improvement was the inhalation sedation unit itself. There had been significant changes made in the method of delivering N_2O-O_2 to the patient since the first clinical use of

agent in 1844. Early in the history of inhalation sedation a bladder bag filled with 100% N_2O was used. A spigot attached to the bag was placed into the patient's mouth, the patient inhaled the gas and lost consciousness, and the procedure was carried out as quickly as was possible.

By 1846 Morton had improved on this method of delivering inhalation anesthetics to the patient. John Snow in England devised and first used an inhaler in 1847 that was quite similar to the full-face masks used today in anesthesia.[18]

As has been mentioned in this chapter, one of the major drawbacks to the use of N_2O was the need for the doctor to manufacture the agent himself. The process was cumbersome and storage of the gas difficult. However, in 1872 the Johnson Brothers, in England, began to produce liquified N_2O on a commercial basis. Approximately 5 years later, the S.S. White Company of Philadelphia began the marketing of liquified N_2O cylinders in the United States. They also manufactured an anesthesia device that administered N_2O gas from the cylinder to the patient. The use of N_2O was greatly enhanced by this innovation.

In 1898 Sir Frederick Hewitt manufactured and sold the first devices for delivering N_2O-O_2 anesthesia. Shortly thereafter the S.S. White Company patented their own similar device. Dr. Charles K. Teter introduced the second N_2O-O_2 anesthesia machine in the United States in 1902. E.I. McKesson perfected the first intermittent-flow N_2O-O_2 anesthesia machine with an accurate means of controlling the percentages of both gases and marketed it in 1910. Also in 1910 the third of the pioneers in the manufacture of anesthesia devices, J.A. Heidbrink, D.D.S., entered the marketplace. His model "OO" appeared, later followed by the model "T." This device included a reducing valve that served as a flowmeter. By 1918 the four major manufacturers of anesthesia devices in the United States were McKesson, Connell, von Foregger, and Heidbrink.

From the designs of these and other pioneers, the modern anesthesia machine has developed. The inhalation sedation apparatus used today for the administration of N_2O-O_2 is modified from this device (Fig. 12-7). The major change required to adapt the anesthesia machine for inhalation sedation was the removal from the unit of all but the O_2 and N_2O gas supplies and flowmeters. However, situations developed in which the cylinder of O_2 became depleted during a procedure, resulting in the delivery of 100% N_2O to the patient. In too many situations serious

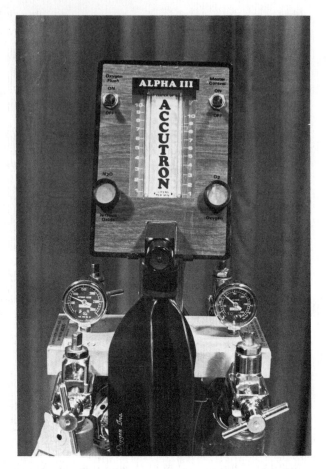

Fig. 12-7. Modern inhalation sedation unit.

morbidity and in some cases mortality occurred. In 1976 the American Dental Association's Council on Dental Materials, Instruments, and Equipment adopted standards for the manufacture of inhalation sedation units in the United States.[39] These standards required inhalation sedation devices to incorporate a series of fail-safe devices into the unit. The primary goal of these devices was to prevent the administration of O_2 in a less than atmospheric concentration.

With more and more scientific information being gathered about the effects of the gases used in inhalation sedation, further modification of these units has occurred. For example, in recent years the nasal inhaler has undergone a change in design because of a potential problem associated with the chronic inhalation of trace amounts of N_2O by dental personnel.[40] The scavenging nasal hood has been introduced. Other refinements in the apparatus for the delivery of N_2O-O_2 may be forthcoming as knowledge of the technique and drugs increases.

in 1985, the author has noticed a significant change in the composition of enrollees in continuing education courses in inhalation sedation. Throughout the 1970s and early 1980s course participants were almost exclusively dentists and other dental personnel. Only occasionally did other health professionals (MDs, podiatrists) enroll in these programs. Indeed, review of course rosters through 1984 reveals but three nondental health professionals (one MD, two podiatrists) of total course enrollment of more than 800 "offices."

The past 8 years have seen a tremendous increase in interest in N_2O-O_2 inhalation sedation (and intravenous sedation) among other health professionals. Of 90 enrolled "offices" in the past 4 years, 39 were nondental. Foremost among these groups are physicians who are engaged in outpatient minor surgical procedures, which are akin to the typical dental treatment. Plastic and reconstructive surgeons, dermatologists, urologists, orthopedic, and general surgeons have become acutely aware of their patients' desire for the management of fear and anxiety as well as for the management of pain (provided by local anesthetics) during these minor surgical procedures.[41] Podiatrists have also begun to use inhalation sedation to a significant degree during many of their surgical procedures that require the administration of local anesthesia. Enrollment by dentists in postgraduate inhalation sedation courses has diminished during this time as ever more recent graduates enter into dental practice having received training and experience in this technique while in dental school. The use of inhalation sedation in the practice of dental hygiene has started to expand as the benefits of this technique for root planing and curettage become increasingly recognized.

In the succeeding chapters in this section we will review the indications for inhalation sedation, the pharmacology of nitrous oxide and oxygen, techniques of their delivery to patients, and complications associated with its use, as well as the components of the armamentarium. All of the material contained in these chapters was in large part first discovered or developed by the men discussed in this chapter. The history of anesthesia to a very large degree is the history of N_2O.

REFERENCES

1. Lee JA, Atkinson RS: *A synopsis of anesthesia,* ed 5. Baltimore, 1964, Williams & Wilkins.

2. Davy H: Researches, chemical and philosophical; chiefly concerning nitrous oxide, 1800. In Fullmer JZ, ed: *Sir Humphry Davy's Published* Works. Cambridge, Mass, 1969, Harvard University Press.

3. Cartwright FF: *The English pioneers of anaesthesia (Beddoes, Davy, and Hickman).* Bristol, 1952, J Wright.

4. Hickman HH: A letter on suspended animation, 1824. Pamphlet.

5. Long C: An account of the first use of sulphuric ether by inhalation as an anaesthetic in surgical operations, *South Med Surg J,* 1849.

6. Raper HR: *Man against pain.* New York, 1945, Prentice-Hall.

7. Archer WH: Life and letters of Horace Wells, discoverer of anesthesia, *J Am Coll Dent* 11:81, 1944.

8. Archer WH: Chronological history of Horace Wells, discoverer of anesthesia, *Bull Hist Med* 7:1140, 1939.

9. Wells H: Letter, *Br Med J,* May 31: 305, 1848.

10. Bankoff G: *The conquest of pain: the story of anesthesia.* London, 1946, MacDonald.

11. Sykes WS: *Essays on the first hundred years of anaesthesia,* vols I and II. Edinburgh, 1961, E & S Livingstone.

12. Driscoll EJ: Dental anesthesiology: its history and continuing evolution, *Anesth Prog* 25:143, 1978.

13. Smith WDA: *Under the influence: a history of nitrous oxide and oxygen anaesthesia.* Park Ridge, Ill, 1982, Wood Library, Museum of Anesthesiology.

14. American Dental Association: Transactions of the fourth annual meeting at Niagara Falls, NY, 1864.

15. Archer WH: Life and letters of Horace Wells, discoverer of anesthesia, *J Am Coll Dent* 11:81, 1944.

16. American Society of Dental Surgeons: Resolutions adopted at Eighth Annual Meeting, *Am J Dent Sci* 9(1):1848.

17. Greenfield W: Anesthesiology in dentistry: past, present and future, *Anesth Prog* 23:104, 1976.

18. Snow J: *On the inhalation of ether.* London, 1858, J Churchill.

19. Snow J: *On chloroform and other anaesthetics.* London, 1858, J Churchill.

20. Sykes WS, *Essays on the first hundred years of anaesthesia,* (Ellis RH, ed) vol III. Edinburgh, 1982, Churchill Livingstone.

21. Levy AG: Sudden death under light chloroform anaesthesia, *J Physiol* 42:3, 1911.

22. *Medical Times,* February 5, 1848, 317.

23. Thomas KB: Some early papers on dental anaesthesia, *Br Dent J* 116:139, 1964.

24. Fowell S: *A treatise on dentistry,* ed 2. London, 1859, J Mitchell.

25. Tomes J: *A course of lecture notes on dental physiology and surgery.* London, 1848, John Parker.

26. Archer WH: *A manual of dental anesthesia: an illustrated guide for student and practitioner.* Philadelphia, 1952, Saunders.

27. Andrews, E: The oxygen mixture: a new anesthetic mixture by E Andrews, *Chic Med Exam* 9:656, 1868.

28. Bert P: Sur la possibilité d'obtenir, a l'aide du protoxyde de d'azote, une insensibilité de longue durée, et sur l'innocuité de cet anesthétique (Concerning the possibility of obtaining, by the aid of the protoxide of nitrogen, an insensibility of long duration and concerning the innocuousness of that anesthetic), *Compte Rendu de e' Académie de Science* (Paris) 87:728, 1878.

29. Archer WH: *The history of anesthesia. Proceedings of the dental centenary celebration.* Baltimore, 1940, Waverly Press.

30. Archer WH: The history of anesthesia. In Archer WH, ed: *A manual of dental anesthesia.* Philadelphia, 1958, Saunders.

31. Nevin M, Puterbaugh PG: *Conduction, infiltration and general anesthesia in dentistry.* New York, 1923, Dental Items of Interest Publishing.

32. Lippe HT: Nitrous oxide analgesia in cavity preparation, *Temple Dent Rev* 14:7, 1944.

33. Seldin HM: *Practical anesthesia for dental and oral surgery,* ed 3. Philadelphia, 1947, Lea & Febiger.

34. Allison ML, Kinney W, Lynch DF et al: The American Dental Society of Anesthesiology: 1953-1978, *Anesth Prog* 25:9, 1978.

35. Greenfield W: Anesthesiology in dentistry: past, present and future, *Anesth Prog* 23:104, 1976.

36. Langa H: *Relative analgesia in dental practice,* ed 2. Philadelphia, 1976, Saunders.

37. American Dental Association Council on Dental Education: Guidelines for teaching the comprehensive control of pain and anxiety in dentistry, *J Dent Educ* 36:62, 1972.

38. American Dental Association Council on Dental Education: *Guidelines for teaching the comprehensive control of pain and anxiety in dentistry,* part I, Chicago, 1992, The Association.

39. American Dental Association, Council on Dental Materials, Instruments and Equipment: Revised guidelines for the acceptance program for nitrous oxide-oxygen sedation machines and devices, Chicago, 1986, The Association.

40. Whitcher C, Zimmerman DC, Piziali RL: Control of occupational exposure to nitrous oxide in the oral surgery office, *J Oral Surg* 36:431, 1978.

41. Cruickshank JC, Sykes SH: Office sedation, *Adv Dermatol* 7:291, 1992.

CHAPTER *13*

Inhalation sedation: rationale

The technique of inhalation sedation with nitrous oxide (N_2O) and oxygen (O_2) possesses many significant advantages over other techniques of pharmacosedation. It is my belief that inhalation sedation represents the most nearly "ideal" sedative procedure. As will be demonstrated in this chapter, the indications for use of N_2O-O_2 in dentistry, and increasingly in other branches of medicine, are constantly expanding.

ADVANTAGES

1. The onset of action of inhalation sedation is more rapid than that of oral, rectal, and intramuscular (IM) sedation. The onset of action of intravenous (IV) medications will be approximately equal to that of inhalation sedation.

Oral	30-minute onset
Rectal	30-minute onset
IM	10- to 15-minute onset
IV	20-second onset (approximate arm-to-brain circulation time); 1 to 2 minutes for clinical actions to develop
Inhalation	<20 seconds pulmonary circulation to brain time; 2- to 3-minute onset for clinical actions to develop

2. Peak clinical effect does not develop in most techniques for a considerable time. Although variations do exist, peak clinical actions do not develop for most orally, rectally, and IM drugs for a period of time that makes titration absolutely impossible. Only inhalation and IV drug administration provide peak clinical actions in a time span permitting titration. For the IV route this time-to-peak effect varies with the drug administered, ranging from 1 minute to approximately 20 minutes (lorazepam).

Oral	60-minute peak action
Rectal	60-minute peak action
IM	30-minute peak action
IV	60-second to 20-minute peak action
Inhalation	3- to 5-minute peak action

3. The depth of sedation achieved with inhalation sedation may be altered from moment to moment, permitting the drug administrator to increase or decrease the depth of sedation. With no other technique of sedation does the administrator have as much control over the clinical actions of the drugs. This degree of control represents a significant safety feature of inhalation sedation.

Oral	Cannot easily deepen or lighten sedation
Rectal	Cannot easily deepen or lighten sedation
IM	Cannot easily deepen or lighten sedation
IV	Sedation level may easily be deepened; however, lessening of sedation is difficult to achieve
Inhalation	Sedation levels *easily* changed either way

4. The duration of action is an important consideration in the selection of a pharmacosedative technique in an outpatient. In situations in which a sedation technique has a relatively fixed duration of clinical activity, dental treatment must be tailored to this, whereas in those techniques with a flexible duration of action the planned procedure may be of any length, for example, a minute or so for the taking of radiographs or 3 to 4 hours for preparation and impression of multiple abutments for fixed bridgework.

198

Oral	Fixed duration of action, approximately 2 to 3 hours
Rectal	Fixed duration of action, approximately 2 to 3 hours
IM	Fixed duration of action, approximately 2 to 4 hours, with significant variation by drug
IV	Fixed duration of action, with significant variation by drug Diazepam, midazolam, 45 minutes Promethazine, 90 minutes Pentobarbital, 2 to 4 hours
Inhalation	Duration variable, at discretion of administrator

5. Recovery time from inhalation sedation is rapid and is the most complete of any pharmacosedation technique. Because N_2O is not metabolized by the body, the gas is rapidly and virtually completely eliminated from the body within 3 to 5 minutes. In all other techniques the recovery from sedation is considerably slower.

Oral	Recovery not entirely complete even after 2 to 3 hours
Rectal	Recovery not entirely complete even after 2 to 3 hours
IM	Recovery not entirely complete even after 2 to 3 hours
IV	Recovery not entirely complete even after 2 to 3 hours
Inhalation	Recovery usually complete following 3 to 5 minutes of inhalation of 100% O_2

6. As discussed, titration is the ability to administer small, incremental doses of a drug until a desired clinical action is obtained. In my opinion the ability to titrate a drug represents the greatest safety feature a technique can possess because it permits the drug administrator virtually absolute control over the actions of the drug. Significant drug overdose will not develop in techniques in which titration is possible as long as the administrator does indeed titrate the drug.

Oral	Titration not possible
Rectal	Titration not possible
IM	Titration not possible
IV	Titration possible
Inhalation	Titration possible

7. In an outpatient setting it is advantageous for the patient to be discharged from the office follow-

ing a procedure with no prohibitions on their activities. Unfortunately, because of the fact that all of the drugs administered for the reduction of fear and anxiety are central nervous system (CNS) depressants, the patient may not be permitted to leave the office unescorted to operate an automobile or to perform tasks requiring mental alertness for a number of hours following the administration of these drugs. To do so is to increase the potential risk to both the patient (physical risk) and the doctor (legal risk). Recovery must be complete, with absolutely no doubt in the mind of the doctor that the patient is able to function normally; if not, the patient should not be permitted to leave the office unescorted.

Oral	Recovery not complete; patient requires escort if less than 3 hours since drug administration
Rectal	Recovery not complete; as usually used in pediatric dentistry, patient will be escorted by parent or guardian
IM	Recovery not complete; patient always requires escort
IV	Recovery not complete; patient always requires escort
Inhalation	Recovery almost always complete; patient usually may be discharged from office alone, with no admonitions about activities

8. No injection is required with inhalation sedation.
9. Inhalation sedation with N_2O-O_2 is safe. There are very few side effects associated with its use, as described in the following chapters.
10. The drugs used in this technique have no adverse effects on the liver, kidneys, brain, or cardiovascular and respiratory systems.
11. Inhalation sedation with N_2O-O_2 can be used instead of local anesthesia in certain procedures. Nitrous oxide does possess analgesic properties when employed in the usual sedative concentrations. The analgesia produced by a 20% concentration of N_2O is equivalent to that of 10 to 15 mg of morphine. However, the degree of analgesia is quite variable from patient to patient and therefore cannot be relied on to provide all of the pain control required for a procedure. Certain procedures, such as those involving

soft tissues (scaling, curettage) may be performed in many instances without using local anesthesia.

DISADVANTAGES

Following are disadvantages associated with N_2O-O_2 inhalation sedation.

1. The initial cost of the equipment required for inhalation sedation is high.
2. The continuing cost of the gases (O_2 and N_2O) used in inhalation sedation is high.
3. The equipment required for inhalation sedation occupies considerable space within the dental surgery suite. Placed in the usual small dental surgery office, a portable N_2O-O_2 unit can be quite cumbersome.
4. Nitrous oxide is not a potent agent. When used in combination with at least 20% O_2 there will be a small percentage of patients in whom the technique will fail to produce the desired clinical actions. In no circumstance should N_2O ever be administered with less than 20% O_2. Inhalation sedation with N_2O-O_2 is not a panacea. Failures will occur, primarily because of the lack of potency of the agent.
5. A degree of cooperation is required from the patient. In order for inhalation sedation to be effective, the patient must be able to inhale the gases through either the nose or the mouth. Should the patient be unable or unwilling to do so, clinical failure will result.
6. All members of the dental staff employing N_2O-O_2 must receive training in its safe and effective use. Ideally this training is acquired in dental, dental hygiene, or dental assisting school. Postgraduate continuing education courses are also available, but quality varies tremendously in these programs. The guidelines established by the American Dental Association (ADA), the American Dental Society of Anesthesiology (ADSA), and the American Association of Dental Schools (AADS) recommend not less than 14 hours of training, to include treatment of dental patients receiving inhalation sedation (see Chapter 20).[1]
7. There is a possibility that chronic exposure to trace amounts of N_2O is deleterious to the health of dental personnel.

CONTRAINDICATIONS

There are no absolute contraindications to the administration of N_2O-O_2 inhalation sedation as long as the percentage of O_2 administered with the N_2O is greater than 20% (atmospheric concentration).

There are, however, several relative contraindications to this technique. As mentioned, a relative contraindication implies that there is an increased potential for an adverse reaction to develop in a certain patient. Whereas the technique in question may be used, if there exists another technique without this contraindication that would prove to be equally successful, it should be used in place of the contraindicated technique. The following are relative contraindications to N_2O-O_2 inhalation sedation.

Patients with a compulsive personality

The use of N_2O-O_2 sedation (or for that matter, any sedation technique) in a person with this personality type would result in a very low probability of success. The person with a compulsive personality is the "take-charge" type of person, one who would not like the feeling of "losing control" associated with the use of sedation. The patient will consciously, or more likely subconsciously, "fight" the effects of the drug(s).

Claustrophobic patients

Inhalation sedation will have a very low success rate in the patient who is unable to tolerate the nasal hood or face mask used in the administration of gaseous agents. Whereas this is not a problem in the patient undergoing general anesthesia because anesthesia may be induced by IV drugs and the face mask applied after unconsciousness is induced, the sedated patient is, of course, conscious throughout the procedure and, if fearful of the mask, will be unable to become comfortable. The nasal cannula is a possible alternative to the nasal hood in these patients; however, with the increased concern over the inhalation of trace levels of N_2O by dental personnel, the nasal cannula has fallen out of favor (see Chapters 14 and 17).

Children with severe behavior problems

The use of N_2O-O_2 in children who are severely disruptive will usually prove to be futile. A degree of patient cooperation is required for this technique to be successful. Patients must accept the nasal hood and be willing and able to breathe through their nose. Precooperative or noncooperative children (or handicapped adult patients) will breathe through their mouth, crying, screaming, or moving about in the chair, thus negating the effects of any N_2O they may inhale. Management of these patients is discussed in Chapter 36.

Patients with severe personality disorders

Patients who are under psychiatric care and are receiving psychotropic drugs, usually mood-elevating antidepressants (see Table 8-3), should be carefully evaluated prior to the administration of any form of sedation. Whereas no serious drug–drug interactions develop between N_2O-O_2 and these psychotropic drugs, it may be prudent to avoid altering the consciousness of persons who have but a tenuous grip on reality. Medical consultation prior to the use of any sedative technique is strongly indicated.

Upper respiratory tract infection or other acute respiratory conditions

Because N_2O-O_2 must be inhaled through the nose during dental treatment, any respiratory problem preventing the use of the nose as a route of entry for the anesthetic gases represents a relative contraindication to using this technique. The common cold, acute or chronic sinus problems, chronic mouth breathing, allergy, tuberculosis, bronchitis, and cough all represent situations in which the technique of inhalation sedation would best be avoided if possible. Other techniques may be substituted effectively. Aside from the difficulty in achieving sedation when the patient is unable to inhale through the nose, there is the distinct possibility of contaminating the rubber goods of the inhalation sedation unit.

Patients with chronic respiratory or other potentially contagious diseases (tuberculosis, HIV/AIDS) who require inhalation sedation may be provided (at cost, of course) with their own "disposable" rubber goods for inhalation sedation. Such disposable systems, consisting of nasal hood, tubing, and reservoir bag, are available at relatively modest cost and will minimize the risk of cross-contamination.

Chronic obstructive pulmonary disease

Chronic obstructive pulmonary disease (COPD) (e.g., emphysema, chronic bronchitis) represents a relative contraindication to inhalation sedation because of the potential effect of administering a gas mixture enriched with O_2 to these patients, many of whom have chronically elevated CO_2 blood levels. Whereas the usual stimulus for breathing in a healthy person is an increase in the blood CO_2 level, patients with COPD have a diminished or absent ability to respond to this stimulus. In its place the stimulus for breathing in these patients is a lowered blood O_2 con-

tent. In the administration of inhalation sedation, an O_2-enriched mixture of gases is always provided, raising the O_2 saturation of the blood. The stimulus for involuntary breathing has now been removed, and apnea should be noted. In the unconscious patient during general anesthesia, such will be the case; however, in the conscious patient (e.g.: during inhalation sedation), where voluntary control over breathing is maintained, prolonged apnea does not develop. These patients should be evaluated quite carefully prior to the planned dental treatment to assess their ability to tolerate dental therapy in general. Most of these patients represent ASA III or IV risks during dental treatment.

The patient who does not want N_2O-O_2

The nasal hood should never be forced onto a patient. Should the adult patient be uncomfortable with the nasal hood, it is often best to remove it. Discuss the reason for the discomfort, and if needed employ a different sedation technique. Because of the light level of conscious sedation produced by N_2O-O_2, it is impossible to overwhelm a patient with the drug against his or her will.

Pregnancy

The use of sedation in the pregnant patient has been discussed in Chapter 5. It is desirable to avoid the use of any drugs (if possible) during the first trimester to avoid increasing the slight possibility of spontaneous abortion or the development of a fetal malformation that might be related to a drug administered at this time. Drugs may be employed in the second trimester if necessary but, as always, with caution, especially CNS depressants. Of the techniques that might be employed for the reduction of anxiety in the pregnant patient, the safest and most recommended is inhalation sedation with N_2O-O_2. The fact that nitrous oxide is not metabolized in the body has virtually no effect on most organ systems, and the fact that it is rapidly and almost totally removed from the body within 3 to 5 minutes is ample evidence of its superiority over other techniques. In the third trimester of pregnancy the major consideration in determining whether or not to treat the patient must be the possibility of the patient giving birth during the dental appointment. As the patient nears term it might be prudent to postpone any nonemergency treatment. However, should emergency care be necessary and if the patient requires sedation, the use of inhalation sedation is suggested. Prior consultation with the patient's obstetrician is advisable whenever sedation is being considered for a pregnant patient.

INDICATIONS

The primary indications for the use of inhalation sedation are the same as those for other sedative techniques—the management of fear and anxiety, the medically compromised patient, and the management of gagging. Over and above these usual indications, the fact that N_2O-O_2 is as readily controllable as it is permits it to be used for aspects of dental care in which the use of conscious sedation might not usually be considered.

There are many procedures generally considered to be nonthreatening or even innocuous that might however prove to be extremely traumatic to some patients. Many of these procedures lend themselves quite readily to the use of N_2O-O_2.

Anxiety

The major indication for the use of N_2O-O_2 inhalation sedation in dentistry is, of course, the management of fear and anxiety related to the dental experience. As discussed in the preceding section on the advantages of inhalation sedation, N_2O-O_2 represents the most nearly ideal sedation technique. Were it not for the fact that some persons are not comfortable with the effects of N_2O-O_2, that some others will not achieve clinically adequate sedation at permissible percentages, and that still others are unable to breathe through their noses, inhalation sedation would be the only technique of sedation required for the management of dental anxieties.

Medically compromised patients

In recent years the use of N_2O-O_2 has become increasingly important in the management of the medically compromised patient. The general evaluation of these patients is discussed in Chapter 5; however, I believe that it is important to review some of these patients and discuss the relevance of their diseases to the use of N_2O-O_2.

Cardiovascular disease

The use of N_2O-O_2 in patients with cardiovascular disease is one of the most valuable methods of minimizing risk to the patient during dental care. In most, if not all, significant cardiovascular disease states, one factor likely to produce an exacerbation of clinical signs and symptoms is an oxygen deficit in the myocardium. Myocardial ischemia is produced in many patients by an increased cardiovascular workload—an increase in the heart rate and in the force of contraction of the heart. In the patient with an underlying cardiovascular disorder that may be asymptomatic while the patient is at rest (nonstressed), this increased workload of the myocardium, leading to ischemia, may precipitate an acute cardiovascular event.

Because oxygen deficit is responsible for the onset of most anginal episodes, an increased severity of heart failure, cardiac dysrhythmias, and possibly myocardial infarction, any sedative technique that decreases myocardial O_2 requirement will decrease the risk to the patient during dental treatment. Therefore, any sedative procedure is appropriate for use in these patients. However, N_2O-O_2 inhalation sedation has several advantages over other techniques; in addition to providing a reduction of anxiety, it also produces an elevation in the pain reaction threshold, as well as providing the myocardium and entire body with a minimum of 30%, but more frequently 50% to 70%, O_2. Therefore, at its very worst the patient is receiving approximately 50% more O_2 than he or she would from atmospheric air, which has an O_2 content of 20.9%.

I have employed N_2O-O_2 inhalation sedation with great success in patients with angina pectoris, congestive heart failure, severe cardiac dysrhythmias, status postmyocardial infarction, and high blood pressure, as well as other cardiovascular disorders.

The use of N_2O-O_2 in patients with severe cardiovascular disease has received considerable attention in the past 20 years. Emergency medical personnel in Wales and Great Britain have employed a premixed combination of N_2O and O_2 in a ratio of 40% to 60% (Entonox) for the management of pain during an acute myocardial infarction.[2] In the past, management of the pain of a myocardial infarction was achieved through the administration of opioid analgesics. The success of N_2O-O_2 in this life-threatening situation was such that paramedical units in a growing number of areas throughout the United States are today incorporating the use of N_2O-O_2 into their armamentarium (Fig. 13-1).[3] In the United States the most commonly used concentration of N_2O to O_2 has been 35% to 65%. At this concentration (available under the proprietary name Dolonox) N_2O has analgesic properties, diminishing or eliminating pain; has sedative properties, helping the victim to relax and become more comfortable, thereby reducing the workload of the myocardium; and provides the patient with 65% O_2—more than three times the volume found in atmospheric air. In a study by Thompson and Lown[2] it was found that 75% of patients receiving 35% N_2O and 65% O_2 dur-

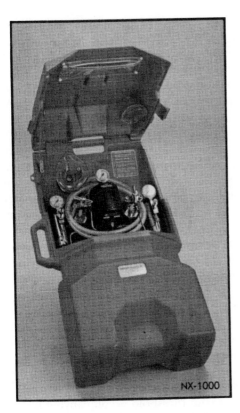

Fig. 13-1. Portable N_2O-O_2 unit, employed by paramedical personnel.

ing acute myocardial infarction have either a distinct decrease in the severity of their pain (36%) or state that the pain was eliminated entirely (39%). Inhalation sedation with N_2O-O_2 has been found to be the most appropriate technique of sedation for the patient with preexisting cardiovascular disease.

Respiratory disease

The use of inhalation anesthetics is frequently contraindicated in patients suffering from acute or chronic respiratory disease. However, N_2O-O_2, is used quite successfully and without untoward incident in many patients with respiratory disease.

Chronic obstructive pulmonary disease represents a relative contraindication to the successful use of N_2O-O_2. Although it is possible for the patient to become apneic during the procedure as a result of the elevation of the O_2 level in the blood, this is rarely a clinical finding. Having been involved with the administration of N_2O-O_2 inhalation sedation since 1969, I have administered it to many patients with respiratory disorders and have never seen this situation develop. The primary concern with patients with respiratory disease is the potential lack of sedative effect of the N_2O-O_2.

Occasionally the dentist will receive a medical consultation that states that the use of N_2O-O_2 is contraindicated in asthmatics. Nitrous oxide may be employed quite safety in patients such as these.[4] The reason behind this medical consultation is the fact that anesthetic gases that are irritating to the respiratory mucosa may precipitate an acute episode of bronchospasm. Many anesthetic gases are in fact contraindicated in asthmatics. However, N_2O is a nonirritating vapor that does not exacerbate asthma. The use of sedation in the asthmatic patient is frequently warranted as increased stress is a potential cause of acute exacerbation of their asthma. Nitrous oxide-oxygen represents a very effective and safe technique of sedation in these patients.

Patients with chronic nasal obstruction, either from anatomic abnormalities (deviated nasal septum) or pathologic conditions (allergy, upper respiratory tract infection) will be difficult to sedate adequately with gaseous agents. In addition, the potential for the infection of other patients through the use of a nasal hood that has become contaminated should be considered before N_2O-O_2 is administered to patients who are ill.

Cerebrovascular disease

The postcerebrovascular accident ("stroke") patient is unable to tolerate levels of O_2 below normal without an increased risk of developing seizure activity or additional neuronal damage. Deep sedation is contraindicated because of the increased (though unlikely) possibility of hypoxia. Whereas other techniques of sedation may be considered for these patients, the one most highly recommended for the status postcerebrovascular accident patient is N_2O-O_2 inhalation sedation. The major recommendation for this technique is the elevated level of O_2 that is routinely provided to the patient. As used in dentistry today, there is little or no likelihood of a hypoxic episode developing.

Hepatic disease

Hepatic disease, such as cirrhosis or hepatitis, represents a contraindication (either relative or absolute) to the use of many of the drugs discussed in this text because most of them undergo biotransformation in the liver. In the presence of significant hepatic dysfunction the rate of biotransformation (half-life) of a drug is slowed, potentially resulting in higher plasma levels, which in turn leads to an increase in the drug effect as well as a prolongation of its clinical activity. However, N_2O does not undergo biotransformation anywhere within the body (see

Chapter 14) and may therefore be used without additional risk and with a high probability of success in the patient with hepatic dysfunction.

Epilepsy and seizure disorders

As with status postcerebrovascular accident, the patient with a history of chronic seizure activity (epilepsy) is more sensitive to hypoxia than is the normal healthy patient. Seizure activity is precipitated more readily in these patients; therefore, hypoxia must be guarded against much more scrupulously. Nitrous oxide is not epileptogenic (it does not increase the risk of seizures developing) and therefore may be administered to these patients as long as hypoxia is avoided. Increased stress and anxiety have been demonstrated to be precipitating causes of seizures. With the sedation machines available today and adherence to the technique of administering N_2O-O_2 presented in Chapter 16, epilepsy does not represent a contraindication to the use of inhalation sedation.

Pregnancy

Nitrous oxide does cross the placenta to the fetus, producing the same degree of CNS depression as in the mother. If delivered in combination with adequate levels of O_2 (greater than 20%), N_2O-O_2 inhalation sedation represents the recommended sedation technique for use during pregnancy. Medical consultation with the patient's physician prior to its use is suggested.

Allergy

There has never been a reported allergy to N_2O.

Diabetes

Diabetes mellitus does not represent a contraindication to the use of N_2O-O_2.

Gagging

Gagging is a potential problem during many dental procedures, especially in the maxillary palatal and mandibular lingual regions. Although there is no absolute solution to this problem, inhalation sedation with N_2O-O_2 has proved to be highly effective in eliminating or at least minimizing severe gagging. Patients are titrated with N_2O-O_2 to their sedation level, at which point impressions, radiographs, or other procedures may be completed. The use of N_2O-O_2 to diminish the gag reflex may require placing the patient in an upright position for some or all of the procedure. Although this position is not usually recommended during sedation (supine is preferred),

some procedures, such as impressions in the maxilla, may require modification of position for increased patient safety. Where other sedation techniques (especially IV sedation) are also effective in decreasing gagging, only N_2O is practical to use for extremely short procedures such as radiographs or impressions.

Besides the three major indications for the use of inhalation sedation—anxiety, medically compromised patient, and gagging—there are a multitude of uses for this technique in other areas of dentistry, including procedures that are usually considered to be too minor or too short to employ sedation. Very often, the doctor or hygienist will advise their patient that the procedure will "hurt just a little." It is this type of procedure that is appropriate for the use of inhalation sedation.

RESTORATIVE DENTISTRY
Initial dental examination

Patients who have come to the dental office in pain may be extremely uncomfortable during the initial examination because of the sensitivity of their soft tissues or teeth. Sedation with N_2O-O_2 and the elevation in pain threshold accompanying it will make this potentially traumatic procedure more tolerable for the patient.

Removal of provisional crowns or bridges

The removal of provisional crowns or bridges from vital teeth is often done without the benefit of local anesthesia because the procedure is short and associated with a minimum of discomfort. This discomfort may be eliminated or minimized through the use of N_2O-O_2. The drying and cleansing of the prepared vital teeth for the cementation of crowns or bridges is also an appropriate area for the use of N_2O-O_2 sedation.

Occlusal adjustment

Occlusal adjustment of crowns, bridges, or natural teeth rarely requires the use of local anesthesia. There are many patients, however, who are quite uncomfortable during this procedure. The sound of the drill or the vibration of the bur on the tooth makes some patients extremely tense. Sedation with N_2O-O_2 can eliminate this response in most patients.

Insertion of matrix bands or wedges

The insertion of matrix bands or wedges between teeth prior to the placement of a restoration may be uncomfortable for the patient if soft-tissue anesthesia is not present. Sedation with N_2O-O_2 provides soft-tissue anesthesia in many patients, thus making this procedure less traumatic.

PERIODONTICS AND DENTAL HYGIENE

Within the speciality of periodontology there is a need for sedation. Surgical procedures in general are more anxiety producing than more routine nonsurgical procedures. The use of inhalation sedation with N_2O-O_2 is especially recommended in periodontics, primarily in its nonsurgical aspect, for in a significant percentage of patients a degree of soft-tissue analgesia will be noted, helping to make the procedure less traumatic.

Initial periodontal examination

The initial periodontal examination and probing can be quite traumatic to the patient, especially patients in whom significant periodontal disease is present. Inflamed, sensitive soft tissues and teeth with deep periodontal pockets will be extremely sensitive during this examination. Inhalation sedation provides both a relaxed patient and a degree of soft-tissue analgesia, which ranges from the total loss of sensation in these tissues to decreased sensitivity so that, although the patient still feels the pain, it no longer bothers her or him.

Scaling, curettage, and root planing

One of the most important uses of N_2O-O_2 within periodontics is for scaling, curettage, and root planing. As mentioned, most patients receiving N_2O-O_2 at sedative levels will develop a degree of soft-tissue analgesia. Scaling, curettage, and root planing are three procedures that, although not normally traumatic, may be so on occasion. The administration of local anesthesia is one means of alleviating this discomfort; however, N_2O-O_2 offers the patient and doctor or hygienist a more pleasant means of achieving essentially the same goal with a technique that is almost immediately reversible on completion of the procedure. A growing number of states in the United States permit trained registered dental hygienists to administer N_2O-O_2 to their patients. The response from hygienists, doctors, and patients has been almost universally positive.

Emergency management of necrotizing ulcerative gingivitis

The management of necrotizing ulcerative gingivitis (NUG) requires debridement of periodontal soft tissues that are extremely sensitive, a situation that can be greatly altered to the benefit of the patient and doctor through the use of N_2O-O_2.

Use of ultrasonic instruments

Ultrasonic instruments are frequently used during periodontal procedures to aid in the removal of calculus from teeth. Some patients may find the use of these devices threatening and uncomfortable. Sedation with N_2O-O_2 is a means of eliminating this fear for most patients.

Periodontal surgery

Patients facing periodontal surgery frequently request the use of sedation because of the nature and length of the surgical procedure. Inhalation sedation with N_2O-O_2 is an appropriate procedure for many of these patients, although IV sedation is also commonly used during periodontal surgery.

ORAL AND MAXILLOFACIAL SURGERY
Lengthy surgical procedures

As discussed in the preceding paragraph, N_2O-O_2 sedation is an acceptable technique for use in the patient undergoing any lengthy procedure as a means of helping to make the procedure more tolerable and of providing analgesia.

Management of abscesses

When an incision and drainage (I & D) procedure is planned to help to relieve the discomfort of an abscess, it is frequently difficult to achieve adequate pain control through the administration of local anesthetics, primarily because of the change in tissue pH brought about by the formation of purulent material within the infected area. Inhalation sedation with N_2O-O_2 may be used to advantage in this situation because of its tendency to provide a degree of soft-tissue analgesia. Titration of the patient to the usual sedative level will almost always provide a degree of soft-tissue analgesia sufficient to permit the I & D procedure to be completed in comfort or with a minimum of discomfort.

Management of postoperative complications

Inhalation sedation can be of great benefit in the management of localized osteitis (dry socket). Most commonly occurring following extraction of third molars, the management of localized osteitis requires irrigation of the socket and the placement of medicated packs into the socket to cover the exposed bone. Local anesthesia is not always used for this procedure, which may produce some patient discomfort.

Inhalation sedation can provide a degree of sedation and analgesia for the brief period necessary to complete the irrigation and packing of the extraction site.

Suture removal

Another potential postoperative use for N_2O-O_2 is as an aid in the removal of sutures, although it is not normally required for this procedure. However, there are occasions when sutures are difficult to locate, and there also is a potential for the scissors to irritate the soft tissues as the sutures are being sought. Inhalation sedation is an excellent means of minimizing potential discomfort.

ENDODONTICS
Cellulitis and pericementitis

Clinically adequate pain control in endodontically involved teeth, although not usually a problem, may occasionally prove to be difficult to achieve. Unfortunately there are no panaceas. An aid to achieving adequate pain control in such cases, however, is N_2O-O_2 sedation. Although the discomfort involved in the opening of a "hot" tooth may not be entirely eliminated, N_2O will raise the pain reaction threshold, thereby modifying the patient's response to it, so that the patient, although still aware of her or his pain, is no longer bothered by it.

Rubber dam clamps

The placement of a rubber dam clamp on the neck of an endodontically involved tooth is almost always entirely atraumatic. However, in those situations in which the clinical crown of a tooth is inadequate to support the clamp, tissue clamping may be required. Either local anesthesia or N_2O-O_2 inhalation sedation may be employed to alleviate patient discomfort in this procedure.

Gaining access to the pulp chamber

It may be difficult to achieve adequate pulpal anesthesia in the vital tooth about to undergo pulpal therapy. As the endodontic access preparation nears the pulp chamber, the patient experiences greater and greater discomfort. Once the pulp chamber has been entered, an intrapulpal injection may be administered that will usually eliminate, once and for all, any further discomfort. However, the greatest problem may be in reaching the point at which an intrapulpal injection can be administered. Should the patient experience great discomfort as the preparation approaches the pulp chamber, N_2O-O_2 in-

halation sedation may be administered to raise the pain reaction threshold, thereby modifying (though not usually eliminating) the discomfort experienced by the patient.

Instrumenting canals

Following extirpation of pulpal tissues, the endodontically involved tooth must be prepared for filling. During instrumentation local anesthetics might not be used, because there should be no discomfort, or at the very most minimal discomfort. Some patients, however, may be quite uncomfortable, and for them the administration of local anesthesia and/or N_2O-O_2 is recommended.

Filling of root canals

As in the instrumentation of the root canal, discomfort is usually nonexistent or at most only minimal during the filling of root canals; therefore, local anesthesia is rarely used. Should patient discomfort or anxiety be present, N_2O-O_2 administration is recommended.

FIXED PROSTHODONTICS
Impression taking

Inhalation sedation may be valuable in two parts of the impression-taking process. First, if local anesthesia has not been administered, N_2O-O_2, through its ability to elevate the pain reaction threshold, will enable the patient to tolerate better any discomfort associated with the procedure. Second, N_2O-O_2 will aid in diminishing the gag reflex so that there will be little or no difficulty in placing the impression materials and trays.

The gingival retraction cord is placed into the sulcus of abutment teeth prior to taking impressions to aid in visualizing and gaining access to the margins of the impression. In the absence of local anesthesia, packing of retraction cord may prove to be quite uncomfortable for the patient, a situation that can be minimized or eliminated by N_2O-O_2.

Removal of provisional crowns and bridges

It is not uncommon for provisional crowns and bridges to be removed without local anesthesia. This will occur prior to the taking of impressions, the trying-in of crowns and bridges, and their cementation. The removal of excess cement from a vital tooth as well as its drying prior to impressions or cementation may be associated with a degree of discomfort. This sensitivity may be decreased or eliminated with N_2O-O_2.

Adjustment of castings

After provisional crowns and bridges are removed, the cast crowns and bridges will be tried in and, if necessary, adjusted. This process may be uncomfortable for some patients, especially if the abutment teeth are vital and if local anesthesia has not been administered (as is frequently the case). Occlusal adjustment of these castings may produce intense vibration and noise, which may bother the patient. Sedation with N_2O-O_2 is recommended in these situations.

REMOVABLE PROSTHODONTICS
Preparation of abutment teeth

Unlike fixed prosthodontics, in which pain control with local anesthetics is normally required for the preparation of abutment teeth, there is usually a minimum of discomfort associated with the preparation of teeth for removable prostheses. Local anesthesia is rarely required for this process, yet some patients will experience a degree of tooth sensitivity or anxiety related to this procedure. Inhalation sedation with N_2O-O_2 is an appropriate means of managing any anxiety or discomfort associated with preparing teeth for the removal of prosthodontic appliances.

Determination of centric relationships

Although it is not a muscle-relaxing drug combination, N_2O-O_2 can aid in determining centric relationship in a patient having difficulty relaxing his or her muscles, help the patient to relax psychologically, thereby taking his or her mind off the procedure and permitting a more accurate tracing of centric relationship.

Occlusal adjustments and impression taking

As in fixed prosthodontics, N_2O-O_2 inhalation sedation may prove to be a valuable help in adjusting occlusion and taking impressions for removable prostheses.

Fitting of immediate dentures

Immediate dentures are placed into the patient's mouth immediately after the extraction of teeth. The tissues in the oral cavity at that time are usually well anesthetized, and there is no discomfort during this procedure. However, at subsequent visits the removal of the immediate full denture may prove to be quite uncomfortable because the underlying soft tissues have not yet fully healed and there may be areas of tissue irritation from the denture itself. When used at this time, N_2O-O_2 sedation can benefit both the patient and the doctor.

ORTHODONTICS

The need for sedation and pain control is minimal in most orthodontic procedures, so much so that many orthodontists rarely, if ever, administer local anesthetics. However, there are occasions when the use of sedation for a brief time may prove to be quite beneficial. These include impression taking, in which excessive gagging can be minimized, and the placement or removal of bands and wires, in which soft-tissue analgesia produced by the N_2O-O_2 can eliminate or modify any discomfort.

PEDIATRIC DENTISTRY

Inhalation sedation with N_2O-O_2 is one of the most valuable sedative techniques available for use in children. The range of procedures in which the use of this technique is appropriate is unlimited. The indications for inhalation sedation in children are the same as those for adults. One complicating factor to be considered is that in order for inhalation sedation to be effective, the patient must be willing to accept the nasal hood and to breathe through his nose. Unfortunately the patient who presents a more severe management problem may be unwilling to accept the nasal hood, condemning the technique to failure. The use of N_2O-O_2 inhalation sedation in pediatric dentistry will be discussed in great detail in Chapters 16 and 36.

REFERENCES

1. American Dental Association, Council on Dental Education: *Guidelines for teaching the comprehensive control of pain and anxiety in dentistry,* part III. Chicago, 1992, The Association.
2. Thompson PL, Lown B: Nitrous oxide as an analgesic in acute myocardial infarction, *JAMA* 235:924, 1976.
3. O'Leary U, Puglia C, Friehling TD et al: Nitrous oxide anesthesia in patients with ischemic chest discomfort: effect on beta-endorphins, *J Clin Pharmacol* 27(12):957, 1987.
4. Rogers MC, Tinker JH, Covino BG et al: *Principles and practice of anesthesiology.* St Louis, 1993, Mosby-Year, p 1073.

CHAPTER 14

Pharmacology, anatomy, and physiology

Pharmacology

NITROUS OXIDE
Preparation

Nitrous oxide (nitrogen monoxide) is prepared commercially through the heating of ammonium nitrate crystals to 240° C, at which point the ammonium nitrate decomposes to N_2O and H_2O.

$$NH_4NO_3 \xrightarrow[240°\ C]{heat} N_2O + 2H_2O$$

The gas is then chemically scrubbed to remove any alkaline and acid substances and is then compressed in stages so that the less easily liquefied gases such as N_2 and O_2 are separated out. Finally it is compressed and stored in metal cylinders, in which approximately 30% of the N_2O in the full cylinder is liquefied. According to the U.S. Pharmacopeia, N_2O must be 97% pure; however, with the manufacturing processes in use today the gas usually approaches a purity of 99.5%.[1]

The most common impurities associated with the manufacture of N_2O are nitrogen (N_2), nitric oxide (NO), nitrogen dioxide (NO_2), ammonia (NH_4), water vapor, and carbon monoxide (CO). NO is the most dangerous impurity because, like CO, it may combine with hemoglobin and prevent the absorption of O_2, or it may react with water vapor to form acids that may damage the pulmonary epithelium and produce pulmonary edema. NO is formed when N_2O is heated above 450° C.

As prepared, N_2O is anhydrous. The absence of water in the gas is of importance because water vapor would freeze as it passes through the reducing valve (see Chapter 15), leading to a drop in the gas pressure.

Properties
Physical properties

N_2O is a nonirritating, sweet-smelling, colorless gas. It is the only nonorganic compound other than CO_2 that has any CNS depressant properties and is the only inorganic gas used to produce anesthesia in humans. The molecular weight of N_2O is 44, and its specific gravity is 1.53, compared with that of air, which is 1. The significance of the specific gravity will be considered in Chapter 17.

N_2O gas is converted to a clear and colorless liquid at 28° C at 50 atm of pressure. The boiling point of N_2O is −89° C. Its oil-water solubility coefficient is 3.2, and the blood-gas solubility coefficient is 0.47.

Chemical properties

N_2O is stable under pressure at usual temperatures. However, NO is formed when N_2O is heated above 450° C. Marketed in cylinders as a liquid under pressure (vapor pressure at room temperature is 50 atm), N_2O returns to the gaseous state as it is released from the cylinder. An interesting phenomenon occurs as the N_2O exits the cylinder. The walls of the cylinder become cold, and in some instances frost may be evident around the exit portal of the gas. This occurs because the liquid N_2O requires heat for vaporization into the gaseous state. The heat required for vaporization is obtained from the walls of the metal cylinder and from the surrounding air, with the result that the cylinder becomes cool to the touch.

Solubility

N_2O is relatively insoluble in the blood (its blood-gas solubility coefficient is 0.47 at 37° C) and is car-

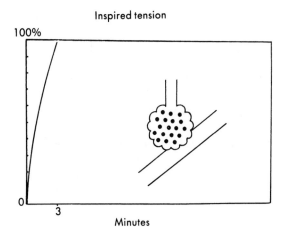

Fig. 14-1. Primary saturation of a gaseous agent with a blood-gas solubility coefficient of 0.00 (totally insoluble) occurs within a very brief period of time. Both onset and recovery are extremely rapid. (Reproduced by kind permission from *A practice of anaesthesia* [2nd ed, 1966], by WD Wylie, FRCP and HC Churchill-Davidson, MD, London: Lloyd-Luke [Year Book Medical Publisher].)

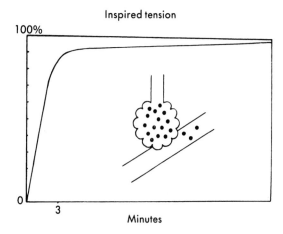

Fig. 14-2. N_2O, with a blood-gas solubility, coefficient of 0.47 (relatively insoluble), demonstrates both rapid onset and rapid recovery. Primary saturation of blood occurs within 3 to 5 minutes. (Reproduced by kind permission from *A practice of anaesthesia* [2nd ed, 1966], by WD Wylie, FRCP and HC Churchill-Davidson, MD, London: Lloyd-Luke [Year Book Medical Publisher].)

ried in the blood in physical solution only, not combining with any blood elements. The oxygen in the N_2O molecule is not available for use by the tissues because N_2O does not break down in the body.

Solubility is a term used to describe how a gas is distributed between two media, for example gas and blood. If the concentration of an anesthetic gas in blood is 2 volumes percent and this is in equilibrium with a concentration in the alveolus of 1 volume percent, the blood-gas solubility would be 2.

When an anesthetic gas is first inspired, blood entering the alveolus by the pulmonary artery contains none of it. When reaching the pulmonary capillary the blood is suddenly exposed to the tension of the gas present in the alveolus. If the gas is totally insoluble in the blood (blood/gas partition coefficient of 0), then none of the agent will be taken up by the circulation and the alveolar concentration will rise rapidly and will soon equal the inspired concentration (Fig. 14-1).

If, on the other hand, the anesthetic is but slightly soluble in blood, then only small quantities will be carried by the bloodstream. Alveolar concentration will again rise rapidly (Fig. 14-2). Since alveolar concentration determines the tension of the anesthetic in the arterial circulation, the tension will also rise rapidly, even though only a small volume of the agent is present in the blood. As the blood travels through the various tissues of the body, the anesthetic is given

Table 14-1. Blood-gas partition coefficients of inhalation anesthetics

Agent	Blood-gas solubility coefficient
Cyclopropane	0.42
Nitrous oxide	0.47
Fluroxene	1.37
Isoflurane	1.40
Enflurane	1.91
Halothane	2.36
Trichloroethylene	9.15
Chloroform	10.30
Diethyl ether	12.10
Methoxyflurane	13.00

up and the venous blood returns to the lungs with a decreased anesthetic gas tension.

N_2O and cyclopropane are examples of anesthetic gases with low blood solubility (Table 14-1). On inhalation these gases rapidly diffuse across the alveolar membrane into the blood. Because of their poor blood solubility only a small quantity is absorbed and the alveolar tension rises rapidly so that the tension of the gas in the blood is also increased quickly (Fig. 14-2). Because of the rich cerebral blood supply, the tension of these gases within the brain also rises rapidly and the onset of clinical actions is quickly apparent. Likewise the rate of recovery from sedation

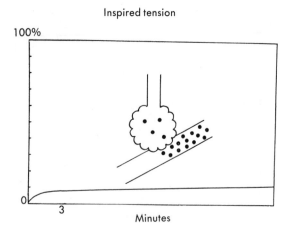

Inspired tension

100%

0

3

Minutes

Fig. 14-3. Primary saturation of a gaseous agent with a high blood-gas solubility coefficient (quite soluble) occurs quite slowly. Both onset and clinical recovery are prolonged. Methoxyflurane is an example of a very soluble agent. (Reproduced by kind permission from *A Practice of Anaesthesia* [2nd ed, 1966], by WD Wylie, FRCP and HC Churchill-Davidson, MD, London: Lloyd-Luke [Year Book Medical Publishers].)

or anesthesia produced by these gases is equally rapid once delivery of the anesthetic ceases.[2,3]

Conversely gases with high blood solubility require longer periods of time for the onset of action to develop. Large volumes of the gas are absorbed by the blood (like a piece of absorbent paper) so that the alveolar tension rises quite slowly (Fig. 14-3). Tension of the gas within the blood also rises slowly in this case, and the induction of sedation or anesthesia is noticeably slower as is the return to the preanesthetic state after termination of drug administration.

N_2O is neither flammable nor explosive; however, it will support combustion of other agents, even in the absence of oxygen, because at temperatures above 450° C N_2O breaks down into N_2 and O_2.

Potency

N_2O is the least potent of the anesthetic gases; however, it remains the most frequently administered inhalation anesthetic. At one time it was thought that any anesthetic effects of N_2O were a result of the exclusion of O_2 from cells in the brain because N_2O is 35 times more soluble in plasma than N_2 and 100 times more soluble than O_2.[4] It has since been demonstrated that N_2O can, in the presence of adequate O_2, produce CNS depression. When a mixture of N_2O-O_2 in a ratio of 65%:35% is administered to patients who have not been premedicated, the second stage of anesthesia is seldom reached. In a few

patients delirium is produced; in even fewer patients is surgical anesthesia (stage III) obtained.

With a MAC (the minimal alveolar concentration of anesthetic that prevents movement in 50% of subjects in response to a standard surgical incision) of 105%, nitrous oxide is unable to produce adequate anesthesia unless it is administered under hyperbaric conditions. More realistically, surgical-depth anesthesia is usually not obtainable unless a more potent inhalation or IV anesthetic is combined with N_2O. Such IV agents include the barbiturates and opioids, and inhalation anesthetics include halothane, isoflurane, and enflurane. These will be discussed in Section Six.

That N_2O in subanesthetic doses produces analgesia—a change in the patient's perception of pain—is no longer doubted. It is estimated that a 20%:80% mixture of N_2O-O_2 produces the analgesic effectiveness of 10 to 15 mg of morphine.[5] The optimal concentration of N_2O for the production of analgesia while still maintaining patient cooperation is approximately 35%. However, biological variability can significantly alter these figures in individual patients.

Pharmacology

After N_2O is inspired through the mouth and/or nose, the gas is transported through the respiratory tract into alveolar sacs, where it is rapidly absorbed into the pulmonary circulation. Because of the high inspired concentration of N_2O and the large gradient of N_2O between the alveolar sacs and the blood, up to 1000 ml of N_2O may be absorbed every minute. N_2O replaces N_2 in the blood, the N_2 being eliminated as the N_2O-O_2 mixture is inhaled. Being 35 times as soluble in the blood as the N_2 it replaces, large volumes of N_2O may be absorbed over prolonged periods of administration.[4,6]

Potential changes may occur within air-filled body cavities during the administration of N_2O because of this degree of absorption of N_2O. During the induction of N_2O-O_2 sedation or anesthesia and during long procedures, N_2O enters a closed air-filled space 35 times more rapidly than N_2 leaves the cavity. This produces an increase in the pressure or volume of that cavity or space. Specific examples of this include increased intestinal distention if bowel obstruction is present; increased pressure in the pleural space aggravating a pneumothorax; and expansion of the middle ear airspace to the point of actually displacing a tympanoplasty graft.[7]

Because of its rapid uptake, two interesting phenomena—the so-called concentration effect and the second gas effect—are seen when N_2O is administered. The *concentration effect* occurs when high concentrations of a gas are administered. The higher the concentration of the gas inhaled, the more rapidly arterial tension of the gas increases. For example, a patient receiving N_2O-O_2 in a ratio of 75%:25% will absorb up to 1000 ml/min of N_2O during the initial stages of induction. As the volume of N_2O is removed from the lungs into the blood, fresh gas is literally sucked up into the lung from the anesthesia machine, thereby increasing the rate at which the N_2O arterial tension increases. If, however, a patient receives only 10% N_2O (a figure more appropriate in dentistry than 75%), the uptake of N_2O by the blood will be only 150 ml/min, which results in no significant change in the rate at which the agent is absorbed or the rate of rise of N_2O arterial tension.[8]

The *second gas effect* occurs when a second inhalation anesthetic is administered along with N_2O-O_2. The second gas effect is also related to the rapid uptake of as much as 1000 ml/min of N_2O-O_2 during the induction of anesthesia. Because of the extremely rapid uptake of a large volume of N_2O, a form of vacuum develops in the alveoli that forces even more fresh gas (N_2O-O_2 plus other inhalation anesthetics) into the lungs. For example, if halothane (1%) is administered along with N_2O-O_2 in a ratio of 75%:25%, its uptake will be more rapid than predicted. This is the second gas effect.[9]

N_2O is absorbed rapidly from the alveolar sacs into the pulmonary circulation. Primary saturation of the blood and brain with N_2O is accomplished by the displacement of N_2 from the alveoli and the blood, and occurs within 3 to 5 minutes of the onset of N_2O-O_2 administration.[10] Clinically this is significant since the patient should be permitted to remain (ideally) at a given level of N_2O for 3 to 5 minutes before the inspired N_2O concentration is increased. This permits the full clinical effect of the given concentration of N_2O to develop before additional gas is added. In actual clinical practice the 3- to 5-minute wait is not necessary. A thorough discussion will be presented in Chapter 16. Tissues with a greater blood flow—including the brain, heart, liver, and kidneys—will receive more N_2O and consequently absorb greater volumes of the gas. The remaining tissues, with a relatively poor blood supply—fat, muscle, and connective tissues—absorb only a small portion of N_2O until primary saturation is completed. At this time these tissues play a predominant role in N_2O absorption. Since the uptake and absorption of N_2O by these tissues is slow (denitrogenation may require 6 to 7 hours), there is no reservoir of N_2O present in

them to impede recovery when N_2O delivery is terminated.

For years it was felt that N_2O did not undergo biotransformation in the body. However, it is demonstrated that anaerobic bacteria in the bowel metabolize N_2O through a reductive pathway with the production of free radicals. There is no convincing evidence that these free radicals cause any specific organ damage.[11] In spite of this the vast majority of inhaled N_2O is exhaled through the lungs within 3 to 5 minutes after termination of its delivery. Approximately 1% of the inhaled N_2O will be eliminated more slowly (over 24 hours) through the lungs and skin.[12]

At the completion of the procedure the N_2O flow is terminated. N_2O diffuses out of the blood and into the alveoli as rapidly as it diffused into the blood during induction. If the patient is allowed to breathe atmospheric air at this time, a phenomenon known as *diffusion hypoxia* (and the Fick principle) may develop.[13] Diffusion hypoxia is responsible for most reports of headache, nausea, and lethargy occurring after N_2O administration—a hangover effect. The alveoli of the patient breathing atmospheric air become filled with a mixture of N_2, O_2, CO_2, water vapor, and N_2O. During the first few minutes the patient breathes atmospheric air, large volumes of N_2O diffuse through the blood into the lungs and are exhaled. As much as 1500 ml of N_2O may be exhaled in the first minute by a patient having breathed N_2O-O_2 in a ratio of 75%:25%. This figure falls to 1200 ml in the second minute and 1000 ml in the third. The concentration effect, discussed previously, is now reversed, and gases rush out of the lungs. More CO_2 is removed from the blood than usual because of this effect, lowering the CO_2 tension of the blood. Decreased CO_2 tension of the blood reduces the stimulus for breathing and produces a depression of respiration.

More important, the rapid diffusion of large volumes of N_2O into the alveoli produces a significant dilution of the O_2 present. In the normal alveolus approximately 14% O_2 is present. This may be reduced to as little as 10% during the first few minutes after termination of N_2O flow. Hypoxia results, producing headache, nausea, and lethargy.

The adverse effects of diffusion hypoxia may be prevented through the routine administration of 100% O_2 for a minimum of 3 to 5 minutes at the termination of the procedure.[14] After N_2O-O_2 inhalation sedation as usually employed in dentistry, diffusion hypoxia is unlikely to develop, and when it does, is usually clinically insignificant.

Recovery from the effects of N_2O is usually rapid and complete. If in the opinion of the drug administrator the patient has fully recovered, the patient may be permitted to leave the office unescorted, to drive his automobile, and to return to his normal activities with no prohibitions. This vitally important aspect of N_2O-O_2 sedation will be discussed thoroughly in Chapter 16.

N_2O is nonallergenic. There has never been a reported allergic reaction to N_2O. It is less toxic than any other inhalation anesthetic.

Central nervous system

The actual mechanism of action of N_2O is unknown, but almost all forms of sensation are depressed (sight, hearing, touch, and pain). Memory is affected to a minimal degree, as is the ability to concentrate or perform acts requiring intelligence.[15] When administered in conjunction with physiological levels of oxygen (greater than 20%), N_2O produces a mild depression of the central nervous system, primarily the cerebral cortex. At therapeutic levels N_2O does not exert any other actions on the central nervous system. The area postrema (the vomiting center) of the medulla is not affected by N_2O unless hypoxia or anoxia is present. Nausea and vomiting occurring after the administration of N_2O are uncommon in the absence of anoxia or hypoxia.[16]

Cardiovascular system

A slight depression of myocardial contraction is produced at a ratio of 80% N_2O:20% O_2 through a direct action of the drug on the heart.[17] The response of vascular smooth muscle to norepinephrine is slightly increased at this level. At levels below this ratio there is no clinically significant effect on the cardiovascular system.

There are no changes in the heart rate or cardiac output directly attributable to N_2O. In the absence of hypoxia or hypercarbia, blood pressure remains stable with an insignificant drop as sedation continues.[18] Cutaneous vasodilation is observed, which produces a degree of flushing and perspiration.[19] The vasodilation can be used to clinical advantage to facilitate venipuncture in patients who are apprehensive or in whom superficial veins are difficult to locate.

Respiratory system

N_2O is not irritating to the pulmonary epithelium; it may therefore be administered to patients with asthma with no increased risk of bronchospasm.[20] Changes in respiratory rate or depth are more likely to result from the sedative relief of anxiety (slower, deeper) or the approach of the excitement stage (rapid, shallow), rather than through a direct action of N_2O on the respiratory system. The resting respiratory minute volume is slightly elevated at a ratio of N_2O-O_2 of 50%:50% without affecting the respiratory response to CO_2.[21]

Gastrointestinal tract

N_2O has no clinically significant actions on the gastrointestinal tract or any organs. In the presence of hepatic dysfunction, N_2O may still be used to effect with no increased risk of overdosage or adverse reaction.[22]

Kidneys

N_2O exerts no significant effects on the kidneys or on the volume and composition of urine.[23]

Hematopoiesis

Nitrous oxide inhibits the actions of methionine synthetase, an enzyme involved in vitamin B_{12} metabolism, leading to impaired bone marrow function.[24] This can affect deoxyribonucleic acid (DNA) synthesis, producing a picture similar to pernicious anemia in laboratory animals exposed to N_2O for prolonged periods. Long-term exposure to N_2O (as in the management of tetanus) can produce transient bone marrow depression. All reported cases have involved exposure to N_2O for more than 24 hours.[25,26]

The effects of repeated short-term exposure to N_2O are of greater concern. A neuropathy resembling vitamin B_{12} deficiency has been reported in dentists using nitrous oxide regularly in their practices and in persons abusing the drug.[27] It is thought that this is a result of the combination of N_2O's actions on methionine synthetase and to the chronic exposure to unusually high N_2O concentrations as the dental team operates in the oral cavity.[28] In addition, there is a consistent finding in retrospective epidemiologic studies that the incidence of spontaneous abortion is increased amongst women working in operating rooms.[29] To date no cause-and-effect relationship has been proved. A recent study has indicated that fertility is decreased in women exposed to N_2O for long periods of time.[30] The important subject of the safety of nitrous oxide use in a dental office, to the dental staff, will be discussed in depth in Chapter 18.

Skeletal muscle

Nitrous oxide does not produce relaxation of skeletal muscles. Any observed effect of this nature during inhalation sedation is attributable to the relief of anxiety rather than to a direct action of N_2O.

Uterus and pregnancy

N_2O and O_2 are frequently used as an aid in the management of discomfort during labor and delivery.[31] Uterine contractions are not inhibited in either amplitude or frequency.[32] N_2O passes easily across the placenta into the fetus, where the O_2 concentration of fetal blood may fall dramatically if less than 20% O_2 is being delivered with the N_2O.[33] Pregnancy does not pose a contraindication to the use of N_2O-O_2 inhalation sedation (see Chapters 5 and 13 for a more complete discussion of the use of sedation during pregnancy).

Physiological contraindications

"There are no contraindications to the use of nitrous oxide in combination with an adequate percentage of oxygen."[34]

"If administered with a minimum of 25% oxygen, it is a safe agent."[35]

"Nitrous oxide is a very safe anesthetic if oxygen is supplied in sufficient concentration."[36]

In the past few years it has become apparent that N_2O is not an innocuous vapor, as it was once considered. Chronic exposure of dental personnel to low levels of N_2O has been associated (though not definitively proved) with increased risk of spontaneous abortion, fetal malformation, and other types of disease.[37-39] On the other hand, chronic exposure of dental personnel (or others) to high levels of N_2O has been demonstrated beyond doubt to be capable of producing a sensory neuropathy that is extremely debilitating to the professional.[40,41] The occurrence of nitrous oxide neuropathy is usually limited to persons who have purposefully abused the drug. These two very important subjects will be discussed in depth in Chapter 18.

OXYGEN

O_2 is the second component of the inhalation sedation technique. First prepared in 1727 by Stephen Hales (who did not recognize it as an element), it was discovered as an element in 1771 by Joseph Priestley (the same man who discovered N_2O 5 years later) and almost simultaneously by Karl Scheele (1771).[42]

Preparation

O_2 is most commonly prepared by the fractional distillation of liquid air. N_2 is the first gas to boil off, with O_2 remaining as a liquid. This method of preparation was first employed in 1895 by Linde. Other methods of preparation of O_2 include the following:
1. Heating of barium peroxide (BaO_2) to 800° C, at which point it forms $BaO + O_2$
2. The electrolysis of water $2H_2O \rightarrow 2H_2 + O_2$
3. The reaction between sodium peroxide and water $2Na_2O_2 + 2H_2O \rightarrow 4NaOH + O_2$

Properties

O_2 is a clear, colorless, odorless gas with a molecular weight of 32. It comprises 20.9% of atmospheric air. Its specific gravity is 1.105, whereas that of air is 1. It is stored in compressed gas cylinders in a gaseous state. A full cylinder has 2000 pounds of pressure per square inch (psi) at room temperature. Its solubility in water is 2.4 volumes percent at 37° C and 4.9 volumes percent at 0° C. The cylinder of O_2 is green in the United States and white internationally as per World Health Organization standards.[43]

O_2 is not flammable (cannot be ignited) but will support combustion. Under high pressure in the presence of oil or grease O_2 may cause an explosion. Therefore, the use of oil and grease should be strictly avoided in and around O_2 cylinders, reducing valves, wall outlets, and cylinder outlets.

Effects of 100% oxygen
Central nervous system

The inhalation of 100% O_2 has no effect on the cerebral cortex. Electroencephalographic (EEG) tracings are unchanged.[44] Cerebral blood flow may be decreased by as much as 10% as a result of constriction of the cerebral blood vessels occurring with 100% O_2 inhalation.[45]

Cardiovascular system

The inhalation of 100% oxygen is associated with a slight fall in both the heart rate (3 to 4 beats/minute) and cardiac output (10% to 20%).[46] Coronary artery blood flow may be decreased up to 10% at this time. There is a slight increase in diastolic, but no change in the systolic, blood pressure with inhalation of 100% O_2.[47] This is a result of increased peripheral resistance secondary to a generalized vasoconstriction that occurs in the systemic, cerebral, renal, and retinal vessels on inhalation of 100% O_2.[48]

The inhalation of greater than 40% O_2 in premature infants may produce retrolental fibroplasia many months later.[49]

Respiratory system

After 2 minutes of inhaling 100% O_2, minute volume is slightly depressed (3%). This occurs because ambient air (20.93% O_2) produces a continuous tonic stimulation of respiration through the chemoreceptors that are located in the carotid and aortic bodies. Inhalation of 100% O_2 abolishes this reflex stimulation, resulting in a decrease in minute volume. Following 6 to 8 minutes of 100% O_2, minute volume exchange actually increases by 7.6%. This increase is produced through stimulation of the lower respiratory passages by O_2, which acts as an irritant, or by dilation of the pulmonary capillaries by O_2 with the production of reflex respiratory stimulation from mild pulmonary congestion.

Anatomy

The anatomy of the respiratory system will be reviewed so that those involved in the use of inhalation sedation will possess a better knowledge of the processes involved in producing the observed state of relaxation.

The respiratory system is composed of a number of parts. These may be divided into two groups: (1) those parts of the respiratory system involved in the transport of gases to and from the outside of the body to and from the respiratory zone of the lungs and (2) those parts involved with the exchange of gases between the blood and the air, variously called the "exchange portion of the lung" and the "respiratory zone." The portion of the respiratory system involved in conduction of gases is termed "anatomic dead space" since there is no exchange of O_2 and CO_2 between the air and the blood.

Structures included in the conducting portion of the respiratory system are as follows (Fig. 14-4):

Nose
Pharynx
  Nasopharynx
  Oropharynx
  Hypopharynx
Larynx
Trachea
Bronchi
Bronchioles

The mouth is considered to be an accessory respiratory passage.

Structures included in the respiratory zone are as follows (Fig. 14-5):

Respiratory bronchioles
Alveolar ducts
Alveolar sacs
Alveoli

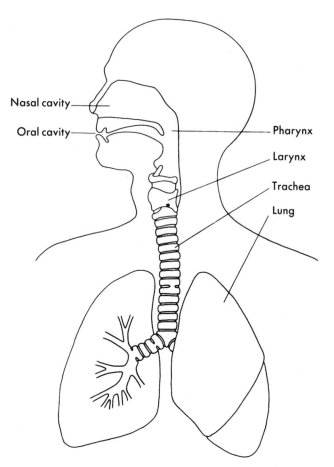

Fig. 14-4. Structures forming the conducting portion of the respiratory system. (From Hammond EC: *Sci Am* 207:48, 1962.)

Nose

The nose, or nasal cavity, is anatomically the most superior part of the respiratory system. It starts as two flexible, flared, rubbery entryways termed "wings" or "alae," enclosing a space on either side called the "vestibule." The nasal cavities continue posteriorly as paired air spaces. The right and left sides are separated by the bony nasal septum. At its posterior aspect above and behind the soft palate the septum ends and the right and left nasal cavities unite to form the uppermost portion of the pharynx, the nasopharynx.

The nose has several functions in respiration.[50,51] Its primary function is to warm and humidify air. The process of warming air is readily accomplished by the mucous membranes of the nose, which are well endowed with an excellent blood supply. This large blood flow through the mucous membranes of the

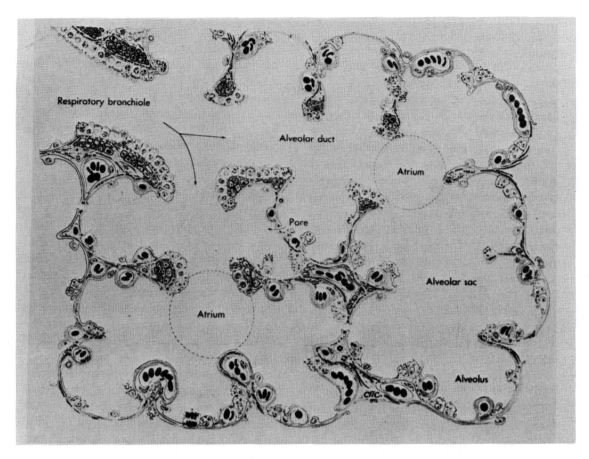

Fig. 14-5. Structures forming the respiratory zone of the respiratory system. (From Sorokin SP: In Greep RO, Weiss L, eds: *Histology.* New York, 1973, McGraw-Hill.)

nose is responsible for warming of the air, a process that continues throughout the respiratory tract.

The nose also serves as: (1) a defense against organisms and foreign materials, a function carried out by cilia found throughout the nose and by the mucous film found throughout the respiratory tract—submucosal glands and goblet cells are responsible for the formation of this mucinous lining; (2) a conduit for air to travel to and from the external environment to the lungs; (3) vocal resonance, a function of both the nose and sinuses (empty air spaces found within the skull, emptying into the nasal cavity); and (4) an organ involved in the sense of smell.

In inhalation sedation as practiced in dentistry, the nose is, of necessity, the prime route of entry of the anesthetic gases into the patient. Situations in which the patient becomes unable to breathe well through the nose, such as deviated septum and chronic or acute sinusitis, will complicate the inhalation sedation procedure.

Mouth

The mouth is considered an accessory respiratory passage. Most people will breathe through the mouth at times, especially during speech and whenever their nasal passages are occluded, such as in respiratory infections. As with the nose, the mouth, because of its mucosal surface and its rich blood supply, serves to warm and humidify the air as it enters the body. The mouth ends at the posterior palatine pillars. These pillars extend superiorly to meet the uvula, a fleshy tab of soft tissue located in the midline, at the posterior border of the soft palate.

The base of the tongue rises out of the hypopharynx to occupy the floor of the mouth. Using the other passive structures of the oral cavity for support, the tongue and the oropharyngeal reflexes actively protect against threats to the airway.[52]

Since the mouth is the region in which dentistry is performed, this area will not be involved in the routine administration of N_2O and O_2; however, the mouth is available for the administration of gases, especially O_2 during emergencies. In such cases both the mouth and nose may be used for the purposes of ventilation.

Pharynx

The pharynx extends from the posterior portion of the nose to the level of the lower border of the cricoid cartilage, where it becomes continuous with the esophagus and the respiratory tract through the larynx.[51] The word pharynx is derived from the Greek for "throat." For anatomical purposes the pharynx is divided into three regions—the *nasopharynx, oropharynx,* and *hypopharynx.* The nasopharynx extends from the back of the nasal cavity to the level of the soft palate. The eustachian tubes open into the nasopharynx connecting with the middle ear. The oropharynx starts superiorly at the level of the soft palate to the level of the cricoid cartilage and the base of the tongue inferiorly. The hypopharynx, also known as the *laryngopharynx,* starts superiorly at the epiglottis to the division of the esophagus and larynx. It is the shortest of the three divisions. The major functions of the pharynx are the conduction, warming, and humidification of air and the removal of foreign materials. The junction of the pharynx and the esophagus represents the narrowest part of the alimentary canal. Foreign bodies trapped at this level may produce aspiration or significant decreases in airflow.[53,54]

Epiglottis

Although not an integral part of the respiratory system, the epiglottis, a platelike structure extending from the base of the tongue backward and upward, must be mentioned. It functions as a flaplike covering over the larynx that closes during swallowing, covering the airway so that swallowed materials enter the esophagus.[50]

Larynx

In the adult the larynx is found at the level of the first through the fifth cervical vertebrae, consisting of a number of articulated cartilages surrounding the upper end of the trachea (Fig. 14-6).[55] "Adam's apple" is another common name for the larynx (more accurately, Adam's apple denotes the thyroid cartilage). The laryngeal cavity extends from just below the epiglottis to the lower level of the cricoid cartilage where it becomes continuous with the trachea.

The primary function of the larynx is phonation, but it also has a protective function, since the airway becomes quite narrow at this point. Structures found

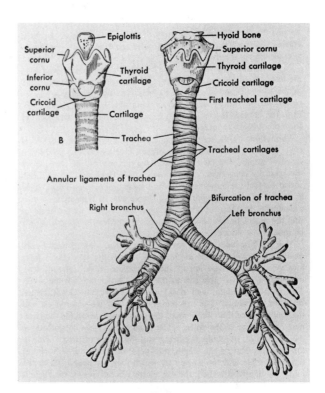

Fig. 14-6. The trachea, bronchi, and bronchioles form a major portion of the conduction system of the respiratory system. (From Kimber DC, Gray CE, Stackpole CE et al: *Textbook of anatomy and physiology,* ed 13. New York, 1955, Macmillan, p 490.)

within the laryngeal cavity include the vestibular folds—the false vocal cords, and the vocal cords—the true vocal cords, which are two pearly white folds of mucous membrane.

The narrowest portion of the larynx in the adult is located at the true vocal cords.[50] Larger aspirated objects will become lodged at this site. They can usually be dislodged by the abdominal thrust or chest thrust. In the child under the age of 10 years the narrowest portion of the larynx occurs at the level of cricoid cartilage.[50,51] Should material be small enough to pass between the vocal cords, in the adult and in most children it will usually enter either the right or left mainstem bronchus, a situation that is serious but not acutely life-threatening.

Trachea

The trachea is a tubular structure that begins at the cricoid cartilage. The tube of the trachea is formed of approximately 16 to 22 C-shaped cartilaginous rings that are incomplete on their posterior surface. A thin muscle band extends between the incomplete posterior ends of the U-shaped cartilages.

The trachea extends through the neck into the mediastinum to a point behind the junction of the upper and middle thirds of the sternum, where it divides into the right and left mainstem bronchi. The carina is the name given to the cartilage that is located at the point of bifurcation. The carina is located approximately 5 cm below the suprasternal notch.[50] The trachea is about 10 to 13 cm long and has an outer diameter of 2.5 cm and an inner diameter of 1.0 to 1.5 cm. This dimension is enlarged in the elderly, and decreased during pregnancy (due to edema).

Bronchi

At the level of the carina the right and left mainstem bronchi branch off from the trachea. Because of the position of the heart in the left side of the mediastinum, the angle formed by the left mainstem bronchus (45 to 55 degrees) is somewhat greater than that formed by the right mainstem bronchus (20 to 30 degrees). This is of importance since aspirated objects will have a greater tendency to enter into the right lung than the left.[50,51]

Each of the mainstem bronchi divides into branches that supply each of the lobes of the lung. The right mainstem bronchus is wider and shorter than the left, giving branches to the upper and middle lobes and then continuing to become the branch to the right lower lobe. The right upper lobe bronchus has its origin about 2 cm from the carina while the left arises about 5 cm from the carina.[51] Each of these bronchi in turn gives off branches.[56] The right upper lobe bronchus gives rise to three main divisions, the right middle lobe bronchus to two divisions, and the right lower lobe bronchus to five or six divisions. The left mainstem bronchus is somewhat longer and narrower than the right. It ends at the origin of the left upper lobe bronchus and continues to become the main bronchus to the left lower lobe. The left upper lobe main bronchus originates at the bifurcation of the left mainstem bronchus and gives off three branches. The left lower lobe main bronchus, the direct continuation of the left mainstem bronchus, gives rise to four branches.[57]

Bronchioles

The bronchi continue to bifurcate and trifurcate well into the periphery of each lung. As these divisions occur the number of bronchi increases significantly, as does the total surface area of the lung. As the bronchi continue to divide they become smaller and their cartilaginous rings gradually recede, becoming irregular plates. Cartilage is found in bronchioles until their diameter is approximately 0.66 to 1 mm, at which point cartilage disappears entirely.[58]

The first 17 divisions of the tracheobronchial tree comprise the conducting zone, since the exchange of O_2 and CO_2—the primary function of the lungs—cannot occur here. This is also termed "dead space." Approximately 150 ml of air is found in the conducting zone in the average-sized adult.[59] From divisions 17 to 23, changes occur in the walls and linings of the airway that dramatically increase their surface area. These airways comprise what is called the "respiratory zone" and include respiratory bronchioles, alveolar ducts, alveolar sacs, and the alveolus (Fig. 14-5). The alveolus represents the final air space and is the unit in which the exchange of gases occurs.

Alveolus

The alveolus is essentially a pocket of air surrounded by a thin membrane containing capillaries (Fig. 14-7). The distance between the air within the alveolus and the capillary is approximately 0.35 and 2.5 μm. This thin wall is essential for the rapid exchange of gases between air and blood. Gases within the alveoli are separated from blood by four thin layers:

1. Mucinous covering
2. Alveolar epithelium (incomplete)
3. Interstitial layer
4. Endothelial cells lining pulmonary capillaries

Blood remains within the pulmonary capillaries for approximately 0.5 second, yet gas exchange is so swift that it is completed by the time the blood has completed only one fourth of its journey through the capillary.

Physiology of Respiration

Gases are inhaled through the nose and/or mouth and are transported to the respiratory zone of the lungs, the more than 300 million alveoli in which the interchange of gases between the alveolus and the pulmonary capillaries occurs. The exchange of gases in the alveoli depends entirely on diffusion of gases across membranes and is controlled by the partial pressures of the respective gases on either side of the alveolar membrane.

Pulmonary capillaries are unique in that they form the most dense capillary network in the entire body. It is estimated that pulmonary capillaries are approximately 10 μm long and 7 μm wide. So finely interlaced are they that they may be considered more of

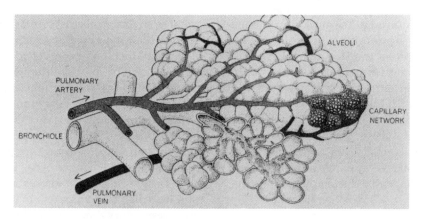

Fig. 14-7. Diagram of alveoli and surrounding vasculature. The capillary bed in this area is the densest vascular network in the entire body. (From Hammond EC: *The effects of smoking.* © 1962 by Scientific American, Inc. All rights reserved.)

a pool of blood vessels than a series of pipes. In adults the surface area of the pulmonary capillary-alveolar interface is about 70 m², or approximately 40 times the surface area of the body.[60] At any given moment, there is approximately 100 to 300 ml of blood within these pulmonary capillaries. Dail has compared this to the spreading of a teaspoon of blood over 1 square meter of surface area.[58]

The gases within the alveoli are separated from the capillaries by approximately 1 to 2 μ of tissue: the mucinous covering of the alveolus, the alveolar epithelium, which in some places is incomplete, an interstitial layer, and the endothelium covering the pulmonary capillary.

MECHANICS OF RESPIRATION

How do gases get into the alveolus from outside the body? Air moves from the external environment to the level of the alveolar capillary membrane because of differences of pressure within the respiratory system. Gases move from a zone of higher pressure to one of lower pressure.

The typical respiratory cycle can be divided into five phases: preinspiration, peak inspiration, end-inspiration, peak expiration, and end-expiration.

At preinspiration the pressure within the pleural cavity is negative: minus 5 cm H_2O, the pressure of the normal resting lung. This negative pressure is produced by the natural tendency of the lung to recoil inward and of the chest wall to recoil outward.

As inspiration begins the muscles of inspiration contract and the chest cavity (thorax) expands, increasing the negative pressure within the thorax to even more than what it was at rest. This results in an expansion of the alveoli as well as the development of negative pressure within them.

With the development of negative pressure within the alveoli—a pressure negative to atmospheric pressure—air begins to flow into the respiratory system through the nose and mouth. As air enters the system a tidal volume develops resulting in the end of inspiration. Pleural pressure reaches its most negative point, alveolar pressure returns to zero as gases enter the alveoli, airflow into the lung ceases, and the maximum inspiratory volume is reached. Expiration now begins.

Pleural pressure begins to return to its original value (minus 5 cm H_2O), resulting in the creation of positive pressure within the alveoli during expiration and maximal expiratory flow out of the respiratory system. At the end of expiration, pleural pressure has returned to baseline, alveolar pressure has returned to zero, flow has ceased, and the expiratory volume has been delivered, returning the lung to its resting lung capacity. Under normal respiratory conditions (quiet breathing), most of the pressure that is generated occurs as a result of the elastic characteristics of the lungs.

Muscles are involved in the process of breathing, helping to produce the increases in negative pressures that draw air into the respiratory system. These muscles are as follows:

1. Diaphragm—primary
2. Intercostals—primary
3. Abdominals—accessory
4. Scalenes—accessory
5. Sternocleidomastoid—accessory
6. Some back muscles—accessory

The *diaphragm* is the primary muscle involved in quiet breathing. In normal breathing a 1-cm downward movement of the diaphragm causes 350 ml of air to enter the lung. The normal 500-ml tidal volume will therefore require approximately a 1.5-cm downward movement of the diaphragm. In quiet breathing the diaphragm is probably the only muscle of respiration working. *Intercostal muscles* do not participate in quiet breathing. *Abdominal muscles* do not participate in quiet breathing or in ventilation up to about 40 lpm. The abdominal muscles take a more active part as the volume of air inspired increases, and above 90 lpm (as seen in strenuous exercise) the abdominals are actively contributing by forceful contraction. The *scalenes* do contract during quiet breathing; however, their contribution to the total volume of air inspired is not great. The *sternocleido-mastoids* do not participate in quiet respiration; however, their actions do become more forceful as ventilation increases. All of the muscles that participate in respiration are attached to the thoracic cage.

COMPOSITION OF RESPIRATORY GASES

The composition of the major gases found in the respiratory system is as follows (percentages):

Gas	Inspired air	Alveolar air	Expired air
O_2	20.94	14.2	16.3
CO_2	0.04	5.5	4.0
N_2	79.02	80.3	79.7

Water vapor constitutes less than 1% of atmospheric air, whereas alveolar air, fully saturated with water vapor, contains 6.2%. The pressure exerted by the water vapor is 47 mm Hg and must be taken into account when determining the partial pressures of the gases within the alveoli.

Barometric pressure	−	Water vapor pressure	=	Alveolar partial pressure
760 mm Hg	minus	47 mm Hg	equals	713 mm Hg

The partial pressure of gases within the alveolus is determined as follows:

Alveolar O_2 tension $= 713 \times 14.2/100 = 103$ mm Hg
Alveolar CO_2 tension $= 713 \times 5.5/100 = 40$ mm Hg
Alveolar N_2 tension $= 713 \times 80.3/100 = 570$ mm Hg
Water vapor $= 47$ mm Hg
Total pressures $= 760$ mm Hg

The speed at which gases diffuse across membranes is controlled by several factors, the most important of which is their partial pressure in each compartment (Table 14-2). For example, the partial pressure of O_2 within the alveolus is 103 mm Hg, whereas in the pulmonary capillary its tension is only 40 mm Hg. O_2 is therefore forced into the capillary from the alveolus.

When arterial blood arrives at the tissues in the

Table 14-2. Partial pressures of gases

Gas (mm Hg)	Air (mm Hg)	Alveolus (mm Hg)	Arterial blood (mm Hg)	Venous blood (mm Hg)
O_2	158.2	103	100	40
CO_2	0.3	40	40	46
N_2	596.5	570	573	573
H_2O vapor	5.0	47	47	47

body it still has an O_2 tension of 100 mm Hg, whereas the O_2 tension within the tissues is only 40 mm Hg. O_2 therefore travels from the plasma into the tissues because of this pressure gradient. The O_2 tension within the plasma falls. In a resting state the tissues remove approximately 30% of the available O_2. Venous blood leaving the tissues still contains quite a bit of O_2; however, during violent exercise the tissues may remove almost all of the available O_2. On returning to the lungs venous blood quickly surrenders its CO_2 (partial pressure, 46 mm Hg) to the alveolus (partial pressure, 40 mm Hg) and O_2 diffuses from the alveolus into the capillary blood (capillary PO_2, 40 mm Hg; alveolar PO_2, 103 mm Hg).

Disease states may alter the rate at which the exchange of gases occurs within the lungs. For example, in emphysema the total surface area of the alveolar membranes is decreased; in pneumonia the alveolar walls become thickened, thereby inhibiting diffusion; and in asthma the increase in bronchial secretions also acts to impede the exchange of gases. In methemoglobinemia the oxygen-carrying capacity of the blood is decreased.

N_2O when inhaled into the lungs will act in the same manner as the gases described previously. When first inhaled the partial pressure of N_2O within the alveolus will be quite high, whereas that within the capillary will be zero. N_2O flow will occur rapidly from the alveolus to the capillary, and the same response will develop within tissues. As the blood becomes saturated with N_2O (3 to 5 minutes), the rate of diffusion into the cardiovascular system decreases. At the termination of the procedure the patient is administered 100% O_2 and N_2O is eliminated. The alveolus now contains little or no N_2O, whereas venous blood returning to the lung is rich in N_2O. N_2O now diffuses out of the blood into the alveolus and out of the body through the respiratory tract.

REFERENCES

1. The National Formulary: *The US pharmacopeia.* Rockville, Md, 1990, US Pharmacopeial Convention.

2. Wood M, Wood AJJ: *Drugs and anesthesia: pharmacology for anesthesiologists.* Baltimore, 1982, Williams & Wilkins.

3. Wollman H, Smith TC: Uptake, distribution, elimination, and administration of inhalational anesthetics. In Goodman LS, Gilman A, eds: *Pharmacological basis of therapeutics,* ed 5. New York, 1975, Macmillan.

4. Gould DB, Lampert BA, MacKrell TN: Effect of nitrous oxide solubility on vaporizer aberrance, *Anesth Analg* 61(11):938, 1982.

5. Gillman MA: Analgesic (sub anesthetic) nitrous oxide interacts with the endogenous opioid system: a review of the evidence, *Life Sci* 39(14):1209, 1986.

6. Longnecker DE, Miller FL: Pharmacology of inhalational anesthetics. In Rogers MC, Tinker JH, Covino BG et al, eds: *Principles and practice of anesthesiology.* St Louis, 1993, Mosby.

7. Taylor E, Feinstein R, White PF et al.: Anesthesia for laparoscopic cholecystectomy: is nitrous oxide contraindicated? *Anesthesiology* 76(4):541, 1992.

8. Severinghaus JW: The rate of uptake of nitrous oxide in man, *J Clin Invest* 33:1183, 1954.

9. Epstein RM, Rackow H, Salanitre E et al: Influence of the concentration effect on the uptake of anesthetic mixtures, *Anesthesiology* 25:364, 1964.

10. Longnecker DE, Miller FL: Pharmacology of inhalational anesthetics. In Rogers MC, Tinker JH, Covino BG et al, eds: *Principles and practice of anesthesiology.* St Louis, 1993, Mosby.

11. Eger EI II: *Nitrous oxide.* New York, 1985, Elsevier.

12. Longnecker DE, Miller FL: Pharmacology of inhalational agents. In Rogers MC, Tinker JH, Covino BG et al, eds: *Principles and practice of anesthesiology.* St Louis, 1993, Mosby.

13. Stewart RD, Gorayeb MJ, Pelton GH: Arterial blood gases before, during, and after nitrous oxide: oxygen administration, *Ann Emerg Med* 15(10):1177, 1986.

14. Quarnstrom FC, Milgrom P, Bishop MJ et al: Clinical study of diffusion hypoxia after nitrous oxide analgesia, *Anesth Prog* 38(1):21, 1991.

15. Ramsey DS, Leonesio RJ, Whitney CW et al: Paradoxical effects of nitrous oxide on human memory, *Psychopharmacol* 106(3):370, 1992.

16. Smiley BA, Paradise NF: Does the duration of N_2O administration affect postoperative nausea and vomiting? *Nurse Anesth* 2(1):13, 1991.

17. Stowe DF, Monroe SM, Marijic J et al: Effects of nitrous oxide on contractile function and metabolism of the isolated heart, *Anesthesiology* 73(6):1220, 1990.

18. Hornbein TF, Martin WE, Bonica JJ et al: Nitrous oxide effects on the circulatory and ventilatory responses to halothane, *Anesthesiology* 31:250, 1969.

19. Moore PA: Nitrous oxide: oxygen sedation: induction and recovery, *Curr Rev Nurse Anesth* 4:35, 1981.

20. Pasternak LR: Outpatient anesthesia. In Rogers MC, Tinker JH, Covino BG et al, eds: *Principles and practice of anesthesiology.* St Louis, 1993, Mosby. *p 2293.*

21. Yacoub O, Doell D, Kryger MH, et al: Depression of hypoxic ventilatory response by nitrous oxide, *Anesthesiology* 45:385, 1976.

22. Ross JA, Monk SJ, Duffy SW: Effect of nitrous oxide on halothane-induced hepatotoxicity in hypoxic, enzyme-induced rats, *Br J Anaesth* 56(5):527, 1984.

23. Eckenhoff RG, Longnecker DE: The therapeutic gases: oxygen, carbon dioxide, helium, and water vapor. In Gilman AG, Rall TW, Nies AS et al, eds: *Goodman and Gilman's the pharmacological basis of therapeutics,* ed 8. New York, 1990, Pergamon, p 332.

24. Deacon R, Lumb M, Perry J et al: Selective inactivation of vitamin B_{12} in rats by nitrous oxide, *Lancet* 2:1023, 1978.

25. Henry RJ: Assessing environmental health concerns associated with nitrous oxide, *JADA* 123(12):41, 1992.

26. Franco G: Occupational exposure to anaesthetics: liver injury, microsomal enzyme induction and preventive aspects, *Ital Medicin Lavoro* 11(5):205, 1989.

27. Layzer RB: Myeloneuropathy after prolonged exposure to nitrous oxide, *Lancet* 2:1227, 1978.

28. Longnecker DE, Miller FL: Pharmacology of inhalational anesthetics. In Rogers MC, Tinker JH, Covino BG et al., eds: *Principles and practice of anesthesiology,* St Louis, 1993, Mosby.

29. Eger EI II: Fetal injury and abortion associated with occupational exposure to inhaled anesthetics, *AANA J* 59(4):309, 1991.

30. Wynn RL: Nitrous oxide and fertility, part I, *Gener Dent* 41(2):122, 1993.

31. Marx GF, Katsnelson T: The introduction of nitrous oxide analgesia into obstetrics, *Obstet Gynecol* 80(4):715, 1992.

32. Arai M, Nishijima M, Tatsuma H: Analgesia and anesthesia during labor in Japan and developed countries, *Asia-Oceania J Obstetr Gynaecol* 15(a3):213, 1989.

33. Landon MJ, Toothill VJ: Effect of nitrous oxide on placental methionine synthase activity, *Br J Anaesth* 58(5):524, 1986.

34. Wylie WD, Churchill-Davidson HC: *A practice of anesthesia,* ed 4. Philadelphia, 1978, Saunders, p 244.

35. Lichtiger M, Moya F: *Introduction to the practice of anesthesia.* New York, 1974, Harper & Row, p 19.

36. Snow JC: *Manual of anesthesia,* Boston, 1977, Little, Brown, p 100.

37. Baden JM, Fujinaga M: Effects of nitrous oxide on day 9 rat embryos grown in culture, *Br J Anaesth* 66(4):500, 1991.

38. Schumann D: Nitrous oxide anaesthesia: risks to health personnel, *Int Nurs Rev* 37(1):214, 1990.

39. Littner MM, Kaffe I, Tamse A: Occupational hazards in the dental office and their control. IV. Measures for controlling contamination of anesthetic gas—nitrous oxide, *Quintess Intern* 14(4):461, 1983.

40. Stacy CB, DiRocco A, Gould RJ: Methionine in the treatment of nitrous oxide-induced neuropathy and myeloneuropathy, *J Neurol* 239(7):401, 1992.

41. Chanarin I: The effects of nitrous oxide on cobalamins, folates, and on related events, *Crit Rev Toxicol* 10(3):179, 1982.

42. Eckenhoff, Longnecker DE: The therapeutic gases: oxygen, carbon dioxide, helium, and water vapor. In Gilman AG, Rall TW, Nies AS et al, eds: *Goodman and Gilman's the pharmacological basis of therapeutics,* ed 8. New York, 1990, Pergamon, p 300.

43. Robiolio M, Rumsey WL, Wilson OF: Oxygen diffusion and mitochondrial respiration in neuroblastic cells, *Am J Physiol* 256:C1207, 1989.

44. Bleiberg B, Kerem D: Central nervous system oxygen toxicity in the resting rat: postponement by intermittent oxygen exposure, *Undersea Biomed Res* 15(5):337, 1988.

45. Bryan RM Jr: Cerebral blood flow and energy metabolism during stress, *Am J Physiol* 259(2):H269, 1990.

46. Voelkel NF: Mechanisms of hypoxic pulmonary vasoconstriction, *Am Rev Respir Dis* 133:1186, 1986.

47. Martindale W: *Extra pharmacopoeia,* ed 29. London, 1989, Pharmaceutical Press.

48. Rothe CF, Maass-Moreno R, Flanagan AD: Effects of hypercapnia and hypoxia on the cardiovascular system: vascular capacitance and aortic chemoreceptors, *Am J Physiol* 259(3):H932, 1990.

49. Weiss NS: Oxygen and retrolental fibrodysplasia: did epidemiology help or hinder? *Epidemiology* 2(1):60, 1991.
50. Morris IR: Functional anatomy of the upper airway, *Emerg Med Clin North Am* 6:639, 1988.
51. Young GP: Clinical airway anatomy. In Dailey RH, Simon B, Young GP et al, eds: *The airway: emergency management.* 1992, St Louis, Mosby.
52. Block C, Vrechner V: Unusual problems in airway management. II. The influence of the temporomandibular joint, the mandible, and associated structures on endotracheal intubation, *Anesth Analg* 50:115, 1971.
53. Danilidis J et al: Foreign body in the airways, *Arch Otolaryngol* 103:570, 1977.
54. Kim IN et al: Foreign body in the airway—a review of 202 cases, *Laryngoscope* 83:347, 1973.
55. Meller SM: Functional anatomy of the larynx, *Otolaryngol Clin North Am* 17:1, 1984.
56. Ellis H, Feldman S: *Anatomy for anesthetists,* ed 4. Oxford, England, 1983, Blackwell Scientific.
57. Clemente CD, ed: *Gray's anatomy of the human body,* ed 30. Philadelphia, 1984, Lea & Febiger.
58. Dail DH: Anatomy of the respiratory system. In Moser KM, Spragg RG, eds: *Respiratory emergencies,* ed 2. St Louis, 1982, Mosby.
59. Benumof JL: The respiratory physiology and respiratory function during anesthesia. In Miller RD, eds: *Anesthesia,* ed 3. New York, 1990, Churchill-Livingstone.
60. Levine S, Kuna ST: Introduction to the respiratory system. In Rose LF, Kaye D, eds: *Internal medicine for dentistry.* St Louis, 1983, Mosby.

CHAPTER *15*

Armamentarium

The armamentarium for the delivery of N_2O-O_2 inhalation sedation is quite simple. Primary equipment consists of a supply of the gases and an apparatus for their delivery to the patient. The modern inhalation sedation unit is a compact, continuous-flow machine used for the administration of compressed gases under controlled conditions. This sedation unit is a modification of the machines used to administer inhalation general anesthesia. These machines (Fig. 15-1) are capable of delivering a number of inhalation anesthetics, whereas the inhalation sedation unit has been altered to deliver only two gases—N_2O and O_2.

TYPES OF INHALATION SEDATION UNITS

There are two basic types of inhalation sedation unit, although only one is recommended for use. These are the continuous-flow machine and the intermittent- or demand-flow unit. Although these devices are similar in design, there are some very significant differences in their operation.

Demand-flow units

The demand-flow type of N_2O-O_2 inhalation sedation unit (Fig. 15-2) does not deliver gas continuously to the patient but instead varies the rate and volume of delivered gas according to the patient's respiratory demands and requirements. In this sense the demand-flow type inhalation sedation unit may be compared to the face mask employed by SCUBA divers, which operates on the same principle. A major advantage of the demand-flow type unit is the economy obtained from the decreased volume of compressed gases used.

In operation the gases delivered are proportioned by the machine. Only one dial, which changes the percentages of gases being delivered, need be adjusted. This dial provides a direct indication of the percentage of O_2 being delivered in the mixture (the remainder of gas is N_2O). The mechanism involved in the demand-flow unit is much more complex than the flowmeter and in clinical practice has been subject to a greater percentage error. Demand-flow units show only what was set, not what is actually delivered. If a discrepancy develops between the dial and the actual gas flow, there is no warning while the unit is in operation.[1]

There are several disadvantages associated with demand-flow units. One is that the volume flow of anesthetic gases per minute is not visible or registered anywhere on the machine. In place of this there is a dial on which the percentages of the gases being delivered are recorded and another on which the pressure at which they are being delivered is visible. The lack of ability to visually monitor the flow of gases to the patient is a major, but not the only, disadvantage of the demand-flow unit.

A second disadvantage of the demand-flow unit was the lack of accuracy of the mixer valve. The percentage of gas being delivered is not accurate over the full range of delivery (0% to 100% N_2O). Gauert and Hustead[2] and Allen[3] demonstrated the lack of accuracy of two demand-flow units, the McKesson Nargraph and Narmatic. At an indicated O_2 percentage of 75% the actual delivered O_2 percentage ranged from 80% to 45%, whereas at 50% indicated O_2 the actual delivered percentage ranged from 75% to 22%. Having to rely on a mixer valve that is inaccurate in a machine in which the flow of the individual gases cannot be visualized provides two significant disadvantages to the use of demand-flow units.

The gas circuit followed by the N_2O and O_2 in the demand-flow machine is as follows:
1. Compressed-gas cylinders
2. Pressure-reducing valves
3. Mixing valve with percentage of N_2O or O_2
4. Pressure regulator (to vary flow of gases)
5. Demand valve

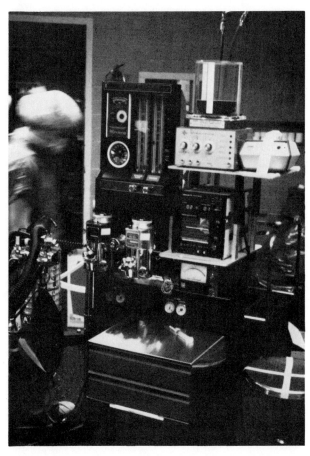

Fig. 15-1. General anesthesia machines can deliver multiple anesthetic gases and contain multiple monitoring devices.

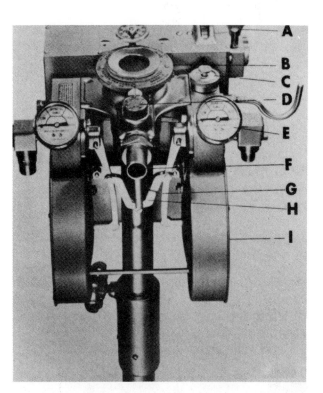

Fig. 15-2. Demand-flow N₂O-O₂ unit. Front view of Nargraf machine. *A*, Pressure adjuster for debreathing device; *B*, mixing top; *C*, oxygen flush valve; *D*, pressure control; *E*, pressure gauge; *F*, outlet; *G*, lever arm; *H*, toggle arm; and *I*, metal drum. (Picture courtesy of McKesson Company, a division of Narco Medical Company.)

6. Conducting tubes
7. Nasal hood
8. Expiratory valve

Clinical examples of demand-flow inhalation sedation/anesthesia units are:

1. Jectaflow
2. Walton (primarily used in United Kingdom)
3. McKesson Euthesor
4. McKesson Nargraph (Fig. 15-2)
5. McKesson Narmatic

Allen has stated that fatalities have resulted from misunderstanding the use of the demand-flow machine.[3] In light of this and the distinct advantages of the continuous-flow machines, primarily their greater accuracy and the fact that the flow of gases can be visualized, use of demand-flow inhalation sedation units cannot be recommended.

Continuous-flow units

In contrast to demand-flow units are the continuous-flow units. These units contain flowmeters and are characterized by the continuous flow of gases, regardless of the respiratory pattern of the patient. Gas continues to be delivered through the machine even as the patient exhales. Whereas continuous-flow machines use a greater volume of gas over a given period of time than the demand-flow unit, this minor disadvantage is more than compensated for by the significantly greater accuracy and safety of continuous-flow units. The two major disadvantages of the demand-flow unit are eliminated in continuous-flow machines. The inability to visualize the flow of gases and the inaccuracy of the mixer valve are eliminated through the incorporation of a flowmeter. Accuracies to within plus or minus 2% can be achieved in gas flow with the flowmeters available today.

The gas circuit utilized in the typical continuous-flow unit consists of the following:

1. Gas cylinders
2. Reducing valves
3. Flowmeters
4. Reservoir bag

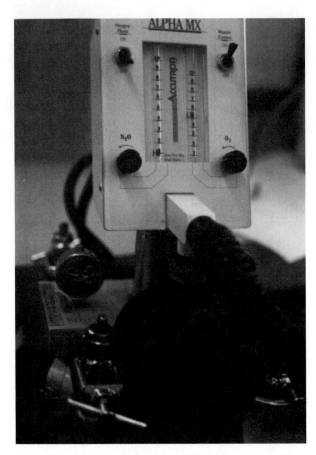

Fig. 15-3. Continuous-flow inhalation sedation unit (portable—front view). *1,* Oxygen flush control; *2,* master control (on/off); *3,* control knobs for N_2O and O_2; *4,* flowmeters; *5,* reservoir bag and tee; *6,* one-way valve; *7,* pressure gauge; and *8,* yoke assembly.

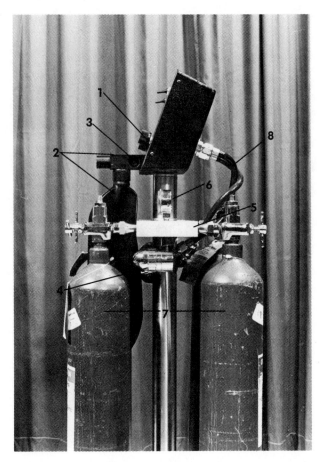

Fig. 15-4. Continuous-flow inhalation sedation unit (portable-side view). *1,* Control knobs for gas flow; *2,* reservoir bag and tee; *3,* emergency air intake valve; *4,* regulator (O_2); *5,* yoke assembly; *6,* pressure gauge; *7,* compressed-gas cylinders; and *8,* low-pressure tubing. Note angle of incline of head and flowmeters.

5. Conducting tubing
6. Nasal hood

All inhalation sedation units contain the same basic components. These are (Figs. 15-3 to 15-5):

1. Compressed-gas cylinders
2. Reducing valves (regulators)
3. Pressure gauges
4. Flowmeters
5. Reservoir bag
6. Conducting tubing
7. Full face mask/nasal hood/nasal cannula

In addition to these, the central storage systems contain manifolds and wall outlets. Modern inhalation sedation equipment is also equipped with safety features, all of which are designed to prevent the inadvertent or accidental administration of less than 20% O_2. These safety features will be discussed in the following paragraphs.

Within the continuous-flow inhalation sedation unit there are three subgroupings. Although each is the same basic unit, the differences between them are the manner in which compressed gases are delivered to the unit and their portability.

Portable system (Fig. 15-6)

In the portable system compressed-gas cylinders are attached to the inhalation sedation unit at the yoke assembly. This system is used in offices where the frequency of N_2O-O_2 use is low or in situations in which the expense of a central storage system is prohibitive.

The primary drawback to long-term use of a portable system lies in its economics. Portable systems require use of smaller compressed-gas cylinders

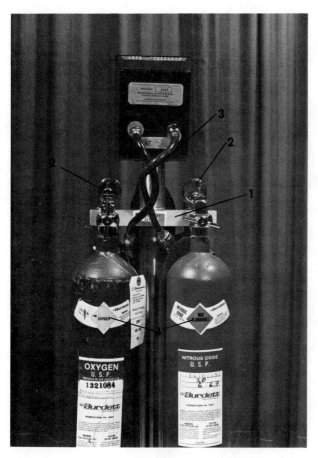

Fig. 15-5. Continuous-flow inhalation sedation unit (portable—from behind). *1*, Yoke assembly; *2*, pressure gauge; *3*, low-pressure tubing; and *4*, compressed-gas cylinders.

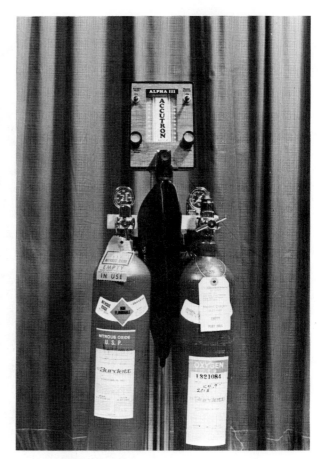

Fig. 15-6. Portable inhalation sedation system. Compressed gases are attached to the unit at the yoke assembly.

("E"), which consequently require replacement more frequently than the larger "G" and "H" cylinders used in central systems. The cost of larger, nonportable cylinders more than justifies their use, especially where N_2O-O_2 is used more frequently.

Central storage system (Fig. 15-7)

In the central storage system the supply of N_2O and O_2 is located at a distance from the area in which the gases are delivered to patients. In the treatment area the inhalation sedation unit (also called the "head") will be present along with the accessory equipment required for the delivery of the gases. The head is usually mounted on a wall or bracket. Gas cylinders are maintained in a storage area and delivered to the treatment area through copper pipes. Because these cylinders are stored in a separate location at a distance from the treatment area larger cylinders are employed in central storage systems.

These cylinders are not portable but they contain significantly more compressed gas than do the smaller cylinders used on portable systems. Multiple treatment areas may be connected through copper piping to this storage area and operated from this bank of cylinders.

The primary advantage of the central system is in offices in which inhalation sedation is used on a more regular basis. The greater initial cost of central storage systems is quickly made up in savings obtained from use of the larger gas cylinders.

Central storage system with mobile heads

Representing a compromise between the portable and central storage systems, this system permits the use of larger compressed gas cylinders while the inhalation sedation unit sits on a portable stand (without the yoke apparatus), which may be moved from treatment area to treatment area as the need for inhalation sedation arises. Quick-connect tubing at-

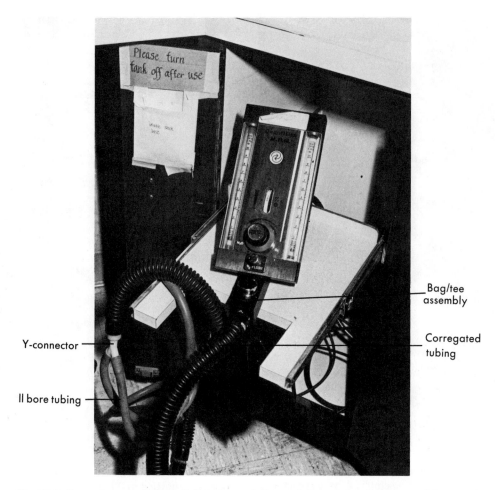

Fig. 15-7. Central storage system. Inhalation sedation unit is contained within a cabinet, and compressed-gas cylinders are stored at a distant site.

taches the unit to the oxygen and nitrous oxide outlets on the wall in each treatment area.

This system is recommended for offices in which the economics of central storage warrant its installation but the frequency of use of inhalation sedation does not justify the purchase of heads for all treatment areas. One head may be used throughout the office, with others being added to the system as increased demand dictates.

Only the continuous-flow unit will be considered in our discussions of inhalation sedation. Major components of these systems will be discussed in depth so that the administrator of inhalation sedation will become knowledgeable about this equipment and comfortable during its clinical use.

Compressed-gas cylinders

Gases dispensed at a pressure of greater than 25 pounds per square inch (25 psig) at 25° C (70° F) are considered to be compressed gases, according to the Hazardous Materials regulations of the United States Department of Transportation (DOT). Such gases are used in the health professions and in non-health professions (construction, automobile racing). Because of the potential for serious injury from improper handling of these cylinders, the DOT has promulgated regulations for these gases, some of which are discussed in the following paragraphs.[4]

Cylinders that are used to store and transport compressed gases are manufactured from ⅜-inch-thick steel. Some cylinders of N_2O have been made from aluminum.

All compressed-gas cylinders are tested by the DOT every 5 years to ensure their integrity. Testing is performed by internal hydrostatic pressure, the pressure to which the cylinder is tested being based upon the size of the cylinder. The shoulder of the cylinder is marked with a metal stamp indicating the date the cylinder was commissioned, dates of testing by the DOT, the pressure for which the cylinder is

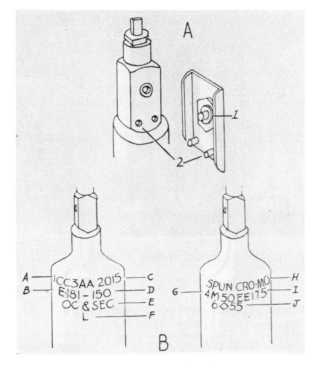

Fig. 15-8. A, Pin index safety system prevents accidental crossing of anesthetic gases (see Figs. 14-10, 14-11). **B,** Compressed-gas cylinders contain much information: *A,* Interstate Commerce Commission specifications; *B,* cylinder size; *C,* maximum working pressure (psi); *D,* manufacturer's serial number; *E,* ownership; *F,* inspector's mark; *G,* manufacturer's mark and date of original test; *H,* composition: chrome-molybdenum (steel); *I,* elastic expansion (ml at 3360 psi); and *J,* retest dates. (From Dripps RD, Eckenhoff JE, Vandam LD: *Introduction to anesthesia,* ed 6. Philadelphia, 1982, Saunders.)

Table 15-1. Color coding of compressed gases

Gas	*Coding color*
O_2	Green (white—international)
N_2O	Light blue
N_2	Gray bottom, orange shoulder
CO_2	Gray
Cyclopropane	Orange
Helium	Brown
Ethylene	Red (violet—international)

2. Store full cylinders in the vertical position.
3. Store cylinders in an area in which the temperature does not fluctuate; heat in particular should be avoided.
4. Handle cylinders with care: especially avoid dropping them.
5. Open cylinder valves slowly in a counterclockwise direction.
6. Close all cylinder valves tightly when not in use. This is important whether the cylinder contains gas or is empty, in order to prevent contamination from water or dirt.
7. Cylinders should be "cracked" before attaching them to the sedation or anesthesia machine. The term "cracked" signifies opening the cylinder just slightly, allowing some gas to escape, thereby blowing out any particles of dust that may have lodged in the orifice of the cylinder.

The importance of keeping grease and oil away from compressed gases is such that additional comment is required. Grease or oil in the presence of a compressed gas forms a potentially explosive mixture. When a cylinder is opened, high-pressure gas (for example O_2 at 2000 psig) is reduced suddenly to approximately 50 psig and atmospheric pressure by the reducing valve (regulator—see p. 230). Sudden expansion of the compressed gas as it exits the cylinder cools the gas to subzero temperatures. The cylinder valve will become cool, with frost possibly forming. However, almost immediately, as more gas rushes from the cylinder into the restricted space of the reducing valve, both the pressure and temperature are increased. The temperature may increase sufficiently, though only for a few seconds, to ignite any combustible materials that may be present (e.g., grease or oil). Temperatures in excess of 1500° F—well above the ignition temperature of grease or oil—can be produced at this time.

Once the grease or oil ignites, either N_2O or O_2, although nonflammable, will support combustion.

designed, the insignia of the testing facility, and the identification of the manufacturer of the cylinder (Fig. 15-8). Cylinders are designed to handle 1.66 times the usual pressure. For example, an O_2 cylinder usually under 2000 psig is designed to hold up to 3400 psig.

In addition, the American Society of Anesthesiologists, the American Hospital Association, and the medical gas industry have adopted a uniform color code that is used on all compressed-gas cylinders (Table 15-1). The agents used in inhalation sedation, N_2O and O_2, are color-coded light blue and green, respectively.

The following are important considerations when handling compressed gas cylinders:

1. Use no grease, oil, or lubricant of any type to lubricate cylinder valves, gauges, regulators, or other fittings that may come into contact with gases. This is extremely dangerous!

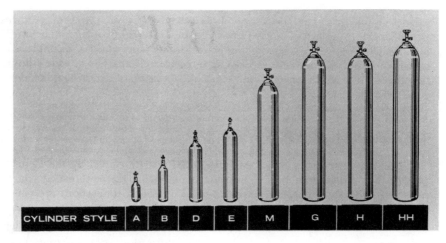

Fig. 15-9. Various sizes of compressed-gas cylinders. (From Williams RH: *Textbook of endocrinology,* ed 6. Philadelphia, 1982, Saunders.)

Temperature and pressure within the cylinder increase even further, producing two grave problems: (1) the rapid increase in pressure will soon exceed the limits of the cylinder, leading to an explosion, and (2) as the temperature within the cylinder increases, the valve stem of the cylinder, composed of an alloy with a melting point of 93° C, will melt, thereby releasing the contents of the cylinder. These processes may occur within 1 to 2 seconds.

Death and serious injuries to doctor, staff, and patients have occurred in this manner.[5]

Compressed-gas cylinders are manufactured in a variety of sizes. They are classified by letter, the "A" cylinder being the smallest and the "HH" the largest (Fig. 15-9). In inhalation sedation with N_2O-O_2 the cylinder sizes employed are the "E," "G," and "H." E cylinders are used for both N_2O and O_2 in portable units, whereas larger cylinders are used in central storage systems—G cylinders for N_2O and H cylinders for O_2. The physical characteristics of these and other compressed-gas cylinders are compared in Table 15-2, and the gas capacities of the E, G, and H cylinders are compared in Table 15-3.

Safety features incorporated in the compressed-gas cylinders include color coding (N_2O, blue; O_2, green) and the pin index safety system (see Fig. 15-31). The pin index safety system is designed so that it becomes physically impossible for an N_2O cylinder to be inadvertently attached to the O_2 portion of the delivery system and vice versa. This is achieved through a series of holes in the stem of the cylinder that have a unique configuration permitting attachment only to the correct yoke on the sedation unit. Fig. 15-10 illustrates the pin index safety system for N_2O and O_2. The large hole on the top of the stem

Table 15-2. Characteristics of compressed-gas cylinders

Cylinder	Dimensions (inches)	Weight of empty cylinder (pounds)
A	3.0 × 10	2.75
B	3.5 × 17	8
D	4.25 × 20	12
E	4.25 × 29.5	21
M	7.12 × 46	74
G	8.5 × 55	130
H	9.0 × 55	130
HH	9.25 × 59	136

is the orifice through which the compressed gas exits the cylinder. The two holes beneath the orifice accept pins found on the yoke of the sedation machine. They are countersunk approximately 0.25 inch. On the appropriate yoke of the inhalation sedation unit are found pins that will permit the attachment of the appropriate compressed-gas cylinder (Fig. 15-11). These pins are welded into the unit. The pin index safety system is designed to prevent the inadvertent attachment of a gas cylinder to the wrong yoke and thus the accidental delivery of 100% N_2O when 100% O_2 is desired, a situation with potentially catastrophic consequences. Errors have been noted in pin indexing of cylinders.[6,7] Careful checking of all compressed-gas cylinders prior to their use is essential to safety.

Oxygen cylinder

O_2 in a compressed-gas cylinder is present in a gaseous state. The gas pressure in a full E cylinder is approximately 1900 psig (pounds per square inch gauge pressure[8]) at 70° F (25° C) (Fig. 15-12, *A*), whereas the pressure within the larger H cylinder is approximately 2200 psig.[9] Oxygen cylinders are color-coded green in the United States and white internationally. One ounce of O_2 liquid is equivalent to 5.22 gallons of O_2 gas.

Table 15-3. Comparison of E, G, and H cylinders

N_2O (Nitrous oxide)

Cylinder size	E	G
Dimensions	4.5″ wide	8.5″ wide
	29.5″ high	55″ high
	21 pounds weight	130 pounds weight
Color of cylinder	Blue	Blue
Psi—full	750-800	750-800
Capacity (liters)	159	13,839
(gallons)	420	3200
Physical state of contents	Gas and liquid	Gas and liquid

O_2 (Oxygen)

Cylinder size	E	H
Dimensions	4.5″ wide	9″ wide
	29.5″ high	55″ high
	21 pounds weight	130 pounds weight
Color of cylinder	Green	Green
Psi—full	2000	2200
Capacity (liters)	625	6909
(gallons)	165	1400
Physical state of contents	Gas	Gas

Because the O_2 cylinder contains only gas, the pressure gauge on the machine yoke reflects the actual contents of the cylinder. In other words, as oxygen leaves the cylinder the pressure within the cylinder will drop accordingly. Therefore, if an O_2 cylinder records a pressure of 1000 psig (Fig. 15-13), the cylinder is 1000/1900, or 52% full. A full E cylinder of O_2 will produce 660 liters of gaseous oxygen. At a flow rate of 6 L/min this tank would empty in 110 minutes (660/6 = 110 minutes). This is an important factor in the safety of inhalation sedation because if an O_2 cylinder became empty during a procedure while the N_2O cylinder still contained gas, it would be potentially possible to administer 100% N_2O. Whereas there are additional safety features designed to prevent this occurrence, the fact that the administrator of the N_2O-O_2 can see the "fuel gauge" for the O_2 permits a new cylinder to be opened before the nearly empty cylinder is depleted. If the sedation machine is equipped with two E cylinders of O_2, only one should be open and in use at any one time so that both tanks are not emptied simultaneously.[10]

Nitrous oxide cylinder

N_2O in compressed-gas cylinders is present in both the liquid and gaseous states. Nitrous oxide cylinders are factory-filled to 90% to 95% capacity with liquid N_2O.[9] Above the liquid in the tank is N_2O vapor. The gas pressure within the cylinder of N_2O is approximately 750 psig at 70° F (25° C) (Fig. 15-12, *B*) within both the E and G cylinders. N_2O compressed-gas cyl-

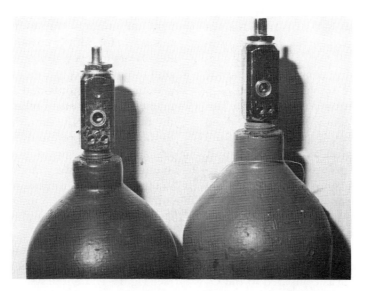

Fig. 15-10. Pin index safety system for O_2 *(left)* and N_2O *(right)*. Large orifice on top of cylinder permits gas to exit cylinder. Smaller holes below are pin-indexed for specific compressed gas.

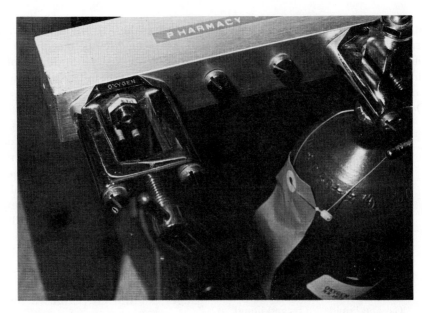

Fig. 15-11. Pins, which are located on yoke of inhalation sedation unit, are aligned to permit attachment of only one compressed gas.

inders are color-coded light blue in the United States and blue internationally. One ounce of N_2O liquid provides 3.88 gallons of N_2O gas. A full E cylinder of N_2O produces approximately 1600 liters of gaseous N_2O at sea level and room temperature, while the larger H cylinder provides approximately 16,000 liters of N_2O gas.[9]

Because of the presence of liquid in the N_2O cylinder, the gas pressure gauge on the cylinder will record "full" (approximately 750 psig) as long as any liquid remains in the cylinder. The pressure of the N_2O vapor floating above the liquid N_2O is 750 psig (Fig. 15-13). As the gaseous N_2O exits from the cylinder, liquid N_2O vaporizes to replace it. The pressure of this "new" gas is 750 psig. This process continues, liquid N_2O becoming converted to gaseous N_2O, with the gas pressure remaining at 750 psig, until no more liquid remains to replace the gas. The pressure gauge for N_2O cannot, therefore, be used as an accurate measurement of the contents of the cylinder. Once all of the liquid N_2O is gone and only gaseous N_2O remains, the pressure gauge will fall in relation to the pressure of gas now remaining (acting now like an O_2 pressure gauge). In normal clinical usage of inhalation sedation it has been our experience that 2.5 O_2 cylinders are used for every N_2O cylinder of the same size. The presence of N_2O in a liquid state is the reason for the increased volume of gas within the N_2O cylinder as compared to the O_2 cylinders.

In central storage systems it is recommended that there be not less than two H O_2 cylinders and one G N_2O cylinder, while in portable systems one or two E cylinders of N_2O and two O_2 cylinders are recommended.

Regulators

Regulators, also called reducing valves, are located between the compressed-gas cylinder and the flowmeter. In central storage systems regulators are commonly placed on the cylinder itself. The regulator functions to reduce the high-pressure gas coming from the cylinder (750 to 2200 psig) to a pressure that is safe for both the patient and the sedation unit. Regulators function to maintain a constant gas pressure to flowmeters and the patient regardless of the pressure of gas contained within the cylinder. By maintaining a constant, relatively low pressure within the body of the N_2O unit, the potential for damage to the machine produced by high-pressure gases is minimized. The actual delivery pressure is set by the manufacturer of the equipment at 45 to 55 psig. When gases enter directly from cylinders the pressure is reduced to 45 psig, while gases entering through a pipeline (central systems) maintain a pressure of 50 to 55 psig.

Regulators on portable units are located between the cylinders of gas and the flowmeters on the yoke (see Fig. 15-4). Central systems commonly have a regulator attached directly to the cylinder, in which case

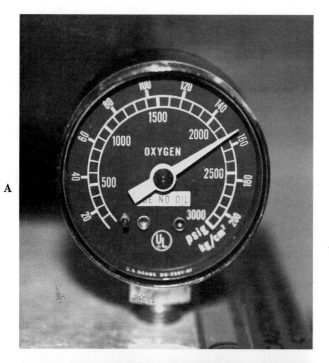

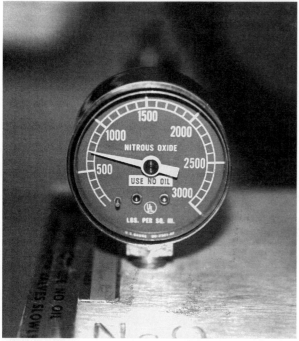

Fig. 15-12. Pressure gauges on inhalation sedation unit. **A,** O₂ pressure gauge. **B,** N₂O pressure gauge.

it frequently has a gas pressure gauge combined with it. This type of system, with individual regulators for each cylinder of compressed gas, requires that the cylinders be switched on and off each day. In addition, when a cylinder of gas empties there is no automatic system for switching to a reserve tank (as is present with the more expensive manifold system; see next section).

It is within the reducing valve that the recompression of gases produces a tremendous increase in temperature to about 1500° to 2000° F. This happens when a cylinder of O_2 at 1900 psig is quickly opened and the high-pressure gas is forced into a reducing valve. Although the reducing valve lowers this pressure to approximately 50 psig, gas backs up in the reducing valve, producing a recompression of gas that leads to a temperature increase. Temperature increases can ignite oil, grease, or Teflon that might be found in this area, leading to explosion and fire. Proper care and handling of cylinders (see the preceding paragraphs) will prevent this potentially disastrous consequence.

Manifolds (central system only)

A manifold serves to join multiple compressed-gas cylinders (Fig. 15-14). For example, twelve N_2O cylinders may be attached to a single manifold. Twelve hoses will enter into the manifold, one from each regulator on the cylinder; but only one hose will exit the manifold, carrying the gas under low pressure (50 psig) to each station outlet in the individual operatories.

A nonautomatic manifold is most commonly used. When a cylinder is empty it must physically be turned off and a new cylinder opened by a staff member. Automatic manifolds are also available. The advantage of these more expensive devices is that they automatically activate a full reserve cylinder of gas when the cylinder in use empties. Other items found on all manifolds include a safety pressure relief valve and an alarm monitor gauge. The latter monitors the pressure of gas in the line (50 psig) and activates a high/low alarm should the pressure exceed 75 psig or fall below 40 psig. A typical manifold in a dental office will operate two O_2 cylinders while a second manifold operates either one or two N_2O cylinders.

Yokes (portable system only)

The yoke assembly holds the cylinder of compressed gas tightly in contact with the nipples of the portable sedation unit (see Fig. 15-8, *top*). Metal pins below the collar of the nipple are situated in such a

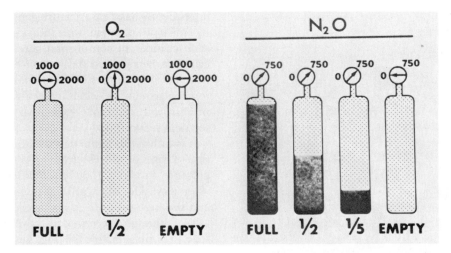

Fig. 15-13. Changes in pressure of compressed-gas cylinders are related to the physical state of its contents (gas or liquid). (From Allen GD: *Dental anesthesia and analgesia,* ed 2. © 1979, the Williams and Wilkins Co., Baltimore).

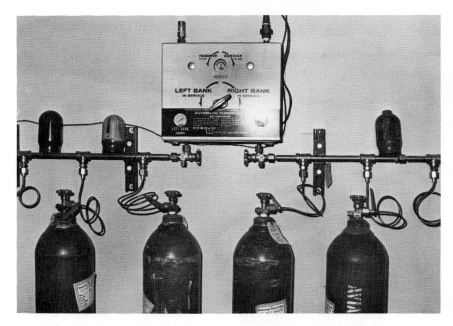

Fig. 15-14. Manifold connecting a series of N_2O and O_2 cylinders for use in a central system. Manifold provides automatic switchover from the cylinder in use.

way that they will accept only one specific type of compressed gas (see Fig. 15-11). This constitutes the pin index safety system.

In the portable inhalation sedation unit the circuit of gases to this point has been from the cylinder through the yoke and into the reducing valve, a portion of the circuit termed the *high-pressure system;* the circuit from the reducing valve to the patient is called the *low-pressure system.* From the reducing valve the

gas enters low-pressure tubing (color-coded for specific gases) that conducts the gas to attachments at the rear of the inhalation sedation unit. It is here that another safety feature of inhalation anesthetic systems is found. The diameter index safety system (DISS) (Figs. 15-15 and 15-31) is designed to ensure that the correct medical gas enters the correct part of the anesthesia (sedation) machine.[11,12] Accidental attachment is prevented in two ways: first, the diam-

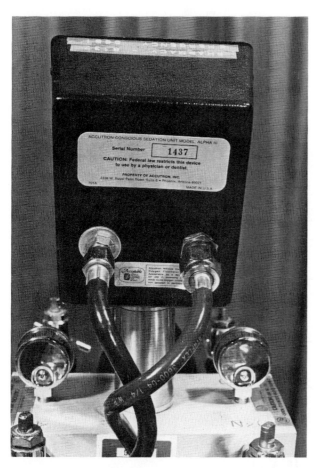

Fig. 15-15. Diameter index safety system. Connectors attaching low-pressure tubing to inhalation sedation unit are of different diameter. O₂ *(left)* is of smaller diameter than N₂O *(right)*, thus preventing accidental crossing of attachments.

eter of the attachments differs considerably, and second, the threading of the attachments differs, making it physically impossible to inadvertently attach tubing to the wrong inlet on the sedation or anesthesia machine. Once in the machine the gases are directed to the appropriate flowmeter, where precise volumes may be delivered to the patient.

The circuit thus far in the central system is similar, with a few important differences. Gas leaving the cylinder enters the reducing valve and the manifold directly, from which it is directed from the storage area through specially prepared copper tubing to the individual treatment areas in the dental office. This tubing may be found in the walls, ceilings, or floors and leads to outlets in the individual treatment room. The outlet station possesses attachments for N₂O and O₂ hoses that are quick-connects, permit-

ting rapid attachment and disconnection of the hoses.[9] To prevent accidental crossing of these hoses, the diameter index safety system is incorporated into the quick-connect for N₂O and O₂.

Flowmeters

From the reducing valves the individual gases are carried through low-pressure tubing into the back of the unit. The gases are then directed to the flowmeters (see Fig. 15-3), which permit the administrator to deliver a precise volume of either gas to the patient. Flowmeters are calibrated only for the gas that will flow through it (N₂O or O₂).[10] Gas flows are calibrated to be read at 25° C at 76 cm Hg (atmospheric pressure). Flowmeters measure the actual quantity of gas in motion rather than static cylinder pressure (as measured by the pressure gauges). If the flow of gas is interrupted, the flow meter will read zero.

The flowmeter is actually a very simple device. Gas enters a tube formed with a tapering lumen that grows wider from the gas inlet at the bottom to the outlet at its top. A float used for measuring the volume is found inside the flowmeter. The float is either a ball or a rotameter. When a ball is used, the precise flow volume of gas is read using the middle of the ball, whereas with the rotameter the flow is read at the top of the bobbin.

Once the flow of gas is started, gas enters the bottom of the flowmeter. The gas forces the float up into the flowmeter. Since the flowmeter is tapered, the area surrounding the float increases in size as the increased flow of gas causes the float to bob at a higher level; the flow rate is proportional to the size of the space surrounding the float.

The calibrations on the flowmeter tubes indicate the flow of gas in liters per minute (lpm). Adjustment of the gas flow is accomplished by means of a fine-needle valve for each flowmeter. The knobs that control the gases are both touch-coded and color-coded. In the United States the O₂ control knob is green in color and fluted while the N₂O control knob is blue and not fluted (Fig. 15-16).[13] In North America the oxygen flowmeter is positioned on the right side of the bank of flowmeters.[14]

There are actually three types of devices—the rotameter, ball, and rod—used inside the flowmeter to measure gas flow. The rod-type flowmeter is seldom used any longer primarily because its accuracy is not as great as that of the ball or rotameter. Accuracy for the rod-type flowmeter is plus or minus 7%.

In the ball-type flowmeter a ball is forced up into

the flowmeter by the gas entering the meter. For best accuracy this type of flowmeter is placed on an inclined plane (Fig. 15-17). The ball-type flowmeter is the most commonly used today. Its accuracy is plus or minus 5%, and it is least accurate at very low flow rates.

The rotameter type of flowmeter is the most accurate, with an accuracy of plus or minus 2%. A metal bobbin, usually aluminum, is pushed upward in the flowmeter by the force of the gas passing through the meter. This stream of gas also causes the rota-

meter to rotate. Flowmeters in this type of unit must be vertical (Fig. 15-18). The three types of flowmeters are compared in Table 15-4.

As the anesthetic gases leave through the top of their respective flowmeters, they are combined in the mixing chamber, which is found within the head of the sedation unit. From this point a combination of the gases flows through the machine. These gases now exit the sedation unit through the outflow tube, which is also known as a bag-tee (see Figs. 15-3 and 15-4), and are carried to the patient.

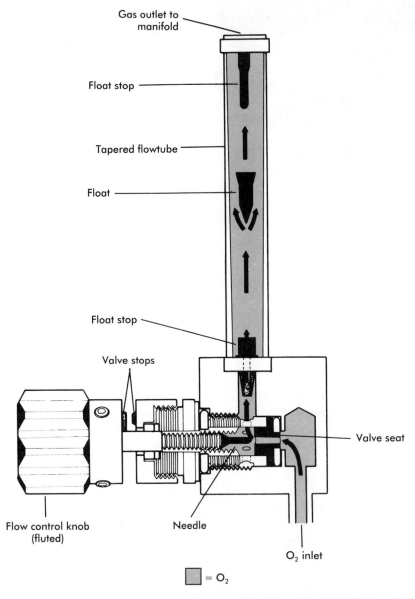

Fig. 15-16. O$_2$ flowmeter and flow control valve. (Modified from Bowie E, Huffman LM: *The anesthesia machine: essentials for understanding.* Madison, Wis, 1985, Ohmeda, BOC Health Care.)

Emergency air intake valve

On the bag-tee, above the reservoir bag, an emergency air valve is located (see Fig. 15-4). It provides the patient a supply of atmospheric air in the event that the sedation unit ceases to function and gas flow from the machine is terminated. During normal use the emergency air valve remains shut, but it opens automatically once gas flow through the machine is terminated. This prevents the patient from experiencing a feeling of discomfort or suffocation as he attempts to breathe through the nasal hood when the unit is not working and the reservoir bag is deflated.

Rubber goods

From the outlet tube the anesthetic gases are carried to the patient. In addition to the reservoir bag, the rubber goods consist of conducting tubes and a face mask, nasal hood, or nasal cannula.

Reservoir bag

Reservoir bags are bladder-type bags, made of rubber or silicone, ranging in size from 1 to 8 liters. The 3-liter reservoir bag is the most frequently used in dentistry. Although commonly used, rubber bags deteriorate more rapidly than silicone bags, especially in areas in which high levels of atmospheric pollutants are found (the planet Earth).

The reservoir bag attaches to the base of the bag-tee, usually immediately below the emergency air inlet valve (see Figs. 15-3 and 15-4). A portion of the gas(es) being delivered through the unit to the patient is diverted into the reservoir bag, where it may be used for any of several purposes.

The primary function of the reservoir bag during inhalation sedation is to provide a reservoir from which additional gas may be drawn should the res-

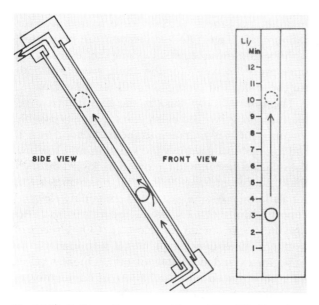

Fig. 15-17. Ball-type flowmeter. (From Allen GD: *Dental anesthesia and analgesia,* ed 2. © 1979, The Williams and Wilkins Co., Baltimore.)

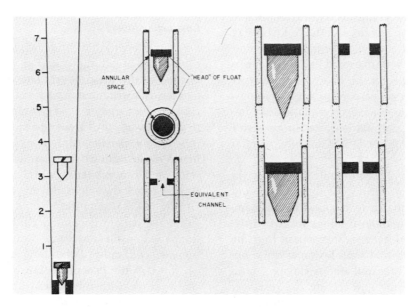

Fig. 15-18. Rotameter-type flowmeter. (From Allen GD: *Dental anesthesia and analgesia,* ed 2. © 1979, the Williams and Wilkins Co., Baltimore.)

Table 15-4. Characteristics of flowmeters

	Rotameter	Ball	Rod
Accuracy	Plus or minus 2%	Plus or minus 5%	Plus or minus 7%
Current use	Intermediate use	Most common	Least common
Flowmeter angle	Vertical	Inclined	Vertical
Material	Aluminum	Plastic	Metal

piratory demands of the patient exceed the gas flow being delivered from the machine. During normal (quiet) respiration the patient receives only fresh gases delivered from the sedation unit, with little or none being taken from the reservoir bag. However, should the patient take an especially deep breath, the machine will be unable to accommodate the necessary volume; in the absence of the reservoir bag the patient will experience a feeling of suffocation. The reservoir bag prevents or minimizes this occurrence.

A second use of the reservoir bag during conscious sedation is to serve as a monitoring device for respiration. Assuming an airtight seal of the nasal hood and no mouth breathing, the reservoir bag will inflate slightly with every exhalation and deflate slightly with each inspiration, permitting the operator to easily determine respiratory rate.

A third potential use for the reservoir bag is its use as a means of providing O_2 during assisted or controlled ventilation. Providing that a full face mask is properly positioned with an airtight seal and a patent airway, the reservoir bag is squeezed and its contents forced into the patient's lungs. It is quite a bit more difficult to ventilate the patient with the reservoir bag when the nasal hood is used. Adequate ventilation can be accomplished with the nasal hood, but this is not likely to be effective in the hands of an inexperienced person (a person who is not anesthesiology-trained). Controlled and assisted ventilation are impossible with a nasal cannula because the reservoir bag is removed from the sedation machine when a cannula is used.

The reservoir bag is of considerable importance in general anesthesia, for during this time the patient is unconscious and unable to respond to the commands of the anesthesiologist. Other means of determining the physical status of the patient must be employed. Monitoring vital signs becomes quite important. Respiratory rate and depth can be monitored easily by observing and feeling the reservoir bag. Should respiratory depth become shallow, the anesthesiologist can assist a patient's breathing by gently squeezing the bag as the patient begins to

breathe spontaneously. Should spontaneous respiration cease, controlled respiration can be started, with the anesthesiologist squeezing the reservoir bag once every 5 seconds for the adult, every 4 seconds for the child, and every 3 seconds for the infant.

The reservoir bag was, in the past, called a rebreathing bag. Not too many years ago it was possible for the patient to exhale into the nasal hood and, if the total flow of gas from the sedation unit was low, the exhaled gases could be forced backward through the conducting tubing to reach the reservoir bag. On inhalation these same gases, now containing elevated concentrations of CO_2, would be rebreathed. Rebreathing gas containing elevated CO_2 levels can lead to unpleasant consequences if permitted to continue for extended periods of time. One-way valves have been placed into the bag-tee of contemporary machines to prevent the possibility of rebreathing.

For the adult patient receiving conscious sedation the 3- or 5-liter reservoir bag is used, whereas in pediatric procedures smaller (1-, 2-, or 3-liter) reservoir bags are used.

Conducting tubes

A variable length of hose called either conducting tubing or a breathing tube (Fig. 15-19) connects the bag-tee to the nasal hood. The hose is of large diameter, is corrugated, and is usually made of black rubber. The large diameter minimizes any resistance to the flow of gases from the machine through the tubes to the patient, while the corrugation prevents inadvertent kinking or occlusion of its lumen. In conscious sedation procedures, the corrugated tubing is less essential than it is during general anesthesia. During N_2O-O_2 sedation, should a hose conducting gas to the patient become occluded by some means, the patient—still conscious—would comment on the increased difficulty of obtaining an adequate gas supply through the nosepiece. During general anesthesia, however, with the patient unconscious and unable to reply, occlusion of the tube carrying gas from the anesthesia machine would produce little or no immediate outward change in appearance, the lack

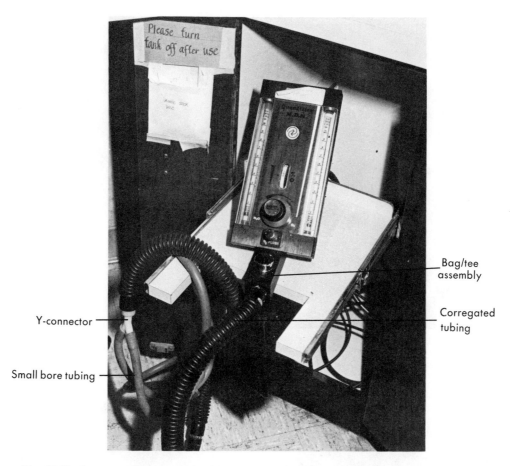

Fig. 15-19. Corrugated conducting tubing connects bag/tee to noncorrugated tubes, which deliver gases to patient.

of O_2 producing a deeper level of "general anesthesia." Only after possibly irreversible brain damage has occurred will changes be noticed by the less than expert observer. Thus the corrugated tubing present on all sedation units is a remnant of the general anesthesia machine from which the modern sedation unit evolved.

The corrugated tubing is attached to one or two noncorrugated tubes that attach directly to the breathing apparatus on the patient (Fig. 15-19). These tubes are of smaller diameter than the corrugated tubing; however, they do not add significantly to the resistance to gas flow to the patient. In those units with one larger-diameter tube flowing to the breathing apparatus, the tube is carried over the top of the patient's head and forehead and then to the breathing apparatus on the patient's nose. More commonly two tubes are attached to the corrugated tubing. These tubes come around the sides of the dental chair and are attached to the breathing ap-

paratus. In both cases the tubing must be secured so that the patient remains comfortable and so that leakage will not occur around the sides of the breathing apparatus. With double tubing there is the possibility that the tubing will be kinked as it comes around the side of the dental chair (Fig. 15-20). Care is required when securing the tubing to prevent this from occurring.

Breathing apparatus

Full face mask. Three types of breathing apparatus may be used to deliver N_2O-O_2 to the patient. The full face mask covers both the mouth and nose of the patient (Fig. 15-21). Although the face mask is the most effective method of delivering gases to the patient, in dentistry the full face mask is impractical since the mouth must remain available for the dental procedure to be completed. However, the presence of a face mask in the dental office is important in emergency situations since the full face mask pro-

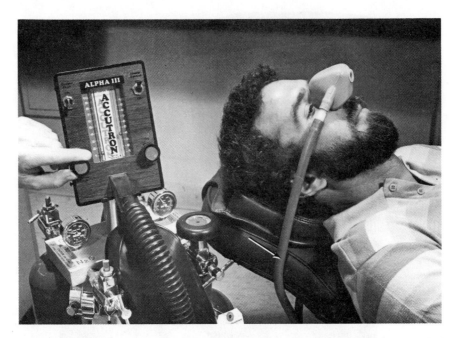

Fig. 15-20. Tubing can become occluded as it bends around the sides of the dental chair *(arrow)*.

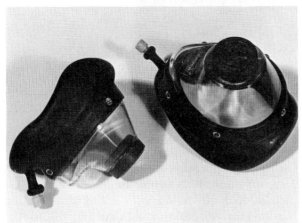

Fig. 15-21. Full face mask covers both nose and mouth of patient. Although inconvenient during dental care, it is appropriate for use in emergency situations.

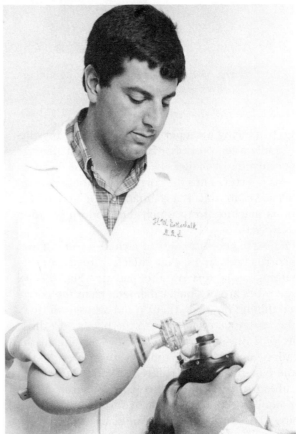

vides the optimal means of delivering O_2 to the patient (provided the person delivering the O_2 has received training in emergency airway management).

Nasal cannula. The nasal cannula (Fig. 15-22) is quite different from the face mask. Made from a softened plastic, the two short (⅛-inch-long) prongs are placed into the nostrils of the patient, and the device is used primarily to provide hospitalized patients with supplemental O_2. It is not possible to obtain an airtight seal with the nasal cannula, a fact that is quite detrimental to its use during N_2O-O_2 sedation since it leads to a significant degree of dilution of the gases being delivered from the machine. To compensate for this air dilution, greater volumes of gases must be delivered to the patient. This is especially relevant for N_2O since significantly greater volumes of N_2O will be needed to produce a desired sedation level. In fact it is often impossible to obtain clinically adequate sedation with the cannula even when maximal volumes of N_2O are being delivered. Because of air dilution and the greater volumes of gases being used, there is considerably greater contamination of the clinical environment with N_2O than is present when a nasal hood is used.

The primary advantages of the nasal cannula include its usefulness in patients with a fear of the full face mask or the nasal hood and in claustrophobic patients. These persons are unable to tolerate the full face mask or nasal hood comfortably, whereas the nasal cannula invariably proves satisfactory to them. A second advantage of the cannula is during treatment of maxillary anterior teeth. Using a traditional nasal hood that rests over the patient's upper lip and against his maxillary anterior teeth, treatment involving the labial soft tissues or the teeth themselves may prove difficult because the nasal hood compresses the upper lip against the soft and hard tissues in this region. One way to minimize this potential difficulty is to place cotton rolls under the patient's upper lip prior to placement of the nasal hood. The cannula, however, does not interfere with dental treatment in this area (Fig. 15-23).

A disadvantage of the nasal cannula is the necessity to remove the reservoir bag from the sedation unit, thereby negating its usefulness as a monitoring or ventilatory device. In its place is a plug, directing all gases from the machine into the cannula.

Since the gases delivered from the sedation unit (O_2 and N_2O) are both anhydrous, they are directed through a humidifier before being sent to the patient (Fig. 15-24). The humidifier is placed on the end of the outlet tube, to which is attached the nasal cannula.

The tubing of the nasal cannula is quite narrow. Gases being delivered to the cannula through the outlet tube and humidifier will therefore gain considerable velocity as they pass from the wider bore of the outlet tube to the narrower space of the cannula. The force of the gas exiting the cannula may in fact prove uncomfortable for the patient.

With today's concern about the potential hazards of trace contamination of the environment with N_2O, the use of the nasal cannula cannot be recommended except in very few cases in which inhalation sedation must be used and other methods of delivering the gases to the patient are unacceptable.

Nasal hood. There are two types of nasal hood, a device designed to fit comfortably and securely over the patient's nose. The traditional nasal hood (com-

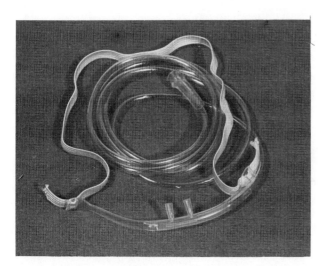

Fig. 15-22. Nasal cannula. Two short plastic prongs are placed in nares of patient.

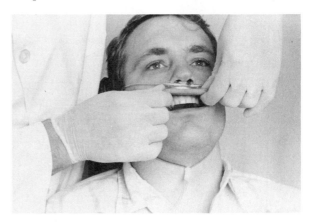

Fig. 15-23. Nasal cannula does not interfere with dental treatment in maxillary anterior region.

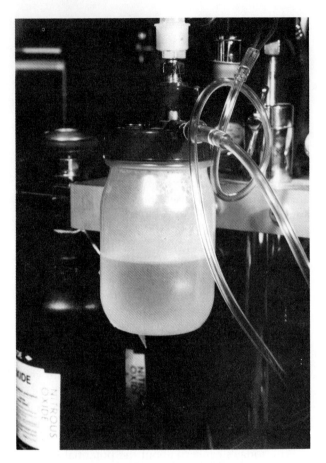

Fig. 15-24. Nasal cannula with humidifier.

monly called a nosepiece) has one or two tubes entering into it (see Fig. 15-20). These tubes deliver gases from the inhalation sedation unit. Exhaled gases are eliminated into the surrounding environment through an exhaling valve located on top of the nasal hood. Along with the exhaling valve, the nasal hood may also possess an air-dilution valve.

The second type of delivery system is the more recently introduced scavenging nasal hood. The prototypical scavenging nasal hood has four tubes entering it. Two tubes deliver fresh gases from the sedation unit, the other tubes carrying exhaled gases away from the treatment area to a safe repository (Fig. 15-25). With concern increasing about the possible deleterious effects on dental staff of prolonged exposure to low levels of nitrous oxide, the scavenging nasal hood is preferred.

The nasal hood is made of rubber or silicone, which readily adapts to the contours of the patient's face, providing an airtight seal (Fig. 15-26). Nasal hoods are designed in a variety of sizes, and it is important that several sizes be available.

The traditional nasal hood contains one or two inlets through which fresh gases are delivered from the sedation unit to the patient. On the top of the mask is an opening into which has been placed one or more valves. When only one valve is present it is an exhaling or one-way valve, permitting the patient to eliminate all exhaled gases into the environment and to inhale only fresh gases from the machine. The exhaling valve contains a thin wafer (Fig. 15-27, *A*) that sits over the opening in the valve. On exhalation

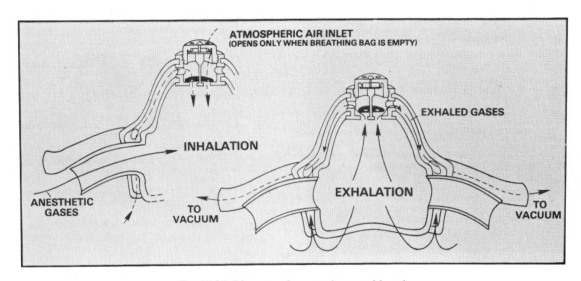

Fig. 15-25. Diagram of scavenging nasal hood.

the wafer is lifted by the force of the gases, and the gases are eliminated. On inhaling the negative pressure created within the nosepiece forces the wafer down into the hole, sealing it shut, thus allowing the patient to inhale only the gases from the machine.

A second valve, present on some nasal hoods, is called the inhaling or air-dilution valve. It consists of an opening from the inside of the nasal hood directly to the atmosphere (Fig. 15-27, *B*). As the patient exhales, gases escape from this valve (as in the exhaling valve); however, on inhalation this valve remains open, permitting the patient to breathe in an unknown quantity of ambient air along with the fresh gases from the sedation unit. It has been estimated that the inspired percentage of N_2O may be diluted by 50% if the air-dilution valve is fully opened. The value of the air-dilution valve is that it permits the patient to breathe comfortably regardless of the volume of gas being delivered from the machine; however, because of dilution, the volume of N_2O must be increased significantly, producing considerably higher concentrations of N_2O in the ambient air, which is undesirable.

The air-dilution valve is capable of being opened or closed, whereas the exhaling valve cannot be closed. If two valves are present on the nasal hood, it is recommended that the air-dilution valve be kept closed. There are virtually no indications for the use of an opened air-dilution valve; in fact, many newer

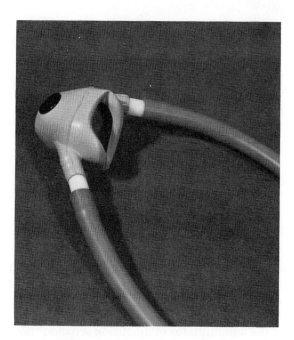

Fig. 15-26. Nasal hood with connecting tubes.

nasal hoods are being manufactured without the air-dilution valve.

The conventional nasal hood is no longer recommended for use with inhalation sedation. Although the absolute risk of chronic inhalation of low concentrations of nitrous oxide is as yet undetermined, evidence indicates that there are no desirable attributes to its being inhaled by health professionals. The scavenging nasal hood should be used whenever possible.

Scavenging nasal hood. With recent concern over the possible long-term effects of trace levels of N_2O on chairside personnel (Chapter 18), it has become expedient to attempt to eliminate exhaled N_2O from the ambient air. To this end the scavenging nasal hood has been developed (see Fig. 15-25). Whereas a number of such devices are currently available, the principle behind their effectiveness is essentially the same. The Brown nosepiece was one of the earliest scavenging devices and will serve as the prototypical scavenging nasal hood (Fig. 15-28).

Scavenging nasal hoods are, quite simply, double nosepieces—a smaller inner mask receiving anesthetic gases from the machine and a slightly larger outer mask that sits directly over the first, which removes exhaled gases from the treatment area. The outer nosepiece is connected to the suction device in the dental operatory, permitting exhaust gases to be vented from the dental operatory through the vacuum system. The effectiveness of this system is in part responsible for the 50 ppm standard for ambient levels of N_2O currently in use today. The scavenging system will be discussed in Chapter 18, but at present the scavenging mask represents the most effective means of minimizing N_2O contamination in the dental or surgical environment.

Other scavenging systems incorporate dual exhaust tubes with a single fresh gas inlet (Allen scavenging mask, Fig. 15-29), while others include a scavenging cone that sits atop the nasal hood (Matrix scavenging nasal hood, Fig. 15-30).

As suggested, it is recommended that scavenging nasal hoods be employed whenever possible during the administration of nitrous oxide oxygen inhalation sedation.

Modern nasal hoods do not contain any metal. This contrasts dramatically with older nasal hoods in which the valves very often contained metal springs or clips. The disadvantage of nasal hoods containing metal became apparent whenever radiographs were taken. Invariably the metal would be superimposed directly above a critical portion of the film. With

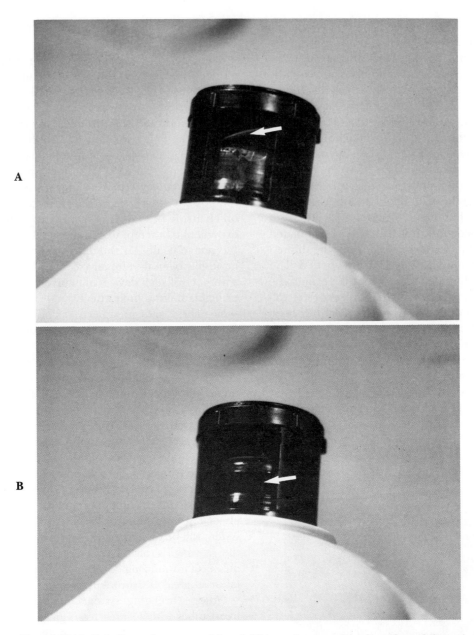

Fig. 15-27. A, Exhaling valve on nasal hood. Thin wafer *(arrow)* seals orifice while patient inhales but is forced off orifice when patient exhales. **B,** Air dilution valve is opening below exhaling valve *(arrow)*, which permits entry of atmospheric air during inhalation.

modern nasal hoods, radiographs may be taken without removing the nasal hood.

SAFETY FEATURES

All inhalation sedation units available in the United States incorporate a series of safety features. The primary purpose of these features is to prevent the delivery, either accidental or intentional, of less than atmospheric levels of oxygen (20.9%).

The Council on Dental Materials, Instruments and Equipment of the American Dental Association has issued guidelines for inhalation sedation units.[15] Although these safety features work well to minimize the occurrence of accidents, it must be emphasized that all mechanical devices are capable of failing, so that the administrator of inhalation sedation should never rely entirely on them for a patient's safety.[5-7] Visual and verbal monitoring of the patient and vi-

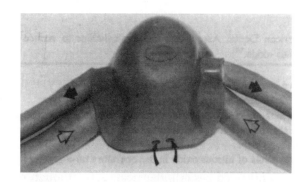

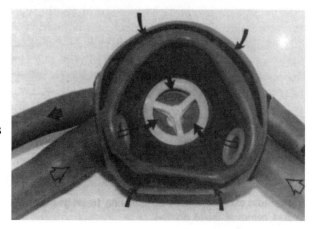

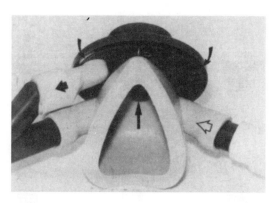

Fig. 15-30. Internal view of Matrix nosepiece demonstrating fresh gas inlet *(open arrow)* and waste gas outflow through the plastic scavenging cone *(solid arrows).* (From Dionne RA, Phero JC: *Management of pain and anxiety in dental practice.* New York, 1991, Elsevier Science Publishing.)

Fig. 15-28. A, An exterior view of a Brown mask. Open arrows indicate gas intake and solid arrows waste gas removal. Smaller solid arrows denote suction intake holes. **B,** An interior view of a Brown mask revealing the double mask construction and gas flow. (From Dionne RA, Phero JC: *Management of pain and anxiety in dental practice.* New York, 1991, Elsevier Science Publishing.)

sual monitoring of the sedation unit are essential at all times.

Pin index safety system

The pin index safety system makes it physically impossible to attach an N_2O compressed-gas cylinder to the yoke attachment for O_2 (or any other compressed-gas yoke except N_2O), which could result in the inadvertent administration of 100% N_2O instead of 100% O_2. The pin index safety system consists of a series of pins, the configuration of which differs for each compressed gas (Fig. 15-31) on the yoke of the sedation unit, and a matching series of holes on the compressed gas cylinders. However, I have seen a blue cylinder (presumably N_2O) with the pin index system for O_2! Beware!

Diameter index safety system

The diameter index safety system makes it impossible to attach a low-pressure hose to the wrong outlet on the sedation unit (Fig. 15-32).[16] The diameter of the couplings differs significantly (the coupling for N_2O being larger than that for O_2). In addition, the threading of the attachments differs. It becomes physically impossible to accidentally cross the low-pressure hoses and deliver the wrong gas to the patient. This system also exists as a safeguard on the larger G and H cylinders.

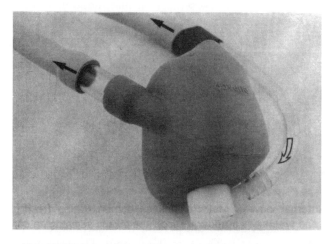

Fig. 15-29. A Dupaco (Allen) scavenging mask with fresh gas inlet *(open arrow)* and waste gas removal *(solid arrows).* (From Dionne RA, Phero JC: *Management of pain and anxiety in dental practice.* New York, 1991, Elsevier Science Publishing.)

Minimum oxygen liter flow

Inhalation sedation units are designed so that once turned on the unit delivers a preset minimum liter flow of O_2 through the flowmeter. In most units this minimum flow is 2.5 or 3.0 L/min of O_2. The

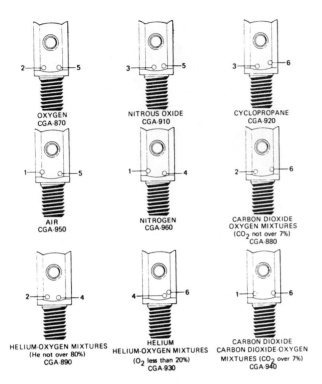

Fig. 15-31. Pin index safety system for compressed-gas cylinders. (Courtesy Puritan-Bennett Corp.)

flow of N_2O cannot start until a flow of O_2 has been established.

Minimum oxygen percentage

Similar to the minimum O_2 liter flow, this safety feature sets a minimum percentage of O_2 that may be delivered to the patient. This minimum O_2 percentage is 30% (some units provide 25%). This allows for a possible error in calibration of the flowmeters of approximately plus or minus 5% while still delivering greater than 20% O_2 to the patient. The ball-type flow meter has a ±5% accuracy rating while the rotameter has a ±2% accuracy.

In a sedation unit in which a minimum O_2 flow of 2.5 L/min is delivered, the N_2O control knob may be turned up as high as the administrator desires, but the flow of N_2O gas will not exceed 5.5 L/min. This provides a 31% oxygen concentration (2.5 L/min/8.0 L/min). If, however, the flow of O_2 is increased above the minimum flow rate, the N_2O flow may also be increased.

Oxygen fail-safe

In either the portable or central systems the cylinder of O_2 will become depleted before the cylinder of N_2O. In fact, approximately 2.5 O_2 cylinders will be used for each N_2O cylinder of comparable size. It

is obvious that a potentially dangerous situation exists, because if the O_2 cylinder becomes depleted during a procedure, the patient might conceivably receive 100% N_2O.

The O_2 fail-safe system is designed to prevent this from happening by automatically terminating the flow of N_2O whenever the delivery pressure of O_2 falls below a predetermined level. For example, both N_2O and O_2 are delivered to the patient at a pressure of approximately 50 psig. When the pressure in the O_2-compressed gas cylinder nears zero (though not quite at zero), the delivery pressure of O_2 through the reducing valve can no longer be maintained at 50 psig. As this pressure falls, to 40 psig, for example, the oxygen fail-safe mechanism is activated and the flow of N_2O gas (from a cylinder that may in fact be almost full) is terminated. The patient at no time receives 100% N_2O. Several other safety devices are activated once the oxygen fail-safe is brought into use. These are discussed in the following paragraphs.

Emergency air inlet

Located on top of the bag-tee outlet, the emergency air inlet is maintained in a closed position as long as O_2 or N_2O-O_2 is delivered through the sedation unit. When the flow of gas ceases, as in the preceding example in which the O_2 fail-safe is activated, the emergency air inlet valve opens, permitting the patient to continue to breathe comfortably, although the gas being inhaled now is atmospheric air (see Fig. 15-4). Should the termination of gas flow through the machine fail to be noticed by the administrator and assistant, the patient will gradually become less and less sedated or may mention an increasing resistance to inhalation.

Alarm

An alarm may be attached to the O_2 fail-safe system that is audible when this system is activated. This will prevent a situation in which the administrator, being so involved in the dental procedure at hand, fails to notice the shutting off of the gas flows on the unit. In central systems an alarm system is placed in an area (such as the reception desk) where personnel are frequently located (Fig. 15-33).

Oxygen flush button

The O_2 flush button permits the rapid delivery of high flows of 100% O_2 to the patient. The button is ideally located on the front of the sedation unit in easy view (see Fig. 15-3). Most O_2 flush buttons permit the delivery of at least 35 L/min of O_2. This is intended for use in emergency situations.

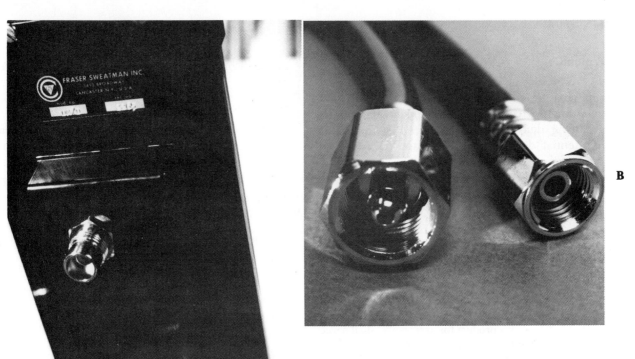

Fig. 15-32. A, Back of inhalation sedation unit. Note different diameters of N_2O *(top)* and O_2 *(bottom two)* connectors. **B,** Diameter index safety system. Diameter and threading of N_2O coupling *(left)* differ from O_2 coupling *(right),* thus preventing accidental attachment to wrong side of inhalation sedation unit.

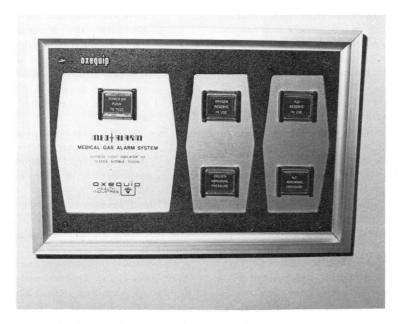

Fig. 15-33. Alarm system for central system. Alarm is activated when O_2 or N_2O pressures are low or high and when reserve tanks are in use.

O₂ monitor

A simple device may be attached to the inhalation sedation unit via the nasal hood to provide a continuous reading of the percentage of oxygen being delivered to the patient. Though not an essential device, an O_2 monitor does add to the level of safety of the inhalation sedation procedure.

Reservoir bag

The reservoir bag may be considered a safety feature since it may be used to aid in assisting or con-

---

REVISED GUIDELINES FOR THE ACCEPTANCE PROGRAM FOR NITROUS OXIDE-OXYGEN SEDATION MACHINES AND DEVICES

A company seeking qualification of its product under the classification system is required to comply with the general guidelines for submission of a product, as well as with the specific guidelines for the device:

A. Installation: The manufacturer, in submitting his product for acceptance, shall agree that the following will be done:
1. The installation of the gas delivery system and the gas storage will be in accordance with the National Fire Protection Association Standards.
2. The complete installation will be supervised by a competent supplier of gases and equipment.
3. The gas cylinders will be stored in locked containers.

The above instructions should be incorporated in the product literature.

B. Fittings:
1. The gas cylinders, hoses, and flow-measuring devices shall be color-coded in accordance with U.S. Standards: green for oxygen and blue for nitrous oxide.
2. Both pin index safety systems and diameter index safety systems are to be used.
3. The pins shall not be press-fitted but shall be attached to the block by a positive means such as welding, screws, or machining out of the block to minimize chances of accidental malfunction of the pin index system.

C. Machine:
1. A fail-safe device shall be installed to close off nitrous oxide supply and sound an audible alarm if oxygen supply fails. The audible alarm shall be on the analgesia head.
2. The machine shall be capable of delivering a flow rate (O_2 and N_2O) of 8 L/min. On activation of the machine a minimal flow of 2.4 L/min O_2 will occur. As a result the maximum percentage of nitrous oxide that can be given will be 70%.

3. Quick-connectors of standard size shall be provided to allow for fitting of resuscitation equipment when gases are supplied centrally.
4. A protection housing shall completely enclose the flow-measuring devices and will be fronted by a transparent safety shield.
5. A reservoir bag shall be provided for delivery of nitrous oxide and oxygen.
6. Flow-measuring devices shall be accurate to plus or minus 5%. The oxygen flow-measuring device should be located on the right side of the machine as viewed from the front. The flow-measuring devices should provide visual monitor of the gas flow.
7. The reservoir bag shall be mounted high enough to allow unrestricted visual monitoring.
8. An on-demand valve shall be available to allow the automatic admission of room air to the system if gas flows are inadequate for the patient's needs.
9. A nonrebreathing valve shall be an integral part of the normal-mode operating system, with the option of being manually disengaged in the event of an emergency.

D. Instructions:
1. Attached to the machine shall be the caution that the equipment is to be used only under the direct supervision of a physician, dentist, or other licensed professional.

The Council has established the effective date for classification of products under these guidelines as 1 year from the date of this announcement. After that date classification of a product will be required before promotion or exhibiting through Association media. Products currently listed on the List of Classified Dental Materials, Instruments, and Equipment as Acceptable or Provisionally Acceptable must show compliance at the time of scheduled renewal of classification.

trolling respiration in emergency situations (see Fig. 15-3). I believe that all inhalation sedation units should have a reservoir bag.

Color coding

Although simple, color coding is an important safety feature of all inhalation sedation units. All parts of the unit that carry or operate O_2 are colored green, whereas tubes, knobs, and other parts handling N_2O are colored light blue.

Lock

Locks may be included in the inhalation sedation unit and on protective caps found on the larger cylinders. As will be discussed in Chapter 18, abuse of N_2O is not uncommon. Although persons in the dental profession are prime candidates for abuse of this technique, there are instances in which nondental persons have gained access to dental systems. The use of a lock on the cylinders makes it less likely that this situation will develop.

Quick-connect for positive-pressure oxygen

All inhalation sedation units have a quick-connect attachment for positive-pressure O_2 located on the head. If it is not present, the units must be adaptable to this device.

AVAILABLE INHALATION SEDATION UNITS

There are many inhalation sedation units currently available for use in the dental or medical office. The underlying mechanism in all is quite similar; however, there are significant differences in appearance. Some units have a wooden veneer, whereas others are made of molded plastic; some are quite large, and others are more compact.

One factor that I believe must be present regarding the inhalation sedation unit is that the unit should have received an acceptable rating from the American Dental Association's Council on Dental Materials, Instruments, and Equipment.[15] The American Dental Association has adopted an Acceptance Program for inhalation sedation units that permits the doctor to better evaluate those units being considered for purchase. The primary emphasis of this program in recent years has been the addition of safety features to these units, which are aimed at making it difficult, if not impossible, to administer less than 20% oxygen to the patient. To receive a satisfactory classification the manufacturer must submit its devices to the Council on Dental Materials, Instruments, and Equipment for evalua-

tion. The Guidelines of the Council are reproduced here.

The Council publishes a listing of acceptable devices, both in the *Journal of the American Dental Association* and in *Dentist's Desk Reference*.[17]

Unit	Manufacturer
Alpha III Nitrous Oxide/Oxygen Sedation Device	Accutron, Inc.
Analor III Sedation Device	McKesson Co.
Chemtron Nitrous Oxide/ Oxygen Flowmeter Chemtron Dental Products; Dupaco Inhalation	Sedation Equipment, Dupaco, Inc.
Mini-3 Nitrous Oxide/Oxygen Sedation Unit	Star Dental Mfg. Co.
NRC-2 Nitrous Oxide/Oxygen Sedation Device	Veriflow Corp.
Parkell Sedatron Model P-1	Parkell Products, Inc.
Porter Nitrous Oxide Sedation Systems	Porter Instruments Co., Inc.
Quantiflex MDM-30, MDM-50, RA	Fraser Sweatman, Inc.
Spica Nitrous Oxide/Oxygen Sedation Device	Spica, Inc.

All of the devices listed have been accepted by the Council on Dental Materials, Instruments, and Equipment of the American Dental Association. The decision as to the most appropriate unit for your dental or medical office should be made after careful consideration of your needs and available space.

In addition the American Dental Association has adopted an Acceptance Program for N_2O-O_2 scavenging and monitoring devices (see box for guidelines).[18] The following devices have been rated acceptable by the Council:

Device	Manufacturer
Blue Mask	Health Care Technology, Inc.
Brown Mask	Summit Services, Inc.
Fraser Harlake Scavenging Nasal Inhaler	Fraser Sweatman, Inc.
Nitrous Oxide Scavenging System	Narco/McKesson

REFERENCES

1. McCarthy FM, Shuken RA: Appraisal of the demand flow anesthetic machine and review of the literature, *J Oral Surg* 27: 624, 1969.
2. Gauert WB, Husted RF: Differences in metered and measured oxygen concentrations during nitrous oxide analgesia, *Anesth Analg* 47:441, 1968.

3. Allen GD: *Dental anesthesia and analgesia,* ed 2. Baltimore, 1979, Williams & Wilkins.

4. Department of Transportation, Office of Federal Regulations, National Archives Administration: Code of Federal Regulations, title 49, section 178, Washington, DC, 1986.

5. Follmer KE: Anesthetic gas fires are preventable, *Anesth Prog* 19:2, 1972.

6. Hogg CF: Pin-indexing failures, *Anesthesiology* 38:85, 1973.

7. Sawhney KK, Yoon YK: Erroneous labeling of a nitrous oxide cylinder, *Anesthesiology* 59:260, 1983.

8. Parbrook GD, Davis PD, Parbrook EO: *Basic physics and measurement in anesthesia,* ed 2. Norwalk, Conn, 1986, Appleton-Century-Crofts.

9. Dorsch JA, Dorsch SE: *Understanding anesthesia equipment,* ed 2. Baltimore, 1984, Williams & Wilkins.

10. Eisenkraft JB: Anesthesia delivery system. In Rogers MC, Tinker JH, Covino BG et al, eds: *Principles and practice of anesthesiology.* St Louis, 1993, Mosby.

11. Compressed Gas Association: Compressed gas cylinder valve outlet and inlet connections, V-1, New York, 1977, The Association.

12. Compressed Gas Association: Diameter-index safety system, New York, 1978, The Association.

13. Bowie E, Huffman LM: *The anesthesia machine: essentials for understanding.* Madison, Wis, 1985, Ohmeda, BOC Health Care.

14. American Society for Testing and Materials: Standard specification for minimum performance and safety requirements for components and systems of anesthesia gas machines, F1161-88, Philadelphia, 1989, The Society.

15. Council on Dental Materials, Instruments and Equipment: Revised guidelines for the acceptance program for nitrous oxide-oxygen sedation machines and devices, Chicago, 1986, American Dental Association.

16. National Fire Protection Association: Standard for health care facilities, Quincy, Mass, 1990, The Association.

17. Council on Dental Materials, Instruments, and Equipment: Dentist's desk reference: materials, instruments and equipment, Chicago, 1981, American Dental Association, p. 335.

18. Council on Dental Therapeutics, American Dental Association: List of accepted products, *JADA* 105:940, 1982.

CHAPTER *16*

Inhalation sedation: techniques of administration

The technique of administration of N_2O-O_2 inhalation sedation is, quite frankly, simple. Because of the multitude of fail-safe devices incorporated into the modern sedation unit, a person with minimal training could safely administer N_2O-O_2 to most patients with expectation of success. However, under no circumstances do I believe that untrained persons should be permitted to administer inhalation sedation, for in spite of the built-in safety features, a number of unpleasant and potentially dangerous complications can still develop. Therefore, the person responsible for the administration of N_2O-O_2 must be aware of these potential problems, and know how to prevent them from occurring, how to recognize them, and how to manage them.

There is much more to the administration of N_2O-O_2 sedation than the mere turning on of a fixed percentage of N_2O and permitting the patient to become sedated. However, the fact that many doctors employ inhalation sedation in this manner without significant difficulty attests to the inherent safety of the gases and devices being employed. When inhalation sedation is employed as described in this chapter, its success rate will be far superior to that of doctors using the fixed percentage type of sedation. When a fixed percentage is used, *all* patients receiving N_2O-O_2 are administered the same concentration of N_2O, usually 40% to 50%, throughout the procedure. Titration is not employed. As will be seen, the normal distribution curve for N_2O-O_2 sedation is such that 40% N_2O will produce clinically adequate sedation in most patients who receive it, but it will prove ineffective in approximately 15%. Additionally, many patients receiving 40% N_2O will be oversedated, feel uncomfortable, and dislike the procedure.

In the technique to be described the principle of titration will be emphasized. All patients will receive the precise amount of N_2O that they require at each appointment to be ideally sedated. In this manner the administrator will be able to achieve a higher clinical success rate with significantly fewer adverse responses (such as nausea, vomiting, and adverse behavioral reactions). N_2O-O_2 sedation used in this manner is more pleasant for both the patients and the dental personnel involved in its administration.

The technique of inhalation sedation with N_2O-O_2 will first be described in general terms. Following this will be presented an in-depth view of the technique, illustrating many of the finer points involved in making it even more effective. We will focus on the cooperative adult patient (the patient who willingly accepts the nasal hood). Management of the more difficult patient, such as the handicapped child or adult and the pediatric patient, will be described in Chapters 36 and 39. In our discussion two basic principles will be strictly followed: (1) N_2O-O_2 procedures will always begin and end with the patient receiving 100% O_2, and (2) N_2O will be titrated.

Although inhalation sedation is not a panacea, administration of N_2O-O_2 in the prescribed manner will produce effective sedation in approximately 90% to 95% of patients receiving it. Inadequate clinical sedation will, of course, occur on occasion. The following factors may produce these failures:

1. A normal distribution curve exists for patient response to N_2O, and inhalation sedation units are unable to provide less than approximately 30% O_2. Some patients will require concentrations of N_2O greater than the inhalation sedation unit is capable of delivering.

249

2. Nasal obstruction or other situations (e.g., common cold, sinus problems, or habitual breathing through the mouth) will prevent some patients from breathing through their nose.

3. Although effective in most patients, N_2O-O_2 will not always be potent enough to provide clinically adequate sedation in extremely anxious patients. For these patients other techniques, such as intravenous sedation or general anesthesia, may be more appropriate.

GENERAL DESCRIPTION

The following is a brief description of the technique of administration of N_2O-O_2 in the cooperative adult patient.

1. A 6 L/min flow of 100% O_2 is established, and the nasal hood is placed on the patient's nose.
2. The appropriate flow rate of gas is established while the patient is breathing 100% O_2.
3. Titration of N_2O is started, with the patient receiving approximately 20% N_2O.
4. The percentage of N_2O is increased approximately 10% every 60 seconds until the ideal level of clinical sedation is reached.
5. The planned dental or surgical procedure is completed.
6. Nitrous oxide flow is terminated, the patient receiving 100% O_2 at a flow equal to the rate established in step 2. Oxygen is administered for a minimum of 3 to 5 minutes or longer if clinical signs and symptoms of sedation persist.
7. The patient may be dismissed from the dental office unescorted if, in the doctor's opinion, recovery from the sedation has been complete.

ADMINISTRATION

The following description of the administration of N_2O-O_2 applies to the adult patient (teenager included) who willingly accepts the nasal hood, is able to breathe through the nose, and is able to sit in the dental chair without involuntary muscular movements interfering with the procedure.

The technique of administration will differ slightly for a patient who has never before received N_2O-O_2. At appropriate points in the technique, these differences will be explained.

Pretreatment visit and instructions

The ideal time to introduce an apprehensive patient to inhalation sedation for the first time is not at an appointment at which actual dental or surgical treatment is scheduled. The patient, fearful about upcoming treatment, will experience a further increase in anxiety if the doctor or hygienist attempts to use N_2O-O_2 without having previously described the technique. There is an inherent fear of anything new (fear of the unknown), and to the patient who has never experienced inhalation sedation, the first sight of the nasal hood might bring back to mind unpleasant experiences that have occurred in the past, such as nausea and vomiting following general anesthesia or a sense of suffocation produced by the nasal hood. The success of N_2O-O_2 when used in this manner, introducing it to the patient immediately before a planned traumatic procedure (i.e., local anesthetic administration), will decrease the likelihood of a successful sedation.

The success of N_2O-O_2 sedation can be better ensured if the patient is initially introduced to the technique at an appointment prior to the beginning of the traumatic aspects of treatment. In the ideal situation the doctor, recognizing the patient's need for N_2O-O_2 sedation (e.g., anxiety, medically compromised states, gagging), will discuss with the patient the reasons for selecting this technique and the benefits to be gained from its use both for the doctor and for the patient. Many nonmedical persons have heard of N_2O but may be unfamiliar with its use in dentistry, thinking of it and the technique of its administration as general anesthesia.

The doctor, dental hygienist, or assistant should describe the technique to the patient in understandable, nonthreatening terms. Nitrous oxide itself is often called by other names, including the historically famous "laughing gas" and "sweet air" because N_2O possesses a sweet odor (to those few who are capable of discerning it). It may be desirable to explain the different levels of sedation, mentioning a tingling sensation of the arms and legs; the warm, floating feeling; and the feeling of either heaviness or extreme lightness that follows. I personally do not describe these feelings to the patient (unless the patient absolutely insists), for as will be evident with experience, not all patients experience the same signs and symptoms during the procedure. I prefer to speak of the experience in more vague, general terms, explaining that the patient will feel much more relaxed and more comfortable than would be the case without the use of N_2O. It is also important to use terms that the patient is comfortable with; for example, the effect of N_2O is often compared to the effect of alcohol (the patient saying that the effect of N_2O-O_2 is similar to that of a "two-beer buzz." However, in a patient who for religious or other personal reasons does not use or like the effects of alcohol, comparing the actions of N_2O to those of alcohol or other drugs will make the patient less willing to try and accept it. Know your patient well before comparing the effects of inhalation sedation to those of alcohol or other drugs.

Following a description of the actions of N_2O-O_2, the patient should be permitted to experience the technique. Slowly titrate the patient to a light level of sedation, and then permit him or her to recover on 100% O_2. There are several sound reasons for this introduction to N_2O-O_2 at a visit prior to the actual dental or surgical treatment appointment:

1. The patient frequently expresses a degree of anxiety toward the sedation technique itself. When N_2O-O_2 is introduced in a less threatening situation than will exist at the treatment appointment, the patient is more likely to accept the experience. If it is not introduced to the patient until the treatment appointment, the fear of the N_2O-O_2 added to the fear of the ensuing dental care may combine to make sedation ineffective.
2. When the patient is sedated at the visit prior to actual treatment the following evaluations can be made that will be of benefit when treatment actually begins: Is N_2O-O_2 effective in the patient? Rather than using an entire appointment period (1 hour approximately) and discovering that the technique is inappropriate for this patient, a 5-minute introductory visit will determine whether another sedative technique should be employed in its place.

If the technique has been successful at the trial visit, the administrator has established several values that will aid in achieving sedation at subsequent visits, such as the total liter volume of gases required for the patient to breathe comfortably and the *approximate* percentage of N_2O required in the patient for sedation.

The recovery of the patient from N_2O-O_2 may also be evaluated. Although most patients recover completely following this technique, some require extended recovery periods or require an escort when they leave the dental office.

If the technique is successful at the trial visit, the patient will actually be somewhat less fearful at the time of the next appointment because of the knowledge that N_2O-O_2 will help to make their dental experience more tolerable.

At this point any preoperative instructions should be given to the patient (see box). Preoperative med-

---

> ### *PREOPERATIVE INSTRUCTIONS: N_2O-O_2*
>
> 1. Preoperative medications (i.e., antibiotics, antianxiety drugs) as indicated.
> 2. Prohibition against eating a heavy meal for 4 hours prior to N_2O-O_2 sedation. Some may prefer to prohibit anything by mouth for 4 hours prior to N_2O-O_2.
> 3. Requirement for an escort to take patient from the dental office following procedure, if desired by the doctor.

---

ications such as prophylactic antibiotics or orally administered antianxiety drugs might be required. Oral antianxiety drugs would be useful in the patient who becomes increasingly fearful as the dental appointment nears. Oral drugs help to reduce these fears. Once in the dental office, the patient may then receive N_2O-O_2 for any additional sedation required during the dental treatment.

For the typical patient about to receive N_2O-O_2 specific preoperative instructions are unnecessary. At one time patients were advised not to have anything by mouth for at least 4 hours prior to treatment (npo 4 hours). However, experience has proven that with N_2O as a sedative agent the presence of food in the patient's stomach does not increase the incidence of nausea or vomiting.[1] Indeed, I have been present on occasions in which patients who have not eaten prior to N_2O-O_2 sedation have become nauseated and have vomited. The patient should be advised, however, to avoid a heavy meal prior to the use of N_2O-O_2 sedation.

Should the doctor desire the patient receiving N_2O-O_2 sedation to be escorted from the office by a companion, this should be stressed at the preliminary appointment and included in the written preoperative instructions.

Day of appointment
Monitoring during inhalation sedation

The following is recommended monitoring for inhalation sedation procedures:

1. Baseline vital signs, preoperatively
2. Verbal communication with patient
3. Vital signs recorded periodically during the procedure
4. Postoperative vital signs

Other monitors, such as the pretracheal stethoscope, pulse oximetry, and the electrocardiogram

(ECG), are considered optional in both the adult and pediatric patient whenever inhalation sedation is employed as a sole technique.

Preparation of the equipment

On the day of the scheduled appointment the dental assistant prepares the unit by opening one O_2 and one N_2O cylinder. The cylinders are opened by turning the knob on the top of the cylinder in a counterclockwise direction. Start by turning the knob only slightly, just barely opening the cylinder, permitting the pressure gauge to rise slowly. Once the pressure reaches its maximal level, the knob may be turned freely until fully open. The purpose of slowly opening the cylinder is to minimize any increase in internal temperature within the reducing valve as gas under high pressure rushes from the cylinder into the reducing valve.

After preparing the cylinders, the nasal hood is checked to be certain that it is clean and the other rubber goods (tubes and reservoir bag) are checked for leaks.

Preparation of the patient

1. Request that the patient visit the restroom and void if necessary prior to the start of the sedative procedure.

COMMENT: Patients receiving N_2O-O_2 sedation do not urinate any more frequently than other persons; however, more urine is produced when a person is in the supine position than when standing. In addition, the patient who has to urinate while receiving N_2O-O_2 must be unsedated (100% O_2), permitted to visit the restroom, and then resedated—a process requiring approximately 10 minutes. This time may be saved by requesting the patient to void, if necessary, prior to treatment.

2. Review the medical history questionnaire, and record preoperative vital signs prior to the start of the N_2O-O_2.

COMMENT: Vital signs to be recorded include blood pressure, heart rate and rhythm, and respiratory rate. Vital signs may be recorded by the doctor, the dental hygienist, the dental assistant, or nurse.

3. Administer the preoperative Trieger test (p. 264) to the patient (Fig. 16-1).

COMMENT: The Trieger test should be completed with the patient seated upright. With the test sheet placed on a firm surface, the patient is advised to connect the dots on the diagram as best as he can.

If the patient wears contact lenses, they should be removed prior to the start of inhalation sedation. Gas leaks from the mask around the bridge of the nose may produce drying of the eyes with potential irritation to the patient.

Technique of administration

1. Position patient in comfortable, reclined position in dental chair.

COMMENT: The preferred position is supine; however, partially reclined position may be used if necessary for the patient's comfort or the convenience of the doctor during the procedure. The upright position is not recommended

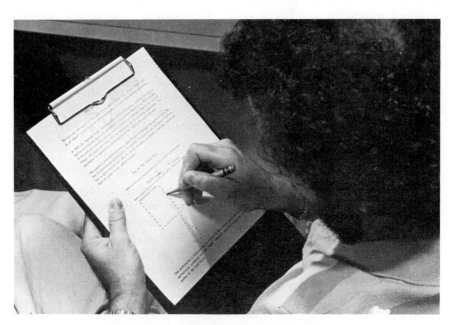

Fig. 16-1. Preoperative Trieger test is completed by patient.

unless essential for the procedure, such as when taking impressions or radiographs.

2. Position the inhalation sedation unit (Fig. 16-2).

COMMENT: This procedure applies only to the use of the portable inhalation sedation unit, as opposed to the fixed, central systems commonly found in dental offices. The N_2O-O_2 unit should always be placed behind the patient out of his or her line of sight. A positive placebo response will occur in a percentage of patients receiving N_2O-O_2, but if the patient can see the unit and watch as the administrator adjusts the controls, this response will be negated.

3. Start the flow of O_2 at 6 L/min, and place the nasal hood over the patient's nose. Remind the patient to breathe through the nose (Fig. 16-3).

COMMENT: Placing the nasal hood on the patient after starting the flow of O_2 will prevent the patient from feeling suffocated when breathing through the nose if the O_2 flow is not begun prior to placing the nasal hood.

Although it may appear ridiculous to remind a patient to breathe through the nose once the nasal hood has been positioned, this is a very important part of the procedure. Many persons will continue to breathe through their mouths unless they are specifically reminded not to do so.

4. Secure the nasal hood (Fig. 16-4).

COMMENT: The nasal hood usually has two hoses coming from the N_2O-O_2 unit. These are placed around the sides of the dental chair, and the nasal hood is secured by adjusting the slip ring behind the headrest. The patient is asked to hold the nasal hood in a comfortable position as this is being done. Care must be taken in adjusting the nasal hood, because one of the tubes is often pulled more than the other, making the nasal hood tilt to one side.

If the nasal hood has only one hose, it is placed over the patient's forehead and secured. The nasal hood should not be too tight or too loose. The patient should have some lateral and up-and-down movement of the head. The *patient* serves as the final check as to whether or not the nasal hood is secure.

Leaks develop on occasion around an ill-fitting mask. Nasal hoods are available in a variety of sizes. The size is checked prior to the start of the procedure. The nasal hood being used should fit the patient's nose. An overly small or overly large mask will leak. Leaks may also develop with masks of the appropriate size. Most often these leaks occur around the bridge of the nose, with the patient complaining of "air" being exhaled into their eyes. Permitting the patient to adjust the nasal hood is frequently all that is needed to correct this situation. If this simple solution is ineffective, the hood is removed, a folded 2-inch square gauze pad is placed over the bridge of the nose, and the nasal hood is replaced. This normally seals the leak (Fig. 16-5).

When a scavenging nasal hood is used, the exhalation tubes must be connected to the vacuum

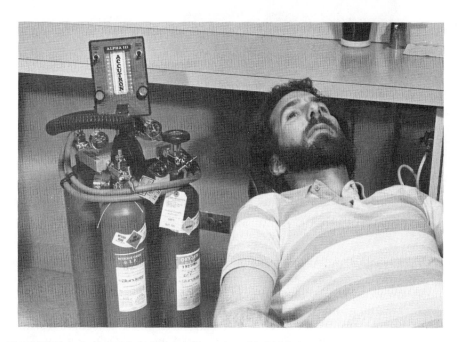

Fig. 16-2. Inhalation sedation unit is best placed behind the patient, out of his line of sight.

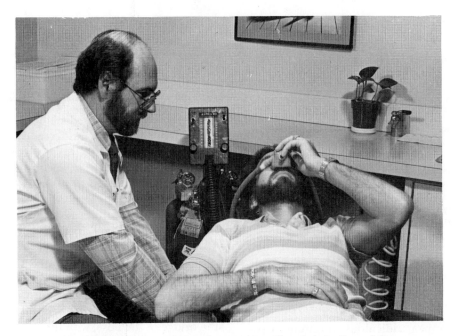

Fig. 16-3. Nasal hood placed on patient. Note L/min flow of O₂.

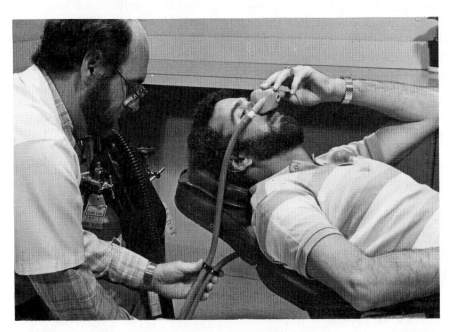

Fig. 16-4. Nasal hood is secured by adjusting slip ring behind back of chair. Patient holds nasal hood in appropriate position.

system. It is important to adjust the vacuum so that the patient is able to exhale and inhale comfortably. If the vacuum is too weak, the patient may experience difficulty in breathing out, and if the vacuum is too forceful, the patient may not receive any nitrous oxide as the gases are rapidly sucked

from the nasal hood into the overly efficient vacuum system.

5. Determine proper flow rate for the patient.

COMMENT: This is one of the most important steps in the successful use of N₂O-O₂ sedation. The patient must be

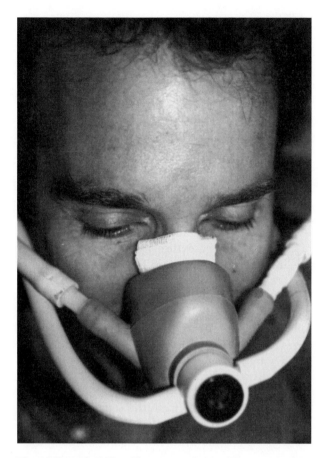

Fig. 16-5. Folded 2″ × 2″ gauze on bridge of nose prevents leaks.

able to breathe comfortably at this point, before the start of N₂O flow, in order to be comfortable throughout the procedure.

At the onset of the procedure a 6-L/min flow of 100% O₂ is initiated for the adult (3 or 4 L/min for smaller pediatric patients), and the nasal hood is placed onto the patient and the patient instructed to breathe only through the nose. In most adult patients (and virtually all children) this minute volume will be more than adequate for the patient to breathe comfortably. Breathing comfortably implies that the patient is able to take a normal breath and feel as though the volume of "air" is adequate, as opposed to the patient who states that the machine is not delivering enough "air," causing her or him difficulty in breathing. I have never seen the opposite situation, in which the patient states that there is too much "air" being delivered.

It is impossible to predict which patient will require a minute volume of greater than 6 L/min.

Larger patients may be quite comfortable at 6 L/min, whereas petite patients may require higher flow rates. Persons who participate in endurance sports, such as marathon running, swimming, and bicycle racing, are more likely to require larger minute volumes. In addition, persons with chronic obstructive pulmonary disease (COPD) or congestive heart failure (CHF) and patients with partial nasal obstruction may also require larger volumes.

The patient is asked, "Can you breathe normally?" or "Are you comfortable?" If the answer is yes, the flow rate is left at 6 L/min; however, if the patient requests a greater volume, the O₂ flow rate is increased to 7 L/min, allowed to remain there for a minute, and the same question is asked. This process is repeated until the patient becomes comfortable.

It is not uncommon for a patient to require a higher flow rate at the beginning of N₂O-O₂ sedation. This is especially so for the patient receiving N₂O-O₂ sedation for the first time. Placing the nasal hood on the patient's nose may pose a subconscious threat, and the individual may overcompensate by breathing more deeply and/or rapidly until satisfied that she or he will not suffocate. This same phenomenon is seen in early training of scuba divers. After the patient becomes sedated on N₂O-O₂ at this elevated flow rate, the doctor might return the flow rate to the original 6 L/min (without the patient being told). In almost all cases the patient will be unable to detect the change.

Establishing the minimal flow rate is important, for if it is assumed that the patient can tolerate 6 L/min comfortably but actually cannot, then the individual will probably never become comfortably sedated with N₂O-O₂ during the procedure. This step is always carried out with the patient receiving 100% O₂ (Fig. 16-6).

6. *Observe the reservoir bag.*

COMMENT: The reservoir bag on the sedation unit will provide an indication of the seal on the nasal hood, in addition to allowing a determination of the adequacy of the minute volume of gas being delivered to the patient. However, the patient is always the most reliable indicator of the signs and symptoms of inhalation sedation, including the seal of the hood and the adequacy of minute volume.

The reservoir bag that remains partially inflated (deflated) (Fig. 16-7, *A*) and deflates and inflates partially with each breath usually indicates that the minute volume is adequate (the bag remains partially inflated throughout the procedure) and that the seal

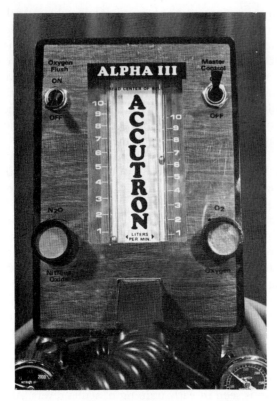

Fig. 16-6. Establishing minimum O₂ flow prior to the start of titration.

of the nasal hood is tight (inflates and deflates with each breath).

A bag that remains totally deflated (Fig. 16-7, *B*) may indicate one of the following:

- The minute volume of gas is inadequate; in this situation the patient will usually complain of not receiving enough "air."
- The nasal hood has relatively large leaks; in this case the patient will have no difficulty breathing, because any lack of gas from the N₂O-O₂ unit is compensated for by ambient air entering through the leaks. The patient may also say, "air is blowing into my eyes every time I breathe."
- The vacuum on the scavenging system is too high, forcing gases directly out of the nasal hood into the vacuum system. The patient will usually complain of not receiving enough "air."

A bag that is overly inflated (Fig. 16-7, *C*), looking like a balloon about to burst, may indicate one of the following:

- The minute volume is too great for the patient. Though an unlikely occurrence, the patient might complain about being unable to breathe against the rapid flow of air into the nasal hood.
- The hoses leading from the sedation unit have become kinked (occluded). In this case the pa-

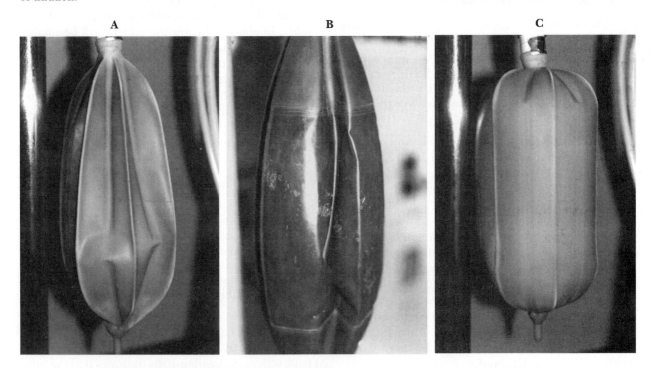

Fig. 16-7. A, Partially inflated reservoir bag usually indicates adequate seal and minute volume. **B,** Deflated reservoir bag usually indicates either a leak around the nasal hood or a deficient minute volume. **C,** Distended reservoir bag indicates either an overly large minute volume or occluded breathing tubes.

tient will complain about being unable to breathe comfortably through the nasal hood. Of these two situations involving an overly inflated bag, the second—occluded tubes—is the more likely to occur.

7. *Begin titration of N₂O.*

COMMENT: Once an adequate minute volume of gas flow for the patient has been determined, the administration of N_2O may begin. Two methods of administering N_2O to the patient will be presented, both of which are quite acceptable. In the first, the total liter flow of gases (N_2O and O_2) per minute will be kept constant throughout the procedure (the *constant liter flow technique*). In the second method, the liter flow of oxygen will remain constant (the *constant O_2 flow technique*), while the volume of N_2O will be adjusted. Advantages and disadvantages of both techniques will be discussed. These techniques are used with inhalation sedation units possessing separate control knobs for the N_2O and the O_2 flows. On inhalation sedation units having a mixing dial, the operator needs only to adjust the dial to the desired concentration of N_2O or O_2. These units operate by keeping the total volume of gas flow constant throughout the procedure (constant liter flow technique).

In all situations, regardless of the type of unit employed or the technique used, the initial percentage of N_2O will be approximately 20%. With the mixing dial units, the administrator needs merely to adjust the percentage dial to either 20% N_2O or 80% O_2. Flows of the individual gases are automatically adjusted. If a 6-L/min O_2 flow is adequate for the patient, when the dial is adjusted to 20% N_2O, the N_2O flowmeter will read 1.2 L/min and the O_2 flowmeter will decrease from 6 to 4.8 L/min.

When operating a unit with individual control knobs for N_2O and O_2 and using the constant liter flow technique, the administrator increases the N_2O flow to 1 L/min and then decreases the O_2 flow rate to 5 L/min (Fig. 16-8). This produces an N_2O percentage of 16.6% (1 L/min N_2O/6 L/min total gas flow). In the constant O_2 flow technique, the O_2 flow is left at its initial rate (6 L/min, in this case), and the N_2O flow is increased to 1 L/min. The N_2O concentration is 14.3% (Fig. 16-9).

In my experience many persons learning to use N_2O-O_2 inhalation sedation have difficulty determining the concentrations of the gases being

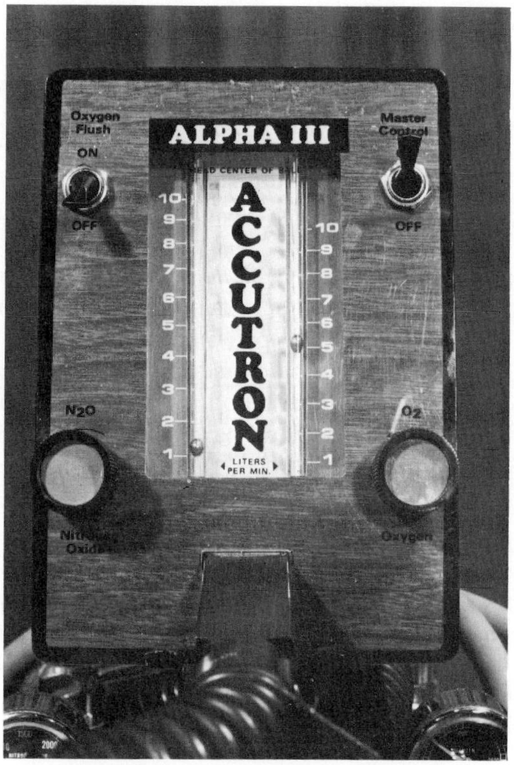

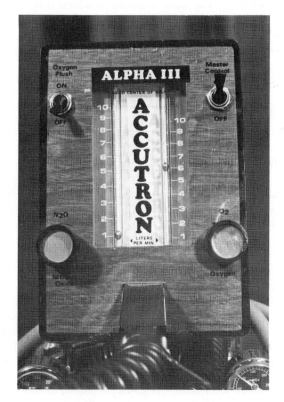

Fig. 16-8. Constant liter flow technique:
O_2 flow decrease 1 L/min to 5 L/min
N_2O flow increase 1 L/min to 1 L/min
N_2O percentage = 16.6%

Fig. 16-9. Constant O_2 flow technique:
O_2 flow remains constant at 6 L/min
N_2O flow raised 1 1pm— to 1 L/min
N_2O percentage = 14.4%

Table 16-1. N_2O percentage chart

Liters per minute O_2	Liters per minute N_2O									
	1	2	3	4	5	6	7	8	9	10
10	9	17	23	29	33	38	41	44	47	50
9	10	18	25	31	36	40	44	47	50	53
8	11	20	27	33	38	43	47	50	53	56
7	13	22	30	36	42	46	50	53	56	59
6	14	25	33	40	45	50	54	57	60	63
5	17	19	38	44	50	55	58	62	64	67
4	20	33	43	50	56	60	64	67	69	71
3	25	40	50	57	63	67	70	73	75	77
2	33	50	60	67	71	75	78	80	82	83
1	50	67	75	80	83	86	88	89	90	91

delivered. One of the most common misconceptions is that the liter flow of the N_2O is equal to the percentage of the gas being delivered. For example, a 2-L/min flow of N_2O equals 20%, a 3-L/min flow equals 30%. The only situation in which this would be the case is when the total gas flow ($O_2 + N_2O$) is 10 L/min. The percentage of a gas being delivered through the N_2O-O_2 unit can readily be determined by dividing the liter flow per minute of the gas by the total volume of both gases being delivered:

$$\text{Percentage } N_2O = \frac{\text{L/min } N_2O}{\text{L/min } O_2 + \text{L/min } N_2O}$$

$$\text{Percentage } O_2 = \frac{\text{L/min } O_2}{\text{L/min } O_2 + \text{L/min } N_2O}$$

Table 16-1 provides an easy method of determining the percentage of N_2O being delivered at common flow rates.

8. Observe the patient.

COMMENT: The patient breathes this concentration of N_2O for approximately 60 to 90 seconds. During this time the administrator should observe the patient, looking for signs or symptoms of sedation. At the end of the 60- to 90-second period, the patient is asked, "What are you feeling?" It is important to ask open-ended questions requiring the patient to respond with more than a simple yes or no. "What are you feeling?" requires the patient to answer in sentences, stating "I feel no different from before," or "I feel a little lightheaded." The question: do you feel good? brings responses of only "yes" or "no."

The typical patient receiving approximately 20% N_2O will have little or no effect after 1 to 1½ minutes. In this case the titration of the N_2O continues.

Two points that may appear minor must be mentioned:

1. *During the titration of N_2O to a patient, the administrator or assistant must remain at all times by the patient, either in visual, physical, or verbal contact.* Otherwise, the patient may think that he or she has been left alone during the procedure and may panic, removing the nasal hood, and become quite agitated. Contact with the patient prevents this.
2. *The patient's legs should be uncrossed during sedation.* The significance of this lies in the fact that once sedated, the patient rarely moves at all. Should the legs be crossed for prolonged periods, circulation of blood to the periphery may be compromised and paresthesia may develop. As blood flow returns, the feeling of hyperesthesia will be quite uncomfortable.

9. Continue titration of N_2O.

COMMENT: If the initial concentration of N_2O proves inadequate, the level of N_2O is increased. Following the initial level of 20% N_2O, all subsequent increases will be smaller, approximately 10%.

With the *mixing dial units*, the administrator simply turns the percentage dial to 30% N_2O (or 70% O_2). The machine will automatically adjust the individual gas flows.

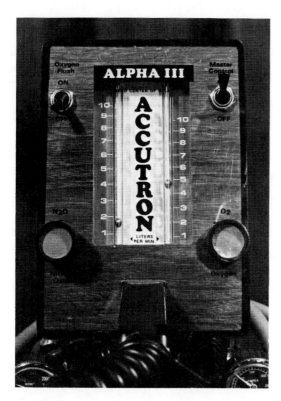

Fig. 16-10. Constant liter flow technique; subsequent changes in gas flow every 60 to 90 seconds are:
0.5 L/min O$_2$ decrease
0.5 L/min N$_2$O increase

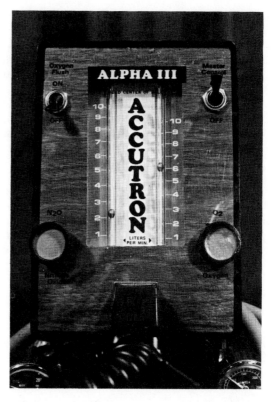

Fig. 16-11. In constant O$_2$ flow technique subsequent changes in gas flow are 1 L/min increase in N$_2$O every 60 to 90 seconds.

In the *constant liter flow technique,* all subsequent increases in N$_2$O and decreases in O$_2$ will be 0.5-L/min changes. Thus with a 6-L/min flow, the N$_2$O is increased to 1.5 L/min and the O$_2$ decreased to 4.5 L/min, giving a concentration of 33% N$_2$O (Fig. 16-10).

Using the *constant O$_2$ flow technique,* the O$_2$ remains at 6 L/min and the N$_2$O is increased to 2 L/min, a N$_2$O concentration of 28.6% (Figure 16-11).

10. Observe the patient.

COMMENT: Questioning the patient after 60 to 90 seconds at approximately 30% N$_2$O is more likely to provide positive responses about the clinical effects of N$_2$O. Table 16-2 lists the usual sequence of signs and symptoms of N$_2$O-O$_2$ inhalation sedation. Following are the more common signs and symptoms.

Light-headedness: The first clinical evidence of the effect of N$_2$O is usually the feeling of light-headedness. Many patients, having never before received N$_2$O, may describe this as dizziness—which they may find uncomfortable. The administrator should im-

mediately tell the patient that this feeling is transient and will pass as the concentration of N$_2$O is increased. The feeling of light-headedness develops at a level that is clinically inadequate for the management of most patients.

Tingling (paresthesia) sensation of arms, legs, or oral cavity: Following the sensation of light-headedness the typical patient will describe a sensation of tingling in the arms, legs, or oral cavity. This symptom also develops at a level that is still inadequate to permit the ideal management of the fearful patient. However, advantage may be taken of the paresthesia that develops. Dental procedures involving soft tissues (i.e., scaling, curettage) can usually be completed without the use of local anesthesia and with minimal, if any, discomfort. The patient receiving N$_2$O-O$_2$ may state that the "pain" is still felt but that it no longer hurts. In other words, the nature of the discomfort has been altered from a sharp, knifelike pain to a duller, much more tolerable one.

Advantage may also be taken of the paresthesia de-

Table 16-2. Signs and symptoms of N_2O-O_2 sedation

Phase	Symptoms	Signs
1. Early to ideal sedation	Light-headedness (dizziness) Tingling of hands and feet Wave of warmth Feeling of vibration throughout body Numbness of hands and feet Numbness of soft tissues of oral cavity Feeling of euphoria Feeling of lightness or heaviness of extremities Analgesia	Blood pressure, heart rate elevated slightly early in procedure, then return to baseline values Respirations are normal, smooth Peripheral vasodilation Flushing of extremities, face Decreased muscle tone as anxiety decreases (arms and legs relax)
2. Heavier sedation/slight oversedation	Hearing, especially of distant sounds, becomes more acute Visual images become confused (patterns on ceiling begin to move) Sleepiness Sweating increases Laughing, crying Dreaming Nausea	Increased movement Increased heart rate, blood pressure Increased rate of respiration Increased sweating Possibly lacrimation
3. Oversedation	Nausea	Vomiting Loss of consciousness

veloping in the patient's arms during intravenous sedation. Nitrous oxide–induced paresthesia will make venipuncture more tolerable for the patient fearful of injections.

Another area of medicine in which peripheral paresthesia is of value is in surgery of the foot. Injections of local anesthetic into the sole of the foot are extremely painful. The use of N_2O-O_2 sedation and the ensuing paresthesia will make this procedure significantly more tolerable.

Feeling of warmth, floating, or heaviness: The next symptoms that develop usually indicate entry into a level of sedation at which the patient is either at or near the ideal for treatment. The ideal sedation level was described as a stage at which the patient is relaxed and comfortable and at which the administrator is also relaxed and able to treat the patient without compromising the quality of care. This ideal level varies from doctor to doctor according to the patient's needs, the training and experience of the doctor and the staff, and the desires of the doctor.

The clinical sensations of heaviness, warmth, and floating usually indicate that the patient is approaching the desired level. Warmth develops first in most cases, the patient stating that he feels warmer. Observation will show the patient to be more flushed, a finding most noticeable on the patient's forehead,

where perspiration may be observed. The patient's hands and arms may also feel warmer. Some few patients may begin to perspire heavily, a situation that may be uncomfortable. If this occurs, the percentage of N_2O should be lowered by approximately 5% (0.5-L/min decrease in N_2O and 0.5-L/min increase in O_2 to attempt to decrease perspiration without significantly altering the sedative action of the N_2O. A feeling of heaviness or floating may also be noted. The patient may state that his arms and legs feel either quite heavy (so heavy that they cannot be moved) or extremely light (so light that they float).

Because clinical signs and symptoms may vary considerably from patient to patient, I rarely describe these symptoms in detail to patients prior to the procedure. Rather, I have found it useful to be purposefully vague, describing the effects of N_2O-O_2 sedation in general terms. Patients are told only that they will feel more relaxed and comfortable. In situations where patients have been told specifically that they will experience light-headedness, tingling, numbness, warmth, and heaviness, it has sometimes been observed that they become quite upset if any of these symptoms fail to develop, as indeed may be the case.

The administrator always observes the patient throughout the sedative technique. Watching the apprehensive patient begin to experience the effects of

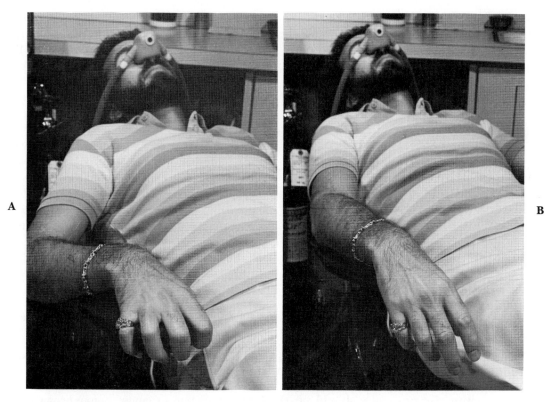

Fig. 16-12. A, "White knuckle" syndrome exhibited by apprehensive patient at start of procedure. **B,** Relaxation of hands is commonly observed when patient becomes sedated.

N_2O is of great benefit in determining the proper level of sedation. As mentioned, a patient who has never before received N_2O-O_2 sedation will prove a little more difficult to sedate than one who has. Patients who have previously achieved ideal sedation (have "been there") can simply tell the administrator when they are "there" again. The patient for whom N_2O-O_2 is being used for the first time finds it somewhat more difficult to gauge the proper level of sedation.

Careful observation of the patient aids in determining this. The appearance of apprehensive patients has been described in Chapter 5. They do not appear comfortable when seated in the dental chair. Hands may firmly clench the armrest in the so-called white-knuckle syndrome, and their legs may appear quite stiff (Fig. 16-12, *A*). As sedation develops, the patient's arms and legs relax, and he or she eventually achieving a "sedated look" (Fig. 16-12, *B*).

The verbal response of the patient will also change as the effect of N_2O increases. Early in the procedure the patient may state that he feels relaxed; however, he may say this in a very rapid, unrelaxed manner.

In fact, the patient does feel somewhat relaxed (compared to their feeling on first entering the dental office). However, should the administrator mistake this level of relaxation for the ideal sedative state and attempt to treat the patient, the result would most likely prove to be less than adequate. As sedation increases, the patient's responses become slower, with an increasing lag time observed between questions and the patient's response to them. It appears almost as though the patient experiences difficulty in phrasing replies. This state is more nearly the ideal.

When asked to describe what they are feeling, some patients will say that the feeling is similar to that produced by alcohol, for example, "It feels like a two-beer buzz." If the administrator is uncertain as to whether the proper sedation level has been reached, he or she asks, "If you were drinking (alcohol) and felt this way, would you stop?" Most people (but unfortunately, not all) will not continue to drink alcohol to a point beyond which they lose control.

The state produced by N_2O-O_2 should not be compared with that of alcohol unless the patient volunteers the com-

parison spontaneously. To compare the effects of N_2O-O_2 to alcohol to patients who do not consume alcohol for religious, medical, or other personal reasons will probably make them less likely to want to try the technique. Before the alcohol comparison is used, the patient's attitudes toward alcohol should be known.

11. Begin dental treatment.

COMMENT: The patient appears quite relaxed at this point. Titration has continued with approximately 10% increases in the level of N_2O until the signs and symptoms associated with adequate sedation have been noted. Despite this the only way of determining with absolute accuracy whether the proper sedative level has been achieved is to begin the planned treatment and observe the patient's response.

If the planned treatment proceeds without any overt signs of discomfort from the patient, it can be assumed that sedation is successful. However, once the procedure begins, it is not unusual for the patient to make movements, especially when potentially traumatic procedures, such as the administration of local anesthetics, are carried out. If the movements are significant or disruptive, the procedure should be halted and the level of sedation increased by approximately 5% N_2O. This apparent lack of adequate sedation can easily be explained when it is realized that the signs and symptoms of ideal sedation observed earlier were produced while N_2O-O_2 was being administered to a patient who was merely sitting in the dental chair. Placing a local anesthetic syringe into a fearful patient's mouth raises her or his anxiety level considerably, potentially to a point beyond which the concentration of N_2O-O_2 being inhaled can effectively manage the patient's fears. Halting the procedure and increasing the percentage of N_2O slightly (5%) will usually eliminate this problem.

Once pain control (via local anesthesia) has been obtained, the procedure will usually procede with little difficulty. The patient may, however, experience periods when the level of sedation may lessen and, conversely, when the level becomes too intense.

One of the prime benefits of inhalation sedation with N_2O-O_2 is the ability to tailor the sedation to the needs of the patient. The administrator and assistant must continually observe the patient for any indication of changes in their level of sedation. The level of sedation may become too light when a particularly traumatic part of the procedure is started. For example, the patient may be quite relaxed until the handpiece is placed in the mouth and turned on. In some patients the sound of the handpiece is quite anxiety provoking. At this point the patient may tell the administrator that the effect of the N_2O is gone, as though the machine were turned off. As before, the procedure should be temporarily halted, the percentage of N_2O increased by approximately 5% (or more, if needed), the patient resedated, and the procedure resumed.

A sedative level that has been particularly effective during therapy will become too intense when the procedure is finished and the patient's anxiety level lessens. The percentage of N_2O being inhaled by the patient is too great for the now diminished anxiety level, and the patient becomes overly sedated. Management of this situation simply requires a decrease of the N_2O flow by approximately 5%. Within 30 to 60 seconds the patient will become less sedated.

12. Observe the patient and inhalation sedation unit during the procedure.

COMMENT: Throughout the procedure the patient and the inhalation sedation unit must be observed by the doctor, hygienist, or assistant. The level of sedation sought with N_2O-O_2 is such that communications between the administrator or assistant and the patient are readily achieved. The patient should be able to respond to any requests or questions posed. Lack of response to any command should indicate to the staff that treatment be terminated immediately and the patient evaluated. In most cases a decrease in the N_2O by 5% to 10% quickly brings about a response from the patient. The assistant or doctor should also observe the N_2O-O_2 unit periodically to reconfirm that the gases are indeed still flowing. All units have fail-safe devices designed to prevent the inadvertent administration of 100% N_2O, and these devices are usually quite effective. However, situations have occurred in which these devices have failed and patients have received 100% N_2O, often with serious consequences. Visual observation of the N_2O-O_2 unit will prevent this from occurring.

13. Terminate the flow of N_2O.

COMMENT: At the completion of treatment or of that part of it requiring sedation, the N_2O flow will be terminated. In all instances the O_2 will be returned to the original flow rate determined at the start of the procedure. (This will not be necessary, of course, in the constant O_2 flow technique.) The patient is permitted to breathe 100% O_2 for not less than 3 to 5 minutes. Longer periods may be necessary should the patient exhibit any clinical signs or symptoms of sedation at the end of this period. There is no formula for determining the length of time to breathe 100% O_2, but for most patients, the longer the N_2O-O_2 sedation procedure, the greater the length of time required to reverse the sedative effects.

Nitrous oxide is not titrated "out of the patient" at the end of the procedure, the way it must be done at the start. The N_2O flow is simply turned to 0 L/min (0%) and O_2 increased to its original level.

It is suggested that the reservoir bag be emptied of any residual gas when the N_2O flow is terminated, the thought being that the reservoir bag contains some N_2O that will be inhaled by the patient, thus slowing the reversal of clinical actions. If the bag is removed from the T-attachment and deflated, when it is placed back onto the unit the O_2 flush should be used to quickly reinflate the bag with 100% O_2.

The proper time to terminate the flow of N_2O will vary from patient to patient. For example, in the extremely fearful patient, whose anxieties relate to all aspects of dental or surgical treatment, it would be advisable to continue the N_2O flow until the entire procedure is completed. However, in the more typical patient, whose apprehensions about dentistry are more specific, such as the administration of local anesthesia or the sound or feel of the handpiece, it is possible to terminate the N_2O flow after the traumatic element of treatment is completed but prior to the end of the entire procedure. There are several benefits to the early termination of the N_2O flow, especially in situations in which the duration of treatment has been prolonged.

When the N_2O flow is terminated before the end of a long procedure (in excess of 1 hour), discharge of the patient from the office is hastened. Rather than waiting until completing the procedure to remove the N_2O and start the 100% O_2 flow, the doctor elects to administer 100% O_2 after completing the preparation of the teeth, but prior to placing the restorations. The doctor or assistant will increase the O_2 flow to its original value and turn off the N_2O. This can be done without the patient being aware of it, if at all possible. The reason for this apparent subterfuge is that when asked how they feel many patients, unaware that the N_2O has been turned off and that they have been breathing 100% O_2 for many minutes, will state that they are still as relaxed as they were before N_2O was terminated. There is a 30% positive placebo response for most drugs, and if approached carefully, this response may be used to advantage in many N_2O-O_2 patients. In the event that the placebo response does not occur in this patient, the patient will simply state that the effect of the N_2O is no longer felt, to which the doctor will reply that it has been turned off because the procedure is almost completed.

In addition, the early termination of N_2O flow will decrease the volume of exhaled N_2O that may be inhaled by the staff in the absence of scavenging equipment (Chapter 18).

For the more apprehensive patient or for shorter procedures N_2O-O_2 may be administered for the entire treatment. On completion, the same procedure of returning the O_2 flow to its original levels and of turning off the N_2O is carried out. The patient inhales 100% O_2 for not less than 3 to 5 minutes.

14. Discharge the patient.

COMMENT: Determination of recovery from the effects of inhalation sedation is quite important, for in many cases the patients will be dismissed from the office and be allowed to resume their normal activities without any prohibitions. For this reason the doctor must be absolutely certain that recovery is complete before considering discharge of the patient. *Not all patients receiving inhalation sedation with N_2O-O_2 will recover adequately enough to permit their discharge from the office without an escort.*

Because it is common practice to permit most patients to leave the office unescorted following inhalation sedation and to operate a motor vehicle or other potentially dangerous machinery, valid criteria must be used to determine the degree of recovery. Several factors are used in evaluating the recovery process: response of the patient to questioning, vital signs, and a test for motor coordination.

The response of the patient to questioning is, in fact, the primary determinant of recovery from sedation. However, because this is a purely subjective response, other, more valid (from a medicolegal standpoint), objective criteria must also be employed. The patient has, at this point in the procedure, received 100% O_2 for at least 3 to 5 minutes. This is adequate to bring about an almost total reversal of symptoms in most patients. Longer periods may be necessary in some patients, particularly those having received N_2O-O_2 longer. The reason for insisting on a minimum of 3 to 5 minutes of 100% O_2 at the end of the procedure is to decrease the possibility of diffusion hypoxia. Diffusion hypoxia will be discussed in Chapter 17.

The position of the patient is altered from the supine or semisupine (during treatment) to a more upright one as recovery continues. The nasal hood remains in position at this time. The patient is asked what she or he is feeling. Any reply other than "I feel perfectly normal" or "I feel the way I did when I arrived in the office" indicates the need for additional O_2. Leave the nasal hood with O_2 on the patient for an additional 2 to 3 minutes, and repeat the question. The patient should not be discharged while any signs or symptoms of sedation remain. In those cases in which N_2O-O_2 was used in combination with other sedation techniques (oral, rectal, IM, IV) the patients should have an adult in attendance to escort them from the office.

Vital signs are valuable adjuncts in the evaluation of recovery from sedation. They are objective parameters indicating the state of function of the patient's cardiorespiratory systems. Vital signs to be measured and recorded on the sedation record include the blood pressure, heart rate and rhythm, and the respiratory rate. It must be understood that vital signs recorded after the procedure will not be exactly the same as those recorded preoperatively or even those obtained at the patient's preliminary visit to the office. Fluctuation in either direction is normal. Parameters that may be employed in determining the degree of recovery following sedation are the following:

- Blood pressure: $\pm$ 20 mm Hg/10 mm Hg from baseline
- Heart rate and rhythm: $\pm$ 15 beats per minute from baseline; same rhythm as baseline
- Respirations: $\pm$ 3 breaths per minute from baseline

Variations in vital signs beyond these parameters are normal or they may indicate a residual effect of the drugs. There may be no correlation between the changed vital signs and the use of inhalation sedation. Significant alteration in one or more of the vital signs should be evaluated prior to discharging the patient.

The third and potentially most valuable criterion in determining recovery from inhalation sedation will be an evaluation of the patient's motor coordination called the Trieger test. This test is an objective measurement of the patient's ability to perform fine motor movements.

The Trieger test was introduced in 1941 as the Bender Motor Gestalt Test and was initially used as an adjunct in the diagnosis and psychotherapy of organic brain damage in children.[2] In 1967 Dr. Norman Trieger modified the original test by selecting one figure and replacing its solid lines with dots (Figs. 16-13 and 16-14). The adaptation of this test for measuring recovery from anesthesia and sedation is based on the fact that fatigue and CNS depressant drugs exaggerate psychomotor dysfunction.[3] Disturbance in motor coordination is determined by successive trials on the test by the same individual.

The patient is requested to complete the test preoperatively. This test provides a baseline with which subsequent tests are compared. The test is supported

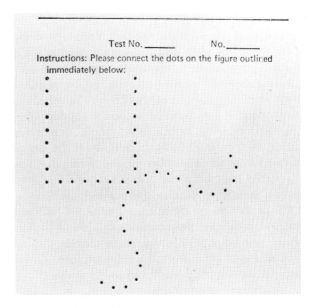

Fig. 16-13. Trieger test for motor coordination.

on a firm surface (e.g., clipboard), and the patient is asked to carefully connect all of the dots. Scoring of the test is based on the number of dots that are missed completely. Two other factors that may be evaluated are (1) the time required for the patient to complete the test (e.g., 10 seconds), and (2) the general quality of the lines (i.e., straight, wavy, or erratic).

Following the administration of 100% O_2 and the patient's subjective response that he or she feels normal, the postsedation Trieger test is administered. The patient is returned to the same position he or she was in for the preoperative test, reminded to carefully complete the test by connecting all the lines, and then the results are evaluated. The patient may miss more or less dots than preoperatively; however, the numbers should be within close proximity. Seven missed dots postsedation with 5 dots having been missed preoperatively is not significant, providing the time and quality of the lines are approximately the same as they were earlier.

It is interesting to employ the Trieger test in patients during their sedation procedure. The degree of motor dysfunction evident at this time is often quite significant. In Trieger's original study, return to the baseline level occurred within 2 to 4 minutes after the termination of the N_2O.[4] If the postsedation Trieger test demonstrates residual effect of N_2O, the patient should recover for several more minutes and then retake the Trieger test.

When it has been determined to the administrator's satisfaction that the patient has fully recovered

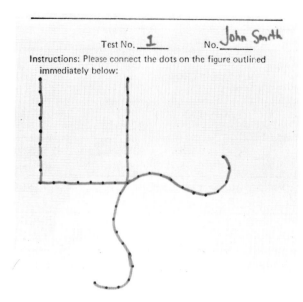

Test No. **1** No. *John Smith*

Instructions: Please connect the dots on the figure outlined immediately below:

Fig. 16-14. Baseline Trieger test. All dots connected and quality of lines good.

from the effects of the N_2O-O_2, the nasal hood is removed and the patient returned to the upright position and permitted to stand. At this point it is important for a member of the office staff (i.e., assistant) to stand in front of the patient so that if the patient should become dizzy or his or her legs weak on standing (possible orthostatic hypotension), the assistant can provide support and return the patient to the chair, avoiding possible injury. This is not more likely to occur with the use of N_2O-O_2 than with other sedation techniques or when no sedation is used. It is merely good practice to be prepared for this potentially dangerous situation that can develop in any patient following prolonged recumbency (the time required varies from patient to patient) or in patients receiving certain drugs, especially antihypertensives.

It is not unusual for a patient to feel quite normal while seated in the dental chair and to feel lightheaded when first standing. Place the patient back in the chair, administer O_2 for several more minutes, and then allow the patient to try standing again. The patient should never be permitted to leave the office if any signs or symptoms of sedation remain. Although virtually all patients will recover fully in a few minutes, some individuals will require significantly longer. I have encountered one patient who after inhaling N_2O (15%) for but 5 minutes required over 60 minutes to recover to an almost normal state. This patient and others like her should neither be dismissed from the office unescorted nor permitted to

drive a car or return to work where mental alertness is required. Provisions must be made for a companion to escort the patient home. Although this negates a major advantage in the use of inhalation sedation, strict adherence to this provision will prevent potential injury to the patient and potential liability to the doctor.

In some situations it may prove prudent to insist on an escort for all patients receiving inhalation sedation. Standard operating procedure in the U.S. Navy for inhalation sedation includes the requirement of an escort for the patient.

Most patients recover completely following inhalation of 100% O_2 for at least 3 to 5 minutes. If the doctor is satisfied that this is the case, the patient may be permitted to leave the office unescorted. This is the only technique of sedation in which this may be considered.

The patient's ability to operate a motor vehicle after receiving inhalation sedation has been studied.[5] Several parameters were evaluated, including steering errors, speeding errors, and braking reaction time (see Table 16-3). Subjects were evaluated before, during, and after the administration of N_2O. In all categories subjects demonstrated a deterioration of ability during the inhalation of N_2O similar to that produced by alcohol. Following the administration of O_2 and then room air, all measured parameters had returned to baseline values or exceeded them. It was concluded that the typical patient may safely operate a motor vehicle following recovery from N_2O-O_2 inhalation sedation.

Postoperative instructions relevant to the dental or surgical procedure are given in written form to the patient, then the patient is dismissed from the office.

15. Record data concerning the sedation procedure.

COMMENT: The assistant should record in the patient's chart that inhalation sedation was employed. A sample entry in the chart follows:

The patient received _____ % N_2O-_____ % O_2 at a total liter flow of _____ L/min. The procedure lasted approximately _____ minutes. At the termination of the procedure the patient received 100% O_2 for minutes at a flow of _____ L/min. The patient tolerated the procedure well and was dismissed from the office in good condition.

Vital signs	Baseline	After procedure
Blood pressure	112/76	118/78
Heart rate	88	82
Respirations	18	16

In addition, any postoperative instructions should be indicated on the chart.

Table 16-3. Recovery from nitrous oxide

	Presedation	*Sedation*	*Postsedation*
Speeding errors Max possible = 11 Mean + s/d	4.33 ± 2.15	3.75 ± 2.05	2.58 ± 1.31
Steering errors Max = 16	9.73 ± 2.87	11.09 ± 3.33	9.09 ± 2.43
Braking errors Max = 35	24.25 ± 4.47	30.42 ± 2.16*	23.42 ± 5.50
Signaling errors Max = 19	7.17 ± 1.85	10.42 ± 4.46**	4.92 ± 1.93
Mean braking time (secs) (range)	0.486 (0.442-0.608)	0.578*** (0.448-0.986)	0.474 (0.412-0.604)

From Jastak JT, Orendurff D: Recovery from nitrous oxide, *Anesth Prog* 22:113, 1975.

A rubber stamp or preglued labels may be prepared with this information and included in the patient's chart, the blanks filled in after the procedure.

16. Cleansing of equipment.

COMMENT: The rubber goods of the inhalation sedation unit are in contact with the patient's skin and exhaled breath and will quite naturally become contaminated with foreign material, bacteria, and viral agents. Serious respiratory infections have resulted from the use of contaminated anesthesia machines in operating rooms.[6-8] Nasal hoods for inhalation sedation have also been demonstrated to be contaminated with multiple human pathogens capable of transmission from one patient to another.[9] In a study by Yagiela et al.[10] 100% of nasal hoods used for 10-minute sedative procedures were inoculated with bacteria.

Cleansing of nasal hoods is mandatory. Simple washing of the nasal hood with soap and water has been shown merely to decrease the number of bacterial and viral contaminants.[11] Other techniques have been employed, including alcohol, gluteraldehyde, iodophor, autoclaving, and microwaving.[8,11-13] All of these techniques have disadvantages when used on nasal masks.

Using the Spaulding classification of inanimate surfaces, nasal hoods are considered semicritical in terms of infection risk.[14] Items in this grouping come into contact with intact mucous membranes and are therefore resistant to infection by common bacterial spores.[8]

The following is the currently recommended procedure for sterilization of nasal hoods:[8,10] After each use the nasal hood is washed with soap and warm water and then immersed in glutaraldehyde solution for 10 minutes. It is then rinsed thoroughly with tap water to remove the disinfectant solution. At the end of each week, all tubing, reservoir bags, and nasal hoods are stored in glutaraldehyde for 10 hours to achieve complete sterilization. Following this 10-hour period the equipment is rinsed in warm tap water for 1 hour.

Subsequent appointments

Once a patient has successfully received inhalation sedation, it is highly likely that the use of N_2O-O_2 will be desired for future treatment. At subsequent visits the same technique should be employed. The experience and information gathered from the initial N_2O-O_2 experience will facilitate any such future procedures. Although the rate at which the sedation is induced will not be increased (increasing the speed of induction frequently leads to increased patient discomfort), the patient will be better able to tell the administrator when "they are there" (at ideal sedation), having been "there" before.

It is important to note that the concentration of N_2O required for ideal sedation may vary somewhat from visit to visit. Ideally this percentage will decrease over time as a patient's level of comfort with treatment increases; however, other, nondental or medical factors will come into play. Factors such as the patient's social life, working life, altered physical condition, and the time of day may decrease or increase the percentage of N_2O required by the patient. Normally, variation from visit to visit is slight (35% today, 40% or 30% at the next visit). Only rarely will significant differences be noted over short periods (for example, 35% to 65%). To use the same concentra-

tion of N_2O at each visit, or not to titrate as a means of "saving time" (see below), is to increase the risk of discomfort to the patient.

COMPARISON OF TECHNIQUES OF ADMINISTRATION

Both the constant liter flow and the constant O_2 flow technique may be used in the delivery of N_2O-O_2, there being little clinical difference between them. The few differences that do exist are presented. The selection of the technique to be used clinically is made at the discretion of the administrator.

Constant liter flow technique
Summary of technique

1. Establish O_2 flow rate.
2. Increase N_2O to 1 L/min, and decrease O_2 by 1 L/min.
3. Subsequently increase N_2O at 0.5 L/min, and decrease O_2 at 0.5 L/min, maintaining same total flow rate during procedure.

Advantages

1. Smaller volumes of gases employed
2. Less costly
3. Decrease in exhaled N_2O contamination

Disadvantages

1. Percentage increments of N_2O are fixed; thus it is easier to oversedate the patient.

Examples of technique

Most inhalation sedation units are incapable of delivering less than a 2.5- or 3-L/min flow of O_2. In this case the O_2 flow rate will remain at 2.5 or 3 L/min, and the N_2O rate will continue to be increased at its usual 0.5-L/min increment, thus converting this to the equivalent of the constant O_2 flow technique:

6.0-L/min flow

N_2O L/min	O_2 L/min	Percentage of N_2O
0	6.0	0
1.0	5.0	16
1.5	4.5	25
2.0	4.0	33
2.5	3.5	41
3.0	3.0	50
3.5	2.5	58
4.0	2.5*	61
4.5	2.5*	64

7.0-L/min flow

N_2O L/min	O_2 L/min	Percentage of N_2O
0	7.0	0
1.0	6.0	14
1.5	5.5	21
2.0	5.0	28
2.5	4.5	35
3.0	4.0	42
3.5	3.5	50
4.0	3.0	58
4.5	2.5	65
5.0	2.5*	67
5.5	2.5*	69

Constant O_2 flow technique
Summary of technique

1. Establish O_2 flow rate.
2. Increase N_2O flow rate to 1 L/min, and leave O_2 constant.
3. Subsequently increase N_2O at 1 L/min.
4. Oxygen flow rate remains constant throughout procedure.

Advantages

1. Slightly easier to use; requires adjustment of one dial
2. Larger volumes of gases employed, thus little difficulty in breathing adequately
3. Percentage increments of N_2O decrease as the percentage of N_2O increases (see charts), minimizing inadvertant oversedation

Disadvantages

1. Larger volumes of gases employed, thus more costly to administer
2. Larger volumes of N_2O employed, thus greater contamination of environment with N_2O

Examples of technique

6.0-L/min O_2

N_2O L/min	O_2 L/min	Percentage of N_2O
0	6.0	0
1.0	6.0	14
2.0	6.0	26
3.0	6.0	33
4.0	6.0	40
5.0	6.0	45
6.0	6.0	50
7.0	6.0	54

*Unable to deliver less than 2.5 L/min.

7.0-L/min O$_2$

N$_2$O L/min	O$_2$ L/min	Percentage of N$_2$O
0	7.0	0
1.0	7.0	12
2.0	7.0	22
3.0	7.0	30
4.0	7.0	36
5.0	7.0	41
6.0	7.0	46
7.0	7.0	50

NORMAL DISTRIBUTION CURVE

As has been stressed throughout this book, patients will vary in their response to drugs. However, if the percentage of N$_2$O required to achieve ideal sedation is summarized for many hundreds or thousands of patients, then a normal distribution curve may be formulated. The following information is a compilation of over 5000 N$_2$O-O$_2$ inhalation sedations administered at the University of Southern Carolina School of Dentistry from 1973 through September 1992.[15] Statistics were obtained at sea level. At higher altitudes (e.g., 5200 ft—Denver, Colorado: 7200 ft—Mexico City, Mexico), greater percentages of N$_2$O will be required to achieve comparable sedation levels.

Percentage of N$_2$O	Percentage of patients achieving ideal sedation
10	<1
15	1
20	4
25	7
30	22
35	24
40	24
45	10
50	4
55	1
60	2
65	<1
70	<1

When divided into larger groups, it can be seen that 70% of patients who achieve ideal sedation with inhalation sedation did so at a N$_2$O percentage between 30% and 40%. Approximately 12% required concentrations of N$_2$O below 30%, whereas 18% required N$_2$O concentrations in excess of 40% to achieve the same level of sedation.

This chart includes only patients who reached ideal sedation with N$_2$O-O$_2$. *Not included are the approximately 3% of patients receiving these agents who did not achieve clinically adequate sedation levels.* For whatever reason (too fearful, required more than 70% N$_2$O, mouth breathing, claustrophobia), the technique failed to achieve its goals. This is to be expected with inhalation sedation as well as with every other technique of sedation.

TITRATION AND TIME

One of the major problems that develops over time in the typical dental practice where inhalation sedation is used is that the doctor stops titrating N$_2$O. Fixed concentrations are delivered to all patients, the percentage of N$_2$O being approximately 40% or 50%. This technique of not titrating N$_2$O cannot be recommended for routine use and will be reviewed in Chapters 17 and 19. The rationale presented for not titrating N$_2$O is that titration takes too long to be done properly and that in the typical dental office such time is not available. Table 16-4 demonstrates that when titrated according to the schedule presented in this chapter (every 60 to 90 seconds) the typical patient requiring approximately 30% to 40% N$_2$O will be sedated within 3 to 6 minutes.

The 3 to 6 minutes required (''wasted'') for sedation to be achieved is compensated for by the fact that, once relaxed, the patient will move little, if at all, during the remainder of the procedure. This is in stark contrast to a fearful, unsedated patient who moves constantly, making treatment more difficult

Table 16-4. Titration times according to percentage of N$_2$O required for sedation

Time (minutes)	Constant liter flow			Constant O$_2$ flow		
	N$_2$O L/min	O$_2$ L/min	Percentage of N$_2$O	N$_2$O L/min	O$_2$ L/min	Percentage of N$_2$O
0	0	6.0	0	0	6.0	0
1.0 to 1.5	1.0	5.0	16	1.0	6.0	14
2.0 to 3.0	1.5	4.5	25	2.0	6.0	25
3.0 to 4.5	2.0	4.0	33	3.0	6.0	33
4.0 to 6.0	2.5	3.5	41	4.0	6.0	40

and stressful for both the staff and themselves. Achieving effective pain control is considerably more difficult (and potentially dangerous) as the patient moves during local anesthetic administration. Once treatment begins, the patient will frequently ask to have it stopped so that he or she may do any number of things that prevent the doctor from completing treatment (such as drinking water or going to the restroom). The few minutes required to achieve ideal sedation with inhalation sedation are worth the effort and time invested.

SIGNS AND SYMPTOMS OF OVERSEDATION

If titration is adhered to, it is unlikely that the patient will become uncomfortable or oversedated. However, it is possible that at various times during treatment the depth of sedation will become greater without the N_2O percentage having been altered. This occurs most often when a part of the treatment is completed and there is a lull (a lack of stimulation of the patient) while additional equipment or materials are prepared for use. During tooth preparation, for example, there is a constant stimulus provided by the sound and vibration of the handpiece. The patient is receiving a concentration of N_2O adequate to produce a calming effect at this time. When, however, the preparation is completed and the restorative material is being prepared and inserted, little or no stimulation of the patient occurs. This same level of N_2O will produce a deepening of the sedation at this time.

The following are some clinical indicators of oversedation.[16] Management of this situation is simply to decrease the level of N_2O by approximately 5% to 10%. There is no need to use the O_2 flush or to terminate the flow of N_2O. Within 30 seconds of decreasing the N_2O flow (approximately 0.5 to 1 L/min) the patient will be more responsive.

Clinical indicators of oversedation
Persistent closing of mouth

Patients receiving N_2O-O_2 sedation should be capable of keeping their mouths open without use of mouth props during the entire procedure. The administrator will tell patients at the start of the sedation that they are to breathe through their nose but are to keep their mouth open. If the patient needs constant reminders to keep the mouth open during dental treatment the percentage of N_2O should be decreased slightly.

Mouth props may be used, but are not recommended for the inexperienced N_2O-O_2 administrator, for they take away one of the earliest signs of oversedation. With clinical experience other clinical clues of oversedation are recognizable to the doctor and assistant, and mouth props may again be recommended.

Most medical procedures in which N_2O-O_2 is used occur away from the mouth. The need for maintaining the mouth in an open position is, of course, nonexistent. In these cases the physician loses an important guide to early detection of oversedation. The doctor or surgical nurse must become more aware of the "other" aspects of patient monitoring.

Spontaneous mouth breathing

Patients receiving N_2O-O_2 have been told by the administrator to breathe only through their nose. A possible sign of oversedation is a spontaneous reversion to mouth breathing, especially in the adult (children are more likely to do this in the absence of oversedation). The first time this occurs, the patient is simply reminded to breathe through the nose; however, after several recurrences, the N_2O flow is decreased by 0.5 L/min.

Mouth breathing is easy for the dentist, hygienist, and dental assistant to detect. Mouth mirrors become fogged, and the exhalation of air through the mouth can be felt. A rubber dam effectively eliminates the potential for mouth breathing.

For physicians and other health professionals working at a distance from the mouth, the occurrence of mouth breathing will be more rare than in dentistry. Patients should be told at the start of the procedure to breathe solely through their nose and not to open their mouth.

Complaints of nausea and effects of sedation felt as too intense or uncomfortable

When a patient says that he or she is uncomfortable, the administrator should immediately decrease the flow of N_2O. Most patients tolerate a degree of discomfort in silence, so at any mention of discomfort, the N_2O flow should be decreased by 0.5 L/min.

If this plea is ignored by the administrator or if the patient does not volunteer the information, it is not unusual for the patient to suddenly and without warning remove the nasal hood. As patients begin to lose control (become oversedated), they respond by attempting to remove the cause of this feeling: the nasal hood. Listening to and watching the patient carefully can prevent these unpleasant situations from arising.

Failure to respond rationally or sluggish responses

The sedated patient becomes distracted from the office environment. To a degree this is desirable; however, when a patient no longer responds to verbal command, the level of sedation should be decreased.

It is not uncommon for a patient to respond more slowly than usual to spoken commands during N_2O-O_2 sedation. However, when the command must be repeated more than twice, decrease the flow of N_2O by 0.5 L/min. The patient receiving N_2O-O_2 conscious sedation should be able to respond rationally and relatively quickly to command.

Sleepiness

As mentioned, a level of sedation will develop at which the patient feels as though he or she is losing control. In the absence of the patient volunteering this information to the administrator, a sudden jerking movement by the patient will be noticed, and the patient may remove the nasal hood. The N_2O flow should be decreased slightly, and within 30 seconds the patient will recover. When questioned about their experience patients will say, "I felt as though I was falling into a bottomless, black hole." This is similar to the feeling that many persons experience when lying down to sleep when quite tired. Commonly, the person will suddenly jerk her or his body upward. This is in response to the feeling of falling into the bottomless hole—an attempt to grab hold of something.

Incoherently speech or dreaminess

Speaking incoherently indicates that the level of sedation is too great. The patient is probably dreaming, and the speaking is a part of the dream. In any case it becomes impossible for dental therapy to be continued at this time. The N_2O flow should be decreased and the patient carefully tended to. The author recently experienced a situation where a Vietnam war veteran returned, under inhalation sedation, to his position as an artillery spotter for the Marines. His demeanor became dramatically intense. The flow of N_2O was decreased and within 30 seconds this negative experience was over.

The patient becomes uncooperative

One of the goals of sedation is for the patient to become more cooperative. As with any technique, this goal will not always be obtainable. In this case the patient, as sedation progresses, becomes more outgoing, verbal, and maybe even somewhat physical (moving about in the chair more than before). Decreasing the level of N_2O may decrease this effect, yet still provide adequate sedation for the planned treatment to continue.

This effect on patients may be seen with any CNS depressant, including N_2O, but is especially common with alcohol. Many persons become more outgoing and friendly after several drinks. Alcohol produces a generalized depression of the cerebral cortex, decreasing inhibitions, allowing the individual to act in an out-of-the-ordinary manner. Unlike the effect of alcohol, this effect of N_2O may be readily reversed by decreasing the flow of N_2O.

The patient laughs, cries, or becomes giddy

Nitrous oxide is commonly known as "laughing gas" because of the propensity of many persons receiving it to begin uncontrollable laughing. Its administration can also lead to uncontrolled crying.

Nitrous oxide does not make a person happy or sad. Nitrous oxide decreases the inhibitions of the patient and increases the intensity of emotions. For example, a person in a very good, happy mood, will feel even better when N_2O is administered. This person will be more likely to enjoy the sedative experience and to start laughing should humorous thoughts come to mind. Conversely, the patient coming to the appointment in a poor mood will be more apt to release these feelings when N_2O-O_2 is administered. Without N_2O-O_2 the person would not cry but does so quite readily once the N_2O is administered.

In either case, laughing or crying, the continuation of dental treatment becomes impossible. The concentration of N_2O must therefore be decreased to a more appropriate level.

The patient has uncoordinated movements

When a patient receiving N_2O-O_2 makes uncoordinated movements, the concentration of N_2O must be decreased. For example, a 20-year-old woman was receiving 40% N_2O for dental treatment because of her fears of dentistry. She was well sedated, but occasionally during the procedure she suddenly, without warning, lifted her legs upward as high as she could, then let them drop back onto the chair. After the N_2O flow was reduced by 0.5 L/min, the patient was asked about this reaction. She stated that she was unaware of lifting her legs but that she did remember that her legs had become extremely light and began to float upward by themselves. She then would "catch them" and bring them back down. Such un-

coordinated movement is potentially injurious. Immediate reduction of the N₂O flow of 0.5 L/min is recommended.

In each of the situations presented, the patient has entered into a level of sedation that is just slightly beyond that which is deemed ideal. Management is not dramatic; the simple reduction of N₂O flow by approximately 5% to 10% corrects the situation. It is very rare indeed when the flow of N₂O must quickly be terminated.

REFERENCES

1. Houck WR, Ripa LW: Vomiting frequencies in children administered nitrous oxide-oxygen in analgesic doses, *J Dent Child* 38:404, 1971.
2. Trieger N, Newman MG, Miller JG: An objective measure of recovery, *Anesth Prog* 16:4, 1969.
3. Trieger NT, Laskota WI, Jacobs AW et al: Nitrous oxide: a study of physiological and psychological effects, *JADA* 82:142, 1971.
4. Newman MG, Trieger NT, Millar JC: Measuring recovery from anesthesia: a simple test, *Anesth Analg* 48:136, 1969.
5. Jastak JT, Orendorff D: Recovery from nitrous oxide sedation, *Anesth Prog* 22:113, 1975.
6. Joseph JM: Disease transmission by inefficiently sanitized anesthetizing apparatus, *JAMA* 149:1196, 1952
7. Olds JW, Kisch AL, Eberle BJ et al: *Pseudomonas aeruginosa* respiratory tract infection acquired from a contaminated anesthesia machine, *Am Rev Resp Dis* 105:628, 1974.
8. Jastak JT, Donaldson D: Nitrous oxide. In Dionne RA, Phero JC, eds: *Management of pain and anxiety in dental practice.* New York, 1991, Elsevier.
9. Hunt LM, Yagiela JA: Bacterial contamination and transmission by nitrous oxide sedation apparatus, *Oral Surg* 44:367, 1977.
10. Yagiela JA, Hunt IM, Hunt DE: Disinfection of nitrous oxide inhalation equipment, *JADA* 98:191, 1979.
11. Christensen RP, Robison RA, Robinson DF et al: Antimicrobial activity of environmental surface disinfectants in the absence and presence of bioburden, *JADA* 119:493, 1989.
12. Rohrer MD, Bulard RA: Microwave sterilization, *JADA* 110:19a4, 1985.
13. Young SK, Graves DC, Rorer MD et al: Microwave sterilization of nitrous oxide nasal hoods contaminated with virus, *Oral Surg* 60:581, 1985.
14. Favero MS: Chemical disinfection of medical and surgical materials. In Block SS, ed: *Disinfection, sterilization and preservation,* ed 3. Philadelphia, 1985, Lea & Febiger, pp 469-492.
15. School of Dentistry, University of Southern California: Statistics from Section of Anesthesia & Medicine, Los Angeles, Calif., Unpublished, 1992.
16. Bennett CR: *Conscious sedation in dental practice,* ed 2. St Louis, 1978, Mosby.

CHAPTER 17

Inhalation sedation: complications

There are but a few significant side effects and complications associated with the use of inhalation sedation as described in Chapter 16. Because of the safety features that have been incorporated into the modern inhalation sedation unit, serious patient-involved problems associated with the use of N_2O-O_2 have been eliminated within the dental profession in the United States. However, several potentially unpleasant side effects and complications of inhalation sedation are worthy of discussion. These include:

- Excessive perspiration
- Expectoration
- Behavioral problems
- Shivering
- Nausea and vomiting

EXCESSIVE PERSPIRATION

Patients may become somewhat flushed during the administration of N_2O-O_2. This is brought about by the peripheral vasodilating properties of N_2O. Minor perspiration may be noted in some patients, usually about the forehead and possibly on the arms or hands. In most instances this is not a problem; some patients, however, will perspire excessively, making them quite uncomfortable. The administrator should slowly decrease the concentration of N_2O (approximately 5% per minute) in an attempt to decrease perspiration. Should this fail and the patient remain uncomfortable, the procedure may need to be aborted.

When perspiration develops by itself, without other unusual signs and symptoms, there is little concern other than that for the comfort of the patient. However, the occurrence of perspiration along with a loss of color (pallor), a drop in blood pressure, and/or increased heart rate is not innocuous and

may indicate any of a number of potentially serious problems. In this situation the flow of N_2O should be terminated, 100% O_2 administered (either through the flowmeters or via the O_2 flush), the patient placed into a supine position with the legs elevated slightly (10 to 15 degrees), and the steps of basic life support instituted as required.

EXPECTORATION

Expectoration quite literally means spitting. During the administration of inhalation sedation there is no increase in the volume of saliva being produced; however, the patient might conceivably experience some difficulty in removing fluids (saliva, water, blood) from her or his mouth. The patient's senses have been altered by N_2O, diminishing the ability to coordinate movements (see Trieger test, Chapter 16). In a dental office in which the aspirating system does not function well, the patient may need to spit on occasion. As the patient bends forward to do so, the potential for injury is increased because he or she will be disoriented and might strike his or her head on a part of the dental unit. In the modern dental office, in which high-volume suction apparatus is available, this is rarely a problem. With a well-trained chairside assistant handling the suction tip, all foreign materials, blood, and saliva are rapidly and effectively removed from the patient's mouth, eliminating this potential cause of injury. Expectoration should not be a problem in procedures occurring in areas away from the oral cavity.

BEHAVIORAL PROBLEMS

Inhalation sedation with N_2O-O_2 is not the appropriate patient management technique for all patients. In the authoritarian-type personality, the loss of control over the body that occurs with sedation will make the patient uncomfortable. This patient, not wanting to lose control, will consciously or subconsciously fight the effects of the agent. Unfortunately, other sedative procedures produce the same effects, so that the success rate of most will be decreased in the authoritarian-type patient.

There is a procedure that can be used to prevent the loss of control from occurring in this patient. I do not recommend its use routinely because some patients may abuse it—to the detriment of both the administrator and themselves. The administrator should consider the use of this procedure in selected patients thought to be unlikely to misuse it. Patients are instructed to regulate the level of sedation with N_2O by altering their breathing. If the patient begins to feel that he is losing control, he breathes through his mouth, thereby decreasing the concentration of inhaled N_2O. When additional N_2O is required, he breathes through the nasal hood. The potential problem is that some patients will desire to get as "high" as they can and will continue to breathe deeply through the nasal hood throughout the procedure. When used judiciously, this technique can help the authoritarian-type personality to adjust to inhalation sedation by allowing a degree of self-control.

Other patients receiving inhalation sedation will talk excessively. These patients become difficult to treat because they are so talkative. Decreasing the concentration of N_2O by 5% to 10% per minute may alleviate the problem; however, the desired depth of sedation may also be lost. Even without decreasing the N_2O level, patients will become less sedated, for as long as they talk they are mouth breathing and receiving less N_2O. By the time patients finish their oration they will be significantly less sedated than when they began. Levels of N_2O in the ambient air will be significantly elevated at this same time.

Behavioral problems of another type may also develop. Patients receiving too much N_2O may experience vivid dreams that may be associated with physical movement of their body. Titration and verbal monitoring of the patient can prevent this potentially serious complication. By adapting the procedure to the patient's needs, rather than adapting the patient to the procedure, oversedation can be virtually eliminated. However, there will be occasions when a "well-sedated" patient may experience this same effect. A high-speed handpiece and high-volume suction device both produce considerable noise and vibration, acting to stimulate the patient. When these

devices are put away and the doctor prepares to insert restorative materials, physical stimulation is reduced. It is at this time that the level of sedation will become deeper and dreaming may occur. A decrease in the level of N_2O by approximately 5% to 10% when the tooth preparation is completed will minimize oversedation. Management of excessive movement by the patient simply involves the prevention of injury and the immediate increase in the O_2 to 100%.

SHIVERING

Although not common, shivering can be quite uncomfortable. Shivering, when it does occur, will almost always develop at the end of the sedative procedure when the N_2O has been terminated and the patient is receiving 100% O_2. In addition, shivering is more likely to develop after longer N_2O-O_2 procedures. Shivering following N_2O-O_2 may be explained by the fact that N_2O produces peripheral vasodilation. Patients will become warmer during the procedure, appear flushed as peripheral blood flow increases, and begin to perspire. The sum of these actions of N_2O is to produce a time-related decrease in the core body temperature of the patient. At the termination of the procedure, N_2O is turned off and its vasodilating effect removed. The patient's body temperature at this time may be somewhat lower than normal. The body responds to this decreased core temperature by returning it to its normal level, an effect achieved in part by peripheral vasoconstriction, piloerection ("gooseflesh"), and skeletal muscle contraction (shivering). Management of the patient during this reaction is purely symptomatic: reassurance that all is fine and placing a blanket over the patient to speed up the warming process.

NAUSEA AND VOMITING

Of all the potential side effects and complications associated with the administration of N_2O-O_2 inhalation sedation, the most frequently mentioned are nausea and vomiting. The incidence of nausea and vomiting associated with N_2O-O_2 inhalation sedation is quite low; however, in the minds of many patients, doctors, and other medical personnel, the perceived incidence is much greater. When N_2O was used as a general anesthetic without O_2 supplementation, the occurrence of nausea and vomiting was considerably greater.[1] During anoxic anesthesia nausea and vomiting was caused by the absence of oxygen rather than the N_2O. When nitrous oxide was combined with atmospheric air and later with oxygen in the technique of relative analgesia, the incidence of nausea and vomiting decreased significantly, primarily as a result of the addition of O_2 to the anesthetic mixture.[2]

With the introduction of the concept of inhalation sedation, the average percentage of N_2O required to achieved ideal sedation was decreased to approximately 30% to 40%. With patients receiving 60% to 70% O_2 the occurrence of nausea and vomiting declined even further. Since 1973 over 5000 inhalation sedation procedures have been performed at the University of Southern California School of Dentistry, with only 15 cases of vomiting reported (less than 0.3%).[3]

Nausea

Although vomiting is not common when N_2O-O_2 sedation is used, nausea will develop somewhat more frequently. However, with prompt recognition, nausea is quickly and effectively eliminated. Nausea that goes unrecognized usually leads to vomiting. Several methods of detecting nausea are available.

Patient response

It is important to tell the patient that it is all right for them to mention any discomfort or unpleasantness they might experience under inhalation sedation to the administrator. I have encountered patients who have "suffered in silence" rather than tell the doctor that they were not feeling well. Their rationale was that they do not feel all that bad and did not want to hurt their doctor's feelings by suggesting that the agent (N_2O) being used was not working as it should. Rather than say anything, the patient lies in the chair feeling uncomfortable. This is one of the reasons why, when patients do vomit, they frequently do so without any apparent warning. All patients receiving N_2O-O_2 should be advised to tell the administrator if they no longer feel comfortable at any time during the sedation procedure.

Patient monitoring

Monitoring the patient during the procedure is the major means of detecting nausea at a time when it may still be treated and vomiting prevented. Both the chairside assistant and the administrator must monitor the patient throughout the procedure. Quite simply this means watching the patient's face, arms, and body for any unusual expressions or movements. A pained expression on the patient's face may indicate that something unpleasant is happening. Pallor and sweating may also indicate the presence of an uncomfortable feeling. The placement of the patient's hands over the abdomen, either pressing or rubbing against it gently, may be another indication of nausea. If any of these indicators are recognized, the patient should be asked, "Are you still comfortable?" not "Are you nauseous?" The manner in which the patient is queried about nausea is quite important, for patients receiving N_2O-O_2 are in a very suggestible state (one akin to hypnosis). To put negative thoughts into a patient's mind at this time may prove counterproductive. A patient who is nauseous will respond to the question, "Are you still comfortable?" with a very emphatic "No!"

Management of nausea

The management of nausea requires that the N_2O concentration be decreased by approximately 5% to 10%. After approximately 1 minute, the patient is asked how he or she feels; if nausea is still present the N_2O is decreased by an additional 5% to 10%. This is continued until the patient feels comfortable again.

Causes of nausea

There are a number of reasons for nausea developing during the use of inhalation sedation, most of which are preventable or correctable.

Depth of sedation. The greater the depth of sedation (the higher the percentage of N_2O), the greater the incidence of nausea. Using volunteers, Parkhouse et al.[4] demonstrated that the incidence of nausea rose with increasing concentrations of N_2O. Little nausea was reported at 20% N_2O, whereas at 40% N_2O, approximately 60% of the volunteers became nauseated. Oversedation is a significant factor in the production of nausea associated with inhalation sedation.

Length of sedation. Although the association is not as great as with the depth of sedation, there is a somewhat greater incidence of nausea when the length of the inhalation sedation procedure is prolonged. This varies from patient to patient.

Patient's emotional status. Patients who are extremely overwrought emotionally prior to the induction of inhalation sedation are more likely to become nauseous than are less fearful patients. A means of eliminating this as a factor would involve the use of other sedation techniques, such as oral, rectal, sublingual or intranasal, to allay the patient's fears about the upcoming procedure.

Inherent tendency to become nauseous. Probably the most significant factor in determining which patients are at greatest risk of developing nausea or of

vomiting during inhalation sedation is the patient's inherent tendency to become nauseous or to vomit. Patients who are likely to become nauseous or vomit or who have had such unpleasant experiences in the past may be premedicated prior to the appointment with an antiemetic medication (Table 17-1).

Houck[5] reported an interesting study of children receiving inhalation sedation. The overall incidence of vomiting among the 67 patients of five administering doctors was 10.4%, a disturbingly high figure. Patients of four of the doctors involved in the study had vomiting incidences of 0%, but seven of seventeen patients (41%) of the fifth doctor vomited. When the treatment characteristics of the five doctors are compared (Table 17-2), it was found that the doctor whose patients experienced all of the vomiting differed from the others only in that his treatment sessions averaged 39 minutes while the next longest was 34 minutes, values well within the norm for the typical dental appointment. **Each of these seven patients was premedicated with an antiemetic prior to their second visit, and still two patients vomited again.** The paper recommended that a preoperative inquiry be made concerning previous vomiting episodes and in the event that such an inquiry proves positive the patient be premedicated with an antiemetic.

Presence of food in stomach. For years it was standard practice in inhalation sedation to preclude the patient from eating for approximately 4 to 6 hours prior to the procedure. It was thought that in this way the incidence of vomiting might be decreased. This rule originated in the operating room, where it is critically important that patients undergoing general anesthesia take nothing by mouth for approximately 8 hours prior to the start of the procedure. As inhalation sedation is but a modification of general anesthesia, many of the rules of general anesthesia were passed down to this technique. It has been determined through many years of experience with inhalation sedation that there is no benefit to be gained by having a patient avoid a meal prior to the procedure. In my experience over the past 20 years at the University of Southern California, several of the patients who have vomited have neither eaten nor had any fluid for at least 8 hours prior to receiving N_2O-O_2. In two of the cases where nausea or vomiting developed the patients stated that they frequently become nauseous when they are hungry, as they were in this situation.

The basic rule I stress in relation to eating and inhalation sedation is that there is no hard and fast rule. Patients are permitted to eat or not eat prior to the procedure, according to their desires. The only thing I ask of a patient is that if they do eat prior to the inhalation sedation procedure they do not over-

Table 17-1. Antiemetics

Generic name	Proprietary name	Adult oral dose (mg)
Dimenhydrinate*	Dramamine	50 to 100
Cyclizine*†	Marezine	50
Meclizine*†	Bonine	25 to 50
Hydoscine, scopolamine	—	0.6 to 1
Hydroxyzine†	Vistaril	25 to 100
Diphenidol†	Vontrol	25 to 50
Trimenthobenzamide	Tigan	100 to 300
Prochlorperazine	Compazine	5 to 10
Promethazine	Phenergan	12.5 to 25

*Nonprescription.
†Should be used with caution, can be teratogenic in pregnancy.

Table 17-2. Vomiting frequency in children administered N_2O-O_2

	Patients			N_2O-O_2 administration		Frequency of vomiting					
			Average			N_2O_2 alone		N_2O-O_2 + premedication		Total	Vomiting
Doctor	#	Age	Range	Average duration (min)	Maintenance concentration N_2O	#	vomiting	#	vomiting	#	%
A	23	7.5	(2-25)	32	50%	20	0	3	0	0	0
B	13	8.1	(4-16)	28	30%	11	0	2	0	0	0
C	5	6.4	(3-10)	16	61%	5	0	0	0	0	0
D	9	7.1	(3-10)	34	38%	6	0	3	0	0	0
E	17	8.8	(4-17)	39	40%	12	5	5	2	7	41%
TOTAL	67					54	5	13	2	7	10.4%

From Houck WR, Ripa WR: Vomiting frequency in children administered nitrous oxide-oxygen in analgesic doses, *J Dent Child* 28:404, 1971.

indulge. If a patient develops nausea or vomits during the ensuing inhalation sedation procedure, then at subsequent appointments with N_2O-O_2 sedation I specifically request the patient to either eat or not to eat, depending on the circumstances surrounding the first visit (i.e., patients eat, become nauseous or vomit, then at next visit they are asked not to eat).

Other factors. Two additional factors that increase the likelihood of the development of nausea are (1) a "roller coaster ride" with N_2O-O_2, and (2) changing the patient's position frequently during the procedure. Frequent changing of the concentration of N_2O during sedation increases the likelihood of nausea developing. As discussed in Chapter 16, there are but few occasions in which the N_2O concentration will be reduced or increased more than 5% to 10%. Minor changes in gas concentration are less likely to produce nausea. However, more significant changes are more likely to provoke nausea and vomiting. Though not as likely to produce nausea and vomiting as changing gas concentrations, significant positional alterations may also increase the risk. Once the patient is placed in a suitable position for treatment (supine is most preferred, reclining is also recommended), there is usually little need for further altering of position.

Vomiting

Vomiting is potentially a serious complication of inhalation sedation. The patient's head will be facing directly upward as he or she lies in the dental chair or surgical bed. Should vomiting occur in this position, there is a greater likelihood that vomitus will be aspirated into the trachea and lungs, potentially producing an obstructed airway, aspiration pneumonitis, lung abscess, or both.

Vomiting may usually be prevented through the prompt recognition and management of nausea, as described. However, there may be cases where even with prompt recognition and management, vomiting will still occur.

Vomiting is much more common in children than adults. Adults are more likely to tell the administrator that they feel uncomfortable, whereas the child, being in most cases less communicative, says nothing, vomiting suddenly without any warning. There are several reasons to explain the greater incidence of vomiting among children. First, children are more difficult to communicate with during the induction of sedation. Therefore, the administrator may be less able to accurately determine the depth of sedation of the child and be more likely to oversedate them.

Second, children are much more likely to mouth-breathe than are adults. Mouth breathing drastically reduces the N_2O concentration of the inhaled gases, producing a lessening of the sedation level. On becoming aware of the mouth breathing the administrator will tell the patient to breathe again through his nose. Once resedated, the patient may again revert to mouth breathing, repeating the sequence again and again. This "roller coaster ride" effect with N_2O-O_2 increases the risk of nausea and vomiting.

Management of vomiting

The signs of impending vomiting are pallor; sweating (usually cold); a cold, clammy feeling of hands; increased salivation; and active swallowing.

Should any of these signs and symptoms appear, the following should be done:

1. Immediately turn off the N_2O flow, permitting the patient to breathe 100% O_2.

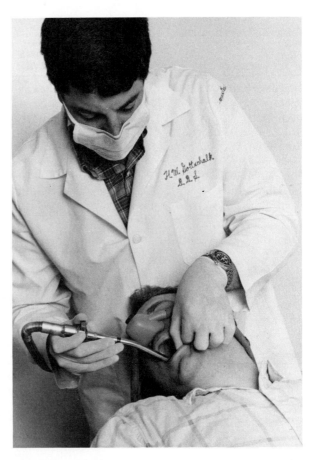

Fig. 17-1. If vomiting occurs, patient's head is turned to side and vomitus removed with suction or finger. Patient should receive 100% O_2.

2. As vomiting begins, remove the nasal hood or other delivery apparatus from the patient's face.
3. Remove the rubber dam, if present, and any other dental equipment from the oral cavity.
4. Turn the patient's head and body to the side. This permits the vomitus to pool in the cheek pouch, thereby not flowing back into the patient's pharynx where it may obstruct the airway. Turn the patient's head away from the side on which the person treating the patient is stationed (Fig. 17-1). A kidney or emesis basin and high-volume suction tip may be used to assist in removing the vomitus from the oral cavity.
5. Following the incident, replace the nasal hood on the patient's nose so that he or she may be permitted to breathe 100% O_2 for at least 3 to 5 minutes. The patient may be somewhat reluctant to have the nasal hood placed back on for fear of becoming sick again. Explain to the patient that she or he will only breathe 100% O_2 and that the reason for so doing is to minimize the chance of becoming sick again.

If the patient does not wish to continue with N_2O-O_2 during treatment, it is best to adhere to these wishes. However, the door should not be closed on the future use of this important technique. It should be stressed to the patient that vomiting is a very unusual occurrence and that it is unlikely to occur again. If deemed necessary, antiemetics may be prescribed preoperatively for this patient.

REFERENCES

1. Seldin HM: *Practical anesthesia and dental and oral surgery: local and general,* ed 3. Philadelphia, 1947, Lea & Febiger, p 425.
2. Langa H: *Relative analgesia in dental practice: inhalation analgesia with nitrous oxide.* Philadelphia, 1968, Saunders, p 164.
3. School of Dentistry, University of Southern California: Statistics from Section of Anesthesia & Medicine, Los Angeles, Calif, unpublished, 1992.
4. Parkhouse J, Henrie JR, Duncan GM et al: Nitrous oxide analgesia in relation to mental performance, *J Pharmacol Exp Ther* 128:44, 1960.
5. Houck WR, Ripa LW: Vomiting frequency in children administered nitrous oxide-oxygen in analgesic doses, *J Dent Child* 38: 404, 1971.

CHAPTER 18

Current concerns: chronic exposure, recreational abuse, and sexual phenomena

Inhalation sedation with N_2O-O_2 has proved to be an extremely effective technique for the reduction of stress in the apprehensive or medically compromised patient. When administered as described in Chapter 16, the incidence of complications and side effects is quite low. The inhalation sedation unit has undergone continual improvement in an attempt to make it as safe as possible. The primary goal of these safety features is to prevent or minimize the possible administration of less than 20% oxygen to any patient at any time. Because of these factors, the use of inhalation sedation with N_2O-O_2 has increased in the medical, dental, and other health professions. Professional education in this technique received a boost in 1971, when standards for educational programs in inhalation sedation were accepted by the Council on Dental Education of the American Dental Association.[1]

Along with the increased use of N_2O-O_2 has come a greater concern for the safety of personnel who are in contact with it for the greatest length of time—the dental office staff. Three major factors must be addressed in this regard:

1. Chronic exposure to trace anesthetic gases
2. Recreational abuse of N_2O
3. Sexual phenomena and N_2O

CHRONIC EXPOSURE TO TRACE ANESTHETICS

It has been known for centuries that exposure to certain chemicals and industrial wastes poses a serious health hazard. Chemicals such as carbon tetrachloride, benzidine, and benzene have been demonstrated to produce disease of the liver, bladder cancer, and leukemia in individuals exposed to them on a long-term basis.[2] In recent years the tranquilizer thalidomide again showed the potential dangers involved in drug use.[3]

Stringent standards have been initiated by several federal departments and agencies in an effort to protect workers from occupational disease. The Occupational Safety and Health Administration (OSHA) of the Department of Labor has been the agency most prominent in this effort in the United States.

In the operating room, however, little or nothing was done to eliminate anesthetic vapors being delivered into the ambient air from anesthesia machines. Indeed, little was known of the possible effects of inhalation of minute amounts of anesthetic vapors until the late 1960s. In 1967 Vaisman[4] published the results of a survey of Russian anesthesiologists in which it was demonstrated that they suffered a higher incidence of irritability, headache, fatigue, nausea, pruritus, spontaneous abortion, and fetal malformation than non–operating room personnel. Other studies followed shortly thereafter,[5-7] confirming Vaisman's results. It must be emphasized that in these studies N_2O was but one of many gases under investigation. Because it is the most commonly used inhalation anesthetic, N_2O will be found in all samples of air taken from operating rooms. It is used in conjunction with O_2 and other more potent inhalation anesthetics such as halothane, methoxyflurane, enflurane, and isoflurane. Therefore it has been impossible to separate the effects of any one of these gases from the others. In other words, the findings presented here are potentially produced by any one of the drugs found in the operating room. Because of the special nature of dental practice, in which virtually the only inhalation anesthetic employed is N_2O, the findings of these operating room studies were not applicable to the dental profession.

The rate of spontaneous abortion among women exposed to inhalation anesthetics on a long-term basis is significantly higher than that of unexposed women.[8] The rate of spontaneous abortion for the American Society of Anesthesiologists was 17.1%, the American Association of Nurse Anesthetists 17.0%, and the Association of Operating Room Nurses and Technicians 19.5%, while the corresponding rates for unexposed women in the American Academy of Pediatrics was 8.9% and that for the American Nursing Association 15.1%. Rates of congenital abnormalities were also significantly elevated in exposed women. Members of the American Society of Anesthesiologists had a congenital malformation rate of 1.24 per 100 live births; the rate for nonexposed members of the American Academy of Pediatrics was but 0.21 per 100 live births.

Other findings of importance included an increased incidence in the development of hepatic disease in persons exposed to inhalation anesthetics on a long-term basis.[9] This is not a surprising finding since it is well established that many of the inhalation anesthetics have the potential to produce liver dysfunction. Specifically, commonly employed anesthetic gases such as halothane are known to produce liver damage in some patients.

Renal disease was also seen more frequently, specifically renal lithiasis. Again some of the commonly employed inhalational anesthetics, specifically methoxyflurane, are known to have the potential to impair renal function.

Nonspecific neurologic disease was another finding in many of the studies just cited. Increased incidences of irritability, headache, and fatigue were not uncommon.

It has been definitely established that long-term exposure to trace concentrations of the potent inhalation anesthetics can indeed lead to the physical findings discussed. That effective methods of minimizing this exposure are available is also known. In a study by Whitcher et al.,[10] the concentration of halothane around an anesthesia machine was determined using different methods of delivery of the gases. The results confirmed that effective elimination of exhaled anesthetic gases was possible (Table 18-1).

In the operating room, because of the availability

Table 18-1. Mean concentrations of halothane determined at various points from exhalation port of an anesthesia machine

Delivery system	Halothane concentration (ppm)
Nonrebreathing	8.69
Partial rebreathing (semiclosed circle system)	4.93
Nonrebreathing with scavenging	0.79
Semiclosed circle system with scavenging	0.73

Modified from Whitcher C, Zimmerman DC, Piziali RL: *J Oral Surg* 36:431, 1978.

of laminar airflow systems, in which there is little or no recirculation of air into the operating room, it is relatively easy to achieve lower concentrations of inhalation anesthetics than in the typical dental office.

The dental profession uses nitrous oxide to the virtual exclusion of other anesthetic gases. None of the previously mentioned studies were able to specify which anesthetic agent was responsible for the disturbing findings. The American Dental Association therefore undertook a survey to compare dentists and dental personnel who use nitrous oxide with those that did not.[11] The information gathered confirmed that women (dentists, dental hygienists, and assistants) exposed to nitrous oxide did indeed have an increased rate of spontaneous abortion, and that spouses of exposed male dentists were likewise affected, presumably due to abnormalities occurring in their sperm.[11,12] Other findings, such as increased rates of liver, renal, and neurologic disorders, were less obvious, with other explanations for the increased rates still being offered. Fertility is also affected by high levels of exposure to nitrous oxide. Dental assistants who were exposed to N_2O-O_2 for more than 5 hours per week were found to be only 41% as likely as unexposed women to conceive during each menstrual cycle.[13] Fortunately, with the removal of N_2O-O_2 from the environment, via scavenging, this problem was eliminated.[14]

Nitrous oxide concentrations in dental offices

In the absence of measures for controlling N_2O concentrations, measurable levels of N_2O are found throughout the dental suite in which N_2O-O_2 inhalation sedation is used without scavenging. Concentrations of N_2O as great as 7000 ppm have been detected in dental treatment rooms where scavenging was not employed.[15] Even the doctor's private office,

Table 18-2. Levels of N_2O (ppm) in breathing zones when using conventional nasal hood with expiratory valve

Categories	Dentist	Assistant	Room average
General dentist's office	775 ± 63	440 ± 52	310 ± 37
Pedodontist's office	940 ± 92	112 ± 23	280 ± 52
Oral surgeon's office	1000 ± 130	1600 ± 250	310 ± 47

Modified from Whitcher CE, Zimmerman DC, Tonn EM et al: *JADA* 95:763, 1977. Copyright by the American Dental Association. Reprinted by permission.

waiting room, closets, and restrooms were found to contain more than 200 ppm of N_2O.[16] Table 18-2 presents N_2O concentrations found in treatment areas in pediatric, oral surgical, and general practice offices. Levels of N_2O were recorded within 12 inches of the mouth and nose of the doctor or assistant (the so-called breathing zone) in situations in which the conventional nasal hood, with an expiratory valve, was employed.

Some explanation of the significant variation among the various types of dentists is necessary. Elevated N_2O levels found in the breathing zone of the pediatric dentist are the result of the propensity of children to mouth breathe. Mouth breathing is one of the more common causes of elevated levels of N_2O in any dental operatory, but especially so in younger patients. In the surgical environment patients often receive inhalation sedation in conjunction with other more potent techniques, such as IV sedation or general anesthesia. It is therefore even more likely that mouth breathing will occur, explaining the elevated levels of N_2O in that environment. In addition, the chairside assistant in the oral surgery office is much more likely to work close to the patient's mouth (aspirating, retracting) than the pediatric assistant. It is noteworthy that the levels of N_2O found in the treatment room at a distance from the patient were quite constant (approximately 300 ppm) regardless of the nature of the dental patient or procedure. Potential sources of N_2O in the dental environment are presented in Table 18-3.

The most important source of N_2O contamination occurs from the normal circuit of gas flow from the inhalation sedation unit to the nasal hood to the patient. During exhalation, gases pass through the exhaling valve and are dispersed into the environment.

Table 18-3. Potential sources of nitrous oxide

1. Normal gas flow
   Exhaling valve
   Around perimeter of nasal hood
2. Patient
   During the procedure—mouth breathing, talking, laughing
   After the procedure—30 liters N_2O exhaled within 3 to 5 minutes
3. Inhalation sedation unit
   High-pressure system:
     Worn wall connectors
     Loose high-pressure hose connections
     Deformed compression fittings
   Low-pressure system:
     Loose, defective, or missing gaskets and seals
     Worn or defective bags and breathing tubes
     Loosely assembled slip joints and threaded connections
     Loose flowmeters
4. Air conditioning

The exhaling valve on most existing sedation units represents the major source of N_2O. Leakage of gases from around the perimeter of a poorly fitted nasal hood is a secondary source of contamination.

The patient is another source of N_2O. During the sedation procedure, mouth breathing, laughing, or talking will lead to increased N_2O concentrations in the ambient air.[17] At the termination of N_2O-O_2 sedation, the patient will exhale approximately 30 liters of N_2O within the first 3 to 5 minutes, representing a significant source of N_2O.

The inhalation sedation unit and its associated hardware (e.g., tubing, hoses) are other sources of N_2O. Rubber goods such as the reservoir bag and the breathing hoses undergo deterioration in polluted environments, leading to cracks and leaks in the rubber. Loosened screws or threaded connectors on the head of the unit are potential sources of leakage.

The role of air conditioning in affecting the concentrations of N_2O is twofold. The fresh air dilution that is a part of an air conditioning system acts to decrease the concentration of N_2O found in the dental suite in areas away from the nasal hood. However, most air conditioning systems found in modern offices are of the recirculating type. In this system a portion of the air that is removed from the room is exhausted into the atmosphere and is replaced by fresh air, while a much larger proportion of the gas is simply recirculated. Any N_2O found in this air will then be recirculated throughout the entire dental office to areas far from the actual source of the N_2O. The levels of N_2O found in such areas as the reception room will, however, be quite low.

Detection of nitrous oxide contamination

Not every dental or medical office employing inhalation sedation has significant concentrations of N_2O in the ambient air. Many factors are at work in determining these levels. Primary among these is the degree to which inhalation sedation is used within an office. It stands to reason that concentrations will be lower in offices in which N_2O is infrequently employed than in offices where N_2O is used more frequently.

A second factor is the size of the treatment area. In small areas the gas concentration will be higher than in larger areas. However, several other factors involving treatment areas will influence N_2O levels. A typical dental treatment room is small. If there is a window, it is usually sealed or closed. In this environment N_2O levels can become quite significant. The addition of air conditioning or improved ventilation of any sort will serve to decrease these levels. Simply opening a window to provide circulation of air through the treatment room will suffice to dramatically decrease N_2O levels. Pediatric dental offices are often arranged not as closed rooms but as large open bays. With this design the concentration of inhalation anesthetics is significantly decreased in the breathing zones of the doctor and assistant because the gas is dispersed into the much larger area of the expanded dental suite. Factors involved in determining N_2O concentrations are summarized here:

FACTORS DETERMINING N_2O
CONCENTRATIONS

1. Incidence of N_2O usage
2. Size of treatment area
3. Ventilation of treatment area
4. Closed treatment area (room) versus open bay area

It is important to determine whether or not high concentrations of N_2O develop in one or more areas of the dental of medical office in which inhalation sedation is employed. Several methods of detection of N_2O are available at this time and will be discussed:

DETERMINATION OF N_2O CONCENTRATIONS

1. Inspection of rubber goods
2. Soapy water solution on all connections
3. Outside service company
4. Infrared (IR) N_2O analyzer

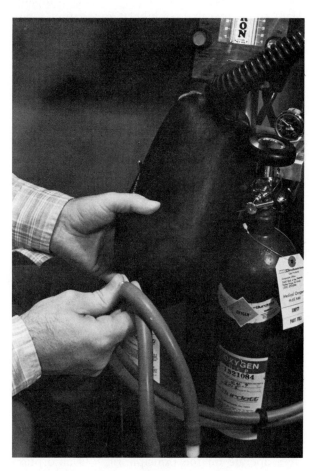

Fig. 18-1. The reservoir bag is checked for leaks by overinflating bag, occluding conducting tubes, and squeezing bag. If the bag deflates, a leak is present in system.

The rubber goods of the inhalation sedation unit should be inspected regularly to determine whether cracks or tears have developed in them. The nasal hood is rarely found to have cracks; however, both the breathing tubes and the reservoir bag do develop cracks. Cracks in the reservoir bag are most frequently found along pleats, where they may be difficult to locate (Fig. 18-1).

A simple method for detecting gas leakage is a

soapy water solution. The solution is painted on various areas of the unit, particularly connections between tubes and the machine, and on screws and knobs. After the gas flow is started, the formation of soap bubbles is evidence of leakage. Such leaks are usually easily corrected by tightening a connection or replacing the rubber goods.

Another means of determining levels of N_2O within a dental office is to employ a service company. Many companies that sell inhalation sedation equipment or supply compressed gas cylinders to the medical and dental professions maintain equipment to monitor nitrous oxide levels, and if elevated levels are detected will determine the source of the N_2O.

The most effective means (though not always readily available) of determining N_2O levels in ambient air is the infrared (IR) N_2O analyzer.[18] IR light is absorbed at different wavelengths by different gases. For N_2O this wavelength is 4.45 μ. The IR analyzer operates by aspirating gas samples into a nozzle-like opening and then transferring them to a sampling cell. Differences in N_2O concentration in the sampled air result in proportional changes in the quantity of IR energy that is transmitted through the sampling cell, sensed by the detector, and then amplified and displayed on the monitor. The response time for the IR analyzer is quite rapid, approximately 2 to 20 seconds. In addition, these analyzers are quite sensitive, responding to a lower limit of 1 ppm and an upper limit of 2000 ppm. Accuracy of the IR analyzer is plus or minus 5%. The IR analyzer is an expensive device, and its purchase is not recommended. However, many service companies and hospitals own such devices and may, for a fee, monitor the dental or medical office.

Other N_2O monitoring systems have been developed for use in medical and dental offices. Such devices operate on the principle of N_2O absorption over a given period of time.[19] A sensor similar to radiation dosimeter badges is worn by staff members (Fig. 18-2). Chemicals within the sensor absorb N_2O. The sensor is sent to a laboratory with a listing of the time of exposure to N_2O. The laboratory returns a time-weighted value of exposure to N_2O. Such devices are convenient to use and serve a useful function in the monitoring of N_2O exposure; however, they are not as effective as the other means already listed.

Elimination of nitrous oxide from air

It has been demonstrated that N_2O does pollute the ambient air within the dental office wherever in-

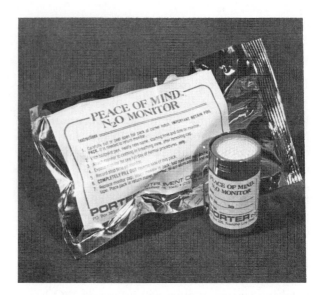

Fig. 18-2. N_2O monitoring device is worn by doctors or auxiliary personnel.

halation sedation is used. That N_2O is capable of long-term undesirable effects on those who inhale it has yet to be fully determined without doubt; however, indications are that such may be the case. It seems quite logical, therefore, that if a mechanism for the removal of N_2O from ambient air exists, it should be employed, regardless of whether trace concentrations of N_2O are ultimately determined to be dangerous or not. Fortunately there are several methods available that act to minimize N_2O levels to which office personnel are exposed:

1. Testing equipment for leaks
2. Venting of waste gases
3. Scavenging nasal hoods
4. Air-sweep
5. Minimizing talking by patient
6. Monitoring of air

Testing equipment for leaks

A self-induced problem encountered by doctors employing inhalation sedation is the lack of routine preventive maintenance of their inhalation sedation units. The overwhelming majority of inhalation sedation units operate effectively for many, many years even in the absence of such maintenance. However, over a period of time small, unnoticeable things can go wrong with the unit, such as the rubber goods becoming brittle and cracks developing, or screws, knobs, and connectors coming loose. These may be the source of small or significant leaks of N_2O. Without specific testing these leaks might never be noticed. It is possible to test both the high- and low-pressure parts of the compressed gas system within an office.

To determine leakage in the high-pressure system, both the flowmeters in the operatories and the cylinder valves in the storage room are turned off at the end of the treatment day. Pressure will remain in the piping between the cylinders and the operatories. The pressure of the gas within the pipes is 50 psi and should remain so overnight if no leaks are present in the high-pressure system. If the overnight pressure drop is less than 10% (45 psi), the system is considered to be airtight. Drops in excess of 10% should be evaluated by a service company.

The low-pressure part of the system is also easily checked. The reservoir bag is evaluated by overfilling it with oxygen (see Fig. 18-1) and then feeling its surface for leaks or cracks. The tubing and nasal hoods may be similarly tested by occluding the tubing at the nasal hood and overfilling the entire system with O_2. Squeezing the reservoir bag should be met with extreme resistance, as the gas cannot exit the system unless leaks are present in the tubing or the reservoir bag. If leaks appear to be present in the low-pressure system use a soapy water solution to locate the source of the leak. If this does not produce satisfactory results, a service company should be consulted.

Venting of waste gases

To prevent waste gases from entering the ambient air, it is recommended that such gases be removed via venting into the atmosphere. Fortunately virtually all dental offices have suction systems that are adequate for scavenging of anesthetic gases and the removal of secretions from patients' mouths. All venting systems are designed to dispose of the gases at a site distant to the dental office. In most instances this is done outside of the building. It is important, of course, to avoid venting outside near windows that might be opened or near air inlets.

Vacuum pumps that are exposed to anesthetic gases must meet any necessary fire codes and safety standards. Turbines that are located in the gas stream are spark-proof, and motor brushes and switches are located outside of the stream of gas.

Scavenging nasal hoods

The greatest single source of trace N_2O in the dental environment is the normal flow of gas from the patient's nose through the exhaling (one-way) valve (see Fig. 15-27, *A, B*) into the air. The conventional nasal hood also provides for the escape of gases around the periphery if an airtight seal is not present.

Once the problem of trace contamination with N_2O became publicized, attempts were made to minimize the loss of N_2O through the nasal hood. Attaching the nasal hood to the suction system found at every dental chair seemed simple enough. Initial efforts at scavenging included the making of an acrylic thimble that fit over the exhaling valve. This acrylic piece was attached to a rubber tube that carried the exhaled gases from the nasal hood to the suction system. Though this system did diminish N_2O levels at chairside, the problem of leakage around the periphery of the hood remained.

The scavenging nasal hood was soon developed. Several such devices are currently available, and the American Dental Association has adopted guidelines for their acceptance by the Council on Dental Materials, Instruments, and Equipment.[20] The scavenging nasal hood is a double mask: an inner mask that is contained within a slightly larger outer mask (Fig. 18-3). Each mask has two tubes entering into it, so that the entire apparatus has four tubes, two on either side of the nasal hood.

The inner mask receives a fresh supply of gases from the inhalation sedation unit and delivers the gas to the nose of the patient through two tubes that are slightly larger in diameter than the other two tubes. The outer, slightly larger, mask connects to two slightly smaller tubes that connect with the vacuum system. Thus a slight vacuum is present in the space between the inner and outer masks. On exhalation through the nose all exhaled gases are vented into the outer nasal hood and then, via the vacuum, are carried away from the patient and the treatment area.

An additional benefit of the scavenging nasal hood is that peripheral leakage of gases resulting from improper fit of the mask is prevented since the outer nasal hood is attached to the vacuum system and will remove any such gases before they reach the ambient air.

Optimal vacuum flow rate for operation of this system is 45 L/min. At this rate, leakage of N_2O into the room is prevented even when the mask is removed from the patient and a gas flow of 4 liters each of N_2O and O_2 is delivered through the nasal hood.[21]

Because the positioning of the scavenging nasal hood on the patient's face is not crucial to its proper functioning, such a device is termed *procedure inde-*

pendent. The nasal hood discussed previously, with the acrylic thimble, and the Bain Littell system (to be discussed next) are termed *procedure dependent* since peripheral leakage occurs when the mask is positioned improperly.

The effectiveness of the scavenging nasal hood cannot be denied. Table 18-4 presents the results of a study reported in the *Journal of the American Dental Association* in 1977.[16] Comparing the scavenging with the conventional mask, the concentration of N_2O is diminished by approximately 97% for the doctor and the assistant and 95% for the room.

A variation on the conventional nasal hood that reduces levels of N_2O is available. This is called the Bain/Littell breathing system and consists of a conventional nasal hood modified so that gas flow through it is one way (Fig. 18-4). Rather than both tubes delivering fresh gases to the patient, the Bain/

Littell system is designed so that one tube delivers fresh gases to the patient while the other carries exhaled gases away from the patient into the vacuum system. Check valves (one-way valves) are placed within the tubing to ensure a one-way flow of gas from the sedation unit to the nasal hood and then from the nasal hood into the other tube, which is attached to the suction system.

The Bain/Littell breathing system derives its effectiveness from an airtight seal between the nasal hood and the patient's face. Peripheral leakage produced by an improperly fitting nasal hood diminishes the effectiveness of this system. Because of its reliance on proper placement of the mask the Bain/Littell system is considered procedure-dependent. Table 18-4 compares the Bain/Littell system with the scavenging system.

The scavenging nasal hood is more effective than

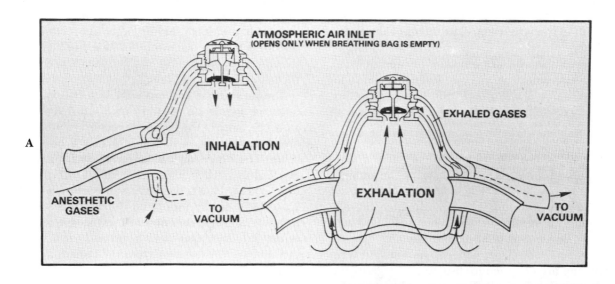

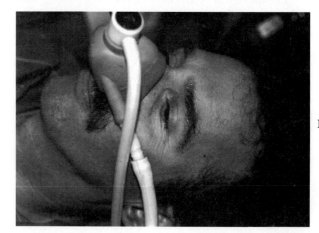

Fig. 18-3. A, Scavenging nasal hood. **B,** Scavenging mask in use.

the Bain/Littell system in decreasing N_2O levels in ambient air; however, the latter system appears to be somewhat more convenient to employ.

Air-sweep

Another device has been employed to decrease the concentration of N_2O being inhaled by dental personnel. The air-sweep is a portable electric fan attached to the light bracket on the dental chair. When operating, it blows the exhaled gases from the patient away from the breathing zones of chairside personnel. The air-sweep is useful in situations where the scavenging system is not being used or where in spite of the use of the scavenging system, unacceptably high levels of N_2O still occur. In the study by Whitcher et al.[16] the air-sweep was able to diminish the N_2O level from 31 ppm to 14 ppm, a 55% decrease.

Minimizing talking by patient

One of the most common sources of trace levels of N_2O is the patient. In spite of the scavenging nasal hood, and in spite of an airtight seal on the conventional nasal hood, significant levels of N_2O might be found if the patient talks a lot.

Unfortunately, some patients receiving inhalation sedation become more talkative as their inhibitions are peeled away through the actions of N_2O on the CNS. Additionally, some patients will begin to laugh or become giddy, to cry or to mouth breathe as the level of sedation produced by N_2O increases. Significant volumes of N_2O are exhaled into the breathing zones of chairside personnel in these circumstances.

Table 18-4. Comparison of Bain/Littell breathing system and scavenging nasal hood

System	N_2O level (ppm)
Bain/Littell	76 ± 8.0
Scavenging	34 ± 13

Modified from Whitcher CE, Zimmerman DC, Tonn EM et al: *JADA* 95:763, 1977. Copyright by the American Dental Association. Reprinted by permission.

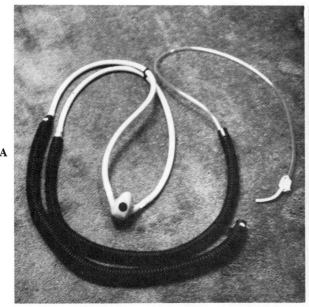

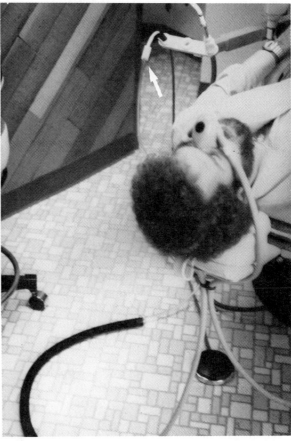

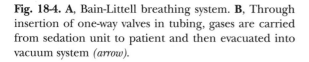

Fig. 18-4. A, Bain-Littell breathing system. **B,** Through insertion of one-way valves in tubing, gases are carried from sedation unit to patient and then evacuated into vacuum system *(arrow).*

Questioning the patient is important so that the operator may accurately determine the level of sedation. However, prolonged conversation is discouraged. Laughing, giddiness, crying, and mouth breathing are frequent indicators that the level of sedation is too great and should be diminished. A highly effective means of minimizing the loss of N_2O through the mouth is to use a rubber dam.

Monitoring of air

In addition to the factors previously mentioned, an ongoing program of monitoring the office environment for N_2O levels is recommended. N_2O leakage into the environment is inevitable and its detection may prove difficult. A regular monitoring system is therefore strongly recommended.

Although a number of nitrous oxide monitoring devices are presently available, the IR N_2O analyzer remains the most highly recommended. These units may frequently be rented from hospitals or service companies. Leaks located anywhere in the central system may be more easily detected with IR analyzers.

The goal of this detection program is to provide the minimal level of ambient air N_2O achievable in a given environment. The lower the level the better, for as stated previously it is not known at what level (if any) of N_2O exposure medical complications may develop. It behooves us therefore to make every effort to minimize our exposure to this highly effective and safe agent. Guidelines have been established stating that N_2O levels of 50 ppm are "reasonably achievable" in a time-weighted sample obtained within 6 to 10 inches of the dentist's nose when the N_2O flowmeter is on.[22] In the study by Whitcher et al.,[16] levels of 31 plus or minus 2.5 ppm and 31 plus or minus 4.8 ppm were obtained when the scavenging nasal hood was used in conjunction with relatively leak-free anesthesia/analgesia equipment. Levels this low are not readily achievable in all situations. Several papers have demonstrated that higher concentrations, below 1800 ppm, failed to produce any reproducible effect on methionine synthetase in chronically exposed dentists.[23] In another study no changes were detected in vitamin B_{12} function when ambient concentrations of N_2O were below 1000 ppm.[24] As a result a more reasonable standard of 400 ppm has been recommended.[23]

In the conclusion to Whitcher's article, the following ADA recommendations are provided[16]:

1. Use of scavenging equipment, such as a nasal hood
2. Venting of the suction unit outside the building
3. Minimizing conversation with the patient
4. Testing of the anesthesia/analgesia equipment for leakage:
   High-pressure system—at least monthly
   Low-pressure system—at least weekly when simple test procedures are applicable; otherwise as often as reasonable
5. Preventive maintenance of anesthesia/analgesia equipment, at least semiannually
6. Use of the air-sweep fan when acceptable concentrations of N_2O are not achieved with the aforementioned measures
7. Air monitoring program to prove the effectiveness of the control measures

Air monitoring should be performed at the beginning of an N_2O control program and at least every 4 months thereafter. A reasonable concentration of N_2O appears to be approximately 50 ppm when the recommended control measures are applied and the air is monitored as discussed. If levels in excess of 50 ppm are found, repairs should be undertaken immediately, with verification by a new air sample.

The ADA's Council on Dental Materials, Instruments, and Equipment has established Guidelines for an Acceptance Program for Scavenging Systems. The following devices were listed as acceptable in the *Dentist's Desk Reference,* edition 2, 1983.[25]

Blue Mask	Health Care Technology, Inc.
Brown Mask	Summit Services, Inc.
Clean Air Pollution Reduction System	Porter Instruments Co.
Fraser Harlake Nitrous Oxide Scavenging System	Fraser Sweatman

RECREATIONAL ABUSE OF NITROUS OXIDE

The use of N_2O for nonmedical purposes by health professionals and others is a second area of concern. Though this has been given the benign-sounding name *recreational abuse,* drug abuse is a more correct term, and it represents a potentially serious situation that can lead to the incapacitation of the health professional.

N_2O has been used for pleasurable, recreational purposes since its discovery in 1772[26]; the potential dangers of its social use were hinted at in 1915 but little or no concern was expressed in this regard until December 1977.[27,28]

That N_2O is a drug with a potential for abuse is well known. Those very same pharmacological properties that make N_2O so valuable as a clinical agent for sedation also make it quite attractive as a source podiatrist, veterinarian, auxiliary personnel, and lay public. Prior to 1977 the author received many telephone inquiries from dental assistants, hygienists, and dentists' spouses in which their concerns over the health and safety of "their dentist" were expressed. Dentists, callers reported, were using N_2O-O_2 as a means of relieving tension after a hard day at the office. In a situation where others might turn to alcohol to relieve their anxieties, these individuals turned to N_2O instead.

A typical question asked was "What danger, if any, is there in the self-administration of nitrous oxide with the inhalation sedation unit?" The response was, "While this type of behavior should not be condoned, there is little danger if the user is careful. Yes, deaths caused by the self-administration of N_2O have occurred.[29] Indeed, life insurance policies available to ADA members specifically exclude payment if the death is a result of the self-administration of N_2O.[30] If the abuser falls asleep (physiologic, not unconscious) in the dental chair while inhaling N_2O-O_2, a partial or total airway obstruction might develop. If the abuser is alone at this time, hypoxic brain damage, leading to prolonged morbidity or to death, might develop." Early in 1987 the deaths of two practicing dentists and one dental student from self-administration of nitrous oxide were reported.[31]

N_2O parties, which were the fashion in Great Britain in the 1830s and 1840s (Fig. 18-5), have once again become popular. Balloons or rubber gloves filled with 100% N_2O are inhaled by party guests until they feel intoxicated.[31] The popularity of this is such that a lay magazine, *High Times,* "the magazine of high society," featured an N_2O party in its centerfold, along with a listing of the dos and don'ts of N_2O etiquette for such occasions.[32] Even a popular television show of the 1970s, *Laverne and Shirley,* featured a segment concerning the pleasurable aspects of N_2O abuse.[33] An interesting book on "laughing gas" was published by Shedlin and Wallechinsky (Fig. 18-6).[34]

Nitrous oxide is legally available in small cylinders called whippets. These are used in the manufacture of whipping cream, N_2O being the propellant gas in whipped cream cylinders (see Fig. 18-7). Used properly, whipping cream is ejected from the cylinder; held improperly, 100% N_2O emerges. On Bourbon Street, in New Orleans, Louisiana, whippets of nitrous oxide are sold in novelty shops as "hits of laughing gas."

Investigation with police, hospital authorities, and

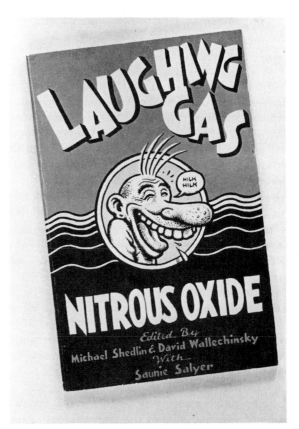

Fig. 18-6. N_2O is a popular drug of abuse among medical and dental professionals, as well as certain segments of the general public. (From Shedlin M, Wallechinsky D: *Laughing gas: nitrous oxide.* Berkeley, Cal, 1973, And/Or Press.)

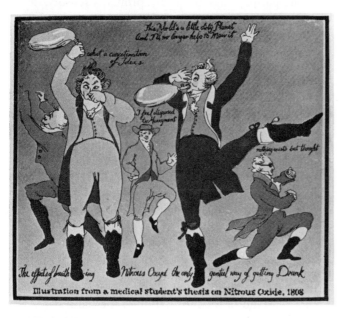

Fig. 18-5. Recreational abuse of N_2O dates back to its discovery in 1772.

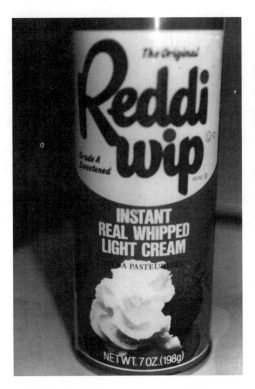
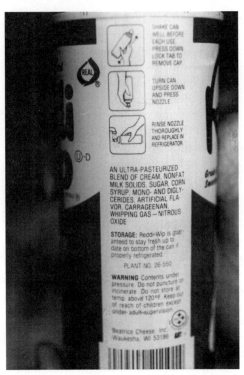

Fig. 18-7. Whipped cream container ultilizes nitrous oxide as its whipping gas *(right).*

N_2O are continually being stolen or reported as missing from hospitals, dental offices, and other medical facilities. Much of this gas is being used recreationally at N_2O parties (Fig. 18-8), and it now appears that much of this abuse is accounted for by health professionals (dentists, physicians, podiatrists, veterinarians), as well as by lay people.

In early 1992 not more than one mile away from this author's home, three teenagers were found dead in the front seat of their truck, asphyxiated while inhaling pure nitrous oxide from a "G" cylinder they had stolen from the loading dock of a local hospital.[35]

Reports have appeared in the medical and dental literature for many years demonstrating the effects of long-term administration of N_2O.[36-38] Most of the studies were on animals and the results may not be entirely transferrable to humans. Kripke et al.[36] reported that prolonged N_2O exposure is toxic to rapidly dividing mammalian cells. Lassen et al.[37] reported severe bone marrow depression in a group of patients receiving N_2O in the management of tetanus. Hayden et al.[38] reported that repeated long-term exposure of rats to N_2O-O_2 produced observable signs of damage to large cortical cells in the parietal and occipital cortices of the brain.

More recent, and significantly more disturbing, are the cases of N_2O-induced neuropathy that have been reported in the medical and dental literature.[39-43] Layzer et al.[39] reported three cases of a disabling peripheral neuropathy, primarily sensory, developing in three health professionals (two dentists, one laboratory technician) who habitually abused N_2O. In one case a 35-year-old dentist took naps 2 to 3 times a week while inhaling N_2O for 30 to 150 minutes at a time. N_2O concentrations were between 60% and 80%. Symptoms that developed included a nearly complete loss of sensation in the toes, followed by reduced tactile sensation in a stocking-glove distribution. Several months of abstention from further N_2O abuse led to a partial improvement in sensation, particularly in the hands. The second dentist, also 35 years old, noted numbness in his arms from the shoulders down and a feeling that his feet were swollen and numb. This doctor had inhaled N_2O for periods of from 10 minutes to 6 hours, 4 to 5 times a week, inhaling approximately 80% N_2O. Six months following cessation of N_2O abuse, mild numbness of the fingers and soles persisted along with mild motor incoordination of the hands.

I have had personal experience with a dentist who abused N_2O. In this case, abuse of N_2O for approxi-

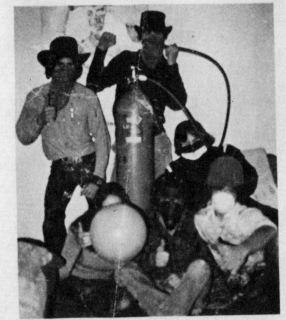

Tanks, I Needed That

Giggle gas kept us laughing through the great blizzards of '77. The 187-pound tank

lasted us three months. It kept us grinning and numb, but not from the cold.
—*Nitrous Freaks of Toledo, Ohio*

Fig. 18-8. Abuse potential of N_2O is illustrated by this letter to the editor. (Courtesy *High Times* magazine.)

mately 6 months led to a peripheral sensory neuropathy of the hands and legs. That N_2O abuse is the likely cause of these signs and symptoms seems probable because of the improvement noted in all victims following cessation of N_2O abuse. In the case I observed, reexposure to N_2O following the return of normal sensation led immediately to a return of the sensory neuropathy. This exposure occurred when the dentist administered N_2O-O_2 to a patient through an unscavenged nasal hood. Following installation of a scavenging device and monitoring of the N_2O-O_2 system for leakage, this doctor was able to administer N_2O to patients without a return of signs and symptoms.

Abuse of N_2O is not a prerequisite for the development of peripheral sensory neuropathy. One of the coauthors of a paper by Malamed et al.[40] noted the development of mild sensory neuropathy (paresthesia of the fingers and toes) after 28 years of exposure to unmonitored trace levels of N_2O in a busy oral and maxillofacial surgery practice. N_2O-O_2 was administered frequently and without a scavenging

device. Elimination of N_2O from this practice led to a marked reversal of symptoms.

It is highly unlikely that the neurological injury described in these papers was produced by hypoxia or anoxia. In all cases the involved doctor used inhalation sedation units that were equipped with fail-safe devices, including minimum O_2 percentages.[41-43] In addition, there were no indications in any reported case of any evidence of cerebral symptoms, which would be expected in the presence of hypoxia or anoxia.

Nitrous oxide inhibits the actions of methionine synthetase, an enzyme involved in vitamin B_{12} metabolism leading to impaired bone marrow function.[44,45]

A direct cause and effect relationship exists between N_2O abuse and the development of peripheral sensory neuropathy. It is important for the dental profession to awaken to the fact that this popular and highly effective technique of conscious sedation is capable of producing serious problems when abused. In response to the question of how large the problem of professional abuse of N_2O is, the answer remains that we are unsure of its magnitude.

Casual observation leads to the belief that a significant number of dentists and dental personnel use N_2O-O_2 for nonprofessional purposes.[46,47] In an attempt to more accurately assess the problem, Orr[46] surveyed dentists concerning the use of N_2O in their practices. Of 881 respondees, 304 employed N_2O to some degree. Forty-nine (18%) reported that they had noted adverse effects on themselves at one time or another during administration of N_2O to patients. These effects included dizziness, lightheadedness or euphoria, headache, nausea or vomiting, and paresthesia of hands or feet.

Abuse of N_2O does occur within the dental profession. Twenty doctors (7%) admitted that they regularly used nitrous oxide for recreational purposes. Abuse of nitrous oxide is not, however, limited to dental personnel. Sahenk et al.[48] reported a case of neuropathy developing with the inhalation of N_2O from whipped cream dispensers. Surveys have indicated that inhalation of N_2O is popular among college students and medical and dental school students.[49]

The problem of N_2O abuse, while not new, has been brought to the surface. Once thought to be the source of a quick "high" associated with no adverse effects, N_2O has been shown to have potentially serious effects on those who abuse it. Sensory loss to the hands in dental professionals is catastrophic.

Is nitrous oxide addictive in the same manner as

opioid analgesics? Gillman[50,51] reported that although it is not possible to state unequivocally that nitrous oxide interacts with the endogenous opioid system to produce addictive behavior, a considerable body of evidence supporting this hypothesis has been presented. It must be emphasized that *the peripheral sensory neuropathies described do not develop in the patient who receives N₂O-O₂ on a controlled basis.* Long-term exposure to high concentrations of N_2O has been implicated as the causative factor in these cases. Common sense and a basic principle of pharmacology state that no drug exerts an action on only one system in the body. All drugs exert multiple actions, some beneficial and some potentially dangerous. N_2O, like all drugs, adheres to these principles. Following many years of darkness, we have today awakened to the fact that N_2O is indeed a drug, not an innocuous vapor, and that as such it cannot and must not be abused.

SEXUAL PHENOMENA AND NITROUS OXIDE

In recent years an increasing number of situations have been reported in which a male doctor has been accused of sexual assault by a female patient who received conscious sedation or general anesthesia during her dental treatment.[52-54] Though some accusations followed the administration of intravenous sedation, the overwhelming majority followed the use of N_2O-O_2 inhalation sedation. Disturbingly, a significant number of these accusations led to formal complaints being lodged with law enforcement agencies. Most have involved formal hearings before state dental boards with a consideration of loss of professional licensure. The possibility of being accused of sexual improprieties, when in fact the patient may have been dreaming, presents a serious problem for the administrator of inhalation sedation as well as all other sedation techniques. Several typical cases will be reviewed.[52]

Case 1. A healthy 28-year-old woman had a chipped tooth restored while under inhalation sedation and local anesthesia. The patient claimed that no one else was present in the dental office during her treatment. She reported that she received too much N_2O and fell asleep. Subsequently she described an experience in which the dentist made sexual advances toward her. Following recovery, the patient left the dental office and after talking about the incident to a friend reported it to authorities. The percentage of N_2O administered to this patient is unknown, having not been recorded on the patient's dental chart.

Case 2. A young woman was seen by a general dentist for placement of a crown. The patient had difficulty in making appointments and finally, out of frustration, the dentist agreed to see the patient after regular office hours. The patient had a history of epilepsy. She received a local anesthetic for pain control and N_2O-O_2 for sedation. She stated that she fell asleep twice during the procedure and awoke when she was stimulated sexually. She experienced mild dizziness and slight amnesia for a few hours after the sedation but otherwise recovered normally. She did not return to this dentist for further care although she did not mention the incident to the dentist at the time of discharge. The record indicates that the patient received 66% N_2O.

Case 3. A healthy 28-year-old woman had been undergoing endodontic treatment for several months. She usually received a local anesthetic and N_2O-O_2 sedation. On several occasions the patient described her reaction to N_2O as "being extremely groggy afterwards." The doctor's records indicate that the patient received approximately 60% N_2O. On the fifth, sixth, and seventh treatments using N_2O, the patient also reported unusual dreams. The patient did not say anything to the doctor immediately after these occurrences because "I kept putting it out of my mind, that it didn't really happen and kept trying to convince myself it was only the influence of the gas making me think it did." The patient returned for additional dental treatment and received N_2O without further incident.

Case 4. An indigent female patient was given free restorative treatments either before or after regular office hours as a charitable gesture. Because of her high degree of apprehension about dental care the dentist prescribed oral diazepam followed by N_2O-O_2 sedation and local anesthesia. On one occasion the patient did not take the diazepam and 70% N_2O was required for sedation. She described being drowsy but was still aware of a feeling of pressure on her breasts and her genital region. After recovering from the sedation she mentioned that she would call the dentist for a follow-up appointment and left the office without any discussion of the experience.

Table 18-5 summarizes the findings in nine cases of sexual phenomena associated with the administration of N_2O-O_2 sedation.[52] All of the cases just reviewed were brought before their state board of dental examiners. In all cases district attorneys were involved in preliminary criminal investigations and one complaint resulted in a closed hearing by a grand jury. Only one of the criminal investigations

Table 18-5. Summary—nine cases of sexual phenomena

Case	Age	% N₂O	Type of phenomenon	Patient comments
1	28	—	Visual*	Fell asleep
2	—	—	Tactile†	Fell asleep
3	28	60	Tactile and visual	—
4	33	70	Tactile and auditory‡	—
5	28	50	Tactile	—
6	15	66	Tactile	Dream state
7	15	66	Tactile and visual	Euphoric state, unable to move
8	29	66	Tactile	Fantasy
9	31	50 to 80	Tactile	Became unconscious

*Dentist reportedly attempted to see patient's breast or pelvic area.
†Dentist reportedly attempted to fondle patient's breast or pelvic area.
‡Suggestive comments reportedly made.

resulted in a jury trial—the dentist was acquitted of all charges. In all other cases and for a variety of reasons criminal charges were ultimately dismissed. Board of dental examiners hearings, however, can be another matter entirely. In one instance the dentist's license was revoked for 1 year, being reinstated at a later time, with restrictions. In another instance, a formal reprimand was issued. Most of the other cases were dismissed after a formal hearing or dropped because of insufficient evidence.

The cases reported here, and another 40 that have been reported since the publication of the Jastak and Malamed[52] paper, have several factors in common:

1. All complaints were from young female patients and involved male dentists.
2. No patient discussed her experience with the doctor after recovery from the sedation.
3. Many of the women commented later on how shocked or stunned they were that this might have occurred.
4. Several patients mentioned that they were unable to think clearly until the next day.
5. Formal complaints to either a law enforcement agency or to a state dental board did not occur until either family members or friends were told of the experience and advice was sought as to how to proceed.
6. No patient gave any indication of distress during treatment, but most mentioned spontaneously that they were frightened by the experience.
7. At the time of the perceived occurrence, the male doctor was alone in the treatment room with the female patient. In only two cases was a dental assistant or any other person present in the treatment room with the doctor and pa-

tient. This appears to be the key factor that allowed these cases to be seriously considered by law enforcement agencies.

8. Concentrations of N₂O in excess of 50% were administered in every situation in which allegations of sexual misconduct were involved.

The incidence of dreaming and hallucinations during the use of N₂O sedation in dentistry is unknown. A study of 1331 cases of inhalation sedation uncovered three cases.[55] It was also determined in this study and corroborated by many other studies that the overwhelming majority of patients will achieve clinically acceptable sedation at levels below 50% N₂O. Many of the reports discussing dreaming and other neuropsychiatric responses with N₂O involve concentrations greater than 50%. Rosenberg found an increased incidence of dreaming from 2% to 29% with the administration of 40% and 80% N₂O respectively in young, healthy females.[56] Other responses noted in this study included paranoid auditory and visual hallucinations, panic, anger, and emotionally kaleidoscopic dreams.

Sexually oriented hallucinations associated with the administration of N₂O-O₂ had not been described in the literature until 1980[52]; however, sexually related responses to N₂O have been known for many years.[57,58] Allen,[59] in his textbook, writes, "A female chaperone is essential in an office where nitrous oxide-oxygen is administered, owing to the propensity of females under nitrous oxide-oxygen to have sexual abreactions." Reports of sexual orgasm while receiving N₂O during routine dental care are available from reliable sources. In a survey of 50 female dental hygiene students 18% expressed a feeling of sexual arousal or increased sexuality while receiving N₂O-O₂ sedation.[60] In a more recent survey

Table 18-6. Summary of findings

	Sexually active	Sexually inactive	Total
Fantasy present	2 (9.5%)	4 (12.9%)	6 (11.5%)
Fantasy not present	19 (90.5%)	27 (87.1%)	46 (88.5%)
Total	21	31	62

Malamed SF et al: Unpublished results of N₂O survey, 1983.

10% of 88 male and female dental students reported feelings of increased sexuality or arousal while receiving N_2O (see Table 18-6).[61] There was no difference in the occurrence of sexual arousal in persons describing themselves as sexually active from those classifying themselves as not sexually active.

It is extremely likely that the incidence of sexually oriented dreams or hallucinations during inhalation sedation is higher than is imagined, but in the typical dental office situation, with both a chairside assistant and a busy office setting, potential complaints by a patient are probably obviated by the relative unlikelihood of the experience having occurred (e.g., "It must have been a dream!"). In addition, patients seem to be somewhat reticent to report such phenomena, although the frequency of such accusations appears to be increasing.

Recommendations

The allegation of sexual impropriety against a health professional is devastating in its potential impact on the livelihood of that person whether the allegation is subsequently proved or disproved. As with all situations involving potential risk it is best to attempt to avoid their occurrence. To do so in this one area is easily accomplished. If put into practice, the following two recommendations related to the administration of N_2O-O_2 inhalation sedation will essentially eliminate the possibility of such allegations:

1. Never sedate any patient with any technique of sedation without an assistant present in the room.
2. Do not routinely use N_2O in concentrations greater than 50%. Always titrate N_2O-O_2.

REFERENCES

1. Council on Dental Education, American Dental Association: Guidelines for teaching the comprehensive control of pain and anxiety in dentistry, *J Dent Educ* 36:62, 1972.
2. Petrelli G, Siepi G, Miligi L et al: Solvents in pesticides, *Scand J Work Environ Health* 19(1):63, 1993.
3. Venning GR: Identification of adverse reactions to new drugs. I: What have been the important adverse reactions since thalidomide? *Br Med J* 286:199, 1983.
4. Vaisman AI: Work in surgical theatres and its influence on the health of anesthesiologists, *Eksp Khir Anestheziol* 3:44, 1967.
5. Askrog V, Harvald B: Teratogen effect of inhalation anesthetics, *Nord Med* 83:498, 1970.
6. Lencz L, Nemes C: Morbidity of Hungarian anesthesiologists in relation to occupational hazard. In Corbett TH: Anesthetics as a cause of abortion, *Fertil Steril* 23:866, 1972.
7. Bruce D, Eide KA, Linde HM et al: Causes of death among anesthesiologists: a 20 year survey, *Anesthesiology* 35:348, 1971.
8. Cohen EN, Belville JW, Brown BW: Anesthesia, pregnancy and miscarriage: a study of operating room nurses and anesthetists, *Anesthesiology* 35:343, 1971.
9. Whitcher CE, Cohen EN, Trudell JR: Chronic exposure to anesthetic gases in the operating room, *Anesthesiology* 35:348, 1971.
10. Whitcher C, Zimmerman DC, Piziali RL: Control of occupational exposure to nitrous oxide in the oral surgery office, *J Oral Surg* 36:431, 1978.
11. Cohen EN, Brown BW Jr et al: A survey of anesthetic health hazards among dentists, *JADA* 90:1291, 1975.
12. Cohen EN, Brown BW Jr, Wu ML et al: Occupational disease in dentistry and chronic exposure to trace anesthetic gases, *JADA* 101:21, 1980.
13. Rowland AS, Baird DD, Weinberg CR et al: Reduced fertility among women employed as dental assistants exposed to high levels of nitrous oxide, *N Engl J Med* 327(14):993, 1992.
14. Scavenging equipment prevents nitrous oxide fertility threat, *JADA* 123(12):18, 1992.
15. Hillman KM, Saloojee Y, Brett I et al: Nitrous oxide concentrations in the dental surgery, *Anaesthesia* 36:257, 1981.
16. Whitcher CE, Zimmerman DC, Tonn EM et al: Control of occupational exposure to nitrous oxide in the dental operatory, *JADA* 95:763, 1977.
17. Allen WA: Nitrous oxide in the surgery; pollution and scavenging, *Br Dent J* 159:222, 1985.
18. Lane GA: Measurement of anesthetic pollution in oral surgery offices, *J Oral Surg* 36:444, 1978.
19. Landauer RS Jr. & Co, Division of Tech Ops Inc, Glenwood Science Park, Glenwood, Ill 40425.
20. Council on Dental Therapeutics, American Dental Association: List of accepted products, *JADA* 105:940, 1982.
21. Borganelli GN, Primosch RE, Henry RJ: Operatory ventilation and scavenger evacuation rate influence on ambient nitrous oxide levels, *J Dent Res* 72(9):1275, 1993.
22. Donaldson D, Orr J: A comparison of the effectiveness of nitrous oxide scavenging devices, *Can Dent J* 55:541, 1989.
23. Sweeney B, Bingham RM, Amos RJ et al: Toxicity of bone marrow in dentists exposed to nitrous oxide, *Br Med J* 291:567, 1985.
24. Nunn JF, Sharer NM, Royston D et al: Serum methinonine and hepatic enzyme activity in anaesthetists exposed to nitrous oxide, *Br J Anaesth* 54:593, 1982.
25. American Dental Association: *Dentists' desk reference: materials, instruments, and equipment*, ed 2. Chicago, 1983, American Dental Association.
26. Davy H: Researches, chemical and philosophical: chiefly concerning nitrous oxide, 1798. In Fullmer JZ: *Sir Humphry Davy's published works*. Cambridge, 1969, Harvard University Press.
27. Talbot F: Psychic disturbances in nitrous oxide analgesia, *Br Dent J* 36:668, 1915.
28. Layzer RB, Fishman RA, Schafer JA: Neuropathy following abuse of nitrous oxide, *Neurology* 28:504, 1978.

29. Wagner SA, Clark MA, Wesche DL et al: Asphyxial deaths from recreational use of nitrous oxide, *J Forensic Sci* 37(4):1008, 1992.

30. American Dental Association. ADA Life Insurance. Chicago, 1994, American Dental Association.

31. Suruda AJ, McGlothlin JD: Fatal abuse of nitrous oxide in the workplace, *J Occup Med* 32(8):682, 1990.

32. Nitrous oxide party, *High Times Magazine* p. 63, June 1977.

33. "Laverne and Shirley" featured a segment concerning the pleasurable aspects of N_2O abuse.

34. Shedlin M, Wallechinsky D: *Laughing gas, nitrous oxide,* Berkeley, Calif, 1973, And/Or Press.

35. Three found dead and laughing gas is blamed (asphyxiation from nitrous oxide inhalation), Los Angeles, Calif, *The New York Times* 141, 1 (March 8, 1992), p 32(L).

36. Kripke BJ et al: Testicular reaction to prolonged exposure to nitrous oxide, *Anesthesiology* 44:104, 1976.

37. Lassen HC, Henriksen E, Neukirch R et al: Treatment of tetanus, severe bone marrow depression after prolonged nitrous oxide anesthesia, *Lancet* 1:527, 1956.

38. Hayden J Jr, Allen GD, Butler LA et al: An evaluation of prolonged nitrous oxide-oxygen sedation in rats, *JADA* 89:1374, 1974.

39. Layzer RB, Fishman RA, Schafer JA: Neuropathy following abuse of nitrous oxide, *Neurology* 28:504, 1978.

40. Malamed SF, Orr DL II, Hershfield S et al: The recreational abuse of nitrous oxide by health professionals, *J Calif Dent Assoc* 8:38, 1980.

41. Ayer WA, Russell EA Jr, Burge JR: Psychomotor responses of dentists using nitrous oxide-oxygen psychosedation, *Anesth Prog* 25:85, 1978.

42. Moore PA: Psychomotor impairment due to N_2O exposure, *Anesth Prog* 30:72, 1983.

43. Stacy CB, DiRocci A, Gould RJ: Methionine in the treatment of nitrous oxide-induced neuropathy and myeloneuropathy, *J Neurol* 239(7):401, 1992.

44. Landon MJ, Creagh-Barry P, McAuthur S et al: Influence of vitamin B12 status on inactivation of methionine synthase by nitrous oxide, *Brit J Anaesth* 69(1):81, 1992.

45. Alston TA: Inhibition of vitamin B12-dependent microbial growth by nitrous oxide, *Life Sci* 48(16):1591, 1991.

46. Orr D: N_2O-O_2 questionnaire, unpublished research for University of Utah Medical Center Department of Anesthesiology, Salt Lake City, 1976.

47. Gillman MA: Nitrous oxide abuse in perspective, *Clin Neuropharmacol* 15(4):297, 1992.

48. Sahenk Z, Mendell JR, Couri D et al: Polyneuropathy from inhalation of N_2O cartridges through a whipped cream dispenser, *Neurology* 28:485, 1978.

49. Heyer EJ, Simpson DM, Bodis-Wollner I et al: Nitrous oxide: clinical and electrophysiologic investigation of neurologic complications, *Neurology* 36(12):1618, 1986.

50. Gillman MA: Nitrous oxide: an opioid addictive agent, *Am J Med* 81:97, 1986.

51. Aston R: Drug abuse: its relationship to dental practice, *Dent Clin North Am* 28(3):595, 1984.

52. Jastak JT, Malamed SF: Nitrous oxide and sexual phenomena, *JADA* 101:38, 1980.

53. Lambert C: Sexual phenomena, hypnosis, and nitrous oxide sedation, *JADA* 105:990, 1982.

54. Gillman MA: Assessment of the effects of analgesic concentrations of nitrous oxide on human sexual response, *Int J Neurosci* 43(1-2):27, 1988.

55. Jastak JT, Paravecchio R: An analysis of 1331 sedations using inhalation, intravenous, and other techniques, *JADA* 91:1242, 1975.

56. Rosenberg P: The effect of nitrous oxide-oxygen inhalation on subjective experiences of healthy young adults, *Ann Chir Gynaecol* 63:500, 1974.

57. Seldin HM: *Practical anesthesia for dental and oral surgery,* ed 3, Philadelphia, 1947, Lea & Febiger.

58. Archer WH: *A manual of dental anesthesia,* Philadelphia, 1952, WB Saunders.

59. Allen GD: *Dental anesthesia and analgesia (local and general),* ed 2. Baltimore, 1979, Williams & Wilkins.

60. Malamed SF, Serxner K, Wiedenfeld AM: The incidence of sexual phenomena in females receiving nitrous oxide and oxygen inhalation sedation, *J Am Analg Soc* 22(2):9.

61. Malamed SF: Results of N_2O survey, Unpublished manuscript, 1983.

CHAPTER *19*

Practical considerations

In previous chapters of this section the technique of administration, complications, and current concerns associated with inhalation sedation have been discussed. In this chapter a number of additional factors are discussed that are not always included in the training of a doctor to administer inhalation sedation. Many of these questions do not usually arise until the doctor has been employing inhalation sedation for a period of time.

DETERMINATION OF PROPER TITRATION AT SUBSEQUENT VISITS

One of the most important factors to consider when using inhalation sedation is that the gases have a very rapid onset of action. Because of this rapid onset, it becomes possible for patients to be titrated to a precise level of sedation. The ability to titrate with inhalation sedation is of considerable importance because it is quite possible that a patient may require different concentrations of N_2O to achieve the same level of sedation at subsequent visits. It is not possible to predict with surety prior to treatment at what level of N_2O the patient will become comfortable. The required concentration of N_2O may be either greater or lesser than that of previous visits. Titration is the only means for the administrator to satisfactorily determine this level. Factors that may influence the concentration of N_2O necessary for adequate sedation include the patient's dental anxiety level, nondental stresses, the time of day, and the patient's level of restfulness.

Dental anxiety

As the patient's dental anxiety decreases, the percentage of N_2O necessary to achieve a given level of sedation will correspondingly decrease, with all other variables remaining equal. With proper patient management by both the doctor and the office staff, a fearful patient should become less apprehensive about the prospect of dental treatment with each succeeding visit. If the patient is titrated carefully to his "ideal sedation level," it will be observed that he will probably require somewhat lower N_2O concentrations as he becomes progressively less phobic over time.

Although this is true for most patients and for most forms of dental treatment, it is also possible that a patient who has been responding quite well at 30% N_2O will have an inadequate clinical effect from that concentration when a different type of dental treatment is undertaken. For example, this patient may respond quite well at 30% N_2O for restorative treatment; however, when undergoing periodontal surgery the patient may require 45% N_2O. This is explained by the increased level of anxiety produced in this patient by the prospect of a surgical procedure in contrast to the more benign (in this patient's mind) restorative treatment.

Nondental stresses

A significant influence on the level of N_2O required for sedation is nondental stress. The patient's state of mind has a significant bearing on the manner in which CNS depressant drugs act. A patient may arrive at the dental office on a day in which things have just not gone well. For example, the patient may have started the day having an argument with a spouse, spent 1 or more hours in heavy traffic, encountered business difficulties, and had to rush to get to the dental office in time for the appointment. If this patient has any degree of dental anxiety, it becomes obvious that our N_2O has a formidable task facing it. Contrast this with the same patient who arrives at the dental office having had a simply wonderful day. Everything that could have gone right for this patient did. The patient arrives in the office in a cheerful mood. The concentration of N_2O required to sedate this patient will probably be lower than that required in the first situation.

It is impossible, and indeed foolhardy, to discount the influence of outside stresses on the dental patient. All practicing dentists, dental hygienists, physicians, and podiatrists have encountered remarkably different behavior patterns from the same patient at different visits. The process of titrating N_2O will help to compensate for the effects of these outside influences.

Time of day

The time of day at which a patient is treated may have considerable bearing on the concentration of N_2O required for sedation. Although this problem is noted primarily in pediatric dentistry, many adult patients will exhibit these same tendencies.

As discussed in Chapter 5, it is recommended that the phobic patient, as well as the medically compromised patient, be scheduled for dental treatment earlier in the day. At this time, presumably following a period of restful sleep, the medically compromised patient is rested and better able to tolerate any additional stresses imposed by dental treatment. The fearful patient ought to be treated early in the day for the simple reason that the patient will want to get ''it'' over with as soon as possible. The dental appointment might well be the most unpleasant part of this patient's day. An appointment scheduled late in the day allows the patient more time to worry and for a level of anxiety to increase. Scheduled later in the day this patient might well require significantly greater levels of N_2O to achieve sedation than would have been necessary if he had been treated earlier in the morning.

Level of restfulness

The level of restfulness has an effect on the patient's pain reaction threshold and therefore on the response to inhalation sedation. Patients who are tired, unable to sleep the night prior to the appointment because of fear of dentistry, overreact to most stimuli. With their ''nerves on edge'' they interpret usually nonpainful stimuli as being painful. N_2O-O_2 inhalation sedation may still prove to be effective; however, the patient may require considerably greater concentrations of N_2O.

When a patient appears to be quite apprehensive about an upcoming treatment, it is prudent for the doctor to address this fact and consider prescribing a sedative-hypnotic for the patient 1 hour before bed-

time the evening before the scheduled treatment. A well-rested patient may require lower concentrations of N_2O to achieve comparable levels of sedation than the overtired patient.

• • •

When the four factors mentioned are considered, it becomes obvious that the same person may respond to N_2O in an entirely different manner at subsequent appointments. Where titration is not employed, it is entirely possible that the level of N_2O used at prior visits will produce either the same level of sedation, decreased levels of sedation, or overly deep sedation of the same patient. The use of titration at each and every dental appointment minimizes the significance of these factors.

WHY NOT A FIXED DOSE?

One of the most frequently heard complaints from doctors who have completed training in inhalation sedation is that the technique worked quite well on their patients for a few months, but then for some unknown reason an ever-increasing number of patients commented that they no longer like N_2O sedation, or more of their patients experienced adverse reactions to it. Some doctors have even ceased using this technique for these reasons. Why does this happen?

The answer is quite simple. The absence of titration leads to increased patient reports of negative reactions to N_2O, and their doctors begin to shy away from its use.

Following a training course in inhalation sedation the doctor goes back to the office and begins the use of N_2O-O_2 as it was taught in the course. The technique works quite well, patients are successfully sedated, and side effects are minimal. Following this initial period of familiarization the doctor seeks to speed up the sedation procedure so that the dental treatment can begin more quickly. To do so the doctor ceases to titrate patients to their proper level of sedation. Arbitrary, fixed concentrations of N_2O are administered instead. Commonly, 40% or 50% N_2O is administered. When administered in this manner, the incidence of adverse responses increases.

To demonstrate the difference achieved between titration and fixed N_2O levels I will carefully titrate a doctor to his or her ideal sedation level, for example, 40% N_2O. After full recovery on 100% oxygen, I administer the same concentration of N_2O to the doctor without titration, simply establishing a 40% N_2O

concentration and putting the nasal hood in place. Though this technique will, on occasion, provide an acceptable level of sedation, more often than not the patient will complain that the effects of the nitrous oxide "came on too fast" and that he or she felt uncomfortable. In clinical practice this effect might be noticed when the patient suddenly pulls the nasal hood off his face.

If 40% or 50% is the most commonly employed concentration of N_2O in this nontitrating technique, it becomes obvious, from looking at the normal distribution curve for inhalation sedation, that many patients receiving N_2O will be oversedated. The bell-shaped curve (Chapter 16) for N_2O is such that most patients achieve ideal sedation with concentrations under 40%. To routinely administer levels of N_2O of 40% to 50% is to invite increased failure. The 3 to 4 minutes required to achieve sedation via titration will minimize the occurrence of unpleasant reactions to N_2O. It is obvious that such time is time well spent.

POOR PATIENT EVALUATION

This factor is somewhat similar to the one discussed previously. I have observed the administration of inhalation sedation by many persons. One of the most disturbing things that I have noticed is that the so-called experienced doctor (with inhalation sedation) will often appear to be sedating the patient to a level that he or she thinks is appropriate for the patient and not a level at which the patient may in fact feel comfortable. In so doing the doctor will be ignoring the many signs and symptoms that the patient will be exhibiting during the procedure. One of the most important safety features of all pharmacosedative techniques is that the patient remains conscious and is able to respond to verbal and physical stimuli. To ignore a patient's input during the important induction phase of sedation is foolhardy. Information imparted by the patient is quite important in the overall assessment of his or her well-being. The patient should be used as a vital component of the overall monitoring of conscious sedation.

PATIENT UNATTENDED DURING SEDATION

Occasions may develop during the treatment of a particular patient when the doctor will be called away for a few moments to attend to some other business. When a patient is undergoing treatment without the concurrent use of sedative medications, leaving him unattended is usually acceptable. However, in any situation in which a patient has received, or is receiving, any CNS depressant drug (e.g., N_2O), the patient must never be left unattended.

This is quite important during inhalation sedation. When N_2O is administered, a constant flow of gases is delivered to the patient. Dental treatment serves as a stimulus to the patient to lighten the level of sedation. When dental treatment stops but the N_2O level is left constant, the depth of sedation will become increasingly deep. The lack of treatment stimulation is the primary reason for this occurrence. This will not normally result in any serious difficulty when someone is present in the treatment room monitoring the patient. However, there have been incidents in which a patient vomited with no one in attendance; other situations have developed in which the airway has been compromised. In the absence of a trained person to monitor the patient and to promptly recognize and manage the situation, significant morbidity or mortality may result.

Should it become essential for the doctor to have to leave a patient receiving N_2O for even a few short minutes, a well-trained assistant should be available to remain with the patient in the treatment area. In addition, because of the lack of treatment-induced stimulation of this patient, the level of N_2O should be decreased by approximately 10% whenever there is a pause in treatment for more than a few minutes. In the absence of a second person to monitor the patient, the doctor must terminate the flow of N_2O, reestablish a flow of 100% O_2, and return the patient to the presedative state before leaving the treatment area. Though this second option is more cumbersome, it should be followed whenever there is no other person available to monitor the patient.

As mentioned in Chapter 18, there is yet another, more important, reason for the doctor to have a second person available during sedative procedures—that of minimizing the possibility of being accused (falsely) of sexual improprieties. It is my recommendation that a second person be present in the treatment area whenever a patient receives any pharmacosedative technique.

SHIVERING DURING RECOVERY

N_2O possesses vasodilating properties, peripheral blood vessels becoming larger than they were prior to the administration of N_2O. Advantage is often taken of this property during attempts at venipuncture: the patient is sedated with N_2O-O_2, the peripheral blood vessels dilate, the venipuncture is established, and the N_2O is terminated.

Vasodilation may also lead to a loss of body heat during the sedative procedure. Such heat is lost through blood vessels near the surface. When these vessels dilate, blood flow through them is increased and heat loss through skin is increased. Some patients may also begin to perspire during N_2O administration, another mechanism through which the body loses heat. Through these mechanisms the body temperature of the patient receiving N_2O-O_2 sedation is artificially lowered. It must be remembered that peripheral vasodilation and perspiration are two of the body's mechanisms for lowering its temperature when it becomes overheated. N_2O activates these mechanisms even though the patient's body is not overheated. Therefore the temperature of the patient may actually become lower than normal during a long inhalation sedation session.

At the conclusion of the procedure, when the flow of N_2O is terminated and 100% O_2 is administered, the vasodilatation and perspiration effects of the N_2O cease. At this time the patient's body is somewhat hypothermic and the body acts to warm itself. Shivering is one method of so doing. Peripheral vasoconstriction and involuntary skeletal muscle contraction occur (shivering). Peripheral vasoconstriction preserves heat, while involuntary skeletal muscle contraction actually produces heat, thus aiding the body in its effort to warm itself.

Management of the patient at this time is simply to explain what has happened so as to minimize any anxiety that may be felt, and to treat the patient symptomatically. Covering the patient with blankets or a plastic apron will usually suffice to speed warming. The duration of the shivering is usually short, about 5 to 10 minutes.

IMPROPER RECOVERY PROCEDURES

Too many doctors will terminate the flow of N_2O and simply remove the nasal hood, permitting the patient to breathe atmospheric air rather than 100% O_2. As will be noted in the following situation, such practice leads to an increased incidence of post-inhalation sedation complications. I have also become aware of the fact that many doctors who do administer 100% O_2 to their patients following N_2O-O_2 sedation do so for a fixed period of time (e.g., 2 minutes) regardless of the length of the inhalation sedation that preceded it. As was discussed in earlier chapters on pharmacology and technique of administration, a minimum period of from 3 to 5 minutes of 100% O_2 is required for the majority of the N_2O to be eliminated from the patient's body. A period of 3 to 5 minutes is considered a minimum. After this period of time the degree of recovery is assessed and if necessary the patient kept on 100% O_2 for an additional period of time.

Discharging the patient without an escort may be permissible when the doctor is assured that patient recovery is complete. Not all patients recover rapidly and completely from inhalation sedation. Doctors who do not use any objective criteria in assessing patient recovery from N_2O-O_2 rely solely on their subjective assessment of how the patient feels. Although this procedure may prove to be adequate for most patients, it is by no means recommended because for some patients it falls far short of being reliable.

Other means of assessing recovery ought to be employed routinely whenever inhalation sedation is used if the patient is to be permitted to leave the office alone. If it is the doctor's habit to require an escort to take the patient home following inhalation sedation, the requirement of complete recovery is not as critical.

Two means of assessment of recovery from sedation are recommended: monitoring of vital signs and the Trieger test. These have been discussed earlier in this section. Vital signs, especially blood pressure, heart rate and rhythm, and respiratory rate, are monitored at a patient's first visit to the dental office to establish baseline vital signs. These same parameters are recorded immediately preoperatively, every 15 minutes during the procedure, and postoperatively after the patient has been receiving 100% O_2 for the number of minutes required for recovery. The postoperative recordings are compared with both the preoperative and baseline values, and if they are reasonably close to these readings it may be assumed that the drugs administered to the patient are no longer producing a depressant action on the cardiorespiratory system. The Trieger test is a test of motor coordination.[1] The patient is given the Trieger test prior to the administration of N_2O to establish a baseline score for motor coordination. At the termination of the recovery phase (when subjectively the patient appears recovered), a second Trieger test is administered. Comparison of the postoperative to the preoperative test provides an objective assessment of the patient's ability to perform fine motor movements.

Both the Trieger test and the monitoring of vital signs are strongly recommended for use in all patients receiving inhalation sedation if the doctor wishes to permit the patients to leave the office unescorted, to drive their automobiles, and to return to work. Though most patients may be able to perform these tasks well following N_2O-O_2 sedation, it must always be remembered that some will not be able to do so, and for the doctor to assume that they are able to function normally is inappropriate.

Proper oxygenation at the end of inhalation sedation and proper assessment of recovery prior to discharge will prevent virtually all of the uncomfortable side effects and potential problems associated with inhalation sedation.

POSTSEDATION NAUSEA, HEADACHE, AND LETHARGY

Following inhalation sedation, the patient, feeling symptom-free and having completed appropriate recovery tests, may be discharged from the office. In most instances the patient will continue to feel normal, with no evidence of any side effects from the N_2O. A few patients will experience a postsedation feeling of being hung over; this effect may act to deter these few from future inhalation sedation appointments. Among the signs and symptoms of this postsedation hangover effect are nausea, headache, and lethargy.

In most cases this effect does not develop within the first few minutes following termination of the sedative procedure. In fact most patients will have returned to their home or business when the symptoms develop. Management is symptomatic. In most cases tincture of time is the recommended treatment.

Causes of these signs and symptoms are not always obvious. One of the more commonly found causes is an inadequate period of oxygenation at the end of the sedative procedure. As mentioned previously, many doctors do not permit their patients to inhale 100% O_2 for at least 3 to 5 minutes. By oxygenating the patient for but 1 to 2 minutes, not as much N_2O is removed from the patient's body, leaving a residuum in the blood. This residual N_2O may be adequate in some patients to produce a CNS depression sufficient to cause the symptoms mentioned. It is also possible for a patient to have received O_2 for the recommended 3 to 5 minutes or even longer, and still encounter these same effects postoperatively. The normal distribution curve provides evidence that there are some persons who still respond to the very low levels of N_2O found in their blood after at least 3 to 5 minutes (or longer) of 100% O_2. It is usually not possible for the doctor to prevent this occurrence the first time that the patient receives inhalation sedation but on subsequent visits the patient, having informed the doctor of this unpleasant experience, will be administered 100% O_2 for a longer period of time. Although this increased period of oxygenation may prove adequate to prevent a recurrence of the signs and symptoms, it is entirely possible that even careful attention to the patient's recovery will fail to produce the desired result in extremely sensitive patients.

The term *diffusion hypoxia* is often mentioned in regard to this situation.[2] As was discussed in Chapter 14, N_2O is rapidly removed from a patient's blood following the cessation of the N_2O gas flow. If the patient breathes atmospheric air rather than 100% O_2 at this time, the alveoli become filled with a mixture of N_2, O_2, CO_2, water vapor, and N_2O. Some N_2O will be reabsorbed into the circulatory system of the patient, and the O_2 present in the alveoli will be diluted to approximately 10% during the first few minutes following termination of the N_2O flow. These factors will produce the signs and symptoms described. It appears that this effect is more frequently noted in cigarette smokers.[3]

One of these symptoms, specifically lethargy, may not be caused completely by the mechanisms just described. A feeling of "not quite being back to normal" does occur in some patients having received N_2O-O_2. When asked to describe this feeling the patient usually describes a feeling similar to that experienced when first arising from a pleasant sleep. The patient, though not tired, is not quite fully awake, feeling perhaps 90% normal. Following a few moments of activity the patient is fully functional once again. This type of postsedation response is not uncommon and will develop immediately following treatment. If this occurs, the patient should be permitted to move about for a few moments. If this added movement does not return the patient to the presedative state, he or she should be placed back into the chair and readministered 100% O_2 for several minutes.

WHO ADMINISTERS NITROUS OXIDE?

The following points are mentioned because of the legalities of inhalation sedation administration within the dental or medical office. It is not at all uncommon within the practice of dentistry for the dental assistant to be the person to administer N_2O to the patient. In some states it is permissible for a dental assistant, under the direct supervision of the dentist (the doctor is physically present in the room at all times), to adjust the flow of gases being delivered to the patient. In this situation the doctor would tell the dental assistant to "raise the N_2O 1 L/min" or "decrease the O_2 by one half a L/min." The doctor controls the sedative process, the assistant being but an extension of the doctor in this case.

However, in other dental offices it is common practice for the dental assistant to administer the

N_2O-O_2 without the doctor being physically present in the treatment area. In this situation it is considered by the parties involved to be acceptable because the dental assistant remains with the patient. In other cases the doctor is the one to place the nasal hood on the patient; however, the doctor will then leave the room, permitting the assistant to complete the sedative procedure alone with the patient.

Because of the legalities involved in the delegation of expanded functions to auxiliaries, such liberties as described cannot be condoned unless (1) such delegation of duty is specifically permitted under the specific state or provincial dental practice act and (2) the auxiliary being permitted to administer the inhalation sedation has received thorough training in all aspects of inhalation sedation, including the recognition and management of side effects and complications. For this reason, dentists employing N_2O-O_2 sedation must be aware of their state's dental practice act and its provisions in this area.

A similar situation involves the use of N_2O-O_2 inhalation sedation by the dental hygienist. Although a number of states permit a certified registered dental hygienist to administer N_2O-O_2 to patients, in all cases the dental practice act specifies that a dentist must be physically present in the dental office. The certified registered dental hygienist is not permitted to administer inhalation sedation to patients when the dentist is not present within the office. Unfortunately such desirable practices do not always develop and in many instances N_2O-O_2 is in fact administered to the patient without the presence of the doctor in the office. Looking at this situation from a purely medico-legal perspective it must be stated that this practice cannot be condoned. It is, at this time, the doctor's ultimate responsibility should any undesirable action develop from the administration of inhalation sedation. Although the well-trained dental hygienist is fully capable of recognizing and managing such situations, the doctor should always be immediately available to direct the patient's management and to render such additional assistance as is deemed necessary under the specific circumstances of the situation.

The doctor should always be present in the office when inhalation sedation is being administered by the certified registered dental hygienist, and the doctor must always be physically present in the treatment area, directing the administration of N_2O-O_2 by the dental assistant if this is permitted in the state or province. As dental practice acts continue to be revised, it is recommended that the doctor, hygienist, and assistant regularly keep abreast of such changes as might effect their practices.

REFERENCES

1. Trieger NT, Laskota WI, Jacobs AW et al: Nitrous oxide: a study of physiological and psychological effects, *JADA* 82:142, 1971.
2. Papageorge MB, Noonan LW Jr, Rosenberg M: Diffusion hypoxia: another view, *APCD* 2(3):143, 1993.
3. Burrows B, Knudson RL, Cline MG et al: Quantitative relationships between cigarette smoking and ventilatory function, *Am Rev Respir Dis* 115:195, 1977.

CHAPTER 20

Guidelines for teaching inhalation sedation

As has been mentioned throughout this section, inhalation sedation with N_2O and O_2 is the safest of all sedation techniques currently available. Factors responsible for this include the nature of the gases being employed, the manner in which they are administered (with not less than 25% O_2), the addition of fail-safe devices to inhalation sedation units and the upgrading of education in the use of inhalation sedation. This last factor will be discussed in this chapter, for although great strides have been taken in improving the educational process in teaching inhalation sedation, there remain many persons who seek an easy way out, looking for shortcuts to make the technique even simpler to learn. In order to maintain the safety of inhalation sedation, high standards for education must be ensured and gradually increased as our knowledge of the technique continues to grow.

As mentioned in Chapter 12, one reason for the failure of inhalation sedation to maintain its popularity among the dental profession in the 1930s and 1940s was the absence of educational programs. Dental schools did not include the use of N_2O in their curricula, and continuing education programs were essentially nonexistent at that time. The few courses offered were usually sponsored by the manufacturer of the anesthesia machine and consisted of a 1-day program held in a hotel room. Out of these courses came doctors who were initially enthused about this technique, but after returning to their dental practices and employing N_2O-O_2 relative analgesia, quickly became disenchanted. Their disenchantment came about because they discovered that patients did not always respond to nitrous oxide in the same manner in which the doctor had been told that they would during the course.

During courses such as these doctors would usually observe a demonstration of the technique, the "patient" being a volunteer from the group of doctors in the course. There being no true dental anxiety present in this volunteer, the technique would usually be quite successful. In some courses the doctors even got a chance to administer N_2O-O_2 to one another, so that they could all experience the sensation of sedation and therefore be better able to describe it to their patients. Although a step in the right direction, even this fell far short of ideal.

In an effort to provide a uniform level of education in the teaching of different techniques of anesthesia and sedation within the dental school curriculum, three groups—the American Dental Society of Anesthesiology (ADSA), American Dental Association (ADA), and the American Association of Dental Schools (AADS)—sponsored four workshops on pain control in 1964, 1965, 1971, and 1977. From these conferences emerged the *Guidelines for Teaching the Comprehensive Control of Pain and Anxiety in Dentistry.*[1,2] The guidelines provide outlines for a curriculum in pain control at three levels: (1) the undergraduate dental student (doctoral student), (2) graduate dental student (postdoctoral student), and (3) in a continuing education program. These guidelines were approved by the ADA's Council on Dental Education in May 1971.[2] In 1977 Part III of the guidelines, relating to continuing education programs, was revised. These revised guidelines were approved by the House of Delegates of the American Dental Association in 1978.[3] Part I of the guidelines underwent revision in 1979[4] with the entire document revised again in 1992.[5] Sections of the most recent revision of the guidelines (1993) relating to inhalation sedation in continuing education programs are reproduced here.[5]

CONSCIOUS SEDATION TECHNIQUES
Course level

Continuing education courses in conscious sedation techniques may be offered at three different levels (intensive, supplemental, and incidental). A description of the intensive course follows:

1. *Intensive courses* in conscious sedation are programs designed to meet the needs of dentists who wish to become knowledgeable and proficient in the safe and effective use of N_2O-O_2 inhalation sedation. . . . They should consist of lectures, demonstrations, and sufficient clinical participation to ensure the faculty that the dentist understands the procedure and can safely and effectively apply them. Faculty must be prepared to assess the individual's competency on successful completion of such training.

2. *Supplemental (or refresher) courses* are designed for persons with previous training in conscious sedation techniques. They are intended to provide a review of the subject and an introduction to recent advances in the field. They should be designed didactically and clinically to meet the specific needs of the participants. Participants must be able to document previous training (equivalent, at a minimum, to the intensive continuing education course described in this document) and current experience in conscious sedation to be eligible for enrollment in a supplemental or refresher course. This does not preclude allied health personnel from attending such courses with the dentist to enhance skills needed for assisting the dentist in the administration of conscious sedation.

3. *Incidental courses* are overview or survey programs designed to provide general information about subjects related to pain and anxiety control. Such courses should be didactic and not clinical in nature, because they are not intended to develop clinical competency. Practitioners seeking to develop clinical competency in any given conscious sedation technique are expected to complete successfully an intensive continuing education course teaching that technique.

Objectives

Upon completion of an intensive continuing education course in conscious sedation techniques, the dentist should be able to

1. Describe the anatomy and physiology of the respiratory, cardiovascular, and central nervous systems (CNS) as they relate to the techniques of conscious sedation.
2. Describe the pharmacologic effects of drugs used for conscious sedation.
3. Describe the methods of obtaining a medical history, and conduct an appropriate physical evaluation of a dental patient.
4. Apply these methods clinically to obtain an accurate evaluation of the dental patient.
5. Use this information clinically for risk assessment.
6. Choose the most appropriate technique of conscious sedation for the individual dental patient.
7. Discuss physiological monitoring and the equipment used in such monitoring.
8. Upon completion of a course in N_2O-O_2 inhalation sedation techniques, the dentist should be able to:
   a. Describe the basic components of inhalation sedation equipment.
   b. Discuss the function of each of these components.
   c. List and discuss the advantages and disadvantages of inhalation sedation with N_2O-O_2.
   d. List and discuss the indications and contraindications for the use of N_2O-O_2 inhalation sedation.
   e. List the complications associated with N_2O-O_2 inhalation sedation.
   f. Discuss the prevention, recognition, and management of these complications.
   g. Administer N_2O-O_2 inhalation sedation to patients in a clinical setting in a safe and effective manner.
   h. Discuss concerns related to use of N_2O-O_2:
      (1) Abuse potential
      (2) Potential occupational hazards
      (3) Hallucinatory effects

Course content

The following course content is generally applicable to both inhalation and parenteral sedation programs:

1. Historical, philosophical, and psychological aspects of pain and anxiety control

2. Patient evaluation and selection through review of medical history, physical diagnosis, and psychological profiling
3. Definitions and descriptions of physiologic and psychological aspects of pain and anxiety
4. Description of the stages of drug-induced CNS depression through all levels of consciousness and unconsciousness, with special emphasis on the distinction between the conscious and the unconscious state
5. Review of respiratory and circulatory physiology and related anatomy
6. Pharmacology of agents used in the conscious sedation techniques being taught, including drug interaction and incompatibilities
7. Indications and contraindications for use of the conscious sedation modality under consideration
8. Review of dental procedures possible under conscious sedation
9. Patient monitoring, with particular attention to vital signs and reflexes related to conscious sedation
10. Importance of maintaining proper records with accurate chart entries recording medical history, physical examination, vital signs, drugs administered, and patient response
11. Prevention, recognition, and management of complications and life-threatening situations that may occur during use of conscious sedation techniques, including the principles of advanced life support
12. Importance of using local anesthesia in conjunction with conscious sedation techniques
13. Course content for programs in inhalation sedation techniques with N_2O should include:
    a. Description and use of inhalation sedation equipment
    b. Introduction to potential health hazards of trace anesthetics and proposed techniques for limiting occupational exposure
    c. Discussion of abuse potential
    d. Discussion of hallucinatory effects

Sequence and length of instruction

The following portions of the intensive pain and anxiety control course may be taken separately, but the first two should be considered prerequisites for the others:
1. Patient evaluation and risk assessment
2. Management of medical emergencies, including the principles of advanced life support

3. Nitrous oxide-oxygen inhalation sedation techniques
4. Parenteral conscious sedation techniques, such as intravenous conscious sedation

Nitrous oxide sedation instruction

Although the length of a course is only one of the many factors to be considered in determining the quality of an educational program, the course should include a minimum of 14 hours, including a clinical component during which competency in N_2O-O_2 inhalation sedation techniques is demonstrated.

Participant evaluation and documentation of instruction

Intensive courses in conscious sedation techniques must afford participants with sufficient clinical experience to enable them to achieve competency. This experience must be provided under the supervision of qualified faculty and must be evaluated. The course director must certify the competency of participants upon satisfactory completion of training in each conscious sedation technique, including instruction, clinical experience, and airway management.

Records of the didactic instruction and clinical experience (including the number of patients managed by each participant in each pain and anxiety control modality) must be maintained and available for review by appropriate credentialing agencies. Such documentation must not be, or resemble, a certificate or diploma.

Faculty

For all facets of training, the course should be directed by a dentist or physician qualified by training. This individual should have had at least three years of experience, including the individual's formal training in general anesthesia. Dental faculty with broad clinical experience in the particular aspect of the subject under consideration should participate. In addition, the participation of highly qualified individuals in related fields, such as anesthesiologists, pharmacologists, internists, cardiologists, and psychologists, should be encouraged.

A participant–teacher ratio of not more than 10 to 1 when inhalation sedation is being used allows for adequate supervision during the clinical phase of instruction; a 1-to-1 ratio is recommended during the early stage of participation. The faculty should provide a mechanism whereby the participant can evaluate the performance of those individuals who will be presenting the course material.

Facilities

Intensive courses should be presented only in a dental or medical school, hospital, dental society–sponsored educational institution, or other institution where adequate facilities are available for proper patient care, including drugs and equipment for the management of emergencies.

Twice a year, the Council on Dental Education of the ADA publishes a list of continuing education courses being sponsored by approved providers. This list appears in June and December. In the January through June 1993 listing there was one intensive inhalation sedation program listed and three courses categorized as either supplemental or incidental relating to inhalation sedation.[6]

REFERENCES

1. Guidelines for postgraduate and continuing education in pain and anxiety control, *Anesth Prog* 20:167, 1973.
2. American Dental Association, Council on Dental Education: Guidelines for teaching the comprehensive control of pain and anxiety in dentistry, *J Dent Educ* 36:62, 1972.
3. American Dental Society of Anesthesiology: Guidelines for the teaching of pain and anxiety control and management of related complications in a continuing education program, part III, *Anesth Prog* 26:51, 1979.
4. American Association of Dental Schools: Curricular guidelines for comprehensive control of pain and anxiety in dentistry, Special Report *J Dent Educ* 44:279, 1980.
5. American Dental Association, Council on Dental Education: *Guidelines for Teaching the Comprehensive Control of Pain and Anxiety in Dentistry,* Chicago, 1992, The Association.
6. American Dental Association, Council on Dental Education: Continuing education course listing for January-June 1993, Chicago, 1992, The Association.

SECTION FIVE

Intravenous sedation

The intravenous (IV) route of sedation is the subject of Section Five. Drugs administered directly into the cardiovascular system produce clinical actions significantly more rapidly than drugs administered via other routes (e.g., oral or intramuscular). Rapid onset of action is both beneficial and of potential danger. It is beneficial because it permits the doctor to effectively titrate the drug to a desired clinical effect; it is potentially dangerous because the effects of intravenously administered drugs develop more rapidly and because their actions are more pronounced than when administered via other routes with slower onsets and less complete absorption. It is therefore of the utmost importance that every person employing the IV route of drug administration or contemplating its use receive thorough training in the procedures involved in its safe and effective use.

The chapters to follow provide the basic didactic material for an intensive course in IV conscious sedation and consist of two parts: The first, a discussion of venipuncture, will include the anatomy for venipuncture, the armamentarium for the continuous IV infusion, and the technique of venipuncture. The second portion of an IV sedation program is the discussion of drugs and specific techniques of IV sedation, including the clinical pharmacology of intravenously administered drugs, the techniques of administering these agents, and the complications associated with the use of this route of drug administration.

Chapter 30 may prove to be the most important chapter in this section. This chapter is titled Guidelines for Teaching, and it is designed to outline the fundamentals of training required for this very valuable, yet potentially dangerous, technique. It is my belief that IV sedation is an important part of the dentist's armamentarium in the management of pain, fear, and anxiety; however, because of the nature of this technique (e.g., its rapid onset of action, more profound effects of drugs), the doctor using it must undergo a degree of training that is beyond that required for employment of many of the techniques already discussed in Sections Three and Four.

Forty-five states have passed legislation requiring a dentist to possess a special permit in order to employ the IV route for sedation.[1] Minimum educational requirements have been established by many of these states and by various organizations (the American Dental Society of Anesthesiology). These requirements will be presented in Chapter 30. It is strongly recommended that all doctors either currently using or contemplating the use of the IV route for conscious sedation read this section carefully. Courses not meeting the requirements presented in this chapter are not considered to be adequate to properly prepare the doctor and the office staff to employ intravenous conscious sedation.

Like the previous section on inhalation sedation, this section is presented in chapters that are shorter than those in other sections. Its purpose is to better enable the reader to locate the specific material that is of importance to him or her.

The IV route of drug administration is extremely valuable. It is only through proper education of those doctors wishing to use the technique that IV sedation can remain a relatively safe procedure. The reader must always keep in mind that this section was designed to be used in conjunction with an intensive course in IV conscious sedation, a course containing both didactic and clinical components. Use of IV conscious sedation after having simply read this section should never even be considered.

REFERENCE

1. American Dental Association, Department of State Government Affairs: Chicago, Unpublished data, 1992.

CHAPTER *21*

Historical perspective

The historical development of intravenous (IV) anesthesia and sedation will be reviewed in this chapter. Though the impact made by the development of the IV route of drug administration was not quite as dramatic as was that of inhalation anesthesia (Chapter 12), the ability to administer medications directly into the cardiovascular system has proved to be a boon to the medical and dental professions.

THE EARLY DAYS

As was true with inhalation anesthetics, it seems as though some of the techniques and drugs had been available for a good many years before it was thought to put them to any therapeutic use. Indeed, with the IV route it was not until well after inhalation anesthesia was developed that the thought of administering drugs directly into the cardiovascular system of a human being occurred.

William Harvey[1] (1578-1657) (Fig. 21-1) provided much of the groundwork for the future of IV medication when he published the results of experiments on the circulation of blood, stating that there was a continuous circulation of blood within a closed system. Prior to Harvey's findings a multitude of theories relating to the flow of blood in the human body were considered. Most of these suggested that blood flowed to tissues within the body in an open system. Harvey was born in England and received his medical training at Oxford. Following graduation he went to Padua, Italy, then the major medical center in the world, where he began to formalize his theories on the circulation of blood. Andrea Cespalino (1519-1603) was an important predecessor of Harvey's. Cespalino was the first person to use the word *circulation* in reference to blood and its travels throughout the body.[2] Cespalino was also first to propose that capillaries connect arteries and veins so that there is no free flow of blood into the tissues of the body, as had

been assumed for many years. The one major drawback to Cespalino's theory was that he also proposed that there were direct connections between major arteries and veins.

On returning to England in 1602, Harvey entered into private medical practice and prospered. He became the court physician for King James I and for King Charles I. Despite his busy practice, Harvey continued to experiment; most of his research involved the circulation of blood. As early as 1615, Harvey spoke of the circulation of blood within a closed system; however, it was not until 1628 that he published one of the most important textbooks in the history of medicine and biology: *Exercitatio Anatomica de Motu Cordis et Sanguinis in Animalibus (On the Movement of the Heart and Blood in Animals)*.[1]

Harvey demonstrated for the first time that because of the presence of valves within the heart and veins, blood flow within the circulatory system was unidirectional. In addition, he discussed capillaries—microscopic vessels that connect smaller arteries and smaller veins, thus providing a closed circulatory system. Harvey, despite his description of capillaries, was never able to see them, for it was not until after his death that Marcello Malpighi (1628-1694) first saw capillaries through the microscope.

Harvey's book produced great controversy following its publication for it attempted to disprove the theories relating to blood that had been held for many years. In fact, controversy over Harvey's book raged for approximately 20 years following its publication. Today, Harvey's work is considered to be the seventeenth century's most significant achievement in physiology and in medicine.

As a logical extension of Harvey's work, the first intravenous administration of a drug occurred in the same century (1657). Sir Christopher Wren and Robert Boyle administered tincture of opium intrave-

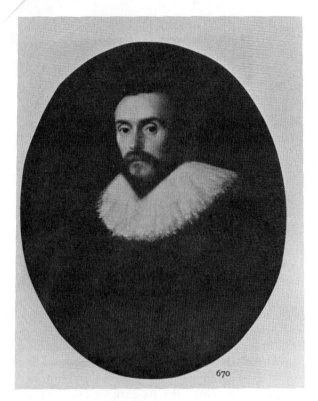

670

Fig. 21-1. William Harvey (1578-1657).

nously into a dog, using a sharpened quill to which a bladder had been attached.[3] Eight years later, Richard Lower successfully transfused blood from one animal to another.

THE 1800s

The late 1700s and early 1800s saw the development of anesthesiology, with the advent of ether, chloroform, and nitrous oxide-oxygen (N_2O-O_2). This history is chronicled in Chapter 12.

In 1839 in New York Isaac E. Taylor and James Augustus Washington administered a solution of morphine in an Anel syringe.[4] The Anel syringe had originally been designed to enter the lacrimal duct, having a finely elongated tapering nozzle instead of a sharp point. Taylor and Washington had to make a skin incision with a knife in order to deposit the morphine under the skin of the patient. This was not an IV injection but more than likely was subcutaneous. By 1842 modifications in syringes had occurred that eliminated the necessity to make a separate skin incision. The Jayne syringe was similar to the earlier Anel syringe; however, a sharp point had replaced the tapered nozzle, permitting a direct puncture of the skin. Charles Gabriel Pravaz (of Lyons, France)

was the first to design a syringe with a separate needle. His syringe, manufactured from glass, was introduced in 1853. The Anel, Jayne, and Pravaz syringes were used primarily to deposit morphine along or near the path of a nerve, in cases of neuralgia.

Professor W. W. Green,[5] from the University of Maine School of Medicine, published in 1868, in the American Journal of Dental Sciences, a paper entitled *The Hypodermic Use of Morphia during Anesthesia*.[5] Green advocated the subcutaneous administration of 0.5 to 1 grain of morphine while the patient was receiving ether anesthesia. Green's reasons for his recommendation included the probability of pain, prevention of shock, a shortening of the anesthetic's influence, and the prevention of delirium and nausea.

Pierre-Cyprien Oré of Bordeaux, France, was the first person to administer a drug intravenously, when he administered chloral hydrate to animals to achieve general anesthesia in 1872.[6] Two years later he administered chloral hydrate general anesthesia to a human being.

THE 1900s

Further development of the IV route was somewhat slow. The major developments in anesthesia during the late 1800s occurred in local anesthesia and in the refinement of the techniques of inhalation anesthesia. However, in 1903 Emil Fisher and J. von Mering synthesized the first barbiturate, barbitone (Veronal).[7] For his part in the discovery of this important drug, Fisher received the Nobel Prize in Medicine in 1903.

In 1929 sodium amobarbital (Amytal) was employed intravenously by L. G. Zerfas.[8] This represented the first IV administration of a rapidly acting barbiturate. However, amobarbital was not administered by Zerfas for the purpose of producing anesthesia. Rather, amobarbital was used primarily as an anticonvulsant. Its function as an anesthetic was limited to those patients in whom inhalation anesthetics could not be administered. A year later, 1930, pentobarbital (Nembutal) was synthesized.

In 1935 John S. Lundy[9] at the Mayo Clinic in Rochester, Minnesota, introduced sodium thiopental (Pentothal).[9] This rapid-acting, short-duration IV anesthetic eventually became the most popular drug (in the United States) for the induction of general anesthesia via the IV route.

At approximately the same time in England, Stanley L. Drummond-Jackson[10] pioneered the use of IV barbiturate anesthesia for both oral surgery and conservative dental procedures.[10] The agent employed by Drummond-Jackson was methohexital, known as Brevital in the United States and Brietal in Europe.

Studying at the Mayo Clinic with Lundy was Adrian Hubbell. Hubbell, along with two others, B. S. Wyckoff and O. K. Bullard, was a pioneer in the administration of IV general anesthesia for ambulatory oral surgical patients.[11] In addition, Hubbell was the first person in North America to use IV general anesthesia without premedication as a sole agent for ambulatory patients having oral operations in a dental office. In 1933 Victor Goldman[12] published the first English-language article dealing with the subject of IV anesthesia for dental surgery.

So far we have discussed the evolution of IV general anesthesia. As also occurred with the use of N_2O general anesthesia in the early to mid-1900s, an evolutionary process was taking place. With the advent of better, more effective local anesthetics for pain control, the requirement of anesthesia and analgesia from IV medications was diminishing.

In 1945 Niels Bjorn Jorgensen became probably the first person to use the IV route to provide what Jorgensen himself termed IV premedication.[13] Jorgensen refined the technique of administering IV barbiturates and combined pentobarbital administration with an opioid (meperidine) and scopolamine. This technique was first used in 1945 at the Loma Linda University School of Medicine. In 1955 this technique for producing IV sedation was first taught to the junior (third-year) dental students at the Loma Linda School of Dentistry, where it has been taught to every succeeding class. This technique gradually became known as the Loma Linda technique and is now known as the Jorgensen technique, after Niels Bjorn Jorgensen, its founder, the father of IV sedation in dentistry.[14]

In 1965 A. Davidau[15] in Paris, France, first employed diazepam (Valium) as a sedative agent in dentistry. Shortly thereafter, D. M. G. Main[16] reported on his first case of diazepam sedation in dentistry. Main employed diazepam as an adjunct to the Jorgensen technique.

R. O'Neil and P.J. Verrill[17,18] used diazepam as the sole sedative agent for patients undergoing oral surgical procedures. The Verrill sign, considered by some as an indicator of the proper level of sedation, came from these studies. Diazepam has become the most commonly employed IV sedative agent within dentistry. Interestingly enough, the Jorgensen technique—the original IV sedative technique—still remains widely used, primarily for longer procedures.

These two techniques remain the backbone of IV conscious sedation in dentistry today. The continued supremacy of diazepam and of the Jorgensen technique is somewhat in doubt at this time. In 1986 midazolam, a water-soluble benzodiazepine, was introduced into clinical practice in the United States following its earlier introduction elsewhere. Although this drug is similar in many respects to diazepam, midazolam has distinct advantages and has become a very popular IV conscious sedative in both medicine and dentistry, rivaling the popularity of diazepam.[19]

Another major change in IV sedation is the increasing attention being placed on patient monitoring during sedation and general anesthesia. An offshoot of the space program in the United States and other countries, several noninvasive forms of monitoring have become available, though for many at a considerable cost. Examples of these devices include automatic vital signs monitors, pulse oximeters, and end-tidal carbon dioxide monitors. The purpose of these devices is to increase safety for the patient receiving IV sedation.[20]

REFERENCES

1. Harvey W: *Exercitatio anatomica de motu cordis et sanguinis in animalibus,* 1628, transl ann CD Leake, Springfield, Ill, 1931, CC Thomas.
2. Lee JA, Atkinson RS: *A synopsis of anesthesia,* ed 5; Baltimore, 1964, Williams & Wilkins.
3. Bankoff G: *The conquest of pain: the story of anesthesia.* London, 1946, MacDonald.
4. Archer WH: *A manual of dental anesthesia.* Philadelphia, 1952, Saunders.
5. Green WW: Hypodermic use of morphia during anaesthesia, *Am J Dent Sc* (third ser) 2:207, 1868 (extracts).
6. Sykes WS: *Essays on the First Hundred Years of Anaesthesia.* Edinburgh, 1960, E & S Livingstone.
7. Driscoll EJ: Dental anesthesiology: its history and continuing evolution, *Anesth Prog* 25:143, 1978.
8. Zerfas LG: Induction of anesthesia in man by intravenous injection of sodium iso-amyl-ethyl barbiturate, *Proc Exp Biol Med* 26:399, February 1929.
9. Lundy JS: Intravenous anesthesia: preliminary report of use of two new thiobarbiturates, *Proc Staff Meetings, Mayo Clinic,* 10: 536, 1935.
10. Drummond-Jackson SL: Evipal anesthesia in dentistry, *Dental Cosmos* 77:130, 1935.
11. Hubbell AO, Adams RC: Intravenous anesthesia for dental surgery with sodium ethyl (1-methylbutyl) thiobarbituric acid, *JADA* 27:1186, 1940.
12. Goldman V: "Evipan" in dentistry, *Dent Mag Oral Top* 50:1153, 1953.
13. Jorgensen NB, Leffingwell FE: Premedication in dentistry, *J Southern Calif Dent Assoc* 21:1, 1953.
14. Jorgensen NB, Hayden J Jr: *Sedation, local and general anesthesia in dentistry,* ed 2. Philadelphia, 1972, Lea & Febiger.

15. Davidau A: New methods in anaesthesiology and their use in dentistry. Treatment of difficult patients and execution of complex procedures, *Rev Assoc Med Israelites* (France) 16:663, 1967.

16. Brown PRH, Main DMG, Lawson JM: Diazepam in dentistry, report on 108 cases, *Br Dent J* 125:498, 1968.

17. O'Neil R, Verrill PJ: Intravenous diazepam in minor oral surgery, *Br J Oral Surg* 7:12, 1969.

18. O'Neil R, Verrill PJ, Aellig WH et al: Intravenous diazepam in minor oral surgery, *Br Dent J* 128:15, 1970.

19. Trieger N: Intravenous sedation in dentistry and oral surgery, *Int Anesth Clin* 27(2):83, 1989.

20. Eichhorn JH, Cooper JB, Cullen DJ et al: Standards for patient monitoring during anesthesia at Harvard Medical School, *JAMA* 256(8):1017, 1986.

CHAPTER *22*

Intravenous sedation: rationale

Intravenous (IV) sedation is a relatively new technique in dentistry. The use of IV general anesthesia has had a long history in dentistry, but it has only been within the past 20 to 30 years that intravenously induced sedation has gained a foothold. Until recently the IV route was employed almost exclusively by oral and maxillofacial surgeons, primarily because their postdoctoral training placed great emphasis on this route of drug administration. Most dental schools in the United States did not (until recently) include training in IV drug administration in their curricula, and there exist today woefully few courses available wherein the postgraduate doctor can receive such training. The past 10 years, however, have seen the implementation of predoctoral courses in IV sedation by a small, but still growing, number of dental schools. Because of this and the present availability of a handful of excellent postgraduate programs in IV sedation, as well as the continuing, though diminished, availability of 1- and 2-year residencies in general anesthesia for dentists, the number of dentists employing IV conscious sedation has continued to grow. It is impossible to even guess at the number of dentists employing the IV route today; however, for the patient who requires this form of therapy it has become somewhat easier to locate a doctor who employs IV sedation for nonsurgical procedures.

Unfortunately, there is another force acting to diminish the number of doctors employing this technique—liability insurance. The 1980s saw a dramatic increase in the cost of liability insurance in all areas of life in the United States, not only in the health professions. However, the fact is that the cost of liability insurance for a dentist using IV sedation has, in many states, become extremely high. This has become a major factor in a doctor's decision whether or not to use this valuable technique of patient management. As we enter the mid-1990s the cost of liability insurance has started to level off and in certain circumstances, for example, for the periodontist using IV sedation (in the state of California), has actually decreased (CDA insurance). It is hoped that as more complete risk-assessment surveys are completed the cost of liability insurance for all doctors using IV conscious sedation will follow this promising path.

ADVANTAGES

1. The onset of action of intravenously administered drugs is the most rapid of all of the techniques discussed in this book. The arm–brain circulation time is approximately 20 to 25 seconds. Although there may be some individual variation in this and in the onset of action for different drugs, overall the IV route of drug administration permits the most rapid onset of action.
2. Because of the rapid onset of action of most intravenously administered drugs, drug dosage may be tailored to meet the specific needs of the patient. Guesswork involved in determining proper dosage of a drug administered orally, rectally, or intramuscularly is eliminated when the IV route is used. As mentioned, this concept of individualizing drug dosages is termed *titration* and represents one of the most important safety factors associated with IV drug administration.
3. Because of the rapid onset of action of most IV drugs, the doctor is able to provide the patient with a suitable level of sedation. The level of sedation must never, of course, exceed that level to which the doctor has been trained. Light, moderate, and deep levels of sedation can easily be achieved via the IV route, and the doctor must always be cognizant of his or her limitations, as based on prior experience and training.

4. The recovery period for most intravenously administered drugs is significantly shorter than that seen for the same drug administered via the oral, rectal, or intramuscular (IM) route. Recovery from intravenously administered drugs will, however, be considerably longer, and less complete, than that following nitrous oxide-oxygen (N_2O-O_2) inhalation sedation.

5. In the continuous IV infusion technique recommended in this book, a patent vein is maintained throughout the procedure. This facilitates the reinjection of any additional drug (though this is rarely necessary). However, the major significance of the patent vein is that through it an avenue exists for the administration of emergency drugs that may be required in the event of a serious medical emergency arising during IV therapy.

6. The side effects of nausea and vomiting are extremely uncommon when drugs are administered intravenously, as recommended.

7. Control of salivary secretions is possible through the IV administration of anticholinergics. This will be of benefit to the doctor during various forms of dental therapy.

8. The gag reflex is diminished. Patients receiving IV conscious sedation rarely experience difficulty with gagging. This action is similar to that occurring with N_2O-O_2 inhalation sedation. If the only requirement in a patient is to decrease their gag reflex, inhalation sedation is preferred over IV therapy. Only in the event that inhalation sedation fails to alleviate gagging should IV sedation be employed solely for this purpose.

9. Many of the medications employed intravenously for sedation effectively diminish motor disturbances (e.g., seizure activity and cerebral palsy).

10. The ability to readily establish an IV infusion may prove to be important in any emergency situation. Although antidotal drug therapy is not recommended as the initial step in the effective management of all emergency situations, the ability to establish an IV line provides immediate access to the cardiovascular system should it become necessary to administer drugs to the victim. By using IV sedation on a regular basis, the doctor is better able to maintain proficiency in venipuncture.

DISADVANTAGES

1. Venipuncture is necessary. Although most patients tolerate venipuncture with little or no difficulty, some patients are psychologically unable to accept needles anywhere in their body. Children may be particularly difficult to manage via this route because veins are proportionally smaller in smaller patients, making the venipuncture itself more difficult. Younger children requiring IV sedation will usually pose severe management problems or be physically unable to control themselves. Not all patients have veins that are easy to visualize and gain access to with a needle. Probably the most significant hurdle facing the doctor learning to use IV sedation is to develop a degree of proficiency at venipuncture. Venipuncture is a learned skill, one that becomes easier to perform as experience is gained.

2. Complications may arise at the site of the venipuncture. As discussed in Chapter 28, there are a variety of minor and some major complications that might arise at the venipuncture site. These include hematoma, phlebitis, and intraarterial injection of a drug.

3. Monitoring of the patient receiving IV sedation must be more intensive than that required in most other conscious sedation techniques. Because intravenously administered drugs act so rapidly, the entire dental team must be trained to assess the physical status of the patient throughout the procedure. The greater the depth of sedation, the greater the significance of increased patient monitoring.

4. Recovery from intravenously administered drugs is not complete at the end of the dental treatment. All patients receiving any intravenously administered central nervous system (CNS) depressant must be escorted from the dental office by a responsible adult companion.

5. Although the depth of sedation provided by intravenously administered drugs can be increased relatively rapidly (by administration of additional drug), the converse is not true. Many intravenously administered drugs cannot be reversed by specific antagonist drugs. Although antagonists do exist for several drug groups, specifically opioids, benzodiazepines, and scopolamine, these possess potentially significant side effects and are not recommended for routine administration.[1,2] Should a patient become overly sedated, the most effective management in all situations is the maintenance of basic life support: check that the patent's airway is unobstructed, assist or support ventilation, and provide for the effective circulation of oxygenated blood. Following these steps consideration may be given to antidotal drug therapy.

Table 22-1. Advantages and disadvantages of intravenous sedation

Advantages	*Disadvantages*
1. Rapid onset of action	1. Venipuncture is necessary
2. Titration is possible	2. Venipuncture complications may occur
3. Highly effective technique	3. More intensive monitoring required
4. Recovery shorter than other techniques (IM, oral)	4. Recovery not complete—escort needed
5. Patent vein is safety factor	5. Most IV agents cannot be reversed
6. Nausea & vomiting uncommon	
7. Control of salivary secretions possible	
8. Gag reflex diminished	
9. Motor disturbances (epilepsy, cerebral palsy) diminished	
10. Ability to perform IV is benefit in serious emergency situations	

Table 22-1 summarizes the advantages and disadvantages of intravenous sedation.

CONTRAINDICATIONS

1. Unless a doctor has received specific training in the administration of CNS depressant drugs to patients under the age of 6 and over 65 years of age, IV conscious sedation is relatively contraindicated in these groups. The primary reason for this recommendation is that in both of these groups there is a greater than usual incidence of overreaction to therapeutic dosages of CNS depressants. In other words, many of these patients will require smaller dosages of a drug to achieve a desired clinical level of sedation. This ought not be a problem as the doctor administering the drug always titrates slowly; however, extreme caution must be exercised whenever the younger or older patient receives CNS depressants via any route. Because of the rapid onset of action of intravenously administered drugs, this route should be reserved for use by the individual specifically trained or experienced in managing these specific patients (e.g., pediatric dentist).

2. Pregnancy represents a relative contraindication to the use of IV conscious sedation because most CNS depressants cross the placenta into the fetus and might produce birth defects in the developing fetus. The subject of sedation in pregnancy is more fully discussed in Chapter 5.

3. A history of significant hepatic disease contraindicates the use of IV sedation. Most intravenously administered drugs are biotransformed in the liver into pharmacologically inactive products. The presence of significant liver damage (ASA III or IV) may alter the rate at which these drugs undergo inactivation. This can lead to both a prolongation of the clinical actions of the drug and a more profound effect from the same dose. Most patients with serious liver impairment (cirrhosis, hepatitis) are not ambulatory; however, when presented with a history of liver disease, the doctor should pursue an in-depth dialogue history and consider medical consultation should any doubt remain as to the patient's physical status.

4. Thyroid dysfunction is a relative contraindication to the use of IV sedation. Patients who are clinically hypothyroid are particularly sensitive to CNS depressants such as sedative-hypnotics, antianxiety agents, and opioid analgesics. Patients exhibiting clinical signs of hypothyroidism should not be administered IV sedation. Table 22-2 lists clinical signs and symptoms of hypothyroidism. This represents a relative (not an absolute) contraindication, for in the event that other sedative techniques (e.g., inhalation sedation) prove to be inadequate, lighter levels of IV conscious sedation may be provided. Titration ought to be carried out even more slowly than is usually recommended. Patients who are hypothyroid but are currently being treated through the administration of thyroid medications can

Table 22-2. Signs and symptoms of hypothyroidism and hyperthyroidism

Hypothyroidism	*Hyperthyroidism*
Weakness	Nervousness
Dry skin	Increased sweating
Lethargy	Hypersensitivity to heat
Slow speech	Palpitation
Sensation of cold	Fatigue
Gain in weight	Eye signs (exophthalmos)
Cold skin	Increased appetite
Thick tongue	Tachycardia
Edema of face	Goiter
Pallor of skin	Tremor
Memory impairment	Weight loss
Decreased sweating	Weakness
Loss of hair	

safely receive IV sedation. Patients who are clinically hyperthyroid are likely to prove extremely difficult to sedate. In addition, drugs such as the anticholinergics atropine and scopolamine ought not be administered to the clinically hyperthyroid patient. Both of these drugs possess vagolytic properties, producing an increased heart rate. As hyperthyroid individuals have a significant increase in heart rate already, any additional increase in the rate of the heart might well prove deleterious to the patient by increasing possible myocardial ischemia and cardiac workload and decreasing cardiac output. Patients with a hyperthyroid history but who through surgery, radiation, or drug therapy are presently euthyroid (normal thyroid function) may receive IV conscious sedation with minimal increase in risk.

5. Adrenal insufficiency is a relative contraindication to the use of IV sedation. Patients receiving chronic corticosteroid therapy or patients suffering from Addison's disease may be less able physiologically to handle the stresses involved in dental care than are patients with normal adrenal cortices. Although these patients require careful management (see stress-reduction protocol—Chapter 5), deeper levels of sedation are not recommended. Intravenous conscious sedation may be employed; however, only light to moderate sedation levels are suggested.

6. Patients receiving either monoamine oxidase inhibitors (MAOIs) or tricyclic antidepressants (TCAs) should be carefully evaluated prior to the administration of any CNS depressant. These drugs are employed in the management of states of depression. Prior to the administration of any other drug that has the ability to alter mental function (e.g., CNS depressants), medical consultation with the patient's psychiatrist or physician is recommended. Opioid agonists and barbiturates are synergistic with these two groups of drugs.

7. Intravenous sedation is not contraindicated in patients with a history of psychiatric disorders; however, it is strongly recommended that medical consultation be obtained prior to the administration of CNS depressant drugs.

8. Patients who are extremely obese present with a variety of potential problems. Because of the excessive amounts of skin and fat it might prove to be extremely difficult to locate and canulate superficial veins. Of greater importance, however, is the fact that in markedly obese persons there is usually a concomitant decrease in cardiovascular and pulmonary reserve. Other forms of sedation, especially inhalation sedation, ought to be considered first, with IV sedation considered only if other techniques prove ineffectual.

9. One of the most significant contraindications to the use of IV sedation in the dental office is a dearth of visible superficial veins. All IV procedures in a dental office environment will be of an elective nature. It seems patently unfair for a patient to have to endure multiple unsuccessful venipuncture attempts so that we can give them a drug to help them to relax. As is discussed in Chapter 25, the preliminary IV visit is used to determine whether or not the patient is an acceptable candidate for the proposed procedure. One of the objectives of this visit is to look for the presence of adequate veins.

10. When employing IV sedation the doctor must specifically question the patient regarding their prior history with each of the drugs being employed in the procedure. Allergic responses and ''hyperresponders'' may be uncovered before the drug is administered. In addition, each drug has specific contraindications to its use. The drug package insert or Chapter 26 of this book should be reviewed for this important information. These contraindications include opioids (specifically meperidine)—asthma; barbiturates—asthma, porphyria; anticholinergics—glaucoma, prostatic hypertrophy.

INDICATIONS

The major indications for the use of IV conscious sedation are essentially those of other sedative techniques. There are, however, a number of indications for IV sedation that are not found for other techniques. These include the control of salivary secretions and the production of amnesia.

Intravenous sedation is not a technique that should be employed as readily as is inhalation sedation. Before employing IV techniques the doctor should carefully consider other procedures, especially inhalation sedation. Intravenous sedation should be considered for use only in those situations in which there exists a specific indication for it.

Anxiety

As with inhalation sedation and the other sedation techniques discussed in this book, the primary indication for use of sedation is the presence of fear and anxiety. Unlike inhalation sedation, however, the use of the IV route ought to be reserved for those patients in whom other techniques have proved inadequate or for patients in whom prior history or the doctor's experience indicates that the IV route is the only method to employ.

In most instances the IV route should be reserved for patients exhibiting rather pronounced levels of apprehension and fear of the dental situation. Inhalation sedation can often effectively manage the patient with a lesser degree of fear and anxiety. However, there will be occasions when IV sedation is required even for these patients.

Amnesia

An advantage of the IV route of drug administration is its ability to provide a degree of amnesia or a lack of recall. Whether amnesia develops following IV drug administration or does not develop depends on several items. Some drugs are much more likely to provide amnesia than others. Diazepam, midazolam, lorazepam, and scopolamine are examples of drugs that have a greater degree of amnesia associated with their administration; meperidine and pentobarbital are less likely to provide an amnestic effect.

The depth of sedation has an effect on whether or not amnesia develops and on the duration of the amnestic period. In general, given the same patient and the same drug (e.g., diazepam), more profound levels of sedation will provide greater degrees of amnesia. This factor is the reason for my considering amnesia to be "the icing on the cake" during a sedation procedure. The major goal of sedation is to relax the patient. In most cases this result can be obtained with the patient only lightly sedated. The patient may tolerate the procedure quite well but at its conclusion may not appear amnesic. In such situations, the sedation procedure must be considered a success. The goal of managing the difficult patient more easily and effectively was accomplished. Should there appear to be a lack of recall of events that occurred during the procedure, so much the better. It is safer to provide the patient comfortable dental treatment with total recall (no amnesia) at a lighter level of sedation than it is to provide comfortable dental treatment with total lack of recall at deeper levels of sedation. With the loss of consciousness, lack of recall (amnesia) is virtually 100%, yet the risk to the patient is significantly greater.

As with all other factors relating to drug response, there is a significant degree of individual variation in the development of amnesia. Some patients will be amnesic following seemingly very light levels of sedation, whereas others may demonstrate no apparent amnesia with deeper levels of sedation. Such response is consistent with normal variation in response to drug administration.

Medically compromised patients

The IV route of sedation is indicated in the management of persons who are medically compromised and unable to tolerate stress in a normal manner. Although inhalation sedation is the preferred technique in most of these patients, light levels of IV conscious sedation may also be employed in many of these situations.

ASA II or III cardiovascular risk patients

Examples of cardiovascular situations in which the IV route should be considered include angina pectoris, previous myocardial infarction, certain dysrhythmias, congestive heart failure, and high blood pressure. The preferred route of sedation for all of these disorders is inhalation sedation with N_2O and O_2. In all of these cardiovascular disorders, the clinical status of the patient will deteriorate should the level of O_2 in the myocardium or in the blood become inadequate to meet the demands of the heart. With N_2O-O_2 sedation the occurrence of such situations is minimized. Whenever IV conscious sedation is employed in the management of the ASA III patient there are two recommendations:

1. Employ only light levels of sedation.
2. Administer 3 L/min of O_2, via nasal cannula or nasal hood, throughout the sedative procedure.

Previous cerebrovascular accident

The patient who has suffered a cerebrovascular accident (CVA—stroke) falls into the ASA II, III, or IV category. The ASA status of the patient is determined by the duration of time since the CVA and by the presence or absence of residual signs and symptoms of CNS dysfunction.

As with the cardiovascular risk patient, the CVA patient may require sedation during dental treatment. Although N_2O-O_2 is the preferred technique because of the increased percentage of O_2 being administered, IV conscious sedation can be employed if these same recommendations (as listed for cardiovascular risk patients) concerning depth of sedation (light only) and the administration of O_2 are adhered to.

Epilepsy

Epileptic patients are acceptable candidates for IV conscious sedation. In most cases the seizure activity of the patient is controlled through the administration of anticonvulsant drugs (many of which, coincidentally, are used intravenously as sedatives) on a daily basis. Such patients will be able to tolerate almost any technique of sedation with little or no difficulty. It is in the patient whose seizure activity has not been controlled effectively that the IV route may prove particularly beneficial. Stress is one factor that acts to precipitate acute seizure activity; therefore, implementation of the stress-reduction protocol is recommended. Although inhalation sedation may prove to be effective, the use of intravenously administered benzodiazepines, particularly diazepam and midazolam, is recommended. The Jorgensen technique, which includes pentobarbital, is also indicated in epileptics. These drugs are effective anticonvulsants, drugs that will be administered intravenously should a protracted seizure develop. Their use as IV sedatives will greatly diminish (though not entirely eliminate) the likelihood of a seizure developing during treatment. Consultation with the patient's physician is recommended prior to IV sedation in these patients. The use of O_2 via nasal cannula or nasal hood is strongly recommended in epileptics, as any degree of hypoxia may precipitate a seizure. Light to moderate levels of sedation may be safely employed in these patients.

Other medically compromised patients

The IV route can also be employed for many other medically compromised patients. ASA IV patients should not receive IV sedation within the dental office, such treatment being relegated to the operating room or the hospital dental clinic where medical consultation and a more controlled treatment environment can be provided. ASA II and III patients are usually acceptable candidates for sedation. Whether or not the IV route is appropriate can be determined through consultation with the patient's physician. The administration of supplemental O_2 throughout the IV procedure is recommended for all ASA II, III, and IV patients.

Control of secretions

There are occasions during dental treatment when it will be beneficial to decrease the volume of salivary secretions. The major indication for this will be impression taking following the preparation of teeth for full coverage. A dry mouth may also prove to be beneficial during restorative dentistry and surgical procedures. Anticholinergics can be administered orally, intramuscularly, and intravenously, but the IV route provides the most effective and reliable results. Agents such as atropine, scopolamine, and glycopyrrolate may be administered intravenously either in conjunction with other CNS depressants or alone.

Analgesia

Although far from being the ideal method of pain control in dentistry, intravenously administered opioid analgesics will assist in obtaining clinically adequate pain control. Local anesthetics remain the ideal drug for eliminating discomfort during dental treatment; however, occasions do arise when these drugs do not provide entirely adequate relief of discomfort. In such situations the administration of CNS depressants, such as N_2O-O_2 or opioid analgesics, will elevate the pain reaction threshold of the patient, thereby decreasing or at least modifying the patient's response to noxious stimulation.

The use of intravenously administered drugs as the sole means of achieving pain control is ineffective in the absence of general anesthesia. General anesthesia should not be considered unless the doctor has completed a residency in anesthesiology (see Section Six).

Diminished gagging

Some dental patients have a significant problem with gagging whenever instruments or fingers are placed in the posterior part of their oral cavity. Whatever the underlying reason for this response, it becomes difficult, if not impossible, for the doctor to treat these patients successfully. Several sedation techniques possess the added benefit of diminishing the gag reflex. Most notable amongst these is IV sedation, followed closely by inhalation sedation with N_2O-O_2.

In most instances, the use of inhalation sedation is recommended to control a hyperactive gag reflex. To obtain a few intraoral radiographs or an impression takes but a few minutes, and IV sedative techniques are too long-acting for these procedures; therefore, inhalation sedation is recommended. If a patient has difficulty whenever anything is placed in his or her mouth (e.g., handpiece, explorer) and treatment is to last for an hour or more, the use of IV conscious sedation becomes more reasonable.

Indications for the use of intravenously administered drugs are quite numerous. Although the obvious indication is fear and apprehension, the doctor should be aware that many other indications for the use of IV sedation do exist.

REFERENCES

1. Brogden RN, Goa ZL: Flumazenil. A reappraisal of its pharmacological properties and therapeutic efficacy as a benzodiazepine antagonist, *Drugs* 42(6):1061, 1991.

2. Reversal of central benzodiazepine effects by flumazenil after intravenous conscious sedation with diazepam and opioids: report of a double-blind multicenter study. The Flumazenil in Intravenous Conscious Sedation with Diazepam Multicenter Study Group II, *Clin Ther* 14(6):910, 1992.

CHAPTER 23

Armamentarium

The equipment required for venipuncture and for intravenous drug administration will be discussed in this chapter. IV drugs can be administered in a variety of ways. These include the following:

1. Direct IV administration; vein not kept patent
2. Needle maintained in the vein without a continuous infusion; patency maintained by periodic flushing
3. Continuous IV infusion; patency maintained by a continuous infusion of solution

Direct intravenous administration

In direct IV administration a tourniquet is placed on the patient's arm, the veins become engorged, the injection site is prepared, and the needle of the syringe containing the drug(s) is placed into the lumen of the vein. After ensuring that the needle is within the vein (aspiration of blood back into the syringe), the doctor or assistant removes the tourniquet and the drug is slowly deposited into the vein. Following drug administration, the needle is removed from the vein, pressure is applied to the site to stop bleeding, and the dental procedure is begun. No access to the vein is maintained during the procedure (Fig. 23-1).

Needle maintained in the vein without continuous infusion

When the needle is maintained in the vein without an infusion being used, the tourniquet is placed, the veins engorged, and the tissues prepared in the usual manner. A winged infusion set or a hollow metal needle is used for venipuncture. Following successful venipuncture the tourniquet is removed and the syringe (without a needle attached) is connected to the needle that has been left in the vein and taped into place. After the drug(s) is titrated to effect, the syringe is detached from the needle and a second syringe containing a solution such as sterile water for injection is attached to the needle. The dental procedure is begun, with the doctor or assistant periodically flushing the needle with 1 ml of solution to keep the vein patent (Fig. 23-2).

Continuous intravenous infusion

In a continuous IV infusion an indwelling needle is attached to a length of tubing that in turn is connected to a bag of infusate. The same venipuncture procedure is carried out that was described for the first two techniques. Following removal of the tourniquet the flow of IV solution is started, and the needle is securely taped. The IV drug(s) is administered through an injection site located on the tubing, and the syringe is then removed. The speed of the IV infusion is adjusted so as to maintain a slow rate that will prevent needle occlusion during the dental procedure, which is then begun (Fig. 23-3).

Advantages and disadvantages of various methods

The first technique, direct IV administration, in which the syringe is removed from the vein following drug administration, cannot be recommended for routine use in intravenous sedation. In fact, the only reasons for considering use of this technique, in my opinion, are:

1. Emergency situations in which IV drug administration is required and time or the lack of equipment does not permit establishment of an IV infusion.
2. Situations in which the needle needs to be maintained in the vein for only a very brief period of time (as in drawing of blood for laboratory analysis).

Why do I believe this technique should not be used? As will be evident in later chapters and during training in IV sedation, the most difficult part of learning

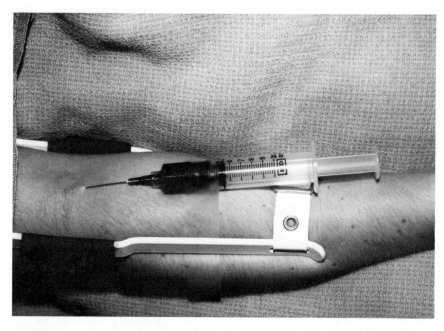

Fig. 23-1. Direct IV drug administration. Blood is aspirated into syringe prior to injection to determine that needle is still within lumen of vein.

ARMAMENTARIUM FOR VENIPUNCTURE AND INTRAVENOUS INFUSION

Basic equipment

IV infusion solution*
IV administration set*
Needle*
IV stand
Tourniquet
Tape*
Sterile gauze pad 2 × 2 inch*
Alcohol wipe*
Armboard
Bandage*

Additional items

Sphygmomanometer
Stethoscope
Monitoring devices
O₂ delivery system
Emergency kit
Antidotal drugs

*Single-use, disposable item.

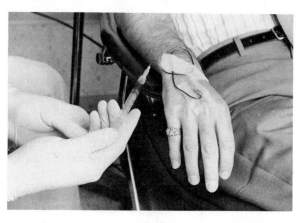

Fig. 23-2. Needle maintained in the vein without continuous infusion.

to use IV sedation is to become proficient in venipuncture. Though not a hard technique to master, venipuncture can be difficult on some occasions in even the most experienced of hands. Why, therefore,

if placing a needle into the vein is the most difficult task in IV sedation, should the needle be removed from the patient's vein following a successful venipuncture? Adherents of this technique claim that the patient is bothered by the needle remaining in the vein, and that the presence of the needle in the vein throughout the procedure reminds the patient of a hospital. However, once the needle is placed into a vein the patient has little, if any, awareness of its being there, be it in for 1 minute or several days. In response to the belief about the hospital setting, I can only state that the presence of a needle within

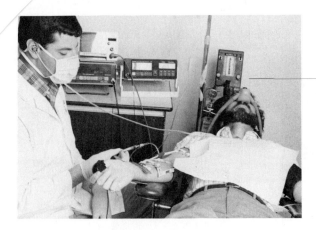

Fig. 23-3. Continuous IV infusion.

the vein throughout the procedure is a routine in hospital practice simply because it adds to the safety of the procedure. Patients will accept as normal most practices within the dental office. A valid argument in favor of this technique is that removal of the needle from the vein makes it difficult for additional drugs to be administered following the initial titration, minimizing the chance of a drug overdosage developing.

Removal of the needle from the vein is illogical because, on occasion, additional IV sedative drugs may be required later in the procedure, or an emergency situation may develop in which antidotal therapy will be needed. Drugs such as flumazenil, naloxone, or physostigmine may be required during or at the end of the IV sedation procedure. In both of these situations a venipuncture will have to be reestablished. Since the venipuncture is the only part of the IV sedation procedure that might be considered difficult, it is not logical not to leave the needle in situ during the entire procedure. In addition, should the patient's blood pressure decrease significantly, superficial veins will become difficult to visualize and to cannulate.

The second technique, in which the needle is left within the vein throughout the procedure, its patency maintained by periodic flushing with some solution, is an improvement on the previous technique. The only drawback to this technique is that periodic flushing of the needle is necessary to prevent clotting of the lumen from occurring. During a busy dental procedure it is not uncommon for the doctor and the assistant to become deeply engrossed in the oral cavity and to neglect to flush the needle, in which case the lumen of the needle becomes clotted with blood and a vein must be recannulated.

Continuous IV infusion is the most highly recommended technique in all situations in which a patent vein is to be maintained for a period of time exceeding but a few minutes. In this technique patency of the needle and vein are maintained by the constant infusion of IV solution from the bag into the needle and patient's vein. The only drawback to this procedure is the possibility of (1) the infusate being contaminated (a highly unlikely occurrence) and (2) the drip rate being too rapid, causing the bag of solution to be emptied during the procedure.

Readministration of sedative or emergency IV drugs is easily done by simply inserting the syringe needle into the injection site on the IV tubing. The ease of maintaining a patent vein and the increased safety afforded the patient by the continuous IV infusion are primary reasons for considering this technique as the ideal for IV drug administration.

The equipment and techniques to be discussed in this section will relate to continuous IV infusion.

INTRAVENOUS INFUSION SOLUTION
Choice of solution

There are a variety of fluids available for IV therapy. Although the type of solution chosen will be of some significance to a hospitalized patient during prolonged intravenous therapy, for a short-duration IV procedure (less than 1 hour to several hours' duration) the choice of infusate becomes academic. Solutions available for IV administration include the following:

Solution	Abbreviation
Sterile water for injection	SW
5% dextrose in water	D5 and W
Sodium chloride injection	¼ NS
Lactated Ringer's solution	LR

Though other infusion solutions are available, these represent the most commonly used solutions.

In the ambulatory ASA I, II, or III patient being considered as a candidate for IV conscious sedation on an outpatient basis there will be no contraindication to the use of any of these solutions. The question of whether a patient with insulin-dependent diabetes should receive 5% dextrose in water often arises—won't this solution add sugar to the patient's blood and induce hyperglycemia?

The answer is that a 5% dextrose and water solution is not contraindicated in the diabetic patient. First, the concentration of dextrose (5%) is not great enough to produce any significant change in the blood sugar level of this patient. Second, as will be

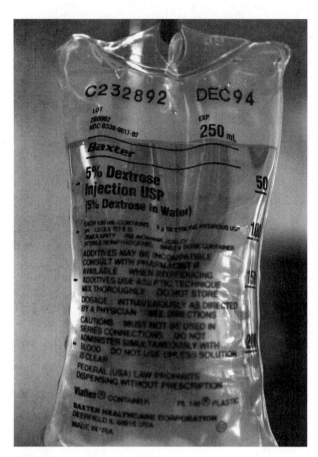

Fig. 23-4. IV infusion solution of 5% dextrose in water (D5W).

stressed in Chapter 27, the patient receiving IV sedation will be requested to take nothing by mouth for approximately 4 hours prior to the planned appointment. The patient will come to the dental office with a decreased blood sugar level, perhaps not quite hypoglycemic, but definitely not hyperglycemic. The addition of 100 to 200 ml of 5% dextrose and water will produce a slight elevation in blood sugar level, a desirable effect at this time. It must be remembered that when a person with diabetes becomes significantly hypoglycemic, treatment of choice in correcting the blood sugar level is the administration of 50% dextrose, a concentration 10 times that which is being infused during IV sedation.

The most commonly used IV infusate is 5% dextrose and water (Fig. 23-4).

Volume of solution

Until recently IV solutions were available in glass bottles. Today, however, all solutions are packaged in plastic bags. Obvious advantages of plastic bags include their unbreakability and the ease of packaging and shipping as compared with glass bottles. An example of a plastic bag of IV solution is shown in Fig. 23-4.

IV solutions are available in a variety of sizes. The more commonly used sizes include 1000 ml, 500 ml, and 250 ml.

The 1000-ml (one-liter) size is commonly employed in the hospital setting when a patient is receiving long-term IV therapy. A patient will usually receive 3 liters of IV solution daily. During general anesthesia 1-liter bags are also commonly used, where the patient must be kept hydrated with fluids during surgery. Use of the 1-liter bag for dental outpatient procedures is not the most highly recommended, although there is no significant reason why it should not be used. However, for the typical IV procedure in the dental office, the 1-liter bag is simply too large. For example, during a 1-hour procedure a patient may receive 125 to 200 ml of infusion solution. At the conclusion of the procedure the infusion bag represents one of the three items in the IV armamentarium that must be discarded. It is a single-use item and must never be reused despite the fact that, in this example, approximately 800 ml of infusate remain. I have seen numerous situations in which well-meaning doctors have reused the bag of IV solution on from 2 to 5 patients, rather than discard it, on the theory that it is extremely unlikely that blood or microorganisms can travel uphill against gravity the 72 inches from the patient's vein to the IV bag. Using a 500-ml bag the same type of situation is likely to arise, as noted with the 1-liter bag. The 500-ml bag is also not recommended for routine use for most dental outpatient IV conscious sedation procedures.

The 250-ml bag of IV solution represents the most nearly ideal size for the typical 1- to 4-hour dental IV conscious sedation procedure. With proper management of the flow rate (as will be discussed in Chapter 27), the 250-ml bag can be made to last for 3 to 4 hours. Discarding the remaining small volume of solution is quite easy, and doctors are less likely to be tempted to reuse this size bag of solution.

The solution found within the IV bag is sterile. However, problems with contaminated solutions have developed in the past, and care must be exercised by the user of such solutions to try to ensure the sterility of the solution.[1] Administration of contaminated solutions directly into the cardiovascular system of the patient can produce bacteremia or sep-

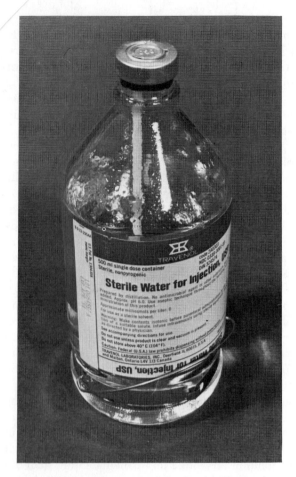

Fig. 23-5. Sterile water for injection in glass bottle.

ticemia and has led to deaths and to significant morbidity.[2]

The following should be checked before using a bag of solution:

1. *All IV infusion solutions are clear.* A solution that has any coloration to it or has any particulate matter floating within it should never be used.
2. The bag of solution has the name of the solution printed on it in addition to its expiration date. *IV infusion solution should never be used after its expiration date has passed* (Fig. 23-4).
3. Once the seal on the bag of infusate has been opened, the solution cannot be stored for any length of time without the possibility of its becoming contaminated. If a bag of solution is prepared for an IV procedure and the appointment is cancelled, the bag could still be used if another procedure is scheduled for that same day. However, the bag should be discarded if it would not be used for a day or more. Bags of

IV solution do not contain any preservatives, and they are excellent culture media for bacterial growth.

4. *If there is ever any doubt as to the sterility of the IV infusion solution, it should not be used.* However, the bag should not be thrown away. On the contrary, the bag should be saved and returned to the manufacturer so that the solution may be assayed. The manufacturer will be very concerned about the possibility of a contaminated IV solution being used clinically.
5. In the rare case in which a glass bottle of IV solution is being employed, there is an additional concern: When the rubber seal on the glass bottle (Fig. 23-5) is punctured, the vacuum within the bottle is dissipated as air is forced into the bottle. The person preparing the IV drip will normally notice air bubbles entering into the glass bottle as the IV tubing is forced into it. Absence of these bubbles or a glass bottle with no seal over the rubber stopper should give the doctor reason to think that perhaps the seal had been broken and the solution is not sterile.

The following checklist summarizes precautions for IV infusion solution:

1. Is the IV solution clear?
2. Has the expiration date of the IV solution passed?
3. Do not store an opened IV bag for more than a few hours.
4. Never use a bag of IV solution when any doubt exists as to its sterility.
5. Is vacuum present? (Glass bottles only)

INTRAVENOUS ADMINISTRATION SET

To deliver the IV infusion solution from the bag to the patient, IV tubing is required. Infusion sets, as they are also known, have several components in common (Fig. 23-6).

The *piercing pin* is that part of the IV tubing that is inserted into the bag or bottle of IV solution. It is a solid plastic piece that should be kept sterile prior to its insertion into the bag of solution.

Located immediately below the piercing pin is the *drip chamber.* The drip chamber is an enlarged chamber into which solution from the bag will drip. The drip chamber has two functions:

1. To prevent air from entering into the IV tubing.
2. To permit regulation of the solution's flow rate.

The drip chamber should be filled approximately halfway with IV solution to prevent the trapping of air bubbles inside

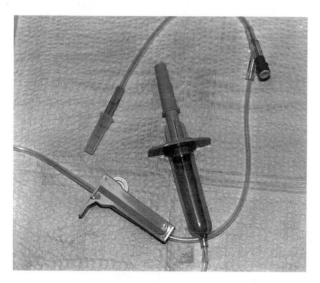

Fig. 23-6. IV administration set: *1*, piercing pin; *2*, drip chamber; *3*, rate adjustment knob; *4*, injection portal; *5*, rubber bulb; and *6*, needle adapter.

the IV tubing. Though isolated air bubbles within the tubing are of little consequence (Chapter 28), the unknowing patient may be quite disturbed to see any bubble of air enter into his body. An unfilled drip chamber or one just barely filled with solution will continue to allow air bubbles to enter the tubing as each drop of solution falls from the bag into the drip chamber.

Conversely an overly filled drip chamber will prevent the doctor from assessing the rate at which IV solution is flowing. Though this factor is not as critical with the ambulatory dental or surgical patient as it is with the hospitalized patient, the rate of flow does require adjustment at times during the procedure (Chapter 27). In addition, in two groups of patients, the smaller child and the patient with serious CHF (ASA III,IV), overhydration is a complication to be avoided. The ability to determine the precise rate of flow will be important in these situations.

When the usual adult IV infusion set is used, 10 drops equal 1 ml of solution. Therefore for a 250-ml bag of IV solution to last for 2 hours (120 minutes) we can adjust the flow rate to 20 drops per minute (2 ml/min × 120 min = 240 ml).

Pediatric infusion sets provide a finer adjustment so that 60 drops equal 1 ml of solution. Use of the pediatric infusion is recommended in the smaller child and in the adult with serious CHF (ASA III) (Fig. 23-7).

Extending from the drip chamber is a length of

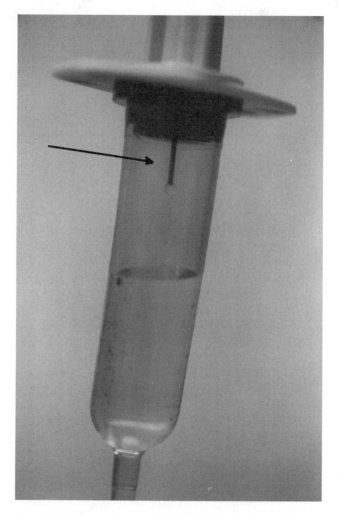

Fig. 23-7. Pediatric IV drip. Note small pin within chamber *(arrow)*.

plastic tubing, usually 72 inches long, that attaches to the IV needle. Along the length of this tubing are found several items (see Fig. 23-6):

    Rate adjustment knob
    Injection portal
    Rubber bulb
    Adapter for needle

The *rate adjustment knob* permits the rate of flow of solution into the drip chamber to be regulated.

The *injection portal* is usually a rubber diaphragm that fits over a hard plastic spur off of the main IV tubing. The needle of the syringe containing the drug to be injected is placed into this portal, and the drug is deposited into the flowing infusion. The rubber diaphragm should not be removed from the plastic prior to injection.

On some, but not all, IV sets, near the distal end of the IV tubing just above the point where the needle adapter is found is a *rubber bulb*. This bulb is larger than the plastic tubing and serves as a means of checking if a needle is still within the lumen of the vein. The bulb need only be squeezed and the pressure released. If the needle tip lies within the lumen of the vein, blood will appear in the tubing just above the entry point of the needle into the patient's skin. A second possible use of the rubber bulb is to serve as an alternate site for injection of a drug. The needle of the syringe may be inserted into the bulb (with care not to perforate the other side of the tubing) and the drug deposited into the infusion. Multiple punctures of the rubber bulb, however, will produce leaking of infusion solution. When present, the injection portal is the recommended site for drug administration on the IV tubing.

At the very end of the IV tubing is the *needle adapter*. As will be seen, a variety of shapes and sizes of needles may be used for venipuncture. In addition, there exists a multitude of manufacturers of each needle. To ensure that needles and tubing from various manufacturers can be used interchangeably, a standard female Luer connector is used. Any IV needle in the following discussion will easily attach onto standard IV tubing. Under no circumstances should the reuse of the IV infusion tubing ever be considered, for the tubing will always become contaminated at its distal end with the patient's blood. This blood may be quite visible as it surges back into the tubing as the needle enters into the lumen of the vein during venipuncture, or it may be quite dilute and perhaps not visible to the eye. Reuse of the IV tubing runs an unacceptably high risk of transmission of potentially very serious diseases. Do not do it!

NEEDLES

To deposit a drug underneath the skin, as in the case of IM or SC injection, or directly into the lumen of a blood vessel, as in the case of IV administration, a needle must be employed. Needles are usually referred to by gauge and type.

Gauge

Gauge usually refers to the outside diameter of the needle. However, in discussions of the hypodermic needle, standard gauge numbers have come to be associated with the size of the lumen. Therefore the gauge number of a needle may refer to the inside diameter (ID) or the outside diameter (OD) of the needle lumen. Needles used for venipuncture gen-

Table 23-1. Needle gauge and function

Gauge	Function
14	Phlebotomy
	Administration of blood
16	Phlebotomy
	Surgical procedures in which blood is likely to be required
18	Common during general anesthesia in which blood administration is unlikely
20, 21	IM drug administration
	Occasionally IV during short procedure on ASA I or II patients
	IV sedation in dentistry
23	IV sedation in dentistry
25, 27	Intraoral local anesthetic administration
30	Intraoral local anesthetic administration
	Acupuncture

erally range from 14 gauge to approximately 23 gauge. The lower (smaller) the gauge number, the larger is the lumen size. Therefore a 16-gauge needle has a larger lumen than a 23-gauge needle.

The term *gauge* is often quite confusing. The term derives from the number of pieces of wire (in this case needles) that can be placed into a 1-mm circle. Therefore only 16 needles of 16 gauge will fit into the same space occupied by 23 23-gauge needles. Table 23-1 lists commonly used needle gauges and their major function.

Types of needles

Several types of needles are available for venipuncture; all have their adherents and their advantages and disadvantages. The following are the three most frequently employed needles (Fig. 23-8):

1. Hollow metal needle
2. Winged needle (scalp vein needle)
3. Indwelling catheter

The *hollow metal needle* is the prototypical needle, that is, the traditional IV needle. This needle represents the basic design from which the other needles in the following discussions have been modified. Components of this needle are shown in Fig. 23-9.

The needle is inserted directly into the vein and then attached via its hub to the IV tubing or directly to the syringe containing the drug to be administered. Since the development of the scalp vein needle and the indwelling catheter, the hollow metal needle has been relegated to use in emergency situations in which other needles are not readily available or situations in which blood is to be drawn from a patient for laboratory analysis.

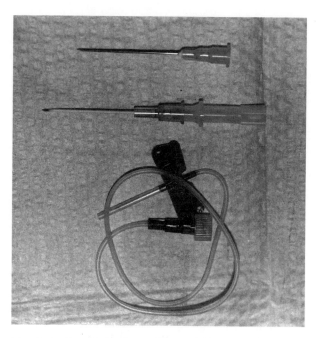

Fig. 23-8. Hollow metal needle *(top)*, indwelling catheter *(middle)*, and winged needles *(bottom)* are available for IV drug administration.

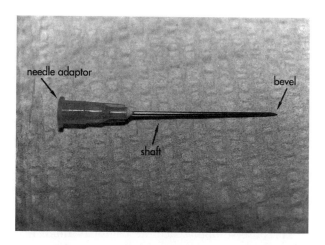

Fig. 23-9. Components of the hollow metal needle.

The hollow metal needle may be used to review the anatomy of the intravenous needle. At one end of the needle is a sharp tip. A triple bevel slopes backward from this tip and ends at the heel of the shaft. The shaft runs from this point to the hub. The length of the shaft varies, but is commonly between ⅝ and 1½ inches in length. The hub is an enlarged metal or plastic portion that permits the needle to be attached to the intravenous tubing or a syringe.

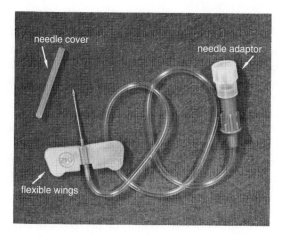

Fig. 23-10. Components of winged needle.

The *winged needle* is probably the most widely used needle for IV conscious sedation procedures in the ambulatory patient within both the dental and medical professions. They are regarded by many as the devices of choice for venipuncture of superficial veins in patients of all ages. Their primary advantage over other types of needles is the ease of manipulation possible with them.

The winged needle (Fig. 23-10) consists of a sharp stainless steel needle, one or two flexible winglike projections mounted to the shaft of the needle, a variable length of flexible tubing, and a female Luer adapter that connects with any standard IV administration set.

The wings permit the user to hold onto the needle more firmly, permitting greater ability to manipulate the needle and to gain greater "feel" during the procedure. Additionally, once the venipuncture is successful, the wings may be taped down to better secure the needle within the vein.

The winged needle has several synonyms: "winged infusion set," "Butterfly needle," and "scalp vein needle."

Butterfly is a proprietary name for the winged infusion set. However, like other proprietary names such as "Ping Pong" and "Linoleum," common usage has turned the proprietary name into the most commonly used name of the device. The term *butterfly needle* is very commonly used and is acceptable, though technically not correct.

The winged infusion set evolved from what was termed the *scalp vein needle*. Superficial veins in most infants are quite small and frequently inaccessible. Frequently the physician had to perform a surgical exposure of a vein (called a venous cutdown) to manually insert a catheter. The scalp vein needle evolved because among the more prominent veins found in the infant are those on their scalp. The scalp vein needle contains a shorter needle, thereby minimizing the problem of needle perforation of the back wall of the vein, which can lead to either an infiltration or a hematoma.

While available in a variety of different gauges, the 21- and 23-gauge winged infusion sets are most commonly used in dentistry, with the 21-gauge needle preferred because it will permit a greater volume of solution to flow through it per minute than the 23-gauge needle (13 ml/min to 3 ml/min).[3] The winged infusion set has been the preferred needle in most instances of outpatient IV conscious sedation in dentistry.

The most recent advance in needle design is the *indwelling catheter.* A potential problem with both the hollow metal needle and the winged infusion set is that they are rigid. Should they be placed into a vein in a mobile area, such as the wrist or the antecubital fossa, special precautions must be observed to prevent the patient from moving that area, or the needle, lying in the lumen of the vein, will perforate the posterior wall, requiring reentry into the vein. Common terminology says that "we have lost the vein."

To minimize this risk the flexible, indwelling catheter was devised. Several types of indwelling catheter are available, among them the catheter-over-needle unit and the catheter-inside-needle unit. Within dentistry only the catheter-over-needle is recommended for use.

Materials used for the plastic catheter include polyvinyl chloride (PVC), Silastic, and Teflon. Modern catheters are made radiopaque so that they may easily be visualized on x-ray examination.

The indwelling catheter, called the "catheter-over-needle," when first designed consisted of a metal hub to which was attached a plastic catheter. The catheter was physically connected to the separate metal hub by means of a piece of plastic. The safety of this design was questioned because the link between the catheter and the hub may not be secure and the catheter could come loose and migrate through the patient's veins. In fact, such occurrences did occur, leading to the development of the modern indwelling catheter in which the catheter is of one-piece design (Fig. 23-11).[4] The potential problem mentioned is virtually nonexistent with the catheter-over-needle unit.

Regardless of the particular design of the indwelling catheter, the basic format is the same. A metal needle, ranging in gauge from 14 to 23, has a tight-fitting plastic catheter placed over it. The catheter, however, is just slightly shorter than the needle so that several millimeters of the metal needle protrude beyond the catheter.

Following successful venipuncture with the metal needle, the catheter is advanced into the vein, the metal needle removed, the appropriate infusion set attached, and the catheter secured with tape. The actual technique of venipuncture using the indwelling catheter is presented in Chapter 25.

The indwelling catheter is recommended for use within the operating room or in most general anesthetic procedures. In situations in which maintenance of a patent vein is essential, indwelling catheters are recommended. The reason indwelling catheters are not taught as the primary venipuncture needle for most ambulatory procedures is that the winged infusion set is somewhat easier for a neophyte to use. After some experience has been gained with the winged infusion set, the student will have little or no difficulty moving to the indwelling catheter.

The IV infusion, the administration set, and the needle are all single-use, disposable items.

OTHER ITEMS

There are a number of other items that are important during venipuncture. An *IV stand* is used to elevate the bag of IV solution. As is discussed in Chapter 25, the height of the bag of IV solution above the patient's heart will, in part, determine the rate of flow of the solution into the patient.

IV poles mounted on a portable stand are commonly used within the operating room. Such devices are usually too cumbersome for use within the dental environment; there simply is not adequate room for the doctor, the assistant, and the IV pole. In addition, portable IV stands are somewhat expensive, whereas the following device is inexpensive but functional.

To conserve floor space the bag of IV fluids may be hung from the ceiling. A bolt and hook, as used for hanging plants, with several links of chain placed on the ceiling to the side of the patient's head, serves quite well as an IV stand.

A *tourniquet* is used to prevent the return of venous blood from the periphery to the heart while allowing the unimpeded flow of arterial blood. A variety of items may be used as tourniquets (Fig. 23-12):

1. Thin rubber tubing (e.g., Penrose drain)
2. Velcro tourniquet
3. Blood pressure cuff (sphygmomanometer)
4. A belt

Tape is needed to secure the needle to the patient's arm (Fig. 23-13). An inexpensive tape such as trans-

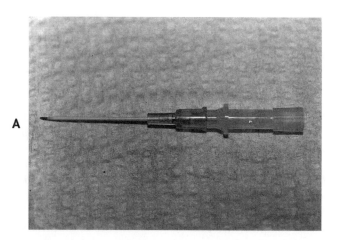

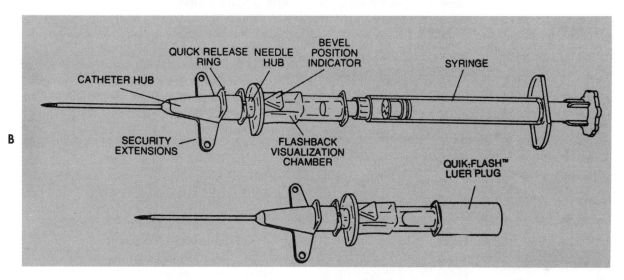

CATHETER HUB

QUICK RELEASE RING

NEEDLE HUB

BEVEL POSITION INDICATOR

SYRINGE

SECURITY EXTENSIONS

FLASHBACK VISUALIZATION CHAMBER

QUIK-FLASH™ LUER PLUG

Fig. 23-11. A, Indwelling catheter. **B**, Components of indwelling catheter. (**B** from Quik-Cath information sheet, Deerfield, Ill, 1983, Travenol Laboratories Inc.).

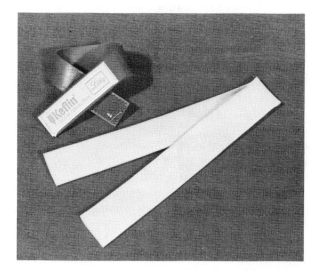

Fig. 23-12. Tourniquets: Velcro tourniquet *(top)* and rubber tubing.

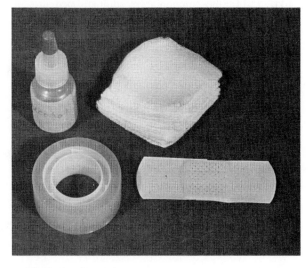

Fig. 23-13. Additional items for venipuncture: alcohol, sterile gauze, transparent tape, and bandages.

parent adhesive tape is usually adequate. Traditional white surgical adhesive tape may be used but is not highly recommended because it is not as easy to work with as are other tapes. Some patients are allergic to the adhesive used on tape and will require the use of a hypoallergenic tape. Always ask this question of the patient prior to the start of the IV procedure.

A simple, inexpensive tape such as transparent tape is recommended since it is easy to manipulate, adheres quite well to skin, and being clear, can be placed in areas where a nontransparent tape should not be placed (e.g., over the point of entry of the needle into the skin).

To cleanse the skin prior to venipuncture and to dry the tissue a number of *sterile 2 × 2 inch gauze wipes* are needed. These gauze squares can also be used as

pressure dressings or to protect the hairs on the hand from adhesive tape.

Prepackaged *alcohol wipes,* or simply a 2 × 2 inch gauze pad moistened with isopropyl alcohol, will be needed to cleanse the skin prior to venipuncture. Alcohol can also be used to cleanse the rubber covering of the injection site on the IV tubing and the rubber stopper on multiple-dose vials of drugs.

An *armboard* is important when IV sedation is contemplated. The armboard will be used to immobilize a portion of the arm, preventing it from being bent by the patient with the needle becoming dislodged from the vein. Armboards are commonly used for the wrist and the antecubital fossa.

A number of devices are available as armboards. A rigid piece of cardboard with a disposable paper sleeve is relatively inexpensive and may be used multiple times, simply replacing the sleeve between uses. It is available in a short length, for use as a wrist immobilizer, and in a longer length for use in the antecubital fossa. Another device is known as an "elbow immobilizer" (Fig. 23-14). It consists of two rigid metal pieces connected at either end by two adjustable plastic straps. In the center is a fabric strap that contains Velcro adhesive that is used to fasten the immobilizer in position. The elbow immobilizer is available in both adult and pediatric sizes, is easy to work with, does an excellent job of immobilizing the antecubital fossa, and is not very expensive. This device does not effectively immobilize the wrist.

Adhesive bandages are used at the end of the procedure to protect the site of venipuncture.

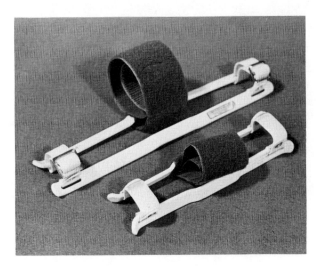

Fig. 23-14. Elbow immobilizers: adult and pediatric.

• • •

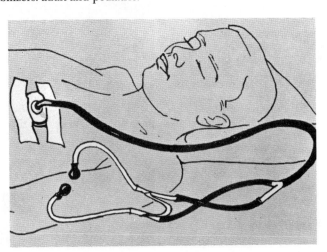

Fig. 23-15. Pericordial stethoscope.

The items just described are the essentials for venipuncture and IV sedation. Several other items should always be available not only for IV sedation but also in every dental office.

A *sphygmomanometer* and *stethoscope* will be required for monitoring of the patient's blood pressure before, during, and after the sedative procedure. Ad-ditionally, the stethoscope may be used to auscultate both the heart and lungs at any time before or during the procedure. A *precordial stethoscope* head taped to the patient's chest either in the precordial region or above the lower border of the trachea will function as a device for continuous listening to the patient's breath and heart sounds (Figs. 23-15 and 23-16).

The blood pressure cuff (sphygmomanometer) can be used as a tourniquet by simply inflating the cuff to a reading above the patient's diastolic pressure but below their systolic pressure.

Patients must be monitored throughout the intravenous sedation procedure. A variety of monitoring devices have become available, ranging from the inexpensive (precordial stethoscope) to the costly (end-tidal CO_2 monitor). The use of these monitors and recommendations for monitoring during sedation are discussed Chapters 6 and 27.

O_2 should be available in all dental offices whether or not IV sedation is being used. Though its primary use will be in the management of emergency situations, the routine administration of O_2 through a nasal cannula or nasal hood (Fig. 23-17) to patients receiving IV sedation is highly recommended (Chapter 27).

An *emergency drug kit* and *emergency equipment* must also be available in all dental offices. The emergency kit in the dental office in which IV sedation is used will contain several drugs that are not considered necessary in the typical emergency drug kit (Fig. 23-18):

1. Opioid antagonist—naloxone or nalbuphine
2. Benzodiazepine antagonist—flumazenil
3. Antiemergence delirium—physostigmine
4. Vasodilator—procaine 1% or 2%

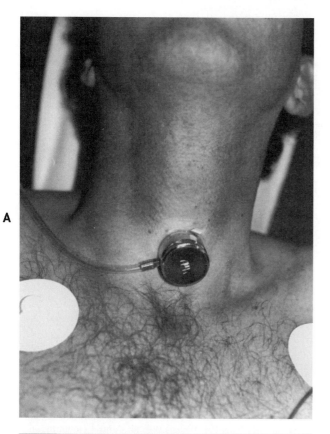

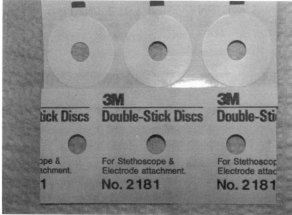

Fig. 23-16. A, Pretracheal stethoscope on patient's trachea. **B**, Double-sided tape for pretracheal stethoscope.

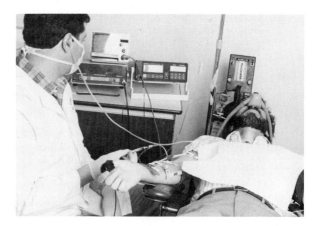

Fig. 23-17. Patient receives O_2 during intravenous sedation.

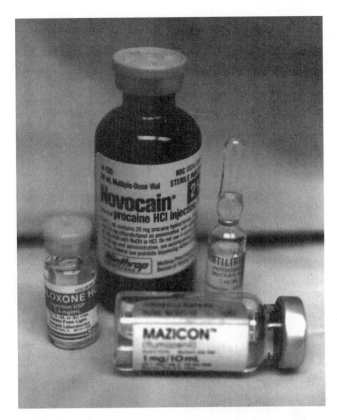

Fig. 23-18. Opioid antagonist [naloxone (*left*)], vasodilator [procaine (*center top*)], antiemergence delirium [physostigmine (*right*)], and benzodiazepine antagonist [flumazenil (*center bottom*)].

These important items and their use are discussed in detail in Chapter 28, while the emergency kit and equipment are reviewed in Chapter 34.

REFERENCES

1. Fleer A et al: Septicemia due to coagulase-negative staphylococci in a neonatal intensive care unit: clinical and bacteriological features and contaminated parenteral fluids as a source of sepsis, *Pediatr Infect Dis* 2(6):426, 1983.
2. Matsaniotis NS, Syriopoulou VP, Theodoridou MC et al: Enterobacter sepsis in infants and children due to contaminated intravenous fluids, *Infect Cont* 5(10):471, 1994.
3. Trieger NT: *Pain control*, ed 2. St Louis, 1994, Mosby.
4. Galdun JP, Paris PM, Weiss LD et al: Central embolization of needle fragments: a complication of intravenous drug abuse, *Am J Emerg Med* 5(5):379, 1987.

CHAPTER 24

Anatomy for venipuncture

Venipuncture is a technique that is separate and distinct from IV sedation. All health professionals should become proficient with this route of drug administration whether IV conscious sedation is practiced or not, for the ability to start an IV line may prove to be important in emergency situations.

The technique of venipuncture is not difficult. Indeed, Malamed[1] has demonstrated that an initial attempt at venipuncture by untrained dental students has a greater than 90% success rate. However, to become proficient requires practice. Once learned, knowledge of the technique remains with the doctor forever, yet being an acquired skill, if it is not used regularly, the level of the doctor's ability will diminish.

In theory, venipuncture may be attempted in any superficial vein of a size sufficient to accommodate the needle. Fig. 24-1 illustrates the major superficial veins in the human body. In practice, however, venipuncture is usually confined to one of the patient's extremities. Either an arm or leg may be used. The usual preference is the arm, with other areas used when arm veins are inadequate or in emergency situations in which the arm may be unavailable or unsuitable for use.

IV sedation in the dental setting in an ambulatory patient is almost always an elective procedure. The selection of a venipuncture site will therefore usually be limited to one of the arms. Use of the leg for venipuncture will usually be reserved for the infant or child, in whom arm veins are small or less superficial than in the adult, and the handicapped adult, in whom the venipuncture site in the foot may be more easily secured than those on the arm.

In this chapter the anatomy of the circulation to the arm will be described in detail. Not only the venous circulation but also the arterial circulation will be discussed, for it is essential to be aware of those sites where anatomically important structures, such as arteries and nerves, lie in close proximity to veins. Knowing where not to attempt a venipuncture is valuable knowledge.

ARTERIES OF THE UPPER LIMB

Blood to the right upper limb leaves the aortic arch through the short, wide brachiocephalic (innominate) trunk, which divides into the right common carotid and right subclavian arteries, the latter delivering arterial blood to the upper limb. On the left side the subclavian artery is a direct branch of the arch of the aorta. From this point onward the arteries of the two sides are symmetrical.[2]

At the outer border of the first rib the *subclavian artery* turns laterally to enter into the axilla. At this point it is termed the *axillary artery*. The axillary artery leaves the axilla at the lower border of the teres major muscle to enter the arm or brachium as the *brachial artery*. Approximately 1 inch below the antecubital fossa the brachial artery bifurcates into the *radial* and *ulnar arteries* (Fig. 24-2), which travel distally in the forearm and terminate in the palm as an *arterial arch*. The ulnar artery forms the *superficial palmar arch*, which travels to the level of the web of the thumb, where it is completed by a small branch arising from the radial artery, the superficial palmar branch. The radial artery crosses the bottom of the so-called snuff box (the hollow at the base of the thumb), reaching the dorsum of the hand and then entering the palm. There it forms the *deep palmar arch*, which is completed by a small branch from the ulnar artery, the deep palmar branch.

The location of these arteries has great clinical significance. Within the antecubital fossa the brachial artery is frequently found beneath the median basilic vein, usually the most prominent vein in the antecubital fossa. The brachial artery is located just me-

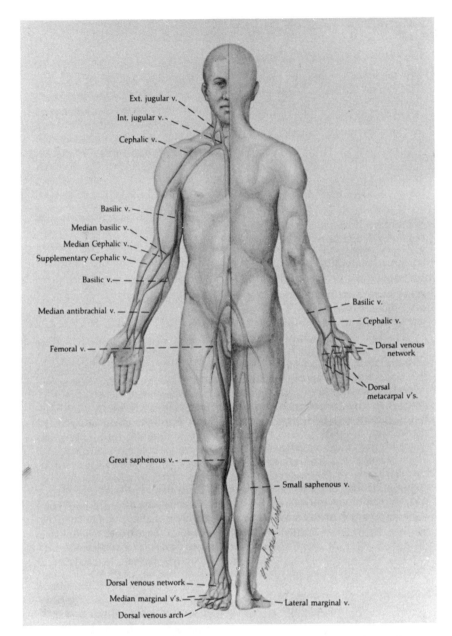

Fig. 24-1. Major superficial veins of the human body. (From Venipuncture and venous circulation. Chicago, 1971, Abbott Laboratories.)

dial of the midline in the antecubital fossa and is the primary reason that the medial aspect of the antecubital fossa is low on my list of preferred venipuncture sites for the neophyte phlebotomist.

Approximately 1 inch below the antecubital fossa, the radial and ulnar arteries arise from the brachial artery. The radial artery lies on the lateral aspect of the ventral surface of the forearm and the ulnar on the medial aspect. Though it is not superficial at its

origin, approximately 5% of the population does possess a recurrent radial artery, which is located on the lateral side of the antecubital fossa and is relatively superficial.

The radial artery continues down the ventral aspect of the forearm not lying near the surface until it reaches the lateral aspect of the wrist, at the base of the snuff box. At this point, on the ventral surface of the wrist, the radial artery is quite superficial. It is

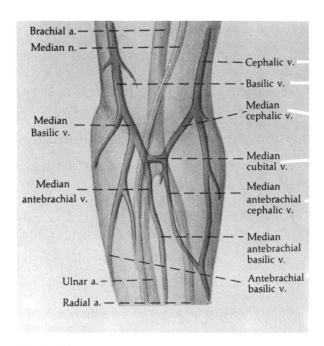

Brachial a.
Median n.
Cephalic v.
Basilic v.
Median cephalic v.
Median Basilic v.
Median cubital v.
Median antebrachial v.
Median antebrachial cephalic v.
Median antebrachial basilic v.
Ulnar a.
Antebrachial basilic v.
Radial a.

Fig. 24-2. Relative location of major arteries in upper arm. (From Venipuncture and venous circulation, Chicago, 1971, Abbott Laboratories.)

at this point that the radial pulse and arterial blood gases may be obtained. Care must be exercised whenever venipuncture is contemplated in this region. Fortunately, venous anatomy does not readily lend itself to venipuncture at this site.

The ulnar artery descends through the forearm lying more deeply within the tissues than does the radial. It lies on the medial aspect of the forearm, but at no point does it become superficial enough to be palpable.

VEINS OF THE UPPER LIMB

The primary venous return from the arm is through the *axillary vein*, which continues as the *subclavian* and *brachiocephalic (innominate) veins* before emptying into the *superior vena cava*.

The veins of the arm may be divided into the deep veins and the superficial veins. The deep veins, for the most part, accompany arteries within the fascial sleeve, while the superficial veins lie for most of their course outside the fascial sleeve.

The deep veins, except for the axillary veins, are arranged in pairs, one on either side of the various arteries. The axillary vein, which is a direct continuation of the basilic vein, crosses the axilla and becomes the subclavian vein at the outer border of the first rib. Its branches correspond to those of the ax-

illary artery, except for the thoracoacromial, which joins the cephalic vein. The axillary vein receives the brachial veins in the lower portion of the axilla, and the cephalic vein in the upper portion of the axilla. The deep veins will not be of significance in venipuncture.

The superficial veins of the upper limb are the veins that will be selected in most elective venipunctures. Their anatomy is discussed below (Fig. 24-1).

Blood to the digits is drained through an anastomosis of *palmar* and *dorsal digital veins*. From the palmar aspect of the hand most blood flows to the dorsum of the hand, especially through the *intercapitular veins* that lie between the heads of the metacarpal bones and around the margins of these heads. Blood from the digits and palm therefore drains primarily into the *dorsal venous network* on the back of the hand. Two major veins arise from this dorsal venous network. The *cephalic vein* arises from the radial aspect of this network, and the *basilic vein* rises from the ulnar side. These veins ascend the forearm, the cephalic on the lateral aspect, the basilic medially. Within the forearm the *median vein of the forearm* arises and ascends the forearm on its medial aspect.

At the antecubital fossa a number of veins are visible. From lateral to medial are the *cephalic vein*, the *median cephalic*, the *median vein*, the *median basilic*, and the *basilic*. The cephalic vein continues upward through the clavipectoral fascia to drain into the *axillary vein*, and the *basilic vein* runs to the axilla, where it continues directly as the axillary vein.

ANATOMY

Clinically the arm provides the phlebotomist with four distinct areas for venipuncture. Starting at the upper part of the arm are found the antecubital fossa, which will be discussed as two separate areas: (1) the medial aspect of the antecubital fossa and (2) the lateral aspect of the antecubital fossa. In the descent down the arm the ventral aspect of the forearm is next, followed by the dorsum of the wrist and of the hand. Each of these potential venipuncture sites presents its own advantages and disadvantages.

Dorsum of the hand

The dorsum of the hand is the most preferred site for venipuncture among anesthesiologists (Fig. 24-3). It has several distinct advantages over other sites and has few disadvantages. It is one of my two preferred sites.

Anatomically it is rare to find arteries on the dorsal aspect of the hand, most arteries being located on

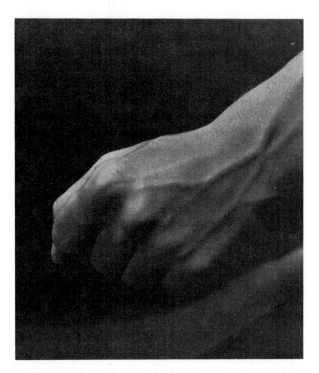

Fig. 24-3. Superficial veins of dorsum of hand and wrist.

the palmar aspect. In addition, most blood returning to the heart is routed into the veins that form the dorsal venous network, a group of superficial veins. Placement of most veins on the dorsum of the hand and of most arteries in the palm obviates the obstructive pressures that occur on the dorsum when a fist is formed, thereby maintaining intact the arterial blood supply to the hand during a "fight or flight" situation. This pattern is similar to the dorsal venous arch of the foot, which is distant from the pressure applied to the sole when a person stands.

The veins within the dorsal venous network have the obvious advantage of being quite superficial. Ease of accessibility is important when an elective venipuncture is being considered. A second advantage of the dorsum of the hand is the anatomical safety of the region. Rarely (but not never) will an artery be found on the dorsal aspect of the hand.

There are two disadvantages to these dorsal veins on the hand. First, the veins are smaller in size than veins found more proximally and second, because these veins are superficial, they tend to be mobile.

As to the first disadvantage, it is common practice within anesthesia to start an IV infusion on the dorsum of the hand using a needle not smaller than 18 gauge. Quite frequently a 16-gauge needle is used in this area. In virtually all children and adults the dorsum of the hand can readily accommodate these large-gauge needles. In dentistry a 21- or, rarely, a 23-gauge needle will be used for venipuncture, needles easily accomodated by the lumens of these smaller veins.

The mobility of veins on the dorsum of the hand can in some cases make venipuncture more difficult to accomplish. There are, fortunately, several techniques available for immobilizing these veins during venipuncture:

1. Holding the hand in a fist during venipuncture.
2. Pulling the skin of the dorsum toward the knuckles during venipuncture.
3. Use of the inverted Y configuration, if present.

These immobilization techniques will be discussed fully in Chapter 25.

It is sometimes said that venipuncture on the dorsum of the hand is more painful for the patient than at other sites. I personally have found that venipuncture in the dorsum is neither more comfortable nor uncomfortable than at any other site on the arm. The most important factor determining comfort or discomfort will be the technical prowess of the doctor attempting the venipuncture. With experience usually comes increasing technical ability and more comfort for the patient.

Wrist

The dorsal venous network continues proximally, draining subcutaneously along the margins of the hand and wrist into two major veins (Fig. 24-3). In most persons the veins of the wrist are not so uniform that they can be assigned names. However, on the lateral (radial) aspect of the wrist, in the snuff box, is found the so-called intern's or resident's vein. This vein becomes the cephalic vein as it ascends the forearm. Though usually visible, this vein has the disadvantage of being quite mobile and of being located in an area that is very difficult to immobilize.

Another vein, which ultimately becomes the basilic vein, is frequently found on the ulnar aspect of the dorsum of the wrist. It too is located in an area where mobility is great and immobilization difficult. Another vein may be found toward the middle of the dorsal aspect of the wrist. Of the three veins, this last represents the most logical choice for venipuncture in this region. It is both superficial and mobile, but immobilization may usually be achieved through the techniques discussed previously.

The ventral aspect of the wrist is not a desirable area for elective venipuncture. Though several veins are usually visible they possess some undesirable characteristics: they are not as large as those on the dorsum of the wrist; the anatomy of the region leaves

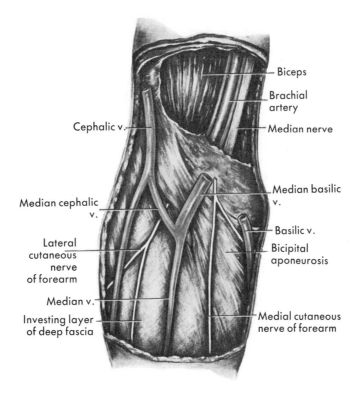

Fig. 24-4. Veins of the ventral forearm and antecubital fossa. (From Drummond-Jackson SL, ed: *Intravenous anaesthesia,* ed 5. London, 1971, Society for the Advancement of Anaesthesia in Dentistry.)

much to be desired—relatively superficial arteries, nerves, and tendons make the region both more sensitive and more risky for attempted venipuncture; and the wrist must be immobilized if a metal needle is to be used. The ventral aspect of the wrist is more difficult to immobilize than the dorsum.

In summary, the dorsum of the wrist is greatly preferred to its ventral aspect. However, significant disadvantages to use of the wrist for venipuncture exist, including vein mobility and the need to immobilize the wrist during the entire IV procedure.

Forearm

The forearm represents one of the two preferred sites for venipuncture on the upper limb (Fig. 24-4). The basilic and cephalic veins are the major veins found in the forearm, the basilic coursing up the medial (ulnar) aspect of the arm, the cephalic on the lateral or radial aspect. The basilic and cephalic veins are not as superficial as the veins found in the dorsum of the hand and the wrist; however, they are usually visible and oftentimes palpable, especially after application of a tourniquet.

A third vein, the median vein of the forearm, runs subcutaneously along the midline of the ventral surface. It lies somewhat deep at the distal end of the forearm, becoming superficial just below the antecubital fossa.

The dorsal aspect of the forearm may also be considered for venipuncture. However, because of a lack of obvious veins and the presence of hair, this site is not of primary importance.

Advantages of the veins of the forearm include the following:

1. The veins are larger than those found in the wrist and dorsum of the hand.
2. Veins, because they are not superficial, do not roll during venipuncture attempts.
3. There is no need to immobilize either the wrist or the antecubital fossa when the forearm is used for venipuncture. This increases patient comfort during the IV procedure.
4. Anatomically, the ventral (and dorsal) aspects of the forearm are devoid of any major arteries or nerves that might lie close to the usual venipuncture sites.

A disadvantage of the ventral aspect of the forearm is the lack of superficiality of the veins, making the venipuncture more difficult to perform in some patients.

Antecubital fossa

The antecubital fossa or elbow joint has for many years been one of the most popular sites for venipuncture. The usual pattern of veins in this region is illustrated in Fig. 24-5.

The cephalic and basilic veins traverse the lateral and medial aspects of the antecubital fossa. They represent relatively large targets for venipuncture. However, in some persons they may be located so far laterally or medially as to make the venipuncture technically difficult to carry out successfully, and where venipuncture is successful, stabilization of the needle is difficult.

The median vein of the forearm usually becomes somewhat more superficial as it approaches the antecubital fossa. It lies almost directly in the midline of the forearm. Just below the border of the antecubital fossa the median vein bifurcates.

In most persons the median vein divides into two major tributaries: the median cephalic and the median basilic veins. The median cephalic, as its name implies, runs laterally to join with the cephalic vein, and the median basilic runs medially, joining with the basilic vein.

In this, the most common pattern, the largest of the veins in the antecubital fossa is the median basilic vein. This is so because a deep vein connects with the median basilic vein in this area. Indeed, the median basilic vein is the first choice of phlebotomists. The median cephalic vein is also large, though not as large as the median basilic vein. The cephalic and basilic veins are also large, but because of their location (lateral and medial respectively), they are more difficult to enter and to secure the needle in.

Though many of the veins of the antecubital fossa appear quite large and therefore inviting targets for

venipuncture, there is a potential problem when venipuncture is carried out on the medial aspect of the antecubital fossa (by the neophyte). The problem lies in the anatomy of the region.

As is evident in a cross-sectional diagram of the antecubital fossa (Fig. 24-5), important structures are located directly below the medial aspect of the fossa. Centrally the biceps tendon passes deeply down to the upper end of the radius. Medial to this lies the bicipital aponeurosis. On the aponeurosis lies the large median basilic vein with the median cutaneous nerve of the forearm on its medial side. This vein is somewhat mobile (though not as mobile as the dorsal wrist veins) and may slip away from the needle tip during venipuncture if it is not immobilized adequately. Should the vessel be nicked, a large hematoma will develop. During immobilization the vein may be flattened, making venipuncture more difficult.

Of far greater importance, however, is the fact that immediately below the bicipital aponeurosis and the median basilic vein lie the median nerve and the brachial artery. It is not impossible for the novice to miss the median basilic vein and enter into the brachial artery or injure the median nerve.

No such potential problem exists on the lateral aspect of the antecubital fossa. The median cephalic vein, though smaller in size than the median basilic, is relatively immobile and can readily accommodate a 21-gauge needle. The lateral cutaneous nerve of the forearm lies nearby, but no important structures lie deep to the fascia. The radial nerve is lateral to the biceps tendon, but it lies in an intramuscular groove deep on the bone, well out of harm's way.

Advantages of the antecubital fossa as a venipuncture site include the following:

1. Veins are larger than other sites on the arm.
2. Veins are not mobile or as mobile as those on the wrist and dorsum of the hand.
3. The lateral aspect of the antecubital fossa is anatomically safe.

Disadvantages of the use of the antecubital fossa for venipuncture are as follows:

1. Veins are not as superficial as in other sites, making venipuncture difficult in some patients.
2. Anatomically the medial aspect of the fossa has important anatomy that should be avoided.
3. The antecubital fossa must be immobilized throughout the time that the needle is within the vein.

It is strongly recommended that the lateral aspect of the antecubital fossa be used preferentially, espe-

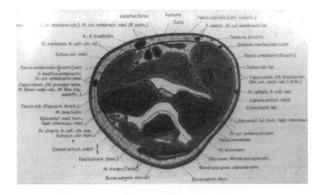

Fig. 24-5. Cross section of antecubital fossa (ventral area on top).

cially by the more inexperienced phlebotomist. As technical prowess increases, the medial aspect may also be employed.

Foot

On a few occasions it may be impractical or impossible to use the arm for venipuncture. Within the dental setting in an elective procedure on an ASA I or II patient, it might be advisable on this occasion to forgo the IV route in lieu of another technique of sedation. However, in pediatric dentistry, where superficial veins of the arm may be small and difficult to locate and cannulate, the foot may be considered for an IV route as more of a necessity than as an elective procedure. Additionally, many younger children are not willing to sit quietly in the chair while the doctor performs a venipuncture on the arm. This is especially so in pediatric patients requiring IV sedation for their management problems. The child can relatively easily move the arm or grab at it with the opposite hand, dislodging the needle. In this situation the foot may prove a more appropriate site for venipuncture.

The superficial veins of the foot are illustrated in Fig. 24-1. Anatomically the dorsum of the foot and the medial and lateral aspects of the ankle offer safe sites for venipuncture. Additionally, the dorsal veins of the foot are usually quite superficial.

The dorsum of the foot contains a dorsal venous network, similar to that found on the dorsum of the hand. As these veins progress toward the ankle, they drain into two major superficial vessels. Located immediately above the medial malleolus is the great saphenous vein, the largest superficial vein in the ankle or foot. On the opposite side, just below the lateral malleolus is found the small saphenous vein.

Advantages of the foot or ankle for venipuncture include the following:
1. Superficial vessels
2. Relatively large vessels
3. Anatomical safety
4. No need to immobilize venipuncture site

Disadvantages of the foot and ankle as a venipuncture site include the following:
1. Accessibility is more limited than upper limb.
2. Veins roll when contacted by needle.

SELECTION OF VENIPUNCTURE SITE

There are several factors to be considered when determining the ideal site for a venipuncture attempt.[3]

Condition of the superficial veins

Veins may appear tortuous, straight, hardened by age, scarred from previous use, sore, or inflamed from recent venipuncture. The preferred vein is one that is unused, easily visible, and relatively straight.

Relation of the vein to other anatomical structures

Potential venipuncture sites in which other anatomical structures of importance might be damaged should be avoided if possible. In the arm the primary area where this is of significance is the medial aspect of the antecubital fossa.

Duration of the venipuncture

During prolonged IV infusion (greater than 2 hours), a site that permits the patient the greatest freedom of movement is important. Thus a vein traversing a joint, such as the antecubital fossa or wrist, is not ideal for prolonged IV therapy because the joint will require immobilization if a rigid metal needle is used. Venipuncture on the dorsum of the hand or the ventral forearm will be better tolerated in this situation. Patients have complained bitterly, during 2- to 4-hour IV sedation, that an elbow has become quite stiff or sore because of the necessity for immobilization. For shorter durations (less than 2 hours), venipuncture may be established at any site on the limb.

Clinical status of the patient

Injury or disease involving one of the limbs may preclude the use of that area for venipuncture. Recent venipuncture in the selected site should lead the doctor to search for another potential site.

A prior history of phlebitis in the patient should forewarn the doctor to either reconsider the use of IV sedation or to search for the largest vein possible in the selected limb.

Age (size) of the patient

In neonates, unlikely to be patients in the dental office, scalp veins are preferred because of their accessibility and to simplify the problem of restraint of the infant. In seriously ill newborn infants the umbilical vein may be used during the first 24 to 48 hours of life.

Smaller children may have superficial veins of the upper limb that are very difficult to visualize. The foot may prove a more acceptable site for venipuncture.

In very obese patients veins may prove difficult or impossible to locate. Careful search of both arms and if necessary the foot will usually be fruitful in locating one or more veins. If the planned dental procedure is elective, the absence of superficial veins should be considered a contraindication to the use of IV sedation. Should it be essential to establish an IV line, hospitalization of the patient, with subsequent surgical cutdown to locate the vein, may be the most prudent course of action.

Type of intravenous procedure

The chemical nature of the drug(s) being administered, the size of the vein to be cannulated, and the size of the needle are important, for they all may produce irritation of the inner wall of the vein, a situation leading to an increased risk of phlebitis.

In general the larger the vein in relation to the size of the needle or catheter, the less likelihood there is that irritation and phlebitis will develop. This is because the drug(s) and infusion solution will undergo more rapid dilution in the blood when the caliber of the vein exceeds the outside diameter of the needle or cannula. Mechanical irritation by the needle or cannula against the endothelial wall of the vein is another cause of phlebitis. Cannulation of larger veins is a means of decreasing risk of venous irritation and subsequent phlebitis.

Two drugs discussed in this section are capable of producing significant venous irritation. These drugs, diazepam and pentobarbital, are also among the more frequently used IV sedatives in dentistry and medicine. Methods of minimizing the risk of phlebitis when these drugs are administered will be discussed in Chapter 27. These drugs should be administered slowly into a rapidly running IV infusion. The use of larger veins will minimize but not eliminate the risk of venous irritation developing.

RECOMMENDED SITES FOR VENIPUNCTURE

Five potential sites for venipuncture in the upper limb have been reviewed in this chapter. Below they are listed in my order of preference (Fig. 24-6):

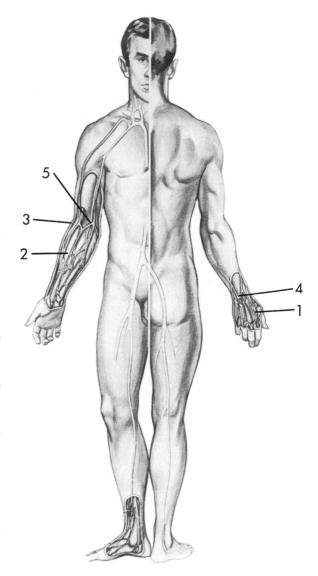

Fig. 24-6. Sites of venipuncture in order of preference: *1*, dorsum of hand; *2*, ventral forearm; *3*, lateral antecubital fossa; *4*, dorsal wrist; and *5*, medial antecubital fossa. (From Venipuncture and venous circulation, Chicago, 1971, Abbott Laboratories.)

Table 24-1. Comparison of venipuncture sites

Order of preference	Site	Proximity to important anatomy	Significant "roll" or movement of vein	Joint immobilization (metal needle only)
1	Dorsum of hand	No	Yes	No
2	Ventral forearm	No	No	No
3	Lateral antecubital fossa	No	No	Yes
4	Dorsal wrist	No	Yes	Yes
5	Medial antecubital fossa	Yes	No	Yes

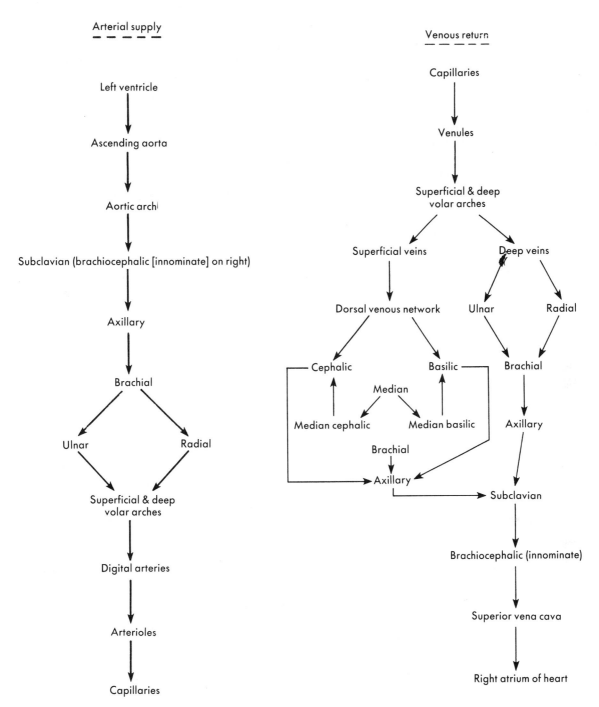

Fig. 24-7. Blood circulation in the upper extremity. Blood leaves the left ventricle; traverses arteries, arterioles, capillaries, venules, and veins; and returns to the right atrium via the superior vena cava.

1. Dorsum of hand
2. Ventral forearm
3. Lateral antecubital fossa
4. Dorsal wrist
5. Medial antecubital fossa

The *dorsum of the hand* is the most preferred because the veins are superficial and because of the anatomical safety of the site. However, the dorsum is not always an appropriate site for drugs that may produce venous irritation. A close second on the list is the *ventral forearm.* This site is the preferred site for longer-duration procedures and when the dorsum of the hand is not available. The absence of a need for immobilization of a joint, anatomical safety, and larger veins make this site suitable for most venipuncture procedures.

Running far behind the first two sites are the *lateral antecubital fossa,* chosen for its larger veins and anatomical safety; the *dorsal wrist,* with its superficial veins; and lastly, the *medial antecubital fossa,* with its larger veins, but with its significant anatomy just below the surface. All three of these sites will also re-quire immobilization of a joint if rigid metal needles are used.

Table 24-1 summarizes some of the important features of the five venipuncture sites on the upper limb. Figure 24-7 summarizes blood flow through the arm.

REFERENCES

1. Malamed SF: Unpublished data, 1993.
2. Grant JCB: *An atlas of anatomy.* Baltimore, 1962, Williams & Wilkins.
3. Abbott Laboratories: Venipuncture and venous cannulation, Chicago, 1971, Abbott Laboratories.

CHAPTER 25

Venipuncture technique

The preparation of the equipment for an intravenous (IV) infusion and the technique of venipuncture will be discussed in this chapter

PREPARATION OF EQUIPMENT

1. The armamentarium discussed in Chapter 24 is laid out and removed from its packaging.
2. The flow-regulating clamp or screw on the IV infusion set is turned to the closed position, so that no fluid will run through the tubing when it is inserted into the bag of IV solution (Fig. 25-1).
3. The winged infusion set is removed from its box and attached to the end of the IV tubing. The needle covering is left on the needle (Fig. 25-2). If an indwelling catheter is to be used, it should not be attached to the IV tubing.
4. The cap or cover is removed from the entry ports on the bag of IV infusion solution (Fig. 25-3).
5. The protective covering over the piercing pin on the IV tubing is removed carefully so as not to contaminate the pin.
6. The IV infusion bag is held securely in one hand while the piercing pin is firmly pushed through the entry port into the IV solution (Fig. 25-4).
7. The bag of IV solution is inverted and suspended from the IV pole.
8. The drip chamber on the IV tubing should be filled approximately halfway with IV solution. If it is not, the chamber is squeezed and released to draw solution into it (Fig. 25-5). If the chamber is filled to the extent that it is impossible to visualize the individual drops of solution as they exit the IV bag, the bag and drip chamber are inverted and the drip chamber is squeezed to force the solution back into the IV bag (Fig. 25-6). Care must be taken to avoid the entry of air bubbles into the IV tubing at this time.

9. The flow-regulating clamp or screw is slowly opened, permitting fluid to run through the entire length of the IV tubing and the attached needle, removing as many air bubbles as possible from the tubing. On occasion it will be impossible to remove every bubble from the tubing. Although there is little significance to a few air bubbles entering the patient's cardiovascular system, it is best to attempt to eliminate them. The potential problem of air embolism will be discussed in Chapter 28.
10. The flow-regulating screw is closed to stop the flow of solution. The IV infusion is now ready for use.

Additional equipment required for venipuncture includes:
- Tourniquet
- Three to five 2- to 3-inch strips of tape
- Alcohol wipe
- Dry 2- × 2-inch gauze squares
- Armboard: wrist or elbow immobilizer
- Bandage
- Sphygmomanometer
- Stethoscope
- Monitoring devices
- O_2 and emergency kit

PREPARATION FOR VENIPUNCTURE

The patient is asked to visit the restroom, if necessary, prior to the start of the venipuncture. Once the IV has been started and sedative drugs administered, it will be more difficult for the patient and office staff to accomplish a visit to the restroom.

The patient is seated in the chair in a comfortable position. A semireclined to supine position is recommended as being physiologically superior to the upright position.

Preoperative vital signs are recorded on the pa-

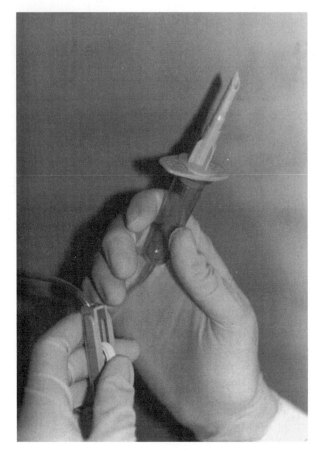

Fig. 25-1. The flow-regulating clamp is placed in the closed position.

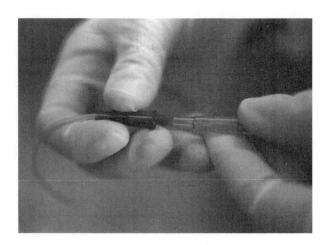

Fig. 25-2. The needle is attached to the infusion set.

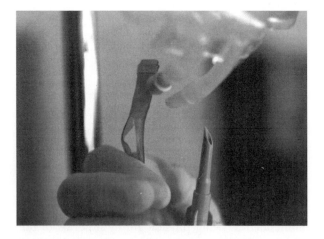

Fig. 25-3. Protective caps are removed from the infusion solution and the piercing pin.

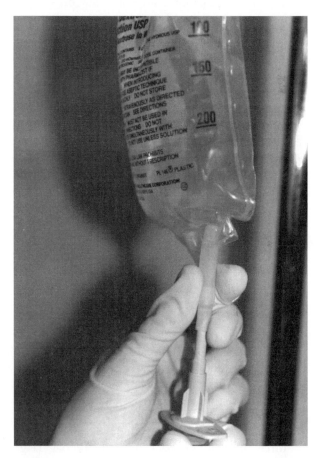

Fig. 25-4. The piercing pin is inserted into the entry port on the IV solution container.

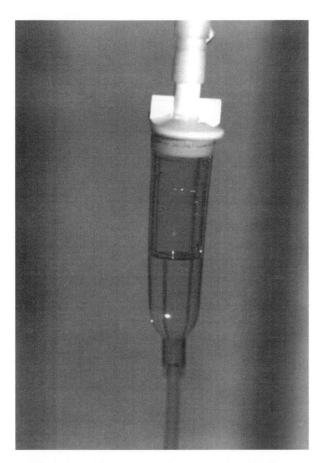

Fig. 25-5. The drip chamber should be approximately half filled with sedation.

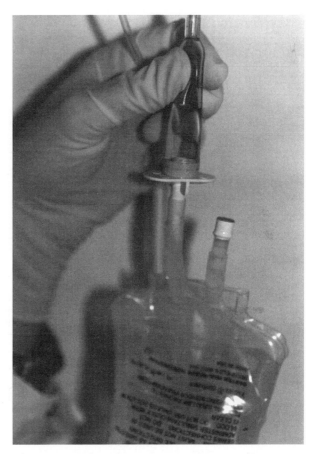

Fig. 25-6. If the drip chamber is overfilled, bag is inverted and chamber squeezed to remove solution.

tient's sedation record sheet (Fig. 25-7). Included should be the blood pressure, heart rate and rhythm, and respiratory rate. The patient's baseline vital signs have been recorded at a prior visit to the dental office.

The blood pressure cuff (sphygmomanometer) is placed on the left arm and permitted to remain in place throughout the IV procedure. The procedure should be reversed if the doctor is left-handed.

The patient's arms (without the tourniquet in place) are scanned for obvious veins. Quite often, veins will be made readily visible if the arm is permitted to hang down below the level of the patient's heart for a few minutes, as this augments venous distention (Fig. 25-8). One of the functions of the preoperative visit is to determine if the patient has suitable veins for the IV procedure.

On occasion, a patient who had very visible, superficial veins at the preoperative visit, will appear in the office on the day of treatment with no obvious veins. This is explained by the presence of a greater degree of anxiety and higher levels of circulating catecholamines. When veins are not readily apparent, the patient should be asked at what site on the arm he has previously had blood drawn successfully. Sometimes a patient will boast that "'they' had to try four times before they found a vein" or that "three people had to try before they succeeded." This should alert the doctor that a more difficult venipuncture might be in the offing. However, such a statement by the patient may also be used to the doctor's advantage. If, by using "special care," the doctor is able to successfully complete the venipuncture on the first or second attempt, the patient will feel more confident in that doctor's overall ability. Several methods of distending veins are available and are discussed later.

If the Trieger test for evaluation of recovery is to be used (see Chapter 6), the baseline Trieger test is now completed by the patient.

Patient's Name:		S.S.#:		Age:		Date: ___/___/___

Medical Hx:	CVS ___	Current Medications: ___	IV started at ___ a.m./p.m.
	Respiratory System ___	___	Venipuncture Site ___
	CNS ___	___	Type of Needle ___
	Liver ___	___	IV d/c'd at ___ a.m./p.m.
	Kidneys ___	Allergy: ___	IV Solution & Volume ___ ML
	Other ___	___	

Base Line Vital Signs:		ASA: I, II, III, IV	DRUGS ADMINISTERED - SUMMARY -
Date of V.S.: ___			
B.P.: ___	P.R.: ___	Reason for Sedation: ___	
R.: ___	T.: ___		
Ht.: ___	Wt.: ___	Evaluator: ___	
Age: ___		Name of Driver: ___	

	PREOPERATIVE	INTRAOPERATIVE					POST-OP	DISCHARGE
	time	time	time	time	time	time	time	time
Blood Pressure								
Heart Rate								
Respirations								
	O₂ LPM							
	N₂O LPM							
	(mg)							
List all drugs	(mg)							
and route of	(mg)							
administration	(mg)							
(IV, IM)	(mg)							
	(mg)							
	(mg)							

DRUGS DISCARDED - SUMMARY -

DENTISTRY TREATMENT

Start_____   Finish_____

Name of person discharged to: _____

Post-Op Medications (if any): _____

Additional Monitoring:	precordial stethoscope _____	pulse oximeter _____
(check as appropriate)	ECG _____	automatic blood pressure _____

COMMENTS

Student Doctor: _____	AMED Faculty: _____	☐ Informed Consent
IV Student: _____	Assistants: _____	☐ Post-Operative Instructions

SAM/USC/SOD
02/85

Fig. 25-7. Sample of a sedation record for IV sedation procedure.

Any other monitoring devices, such as the pulse oximeter, precordial stethoscope, or electrocardiograph, are now placed on the patient.

Because of the possibility of accidental inoculation of health professionals with viral and other organisms found in some patients' blood, precautions are essential in situations that involve potential contact with blood. All persons working with the venipuncture should wear gloves throughout the procedure, from the point of preparation until the IV is removed, the bleeding stops, and a bandage is in place. For doctors and personnel who have performed venipuncture for many years without using gloves this may present a little difficulty at first. However, with perseverance, the wearing of gloves will no longer be an added burden, only an additional safety measure.

CAUTION

Latex gloves should *always* be worn by all personnel while preparing for and performing venipuncture.

A tourniquet is next applied to the limb (arm or leg) selected for venipuncture. On the arm the tourniquet is applied superior to the antecubital fossa. The commonly used soft rubber tubing is applied in a slipknot (Fig. 25-9). The tourniquet should be sufficiently tight as to obstruct venous drainage without obstructing arterial flow into the limb. A radial pulse should still be present if the arm is used.

When a blood pressure cuff is used as a tourniquet, the pressure in the cuff is raised and locked at a point between the patient's systolic and diastolic pressures (e.g., 120 mm Hg if the blood pressure is 140/90). This produces venous distention in the same manner as the tourniquet.

The patient is asked to repeatedly open and close her or his hand. This muscular activity forces more blood into the veins, allowing additional arterial blood to enter into the limb and further distend the veins. Once the veins have been distended, the patient is asked to keep the fist clenched until the venipuncture has been successfully completed.

At this point, most persons will have one or more readily visible veins; however, some others will as yet have no visible or even palpable veins. Several methods are available to increase venous distention.

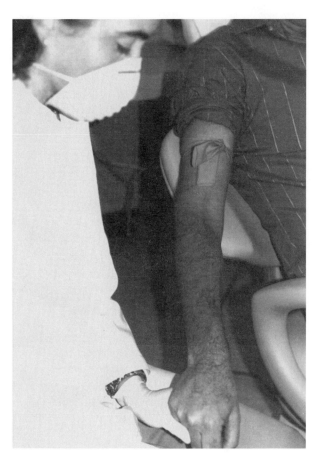

Fig. 25-8. Distention of veins may be augmented by permitting the arm to hang below heart level.

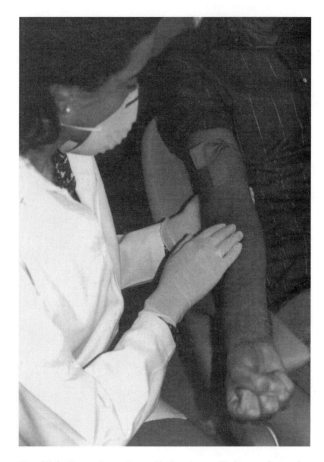

Fig. 25-9. Tourniquet is applied, using a slipknot, above the antecubital fossa. Opening and closing of the hand further aids venous distention.

1. *Light slapping* or *rubbing of the skin* over the vessel will aid in venodilation.
2. Anything that produces heat aids in dilating the blood vessel. The direct application of heat to the area is also a great aid.
   a. A *warm, moist towel* should be applied for several minutes to the entire region proximal and distal to the proposed venipuncture site.
   b. It had been suggested that an *electric hairdryer* can be used as a quick method to produce vasodilation at almost any site.
3. Another means of producing vasodilation is to use nitrous oxide-oxygen (N_2O-O_2) sedation, which produces the following beneficial effects during venipuncture:
   a. Peripheral vasodilation
   b. A degree of analgesia, making the venipuncture less traumatic

When N_2O-O_2 is used as an aid during venipuncture, the patient should be sedated as in Chapter 16 and returned to a nonsedated state prior to the administration of any IV medications.

Once the vein chosen for cannulation has been adequately distended the site must be prepared. Physical restraints are seldom required, as most patients rarely object strenuously to venipuncture (although they may not "like it"). When a vein in the antecubital fossa is selected, an elbow immobilizer should be placed prior to start of the venipuncture (Fig. 25-10). When the wrist is selected, the wrist immobilizer is applied after the venipuncture.

Some experts recommend that any solution used to cleanse the injection site be warmed to body temperature. Because the arm is warm, it is more sensitive to cold, so that the blood vessel may contract (e.g., disappear or "collapse") almost immediately on exposure to a cold or rapidly evaporating solution such as alcohol.

When using needles larger than 21 gauge (18, 16,

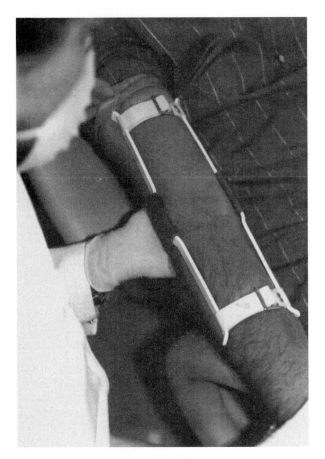

Fig. 25-10. Elbow immobilizer is placed prior to the venipuncture.

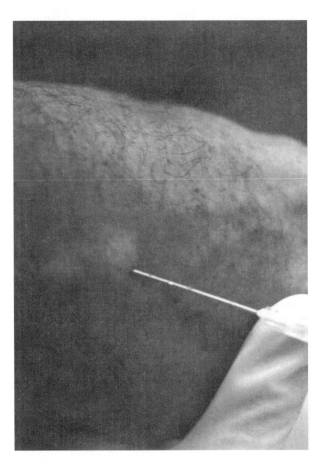

Fig. 25-11. One percent lidocaine wheal is raised at site of venipuncture.

or 14 gauge), venipuncture can be rendered virtually painless by simply raising a wheal in the skin over the vein by injecting 0.2 to 0.3 ml of a 1% lidocaine hydrochloride solution (Fig. 25-11). A 25-gauge needle should be used. However, use of needles of 21 gauge or smaller is not associated with excessive discomfort so that the preceding technique is not necessary. Indeed, the injection of lidocaine itself produces a stinging sensation.

Patients who are fearful about both the dental and the IV procedure should have received preoperative oral sedative drugs approximately 1 hour prior to the planned start of the procedure. Sedation with N_2O-O_2 should also be considered at this time.

The venipuncture site must now be cleansed. In many large hospitals it is common practice to prepare the venipuncture site by using both a defatting agent and an antibacterial agent. Commonly available preparations are benzalkonium chloride tincture and 70% alcohol solution and 99% isopropyl

alcohol and Betadine (povidone-iodine). Povidone-iodine solution is preferred to tincture of iodine because it is considerably less irritating and equally effective; on the other hand, tincture of iodine is more rapid acting. In most short-term IV situations, the traditional alcohol wipe is still used and is considered to be the minimal preparation recommended at the IV site. The site is thoroughly cleansed with the alcohol wipe and then permitted to air-dry, or a sterile, dry 2- × 2-inch gauze wipe may be used to dry the area prior to venipuncture.

WINGED INFUSION SET
Dorsum of hand

The wings of the needle are held by the thumb and middle fingers, the index finger placed between the wings (Fig. 25-12).[1] This permits the operator the greatest control over the needle. Holding the needle as illustrated in Fig. 25-13 is improper, as the finger beneath the needle will interfere with the attempted

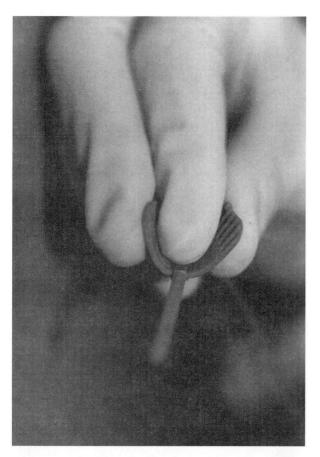

Fig. 25-12. The index finger is placed between wings of needle and the wings are folded over by thumb and middle fingers. This provides doctor with increased tactile sensation during venipuncture.

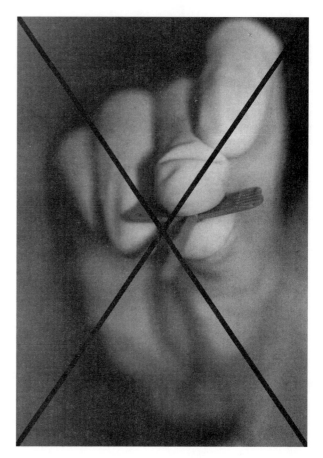

Fig. 25-13. The thumb and index finger are placed on either side of the wings of the needle. This technique makes it more difficult to successfully complete venipuncture.

venipuncture. The sheath over the needle is removed and care taken from this point on not to contaminate the needle by touching it to any object. Should this occur, the needle is immediately replaced with a new, sterile one. Air in the tubing of the new needle must be removed by running the IV infusion solution through the needle.

The patient's hand is kept in a clenched fist until the venipuncture is completed. The patient's fist is supported in the doctor's left hand, the thumb of the doctor's left hand placed below the patient's knuckles, and the skin of the dorsum of the hand pulled toward the doctor (Fig. 25-14).

These two techniques aid in minimizing the mobility of the vein during venipuncture. Should this be ineffective, the patient bends the fist down, further immobilizing the vein. Care is taken in these techniques, as in some patients the vein may actually collapse when attempts are made to immobilize it.

When the dorsum of the hand is used for venipuncture, the site of needle entry into the skin will be lateral to the vein and approximately ¼ inch below the desired point of entry of the needle into the vein (Fig. 25-15). This takes into account the mobility of these veins. Should the needle be placed directly atop the vein, as pressure is applied on the needle, the vein will invariably roll out from under the needle.

The optimal angle of entry of the needle through the skin is 30 degrees (Fig. 25-16). Angles greater than this increase the risk of the needle penetrating through the entire vein, and angles of less than 30 degrees lead to increased discomfort during passage through the skin. *The bevel of the needle will always be facing up.* The point of the needle is placed gently against the skin at the site of entry and the needle directed parallel to the course of the vein.

With the skin of the dorsum still pulled over the

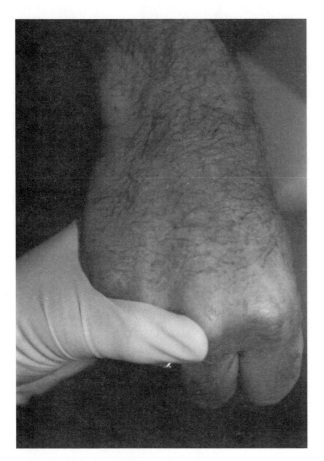

Fig. 25-14. The doctor supports the patient's hand and pulls the skin of the hand over the knuckle.

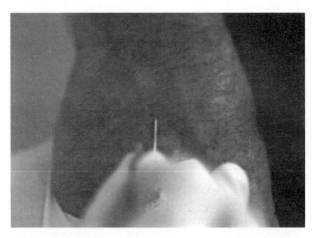

Fig. 25-15. Entry point of the needle is just lateral to vein.

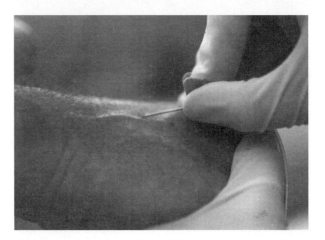

Fig. 25-16. Optimum angle of needle entry is 30 degrees.

knuckles, the point of the needle penetrates the skin just to the side of the vein. Resistance to the needle will be noted as it passes through the skin. Once through the skin, resistance decreases markedly. At this point, the angle of the needle is decreased so that the shaft of the needle is held parallel to the skin (Fig. 25-17). The veins of the dorsum are quite superficial, and if the needle is passed deeper, the vein may be missed entirely. Direction of the needle is also altered at this time. The needle should be angled toward the spot on the vein where the needle tip is about to enter the lumen of the vessel. Angulation should be gentle, so that the needle meets with the vein about 10 mm above the point of entry into the skin.

The needle is gently advanced toward the vein. There should be little resistance and no discomfort to the patient at this time. As the needle tip comes into contact with the vein wall on the dorsum of the hand, the doctor will observe the vein move as it is pushed by the needle. This is a common occurrence,

and it is easily managed. The needle tip has yet to enter into the lumen of the vein, but the tip has come into contact with the vein wall. As the needle continues to move in the same direction, the vein may continue to be pushed along with the needle. Because the vein cannot move indefinitely within the confines of the skin, it will soon appear to "pop" and to fall back to its original position on the hand. (This is similar to increasing pressure being applied to the outside of an inflated balloon until the balloon finally pops). This occurs as the needle enters into the lumen and resistance is lost. On some occasions, the patient may also be aware of this "popping" feeling.

A backflow of blood into the tubing is the one sure sign of a successful venipuncture (Fig. 25-18). The needle is redirected so that it lies parallel to the direction of the vein, and the needle is advanced very gently several more millimeters into the lumen of the vessel.

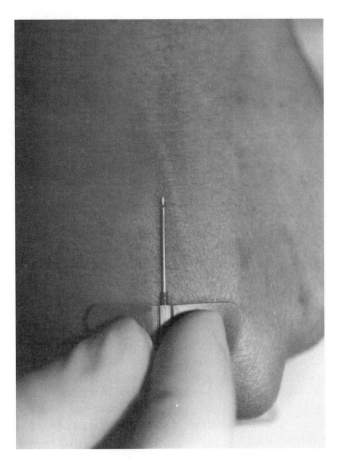

Fig. 25-17. Angle of needle decreased and needle tip directed toward vein.

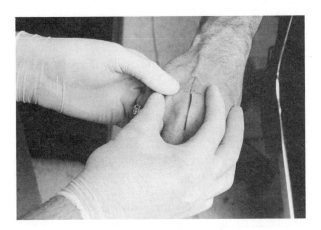

Fig. 25-18. Return of blood into IV tubing signifies successful venipuncture. Doctor holds wing securely until needle is secured.

This minimizes the risk of a needle that is tenuously placed within a vein becoming dislodged as it is being secured or if the patient accidentally moves his or her hand.

Care must be taken during this procedure so that the point of this rigid needle does not puncture or perforate the inferior wall of the vessel. To prevent this, the needle tip is angled so that it is held upward within the lumen of the vein as the needle is being advanced. The shaft of the needle need be placed only a few millimeters into the lumen of the vessel. Attempts to advance the entire needle shaft into the vessel frequently result in loss of the vein through puncture of the wall and in the formation of a hematoma.

Once in the vein, the plastic wings of the needle are placed against the patient's skin and held in position by the doctor while the assistant performs several important tasks. The doctor's primary job at this time is to maintain the needle within the vein.

The assistant releases the tourniquet on the patient's arm. This results in a significant drop in the venous blood pressure, and the blood leaves the IV tubing, and reenters the patient's blood vessels. The tourniquet is removed and the IV infusion started.

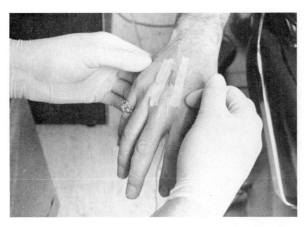

Fig. 25-19. Tape is placed across each wing, being secured from below needle proximally.

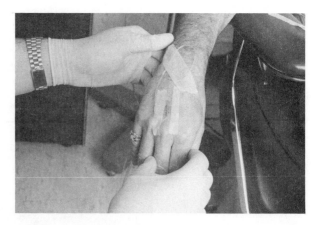

Fig. 25-20. Loop of tubing is secured with the third piece of tape, and the fourth piece is placed at the site of needle penetration of the skin.

The assistant opens the flow screw or knob on the tubing, and drops of solution should appear in the drip chamber. This is done immediately so as to prevent the clotting of blood within the needle or tubing. The next task is to secure the needle within the vein by taping the needle into position.

Many variations on taping exist, and only one is offered here. The goal in taping, of course, is to secure the needle in position for the duration of the planned procedure. With the doctor holding the needle gently against the patient's skin a 2-inch piece of tape is placed across one of the wings, parallel to the direction in which the needle is pointing. A second piece of tape is placed on the other wing in the same exact manner. It is strongly recommended that as the tape is being secured against the skin, it be applied from the site away from the needle entry point into the skin toward the needle tip (Fig. 25-19). Although this may seem a trivial point, I have observed many doctors accidentally dislodge the needle from the vein as they sought to secure it with tape, pressure being applied from the needle tip toward the wings.

A 3- to 4-inch length of tape is next placed across a loop made in the IV tubing. This loop serves as a shock absorber in the event that the IV tubing is accidentally pulled. The loop of tubing serves to prevent the needle from being easily pulled out of the vein should this occur.

A fourth piece of tape, about 2 inches long, is placed over the site at which the needle enters the skin to keep the site clean. This is done only if the tape is transparent. The site of needle entry into the skin should remain visible during the procedure in the event of swelling or discomfort at the site (Fig.

25-20). The patient is now ready for the administration of IV medications.

The most pressing problem in establishing an IV infusion on the dorsum of the hand is the mobility of the veins; any method of immobilization is appreciated. Three means of so doing have been described (clenched fist, bending hand, and thumb pulling skin over knuckles). A fourth, a naturally occurring anatomical configuration of veins, may also be used to advantage. This configuration involves the formation of an inverted *Y*, formed from the merging of two smaller veins to form a larger one. Frequently this configuration is located just above the knuckles as two digital veins converge (Fig. 25-21). Basic venipuncture technique is identical to that just described. The primary difference is that the entry of the needle into the vein will occur at the point of confluence of these three vessels. By inserting the needle between the two digital veins and aiming for the point at which they merge, the veins are prevented from rolling away from the needle.

The needle enters into the skin about ¼ to ½ inch below the convergence of the veins and is directed toward that spot. Pressure is exerted on the needle, which then enters the lumen of the vein, and the needle is advanced and then secured, as previously described. The inverted *Y* is a highly recommended site for venipuncture on the dorsum of the hand.

Following successful completion of the venipuncture on the dorsum of the hand, immobilizing the wrist should be considered if the needle tip is located in its proximity. Needles placed further away from the wrist do not require the use of an arm immobilizer (Fig. 25-22).

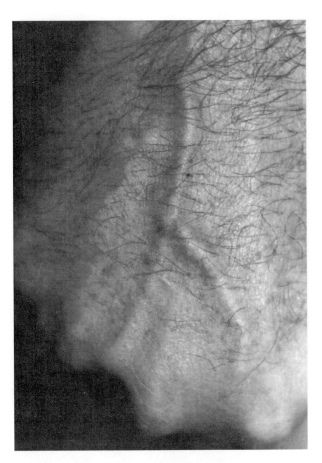

Fig. 25-21. Y formed by merging of two veins is ideal configuration for venipuncture. Needle is placed approximately ¼" to ½" below convergence of veins.

The patient holds the armboard securely while tape is placed around the fingers and the armboard. The proximal end of the armboard is then taped to the patient's forearm. A piece of gauze placed between the patient's skin and the tape will prevent hairs from sticking to the tape, thereby minimizing patient discomfort when the tape is removed.

Dorsum of wrist

The technique of venipuncture on the dorsum of the wrist with the winged infusion set is identical to that just described for the dorsum of the hand. It is extremely rare to find the inverted Y configuration on the wrist; however, when it is present, its use is recommended. The use of an armboard is necessary whenever a rigid needle tip is located in the wrist.

Ventral forearm

The ventral aspect of the forearm and the dorsum of the hand are the most recommended sites for ve-

nipuncture. Because veins at this site are less superficial than those of the dorsum of the hand and wrist, they tend to be somewhat less mobile. Because of this decreased mobility, there is a slight variation in the venipuncture technique on the ventral forearm.

Needle placement on the skin of the forearm will be directly atop the vein to be entered rather than on the side of the vein. Held in the same 30-degree angle, the needle is directed into the skin and then directly into the vein. Once blood returns into the tubing, signifying successful entry into the vein, the angle of the needle is decreased so that it is held almost parallel to the skin and slowly advanced several millimeters into the vein.

During venipuncture, the thumb of the opposite hand of the doctor should be placed on the skin several inches below (distal to) the planned entry site, pulling skin at the site in a direction opposite to that of the needle (Fig. 25-23). This facilitates entry of the needle through the skin. All other components of venipuncture at this site are identical to the basic procedure described. Immobilization of the wrist or antecubital fossa is not required when the forearm is used for venipuncture.

Antecubital fossa

The technique of venipuncture at either the medial or lateral antecubital fossa is identical to that of the ventral forearm with the important exception that the elbow must be immobilized. It is suggested that immobilization of the joint occur *prior* to venipuncture rather than after, when accidental movement by the patient might dislodge the needle (Fig. 25-24).

Occasionally veins in the antecubital fossa will be superficial. In this case it is possible that the vein will roll out from under the needle as venipuncture progresses. Should this occur, the attempt is continued using the technique described for the dorsum of the hand, with the needle entering from the side of the vein.

INDWELLING CATHETER
All injection sites

The indwelling catheter requires a somewhat different venipuncture technique from that just described for the winged infusion set, a device that is somewhat more manageable by the beginner. The IV infusion is prepared for use as described previously, with the exception that the catheter is not attached to the IV tubing.

The vein is selected, distended, and prepared for venipuncture as usual. The indwelling catheter is

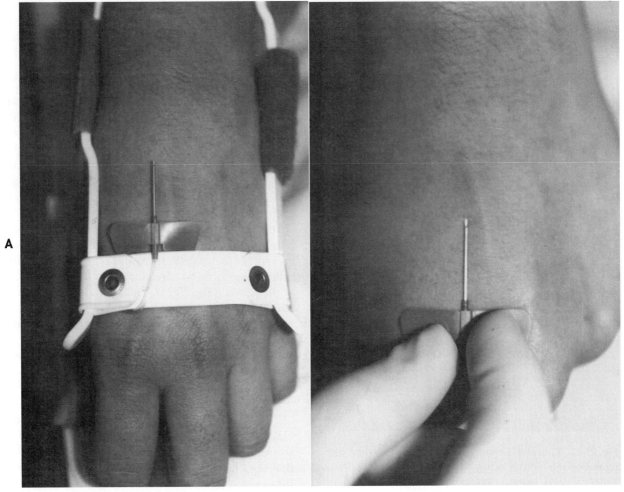

Fig. 25-22. Needle placed in dorsum of wrist requires wrist to be immobilized (**A**) while needle placed in dorsum of hand does not (**B**).

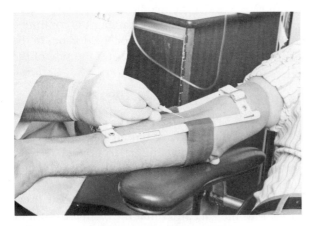

Fig. 25-23. Angle of penetration of skin is 30 to 45 degrees. Skin is retracted by fingers of other hand.

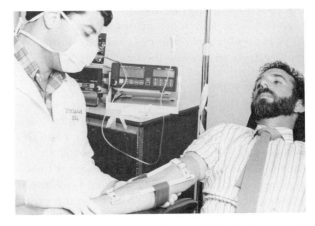

Fig. 25-24. Antecubital fossa is immobilized prior to venipuncture.

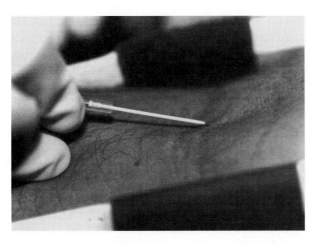

Fig. 25-25. Needle is inserted into vein at angle of 30 degrees until blood return is observed in plastic window *(arrow)*.

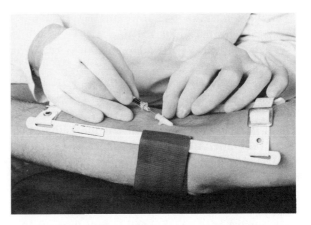

Fig. 25-26. Once vein is entered, decrease needle angle, advance needle several millimeters into vein, and advance catheter to its hub.

held at a 30-degree angle to the skin, either lateral to the vein or directly atop it, depending on the site of venipuncture.[2,3] The skin is pulled in the direction opposite to which the needle is being advanced to facilitate passage through the skin. Resistance is lost once skin is penetrated, the angle of the needle is decreased, and the needle directed toward the vein. On entry of the needle into the vein, blood will be noted in the needle (Fig. 25-25). The needle is angled parallel to the course of the vein and advanced a few more millimeters into the vessel. It is at this point that the technique of venipuncture with the indwelling catheter differs from the technique with the winged infusion set.

The hub of the metal needle is held securely in one hand while the other hand is placed onto the catheter hub. The entire length of the plastic catheter is slowly and gently advanced into the vein (Fig. 25-26). It is important that *the catheter not be forced if any resistance is encountered.* It is also important that *only the catheter be advanced into the vein and that the metal introducer (the metal needle) not be withdrawn from the catheter.*

The tourniquet is removed to decrease venous pressure. The assistant holds the needle adapter end of the IV tubing while the doctor removes the metal introducer needle from the indwelling catheter. The needle adapter is expeditiously connected to the catheter hub and the IV flow begun (Fig. 25-27). The needle adapter and catheter must not be released at this time because they have yet to be secured. Once the introducer needle is removed from the catheter, blood will flow back into the catheter and, if the cath-

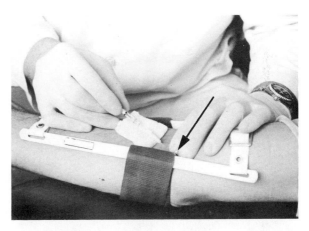

Fig. 25-27. The catheter is inserted slowly into the vein and the metal needle is removed. Note placement of the doctor's finger over the tip of the catheter *(arrow)*. This prevents any bleeding when the metal needle is removed.

eter is not attached to the IV tubing, onto the patient. The importance of removing the tourniquet prior to this step is obvious, for what amounts to a mere oozing of blood out of the catheter without the tourniquet would be a torrent of blood if the tourniquet were left in place. Even for experienced hands this step can become untidy. To minimize this possibility the following is suggested:

1. Release the tourniquet.
2. Place a dry 2- × 2-inch gauze wipe beneath the end of the catheter (Fig. 25-27). This will absorb the small volume of blood that might be lost.
3. Press your fingertip onto the skin directly above the tip of the catheter within the vein. This oc-

cludes the catheter, preventing any blood loss through the catheter.

4. Connect the needle adapter and the catheter (Fig. 25-28).

If step 3 is done properly, this entire process can be completed at a leisurely pace, without the loss of any blood.

The IV drip is now started and the catheter secured with tape. Although several taping techniques are available, just one will be presented. A 5- or 6-inch piece of narrow tape is used for taping the catheter (This tape is prepared by tearing a full piece of tape in half lengthwise.) Standard-size Scotch-brand tape (uncut) is of suitable width (not more than 1 inch wide). The center of the tape is placed beneath the catheter just below the needle adapter with the adhesive side of the tape facing upward (away from the skin). One end of the tape is then crossed over the top of the catheter and secured against the skin (Fig. 25-29). The same process occurs for the other end of the tape, crossing the catheter and the first piece of tape. This technique results in the catheter being securely placed within the lumen of the vein with little possibility of its being accidentally removed.

The connection between the needle adapter and the catheter is checked to ensure that it is secure, and a 3- to 4-inch piece of tape is placed over the connection (Fig. 25-30).

A loop is made with the IV tubing and taped against the skin. Whenever tape is used to secure a venipuncture, it should be secured to the patient's skin, not to another piece of tape. If one piece of tape becomes loose, any tape that is attached to it will also become loose, jeopardizing the venipuncture.

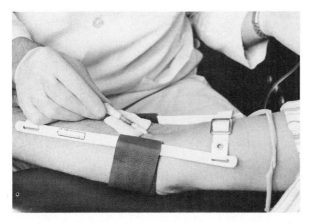

Fig. 25-28. IV tubing is attached to the catheter, drip is started, and flashbulb is squeezed to check adequacy of venipuncture.

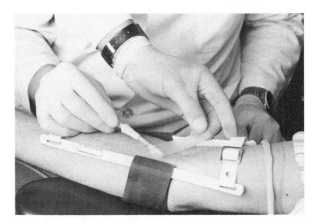

Fig. 25-29. Adhesive is placed beneath the catheter and then brought forward onto the skin.

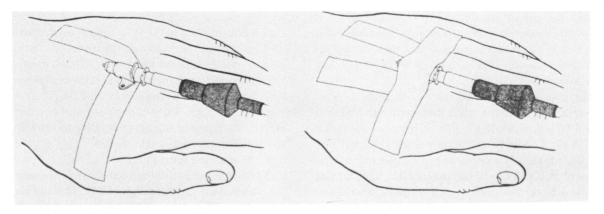

Fig. 25-30. A second piece of tape is placed over the catheter hub. (From Quik-Cath information sheet, Deerfield, Ill, 1983, Travenol Laboratories.)

Because of the flexible catheter within the vein, armboards and elbow immobilizers are not necessary. The patient is now ready for the administration of the IV medications.

HOLLOW METAL NEEDLE
Dorsum of hand and ventral forearm

Although not recommended for use in routine IV sedation, the hollow metal needle may be used for venipuncture in emergency situations or in short-term procedures, such as the drawing of blood samples for laboratory analysis. The hollow metal needle will almost always be attached to a syringe, which contains a drug to be injected or into which blood is to be drawn.

The basic technique of venipuncture is the same as that described earlier for the winged infusion set. Once the metal needle has entered the vein, however, great care must be taken in advancing the needle because it is often difficult to obtain the correct needle angulation within the vein with a syringe attached (syringes are available that have an excentrically placed needle, making venipuncture somewhat easier). The tourniquet is removed and the syringe held securely in place.

Prior to the administration of the drug, an aspiration test must be performed to confirm that the needle tip still lies within the vessel's lumen. With one hand holding the syringe in position, the other hand gently pulls the plunger of the syringe back until a backflow of blood is observed. This technique (drawing of blood into syringe) is called *barbitage*. (Fig. 25-31). The drug is then administered.

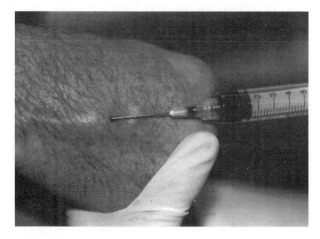

Fig. 25-31. Barbitage. Blood pulled into syringe to dilute drug.

Dorsal wrist and antecubital fossa

Venipuncture with the hollow metal needle on the dorsum of the wrist or the antecubital fossa differs from the technique described above only in that movement of the joint must be prevented. An elbow immobilizer or armboard may be used.

Before discussing the termination of the intravenous infusion, a few comments are warranted concerning the technique of venipuncture:
1. Experienced phlebotomists spend more time locating a suitable vein than in actually doing the venipuncture. Time spent in distending veins is usually time well spent, as the likelihood of successfully entering a larger diameter vein is greater than of penetrating a small vein.
2. If the tourniquet is placed on the leg or arm for an extended time, the skin will become mottled, then purple, and will feel cool. The patient will probably complain of discomfort as a period of hyperesthesia develops. Should this occur, remove the tourniquet and permit the circulation in the tissue to be restored. After 2 to 3 minutes, the tourniquet may be reapplied and the procedure restarted. Venipuncture should not take long to complete. Each of the steps described is performed sequentially. As experience and technical ability are acquired, the speed with which venipuncture is completed will increase.
3. If the needle gets "lost" within the tissues during attempted venipuncture (e.g., the needle should be in the vein, but it is not), do not use the needle as a probe in an attempt to locate the vein. Using the needle as a probe will simply traumatize the tissues, increase patient discomfort, and greatly increase the risk of accidentally puncturing the vein and producing a hematoma. The following sequence is recommended in this situation:
    a. Locate the tip of the needle by lifting the needle tip up and looking for the imprint it makes under the skin.
    b. If the tip is located under and beyond the vein, withdraw the needle slightly so that the tip is pulled back on the other side of the vein. Elevate the tip of the needle and readvance it toward the vein.
    c. If the needle tip has advanced over and beyond the vein, withdraw the needle slightly so that the tip is pulled back to the original side of the vein. Readvance the needle with

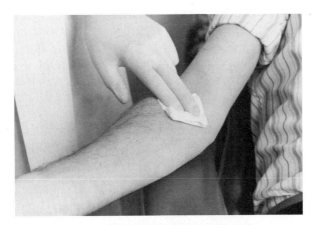

Fig. 25-32. Firm, direct finger pressure over the site of venipuncture prevents postoperative hematoma.

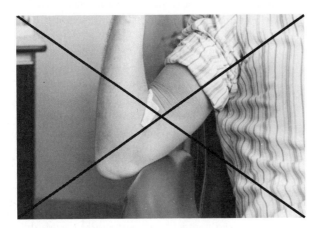

Fig. 25-33. Placing gauze over the injection site and bending the elbow does *not* provide adequate pressure and frequently results in hematoma formation.

the tip pointed more parallel to the vein than in the previous attempt.

TERMINATING THE INTRAVENOUS INFUSION

At the conclusion of the IV procedure, the needle or catheter must be removed prior to discharge of the patient from the office. Criteria for terminating the IV infusion are discussed in Chapter 27. It is assumed here that all criteria have been satisfactorily met by the patient.

1. If an IV infusion is being used, the drip is stopped by tightening the rate control screw or knob.
2. The needle or catheter is held gently in position while the tape is carefully removed from the skin.
3. A sterile 2- × 2-inch gauze square is placed over

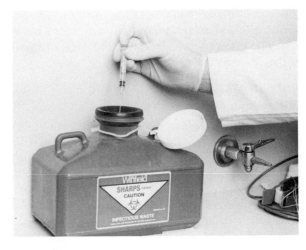

Fig. 25-34. An appropriate disposal unit should be available for used needles.

the site of needle entry into the skin. No pressure is exerted because pressure on the skin while the needle is still within the vein will be uncomfortable for the patient and might well injure the vein as the needle is withdrawn.

4. The needle or catheter is carefully withdrawn from the vein. The assistant should cap the needle immediately so that no one will be accidentally stuck with a contaminated needle.
5. As soon as the needle is withdrawn from the skin firm, direct finger pressure is applied onto the gauze square over the site of penetration of the skin (Fig. 25-33). Pressure is maintained for at least 3 to 5 minutes. Failure to do so may result in the formation of a hematoma.
6. When the antecubital fossa is used for venipuncture, a common mistake is to place a gauze square on the site and have the patient bend his elbow (Fig. 25-34), assuming that this will provide pressure adequate to stop the bleeding. *Bending of the elbow does not provide adequate pressure and will result in a hematoma!* Regardless of the location of the venipuncture, it is important that firm, direct pressure with a gloved hand be applied for at least 3 to 5 minutes.
7. A bandage is placed over the puncture site.
8. The needle is destroyed (Fig. 25-35), and the IV needle, tubing, and bag are discarded.

REFERENCES

1. Abbott Laboratories: *I.V. Tips #6: how to use the butterfly infusion set,* Chicago, 1972, Abbott Laboratories, Inc.
2. Travenol Laboratories: *Quik-Cath, product information sheet,* Deerfield, Ill, 1978, Travenol Laboratories, Inc.
3. Abbott Laboratories: Venipuncture and Venous Cannulation, Chicago, 1971, Abbott Laboratories, Inc.

CHAPTER 26

Pharmacology

A significant number of drugs are available for conscious sedation via the intravenous (IV) route. These include a number of categories, primarily sedative-hypnotics, opioids, and the anticholinergics. The drugs used most frequently in IV sedation are listed in Table 26-1. Also listed in Table 26-1 are several drugs (indicated by an asterisk) that are not recommended for IV use by doctors who have not completed a residency in anesthesiology. These drugs are discussed briefly in this chapter so that the doctor may fully understand the rationale for their not being recommended.

BENZODIAZEPINES

The benzodiazepines have become the most commonly used IV sedative drugs in dentistry and perhaps also in medicine. Five benzodiazepines will be discussed (Table 26-2), four of which are presently available in the United States and one (flunitrazepam) that is available outside the United States.

Diazepam

Diazepam was synthesized in 1959 by Sternbach and Reeder. The drug became available as Valium (Hoffmann-LaRoche) in 1963 and shortly thereafter became the most prescribed oral drug in the Western world, a position it only recently relinquished to cimetidine (Tagamet).[1] Diazepam is also available in a parenteral preparation for intramuscular (IM) and IV use (Chapter 11).

Intravenous administration of diazepam appears to have begun with the work of Davidau[2] in Paris in 1965. This was followed shortly thereafter by a report by Main[3] in 1967, who used diazepam as an adjunct to the Jorgensen technique. In 1968 Brown[4] reported on 40 cases in which diazepam was used alone, the drug being administered until the patient felt sleepy.

In 1969 O'Neill and Verrill[5] reported on the use of IV diazepam for the production of sedation in minor oral surgical procedures, with good to excellent results in 51 of 52 patients treated. The following year O'Neill et al. reported on 55 patients undergoing dental surgical procedures lasting between 20 and 45 minutes. Intravenous diazepam provided successful sedation and cooperation in 49 patients, four others moved and spoke occasionally but were able to be treated, and two patients required additional IV medications (methohexital) for treatment to be completed successfully.[6]

The dosage used in these patients was that required to produce marked ptosis (drooping of the upper eyelid). Halfway ptosis of the upper eyelid is now recognized as the Verrill sign.[7] The practice of administering diazepam until the appearance of the Verrill sign produces a sedative level that is considered by some to be more profound than is necessary and is therefore not recommended for routine use.[8]

Peter Foreman[9] in New Zealand used diazepam in combination with atropine and incremental doses of methohexital. Although successful, he stated that the addition of even small amounts of methohexital greatly increased the risk of overdosage. In his next study Foreman used diazepam alone for a variety of dental therapies, finding that although the degree of amnesia produced by diazepam varied significantly from patient to patient, virtually all patients agreed that dental treatment had been at least tolerable rather than an ordeal. He found that IV diazepam had made it possible to treat those patients who may not have received proper treatment in the past because of fear. Foreman stated, "Diazepam has become the drug of choice for the trained general dental practitioner, as well as for the introduction of dental students to intravenous sedation."[10]

Table 26-1. Drugs available for IV sedation

Sedative-hypnotics and antianxiety drugs

 Benzodiazepines
  Diazepam
  Midazolam
  Lorazepam†
  Flunitrazepam‡
  Chlordiazepoxide†
 Barbiturates
  Pentobarbital
  Secobarbital
  Methohexital*
  Thiopental*
  Thiamylal*

Antihistamines

 Promethazine
 Hydroxyzine†

Opioid agonists

 Meperidine
 Morphine
 Alphaprodine‡
 Fentanyl

Opioid agonist/antagonists

 Pentazocine
 Nalbuphine
 Butorphanol

Opioid antagonist

 Naloxone

Anticholinergics

 Atropine
 Scopolamine
 Glycopyrrolate

Antidotal drugs

 Flumazenil
 Naloxone
 Nalbuphine
 Physotigmine
 Procaine

Others

 Innovar (droperidol with fentanyl)*
 Ketamine*
 Propofol

*Not recommended for use in IV sedation without anesthesiology training.
†Not recommended for use in IV conscious sedation.
‡Not available for clinical use in United States (7/94).

Chemistry

Diazepam is a member of the 1,4-benzodiazepine group of compounds. The chemical formula for diazepam is 7-chloro-1,3-dihydro-1methyl-5-phenyl-2H-1,4-benzodiazepin-2-one. It is a pale yellow-white crystalline powder with virtually no odor. It is considerably soluble in chloroform and acetone, moderately soluble in ethanol and ether, and poorly soluble in water.[11]

General pharmacology

It is believed today that emotions are largely controlled by the limbic system, that portion of the brain composed of the amygdala, hippocampus, and septal areas.[12] The midbrain reticular formation, hypothalamus, and thalamus are also involved with the experience or transmission of emotions.

Diazepam in very small doses appears to act on the hippocampus, whereas other areas of the brain remain unaffected and the patient remains alert.[13] After oral diazepam this action of the drug would be appropriate; however, when administered intravenously a greater effect of diazepam is desired. When administered to the point at which sedation and ataxia (loss of muscular coordination) occur, a more generalized depression of the central nervous system is noted.

More specifically, research has suggested that the anxiolytic properties of benzodiazepines are mediated by increased inhibitory nerve transmission.[14] Aminobutyric acid (GABA) is an important inhibitory neurotransmitter in the brain. Glycine (aminoacetic acid), the simplest nonessential amino acid, may be the major inhibitory transmitter of the spinal cord. The anticonvulsant and sedative properties of benzodiazepines may result from a direct agonist effect on stereospecific benzodiazepine receptors, which in turn facilitate the inhibitory action of GABA on its own postsynaptic receptors.

Fate of intravenous diazepam

Following IV administration diazepam reaches a peak blood level in approximately 1 to 2 minutes. The onset of clinical activity is therefore quite rapid.[15] Blood levels of approximately 1.0 μg/ml may be achieved after an IV dose of 10 to 20 mg of diazepam.[16] Clinically this would equate with a deeper level of sedation and a period of anterograde amnesia.

As has been mentioned in Chapters 8 and 11, diazepam has a plasma half-life of approximately 30 hours.[17] A commonly held misconception is that a

Table 26-2. Benzodiazepines for IV administration

Generic name	Proprietary name	Mg/ml	Duration of action (minutes)	Average sedative dose, (mg)
Diazepam	Valium	5	45	10-12
Lorazepam	Ativan	2, 4	6-8 hours	2-4
Midazolam	Versed, Dormicum	1	45	2.5-7.5

drug with a long half-life will possess a long duration of action, whereas one with a shorter half-life will have a shorter duration of action. This is not true, and diazepam is an excellent example of this. The β–half-life of a drug simply indicates the rate at which the drug undergoes biotransformation in the liver, whereas the factor most responsible for a drug's duration of action is its degree of receptor-site (protein) binding.

Over a period of approximately 45 minutes after the administration of an appropriately titrated dose of diazepam, the patient will remain sedated and free of anxiety. In many patients the following distinct phases of this sedation can be observed, each lasting approximately 15 minutes.

Phase 1. Zero to 15 minutes. During this period the patient is sedated to his or her maximal degree, because the cerebral blood level of diazepam is at its peak level. The patient remains responsive to verbal and physical stimulation, but response time is increased, speech is slurred, and the patient may have difficulty enunciating words. The patient may not appear to be aware of the presence of the doctor or the assistant during this phase. Amnesia, if it is to occur, usually involves procedures occurring at this time.

Phase 2. 16 to 30 minutes. The level of sedation is somewhat diminished (the patient is more aware of his surroundings than in phase 1; however, he or she is definitely still sedated, as the cerebral blood level of diazepam begins to decrease as the drug undergoes redistribution: (α–half-life) to those organs and parts of the body that are less vessel rich than the brain. Response from the patient is more rapid, the slowing down of responses from phase 1 having diminished or disappeared. Patients can usually recall events occurring during this phase, although in isolated cases amnesia may occur in this phase too.

Phase 3. 31 to 45 minutes. During this period the typical patient will state that he or she feels normal again; in other words the feeling of sedation has dis-

sipated. Many doctors may be tempted to administer additional diazepam to the patient; however, this is normally not necessary. Although no longer feeling sedated, the patient is also no longer apprehensive. The now decreasing cerebral blood level of diazepam is no longer adequate to maintain the earlier depth of sedation, but it is sufficient to provide an anxiolytic state (similar to the desired actions of oral diazepam). With treatment nearing completion and the patient free of pain as a result of the administration of local anesthetics, there is usually no need for the readministration of diazepam at this time.

Phase 4. 46 to 60 minutes after receiving diazepam, virtually all patients will feel, and in fact look, recovered. This is not a result of the β-half-life of the drug (30 hours) but because of redistribution: α-half-life. The blood level of diazepam at 60 minutes after administration of 20 mg intravenously is 0.25 µg/ml.[16] The patient is not recovered at this time, and under no circumstances should the doctor think that this patient is capable of operating a car or leaving the dental or surgical office unescorted.

As redistribution of diazepam continues during this first hour after IV administration, the level of the drug increases in several storage sites—the fat, the walls of the intestines, and the gallbladder. Diazepam stored in fat will usually be retained there because the drug is quite lipid-soluble and the blood supply of fat is relatively poor.

A clinically significant phenomenon can arise at this point, produced by the diazepam now stored in the gallbladder and intestinal walls. Known as the *rebound effect* or *second peak effect,* it involves a recurrence of symptoms of sedation and drowsiness approximately 1 hour after the first meal taken after the patient leaves the treatment site.[18] In most cases this will be about 4 to 6 hours after the procedure began. After a meal, particularly one rich in lipids, the gallbladder constricts, releasing its contents of bile and unmetabolized diazepam into the small intestine, where over the next hour or so the diazepam is reabsorbed into the cardiovascular system. In some patients the diazepam blood level may reach a level at which clinical signs and symptoms of sedation recur. In most instances the patient feels quite tired and will want to lie down for a few minutes. It becomes absolutely essential, therefore, that the patient receiving diazepam, as well as his or her escort, be advised of this possibility prior to discharge from the dental office. The rebound effect is less likely to be observed in patients whose gallbladder has been removed.

Because diazepam is extremely lipophilic, it cannot be excreted through the kidneys and must therefore undergo biotransformation in the liver.

Biotransformation

Diazepam is biotransformed by one of two pathways. In the first the diazepam molecule undergoes demethylation to desmethyldiazepam, which possesses anxiolytic, but not sedative, effects. Desmethyldiazepam is too lipophilic to permit its excretion by the kidney. Desmethyldiazepam has a half-life of 96 hours and eventually undergoes hydroxylation to oxazepam.[19]

The second pathway involves the hydroxylation of the diazepam molecule to 3-hydroxydiazepam, another pharmacologically active metabolite also known as temazepam. Temazepam undergoes demethylation into oxazepam.

Oxazepam is yet another water-insoluble, anxiolytic benzodiazepine. It is used as an anxiolytic agent by the oral route of administration. The pharmacology of oxazepam (Serax) was discussed in Chapter 8. The half-life of oxazepam is short, ranging between 3 and 21 hours. It is rapidly biotransformed into its major metabolite, oxazepam glucuronide.

Effects of age and disease

It is frequently stated that drug dosages should be decreased in the very young and the elderly patient as well as in patients with significant liver disease. The clinical properties of diazepam have been well studied in these groups of patents.[20-23] The following is presented as a summation of that research:

In patients age 2 years and older, diazepam is handled as in the adult. The only significant clinical advice is to adjust the dose of the drug appropriately. With titration via the IV route, clinical results are usually achieved at smaller doses than in adults.

In the older patient the dose of diazepam by the IV (or any other) route should be decreased for several reasons. The rate at which the drug undergoes

biotransformation is decreased in older patients. In addition, when administered orally, the drug will be absorbed in the gastrointestinal tract somewhat more slowly. However, the most important reason for the apparent increased sensitivity of older patients to diazepam and other drugs is related primarily to protein binding. Older patients exhibit decreased protein binding of drugs.[20] This means that there will be more of the free, unbound drug available within the blood to cross the blood-brain barrier and produce central nervous system (CNS) depression. Diazepam is offered as an example: In the younger patient diazepam is approximately 98.5% protein bound.[21] Therefore, the clinical effects of diazepam will be produced by but 1.5% of the dosage administered—the non–protein-bound diazepam. In the older patient, in whom protein binding has decreased, diazepam may be 97% protein bound, still a significant figure, but one permitting 3% (or twice as much) non–protein-bound diazepam to be available to produce CNS depression. It becomes obvious that when administered the same dose of the drug, the clinical actions on the older patient will be exaggerated. The dosages of diazepam by the oral and IM routes must be decreased in older patients. With IV administration, titration will provide effective sedation at what will probably be a smaller dose of the drug than is usually given.

Skeletal muscle relaxation

Diazepam, as well as the other benzodiazepines, produces skeletal muscle relaxation. Research has demonstrated that the muscle-relaxant properties of benzodiazepines are caused by central rather than peripheral effects.[24] Monosynaptic reflexes such as the knee jerk reflex are essentially unaffected by even large doses of diazepam, whereas polysynaptic reflexes are depressed by rather small doses.

Anticonvulsant activity

Benzodiazepines have important anticonvulsant properties. Diazepam, midazolam, chlordiazepoxide, nitrazepam (as well as other benzodiazepines) have the ability to antagonize the convulsive effects of local anesthetic overdose produced by lidocaine, mepivacaine, bupivacaine, cocaine, and procaine.

In one study the seizure threshold for lidocaine-induced tonic-clonic seizure activity was 8.5 mg/kg.[25] When IM diazepam was administered 60 minutes before treatment in a dose of 0.25 to 0.5 mg/kg, the seizure threshold was elevated to 16.8 mg/kg of lidocaine. Although barbiturates also provide protection (e.g., pentobarbital, 10 mg/kg), they also produce profound behavioral, cardiovascular, and respiratory depression compared to the minimal effects produced by the benzodiazepines.[26]

In the management of generalized tonic-clonic seizures the benzodiazepines have not supplanted phenytoin and phenobarbital as oral maintenance anticonvulsants. Intravenous diazepam is the drug of choice, however, in the management of status epilepticus and acute seizure activity.[27] Once the seizure has been controlled, maintenance therapy with other anticonvulsants is initiated.

Cardiovascular system

Hemodynamic studies show that diazepam produces little effect on the cardiovascular system of healthy human subjects.[28] Intravenous diazepam, in a dose of 0.3 mg/kg, produces no clinically significant changes in either blood pressure or cardiac output.

Diazepam has been compared with thiopental as a preanesthetic induction agent in the cardiovascularly compromised patient (ASA III and IV).[29] Administered intravenously in a dose of 0.2 mg/kg, fewer than 1% of the patients studied experienced a reduction of cardiac output of more than 15%, and none had a mean blood pressure reduction of more than 15%. In contrast, on receiving 2 mg/kg of thiopental, 85% of the patients exhibited more than a 15% reduction in cardiac output, whereas 68% demonstrated more than a 15% reduction in blood pressure.

Adverse hemodynamic effects attributable to the benzodiazepines are rare in humans, even in patients with significant cardiac or pulmonary disease.[30]

Respiratory system

All sedative-hypnotics, including the benzodiazepines, are potential respiratory depressants. When studied in patients without pulmonary disease, respiratory depression produced by intravenously administered benzodiazepines is barely detectable.[31] In addition, and quite significantly, the benzodiazepines do not potentiate the respiratory-depressant actions of opioids.[32]

Hepatic disease

Agitation and combativeness are not infrequently encountered among patients with liver disease. Murray-Lyon et al.[33] in a study of patients with severe parenchymal liver disease administered diazepam intravenously.[33] Adequate sedation was achieved in all patients with no deterioration of their clinical status. Diazepam, when administered with care, is an appropriate sedative for patients whose liver function is impaired.

Pain

In general, studies have failed to demonstrate specific analgesic properties of the benzodiazepines; however, high doses of these agents will impair motor response to painful stimulation.[34] These studies show that benzodiazepines are much more capable of attenuating the emotional response to pain than of altering the actual sensation of pain.

More recent studies have demonstrated that diazepam may possess some slight analgesic properties.[35] These properties do not, however, alter the fact that in clinical situations in which pain control is a factor during dental treatment local anesthetics must still be administered in the usual manner.

Amnesia

Intravenously administered diazepam produces what is termed *anterograde amnesia*.[36] This is a lack of recall occurring from the time of injection onward. Retrograde amnesia, a lack of recall of events occurring prior to drug administration, is quite rare. Amnesia following diazepam administration is infrequent after IM administration and essentially nonexistent after oral administration.

After IV administration of diazepam the duration of the amnesic period is approximately 10 minutes; however, considerable variation is noted. During this time patients respond normally to stimulation, but at a later time (immediately postoperatively or 24 hours later) they will be unable to recall the event.

In my experience with IV diazepam sedation, amnesia has developed in approximately 75% of patients. Whereas the length of amnesia has varied, it has been limited in most persons to the first 10 to 15 minutes after diazepam administration. In fewer patients the amnesic effect has lasted through the entire appointment.

The importance of the amnesic phase is that traumatic procedures may be completed, with the patient responding normally to them. However, at the termination of the procedure the patient will have no recall of the procedure. The most commonly employed procedure at this time is the administration of local anesthetic. It is quite common for the patient to respond to the initial administration of the local anesthetic (although administration should be performed as atraumatically as possible). At the end of the dental or surgical procedure patients will often question the doctor to find out either how their lips or tongue became numb without a "shot" or how the drug that was injected into their arm (the diazepam) kept them from feeling the procedure. Unfortunately the amnesic period will not include the time period prior to the administration of the diazepam (retrograde amnesia); therefore, the patient will almost always remember the venipuncture attempt or attempts.

Although amnesia is usually a welcome benefit of IV conscious sedation, the absence of amnesia does not imply that the procedure was a failure. The goal of sedation is the relaxation of the patient so that treatment can be completed in a more ideal manner. The presence or absence of amnesia does not alter this fact. Lack of recall should be considered to be the "icing on the cake."

Contraindications

Injectable diazepam is contraindicated in patients with the following: Known allergy to diazepam or other benzodiazepines and acute narrow-angle glaucoma and open-angle glaucoma, unless the patient is receiving appropriate therapy.

Warnings

Probably the most significant side effect of intravenously administered diazepam is the occurrence of venous thrombosis, phlebitis, local irritation, or swelling. Although these complications are quite rare with the administration of IV diazepam as recommended in Chapter 27, one of the manufacturers of diazepam, Roche Laboratories, Inc., recommends the following as a means to minimize this possibility[37]:

1. The solution should be injected slowly, taking at least 1 minute for each milliliter (5 mg).
2. Small veins, such as those on the dorsum of the hand or wrist, should not be used.
3. Extreme care should be taken to avoid intraarterial administration or extravasation.
4. Diazepam should not be mixed or diluted with other solutions or drugs in a syringe or infusion flask.
5. If it is not feasible to administer diazepam directly intravenously, it may be injected slowly through the infusion tubing as close as possible to the vein insertion.

Other warnings include the following:

1. Extreme care must be exercised when diazepam is administered to elderly or debilitated patients and to those with limited pulmonary reserve because of the possibility of apnea or cardiac arrest or both.
2. Concomitant use of barbiturates, alcohol, or other CNS depressants increases depression with increased risk of apnea.
3. When diazepam is administered with an opioid analgesic, the dosage of the opioid should be reduced by at least one-third and should be administered in small increments.

The administration of IV diazepam as recommended in Chapter 27 takes into account these warnings. Titration will prevent accidental overdose in the preceding situations.

Use in pregnancy

Any drug that crosses the blood-brain barrier also crosses the placenta into the fetus. An increased risk of congenital malformation associated with the administration of benzodiazepines during the first trimester of pregnancy has been suggested in several studies.[38] Because the administration of these drugs in dentistry is rarely a matter of urgency, their use at this time cannot be recommended. The possibility that a woman of childbearing potential may be pregnant at the time diazepam is used should always be considered.

Pediatric use

Children 2 years of age and older handle diazepam as adults do. The major consideration is the dosage, which in all likelihood will be smaller than that for the typical adult. If administered intravenously, titration will provide the proper safeguard to prevent overdosage.

The administration of IV diazepam alone to younger children in the dental setting has not always provided ideal sedation. Difficulties exist in establishing venipuncture in any of these patients. Even more significant, however, is the child's response to the feeling of being lightly sedated. Whereas the adult will become more relaxed and cooperative as the effect of the diazepam increases, many younger children will appear to "fight" the effect, becoming increasingly agitated and uncomfortable. Some persons will term this a paradoxical reaction to the drug. It is my feeling that the child is responding to the altered sensations occurring in his head. Being unaccustomed to this feeling, the child moves around so as to "get away" from it. Intravenous diazepam used alone in younger children does not provide a consistently adequate level of sedation.

Precautions

When diazepam is combined with other psychotropic agents, careful consideration must be given to possible potentiation of drug effect.[37] Categories such as the phenothiazines, opioids, barbiturates, monoamine oxidase inhibitors (MAOIs), and other antidepressants are included.

Because metabolites of diazepam are excreted in the kidneys, the administration of diazepam in patients with compromised renal function should be undertaken with care. Lower dosages may be required for the elderly or debilitated patient.

Patients receiving diazepam intravenously must be cautioned against engaging in hazardous occupations requiring complete mental alertness, such as operating machinery or driving a motor vehicle. Patients should also be advised against the use of alcoholic beverages after the administration of IV diazepam. As a general rule it is my policy to recommend that patients neither drive their car nor consume alcohol for the remainder of the treatment day at least, and not the next day if recovery at that time is not complete.

Adverse reactions

The most frequently reported adverse reaction to intravenously administered diazepam is phlebitis at the site of injection. This will be discussed in Chapter 28. Other less frequently occurring adverse reactions include:

Hyperactivity

Confusion

Nausea (extremely rare)

Changes in libido

Hiccoughs (not uncommon; more annoying than anything)

Decreased salivation (a benefit in dental treatment)

Paradoxical reactions such as acute hyperexcited states, anxiety, hallucinations, increased muscle spasticity, rage, and stimulation are also seen. The general term for this phenomenon is *emergence delirium*. It is seen more frequently with scopolamine administration and will be discussed thoroughly in Chapter 28.

Dosage

The following directions regarding recommended dosage are taken from the diazepam package insert[37]:

Dosage should be individualized for maximal beneficial effect. The usual recommended dose in older children and adults ranges from 2 to 20 mg IV, depending on the indication and its severity. Lower doses, usually 2 to 5 mg . . . should be used for elderly or debilitated patients.

The dose of intravenously administered diazepam will always be determined by titrating the drug slowly into a rapidly running IV infusion. In this manner each patient will receive the dose appropriate for sedation, and overdosage should not occur.

Availability

Valium (Roche): 5 mg/ml in 2-ml ampules, 10-ml multiple-dose vials, and 2-ml preloaded syringe. Injectable diazepam consists of the following ingredients[37]:

40% propylene glycol

10% ethyl alcohol

5% sodium benzoate and benzoic acid as buffers

1.5% benzyl alcohol as preservative

Diazepam is classified as a Schedule IV drug. Propylene glycol and ethyl alcohol are included because diazepam is lipid soluble and relatively water insoluble; therefore, it requires a nonaqueous solvent system. Many of the complications and side effects attributed to diazepam, especially phlebitis, are in fact produced by the propylene glycol, which is also a major component of antifreeze.[39]

The IV administration of diazepam can produce a sensation of burning in some patients. This is caused not by the diazepam but rather by the propylene glycol vehicle. It is recommended that the patient be advised of this possibility as the drug is administered. The doctor will tell the patient that "there may be a feeling of warmth as the drug is administered. This is entirely normal and will pass within a few minutes." As the drug is carried by the blood away from the injection site, this sensation fades. Its occurrence may be minimized by opening the IV infusion to a rapid rate prior to the injection of the diazepam. Some persons recommend the administration of 1 ml of 1% lidocaine or procaine into the IV line immediately prior to the administration of diazepam. The analgesic properties of lidocaine and procaine prevent the burning sensation from occurring. In my experience with diazepam, slow injection of the drug (diazepam) into a rapidly running infusion will prevent this sensation from arising. Lidocaine administration is not necessary.

The search for a water-soluble benzodiazepine with clinical properties similar to diazepam but without its potential for venous irritation has led to the development of midazolam. Diazepam is presently the most frequently used IV sedative within dentistry. When used as recommended it is quite safe and extremely effective in the management of severe apprehension and fear of the dental or surgical situation. Intravenous diazepam is recognized as one of the two "basic" intravenous sedation techniques in dentistry.

DIAZEPAM

The medical history of patients receiving diazepam should be checked for the following:
Allergy or hypersensitivity to benzodiazepines
Glaucoma (untreated)
Phlebitis, thrombophlebitis

DIAZEPAM

Proprietary name	Valium
Classification	Benzodiazepine
Availability	5 mg/ml
Average sedative dose	10-12 mg
Maximal single dose	20 mg
Maximal total dose	30 mg

Midazolam

Midazolam is a 1,4-benzodiazepine compound that is similar in most pharmacological aspects to diazepam. It possesses several attributes, however, which appear to make it somewhat more attractive than diazepam in certain clinical situations.

Midazolam was synthesized in 1975 by Walser and Fryer at Hoffmann-LaRoche, Inc. Midazolam was available in many parts of the world in the early 1980s and was released for use in the United States in 1986. The chemical formula is 8-chloro-5(2′fluorophenyl)-1-methyl-4H-imidazo (1,5-a)(1,4) benzodiazepine maleate. It is a colorless crystal in an aqueous solution. Each milliliter contains either 1 or 5 mg midazolam maleate buffered to a pH of 3.3.[40] The acidic pH maintains the benzodiazepine ring in an open configuration, which is required for its water solubility (the diazepam ring is closed, and it is insoluble in water). Once in the body, the physiologic pH (7.4) acts to close the ring, providing the chemical structure of the drug that is required for its clinical efficacy.

Its water solubility differentiates midazolam from other parenteral benzodiazepines—diazepam, lorazepam, and chlordiazepoxide. The requirement for potentially irritating solvents, such as propylene glycol, is eliminated with midazolam. The water solubility of midazolam is produced by the substitution of imidazole at the 1,2 position of the 1,4 benzodiazepine ring structure and is aided because midazolam is the salt of an acid. This water solubility is responsible for the positive findings of a lack of burning sensation on injection and the absence of phlebitic sequelae at the injection site.

Pharmacokinetics and biotransformation

Midazolam undergoes metabolism in the liver by hydroxylation into three major metabolites.[41] Whereas the major metabolites of diazepam are pharmacologically active anxiolytics, the major metabolites of midazolam have no pharmacologic activity. In addition, because of the lack of active metabolites and its shorter half-life, a rebound effect is not evidenced with midazolam.

The α–half-life (produced by distribution and redistribution) of midazolam has been recorded as 4 to 18 minutes. The β–half-life (the result of metabolism and excretion) is 1.7 to 2.4 hours. By contrast, diazepam's β–half-life is 31.3 hours.[42] The shorter half-lives of midazolam make the drug more suitable for ambulatory sedation procedures—a relatively short duration of action combined with a relatively rapidly inactivated and excreted drug.

Midazolam is 94% protein bound, binding occurring primarily in the serum albumin. Midazolam possesses a relatively rapid onset of action, the induction of general anesthesia having ranged from 55 to 143 seconds.[43]

Amnesia

Midazolam, like the other parenteral benzodiazepines, has the ability to produce anterograde amnesia. Conner et al.[44] demonstrated the following incidence of amnesia in patients receiving IV midazolam[44]:

Time after injection (minutes)	Amnesic patients (%)
2	96
30	87.5*
32	69
43	57

---

*From Fragen RJ and Caldwell NJ: Recovery from midazolam used for short operations, *Anesthesiology* 153:511, 1980.

These results indicate that midazolam is superior to other benzodiazepines or IV drug combinations in providing anterograde amnesia. In one study 71% of the patients did not recall being in the recovery room.[44] Other studies have not demonstrated these same remarkable results, but in all cases the degree of anterograde amnesia provided by midazolam was at least equal to that produced by diazepam.[45] Retrograde amnesia is not produced by midazolam.

Since the introduction of midazolam to clinical use in the United States, the author has seen the dramatic effects of midazolam-induced amnesia; most are beneficial, but some are potentially dangerous. For the typical 1-hour IV conscious sedation procedure in dental or outpatient surgical practice, most patients have little recall of most of the procedure, and for most patients this is quite acceptable and positive. One case, however, must be mentioned as a caution:

A young, healthy (ASA I) woman received IV midazolam and local anesthesia for the removal of 3 third molars. Following the 20-minute procedure, the patient appeared alert and was quite responsive to questions. Gauze packs had been placed at the sites of extraction, and the patient had been told to bite down hard on the gauze and not to swallow. She responded verbally that she would do as directed. Within 2 minutes the patient was complaining of a lump in her throat. Observation of the mouth indicated that all gauze packs had disappeared—the patient had swallowed them. Fortunately, they were located in the esophagus and were of no great consequence. However, when questioned, the patient had absolutely no recall either of receiving the instructions given her by the doctor or of swallowing the gauze pads.[46]

It becomes imperative, therefore, for the patient to be observed much more carefully during the in-office recovery period, that special precautions be taken to prevent such events from recurring, and that postoperative instructions (verbal and written) be given to both the patient and the escort. The benzodiazepine antagonist flumazenil, which has been recently approved for clinical use, has been shown to decrease the duration of midazolam's amnesic period.[47]

Duration of clinical activity

Because of its short α–half-life, the duration of clinical sedation noted with midazolam is somewhat shorter than that of diazepam. Its duration of action is therefore quite compatible with the typical 1-hour dental or surgical procedure.

Midazolam differs in another manner from diazepam. It appears that midazolam is much more effective than diazepam when amnesia is a desired result of the drug's administration. However, when sedation is of higher priority, diazepam appears to be the more effective agent. These are personal observations that have not received the careful scientific study required to make a categorical statement.

Cardiorespiratory activity

Midazolam, as a typical member of the benzodiazepines, has minimal effect on the cardiovascular and respiratory dynamics of the ASA I or II patient in usual doses. Intravenous doses of 0.15 mg/kg of midazolam in healthy persons have produced statistically significant, but clinically insignificant, decreases in arterial blood pressure and increases in heart rate.[48] However, other researchers noted no untoward cardiovascular response with similar doses.[49] In fact, Gath et al.[50] recommends midazolam as an induction agent for patients with ischemic heart disease because of its rapid onset of action and minimal effects on the cardiovascular system.

Diazepam and midazolam both produce the same effects on the respiratory system. A dose of 0.3 mg/kg of diazepam and 0.15 mg/kg of midazolam produced comparable depression of respiratory response to CO_2 in healthy volunteers.[48] It was concluded that midazolam and diazepam injected intravenously in equipotent doses depress respiration significantly and similarly. The results of the study indicate that this is a result of a direct depression of central respiratory drive rather than being caused by a simultaneous depression of the muscles of respiration, although this cannot be excluded. In the doses administered, equivalent to 21 mg of diazepam and 10 mg of midazolam for the typical 70-kg adult male, such a response might be expected. Since publication of this study in 1980, it has been demonstrated that equipotent doses of midazolam are approximately one-fourth of the diazepam dose.

In all cases the cardiovascular and respiratory depression noted with midazolam were typical for parenteral benzodiazepines and significantly less than those observed following equipotent doses of barbiturates (thiopental, pentobarbital). No cardiac dysrhythmias were provoked by midazolam administration.

In November 1987 Roche Laboratories, the manufacturer of midazolam, sent a warning to doctors about the use of midazolam in conscious sedation.[51] It stated that the administration of midazolam had been associated with respiratory depression and respiratory arrest. Guidelines for the safe administration of this agent were offered (see *"Dosage and Ad-*

ministration"). These guidelines emphasized the need for the slow titration of midazolam to all patients, especially the medically compromised.

Side effects

The most frequently noted complaint after midazolam administration is dizziness. In the study by Conner[44] et al., 46% of patients mentioned experiencing dizziness. Despite this, 92% stated that they enjoyed the feeling produced by midazolam and 100% said that they would accept the drug again if they required another operation.

MIDAZOLAM

The medical history of patients receiving diazepam should be checked for the following:
Allergy or hypersensitivity to benzodiazepines
Acute pulmonary insufficiency
Respiratory depression

MIDAZOLAM

Proprietary name	Versed (United States)
	Hypnovel, Dormicum
	(United Kingdom)
Classification	Benzodiazepine
Availability	1 mg/ml, 5 mg/ml
Average sedative dose	2.5-7.5 mg
Maximal single dose	6-8 mg
Maximal total dose	10 mg

Dosage and administration

When midazolam was introduced, initial reports implied that midazolam was 1.5 times as potent as diazepam. Subsequent clinical experience with midazolam has shown it to be approximately two to four times as potent as diazepam. The mean effective dose for 50% of subjects (MED_{50}) for the induction of general anesthesia is 0.2 mg/kg, although significant patient variation exists.[52] Clinically adequate conscious sedation with intravenously administered midazolam should always be achieved by slow titration. In its recent letter, Roche recommends "an initial intravenous dose for conscious sedation as little as 1 mg, but not exceeding 2.5 mg for a normal, healthy adult."[51] "Lower doses are necessary for older (over 60 years) or debilitated patients and in patients receiving con-

comitant opioids or other CNS depressants. The initial dose and all subsequent doses should never be given as a bolus; administer over at least 2 minutes and allow an additional 2 or more minutes to fully evaluate the sedative effect. The use of the 1 mg/ml or dilution of the 5 mg/ml formulation is recommended to facilitate slower injection."[51]

Doses of midazolam administered to normal, healthy (ASA I) adult patients at the University of Southern California School of Dentistry have ranged from as little as 2 to 10 mg for an initial titrating dose. As with all drugs, there is significant patient variation in response to dosage.

Availability

Versed (Roche Laboratories): 1 and 5 mg/ml in 2- and 10-ml vials. (Hypnovel, Dormicum [Roche Laboratories] in the United Kingdom and other parts of the world.) Midazolam is classified as a Schedule IV drug.

As with other CNS depressants, the dose of midazolam must be decreased when other CNS depressants are being administered concomitantly. In addition, following IV sedation the patient must be escorted from the dental office in the company of a responsible adult and be advised not to have any alcohol and not to engage in any hazardous occupation requiring complete mental alertness, such as operating machinery or driving a motor vehicle, for approximately 24 hours.

Lorazepam

Lorazepam is a benzodiazepine with sedative and antianxiety effects. It may be administered either intramuscularly or intravenously. Chemically it is 7-chloro-5-(o-chlorophenyl)-1,3-dihydro-3hydroxy-2H-1,4-benzodiazepin-2-one. Lorazepam, like diazepam, is virtually insoluble in water. Although available for IV use, lorazepam is seldom used in the outpatient ambulatory patient because of the relative inability to titrate the drug and its prolonged duration of action.[53]

Lorazepam differs from most IV drugs in that its onset of clinical action is quite slow. After IV administration lorazepam produces little or no clinical effect for about 5 minutes, with its maximal effect noted approximately 20 minutes after administration. Because of this extremely slow onset of action, lorazepam cannot be titrated to effect. "Average" dosages must be administered—a situation that takes away one of the most important safety features of the IV route of drug administration.

From personal experience with IV lorazepam I have found that it is rather easy to oversedate the patient. Administration of 1 or 2 mg of lorazepam will usually provide adequate sedation, but because of the bell-shaped curve, many patients will become overly sedated at this same dose.

The duration of clinical action of lorazepam is too long for the typical dental procedure. The usual duration of sedative effects of lorazepam is 6 to 8 hours; however, some degree of unsteadiness and sensitivity to the CNS-depressant effects of other drugs (e.g., opioid analgesics prescribed for postsurgical pain control) may persist for as long as 24 hours. I vividly recall the patient who contacted me 36 hours after having received 2 mg of lorazepam intravenously and asked me when the effect of the drug would go away.

The introduction of flumazenil offers a means of reversing the sedative effects of lorazepam at the conclusion of the procedure. However, the clinical actions of flumazenil, especially following IV administration, will be shorter than the clinical actions of lorazepam, leading to a possible recurrence of sedation after the patient is discharged from the office, a possibly dangerous situation. As will be discussed in the sections on flumazenil, antidotal drugs and complications (Chapter 28), consideration should be given for IM flumazenil administration whenever IV flumazenil is used.

The amnesic properties of lorazepam are impressive and include both anterograde and a degree of retrograde amnesia. Lack of recall is maximal approximately 15 to 20 minutes after IV administration and may include events occurring throughout the treatment day. This feeling of "losing a day" may not be very comfortable for the ambulatory patient.

Lorazepam is more highly recommended for use in the hospitalized patient as a preoperative IM or IV drug than in the ambulatory outpatient.

Warnings and precautions

Patients receiving lorazepam must be warned against operating a motor vehicle or machinery or engaging in hazardous occupations for 24 to 48 hours after its administration. Dosages of lorazepam should be decreased in patients over the age of 50 years to minimize the risk of oversedation.[54]

The use of scopolamine with lorazepam is not recommended as there is no beneficial effect to be gained; however, additive CNS depression, hallucination, and irrational behavior may be more likely to occur.

Patients must be advised that getting out of bed unassisted may result in falling and injury if undertaken within 8 hours of receiving parenteral lorazepam. Alcohol should not be used for at least 24 to 48 hours after lorazepam injection. Other warnings and precautions for lorazepam are similar to those for diazepam and other benzodiazepines.

Pediatric use

There are insufficient data to support the use of lorazepam in patients under the age of 18 years. Its administration in outpatient pediatric dentistry appears unwarranted at this time, especially in light of its prolonged clinical action.

Adverse reactions

The most frequently noted adverse reactions to lorazepam are caused by a direct extension of its CNS–depressant properties and include[55]:

1. *Excessive sleepiness* that interfered with regional nerve block developed in 6% of patients studied. Patients over the age of 50 years had a significantly greater incidence of excessive sleepiness than did younger patients.
2. Restlessness, confusion, depression, and delirium occurred in 1.3% of patients.
3. Visual and self-limiting hallucinations developed in 1% of patients.

Because of its lack of water solubility, lorazepam may produce a burning sensation at the site of IV administration similar to that of diazepam. This occurred in 1.6% of patients receiving the drug. At 24 hours after injection 0.5% still complained of discomfort. Patients should be advised that there may be a slight warmth felt at the injection site as the drug is administered and that this is entirely normal and will pass within a few minutes. Slow injection of lorazepam into a rapidly running IV infusion will minimize this reaction.

Dosage

The following directions regarding recommended dosage are taken from the lorazepam package insert:

For the primary purpose of sedation and relief of anxiety, usual recommended initial IV dose of lorazepam is 2 mg total, or 0.02 mg/lb (0.044 mg/kg), whichever is smaller. This dose will suffice for sedating most adults, and should not ordinarily be exceeded in patients over 50 years.[54]

Administration

Lorazepam should be diluted immediately prior to IV administration with an equal volume of a compatible solution. When properly diluted lorazepam may be administered directly into a vein or into the tubing of an existing IV infusion. The rate of injection of lorazepam should not exceed 2.0 mg/minute. Lorazepam may be diluted with the following:

    Sterile water for injection
    Sodium chloride injection
    5% Dextrose injection[54]

Availability

Ativan (Wyeth): 2 and 4 mg/ml in 10-ml vials and 1-ml preloaded syringes. Each milliliter of solution consists of:

    2 or 4 mg lorazepam
    0.18 ml polyethylene glycol 400 in propylene glycol
    2% benzyl alcohol as a preservative

Lorazepam is not highly recommended for use in outpatient sedation because of its prolonged clinical action, its extreme amnesic properties, and primarily the lack of ability of the administrator to titrate the drug to clinical effect.

Lorazepam is classifed as a Schedule IV drug.

Lorazepam is an excellent IV sedative for nonambulatory, hospitalized patients for whom close post-treatment monitoring is available for extended periods.

LORAZEPAM

Proprietary name	Ativan
Classification	Benzodiazepine
Availability	2 and 4 mg/ml
Average sedative dose	2 mg
Maximal single dose	2 mg
Maximal total dose	4 mg

LORAZEPAM

The medical history of patients receiving lorazepam should be checked for the following:
Allergy or hypersensitivity to benzodiazepines

Flunitrazepam

Flunitrazepam is a water-soluble benzodiazepine derivative that is chemically and pharmacologically related to diazepam and other drugs of this group. The chemical formula for flunitrazepam is 5-(o-fluorophenyl)-1,3-dihydro-1-methyl-7-nitro-2H-1,4-benzodiazepin-2-one. The sedative, antianxiety, amnesic, and muscle-relaxing properties of flunitrazepam are similar to those of diazepam except that its sedative and sleep-inducing properties are more pronounced and long-lasting than those of diazepam.[56] Foreman[56] reported flunitrazepam to be approximately 15 times as potent as diazepam and suggested that the drug be diluted prior to administration to ensure precise titration.

Flunitrazepam is available in a 1-ml ampule containing 2 mg. The manufacturer suggests diluting the drug with 1 ml of sterile water for injection prior to use, providing a solution of 1 mg/ml.[57] Foreman, however, suggests that further dilution is warranted, recommending the dilution of 2 mg (1 ml) of flunitrazepam in 9 ml of sterile water, providing a solution of 0.2 mg/ml.[56]

Following IV administration for the induction of general anesthesia, flunitrazepam produces its clinical effects within 1 to 3 minutes, the peak effect noted in 5 minutes. The duration of clinical action ranged from 10 to 60 minutes, with significant variation with dosage (1 to 6 mg). The α– and β–half-lives of flunitrazepam are 19 and 34 hours.

Side effects and complications associated with flunitrazepam administration are similar to those of other benzodiazepines. As with most benzodiazepines, flunitrazepam is remarkably free of respiratory- or cardiovascular-depressant effects. The most frequently reported side effects associated with flunitrazepam administration are diaphoresis, ataxia, erythema, blurred vision, hypersalivation, dry mouth, weakness, hypothermia, hypoventilation, and prolonged drowsiness.[57] The dosage of flunitrazepam should be decreased in elderly and debilitated patients. The use of alcohol and driving should be prohibited for 24 hours after the administration of flunitrazepam.

Flunitrazepam sedation in dentistry

Foreman[56] reported on 10 patients who received IV flunitrazepam for conscious sedation.[56] The dosages ranged from 1.4 to 2 mg. Treatment conditions ranged from good to excellent in 8 of the 10 patients. No patient recalled receiving a local anesthetic during treatment (although they all did receive local anesthetics), nor in fact did they recall any of the dental treatment. They did remember being escorted to the recovery area and being driven home after discharge from the office.

The duration of sedation produced by flunitrazepam is somewhat longer than that produced by diazepam. This would contraindicate its use in shorter procedures (those lasting less than 1 hour) but would be an indication for its administration in longer procedures. Recovery from sedation was less complete than that seen with diazepam, even at 24 hours. In cases in which a more rapid patient recovery is important, flunitrazepam may not be the desired drug for IV sedation.

Availability

Rohypnol (Roche Laboratories): 2 mg in 1-ml ampules. Flunitrazepam is not available in the United States at this time. It is available in both oral and parenteral preparations in the United Kingdom and other countries under the proprietary name Rohypnol.

Chlordiazepoxide

Chlordiazepoxide is also available for injectable use; however, because of the more ready accessibility of other benzodiazepines, it is rarely used parenterally, especially intravenously.

Because of the instability of parenteral forms of chlordiazepoxide, chlordiazepoxide for IV and IM use must be prepared immediately prior to its administration by mixing a 5-ml dry-filled ampule containing 100 mg of chlordiazepoxide with 5 ml of either sterile physiological saline or sterile water for injection.[58] This produces a concentration of chlordiazepoxide of 20 mg/ml, which is then injected at a rate of 1 ml/minute.

In view of the current availability and efficacy of diazepam, midazolam, and flunitrazepam, there appears to be little reason for considering the IV administration of chlordiazepoxide.

Summary

The benzodiazepines represent the most nearly ideal agents for IV sedation in the ambulatory patient. Pharmacologically they normally have little significant effect on the cardiovascular and respiratory systems when administered in recommended doses via recommended techniques. Diazepam and midazolam are the drugs of choice for IV conscious sedation procedures with a duration of 60 minutes or less. Midazolam appears to possess several significant advantages over diazepam, most important of which are its amnesic qualities, lack of irritation to blood vessels, and the lack of a rebound or second peak effect.

Flunitrazepam is recommended for administration where procedures in excess of 1 hour are contemplated, whereas lorazepam should be reserved, in most instances, for nonambulatory well-monitored patients undergoing longer procedures.

BARBITURATES

The barbiturates have served as an important group of sedative drugs in dentistry for almost 50 years. Niels B. Jorgensen,[59] the father of intravenous sedation in dentistry, utilized a barbiturate in his technique of IV premedication, now known worldwide as the Jorgensen technique.[59]

Although several barbiturates are available for IV administration (Table 26-3), only one—pentobarbital—has retained any popularity.

Secobarbital is used intravenously in the Berns technique.[60] Other barbiturates used intravenously include the ultrashort-acting general anesthesia–induction agents methohexital, thiopental, and thiamylal.

Pentobarbital sodium

Chemically pentobarbital sodium is sodium 5-ethyl-5-(1-methylbutyl) barbiturate. The sodium salt is freely soluble in water and alcohol. Pentobarbital is classified as a short-acting barbiturate. It possesses characteristics of the entire group of barbiturates, which will now be discussed.

Table 26-3. Barbiturates for intravenous administration

Generic name	Proprietary name	Usual concentration (mg/ml)	Duration of action	Average sedative dose (mg)
Pentobarbital	Nembutal	50	2-4 hours	125-175
Secobarbital	Seconal	50	2-4 hours	100-150
Methohexital	Brevital (United States)			
	Brietal (United Kingdom)	10	5-7 minutes	*
Thiopental	Pentothal	25	—	*
Thiamylal	Surital	25	—	*

*Not recommended for IV sedation.

Pharmacology

Barbiturates are frequently classified according to their duration of clinical action following oral administration (see Table 8-5). After oral and IV administration, the clinical actions of pentobarbital will be observed for approximately 2 to 4 hours.

All barbiturate sedative-hypnotics are generalized depressants, with the CNS being the most sensitive system. Barbiturates produce a characteristic pattern of CNS depression: The cerebral cortex and the reticular activating system (RAS) are most sensitive to the actions of the barbiturates; the cerebellar, vestibular, and spinal systems less so, and the medulla least sensitive of all.[61]

The RAS is important in the maintenance of a conscious alert state. Sedative doses of barbiturates act on this system to depress ascending neuronal conduction to the cerebral cortex; as a result consciousness is diminished or lost.

Unlike true analgesic drugs, such as the opioids or nonsteroidal antiinflamatory drugs (NSAIDs), barbiturates have no effect on pain threshold except in doses that affect the level of consciousness (as in deep IV sedation). In the presence of severe pain it is found that barbiturates often render the patient restless and more difficult to manage. This occurs because of a decreased control over emotions by the cortical centers of the brain. In other words, the patient becomes less inhibited and more likely to respond to a noxious stimulus as would the typical uninhibited child. Barbiturates should not be used as the sole agent for sedation when a painful procedure is planned. Analgesics, such as meperidine and local anesthetics, are almost always used when IV barbiturates are administered in order to counteract this negative effect on pain reaction.

The parenteral barbiturates are effective anticonvulsants and are administered in the management of seizures produced by tetanus, epilepsy, and local anesthetic overdose. However, with the introduction of the benzodiazepines, which are equally effective anticonvulsants with a decreased potential for respiratory depression, the use of barbiturates as anticonvulsants has declined.

Respiratory system

The barbiturates produce respiratory depression by a direct action on the medullary respiratory center. The degree of respiratory depression is dose related.[62] Respiratory arrest (failure) is the usual cause of death from barbiturate overdose. As respiratory depression develops from barbiturate administra-

tion, the rate of respiration increases while the tidal volume decreases. Respiratory reflexes, such as coughing, sneezing, hiccoughing, and laryngospasm, are only slightly depressed until the degree of CNS depression is pronounced. Laryngospasm is one of the chief respiratory complications of IV barbiturate general anesthesia (see Chapter 32).

Cardiovascular system

In comparison to the respiratory system, the cardiovascular system is relatively resistant to the depressant actions of barbiturates. Normal hypnotic doses are associated with only a slight fall in heart rate and blood pressure, similar to that seen in normal sleep. Intravenous thiopental anesthesia will produce more significant depression of the cardiovascular system.[63] The slight drop in blood pressure observed with IV barbiturate sedation or anesthesia is a result of depression of the vasomotor center with consequent peripheral vasodilation. Larger doses of the barbiturates act directly on smaller blood vessels to produce dilation and increased capillary permeability.

Absorption, metabolism, and excretion

The parenteral barbiturates are highly lipid soluble, a property that facilitates their rapid redistribution from the blood to other tissues within the body. When administered intravenously, the ultrashort-acting barbiturates reach peak concentration in the brain within 30 seconds. During this time the other so-called vessel-rich tissues—heart, liver, and kidneys—also reach saturation levels. Lipid solubility and plasma protein binding of the barbiturates vary (Table 26-4) and are responsible for onset and duration of action. Drugs with greater lipid solubility (greater partition coefficient) have a more rapid on-

Table 26-4. Characteristics of intravenous barbiturates

Drug	Partition coefficient	Plasma protein binding	Delay in onset of action (minutes)
Barbital	1	0.05	22
Phenobarbital	3	0.20	12
Pentobarbital	39	0.35	0.1
Secobarbital	52	0.44	0.1
Thiopental	580	0.65	Less than 0.1

Modified from Goodman LS, Gilman A: *The pharmacological basis of therapeutics,* ed 5. New York, 1975, Macmillan.

set of action, whereas protein binding relates to the relative duration of action of the agent.

The barbiturates rapidly diffuse out of the blood and are redistributed to all tissues. This leads to a rapid decrease in the blood level of the drug and a termination of clinical activity (α–half-life). The liver and muscles account for most of the volume of barbiturate that is withdrawn from the blood. Body fat, with a sparse blood supply, requires approximately 1.5 to 2 hours to become saturated. When equilibrium between the barbiturate in the tissues and the blood occurs, the decline in barbiturate blood level is slowed and becomes a measure of the rate of metabolism of the drug.

It is this rapid removal (redistribution) from the blood that accounts for the brief action of the so-called ultrashort-acting barbiturates, not their rapid metabolism. Thiopental, for example, undergoes metabolism at the rate of 15% per hour. This important aspect of barbiturate pharmacology will be discussed more fully in Chapter 32.

Barbiturates are eliminated in one of two methods: biotransformation in the liver and excretion through the kidneys. A few barbiturates are largely excreted, others are almost completely inactivated by the liver, and still others are partially excreted and partially metabolized (Table 26-5).

The liver is the most important organ for metabolism of barbiturates, although other organs such as the kidneys, brain, and muscle are also involved. Any form of liver disease or dysfunction may tend to prolong the action or intensify the depth of depression produced by the barbiturate and should be considered a relative or absolute contraindication to barbiturate administration.

The β–half-lives (the time required for biotransformation and excretion) of some of the barbiturates are listed in Table 26-6. The slow release of the barbiturates from these tissue depots may be somewhat responsible for the hangover effects so often noted after barbiturate administration.[64] The day after the administration of IV pentobarbital, some patients will still exhibit clinical signs of CNS depression.

Unwanted effects

The most commonly observed unwanted effects from barbiturate administration are hangover and excitement. Hangover, or unwanted posttreatment lethargy, is produced by the slow reabsorption of the barbiturate from tissue depots (fat, muscle) into the blood and is more likely to develop with the longer-acting barbiturates.

In some patients the barbiturates produce excitation rather than depression, and the patient will appear to be inebriated, becoming quite talkative. This represents an idiosyncratic response and is more likely after administration of phenobarbital, although it may develop with other barbiturates.

Patients with a personal or familial history of acute intermittent porphyria represent one of the few absolute contraindications to barbiturate administration. (See Chapter 5 for a discussion of acute intermittent porphyria.)

Allergy to barbiturates, although uncommon, is more likely to develop in patients with histories of allergy, urticaria, and angioedema. Barbiturate use, especially chronic, can produce drug dependence and tolerance. In addition, drug-drug interactions with other CNS depressants must be considered whenever concomitant drug therapy is used.

Warnings

Patients receiving pentobarbital must be advised against performing any potentially hazardous tasks such as driving a vehicle or operating machinery. It has been my clinical experience that patients who have received IV pentobarbital do not want to do

---

Table 26-5. Method of elimination of barbiturates

Primarily excreted by kidney
  Barbital
  Phenobarbital
Degraded by liver and excreted by kidney
  Aprobarbital
Primarily metabolized by liver
  Amobarbital
  Pentobarbital
  Secobarbital
Distributed to body fat, eventually dependent on liver
  and kidney
  Thiopental
  Thiamylal

Table 26-6. β–Half-lives of selected barbiturates

Drug	β–half-life (hours)
Hexobarbital	4.35
Amobarbital	21.1
Pentobarbital	21.8
Secobarbital	28.9
Phenobarbital	86

anything other than return home and go to sleep in the immediate postsedation period. Patients are advised that the next day they will probably be fully capable of functioning normally; however, in some few instances signs and symptoms may persist and the patient is advised to continue resting.

The use of alcohol or other CNS depressants after pentobarbital administration must be cautioned against because potentially significant additive effects may develop. Prescriptions for postoperative analgesics must take this into consideration. The use of a long-acting local anesthetic, such as bupivacaine or etidocaine, as well as nonsteroidal antiinflammatory drugs, are recommended. Chronic use of barbiturates induces liver microsomal enzyme activity and may influence the dosage of pentobarbital required for sedation. Because pentobarbital crosses the placenta, its use is contraindicated in pregnancy.

Precautions

Pentobarbital should be used with caution in patients with impaired liver function or a history of drug dependence or abuse. A history of cirrhosis or recent hepatitis represents a relative contraindication to pentobarbital administration, as does recent or chronic alcoholism. The alcoholic may respond in one of three ways to administration of the barbiturate: In most instances the response will approximate the usual response with doses within the normal range. In the second posssible response the alcoholic's liver will have produced a greater volume of hepatic microsomal enzymes, which will decrease the patient's response to the usual barbiturate dosage. Significantly larger doses may be required to provide a sedative effect with pentobarbital. This response is usually noted in the "early" alcoholic, prior to the development of liver dysfunction—fatty degeneration (cirrhosis)—making the patient less able to manage the usual dose of barbiturates. In this third situation the alcoholic patient will overrespond to usual dosages of pentobarbital and other barbiturates.

Patients with any respiratory disorder, especially asthma, should be administered pentobarbital with caution. Because barbiturates are potent respiratory depressants, they should be administered carefully in all patients with a suspicion of pulmonary dysfunction. The parenteral solution of pentobarbital is quite alkaline (pH of 9.5). Extravascular injection of the drug may produce tissue irritation and possible damage, such as sloughing or sterile abscess formation (see Chapter 28). Hypotension may occur following rapid IV administration of pentobarbital. When the agent is administered at the recommended rate of 1 ml/minute, such response is rare.

Patients must be warned against operating a motor vehicle for the remainder of the day on which the drug is administered. As mentioned, most patients receiving pentobarbital have no desire to drive a car.

Adverse reactions

Possible adverse reactions to pentobarbital administration include the following[65]:

Respiratory depression
Apnea
Circulatory collapse
Pain
Skin rash
Allergic reaction
Residual sedation (hangover)
Nausea and vomiting
Paradoxical excitement

Coughing, hiccoughing, laryngospasm, and chest-wall spasm have been observed after IV pentobarbital sedation. Slow administration minimizes the occurrence of these effects. With over 1250 administrations of pentobarbital (at the University of Southern California School of Dentistry), laryngospasm and chest-wall spasm have never been encountered. Bronchospasm may occur, particularly in patients with a history of asthma. This represents a relative contraindication to pentobarbital. Thrombophlebitis may also occur at the site of drug administration, although its incidence from pentobarbital is quite insignificant.

Dosage

When administered intravenously, pentobarbital must be titrated to effect. As used in the Jorgensen technique, pentobarbital will be used to provide the suitable level of sedation. The dosage range observed with pentobarbital is quite wide—as little as 30 mg to as much as 300 mg, providing the same clinical signs and symptoms in different patients. This wide range of safety with pentobarbital is one of the reasons why this drug may be recommended in IV conscious sedation procedures. Other barbiturates do not possess the same relatively flat dose-response curve and are therefore not recommended for sedative use by any doctor not trained in general anesthesia.

Although doses of pentobarbital as high as 500 mg have been used to achieve sedation in some patients, it is my recommendation that a single dose not exceed 300 mg. Repeat titrations (if needed) could bring the dose up to a maximum of 500 mg for one appointment. The average dose of pentobarbital required for adequate sedation in the Jorgensen technique is 125 to 175 mg.[66]

Availability

Nembutal (Abbott): 50 mg/ml of 2-ml ampules and 20- and 50-ml multidose vials. Each milliliter of pentobarbital sodium contains:

40 mg pentobarbital sodium
40% propylene glycol
10% alcohol
Water for injection
pH adjusted to 9.5 with hydrochloric acid and/or sodium hydroxide
Air in container displaced by nitrogen

Pentobarbital is classified as a Schedule II drug.

```
┌─────────────────────────────────────────┐
│              PENTOBARBITAL               │
│                                          │
│   The medical history of patients        │
│   receiving pentobarbital should be      │
│   checked for the following:             │
│     Allergy or hypersensitivity to       │
│       barbiturates                       │
│     Porphyria                            │
│     Liver disease                        │
│     Asthma                               │
│     Respiratory depression               │
│     Alcoholism                           │
└─────────────────────────────────────────┘
```

```
┌─────────────────────────────────────────┐
│              PENTOBARBITAL               │
│                                          │
│   Proprietary name        Nembutal       │
│   Classification          Barbiturate    │
│   Availability            50 mg/ml       │
│   Average sedative dose   125-175 mg     │
│   Maximal single dose     300 mg         │
│   Maximal total dose      500 mg         │
└─────────────────────────────────────────┘
```

Secobarbital

Secobarbital is a short-acting barbiturate similar in action to pentobarbital that is used intravenously in the Berns technique, a combination of secobarbital with an opioid and ultrashort-acting barbiturate.[60] The basic pharmacology, warnings, precutions, and side effects of secobarbital are similar to those for pentobarbital.

Dosage

In the Berns technique, when used in combination with other drugs, the maximal recommended dose of secobarbital is 50 mg.[60] When used as the sole agent for sedation, doses of 100 to 150 mg may be used, injected slowly.

Availability

Seconal (Lilly): 50 mg/ml in 1-, 2-, 10-, 20-, and 30-ml vials. Secobarbital sodium is available as a powder that is diluted with sterile water for injection. Bacteriostatic water and Ringer's lactate solutions are incompatible with secobarbital sodium. As a powder it comes in ampules containing 250 mg of the drug. It is diluted with 5 ml of diluent to produce a concentration of 5%, or 50 mg/ml. It is also available generically.

Secobarbital is classified as a Schedule II drug.

```
┌─────────────────────────────────────────┐
│              SECOBARBITAL                │
│                                          │
│   The medical history of patients        │
│   receiving secobarbital should be       │
│   checked for the following:             │
│     Allergy or hypersensitivity to       │
│       barbiturates                       │
│     Porphyria                            │
│     Liver disease                        │
│     Asthma                               │
│     Respiratory depression               │
│     Alcoholism                           │
└─────────────────────────────────────────┘
```

```
┌─────────────────────────────────────────┐
│           SECOBARBITAL SODIUM            │
│                                          │
│   Proprietary name        Seconal        │
│   Classification          Barbiturate    │
│   Availability            50 mg/ml       │
│   Average sedative dose   50-150 mg      │
│   Maximal single dose     150 mg         │
│   Maximal total dose      250 mg         │
└─────────────────────────────────────────┘
```

Methohexital sodium

Methohexital sodium is an ultrashort-acting barbiturate most frequently used for the rapid induction of general anesthesia (stage III) or the production of short-duration ultralight general anesthesia as frequently used for oral surgical procedures (Guedel stage II). Methohexital was synthesized by Stoelting in 1957 and popularized as an agent for outpatient dental anesthesia by Adrian Hubbell in the early 1960s.[67]

Although primarily used as a general anesthetic, methohexital sodium may be used in smaller doses as a sedative-hypnotic. Several IV sedation techniques have been developed in which methohexital is used—intermittent methohexital sedation, the Berns technique (secobarbital, meperidine, and methohexital), the Shane technique (hydroxyzine, alphaprodine, and methohexital), and diazepam and methohexital sedation. These techniques will be discussed in the following chapter, but the use of methohexital by any person not trained in general anesthesia cannot be recommended.

The chemical formula for methohexital sodium is sodium-a-dl-1-methyl-5-ally 1-5-(1-methyl-2-pentyl) barbiturate. It differs from other barbiturate anesthetics in that it does not contain any sulfur. When compared to the actions of other IV barbiturate anesthetics (thiopental, thiamylal), methohexital possesses several advantages:

Shorter duration of action

Faster clinical recovery

Relative absence of local complications

Amnesia

Relatively stable solution

The usual duration of action of a induction dose of methohexital is 4 to 7 minutes. It is therefore suitable for short procedures requiring less than 20 minutes. Foreman[56] recommends its use as a sedative only for restorative and minor oral surgical procedures of short duration and says that if this limitation is observed and if the patency of the airway is ensured at all times by effective mouth packing, intermittent methohexital sedation is a safe and useful technique.[9] Because of the steeper dose-response curve of methohexital, it is possible to produce overly deep sedation or light general anesthesia quite by accident. This relative lack of safety with methohexital is the basis for my recommendation against its use as a sedative by anyone without advanced training in general anesthesia. Methohexital is used as a 1% (10 mg/ml) solution. Contraindications and warnings for methohexital are similar to those for pentobarbital.

Adverse reactions

The following are the major adverse reactions observed after the administration of methohexital sodium[68]:

Circulatory depression: most often seen after overly rapid administration of larger doses (>10 to 20 ml)

Thrombophlebitis: not a significant problem

Respiratory depression, apnea: probably the most significant adverse responses to use of methohexital sodium; usually dose related; however, in sensitive individuals respiratory depression or apnea may develop at unusually small doses

Laryngospasm: a serious complication that will develop as the patient becomes more deeply sedated if the pharynx contains fluid or foreign matter

Bronchospasm: much more likely to develop in the patient with a history of asthma

Hiccoughs: usually associated with rapid administration

Skeletal muscle hyperactivity: not uncommon as the patient enters stage 2 of anesthesia; this should not develop with the small doses (10 to 20 mg) recommended for sedation

Emergence delirium

Nausea and vomiting

Acute, life-threatening allergic reactions, although rare, have developed after administration of methohexital sodium

Dosage

When used as a sedative in dentistry, methohexital sodium must always be titrated in extremely small doses not exceeding 10 mg. On rare occasion a 20-mg dose may be used by the experienced individual, but this is never to be exceeded.

Because dental procedures in which methohexital sodium is used for sedation should not exceed 20 minutes, the maximum suggested total dose of methohexital is 100 mg. In procedures expected to require more than 20 minutes, other IV drugs should be considered for use.

In both the Berns and Shane techniques, 10- to 20-mg increments of methohexital sodium are administered after the injection of other IV drugs.[60,69]

Availability

Brevital (Lilly), Brietal: 500 mg in 50-ml vials. Methohexital is prepared prior to use by adding 50 ml of suitable diluent to the vial to produce a 1%, or 10 mg/ml, solution. Suitable diluents include sterile water for injection, in which case the solution may be stored for up to 6 weeks, and 5% dextrose in water or isotonic (0.9%) sodium chloride solution, in which case the solution is only stable for 24 hours. Each vial of methohexital sodium contains:

500 mg methohexital sodium
30 mg anhydrous sodium carbonate
It contains no preservative.

Methohexital is classified as a Schedule IV drug.

METHOHEXITAL

The medical history of patients receiving methohexital should be checked for the following:
Allergy or hypersensitivity to barbiturates
Porphyria
Liver disease
Asthma
Respiratory depression
Alcoholism

METHOHEXITAL SODIUM

Proprietary name	Brevital (United States)
Classification	Brietal (United Kingdom)
Availability	Barbiturate
Average sedative	10 mg/ml
dose	10- 20-mg increments
Maximal single	20 mg
dose	
Maximal total dose	Approximately 100 mg*

*Procedure should not require more than 20 minutes to complete.

Thiopental and thiamylal

Two other ultrashort-acting barbiturates—thiopental and thiamylal—are available for IV administration. Thiopental (Pentothal [Abbott]) and thiamylal (Surital [Parke-Davis]) are used for the induction of general anesthesia (stage 3) and as solo agents for general anesthesia in surgical procedures requiring 30 minutes or less. Thiopental was introduced into clinical practice by Lundy in 1934, whereas thiamylal was first described in 1935 by Volwiler and Tabern.[70] Thiopental is the most widely used ultrashort-acting barbiturate in current anesthesia practice. The duration of action of both thiopental and thiamylal is longer than that of methohexital. These drugs are rarely used in sedative procedures and cannot be recommended for use in this regard. They will be discussed further in Chapter 32.

Summary

Although a number of barbiturates are available for IV administration, there are some important reasons for not recommending some of them for use in IV conscious sedation. The potent respiratory depressant properties of the barbiturates, combined with the steep dose-response curves of methohexital, thiopental, and thiamylal, are reason enough to recommend against their use by any doctor not extensively trained in general anesthesia and in the management of the airway of the unconscious patient. It is simply too easy to get into trouble (e.g., inadvertent unconsciousness and airway obstruction) with these drugs. There are, however, two barbiturates—pentobarbital and secobarbital—that are recommended for use as IV sedatives. Although pharmacologically similar, pentobarbital is the more commonly used. Possessing a relatively flat dose-response curve, pentobarbital is an excellent drug for sedative procedures requiring 2 to 4 hours.

ANTIHISTAMINES

Two drugs that are classified as antihistamines—promethazine and hydroxyzine—are also used occasionally as IV sedatives. The basic pharmacology of these two drugs has already been discussed in Chapters 8 and 11. In this section only those aspects of their pharmacology relevant to IV administration will be reviewed.

Promethazine

Promethazine is a phenothiazine derivative that is frequently used in dentistry, primarily in pediatric dentistry, as a sedative-hypnotic administered either orally or intramuscularly. Promethazine may also be administered intravenously either as a solo drug or in combination with an opioid.

The clinical duration of action of promethazine after IV administration is approximately 1 to 2 hours. Clinical recovery of the patient at this time is somewhat greater than that observed after pentobarbital administration; however, it is significantly less than that seen with diazepam or midazolam. Promethazine fills the void between the diazepam/midazolam sedative actions of less than 1 hour and the 2- to 4-hour sedation provided by pentobarbital.

The most significant adverse reaction to the administration of promethazine is the occurrence of extrapyramidal reactions. Clinical signs and symptoms of extrapyramidal reactions and their management have been discussed in Chapter 8.

Dosage

The usual dose of promethazine required for sedation following intravenous administration is approximately 25 to 35 mg. This drug should be administered in a concentration of 25 mg/ml. Promethazine may be administered intravenously to children. The drug should be titrated to clinical effect. In most cases the pediatric dose will not exceed that for the average adult.

Availability

Phenergan (Wyeth), Fellozine (O'Neal, Jones & Feldman), Lemprometh (Lemmon), Provigan (Reid-Provident), and Zipan (Savage): 25 mg/ml in 1-ml ampules and 10-ml vials. It is also available in a 50 mg/ml concentration that is recommended for IM use only. Promethazine is not a scheduled drug.

PROMETHAZINE

The medical history of patients receiving promethazine should be checked for the following:
Allergy or hypersensitivity to promethazine
Glaucoma
Prostatic hypertrophy
Stenosing peptic ulcer
Bladder neck obstruction

PROMETHAZINE

Proprietary name	Phenergan
Classification	Antihistamine
Availability	25 mg/ml
Average sedative dose	25-35 mg
Maximal single dose	50 mg
Maximal total dose	75 mg

Hydroxyzine

Hydroxyzine is an antihistaminic drug that has potent sedative properties, although not as potent as those of promethazine. The chemical formula for hydroxyzine is 1-(p-chlorobenzhydryl)4-(2-[2-hydroxyethoxy]ethyl) piperazine hydrochloride. The pharmacology of hydroxyzine has previously been discussed in Chapters 8 and 11.

Clinically important properties of hydroxyzine include its antiemetic actions and its ability to potentiate the actions of other CNS depressants, such as opioids and barbiturates. Hydroxyzine has been recommended for IV use in the Shane technique (which involves the administration of hydroxyzine, alphaprodine, and methohexital).[69] In spite of the reported success of the Shane technique there are limitations to its use, not least of which is the fact that hydroxyzine is not recommended by its manufacturer for intravenous use.[71]

The drug package insert accompanying hydroxyzine lists the following as contraindications[71]:

Hydroxyzine hydrochloride intramuscular solution is intended only for intramuscular administration and should not, under any circumstances, be injected subcutaneously, intraarterially, or intravenously.

Hydroxyzine appears to be quite irritating to blood vessel walls, producing a high incidence of local complications ranging from mild phlebitis to more serious thrombosis. Because of the availability of other equally effective intravenous sedative-hypnotics that are not associated with the same degree of complications and adverse effects, the administration of hydroxyzine intravenously cannot be recommended.

Summary

Promethazine is an effective IV sedative. Its primary indication is for IV procedures requiring more than 1, but less than 2, hours to complete.

Hydroxyzine, although an effective sedative, is associated with an unacceptably high rate of localized complications and is not recommended for use intravenously.

PROPOFOL

Propofol, a 2,6-diisopropylphenol compound, is virtually insoluble in aqueous solution. Following its initial introduction in a chromophore EL formulation, propofol was withdrawn from clinical usage because of a high incidence of anaphylactic reactions to the chromophore solvent (1 in 1000 administrations). Propofol has subsequently been reintroduced as a 1% solution in an egg lecithin emulsion formulation consisting of 10% soya bean oil, 2.25% glycerol, and 1.2% egg phosphatide.[72] Pain on injection into small veins occurs in a high proportion of patients, but injection into larger veins or prior administration of lidocaine or an opioid analgesic ameliorates the pain.[73]

Propofol may be administered into an IV infusion

of dextrose or saline but should not be mixed with other drugs or IV fluids.

Pharmacodynamics

Central nervous system

Propofol decreases cerebral metabolism, blood flow, as well as intracranial pressure.[74,75] However when larger doses are administered, marked lowering of systemic arterial pressures can significantly diminish cerebral perfusion.[76]

Respiratory system

Propofol, like most other IV CNS depressants, possesses respiratory depressant properties. Propofol depresses respiration similarly to the barbiturates in normal patients (ASA I) but to a greater degree than the benzodiazepines.[77]

Cardiovascular system

Propofol's cardiovascular depressant effects are more profound than those of thiopental.[78] Both a direct myocardial depression and decreased systemic vascular resistance have been implicated in producing profound hypotension following large bolus doses of propofol.[78,79] Age also affects cardiovascular response to propofol, and caution is mandatory when propofol is administered to the elderly.[80]

Miscellaneous effects

Propofol may have antiemetic effects. Studies have demonstrated an extremely low incidence of emetic sequelae after outpatient anesthesia with propofol.[81] Propofol has a distribution half-life of 2 to 4 minutes and an elimination half-life of 1 to 3 hours.[77]

Like most IV anesthetics, propofol is eliminated via hepatic metabolism followed by renal excretion of the more water-soluble metabolites. There is some evidence that an extrahepatic route of elimination, such as the lungs, contributes to the clearance of propofol.[77] Propofol is rapidly and extensively metabolized to inactive, water-soluble sulphate and glucuronic acid conjugates that are eliminated by the kidney.[82] No changes in propofol's pharmacokinetics have been reported to date in the presence of hepatic or renal disease.

Clinical use

Intravenous administration of propofol results in a rapid onset of action that is comparable to that of barbiturates.[83,84] Recovery from propofol's sedative-hypnotic effects is equally rapid.[85] The duration of propofol's central depressant effects increases in a dose-dependent fashion.[86] In contrast to the barbiturates there appears to be less residual postoperative sedation, fatigue ("hangover"), and cognitive and psychomotor impairment with propofol.[87]

Propofol has received extensive interest in the area of conscious sedation and may offer advantages over other sedative-hypnotics because of its short duration of effect, rapid recovery, and minimal side effects.[88-90]

A carefully titrated subhypnotic dose of propofol (0.5 to 1 mg/kg followed by 3 to 4.5 mg/kg/h) produces excellent sedation with minimal respiratory depression and a short recovery period.[91]

Warnings

Propofol is not recommended for use in pediatric patients because safety and effectiveness have not been established.[92] Propofol administration is contraindicated in patients with a known hypersensitivity to the drug or its components.

Patients receiving propofol should be continuously monitored by persons not involved in the conduct of the surgical or diagnostic procedure; oxygen supplementation should be immediately available and provided where clinically indicated; and oxygen saturation should be monitored in all patients.[92]

Adverse reactions

The most common adverse reactions, which occurred in more than 3% of patients receiving propofol, included hypotension, nausea, headache, and injection site pain or hotness.

Dosage and administration

Drug dosages should always be individualized. The following are general dosage guidelines[92]:

Induction of anesthesia:

Adults: 2 to 2.5 mg/kg or approximately 40 mg every 10 seconds until induction

Elderly, debilitated: 1 to 1.5 mg/kg or approximately 20 mg every 10 seconds until induction

Variable rate infusion: titrated until the desired clinical effect is obtained

Maintenance of anesthesia:

Variable rate infusion: titrated to desired clinical effect

Adults: Most patients require 100 to 200 µg/kg/min, or 6 to 12 mg/kg/h

Elderly and debilitated and ASA III or IV: most require 50 to 100 µg/kg/min, or 3 to 6 mg/kg/h

With an intermittent bolus of propofol a dose of 25 to 50 mg as needed is suggested

Sedation

Dosage and rate should be individualized. A slow infusion or slow injection is preferred to rapid bolus administration. Most require an infusion of 100 to 150 μg/kg/min (6 to 9 mg/kg/h) or a slow injection of 0.5 mg/kg over 3 to 5 minutes.

Elderly and debilitated and ASA III or IV patients: Most require doses similar to healthy adults but must be given as a slow infusion or slow injection and not as a rapid bolus.

Bolus and rate should be titrated to clinical effect. A variable rate infusion technique is preferred over an intermittent bolus technique. Most patients require an infusion of 25 to 75 μg/kg/min (1.5 to 4.5 mg/kg/h) or incremental bolus doses of 10 or 20 mg.

Elderly and debilitated and ASA III or IV patients require a 20% reduction of the adult dose. A rapid (single or repeated) bolus dose should not be used.

Propofol has been shown to be compatible with the following IV fluids when administered into a running IV catheter:

5% dextrose injection

Lactated Ringers injection

Lactated Ringers and 5% dextrose injection

5% dextrose and 0.45% sodium chloride injection

5% dextrose and 0.2% sodium chloride injection

Strict aseptic technique must always be maintained during handling as propofol is a single-use parenteral preparation and contains no antimicrobial preservative. The vehicle is capable of supporting rapid growth of microorganisms. Failure to follow recommended handling procedures may result in microbial contamination causing fever, infection or sepsis, or other adverse consequences that could lead to life-threatening illness. Propofol should be prepared for use just prior to administration. Administration should be completed within 6 hours after opening of the ampules or vials.

Availability

Propofol (Diprivan—Stuart Pharmaceuticals) is available in ready to-use 20-ml ampules and 50-ml

---

PROPOFOL	
Proprietary name	Diprivan
Classification	Intravenous anesthetic/sedative-hypnotic
Availability	10 mg/ml
Average sedative dose	An infusion of 100 to 150 μg/kg/min (6 to 9 mg/kg/h) or a slow injection of 0.5 mg/kg over 3 to 5 minutes
Maximal single dose	Remains to be determined
Maximal total dose	Remains to be determined

---

infusion vials containing 10 mg/ml of propofol. Propofol is not a scheduled drug.

OPIOID ANALGESICS

Opioids are administered primarily for their analgesic properties. They are excellent drugs for the relief of moderate to severe pain.[93] Although they affect many systems throughout the body, their primary therapeutic actions derive from their effects on the CNS. Opioids are able to produce analgesia, drowsiness, changes in mood, and mental clouding. Of significance is the fact that analgesia is produced without the loss of consciousness. The use of these drugs by the oral and IM routes has been discussed in Chapters 8 and 11, with relevant pharmacology reviewed in Chapter 11. In this section the potential use of these drugs in IV sedation will be discussed.

Opioid analgesics may be divided into the following categories: (1) opioid agonists, (2) opioid antagonists, and (3) opioid agonist/antagonists. Opioid agonists are those drugs that interact with an opioid receptor producing a physiologic change. An opioid antagonist is a drug that occupies a receptor site with no resultant pharmacologic effect. Opioids of the third group, opioid agonist/antagonists, possess properties of opioids of both of the preceding groups. With the appearance in the 1960s of drugs such as pentazocine, which had both agonist and antagonist properties, it became necessary to formulate a concept of multiple-opioid receptors in the CNS.

In 1976 Martin et al.[94] proposed a theory of multiple receptors rather than a single target for opiate agonists. Three separate opioid receptors—mu (μ),

---

PROPOFOL
The medical history of patients receiving propofol should be checked for the following: Nursing females   Allergy or known hypersensitivity to propofol or its components

Table 26-7. Opioid receptor activation and physiological effects

Mu (μ) receptor	Kappa (κ) receptor
Euphoria	Sedation
Supraspinal analgesia	Spinal analgesia
Indifference to stimuli	Miosis
Respiratory depression	Limited respiratory depression
Catalepsy	Depressed flexor reflexes
Locomotion	
Hypothermia	
Muscular rigidity	
Dependence	

Sigma (σ) receptor	Delta (δ) receptor
Dysphoria	Sedation
Hallucinations	Euphoria
Catatonia	
Mydriasis	
Tachycardia	
Respiratory stimulation	
Vasomotor stimulation	

From Pallasch TJ, Gill CJ: Butorphanol and nalbuphine: a pharmacologic comparison, *Oral Surg* 59:15, 1985.

kappa (κ), and sigma (σ)—were defined. A fourth, delta (δ), has since been identified. Table 11-4 lists the opioid receptors as well as agonist and antagonist drugs for each. Table 26-7 lists the various physiologic responses attributed to the various opioid receptors.[95,96]

OPIOID AGONISTS

A number of opioid agonists—meperidine, morphine, alphaprodine, fentanyl, alfentanil, and sufentanil—are used intravenously during sedation in dentistry.

Meperidine

Meperidine is the most frequently used IV opioid in dentistry. The basic pharmacology of meperidine has been discussed in Chapter 11. After IV administration meperidine will exhibit clinical actions in 2 to 4 minutes. Its duration of action is approximately 30 to 45 minutes, with considerable variation noted between patients and with administration of larger doses.

Meperidine has atropinelike properties, having been synthesized in the 1930s as an anticholinergic (see the following paragraph).[97] Patients receiving meperidine may demonstrate decreased salivary secretions and an increased heart rate because of its vagolytic properties. In the doses recommended here, these responses are normally quite minimal.

Meperidine may also produce a localized histamine release, resulting in the phenomenon of "tracking" at the site of meperidine administration. The skin overlying the vein into which meperidine is injected will appear red, and the patient may mention that itching is present. As meperidine is carried by venous blood up the patient's arm toward the heart, the reddening may continue to follow the path of the vein. It is important to remember that this is a normal response to meperidine administration, not an allergic reaction. Meperidine-induced histamine release will be localized to the path of the vein, whereas an allergic response will be more generalized over the entire region. Management of meperidine-induced histamine release is simply to allow it to dissipate spontaneously, which occurs over the next 10 to 15 minutes.

Dosage

When meperidine is administered intravenously during conscious sedation in most dental situations the recommended maximal dose is 50 mg. Administered in this dose the usual patient response will be an increase in the pain reaction threshold (analgesia) without any significant change in the depth of sedation. Opioids are usually administered *following* administration of a sedative-hypnotic (the primary drugs used to produce sedation). At a maximal dose of 50 mg, meperidine produces virtually no cardiovascular or respiratory depression in the typical patient.[98] Meperidine should be administered in a concentration not exceeding 10 mg/ml. When using the 50-mg/ml concentration, 1 ml of meperidine is placed into a 5-ml syringe and 4 ml of diluent (e.g., 5% dextrose and water) is added. The resulting solution contains 50 mg of meperidine in 5 ml of fluid, or 10 mg/ml.

Availability

Demerol (Winthrop) (Pethidine in the United Kingdom): 10 mg/ml in 1-ml ampules, 25 mg/ml in 0.5- and 1-ml ampules, 50 mg/ml in 0.5- and 1-ml ampules and 30-ml vials, 75 mg/ml in 1- and 1.5-ml ampules, and 100 mg/ml in 1- and 2-ml ampules and 20- and 30-ml vials. Meperidine is classified as a schedule II drug (FDA). Each milliliter of solution contains:

x mg Meperidine

pH adjusted to 3.5 to 6 with sodium hydroxide or hydrochloric acid

Multidose vials contain 0.1% metacresol as a preservative. No preservatives are added to the ampules.

It has been my clinical experience that the 50-mg/ml dosage form of meperidine is the most convenient to work with. More concentrated solutions are potentially dangerous because it is too easy for a mistake in calculation to lead to the administration of an overly large dose. The 10- and 25-mg/ml dosage forms are also appropriate; however, with the 10-mg/ml form larger volumes of solution will be used.

Single-use 1-ml ampules are recommended instead of multidose vials unless meperidine is used on a regular basis. The 20- or 30-ml vial may become contaminated if permitted to remain unused for a considerable time. Because meperidine (and other opioid analgesics) are schedule II drugs, precise records must be kept of the drug's administration. Use of 1-ml ampules simplifies this task considerably.

MEPERIDINE

The medical history of patients receiving meperidine should be checked for the following:
Allergy or hypersensitivity to opioid analgesics
MAOIs taken within 14 days
Chronic obstructive pulmonary disease (COPD) and decreased respiratory reserve

---

MEPERIDINE

Proprietary name	Demerol
Classification	Opioid agonist
Availability	10, 25, 50, 75, and 100 mg/ml
Average sedative dose	37.5-50 mg
Maximal single dose	50 mg
Maximal total dose	50 mg

Morphine

Morphine sulfate is the classical opioid agonist. It is useful but rarely employed for IV conscious seda-

---

MORPHINE

The medical history of patients receiving morphine should be checked for the following:
Asthma
Allergy or hypersensitivity to opioid analgesics
MAOIs taken within 14 days
COPD and decreased respiratory reserve

MORPHINE

Proprietary name	Morphine
Classification	Opioid agonist
Availability	2, 4, 8, 10, 15 mg/ml
Average sedative dose	5-6 mg
Maximal single dose	8 mg
Maximal total dose	8 mg

---

tion in outpatient situations because of its long duration of action (1.5 to 2 hours). The pharmacology of morphine is discussed in Chapter 11.

Dosage

When administered for IV conscious sedation in dentistry, the maximal dose of morphine should not exceed 8 mg. The drug is diluted to a concentration of 1 mg/ml prior to use. Little change in the depth of sedation will normally occur at this dose level, yet the patient's pain reaction threshold will be elevated.

Availability

Morphine sulfate: 2, 4, 8, 10, and 15 mg/ml. Morphine sulfate is classified as a Schedule II drug. The use of morphine sulfate should be restricted to dental procedures requiring more than 2 hours.

Alphaprodine

In response to a number of unfortunate incidents involving its administration, the manufacturer of alphaprodine (Roche Laboratories) removed the agent from the United States market in 1986.[99] This was the second time in recent years that this action had been taken and probably represented the end of alphaprodine's clinical use in the United States. The agent is still available, and used successfully, in many other parts of the world.

Alphaprodine is a rapid-onset, short-acting opioid agonist used primarily in pediatric dentistry by the submucosal (SM) route of administration.[100] Its pharmacology has been reviewed in Chapter 11. Onset of action after IV administration is 1 to 2 minutes. Duration of action of IV alphaprodine is approximately 30 minutes, which makes this a potentially very useful drug in dentistry.

Dosage

Although titration to effect is always recommended, the usual IV dose for adults is based on 0.4 to 0.6 mg/kg. For an average 70-kg patient, this is a dose of 28 to 42 mg. The lower dosage range is recommended initially to assess properly the patient's response. The initial IV dose should not exceed 30 mg, with a maximal total dose of 40 mg recommended.

Availability

Nisentil (Hoffmann-LaRoche): 40 mg/ml in 1-ml ampules and 60 mg/ml in 10-ml vials. Each milliliter of the 1-ml ampule contains:
  40 mg alphaprodine hydrochloride
  0.875% citric acid and sodium citrate to adjust pH to 4.6
Each milliliter of the 10-ml vial contains:
  60 mg alphaprodine hydrochloride
  0.875% citric acid and sodium citrate to adjust pH to 4.6
  0.45% phenol as preservative
Caution: Doctors using alphaprodine must be acutely aware of the difference in drug concentration between the 1-ml (40 mg/ml) and 10-ml (60 mg/ml) forms. Accidental overdosage might occur should the drug be administered from the multidose vial instead of the 1-ml ampule. The label of the drug being administered should always be read.

Alphaprodine is no longer available in the United States. When available, it was classified as a Schedule II drug.

ALPHAPRODINE

The medical history of patients receiving alphaprodine should be checked for the following:

Allergy or hypersensitivity to opioid analgesics
Asthma
MAOIs taken within 14 days
COPD and decreased respiratory reserve

ALPHAPRODINE

Proprietary name	Nisentil
Classification	Opioid agonist
Availability	40 and 60 mg/ml
Average sedative dose	15-20 mg
Maximal single dose	30 mg
Maximal total dose	40 mg

Fentanyl

Fentanyl is a rapid-onset, short-acting opioid agonist that is approximately 100 times more potent than morphine (0.1 mg of fentanyl is equianalgesic to 10 mg of morphine).[101] It was originally synthesized and introduced as one of the components of the drug combination known as Innovar.

After IV administration the onset of analgesia and sedation occurs almost immediately (less than 1 minute), although the maximal analgesic and respiratory depressant effects of fentanyl do not develop for several minutes. Average duration of clinical action is 30 to 60 minutes, which makes fentanyl an almost ideal drug for outpatient procedures requiring approximately 1 hour to complete.[102]

Respiratory depression is a side effect of all opioid agonists, with the respiratory depressant effect of fentanyl lasting longer than its analgesic properties. This potential must always be considered prior to discharge of an apparently "recovered" patient from the office in the custody of a person who is not trained to recognize respiratory depression and to manage it.

As with other opioid agonists, fentanyl slows the respiratory rate. This action of fentanyl is rarely observed for more than 30 minutes after the drug's administration. After IV administration of a single dose of fentanyl, peak respiratory depression is noted 5 to 15 minutes later.[103] Depression of breathing (decreased sensitivity to CO_2 stimulation) has been demonstrated for up to 4 hours in healthy volunteers.

Indications

Fentanyl is indicated for use:
1. As an analgesic in short anesthetic procedures and in the recovery room.
2. As an analgesic to supplement general or regional anesthesia.
3. In combination with a neuroleptic as a premedication for the induction of anesthesia and as an adjunct in the maintenance of general and regional anesthesia.

Contraindications

Fentanyl is contraindicated for use in patients with known allergy or intolerance to it.

Warnings

Fentanyl may cause muscular rigidity, especially involving the muscles of respiration (thoracic and abdominal).[104] This action appears to be related to rate of injection, occurring more frequently when the drug is administered rapidly. This can usually be prevented by the slow IV administration of the drug.

Should muscular rigidity develop, management consists of assisted or controlled ventilation or, if necessary, the administration of a neuromuscular blocking agent such as succinylcholine. This latter step must never be considered unless the doctor has been trained to administer skeletal muscle relaxants and is intimate with the technique of controlled ventilation. Patients who have received MAOIs within the past 14 days should not receive fentanyl or any other opioid agonist because of the potential for severe and unpredictable potentiation of the opioid effect.[105]

The safety of fentanyl in patients under the age of 2 years has not been established; therefore, it cannot be recommended for use in dental outpatient sedation in this population. Fentanyl should not be administered to pregnant patients unless the benefits of its administration clearly outweigh the potential hazards of opioid administration.[106]

Precautions

Fentanyl should be administered with caution to patients with COPD and to patients with decreased respiratory reserve (ASA III-V). In these patients opioids may decrease respiratory drive to an even greater degree than usual. Significant liver and renal dysfunction also represents relative contraindications to fentanyl administration.

Adverse reactions

The most frequently noted adverse reactions to fentanyl administration include respiratory depression, apnea, muscular rigidity, and bradycardia. If untreated, these may progress to respiratory arrest, circulatory depression, or cardiac arrest. Other adverse reactions include hypotension, dizziness, blurred vision, nausea and vomiting, laryngospasm, and diaphoresis.[106]

Dosage

Fentanyl is administered in conjunction with other antianxiety or sedative-hypnotic medications for sedation. The recommended dose of fentanyl is therefore predicated on the fact that the patient has already received one or more other CNS depressants. The maximal dose of fentanyl recommended for use in outpatient sedative procedures is 0.05 to 0.06 mg (1.0 to 1.2 ml). This dose is equivalent to approximately 8 mg morphine and about 50 mg of meperidine.

Fentanyl should always be diluted from its initial concentration of 0.05 mg/ml by adding 4 ml of diluent (e.g., 5% dextrose and sterile water) to produce a final concentration of 0.01 mg/ml.

Availability

Sublimaze (Janssen) (McNEILAB): 0.05 mg/ml in 2-, 5-, 10-, and 20-ml ampules. Each milliliter of solution contains:
0.05 mg fentanyl citrate
Sodium hydroxide for adjustment of pH to 4.0 to 7.5
Fentanyl (Abbott) (Elkins-Sinn): 0.05 mg/ml in same forms as Sublimaze. Fentanyl is classified as a Schedule II drug.

FENTANYL

The medical history of patients receiving fentanyl should be checked for the following:
Allergy or hypersensitivity to opioid analgesics
MAOIs taken within 14 days
COPD and decreased respiratory reserve

FENTANYL

Proprietary name	Sublimaze
Classification	Opioid agonist
Availability	0.05 mg/ml
Average sedative dose	0.05-0.06 mg
Maximal single dose	0.08 mg
Maximal total dose	0.08 mg

Alfentanil and sufentanil

Two analogs of fentanyl, alfentanil and sufentanil, are in clinical use in the United States. Clinical actions of both drugs are similar to those of fentanyl, but there are some significant differences. Although the onset of clinical action of alfentanil is very rapid, occurring within 1 minute after injection, its duration is very short (11 minutes at twice its MED$_{50}$).[107] The elimination half-life of alfentanil is 97 ± 22 minutes in adults, whereas in geriatric patients and persons with liver dysfunction, clearance rates are slower.[108,110] Alfentanil is a tetrazole derivative of fentanyl with many pharmacologic actions similar to those of fentanyl and sufentanil; however, alfentanil has a quicker onset of action than fentanyl and a shorter duration of action than either fentanyl or sufentanil.[111] In addition, alfentanil has a shorter half-life and may produce a lesser degree of respiratory depression than either fentanyl or sufentanil.

The use of these two drugs in general anesthesia

has been evaluated in depth[112,113]; they are now quite well accepted, especially for short surgical procedures. Alfentanil has received considerable attention in dentistry and other outpatient surgical procedures.[114-116] Alfentanil is frequently administered in conjunction with propofol.[117] Both drugs are opioid agonists and as such should be managed with the same care as other members of this group.

Availability

Alfenta (Janssen): 500 μg (as hydrochloride) per milliliter in 2-, 5-, 10-, and 20-ml ampules.

Sufenta (Janssen): 50 μg (as citrate) per milliliter in 1-, 2-, and 5-ml ampules.

Alfentanil and sufentanil are classified as Schedule II drugs.

OPIOID AGONIST/ANTAGONISTS

Because of the potentially significant side effects associated with administration of opioid agonists considerable research has been conducted to find a potent analgesic that possesses the efficacy of morphine but lacks its respiratory depressant actions, its drug dependence, and abuse liability.

In the 1960s some success was attained with the introduction of pentazocine, the first drug with both opioid agonist and opioid antagonist properties to be marketed (1967).[118] In succeeding years some of the initial fervor for pentazocine waned as significant side effects were reported.[119,120] Two other drugs in this same category—nalbuphine and butorphanol—recently became available and are gaining popularity in IV sedation in both dental and medical outpatient procedures.[121,122] The three drugs classified as opioid agonist/antagonists are pentazocine, nalbuphine, and butorphanol.

Pentazocine

The chemical formula for pentazocine is 1,2,3,4,5,6-hexahydro-6,11-dimethyl-3-(3-methyl-2-butenyl)-2,6-methano-3-benzazocin-8-ol lactate. Pentazocine was introduced in 1967 as a nonnarcotic opioid in both oral and parenteral formulations.[118]

A dose of 30 mg of pentazocine is equivalent to approximately 10 mg of morphine or 75 mg of meperidine. Administered intravenously, pentazocine's onset of action is 1 to 2 minutes with a duration of approximately 1 hour, although the patient may still exhibit alterations in consciousness for a number of hours following discharge from the office.

Pentazocine has opioid antagonist effects as well as sedative properties. Administered to patients re-

ceiving morphine-type opioids, pentazocine weakly antagonizes the analgesic, cardiovascular, respiratory, and CNS–depressant effects produced by these agents.[123] The sedative effect of a 30-mg IV dose of pentazocine is equivalent to approximately 10 mg of IV diazepam.[124] Pentazocine, however, does not provide the same degree of amnesia as does diazepam.

Pentazocine is indicated for use in the management of moderate to severe pain (usually administered orally or intramuscularly), as well as a preoperative or preanesthetic medication (usually administered intramuscularly), and as a supplement during general anesthesia (administered intravenously). Pentazocine initially gained some popularity within dentistry as an alternative to the opioid agonists.[125] However, with the introduction of butorphanol and nalbuphine, the dental use of pentazocine decreased substantially.

Contraindications

Pentazocine is contraindicated for use in patients with documented allergy to it.

Warnings

Despite early claims to the contrary, experience with pentazocine has demonstrated that both psychological and physical dependence can develop.[126] Abrupt discontinuance of pentazocine has produced a clinical syndrome exhibiting abdominal cramps, elevated temperature, rhinorrhea, restlessness, anxiety, and lacrimation.[127] Pentazocine is a drug with significant abuse potential, being combined (orally) with the antihistamine pyribenzamine in a combination called "Ts and blues."[128]

In the 1980s the manufacturers of oral pentazocine (Talwin) reformulated its compound, taking into account this abuse potential. Its new formulation, Talwin Nx, combines pentazocine (50 mg) with the opioid antagonist naloxone (0.5 mg). The intent of this combination is obvious, but its effectiveness is not yet known.[129]

Pentazocine should only be administered to the pregnant patient in situations in which the benefits of administration clearly outweigh its potential hazards. For routine outpatient sedation in a typical dental setting, there is little indication for pentazocine administration in pregnant patients.

Another significant untoward effect of pentazocine is the occurrence of acute neuropsychiatric manifestations, such as visual hallucinations, disorientation, confusion, mental depression, disturbing dreams, and dysphoria.[130] These responses usually resolve spontaneously within a few hours. The responsible mechanism is as yet unknown. Administration of naloxone may end in recovery. Management of reactions that do occur is symptomatic, with vital signs being monitored and recorded on a regular basis during the reaction, although stimulation of the sigma receptor will produce these same responses. Readministration of pentazocine to this same patient at future dates should be avoided if at all possible to minimize the possibility of recurrence.

The administration of pentazocine to patients under the age of 12 years is not recommended because of a lack of clinical data. The drug package insert for pentazocine recommends that ambulatory patients receiving parenteral pentazocine be cautioned not to operate machinery, drive cars, or unnecessarily expose themselves to hazards.[131]

Precautions

Patients with asthma, COPD, or other conditions associated with decreased respiratory reserve should be given pentazocine with caution, if at all. Patients with extensive liver disease appear to exhibit a greater number of adverse side effects from the usual clinical dose, a response indicating a decreased rate of metabolism of the drug by the liver. The plasma half-life of pentazocine is approximately 2 hours.

Pentazocine should be administered with caution to patients with seizure disorders. Seizures have developed after administration of pentazocine, although a direct cause-and-effect relationship has never been established.[132]

Adverse reactions

Pentazocine exhibits the same adverse reactions as the opioid agonists discussed, including nausea and vomiting, xerostomia, diarrhea, constipation, blurred vision, euphoria, dysphoria, respiratory and cardiovascular depression, and allergic reactions. In addition, pentazocine produces the neuropsychiatric reactions noted.

Dosage

Pentazocine is commonly administered in conjunction with an antianxiety or sedative-hypnotic agent for conscious sedation. It is, therefore, usually administered after the patient has received one or more drugs. The maximal recommended dose of pentazocine in IV conscious sedation is 30 mg. When titrated slowly, the usual dose required (in combination with other drugs) for sedation is approximately 20 mg.

Availability

Talwin (Winthrop): 30 mg/ml in 1-ml, 1.5-ml, and 2-ml ampules and in 10-ml vials. Each milliliter of solution in the ampule contains:
  30 mg pentazocine lactate
  1 mg acetone sodium bisulfite
  2.2 mg sodium chloride
  Water for injection
Each milliliter of solution in the vial contains:
  30 mg pentazocine lactate
  2 mg acetone sodium bisulfite
  1.5 mg sodium chloride
  1 mg methyl paraben as preservative
  Water for injection
The pH of both solutions is adjusted to 4 to 5 with lactic acid or sodium hydroxide. Air in both the ampules and vials has been displaced with nitrogen. Pentazocine is classified as a Schedule IV drug.

PENTAZOCINE

Proprietary name	Talwin
Classification	Opioid agonist/ antagonist
Availability	30 mg/ml
Average sedative dose	20 mg
Maximal single dose	30 mg
Maximal total dose	30 mg

PENTAZOCINE

The medical history of patients receiving pentazocine should be checked for the following:
  Allergy to pentazocine
  Suspected drug dependence
  Prior adverse CNS reaction to pentazocine
  Asthma
  COPD or decreased respiratory reserve

Nalbuphine

Nalbuphine, 17-(cyclobutylmethyl)-4,5a-epoxymorphinan-3,6a,14-triol hydrochloride, was synthesized in 1965. The chemical incorporates the molecular features of the opioid agonist oxymorphone hydrochloride (Numorphan) with that of the opioid antagonist naloxone hydrochloride (Narcan).[133]

Pharmacology

Nalbuphine is a potent analgesic with an analgesic potency approximately 0.8 to 0.9 times that of morphine. In clinical practice nalbuphine is considered to be equianalgesic to morphine when administered in equal doses (e.g., 10 mg of nalbuphine is equal to 10 mg of morphine).[134]

Following IV administration nalbuphine's onset of action is 2 to 3 minutes. Its duration of action is slightly longer than that of morphine (approximately 3 to 6 hours). A 10-mg dose of nalbuphine is equivalent to approximately 50 to 75 mg of meperidine.[135]

Studies of the effectiveness of nalbuphine as a preoperative sedative agent are lacking, and there are few studies evaluating IV nalbuphine in dental procedures.[136,137] To date I have used nalbuphine several hundred times in IV procedures on dental outpatients, usually with acceptable results.

Nalbuphine possesses opioid antagonist effects at the μ-opioid receptor. Nalbuphine is 10 times as effective as pentazocine as a opioid antagonist and one fourth as potent as nalorphine in morphine-dependent subjects. Quite interesting, and potentially very significant, is the fact that nalbuphine may be used as a opioid antagonist in place of naloxone. Magruder et al.[138] substituted nalbuphine (0.1 mg/kg) for naloxone to reverse respiratory depression produced by oxymorphone or hydromorphone. They noted a dramatic reversal of respiratory depression and a restoration of normal ventilation within 5 minutes. Of greater importance is the fact that nalbuphine provided substantial analgesia *after* reversal of the opioid-induced respiratory depression, which extended well into the postoperative period. These differential μ- (opioid antagonism) and κ- (agonist analgesia) opioid receptor actions of nalbuphine may be of value in avoidance of the adverse cardiovascular stimulation observed in some patients suffering from surgical pain when naloxone is administered to reverse opioid-induced CNS depression; unfortunately, however, naloxone also acts to reverse the analgesia produced by the opioid.[139] Although not yet recommended as the drug of choice for reversal of opioid-induced respiratory depression, nalbuphine is being increasingly used in place of naloxone for this purpose.

Pharmacokinetics

After IV administration the analgesic effects of nalbuphine appear in 2 to 3 minutes. The analgesic effects of the drug last for approximately 3 to 6 hours. The plasma half-life of nalbuphine is 5 hours. The drug undergoes metabolism in the liver; oral doses of nalbuphine undergo a significant hepatic first-pass effect, with only 20% of an orally administered dose being biologically available.[140]

Nalbuphine is physically compatible with most aqueous drugs and can thus be combined in the same syringe. Nalbuphine cannot, however, be combined with either diazepam or pentobarbital because a milky white precipitate forms.

Adverse effects

When used solely as an analgesic, the most frequently noted adverse effect is sedation, which is reported in 36% of patients treated with nalbuphine.[141] This "side effect" is used to advantage in IV conscious sedation procedures. Other common adverse responses (occurring in more than 3% of patients) include the following:

Sweaty, clammy feeling	9%
Nausea and vomiting	6%
Dizziness, vertigo	5%
Dry mouth	4%
Headache	3%

Psychotomimetic effects occurred only rarely and included depression, confusion, dysphoria, euphoria, feelings of unreality, feelings of hostility, and hallucinations. The incidence of these is significantly less than that seen with pentazocine.[141]

Possibly the most potentially serious adverse effect associated with nalbuphine administration is respiratory depression. When the classic opioid agonists (morphine, meperidine) are administered, both the rate and depth of respiration are depressed in a dose-related manner until apnea occurs. For outpatient ambulatory procedures, respiratory depression is usually the factor that most limits the use of opioid agonists. Nalbuphine possesses ceiling effects for respiratory depression, whereas its analgesic effects may become more pronounced with increasing doses. Gal et al.[142] demonstrated a plateau effect for both respiratory depression and analgesia for nalbuphine at doses up to 0.6 mg/kg. In other studies it was demonstrated that the normal dose of nalbuphine (7 to 10 mg/70 kg) produced the same degree of respiratory depression as an equivalent dose of morphine; however, nalbuphine-induced respiratory depression peaked at 30 mg/70 kg (equivalent to 20 mg/70 kg morphine) and remained the same even at nalbuphine doses of 3 mg/kg (210 mg/70 kg), whereas morphine-induced depression continued in a dose-related manner.[143,144]

Larger doses of nalbuphine do not extend the duration of respiratory depression beyond the usual 3 hours. Nalbuphine therefore possesses a ceiling effect to both the degree and the duration of respiratory depression. This is in contrast to butorphanol, which has a ceiling effect only for the degree of respiratory depression, not its duration.[145]

In the area of administration to medically compromised patients, especially the cardiovascular risk patient, nalbuphine produces a slight decrease in the cardiac workload, a potentially beneficial effect. Romagnoli and Keats[146] considered nalbuphine an ideal drug for patients with heart disease because it was devoid of hemodynamic effects except those associated with the relief of pain and anxiety.

One of the potential benefits of the opioid agonist-antagonist analgesics is a limited or absent drug dependence and abuse liability (psychic dependence, physical dependence, tolerance) as a result of their opioid antagonist actions when compared to complete μ-receptor agonists such as morphine.[147] It appears at this point that this hope is fulfilled to some extent with nalbuphine and butorphanol.

Overdose

Overdose of nalbuphine is exceptionally rare but potentially possible. Signs and symptoms of overdose would include CNS depression and respiratory depression, both of which are managed with basic life support and completely reversed with the IV administration of naloxone.

Contraindications

Nalbuphine is contraindicated for use in patients who are allergic or hypersensitive to it.

Warnings

Because nalbuphine produces CNS depression, patients receiving this drug must be cautioned against the performance of potentially dangerous tasks such as driving a car and operating machinery.[133] Nalbuphine is not recommended for administration to patient's under the age of 18 years because of a lack of clinical experience in patients in this age group. Pregnant patients should not receive nalbuphine unless the advantages of its administration clearly outweigh its potential disadvantages.

Nalbuphine may exhibit additive effects with other CNS depressants administered concurrently. The dosage of one or both of the drugs should be reduced. This should not be a significant problem with intravenous administration if the drugs are titrated to effect.

Precautions

Nalbuphine should be administered with caution, at reduced doses, to patients with impaired respiratory drive, including asthma and COPD (ASA III, IV, V). Because nalbuphine is metabolized in the liver and excreted through the kidneys, it is possible that patients with impaired hepatic or renal function may overrespond to the usual dose of the drug. Doses should be reduced in these patents. Titration minimizes this risk.

Dosage

When administered intravenously, nalbuphine should be titrated to clinical effect. The maximal dose of nalbuphine recommended for IV conscious sedation is 10 mg. This represents both the maximal single and total doses. Onset of action after IV administration is 2 to 3 minutes, with a duration of analgesic effect of 3 to 6 hours. The average IV dose of nalbuphine is approximately 7 to 8 mg.

When nalbuphine is administered following diazepam or midazolam, the depth of sedation is rarely increased; however, recovery from sedation will be somewhat less complete than that observed when diazepam or midazolam are administered alone.

Because of the doses recommended here, the beneficial effects of nalbuphine's ceiling level for respiratory depression will not be observed. It is only at doses considerably greater than these that the ceiling effect on respiratory depression will be noted. In doses up to 10 mg of nalbuphine the degree of respiratory depression should not be profound but will be equivalent to that induced by 10 mg of morphine or 50 to 75 mg of meperidine.

Availability

Nubain (Endo): 10 mg/ml in 1- and 2-ml ampules and 10-ml vials. Each milliliter of solution contains:
10 mg nalbuphine hydrochloride
0.1% sodium chloride
0.94% sodium citrate

NALBUPHINE	
Proprietary name	Nubain
Classification	Opioid agonist/antagonist
Availability	10 mg/ml
Average sedative dose	7-8 mg
Maximal single dose	10 mg
Maximal total dose	10 mg

1.26% citric acid anhydrous
0.1% sodium metabisulfite
0.2% 9:1 mixture of methylparaben and propyl-
    paraben as a preservative
Hydrochloric acid to adjust pH
Nalbuphine is not a scheduled drug.

Butorphanol

Butorphanol was synthesized in 1971 by Monkovic
and introduced in 1978. Butorphanol is a synthetic
agonist/antagonist analgesic similar in pharmacology to nalbuphine. The chemical formua of
butorphanol is levo-N-cyclobutylmethyl-6,10a,b-
dihydroxy-1,2,3,9,10,10a-hexahydro-(4H)-10,4a-imi-
noethanophenanthrene tartrate.

Pharmacology

Comparing butorphanol to morphine for analgesia, 2 mg of butorphanol (administered intramuscularly) is approximately as effective as 10 mg of morphine, 80 mg of meperidine, and 40 mg of
pentazocine. Data indicate that butorphanol is approximately 3.5 to 7 times as potent as morphine; 15
to 20 times more potent than pentazocine; and 30 to
40 times more potent than meperidine on a weight
basis.[148]

Pharmacokinetics

After IV administration, analgesic actions are
noted within minutes. Maximal blood levels occur in
5 minutes and thereafter decline in a biphasic manner. The α–half-life of rapid elimination (distribution) is approximately 0.1 hour, and the β–half-life
(metabolism and excretion) is 2.15 to 3.5 hours. Duration of analgesic properties is 3 to 4 hours.[149]

Butorphanol undergoes extensive metabolism in
the liver prior to excretion through the kidneys. Less
than 5% of a dose is excreted unchanged in the
urine. The major route of elimination of butorphanol and its metabolites is through the kidney
(75%), with biliary excretion accounting for 15% of

the dose. It is 80% bound to human serum protein
and distributed extensively to tissues. Butorphanol is
highly lipid soluble and concentrates in adipose tissue and excretory organs. Cumulation may occur
with repeated doses of the drug.[148]

Effect on respiration

Butorphanol has properties similar to those of pentazocine and nalbuphine with respect to respiratory
depression and opioid antagonist properties. As an
antagonist, butorphanol is 30 times as potent as pentazocine but only one-fortieth as potent as naloxone.
In a study by Nagashima et al., 2- and 4-mg IV doses
of butorphanol were compared to 10- and 20-mg
doses of morphine.[150] Respiratory depression produced by 4 mg of butorphanol was found to be statistically and clinically equivalent to that produced by
2 mg of butorphanol or 10 mg of morphine. This as
well as other studies have demonstrated that butorphanol does not produce a dose-related effect on respiration in contrast to that observed with opioid agonists such as morphine and meperidine.

Increasing doses of butorphanol did, however,
produce a longer duration of respiratory depression,
although the degree of depression did not increase.[151] Butorphanol possesses a ceiling effect only
for the degree of respiratory depression but not for
its duration, whereas nalbuphine possesses a ceiling
effect for both the depth and duration of respiratory
depression. As with other opioid agonists and opioid
agonist/antagonists, these respiratory-depressant
properties of butorphanol are reversible with naloxone.

Cardiovascular effects

Unlike nalbuphine, butorphanol does possess cardiovascular effects similar to, but less intense than,
those of pentazocine. These include increased pulmonary artery pressure, increased pulmonary wedge
pressure, increased left ventricular end-diastolic
pressure, increased systemic arterial pressure, and increased pulmonary vascular resistance. Both the cardiac index and cardiac workload are increased with
butorphanol.[152]

Butorphanol as well as pentazocine administration
should be restricted in patients with acute myocardial infarction, coronary insufficiency or ventricular
dysfunction, and high blood pressure (ASA IV and
V).

Butorphanol, like nalbuphine, is an agonist/an-
tagonist analgesic with a low physical-dependence liability, which distinguishes it from traditional potent
opioid agonists.

When butorphanol is administered in large doses, the incidence of unpleasant psychotomimetic effects is increased. This factor may serve to limit the abuse potential of butorphanol.

Side effects

Side effects reported after butorphanol administration are similar to those for other parenteral analgesics. The most frequently reported side effect was sedation (37%), a side effect that is used to advantage during IV sedation. Other common side effects were:

Nausea	7%
Clamminess, sweating	5%
Headache	2%
Vertigo	2%
Floating, pleasant feelings	2%
Dizziness	2%
Lethargy	2%

Overdosage

Overdose of butorphanol is extremely unlikely to develop; however, it is a clinical possibility. Signs and symptoms relate to exaggerated CNS and respiratory depression. Management consists of basic life support, with consideration for airway patency and ventilation, followed by the administration of naloxone or other opioid antagonists.

Warnings

Because of its opioid antagonist properties, the use of butorphanol is not recommended in patients known to be physically dependent on opioids. Administration in such patients may induce an acute abstinence syndrome (withdrawal).[153]

Because of the increased workload of the heart occurring with butorphanol administration, this drug is not recommended in patients with ventricular dysfunction or coronary insufficiency.

Precautions

Because butorphanol produces some respiratory depression, it should be administered with caution to patients with preexisting respiratory depression, such as patients receiving other CNS depressants, patients with asthma, COPD, or other types of decreased respiratory reserve, or patients with high blood pressure (ASA III, IV, V).

Patients with hepatic or renal dysfunction may overrespond to usual doses of butorphanol. If administered to these patients, the dose should be adjusted to account for this response. With IV administration, slow titration will minimize this possibility.

Use of butorphanol in patients under 18 years of age or in pregnant patients is not recommended because of a lack of clinical experience to indicate its safety in these groups. Ambulatory patients receiving butorphanol must, of course, be cautioned against possible hazardous situations such as driving a car or operating machinery.

Dosage

My experience with butorphanol administered for IV sedation has been limited to approximately 95 cases at this time (August 1994). However, it has been my impression that butorphanol may effectively be substituted for the traditional opioid agonists with no decrease in effectiveness and with the possible addition of decreased risk of respiratory depression. The doses recommended for IV use should preclude significant respiratory depression regardless of the pharmacologic properties of butorphanol.

After IV administration of 1 to 2 mg, onset of analgesic and sedative actions is quite rapid (1 to 2 minutes). Administered following diazepam, titrated butorphanol usually will not deepen the sedative level of the patient; therefore, the maximal recommended dose (2 mg) is usually given. Recovery from diazepam-butorphanol sedation is not as complete clinically as from diazepam sedation alone.

Availability

Stadol (Bristol): 1 mg/ml in 1-mg single-dose vial and 2 mg/ml in 1-, 2-, and 10-ml vials. Each milliliter of solution contains: Sodium chloride, sodium citrate, and citric acid as buffers.

The 10-ml multidose vial also contains the preservative benzethonium chloride. Butorphanol is not a scheduled drug.

BUTORPHANOL

The medical history of patients receiving butorphanol should be checked for the following:
Allergy or hypersensitivity to butorphanol
Known or suspected opioid dependence
Asthma, COPD, or decreased respiratory reserve
High blood pressure
Cardiovascular disease

```
┌─────────────────────────────────────────────┐
│                                             │
│              BUTORPHANOL                    │
│                                             │
│   Proprietary name      Stadol              │
│   Classification        Opioid agonist/antag-│
│                           onist             │
│   Availability          1 and 2 mg/ml       │
│   Average sedative dose 1.5 mg              │
│   Maximal single dose   2 mg               │
│   Maximal total dose    2 mg               │
│                                             │
└─────────────────────────────────────────────┘
```

Summary

The opioid agonist/antagonists offer several advantages over traditional opioid agonists such as meperidine, alphaprodine, fentanyl, and morphine. Where respiratory depression was a significant factor in drug administration, this risk has been reduced (although not eliminated). Problems may still develop with administration of these newer agents, but they appear to be less common.

Pentazocine has been available for almost 20 years. Its use intravenously in sedation is not common, primarily because of the significant incidence of negative psychotomimetic effects. In addition it is known today that physical dependence to pentazocine does occur.

Butorphanol, a more recent addition to the armamentarium, appears to have fewer significant adverse effects than pentazocine; however, it produces an increase in cardiovascular workload, which mitigates against its use in cardiovascular risk patients.

Nalbuphine appears to have all the advantages of butorphanol, with the additional advantages of not increasing cardiovascular workload and of being an excellent opioid antagonist. One additional benefit of butorphanol and nalbuphine is that they are nonscheduled drugs, requiring no special forms or paperwork for their purchase or administration. Pentazocine is a schedule IV drug, whereas the opioid agonists are schedule II drugs.

Note: Throughout this discussion of the opioid agonists and opioid agonist/antagonists, it has been mentioned in the "Warnings" and "Precautions" sections that the use of these agents in patients with significant liver or renal dysfunction, or both, and in patients with significant pulmonary disease (COPD) is contraindicated. Please bear in mind that the use of intravenous sedation was earlier recommended for patients who have been categorized as ASA physical status classifications I and II, with only a selected few ASA III patients being considered acceptable.

The patients mentioned in the "Warnings" and "Precautions" sections are considered to be at best ASA III and are usually ASA IV. Adherence to basic tenets of patient selection for IV conscious sedation will minimize the number of problems that may develop in these patients.

OPIOID ANTAGONISTS

The only drug presently available possessing pure opioid-antagonist properties is naloxone. The pharmacology and clinical importance of this drug will be reviewed in the section on antidotal drugs (p. 398).

ANTICHOLINERGICS

The anticholinergics, also known as belladonna alkaloids and cholinergic blocking agents, are important to the practice of anesthesia and are valuable adjuncts to intravenously administered sedatives. Indications for the use of anticholinergics in the practice of anesthesia and IV sedation include the following: (1) as preoperative medication to reduce salivary secretions, (2) to correct vagally induced bradycardia, and (3) to reverse curarization (in general anesthesia) when administered with neostigmine. Three anticholinergics—atropine, scopolamine, and glycopyrrolate—will be discussed. These drugs are very popular during IV conscious sedation in dentistry, administered primarily for their antisalivary actions.

Pharmacology

The belladonna alkaloids are widely distributed in nature. **Atropine,** chemically a racemic mixture of levo- and dextrohyoscyamine (only the levo form is pharmacologically active), is found in the following botanicals:

Atropa belladonna—known as the deadly nightshade

Datura stramonium—Jamestown weed, jimson weed, stinkweed, thorn-apple, and devil's apple

Scopolamine, chemically levo-hyoscine, is found in the following:

Hyoscyamus niger—black henbane

Scopolia carniolica

Glycopyrrolate, a synthetic anticholinergic, was introduced in 1961. It is a quaternary ammonium compound with the chemical name 1-methyl-3-pyrrolidyl-phenyl-cyclopentane-glycolate methobromide.

Mechanism of action

The anticholinergics act as competitive antagonists to acetylcholine at the postganglionic receptor located at the neuroeffector junction of the parasympathetic nervous system. Although the actions of these drugs are essentially similar, the degree to which the individual drug possesses a certain property may differ. For example, scopolamine has a greater effect on salivary glands than does atropine, but atropine has a greater effect on the heart and bronchial musculature. In clinical doses atropine does not produce CNS depression; however, scopolamine does and is therefore used quite commonly for preoperative medication.

Central nervous system

Atropine produces a stimulation of the medulla and higher cerebral centers. In clinical doses of 0.5 to 1.0 mg this effect is noted as a mild vagal stimulation in which both the rate and depth of breathing are increased.[154] This effect is a result of bronchiolar dilation and increased physiologic dead space. Atropine is not effective in reversing significant respiratory depression.

Scopolamine in therapeutic doses produces a degree of CNS depression, clinically noted as drowsiness, euphoria, amnesia, fatigue, and dreamless sleep. Unfortunately, in some patients the same clinical dose may produce excitement, restlessness, hallucinations, and delirium, and is more likely to occur in the presence of pain.

Glycopyrrolate, a quaternary ammonium compound, does not cross the blood-brain barrier and does not produce the CNS actions noted for atropine and scopolamine.

In cases in which sedation is a desirable effect, the administration of scopolamine is preferred to either atropine or glycopyrrolate. Scopolamine provides 5 to 15 times the sedative effects of the other two drugs.[155]

Amnesia may be a desirable action of an anticholinergic drug. Of the three, only scopolamine produces this effect. Although amnesia may occur after scopolamine administration, it is not as consistent a finding as it is with diazepam or midazolam. When present, however, amnesia tends to be prolonged, often persisting for 2 to 4 hours. Although anterograde amnesia—lack of recall of events occurring after administration of scopolamine—is most common, retrograde amnesia—the lack of recall of events occurring prior to administration of the drug—may also occur.[156]

Eye

Anticholinergics block the responses of the sphincter muscle of the iris and the ciliary muscle of the lens to cholinergic stimulation. They therefore produce mydriasis (dilation of the pupil) and cycloplegia (paralysis of accommodation). Administered in therapeutic doses, atropine (0.4 to 0.6 mg) produces little ocular effect. However, scopolamine in therapeutic doses produces significant mydriasis and cycloplegia.

Administered parenterally, the anticholinergics have little effect on intraocular pressure, except in patients with acute narrow-angle glaucoma, in whom dangerously high intraocular pressures may develop. This occurs when the iris, which is crowded back into the angle of the anterior chamber of the eye, interferes with drainage of the aqueous humor.[157] In the more commonly seen wide-angle glaucoma, such an increase in intraocular pressure seldom occurs, and the anticholinergics may be used with little increase in risk to the patient. The administration of anticholinergics is contraindicated for patients who wear contact lenses.

Respiratory tract

The anticholinergic drugs decrease secretions of the nose, mouth, pharynx, and bronchi, thereby drying the mucous membranes of the respiratory tract. This of course represents one of the indications for administration of these drugs as preanesthetic medications. Clinically the antisialagoric actions of 0.4 mg of atropine are equal to a dose of 0.2 mg of glycopyrrolate.

Bronchial smooth muscle is also dilated following administration of anticholinergic drugs, atropine being considerably more potent in this regard than either scopolamine or glycopyrrolate. Atropine, scopolamine, and glycopyrrolate decrease the incidence of laryngospasm during general anesthesia. This is because of the decrease in respiratory tract secretions that might precipitate reflex laryngospasm, which is produced by contraction of laryngeal skeletal muscle.

Cardiovascular actions

The principal effect of the anticholinergics on the heart is an alteration in rate. Clinical doses of 0.4 to 0.6 mg of atropine produce a decrease in heart rate of 4 to 8 beats/minute. This effect is not seen if the drug is administered rapidly intravenously. Larger doses produce a tachycardia by blocking the effects of the vagus nerve at the S-A pacemaker. The rate may rise as much as 35 to 40 beats above the resting rate (in a study with young men receiving 2 mg of atropine intramuscularly).[158] This action of the anticholinergics is most notable in young healthy adults in whom vagal tone is great. In very young patients and geriatric patients atropine may fail to accelerate the heart rate.

Scopolamine in small doses, 0.1 to 0.2 mg, produces even more profound cardiac slowing than atropine. With higher doses, the resultant tachycardia is equal to that of atropine but shorter lived. The heart rate will return to baseline or perhaps result in a bradycardia.

Glycopyrrolate produces less tachycardia than either atropine or scopolamine and thus is indicated for use in patients in whom atropine- or scopolamine-induced tachycardia is not desirable. Conversely, in situations in which significant bradycardia has developed, the administration of glycopyrrolate will not provide the desired increase in heart rate. Atropine or scopolamine are necessary at this time.

Gastrointestinal tract

Therapeutic doses of anticholinergics do not greatly affect gastric secretion. Doses in excess of 1 mg (atropine) must be administered to alter gastric secretion significantly. The anticholinergics have little effect on the secretion of pancreatic juice, bile, or succus entericus.

On the other hand, anticholinergics have profound actions on gastrointestinal motility. In both healthy patients and in those with gastrointestinal disease, therapeutic doses inhibit the motor activity of much of the small and large intestine. Motility is reduced along with muscle tone, as well as the amplitude and frequency of peristaltic activity. This is termed the antispasmodic effect of the anticholinergics.[159]

Secretory glands

The actions of the anticholinergics on respiratory and digestive tract secretions have been discussed. Even small doses inhibit the activity of sweat glands. The skin becomes hot and dry. If sweating is depressed enough, body temperature may rise, but this is usually noted only after toxic doses. The lacrimal glands are also inhibited by the anticholinergics, but to a smaller extent than other secretory glands. The secretion of milk is not significantly affected.

Biotransformation

The anticholinergics are rapidly removed from the blood and are distributed throughout the body. Atropine is approximately 50% protein bound in the blood. The metabolism of the anticholinergics is not very well understood. Approximately 13% to 50% of a dose of atropine is found unchanged in the urine.

The liver is the primary organ of biotransformation. A small amount of the drug is found in the feces, and an even smaller amount is found in expired air.[160] Less than 1% of a dose of scopolamine is recovered unchanged in the urine.

Atropine

In clinical doses (0.5 to 1 mg), atropine produces stimulation of the medulla and higher cerebral centers, resulting in a mild central vagal stimulation and moderate respiratory stimulation. Its primary IV use is for the reduction of salivary and bronchial secretions.[161]

Contraindications to the administration of atropine include glaucoma, adhesions (synechiae) between the iris and the lens of the eye, and asthma.[162]

The effects of atropine on the developing fetus are not known with any degree of certainty; therefore, the use of atropine during pregnancy should be reserved for those cases in which its effects are truly important. This will rule out its use in most dental situations.

Adverse reactions

Although systemic tolerance to drug effects varies greatly, the following is the "normal" response to increasing doses of atropine:

Dose (mg)	Effect
0.5	Slight dryness of nose and mouth
	Bradycardia
1	Greater dryness of nose and mouth, with thirst
	Slowing, then acceleration, of the heart
	Mydriasis
2	Very dry mouth
	Tachycardia with palpitation
	Mydriasis
	Slight blurring of near vision
	Flushed, dry skin
5	Increase in the preceding symptoms plus the following:
	Disturbance of speech
	Difficulty in swallowing
	Headache
	Hot, dry skin
	Restlessness with asthenia (lack of energy)
10	The preceding symptoms to an extreme degree plus the following:
	Ataxia
	Excitement
	Disorientation
	Hallucinations
	Delirium
	Coma

Intoxication to atropine has been described as follows: "Dry as a bone, red as a beet, and mad as a hatter." Fortunately, atropine intoxication is rarely fatal if rapidly diagnosed and antidotal therapy instituted. Physostigmine, 1 to 5 ml of a dilution of 1 mg of physostigmine in 5 ml (0.2 mg/ml) administered intravenously, is the drug of choice in the management of this reaction. The dose may be repeated every 5 minutes if necessary for a total dose of 2 mg in children and 6 mg in adults.[163]

Dosage

The usual adult dose of atropine is 0.4 to 0.6 mg. In children the following doses are recommended:

Weight (pounds)	Dose (mg)
7-16	0.1
17-24	0.15
25-40	0.2
41-65	0.3
66-90	0.4
More than 90	0.4-0.6

Availability

Atropine sulfate: 0.3, 0.4, 0.5, 0.6, 1, and 1.3 mg/ml. Each milliliter of atropine sulfate solution contains:

0.4 mg atropine sulfate
0.5% chlorobutanol as a preservative

Atropine is not a scheduled drug.

ATROPINE SULFATE

The medical history of patients receiving atropine sulfate should be checked for the following:
Glaucoma
Prostate disease
Asthma
Adhesions between iris and lens of eye
Myasthenia gravis
Contact lenses

ATROPINE SULFATE

Classification	Anticholinergic
Availability	0.3-1.3 mg/ml
Average therapeutic dose	0.4-0.6 mg
Maximal single dose	0.4-0.6 mg
Maximal total dose	0.4-0.6 mg

Scopolamine hydrobromide

Scopolamine hydrobromide differs in several significant ways from atropine. It can produce a degree of CNS depression, whereas atropine does not. Scopolamine is a frequently used constituent of preanesthetic medication. In this regard scopolamine provides the following three beneficial effects:

Decreases in salivary and bronchial secretions
Some sedative effect (minor)
Anterograde amnesia

The latter two effects are unique to scopolamine and form the basis for its widespread use in anesthesia practice.[164] Unfortunately, scopolamine is also more apt to produce the phenomenon known as emergence delirium than either atropine or glycopyrrolate. Because this reaction, which involves vivid dreaming, nightmares, and hallucinations, develops most often in very young and elderly patients, the use of scopolamine in patients under the age of 6 years and over the age of 65 years is discouraged.[165]

Dosage

The usual adult therapeutic dose is 0.32 to 0.65 mg. The following dosage scale is recommended for children[166]:

Age	Dose (mg)
6 months to 3 years	0.1-0.15
3-6 years	0.15-0.2
6-12 years	0.2-0.3

Availability

Scopolamine hydrobromide: 0.3 mg/ml, 0.4 mg/ml in 0.5- and 1.0-ml ampules, and 0.6 mg/ml. Each milliliter of scopolamine hydrobromide solution contains:

0.3 mg scopolamine hydrobromide
1% alcohol

SCOPOLAMINE HYDROBROMIDE

The medical history of patients receiving scopolamine hydrobromide should be checked for the following:
Glaucoma
Adhesions between iris and lens
Asthma
Prostatic disease
Myasthenia gravis
Contact lenses

```
┌─────────────────────────────────────────────┐
│         SCOPOLAMINE HYDROBROMIDE            │
│                                             │
│   Classification          Anticholinergic   │
│   Availability            0.3-0.6 mg/ml     │
│   Average therapeutic dose 0.3 mg           │
│   Maximal single dose     0.3 mg            │
│   Maximal total dose      0.3 mg            │
│                                             │
└─────────────────────────────────────────────┘
```

10% mannitol
Water for injection
Scopolamine is not a scheduled drug.

Glycopyrrolate

Glycopyrrolate is a relatively recent addition to the anticholinergic armamentarium. Because it is a quaternary ammonium compound, glycopyrrolate does not cross lipid membranes, such as the blood-brain barrier, in contrast to both atropine and scopolamine. Glycopyrrolate is less likely to produce unwanted CNS depression or delirium-type reactions.

Following IV administration the onset of clinical action develops within 1 minute. Glycopyrrolate has a duration of action of vagal blocking effects for 2 to 3 hours and antisialagogue effects for up to 7 hours.[167] This latter effect may be undesirable in the ambulatory patient.

Warnings

Ambulatory patients receiving glycopyrrolate must be advised not to perform hazardous work, operate machinery, or drive a motor vehicle, because the drug may produce drowsiness or blurred vision.[168] In the presence of a high environmental temperature, heat prostration (heat stroke and fever caused by decreased sweating) can occur with the use of glycopyrrolate.

Precautions

Glycopyrrolate should be used with caution in patients with tachycardia because the drug may cause a further increase in the heart rate.[168] In addition, patients with ischemic heart disease, coronary artery disease, heart failure, dysrhythmias, hypertension, or hyperthyroidism should be evaluated carefully prior to administration of glycopyrrolate.

Although glycopyrrolate has been shown to be nonteratogenic in animal studies, its effect on the human fetus is unknown; therefore, the use of glycopyrrolate in pregnancy is not recommended and should be reserved for those cases in which it is truly required.

Dosage

The usual therapeutic dose of glycopyrrolate in adults is 0.1 mg (0.5 ml) as needed and may be repeated every 2 to 3 minutes. In children the IV dose of glycopyrrolate is 0.02 mg (0.1 ml) per pound of body weight, not to exceed a dose of 0.1 mg (0.5 ml) in a single dose. As with the adult, this dose may be repeated every 2 to 3 minutes as needed.

Availability

Robinul (Robins): 0.2 mg/ml in 1-, 2-, 5-, and 20-ml ampules and vials. Each milliliter of glycopyrrolate contains:

0.2 mg glycopyrrolate
Water for injection
0.5 to 0.9% benzyl alcohol as preservative
pH adjusted to 2 to 3 with sodium hydroxide or hydrochloric acid

Glycopyrrolate is not a scheduled drug.

```
┌─────────────────────────────────────────────┐
│              GLYCOPYRROLATE                 │
│                                             │
│   The medical history of patients receiving │
│   glycopyrrolate should be checked for the  │
│   following:                                │
│     Allergy to glycopyrrolate               │
│     Glaucoma                                │
│     Prostatic disease                       │
│     Asthma                                  │
│     Myasthenia gravis                       │
│     Ischemic heart disease                  │
│     Contact lenses                          │
│                                             │
└─────────────────────────────────────────────┘
```

```
┌─────────────────────────────────────────────┐
│              GLYCOPYRROLATE                 │
│                                             │
│   Proprietary name         Robinul          │
│   Classification           Anticholinergic  │
│   Availability             0.2 mg/ml        │
│   Average therapeutic dose 0.1 mg           │
│   Maximal single dose      0.1 mg           │
│   Maximal total dose       0.2 mg           │
│                                             │
└─────────────────────────────────────────────┘
```

Summary

The anticholinergics serve primarily as adjunctive drugs during IV conscious sedation in outpatients.

The selection of the appropriate anticholinergic will be based on the indication for its use, for example:

Longer procedures (more than 2 to 3 hours): glycopyrrolate

Amnesia: scopolamine

Sedation: scopolamine

Decreased cardiovascular action: glycopyrrolate

Short procedure, no amnesia, no sedation: atropine

Anticholinergics may be administered in combination with any of the drugs discussed in this section, with the notable exception of lorazepam (Ativan). The use of scopolamine is not recommended in conjunction with lorazepam because of the intense amnesic effect and the increased possibility of emergence delirium produced by this combination.[169]

INNOVAR

Innovar is the proprietary name of a combination of two drugs, the long-acting, potent, nonphenothiazine tranquilizer of the buterophenone type, droperidol, and the potent, short-acting opioid agonist, fentanyl. When administered intravenously this combination of drugs produces a state termed neuroleptanesthesia or neuroleptanalgesia, dependent on the dosage of drugs administered.[170]

The term *neuroleptic* is defined as a state of consciousness in which the patient has the following characteristics:

Is sleepy but not unconscious

Is psychologically detached from the environment

Retains the ability to obey commands

Has diminished motor activity

The concept of neuroleptanesthesia, introduced in 1959, proposed combining the neuroleptic state with analgesia and amnesia to provide ideal circumstances for surgery.[171]

The combination of droperidol and fentanyl provides neuroleptanalgesia, a state in which the patient retains consciousness, yet is detached from the environment. The addition of nitrous oxide (N_2O) and oxygen (O_2) renders the patient unconscious in a state called neuroleptanesthesia.

Within the operating room neuroleptanesthesia is a popular technique of general anesthesia, especially in medically compromised patients (ASA III and IV). In the hospital environment in which the patient is nonambulatory the use of Innovar is rational. In typical ambulatory outpatient dental situations or in short-stay surgery centers, however, the use of Innovar makes less sense. The pharmacology of the component drugs will demonstrate this point.

Droperidol

Droperidol was synthesized in 1962 by Janssen Pharmaceutica in Belgium.

Pharmacology

Droperidol produces marked tranquilization and sedation. Other pharmacologic actions of droperidol include the following[172]:

1. Antiemetic actions
2. Potentiation of CNS-depressant drugs
3. Mild α-adrenergic blockade (producing peripheral vasodilation) and a decrease in the pressor effects of epinephrine; droperidol can produce hypotension and a decrease in peripheral vascular resistance; however, this effect is not usually observed in therapeutic doses
4. The incidence of epinephrine-induced cardiac dysrhythmias is reduced by the α-adrenergic properties of droperidol; however, there is no effect on the incidence of other types of dysrhythmias

Following IV administration the clinical actions of droperidol are noted within 3 to 10 minutes; however, the full effect may not be observed for as long as 30 minutes. This is a negative factor in the use of droperidol for ambulatory, outpatient procedures, which are usually short. Even more significant than the relatively slow onset is the fact that although the duration of clinically evident sedation and tranquilization produced by droperidol usually lasts for 2 to 4 hours, alterations in the patient's state of consciousness may persist for up to 12 hours. This is the primary reason for not recommending this drug for use in outpatient procedures.

Indications

The following three indications are listed in the drug package insert for droperidol[173]:

1. To provide tranquilization and reduce the incidence of nausea and vomiting in surgical procedures
2. For premedication, induction, and as an adjunct in the maintenance of general and regional anesthesia
3. In neuroleptanalgesia, in which droperidol is administered concurrently with fentanyl to aid in tranquilization and decrease pain and anxiety

Warnings

Fluids and other countermeasures must be readily available to counteract hypotension if it should develop after administration of droperidol. Droperidol potentiates the CNS-depressant properties of other drugs, including opioid agonists such as fentanyl. The initial dose of opioid should be decreased to about one fourth or one third of the usually recommended dose.

Droperidol may be used safely in children over the age of 2 years; however, there are insufficient data to recommend its use in younger patients.

The safety of droperidol in pregnancy has not been established with respect to its possible effect on the fetus. Droperidol, therefore, should be reserved for use in pregnant women and women of childbearing potential only when the benefits clearly outweigh the potential hazards of its use. In elective, ambulatory, outpatient procedures, the use of droperidol is rarely indicated.

Precautions

The initial dose of droperidol should be reduced appropriately in the elderly, debilitated, and other high-risk patients (ASA III, IV). Other CNS-depressant drugs (opioids, phenothiazines, barbiturates) have additive or potentiating effects when administered in conjunction with droperidol. When a patient has received one of these prior to droperidol, the dose of droperidol should be reduced. In the same manner, the dose of the other CNS depressant is decreased when it is administered following droperidol. Patients with significant liver or kidney disease should receive droperidol with caution because it is metabolized and excreted through these organs.

Adverse reactions

The most frequently reported adverse reactions to droperidol are hypotension and a mild tachycardia. Both of these effects usually resolve without drug management. The management of hypotension, if severe or prolonged, is to administer IV fluids to the patient in an effort to increase fluid volume. Other adverse reactions include the following:

Postoperative drowsiness

Extrapyramidal symptoms, such as dystonia, akathisia, and oculogyric crisis; management requires IV administration of diphenhydramine

Restlessness, hyperactivity, anxiety

Dizziness

Chills, shivering, or both

Laryngospasm, bronchospasm

Postoperative hallucinations

Respiratory depression, apnea, and muscular rigidity can develop when droperidol is adminis-

tered with fentanyl. If permitted to remain untreated, these may lead to respiratory arrest.

The use of droperidol in the ambulatory outpatient is not recommended.

Droperidol is combined with the short-acting opioid agonist fentanyl to produce the combination marketed as Innovar. Fentanyl has previously been discussed (see p. 381).

Effects of Innovar

The administration of Innovar alone does not normally produce loss of consciousness. It does produce the state of neuroleptanalgesia, which was described at the beginning of this section.

When Innovar is administered, both pharyngeal and laryngeal reflexes are obtunded, and care must be taken to protect the patient's airway. Fentanyl possesses mild emetic properties that are effectively counterbalanced by the potent antiemetic properties of droperidol.

One of the most significant concerns when Innovar is used is the potential for the production of respiratory depression. Innovar produces depression of the medullary respiratory center, raising the threshold to arterial carbon dioxide (CO_2) tension.[174] Large doses of fentanyl may produce apnea.

The fentanyl component may also produce skeletal muscle rigidity of the thoracic and abdominal walls. Although not common, this action is most often related to the speed of administration of the drug and may be effectively prevented by the slow injection of Innovar or fentanyl. Should it develop, assisted or controlled ventilation is required, with the possible need for a neuromuscular blocking agent such as succinylcholine.

Contraindications

Contraindications to the administration of Innovar are allergy or hypersensitivity to either the droperidol or fentanyl component.

Warnings

The safety of fentanyl in patients who have received MAOIs within 14 days has not been established and is therefore not recommended.[175] The safety of Innovar in patients under 2 years of age has not been established and is therefore not recommended.

Pregnant patients should not be administered Innovar unless the benefits of its administration clearly outweigh the potential hazards of its use. For this reason the use of Innovar cannot be recommended

---

DROPERIDOL

The medical history of patients receiving droperidol should be checked for the following:
Possible hypovolemia (increases risk of hypotension with droperidol)
Allergy or hypersensitivity to droperidol

---

for the pregnant patient in the outpatient environment.

Adverse reactions

Adverse reactions to Innovar are the same as those previously discussed for droperidol and fentanyl. The two most common adverse reactions are hypotension and respiratory depression.

Orthostatic hypotension, primarily caused by the droperidol, is another factor to consider in the ambulatory patient. Positional changes (from supine to upright) may produce dramatic decreases in the patient's blood pressure after droperidol administration. Droperidol's duration of activity is approximately 8 hours, requiring the patient and the escort to be made fully aware of this possibility.

Dosage

As with all intravenously administered drugs, the dose of Innovar should be individualized. Anesthesia is induced with a dose of 1 ml of Innovar per 20 to 25 pounds (1 ml/9 to 11 kg). This dose must be administered slowly (over 5 to 6 minutes) to minimize the risk of muscular rigidity. Once the patient is heavily sedated with Innovar, N_2O-O_2 is added, unconsciousness occurs, and other general anesthetic drugs may be added. In the absence of N_2O-O_2, the patient remains conscious, yet sedated.

Availability

Innovar (McNEILAB): 0.05 mg/ml fentanyl citrate (Sublimaze) and 2.5 mg/ml droperidol (Inapsine) in 2- and 5-ml ampules. Lactic acid is added to adjust the pH of the solution to 3.5 ± 0.3. Innovar is classified as a Schedule II drug.

Summary

Innovar is a popular drug combination for the production of neuroleptanalgesia or neuroleptanesthesia. As used in the hospitalized patient in whom postoperative recovery can be carefully monitored, neuroleptanesthesia and neuroleptanalgesia are excellent techniques. For outpatient procedures, on

---

INNOVAR

Proprietary name	Innovar
Classification	Neuroleptic
Availability	Droperidol, 2.5 mg/ml
	Fentanyl, 0.05 mg/ml
Average sedative dose	1-2 ml
Maximal single dose	0.5-1 ml
Maximal total dose	0.5-1 ml

Note: *Innovar is not recommended for use in outpatient procedures.*

---

the other hand, the use of Innovar cannot be recommended because the duration of action of one of its components—droperidol—is 8 hours, entirely too long for ambulatory patients. Innovar cannot, therefore, be recommended for use in the typical outpatient environment.

The combination of droperidol and fentanyl appears to be illogical. Fentanyl, with its 45-minute duration of action, combined with droperidol's 8-hour duration of action, does not seem logical. In the hospital a patient will receive an initial dose of the Innovar combination, after which there is no longer a need to readminister droperidol for approximately 2 to 4 hours (usual duration of its sedative actions); however, the opioid actions of fentanyl will disappear within 45 minutes. Individual doses of fentanyl are therefore readministered, as needed, during the procedure. In surgical procedures of longer duration an initial dose of Innovar or droperidol is administered and a longer-acting opioid such as morphine substituted for fentanyl.

A word of caution is needed before this discussion on Innovar is concluded. Many doctors employ nurse anesthetists to administer outpatient sedation or general anesthesia in their offices. Many of these hospital-based persons favor the use of Innovar in the dental patient. Remember that most of the procedures that these persons usually perform are on hospitalized patients in whom postoperative recovery is closely monitored for however many hours are required. Such is not the case in the typical dental patient. The use of Innovar should be discouraged in this environment. Other highly effective drugs for IV sedation are available in its place.

KETAMINE

Ketamine hydrochloride is a cyclohexane derivative closely related chemically and pharmacologically to phencyclidine, a veterinary anesthetic and prominent drug of abuse (known as "angel dust").

NALOXONE

Proprietary name	Narcan
Classification	Opioid antagonist
Availability	0.02 and 0.4 mg/ml
Average therapeutic dose	0.4 mg (adult)
Maximal single dose	0.4 mg (adult)
Maximal total dose	1.2 mg (adult)*

*k of improvement after two or three doses usually indicates
respiratory depression is not produced by opioids

0 mg methylparaben and propylparaben in a ratio of 9:1 as preservatives
H adjusted with hydrochloric acid
oxone is not a scheduled drug.

buphine

s mentioned in the introduction to opioid antag-
sts, nalbuphine, an opioid agonist/antagonist,
been used to reverse opioid-induced respiratory
ression. It appears to be as effective as naloxone
possesses the added benefit of not reversing an-
esia when used in large doses. The dosage of nal-
ohine used by Magruder et al.[184] was 0.1 mg/kg.
hough nalbuphine is a very promising addition to
armamentarium of opioid antagonists, addi-
nal research is required before it can be recom-
nded over naloxone.

mmary

The availability of drugs capable of reversing sig-
icant undesirable effects of opioids is quite im-
rtant. However, it is significantly more important
remember that the occasion to use these drugs will
nost never develop if IV sedatives and opioids are
ministered reasonably. The maximal doses of
ioids recommended in this and in succeeding
apters will not produce respiratory depression in
y but the most debilitated or acutely sensitive pants. However, maximal doses rarely need be ad-
inistered. Adequate clinical effects will usually be
otained with doses below these maximal doses. The
cret to success and safety with opioids, as with all
ugs, is the slow titration of the drug to the desired
fect.

In 20 years of teaching IV sedation on the doctoral,
ostdoctoral, and continuing education levels, I have
ever treated a patient who required an opioid an-
gonist for reversal of opioid-induced respiratory
epression. Having the drug readily available is ab-

solutely essential if opioids of any type are administered by any route. Routine opioid reversal, recommended by some, is unnecessary and may in some
cases increase patient risk (as in cases in which postoperative pain is present, overstressing the cardiovascular system).

BENZODIAZEPINE ANTAGONIST

Although the benzodiazepines have been described as the most nearly ideal drugs for anxiety
control and sedation, there are still adverse reactions
associated with their administration. Emergence delirium, excessive duration of sedation, and possible
respiratory depression are but a few of these. Although rare, their occurrence can wreak havoc on a
procedure. Until recently, no antidotal drug was
available to reverse the undesirable actions of benzodiazepines. Since publication of the first edition of
this book, a specific benzodiazepine antagonist has
been identified. Flumazenil was introduced into clinical practice in the late 1980s and in the United
States in 1992.

Flumazenil, administered intravenously following
the IV administration of diazepam or midazolam,
produces a rapid reversal of sedation and improved
ability to comprehend and obey commands.[187] Flumazenil also reduces the duration of anterograde
amnesia produced with midazolam—91 minutes
(with flumazenil) compared with 121 minutes (no
flumazenil).[188,189] When administered in a geriatric
population (72 ± 9 years) following midazolam sedation, patients required less recovery time from sedation, demonstrated increased alertness and a decreased amnesic effect. Two patients became
somewhat anxious following flumazenil administration.[189]

The dose administered in trials has varied considerably, from 0.5 mg to 0.6 to 1 mg to 20 to 40
mg.[190-192] The elimination half-life of flumazenil is
short, less than 1 hour, and there appear at this time
to be a few side effects, aside from the possibility of
producing anxiety states in the patient after use of
flumazenil.[192] Sage et al.[190] concluded that "in doses
up to 0.5 mg [flumazenil] provided safe and effective
antagonism of midazolam-induced sedation in a clinical setting."[190]

How flumazenil will be used clinically remains to
be seen. It will definitely be a means of terminating
any undesirable actions of injected benzodiazepine
However, the need for the "routine" administrati
of flumazenil at the termination of every IV be
diazepine procedure will likely be unnecessary

The type of anesthesia produced by ketamine has
been termed dissociative anesthesia.[176] It is a state in
which the patient appears to be awake, has his or her
eyes open, and is capable of muscular movement but
appears to be unaware of, or dissociated from, the
environment. Another term for the type of state induced by ketamine is *cataleptic anesthesia*. Profound
analgesia and amnesia are associated with ketamine
administration.

The dissociative state produced by ketamine is an
excitatory state, completely dissimilar from that seen
after administration of traditional general anesthetics such as halothane, thiopental, and meperidine.
Blood pressure and heart rate, usually somewhat depressed during general anesthesia, are elevated following ketamine administration. Respiration is spontaneous, and the airway is affected very little by the
drug, the patient retaining the ability to maintain a
patent airway throughout the procedure. Laryngeal
and pharyngeal reflexes are intact or even hyperactive during ketamine anesthesia. When used in dental procedures it is important to place an oropharyngeal pack to prevent contamination of the pharynx
and/or larynx with debris.

In the operating room IV ketamine is used for
short procedures, such as dilatation and curettage (D
& C), surgical procedures on the skin, or dental procedures such as extraction or restorative dentistry in
pediatric patients. Another use of ketamine is in patients in whom multiple surgical procedures will be
required, such as burn victims requiring multiple de-
bridements and skin grafts over a brief time.

The onset of action of ketamine after IV administration is rapid (less than 1 minute), with a duration
of clinical effect of approximately 10 minutes.[177] The
usual IV induction dose of ketamine is 1 to 4.5 mg/
kg (approximately 0.5 to 2 mg/pound) administered
over 1 minute. More rapid administration results in
respiratory depression and an exaggerated pressor
response. The duration of anesthesia may be extended with the readministration of ketamine in
doses of 0.5 mg/kg. Recovery from ketamine anesthesia is prolonged the larger the dose of ketamine
administered. An even more effective method of prolonging the anesthesia from ketamine is by administering local anesthesia for pain control and N_2O-
O_2 for additional CNS depression. Administration of
these drugs along with ketamine reduces the dose of
ketamine required, speeds recovery, and minimizes
adverse recovery room phenomena (hallucinations).

Recovery from ketamine-induced anesthesia is
prolonged and is frequently associated with vivid
dreams, hallucinations, and delirium.[178] These emer-

gence reactions are significantly more common in
adults than in children and may last from minutes to
hours. Flashbacks—recurrence of these experiences—have occurred months after the administration of ketamine. This is somewhat similar to flashbacks occurring after administration of LSD.
Sussman reported that 24% of patients over 16 years
of age reported emergence reactions, whereas only
8% of those under 16 years of age had the same response.[179] Patients over the age of 65 years have decreased incidence of adverse emergence phenomena. The incidence of recovery phenomena may be
minimized if the patient is permitted to remain un-
disturbed in a quiet, darkened recovery area.[180] Intramuscular administration of ketamine is associated
with a decreased incidence of these reactions.

Ketamine is frequently used in the younger patient
as an induction agent (via IM administration), after
which an IV infusion is started and the patient maintained with IV ketamine as needed. Ketamine is also
used as an anesthetic agent for diagnostic procedures, for minor operations of shorter duration, and
for patients undergoing multiple procedures under
general anesthesia.

Having considerable experience with ketamine anesthesia with both inpatients and outpatients, I believe that ketamine use should be limited to those
doctors who have completed a residency in anesthesiology, have experience with ketamine (because it is
so different from "traditional" general anesthetics),
and have adequate recovery room facilities and monitoring available in the office.

KETAMINE

The medical history of patients receiving keta-
mine should be checked for the following:
Elevated blood pressure
Allergy or hypersensitivity to ketamine

KETAMINE

Proprietary names	Ketaject, Ketalar
Classification	Dissociative anesthetic
Availability	10, 50, 100 mg/ml
Average sedative dose	Not recommended
Maximal single dose	Not recommended
Maximal total dose	Not recommended

Note: *Administration of ketamine for outpatient sedation is not recommended.*

ANTIDOTAL DRUGS

In concluding this section on the pharmacology of IV sedation drugs, several additional agents must be mentioned. These drugs will be used but rarely; however, like an umbrella on a cloudy day, their presence is important. This group may be called antidotal drugs, for their use will be reserved for reversing adverse effects of drugs that have been previously administered. The following categories of drugs are included:

Opioid antagonist
Benzodiazepine antagonist
Agent for reversal of emergence delirium
Vasodilator for extravascular or intraarterial drug administration

Each of these categories should be represented in the emergency kit of doctors administering parenteral sedation by the SC, IM, or IV routes or by IV general anesthesia.

Opioid antagonists

The most significant side effect of opioid analgesics is respiratory depression. This, more than anything else, limits the use of these potentially valuable drugs in dentistry. Less than adequate monitoring of respiratory efforts in the sedated patient has led to significant morbidity and death.[181] Management of respiratory depression is reviewed in Chapter 28 and includes the administration of an opioid antagonist. Intravenous administration of an opioid antagonist rapidly reverses the respiratory-depressant effects of the opioid agonist.

The first opioid antagonist—nalorphine—became available in 1951, followed a year later by levallorphan. Both of these drugs reverse the analgesic effects of opioids as well as their respiratory-depressant properties. Administered to an opioid-dependent individual, these drugs induce acute abstinance syndrome (withdrawal). When administered in the absence of opioid-induced respiratory depression, both nalorphine and levallorphan are capable of producing respiratory depression and of enhancing respiratory depression produced by barbiturates.[182]

In the late 1960s naloxone was introduced and has replaced both levallorphan and nalorphine as the drug of choice in reversing opioid-induced respiratory depression. It is the only opioid antagonist currently available that is free of opioid agonist effects.[183]

Nalbuphine is an opioid agonist/antagonist analgesic that is used in both anesthesia and sedation. Magruder et al.[184] used nalbuphine in place of naloxone for reversal of opioid-induced respiratory depression, noting dramatic improvement within minutes without any reversal of analgesia or euphoria.[184] Further study is necessary before nalbuphine can be recommended as the drug of choice for reversal of opioid-induced respiratory depression.

Naloxone

Naloxone is a synthetic congener of the opioid analgesic oxymorphone from which it differs by the replacement of the methyl group on the N_2 atom by an allyl group.[183] Naloxone hydrochloride is soluble in water and dilute acids and strong alkali. It is only slightly soluble in alcohol and practically insoluble in ether and chloroform.

Naloxone hydrochloride is an essentially pure opioid antagonist. It does not possess any "agonistic" or opioid-type properties. Naloxone does not produce respiratory depression, as did levallorphan and nalorphine, nor does it produce psychotomimetic effects or miosis. When administered in the absence of opioids, naloxone exhibits essentially no pharmacologic activity. Administered to a patient who is physically dependent on opioids, naloxone induces withdrawal symptoms. Naloxone in and of itself does not produce tolerance or lead to physical or psychological dependence.

After IV administration, improvement in respiration may be observed within 2 minutes. The duration of naloxone's effect is relatively short after IV use (about 30 minutes). The duration of respiratory depression produced by the opioid will vary considerably with different opioids. It is therefore possible for naloxone to reverse successfully opioid-induced respiratory depression, only to have respiratory depression recur later after the clinical activity of naloxone has regressed. For this reason, it has become common practice to administer an IM dose of naloxone immediately following the IV dose. The IM dose provides a longer duration of clinical action. After the administration of naloxone the patient should not be discharged from the office for approximately 1 hour so that any recurrence of respiratory depression may be recognized and managed by readministration of naloxone, if necessary.

Naloxone is indicated for use in opioid depression, including respiratory depression, induced by any of the natural or synthetic opioids, propoxyphene, and the opioid agonist/antagonists pentazocine, nalbuphine, and butorphanol.

Contraindications

Naloxone is contraindicated for use in patients who are allergic or hypersensitive to it.

Warnings

Naloxone must be administered with extreme care to persons with known or suspected physical dependence on opioids. The abrupt and complete reversal of opioid agonist effects may precipitate an acute abstinence syndrome. After naloxone reversal of opioid-induced respiratory depression, the patient must be kept under surveillance in the event that repeated doses of naloxone might be needed. Respiratory depression produced by nonopioids (e.g., barbiturates) is not reversible by naloxone or other opioid antagonists.

Precautions

In the event of opioid-induced respiratory depression, naloxone is neither the most important nor the first step in patient management. Of greater importance is patency of the airway and adequate ventilation. All persons administering opioid analgesics parenterally must be capable of maintaining the airway of the unconscious patient and of assisting or controlling the ventilation of the patient.

Adverse reactions

Administered to patients in the absence of opioids, naloxone is essentially free of any side effects. In the presence of opioids, abrupt reversal of opioid depression may produce the following:

Nausea and vomiting
Sweating
Tachycardia
Increased blood pressure
Tremulousness

In the presence of pain, reversal of opioid depression by large doses (greater than 0.4 mg) of naloxone may also significantly reverse analgesia, resulting in extreme discomfort and excitement. It has been reported in cardiac risk patients that rapid reversal of opioid-induced respiratory depression by large doses of naloxone has produced tachycardia and dramatic elevations in blood pressure, resulting in left ventricular failure and pulmonary edema.[185]

Dosage

Naloxone may be administered subcutaneously, intramuscularly, or intravenously. As mentioned, the onset of action after IV administration is within 2 minutes. After IM or subcutaneous administration,

approximately 10 minutes may ⎯
of action. Duration of action ⎯
administration and 1 to 4 hou⎯
cutaneous administration. The⎯
will be greater after IV admini⎯

For the adult naloxone is d⎯
concentration. This is accomp⎯
of the 0.4-mg/ml concentratio⎯
diluent (e.g., 5% dextrose an⎯
minutes 0.1 to 0.2 mg should ⎯
travenously while observing the⎯
reversal of respiratory depress⎯
lation effort and increased ale⎯
cant pain or discomfort.

Additional doses of naloxon⎯
some patients, depending on ⎯
opioid administered and the ⎯
naloxone. If repeated adminis⎯
necessary, it is recommended ⎯
given serious consideration sin⎯
tion of naloxone will be prolo⎯
administration.

In children the initial dose of ⎯
kg of body weight administered⎯
muscularly, or subcutaneously. ⎯
peated every 2 to 3 minutes ⎯
response, or lack of response, ⎯
tion.

If for some reason naloxone ⎯
subcutaneously or intramuscul⎯
0.4 mg and the pediatric dose⎯
onset of action is slower; how⎯
action will be significantly long⎯
ing IV administration.

Availability

Narcan (Endo): adults and ⎯
in 1-ml ampules and 10-ml vials;⎯
ml in 2-ml ampules. Each milli⎯
tains:

Either 0.02 or 0.4 mg/ml nal⎯
8.6 mg sodium chloride

NALOXONE⎯

The medical history of pati⎯
oxone should be checked for t⎯
Allergy or hypersensitivity to⎯
Opioid dependence

Dosage

Initial IV dose of 0.2 mg (2 mL) with subsequent doses administered every minute as needed, to a maximum dosage of 1.0 mg.

Availability

Romazicon (Roche) is supplied in 5 mL multiple-use vials containing a 0.1 mg/mL flumazenil.

FLUMAZENIL

The medical history of patients receiving flumazenil should be checked for the following:
Known allergy or hypersensitivity to flumazenil or benzodiazepines
Patients who have been given benzodiazepines for control of a life-threatening condition, such as status epilepticus or control of intracranial pressure

---

FLUMAZENIL

Proprietary name	Romazicon
Classification	Benzodiazepine antagonist
Availability	0.1 mg/ml
Average therapeutic dose	0.2 mg
Maximal single dose	0.2 mg every 60 seconds
Maximal total dose	1 mg

AGENTS FOR REVERSAL OF EMERGENCE DELIRIUM

Several of the drugs previously discussed in this chapter have the disturbing ability to produce what is known as emergence delirium.[193] During recovery from clinical sedation with a benzodiazepine or scopolamine (the two drugs most likely to produce this action), the patient appears to lose contact with reality. There may be increased muscular activity, and the patient may be speaking, but the sounds are unintelligible. A variety of clinical responses may be noted; however, in all of them it is apparent that the patient is not returning to his "normal" state of consciousness. Until the mid-1970s management of this situation consisted of monitoring of the patient and

symptomatic treatment. Antidotal therapy was not available.

Physostigmine

Physostigmine is a reversible anticholinesterase similar in action to neostigmine, with the important difference that neostigmine, a quaternary compound, cannot cross the blood-brain barrier, whereas physostigmine, a tertiary ammonium compound, readily crosses it.

Actions

Physostigmine is extracted from the seeds of *Physostigma venenosum* (Calabar bean). It is a reversible anticholinesterase that increases the concentration of acetylcholine (ACh) at cholinergic transmission sites. The action of ACh is normally quite transient because of its rapid hydrolysis by the enzyme anticholinesterase. Physostigmine inhibits this action of anticholinesterase and thereby prolongs and intensifies the actions of ACh.[194]

Being a tertiary ammonium compound, physostigmine crosses the blood-brain barrier to reverse the central toxic effects of anticholinergia and emergence delirium—anxiety, delirium, disorientation, hallucinations, hyperactivity, and seizures. Physostigmine is rapidly metabolized (60 to 120 minutes).

Contraindications

Physostigmine should not be administered to patients with asthma, diabetes, cardiovascular disease, or mechanical obstruction of the gastrointestinal or genitourinary tracts.[195]

Warnings

Physostigmine may produce excessive salivation, emesis, urination, and defecation. These are unlikely to develop if the drug is administered slowly intravenously at a rate of 1 mg/minute. More rapid administration can produce the preceding signs and symptoms as well as bradycardia, hypersalivation, leading to respiration difficulties and possibly convulsions.

Precautions

Atropine sulfate should always be available whenever physostigmine is administered because it is an antagonist and antidote for physostigmine.

Dosage

The usual adult dose of physostigmine for reversal of emergence delirium is 0.5 to 2 mg. The drug is administered slowly through the IV infusion at a rate of not more than 1 mg/minute. Maximal dose should not exceed 4 mg.

Availability

Antilirium (O'Neal, Jones & Feldman) 1.0 mg/ml in 2-ml ampules. Each milliliter of solution contains:
1.0 mg physostigmine salicylate
0.1% sodium bisulfite
2.0% benzyl alcohol
Water for injection
Physostigmine is not a scheduled drug.

Summary

Although emergence delirium is an uncommon complication of sedative procedures, it can occur. It is most often seen after the administration of scopolamine to a younger (less than 6-year-old) or older (more than 65-year-old) patient. Management of emergence delirium is based primarily on symptomatic treatment. Physostigmine administration hastens the reversal of signs and symptoms.

Agitation and excessive movement during or after sedation may also be a sign of hypoxia. The patency of the patient's airway and oxygenation of the lungs must always be considered prior to administration of a drug for what is presumed to be emergence delirium.

PHYSOSTIGMINE

Proprietary name	Antilirium
Classification	Reversible anticholinesterase
Availability	1.0 ml/ml
Average therapeutic dose	0.5 to 2.0 mg
Maximal single dose	2 mg
Maximal total dose	4 mg

PHYSOSTIGMINE

The medical history of patients receiving physostigmine should be checked for the following:
Asthma
Diabetes mellitus
Cardiovascular disease
Mechanical obstruction of gastrointestinal or genitourinary tract

---

VASODILATOR FOR EXTRAVASCULAR OR INTRAARTERIAL DRUG ADMINISTRATION
Procaine

Procaine, the last of the antidotal drugs recommended for the emergency kit of the doctor administering parenteral sedation or general anesthesia, is a local anesthetic with considerable vasodilating properties. The following are indications for use of this drug:
Extravascular administration of an irritating chemical
Intraarterial administration of a drug
In both cases the major problem is that of compromised circulation to either a localized area of tissue (extravascular injection) or a limb (intraarterial). Management requires the restoration of blood flow.

A property of all injectable local anesthetics (with the notable exception of cocaine) is vasodilation. Of the available injectable local anesthetics, procaine (Novocain) is the most vasodilating. This property makes procaine less effective as an anesthetic drug (without the addition of a vasopressor), but makes it eminently suitable for the reversal of blood vessel spasm.

Procaine should be used in a 1% concentration without vasopressor. More detailed discussion of management of these problems is found in Chapter 28.

Dosage

For management of extravascular drug administration, 1 to 5 ml of 1% procaine is administered as described in Chapter 28. For intraarterial administration, 1 to 2 ml of 1% procaine will usually be sufficient.

Availability

Novocain (Breon): 1% procaine in 2- ml and 6- ml ampules and 30-ml vials. Each milliliter of solution of 1% procaine contains:

PROCAINE

The medical history of patients receiving procaine should be checked for the following:
Allergy to ester-type local anesthetics
Familial history of atypical plasma cholinesterase

Dosage

Initial IV dose of 0.2 mg (2 mL) with subsequent doses administered every minute as needed, to a maximum dosage of 1.0 mg.

Availability

Romazicon (Roche) is supplied in 5 mL multiple-use vials containing a 0.1 mg/mL flumazenil.

FLUMAZENIL

The medical history of patients receiving flumazenil should be checked for the following:
Known allergy or hypersensitivity to flumazenil or benzodiazepines
Patients who have been given benzodiazepines for control of a life-threatening condition, such as status epilepticus or control of intracranial pressure

---

FLUMAZENIL

Proprietary name	Romazicon
Classification	Benzodiazepine antagonist
Availability	0.1 mg/ml
Average therapeutic dose	0.2 mg
Maximal single dose	0.2 mg every 60 seconds
Maximal total dose	1 mg

AGENTS FOR REVERSAL OF EMERGENCE DELIRIUM

Several of the drugs previously discussed in this chapter have the disturbing ability to produce what is known as emergence delirium.[193] During recovery from clinical sedation with a benzodiazepine or scopolamine (the two drugs most likely to produce this action), the patient appears to lose contact with reality. There may be increased muscular activity, and the patient may be speaking, but the sounds are unintelligible. A variety of clinical responses may be noted; however, in all of them it is apparent that the patient is not returning to his "normal" state of consciousness. Until the mid-1970s management of this situation consisted of monitoring of the patient and

symptomatic treatment. Antidotal therapy was not available.

Physostigmine

Physostigmine is a reversible anticholinesterase similar in action to neostigmine, with the important difference that neostigmine, a quaternary compound, cannot cross the blood-brain barrier, whereas physostigmine, a tertiary ammonium compound, readily crosses it.

Actions

Physostigmine is extracted from the seeds of *Physostigma venenosum* (Calabar bean). It is a reversible anticholinesterase that increases the concentration of acetylcholine (ACh) at cholinergic transmission sites. The action of ACh is normally quite transient because of its rapid hydrolysis by the enzyme anticholinesterase. Physostigmine inhibits this action of anticholinesterase and thereby prolongs and intensifies the actions of ACh.[194]

Being a tertiary ammonium compound, physostigmine crosses the blood-brain barrier to reverse the central toxic effects of anticholinergia and emergence delirium—anxiety, delirium, disorientation, hallucinations, hyperactivity, and seizures. Physostigmine is rapidly metabolized (60 to 120 minutes).

Contraindications

Physostigmine should not be administered to patients with asthma, diabetes, cardiovascular disease, or mechanical obstruction of the gastrointestinal or genitourinary tracts.[195]

Warnings

Physostigmine may produce excessive salivation, emesis, urination, and defecation. These are unlikely to develop if the drug is administered slowly intravenously at a rate of 1 mg/minute. More rapid administration can produce the preceding signs and symptoms as well as bradycardia, hypersalivation, leading to respiration difficulties and possibly convulsions.

Precautions

Atropine sulfate should always be available whenever physostigmine is administered because it is an antagonist and antidote for physostigmine.

Dosage

The usual adult dose of physostigmine for reversal of emergence delirium is 0.5 to 2 mg. The drug is administered slowly through the IV infusion at a rate of not more than 1 mg/minute. Maximal dose should not exceed 4 mg.

Availability

Antilirium (O'Neal, Jones & Feldman) 1.0 mg/ml in 2-ml ampules. Each milliliter of solution contains:
1.0 mg physostigmine salicylate
0.1% sodium bisulfite
2.0% benzyl alcohol
Water for injection
Physostigmine is not a scheduled drug.

Summary

Although emergence delirium is an uncommon complication of sedative procedures, it can occur. It is most often seen after the administration of scopolamine to a younger (less than 6-year-old) or older (more than 65-year-old) patient. Management of emergence delirium is based primarily on symptomatic treatment. Physostigmine administration hastens the reversal of signs and symptoms.

Agitation and excessive movement during or after sedation may also be a sign of hypoxia. The patency of the patient's airway and oxygenation of the lungs must always be considered prior to administration of a drug for what is presumed to be emergence delirium.

PHYSOSTIGMINE

Proprietary name	Antilirium
Classification	Reversible anticholinesterase
Availability	1.0 ml/ml
Average therapeutic dose	0.5 to 2.0 mg
Maximal single dose	2 mg
Maximal total dose	4 mg

PHYSOSTIGMINE

The medical history of patients receiving physostigmine should be checked for the following:
Asthma
Diabetes mellitus
Cardiovascular disease
Mechanical obstruction of gastrointestinal or genitourinary tract

---

VASODILATOR FOR EXTRAVASCULAR OR INTRAARTERIAL DRUG ADMINISTRATION

Procaine

Procaine, the last of the antidotal drugs recommended for the emergency kit of the doctor administering parenteral sedation or general anesthesia, is a local anesthetic with considerable vasodilating properties. The following are indications for use of this drug:
Extravascular administration of an irritating chemical
Intraarterial administration of a drug

In both cases the major problem is that of compromised circulation to either a localized area of tissue (extravascular injection) or a limb (intraarterial). Management requires the restoration of blood flow.

A property of all injectable local anesthetics (with the notable exception of cocaine) is vasodilation. Of the available injectable local anesthetics, procaine (Novocain) is the most vasodilating. This property makes procaine less effective as an anesthetic drug (without the addition of a vasopressor), but makes it eminently suitable for the reversal of blood vessel spasm.

Procaine should be used in a 1% concentration without vasopressor. More detailed discussion of management of these problems is found in Chapter 28.

Dosage

For management of extravascular drug administration, 1 to 5 ml of 1% procaine is administered as described in Chapter 28. For intraarterial administration, 1 to 2 ml of 1% procaine will usually be sufficient.

Availability

Novocain (Breon): 1% procaine in 2-ml and 6-ml ampules and 30-ml vials. Each milliliter of solution of 1% procaine contains:

PROCAINE

The medical history of patients receiving procaine should be checked for the following:
Allergy to ester-type local anesthetics
Familial history of atypical plasma cholinesterase

```
┌─────────────────────────────────────────┐
│              PROCAINE                     │
│                                           │
│  Proprietary name        Novocain         │
│  Classification          Local anesthetic │
│  Availability            1% (10 mg/ml)     │
│  Average therapeutic dose 1-5 ml           │
│  Maximal single dose     1-5 ml            │
│  Maximal total dose      5 ml              │
└─────────────────────────────────────────┘
```

10 mg procaine
Less than 1 mg acetone sodium bisulfite as preservative
Less than 2.5 mg chlorobutanol (in vial form only) as preservative

REFERENCES

1. Giovannitti JA, Trapp LD: Adult sedation: oral, rectal, IM, IV. In Dionne RA, Phero JC, eds: *Management of pain and anxiety in dental practice.* New York, 1991, Elsevier, p. 211.
2. Davidau A: New methods in anaesthesiology and their use in dentistry: treatment of difficult patients and execution of complex procedures, *Rev Assoc Med Israelites* (France) 16:663, 1967.
3. Main DMG: The use of diazepam in dental anaesthesia. In Knight PF, Burgess CG, eds: *Diazepam in anaesthesia.* Bristol, 1968, John Wright, p. 85.
4. Brown PRH, Main DMG, Wood N: Intravenous sedation in dentistry: a study of 55 cases using pentazocine and diazepam, *Br Dent J* 139:59, 1975.
5. O'Neill R, Verrill P: Intravenous diazepam in minor surgery, *Br J Oral Surg* 7:12, 1969.
6. O'Neill R, Verrill PF, Aellig WH et al: Intravenous diazepam in minor oral surgery, *Br Dent J* 128(1):15, 1970.
7. Trieger N: Intravenous sedation in dentistry and oral surgery, *Int Anesthesiol Clin* 27(2):83, 1989.
8. Trieger N: *Pain control.* Chicago, 1974, Quintessence, p. 94.
9. Foreman PA: Diazepam in dentistry: clinical observations based on the treatment of 167 patients in general dental practice, *Anesth Prog* 15:253, 1968.
10. Foreman PA: Intravenous diazepam in general dental practice, *N Z Dent J* 65:243, 1969.
11. Danneberg P, Weber KH: Chemical structure and biological activity of the diazepines, *Br J Clin Pharmacol* 16(suppl 2):231S, 1983.
12. Joseph R: The limbic system: emotion, laterality and unconscious mind, *Psychoanal Rev* 79(3):405, 1991.
13. Medina JH, Novas ML, DeRoberts E: Chronic RO 15-1788 treatment increases the number of benzodiazepine receptors in rat cerebral cortex and hippocampus, *Eur J Pharmacol* 90(1):125, 1983.
14. Haefely W: The biological basis of benzodiazepine actions, *J Psychoactive Drugs* 15(1-2):19, 1983.
15. Jack ML, Colburn WA, Spirt NM et al: A pharmacokinetic/pharmacodynamic/receptor binding model to predict the onset and duration of pharmacological activity of the benzodiazepines, *Prog Neuro-Psychopharmacol Biol Psychiatr* 7(4-6):629, 1983.
16. Ghoneim MM, Mewaldt SP, Hinrichs JV: Behavioral effects of oral versus intravenous administration of diazepam, *Pharmacol Biochem Behav* 21(2):231, 1984.
17. Colburn WA, Gibson M: Composite pharmacokinetic profiling, *J Pharm Sci* 73(11):1667, 1984.
18. Baird ES, Hailey DM: Delayed recovery from a sedative: correlation of the plasma levels of diazepam with clinical effects after oral and intravenous administration, *Br J Anaesth* 144:803, 1972.
19. Vree TB, Hekster CA, vander Kleijn E: Significance of apparent half-lives of a metabolite with a higher elimination rate than its parent drug, *Drug Intell Clin Pharm* 16(2):126, 1982.
20. Salzman C, Shader RI, Greenblatt DJ et al: Long v. short half-life benzodiazepines in the elderly. Kinetics and clinical effects of diazepam and oxazepam, *Arch Gen Psychiatr* 40(3):293, 1983.
21. Greenblatt DJ, Divoll M, Abernethy DR et al: Benzodiazepine kinetics: implications for therapeutics and pharmacogeriatrics, *Drug Metab Rev* 14(2):251, 1983.
22. Pacifici GM, Cuoci L, Placidi GF et al: Elimination of kinetics of desmethydiazepam in two young and two elderly subjects, *Eur J Drug Metab Pharmacokinet* 7(1):69, 1982.
23. Pomara N, Stanley B, Block R et al: Adverse effects of single therapeutic doses of diazepam on performance in normal geriatric subjects: relationship to plasma concentrations, *Psychopharmacology* 84(3):342, 1984.
24. Zbinden G, Randall LO: Pharmacology of benzodiazepines: laboratory and clinical correlations, *Adv Pharmacol* 5:213, 1967.
25. Ausinch B, Malagodi MH, Munson ES: Diazepam in the prophylaxis of lignocaine seizures, *Br J Anaesth* 48:309, 1976.
26. de Jong RH: Clinical physiology of local anesthetic action. In Cousins MJ, Bridenbaugh PO, eds: *Neural blockade,* ed 2. Philadelphia, 1988, Lippincott.
27. Ramsay RE: Treatment of status epilepticus, *Epilepsia* 34(suppl 1):S71, 1993.
28. Darmansjah I, Muchtar A: Dose-response variation among different populations, *Clin Pharmacol Ther* 52(5):449, 1992.
29. Luo A, Huang Y, Liu Y et al: Midazolam as a main anesthesia induction agent—a comparison with thiopental and diazepam, *Chin Med Sci J* 6(3):172, 1991.
30. Jacka MJ, Johnson GD, Milne B: Diazepam's effect on systemic vascular resistance during cardiopulmonary bypass is not caused by its vehicle (alcohol-propylene glycol), *J Cardiothorac Vasc Anesth* 7(I):28, 1993.
31. Taburet AM, Tollier C, Richard C: The effect of respiratory disorders on clinical pharmacokinetic variables, *Clin Pharmacokinet* 19(6):462, 1990.
32. Paakkari P, Paakkari I, Landes P et al: Respiratory μ-opioid and benzodiazepine interactions in the unrestrained rat, *Neuropharmacology* 32(4):323, 1993.
33. Murray-Lyon IM, Young J, Parkes JD et al: Clinical and electroencephalographic assessment of diazepam in liver disease, *Br Med J* 4:265, 1971.
34. DeFeudis FV: GABA-ergic analgesia—a naloxone-insensitive system, *Pharmacol Res Comm* 14(5):383, 1982.
35. Sawynok J: GABAergic mechanisms of analgesia: an update, *Pharmacol Biochem Behav* 26(2):463, 1987.
36. Unrug-Neervoort A, van-Luijtelaar G, Coenen A: Cognition and vigilance: differential effects of diazepam and burspirone on memory and psychomotor performance, *Neuropsychobiology* 26(3):146, 1992.

37. Roche Laboratories: *Valium. Drug package insert,* Nutley, NJ, Roche Laboratories, 1990.

38. Bergman U, Rosa FW, Baum C et al: Effects of exposure to benzodiazepines during fetal life, *Lancet* 340:694, 1992.

39. Doenicke A, Lorenz W, Hoernecke R et al: Histamine release after injection of benzodiazepines and of etomidate. A problem associated with the solvent propylene glycol, *Ann Fr Anesth Reanim* 12(2):166, 1993.

40. Amrein R, Hetzel W: Pharmacology of drugs frequently used in ICU's: midazolam and flumazenil, *Intensive Care Med* 17:S1, 1991.

41. Fraser AD, Bryan W, Isner AF: Urinary screening for midazolam and its major metabolites with the Abbott ADx and TDx analyzers and the EMIT d.a.u. benzodiazepine assay with confirmation by GC/MS, *J Anal Toxicol* 15(1):8, 1991.

42. Jones RD, Chan K, Rouolson CJ et al: Pharmacokinetics of flumazenil and midazolam, *Br J Anaesth* 70(3):286, 1993.

43. Ouellette RG: Midazolam: an induction agent for general anesthesia, *Nurse Anesth* 2(3):134, 1991.

44. Conner JT, Katz RL, Pagano RR et al: RO 21-3981 for intravenous surgical premedication and induction of anesthesia, *Anesth Analg* 57:1, 1978.

45. Hennessy MJ, Kirkby KC, Montgomery IM: Comparison of the amnesic effects of midazolam and diazepam, *Psychopharmacology* 103:(4):545, 1991.

46. Malamed SF, Nikchevich D Jr, Block J: Anterograde amnesia as a possible postoperative complication of midazolam as an agent for intravenous conscious sedation, *Anesth Prog* 35(4):160, 1988.

47. Longmire AW, Seger DL: Topics in clinical pharmacology: flumazenil, a benzodiazepine antagonist, *Am J Med Sci* 306(1):49, 1993.

48. Forster A, Gardaz JP, Suter PM et al: Respiratory depression by midazolam and diazepam, *Anesthesiology* 53:494, 1980.

49. Brown CR, Sarnquist FH, Canup CA et al: Clinical, electro-encephalographic, and pharmacokinetic studies of a water-soluble benzodiazepine, midazolam maleate, *Anesthesiology* 50:467, 1979.

50. Gath I, Weidenfeld J, Collins GI et al: Electrophysiological aspects of benzodiazepine antagonists, Ro 15-1788 and Ro 15-3505, *Br J Clin Pharmacol* 18(4):541, 1984.

51. Roche Laboratories: Important new information on the administration of VERSED (midazolam hydrochloride/Roche) injection for conscious sedation, Letter, November 1987.

52. Jones RD, Lawson AD, Andrew LJ et al: Antagonism of the hypnotic effect of midazolam in children: a randomized, double-blind study of placebo and flumazenil administered after midazolam-induced anaesthesia, *Br J Anaesth* 66(6):660, 1991.

53. Saano V, Hansen PP, Paronen P: Interactions and comparative effects of zopiclone, diazepam and lorazepam on psychomotor performance and on elimination pharmacokinetics in healthy volunteers, *Pharmacol Toxicol* 70(2):135, 1992.

54. Wyeth-Ayerst Laboratories: *Ativan. Drug package insert.* Philadelphia, 1992, Wyeth-Ayerst Laboratories.

55. Eldor J: High dose flunitrazepam anesthesia, *Med Hypotheses* 38(4):352, 1992.

56. Foreman PA: Flunitrazepam in outpatient dentistry, *Anesth Prog* 29:50, 1982.

57. Dixon RA, Bennett NR, Harrison MJ et al: I.V. flunitrazepam in conservative dentistry: a cross-over trial, *Br J Anaesth* 52:517, 1980.

58. Steen SN, Martinez LR: Some pharmacologic effects of intravenous chlordiazepoxide, *Clin Pharmacol Ther* 5:44, 1964.

59. Jorgensen NB: Local anesthesia and intravenous premedication, *Anesth Prog* 13:168, 1966.

60. Berns J: Twilight sedation—a substitute for lengthy office intravenous anesthesia, *J Conn State Dent Assoc* 37:4, 1963.

61. Andrews PR, Mark LC: Structural specificity of barbiturates and related drugs, *Anesthesiology* 57:314, 1982.

62. Harvey SC: Hypnotics and sedatives: the barbiturates. In Goodman LS, Gilman A, eds: *Pharmacological basis of therapeutics,* ed 8. Elundford, NY, 1990, Pergamon.

63. Lebowitz P, Cote W, Daniels AL et al: Comparative cardiovascular effects of midazolam and thiopental in healthy patients, *Anesth Analg* 61:771, 1983.

64. Burch PG, Stansk DR: The role of metabolism and protein binding in thiopental anesthesia, *Anesthesiology* 58:146, 1983.

65. Abbott Laboratories: *Nembutal. Drug package insert.* Chicago, 1992, Abbott Laboratories.

66. Everett GB, Allen GD: Simultaneous evaluation of cardiorespiratory and analgesic effects of intravenous analgesia using pentobarbital, meperidine, and scopolamine with local anesthesia, *JADA* 83:155, 1971.

67. Breimer DD: Pharmacokinetics of methohexitone following intravenous infusion in humans, *Br J Anaesth* 48:643, 1976.

68. Lilly Laboratories: *Brevital. Drug package insert.* Indianapolis, 1989, Eli Lilly Laboratories.

69. Shane SM: Intravenous amnesia for total dentistry in one sitting, *Oral Surg* 24:1,27, 1966.

70. Van Hemelrijck J, Gonzales JM, White PF: Pharmacology of intravenous anesthetic agents. In Rogers MC, Tinker JH, Covino BG et al, eds: *Principles and practice of anesthesiology.* St Louis, 1993, Mosby, p 1143-1144.

71. Roerig Laboratories: *Vistaril. Drug package insert.* New York, 1992, Roerig Laboratories.

72. Briggs LP, White M: The effects of premedication on anaesthesia with propofol (Diprivan), *Postgrad Med J* 61(3):35, 1985.

73. Briggs LP, Clarke RS, Dundee JW et al: Use of diisopropylphenol as main agent for short procedures, *Br J Anaesth* 53:1197, 1981.

74. Vandesteene A, Trempont V, Engelman E et al: Effect of propofol on cerebral blood flow and metabolism in man, *Anaesthesia* 43:37, 1988.

75. Van Hemelrijck J, Fitch W, Mattheussen M et al: Effect of propofol on the cerebral circulation and autoregulation in the baboon, *Anesth Analg* 71:49, 1990.

76. Van Hemelrijck J et al: The effects of propofol on ICP and cerebral perfusion pressure in patients with brain tumors, *Anesthesiol Rev* 15:67, 1988.

77. Hemelrijck JV, Gonzales JM, White PF: Pharmacology of intravenous anesthetic agents. In Rogers MC, Tinker JH, Covino BG et al, eds: *Principles and practice of anesthesiology.* St Louis, 1993, Mosby.

78. Grounds RM, Twigley AJ, Carli F et al: The haemodynamic effects of intravenous induction, comparison of the effects of thiopentone and propofol, *Anaesthesia* 40:735, 1985.

79. Patrick MR, Blair IJ, Feneck PO et al: A comparison of the hemodynamic effects of propofol (Diprivan) and thiopentone in patients with coronary artery disease, *Postgrad Med J* 61:23, 1985.

80. Dundee JW, Robinson FP, McCollum JS et al: Sensitivity to propofol in the elderly, *Anaesthesia* 41:482, 1986.

81. McCollum JSC, Milligan KR, Dundee JW: The antiemetic action of propofol, *Anaesthesia* 43:239, 1988.

82. White PF: Propofol, pharmacokinetics and pharmacodynamics, *Semin Anesth* 7:4, 1988.

83. Rogers KM, Dewar KM, McCubbin TD et al: Preliminary experience with ICI 35868 as an IV induction agent: comparison with althesin, *Br J Anaesth* 52:807, 1980.

84. Rutter DV, Morgan M, Lumley J et al: ICI 35868 (Diprivan): a new intravenous induction agent, *Anaesthesia* 35:1188, 1980.

85. Weightman WM, Zacharias M: Comparison of propofol and thiopentone anaesthesia (with special reference to recovery characteristics), *Anaesth Intensive Care* 15:389, 1987.

86. Kay B, Stephenson DF: Dose-response relationship for disoprofol (IC 135868; Diprivan), *Anaesthesia* 36:863, 1981.

87. MacKenzie N, Grant IS: Comparison of the new emulsion formulation of propofol with methohexitone and thiopentone for induction of anaesthesia in day cases, *Br J Anaesth* 57:725, 1985.

88. MacKenzie N, Grant S: Comparison of propofol with methohexitone in the provision of anesthesia for surgery under regional blockade, *Br J Anaesth* 57:1167, 1985.

89. MacKenzie N, Grant IS: Propofol for intravenous sedation, *Anaesthesia* 42:3, 1987.

90. MacKenzie N, Grant IS: Propofol infusion for sedation in the intensive care unit, *Br Med J* 294: 774, 1987.

91. White PF, Negus JB: Sedative infusions during local or intravenous regional anesthesia—a comparison of propofol and midazolam, *J Clin Anesth* 3:32, 1991.

92. Stuart Pharmaceuticals: *Diprivan, drug package insert*. Wilmington DE, 1992, Stuart Pharmaceuticals.

93. Stanley TH: Opiate anaesthesia, *Anaesth Intensive Care* 15:38, 1987.

94. Yaksh TL, Howe JR: Opiate receptors and their definition by antagonists, *Anesthesiology* 56:246, 1982.

95. Phillips WJ: Central nervous system pain receptors. In Faust RJ, ed. *Anesthesiology review*. New York, 1991, Churchill Livingstone.

96. Shields SE: Pharmacokinetics of epidural narcotics. In Faust RJ, ed. *Anesthesiology review*. New York, 1991, Churchill Livingstone.

97. Pallasch TJ: *Clinical drug therapy in dental practice*. Philadelphia, 1973, Lea & Febiger.

98. Rosow C: Pharmacology of opioid analgetic agents. In Rogers MC, Tinker JH, Covino BG et al, eds: *Principles and practice of anesthesiology*. St Louis, 1993, Mosby, p. 1158.

99. Lambert LA, Nazif MM, Moore PA et al. Nonlinear dose-response characteristics of alphaprodine sedation in preschool children, *Pediatr Dent* 10(1):30, 1988.

100. Lunt RC, Howard HE: A descriptive study of 201 uncombined alphaprodine HCl conscious sedations in pediatric dental patients (1982-1985), *Pediatr Dent* 10(2):121, 1988.

101. Wedell D, Hersh EV: A review of the opioid analgesics fentanyl, alfentanil, and sufentanil, *Compendium* 12(3):184, 1991.

102. Gracely, RH, Dubner R, McGrath PA: Fentanyl reduces the intensity of painful tooth pulp sensations: controlling for detection of active drugs, *Anesth Analg* 61:751, 1982.

103. Shook JE, Watkins WD, Camporesi EM: Differential roles of opioid receptors in respiration, respiratory disease, and opiate-induced respiratory depression, *Am Rev Respir Dis* 142(4): 895, 1990.

104. Rosenberg M: Muscle rigidity with fentanyl: a case report, *Anesth Prog* 24:50, 1977.

105. Mackenzie JE, Frank LW: Influence of pretreatment with a monoamine oxidase inhibitor (phenelzine) on the effects of buprenorphine and pethidine in the conscious rabbit, *Br J Anaesth* 60(2):216, 1988.

106. Elkins-Sinn: *Fentanyl citrate injection. Drug package insert.* Cherry Hill, NJ, 1992, Elkins-Sinn.

107. Janssens F, Torremans J, Janssen PA: Synthetic 1,4-disubstituted-1, 4-dihydro-5H-tetrazol-5-one derivatives of fentanil: alfentanil (R 39209), a potent, extremely short-acting narcotic analgesic, *J Med Chem* 29:2290, 1986.

108. Meistelman C, Saint-Maurice C, Lepaul M et al: A comparison of alfentanil pharmacokinetics in children and adults, *Anesthesiology* 66:13, 1987.

109. Helmers JH, Noordiun H, van-Leeuwen L: Alfentanil used in the aged: a clinical comparison with its use in young patients, *Eur J Anaesthesiol* 2:347, 1985.

110. Shafer A, Sung ML, White PF: Pharmacokinetics and pharmacodynamics of alfentanil infusions during general anesthesia, *Anesth Analg* 65:1021, 1986.

111. Reitz JA: Alfentanil in anesthesia and analgesia, *Drug Intell Clin Pharm* 20:336, 1986.

112. Fone KC, Wilson H: The effects of alfentanil and selected narcotic analgesics on the rate of action potential discharge of medullary respiratory neurones in anesthetized rats, *Br J Pharmacol* 89:67, 1986.

113. Bagshaw ON, Singh P, Aitkenhead AR: Alfentanil in daycase anaesthesia. Assessment of a single dose on the quality of anaesthesia and recovery, *Anaesthesia* 48(6):476, 1993.

114. Phitayakorn P, Melnick BM, Vuicinie AF: Comparison of continuous sufentanil and fentanyl infusions for outpatient anaesthesia, *Can J Anaesth* 34(3)242, part 1, 1987.

115. Davis PJ, Chopyk JB, Nazif M et al: Continuous alfentanil infusion in pediatric patients undergoing general anesthesia for complete oral restoration, *J Clin Anesth* 3(2):125, 1991.

116. Edgin WA, Ford ML, Mansfield MJ: Alfentanil for general anesthesia in oral and maxillofacial surgery, *Oral Maxillofac Surg* 47(10):1039, 1989.

117. Bostek CC, Fiducia DA, Klotz RW et al: Total intravenous anesthesia with a continuous propofol-alfentanil infusion, *CRNA* 3(3):124, 1992.

118. Goldstein G: Pentazocine, *Drug Alcohol Depend* 14(3-4):313, 1985.

119. Burstein AH, Fullerton T: Oculogyric crisis possibly related to pentazocine, *Ann Pharmacother* 27(7-8):874, 1993.

120. Wilkinson DJ: Opioid agonist/antagonists in general anaesthesia, *Br J Hosp Med* 38(2):130, 1987.

121. Pallasch TJ, Gill CJ: Butorphanol and nalbuphine: a pharmacologic comparison, *Oral Surg* 59(1):15, 1985.

122. Zallen RD, Cobetto GA, Bohmfalk C et al: Butorphanol/diazepam compared to meperidine/diazepam for sedation in oral and maxillofacial surgery: a double-blind evaluation, *Oral Surg* 64(4):395, 1987.

123. Woolverton WL, Schuster CR: Behavioral and pharmacological aspects of opioid dependence: mixed agonist/antagonists, *Pharmacol Rev* 35(1):33, 1983.

124. Donadoni R, Rolly G, Devulder J et al: Double-blind comparison between nalbuphine and pentazocine in the control of postoperative pain after orthopedic surgery, *Acta Anaesthesiol Belg* 39(4):251, 1988.

125. Davidson-Lamb R: Nalbuphine hydrochloride (Nubain) versus pentazocine for analgesia during dental operations. A double blind, randomized trial, *SAAD Dig* 6(4):76, 1985.

126. Baum C, Hus JP, Nelson RC: The impact of the addition of naloxone on the use and abuse of pentazocine, *Public Health Reports* 102(4):426, 1987.

127. Kewitz H: Rare but serious risks associated with non-narcotic analgesics: clinical experience, *Med Toxicol* 1 (suppl 1):86, 1986.

128. Schnoll SH, Chasnoff IJ, Glassroth J: Pentazocine and tripelennamine abuse: T's and Blues, *Psychiatr Med* 3(3):219, 1985.

129. Challoner KR, McCarron MM, Newton EJ: Pentazocine (Talwin) intoxication: report of 57 cases, *J Emerg Med* 8(1):67, 1990.

130. Jago RH, Restall J, Stonham J: The effect of naloxone on pentazocine induced hallucinations, *J Royal Army Med Corps* 130(1):64, 1984.

131. Winthrop Laboratories: *Talwin. Drug package insert.* New York, 1992, Winthrop Laboratories.

132. Roytblat L, Bear R, Gesztes T: Seizures after pentazocine overdose, *Isr J Med Sci* 22(5):385, 1986.

133. Facts and Comparisons: *Nalbuphine,* St Louis, 1982, Facts and Comparisons, Inc.

134. Miller RR: Evaluation of nalbuphine hydrochloride, *Am J Hosp Pharm* 37:942, 1980.

135. Lefevre B, Freysz M, Lepine J et al: Comparison of nalbuphine and fentanyl as intravenous analgesics for medically compromised patients undergoing oral surgery, *Anesth Prog* 39(1-2):13, 1993.

136. Hunter PL: Use of nalbuphine for analgesia in combination with methohexital sodium, *Anesth Prog* 36(4-5):150, 1989.

137. Dolan EA, Murray WJ, Ruddy MP: Double-blind comparison of nalbuphine and meperidine in combination with diazepam for intravenous conscious sedation in oral surgery outpatients, *Oral Surg* 66(5):536, 1988.

138. Magruder MR, Delaney RD, DiFazio CA: Reversal of narcotic-induced respiratory depression with nalbuphine hydrochloride, *Anesth Rev* 9(4):34, 1982.

139. Pallasch TJ, Gill CJ: Naloxone-associated morbidity and mortality, *Oral Surg* 52:602, 1981.

140. Schmidt WK, Tam SW, Shotzberger GS et al: Nalbuphine, *Drug Alcohol Depend* 14(3-4):339, 1985.

141. Hameroff SR: Opiate receptor pharmacology: mixed agonist/antagonist narcotics, *Contemp Anesth Pract* 7:27, 1983.

142. Gal TJ, DiFazio CA, Moscicki J: Analgesic and respiratory depressant activity of nalbuphine: a comparison with morphine, *Anesthesiology* 57:367, 1982.

143. Errick JK, Heel RC: Nalbuphine. A preliminary review of its pharmacological properties and therapeutic efficacy, *Drugs* 26(3):191, 1983.

144. Crul JF, Smets MJ, van Egmond J: The efficacy and safety of nalbuphine (NUBAIN) in balanced anesthesia. A double blind comparison with fentanyl in gynecological and urological surgery, *Acta Anaesthesiol Belg* 41(3):261, 1990.

145. Bowdle TA: Clinical pharmacology of antagonists of narcotic-induced respiratory depression. A brief review, *Acute Care* 12(suppl 1):70, 1988.

146. Romagnoli A, Keats AS: Ceiling effect for respiratory depression by nalbuphine, *Clin Pharmacol Ther* 27:478, 1980.

147. Preston KL, Jasinski DR: Abuse liability studies of opioid agonist-antagonists in humans, *Drug Alcohol Depend* 28(1):49, 1991.

148. Vandam LD: Butorphanol, *N Engl J Med* 302:381, 1980.

149. Vagelsang J, Hayes SR: Butorphanol tartrate (Stadol): a review, *J Post Anesth Nurs* 6(2):129, 1991.

150. Nagashima H, Karamanian A, MaLovany R et al: Respiratory and circulatory effects of intravenous butorphanol and morphine, *Clin Pharmacol Ther* 19(6):738, 1976.

151. Roscow CE: Butorphanol in perspective, *Acute Care* 12 (suppl 1):2, 1988.

152. O'Hair KC, Dodd KT, Phillips YY et al: Cardiopulmonary effects of nalbuphine hydrochloride and butorphanol tartrate in sheep, *Lab Animal Sci* 38(1):58, 1988.

153. Facts and Comparisons: *Butorphanol (package insert).* St Louis, 1982, Facts and Comparisons, Inc.

154. From RP: Substance dependence and abuse by anesthesia care providers. In Rogers MC, Tinker JH, Covino CG et al, eds: *Principles and practice of anesthesiology.* St Louis, 1993, Mosby.

155. Finder RL, Bennett CR: Use of scopolamine for dental anesthesia and analgesia techniques, *J Oral Maxillofac Surg* 42(12):802, 1984.

156. Izquierdo I: Mechanism of action of scopolamine as an amnestic, *Trends Pharmacol Sci* 10(5):175, 1988.

157. Fassi A, Rosenberg M: Atropine, scopolamine and glycopyrrolate, *Anesth Prog* 26:155, 1979.

158. Das G: Therapeutic review. Cardiac effects of atropine in man: an update, *Int J Clin Pharmacol Ther Toxicol* 27(10):473, 1989.

159. Noronha-Blob L, Lowe VC, Peterson JS et al: The anticholinergic activity of agents indicated for urinary incontinence is an important property for effective control of bladder dysfunction, *J Pharmacol Exp Ther* 251(2):586, 1989.

160. Kanto J, Klotz U: Pharmacokinetic implications for the clinical use of atropine, scopolamine and glycopyrrolate, *Acta Anaesth Scand* 32(2):69, 1988.

161. Bryant DH: Anti-cholinergic drugs and their use in asthma, *Prog Clin Biol Res* 263:379, 1988.

162. Astra Pharmaceuticals: *Atropine. Drug package insert,* Westboro, Mass, 1987, Astra Pharmaceuticals.

163. Reprecht J: The central muscarinic transmission during anaesthesia and recovery—the central anticholergic syndrome, *Anaesth Reanim* 16(4):250, 1991.

164. Nuotto E: Psychomotor, physiological and cognitive effects of scopolamine and ephedrine in healthy man, *Eur J Clin Pharmacol* 24(5):603, 1983.

165. Schneck HJ, Rupreht J: Central anticholinergic syndrome (CAS) in anesthesia and intensive care, *Acta Anaesthesiol Belg* 40(3):219, 1989.

166. Helfaer MA, Rock P: Formulary: Guide to physiologic assessment and pharmacologic dosing in common anesthetic practice. In Rogers MC, Tinker JH, Covino CG et al, eds: *Principles and practice of anesthesiology.* St Louis, 1993, Mosby, p. 2591.

167. el-Hakim M: Cardiac dysrhythmias during dental surgery, comparison of hyoscine, glycopyrrolate and placebo medication, *Anaesth Reanim* 16(6):393, 1991.

168. AH Robins: *Robinul Injectable. Drug package insert.* Richmond, 1992, AH Robins.

169. Preston GC, Broks P, Traub M et al: Effects of lorazepam on memory, attention and sedation in man, *Psychopharmacology* 95(2):208, 1988.

170. Henschel WF: 30 years of neuroleptanalgesia—the current status, *Anaesth Reanim* 15(5):267, 1990.

171. Greenfield W: Neuroleptanalgesia and dissociative drugs, *Dent Clin North Am* 17:263, 1973.

172. Mehrotra RG, Gupta NR: Neuroleptanalgesia with fentanyl-droperidol: an appreciation based on 100 anesthetics for dental surgery on ambulatory patients, *J Indian Dent Assoc* 54(3):95, 1982.

173. Janssen: *Inapsine injection. Drug package insert.* Piscataway, NJ, 1986, Janssen.

174. Dangers of Innovar, *Med Lett Drugs Ther* 16:42, 1974.

175. Janssen: *Innovar. Drug package insert,* Piscataway, NJ, 1988, Janssen.

176. Reich DL, Silvay G: Ketamine: an update on the first twenty-five years of clinical experience, *Canad J Anaesth* 36(2):186, 1989.

177. Haas DA, Harper DG: Ketamine: a review of its pharmacologic properties and use in ambulatory anesthesia, *Anesth Prog* 39(3):61, 1992.

178. Becsey L, Malamed SF, Radnay P et al: Reduction of the psychotomimetic and circulatory side effects of ketamine by droperidol, *Anesthesiology* 37:536, 1972.

179. Sussman DR: A comparative evaluation of ketamine anesthesia in children and adults, *Anesthesiology* 40:459, 1974.

180. White PF, Way, WL, Trevor AJ: Ketamine—its pharmacology and therapeutic uses, *Anesthesiology* 56:119, 1982.

181. Goodson JM, Moore P: Life-threatening reactions following pedodontic sedation: an assessment of narcotic, local anesthetic and antiemetic drug interaction, *JADA* 107:239, 1983.

182. Lasagna L, Beecher HK: The analgesic effectiveness of nalorphine and nalorphine-morphine combinations in man, *J Pharmacol Exp Ther* 112:356, 1954.

183. Sharts-Engel NC: Naloxone review and pediatric dosage update, *Am J Maternal Child Nurs* 16(3):182, 1991.

184. Magruder MR, Delaney RD, DiFazio CA: Reversal of narcotic-induced respiratory depression with nalbuphine hydrochloride, *Anesth Rev* 9(4):34, 1982.

185. Wride SR, Smith RE, Courtney PG: A fatal case of pulmonary edema in a healthy young male following naloxone administration, *Anaesth Intensive Care* 17(3):374, 1989.

186. DuPont: *Narcan. Drug package insert.* Wilmington DE, 1988, DuPont Multi-Source Products.

187. Rodrigo MR, Rosenquist JB: The effect of Ro 15-1788 (Anexate) on conscious sedation produced with midazolam, *Anaesth Intensive Care* 15:185, 1987.

188. Wolff J, Carl P, Clausen TG et al. Ro 15-1778 for postoperative recovery. A randomized clinical trial in patients undergoing minor surgical procedures under midazolam anaesthesia, *Anaesthesia* 41:1001, 1986.

189. Ricou B, Forster A, Bruckner A et al: Clinical evaluation of a specific benzodiazepine antagonist (Ro 15-1788). Studies in elderly patients after regional anaesthesia under benzodiazepine sedation, *Br J Anaesth* 58:1005, 1986.

190. Sage DJ, Close A, Boas RA: Reversal of midazolam sedation with Anexate, *Br J Anaesth* 59:459, 1987.

191. Kirkegaard L, Knudsen L, Jensen S et al: Benzodiazepine antagonist Ro 15-1788. Antagonism of diazepam sedation in outpatients undergoing gastroscopy, *Anaesthesia* 41:1184, 1986.

192. Roncari G, Ziegler WH, Guentert TW: Pharmacokinetics of the new benzodiazepine antagonist Ro 15-1788 in man following intravenous and oral administration, *Br J Clin Pharm* 22:421, 1986.

193. Olympio MA: Postanesthetic emergence delirium: historical perspective, *J Clin Anesth* 3(1):60, 1991.

194. Lauven PM, Stoeckel H: Flumazenil (Ro 15-1788) and physostigmine, *Resuscitation* 16(suppl):S41, 1988.

195. Forest Pharmaceuticals: *Antilirium. Drug package insert.* St Louis, 1992, Forest Pharmaceuticals.

CHAPTER 27

Techniques of intravenous sedation

In this chapter techniques of IV conscious sedation will be discussed. These techniques employ many of the drugs discussed in Chapter 26 and will be grouped into four different levels. These levels are based upon the degree of complexity, the level of training required by the doctor prior to considering use of the technique, and the requirement for patient monitoring during the procedure. These four categories are (1) basic techniques, (2) modifications of basic techniques, (3) advanced techniques, and (4) other techniques.

INTRAVENOUS SEDATION TECHNIQUES

Basic techniques
1. Benzodiazepine
2. Jorgensen technique
3. Promethazine

Modifications of basic techniques
Benzodiazepine with anticholinergic agent

Advanced techniques
1. Benzodiazepine with opioid plus anticholinergic agents
2. Promethazine with opioid
3. Jorgensen plus benzodiazepine
4. Opioid with group A drug

Others
1. Diazepam with methohexital (Foreman technique)
2. Berns technique
3. Shane technique

On this and the following page the categories and the techniques are discussed.

MONITORING INTRAVENOUS SEDATION

Whenever drugs are administered parenterally it is of paramount importance that the patient be monitored more closely than following oral or inhalation sedation. Guidelines for monitoring during conscious sedation have been developed.[1] The following regimen is suggested by the author for monitoring during intravenous conscious sedation:

1. Baseline vital signs are recorded at preliminary appointment.
   a. Blood pressure
   b. Heart rate and rhythm
   c. Respiratory rate
   d. Height/weight (optional)
   e. Temperature (optional)
2. Vital signs are recorded preoperatively on day of treatment.
3. Immediately following IV drug administration, vital signs are recorded.
4. Every 10 to 15 minutes, vital signs should be recorded.
5. Postoperatively, vital signs are recorded.
6. Following recovery and immediately prior to patient discharge from the office, a final set of vital signs is recorded.

In addition, the protocol for intravenous conscious sedation at the University of Southern California requires the use of two continuous monitors during IV procedures.[2] The following methods are available (see discussion in Chapter 6):
1. Precordial/pretracheal stethoscope
2. Pulse meter

3. Pulse oximeter
4. End-tidal CO_2 monitor
5. Electrocardiograph (ECG)
6. Vital signs monitor

A pretracheal stethoscope should be required in all IV procedures. It is very effective, and inexpensive as well. The pulse oximeter has become an essential monitoring device for IV procedures. Functioning as a continuous monitor of arterial oxygen saturation as well as heart rate, the pulse oximeter is considered the standard of care in parenteral sedation. As an aside, recent graduates from United States dental schools who employ IV sedation would never consider starting an IV case in the absence of an oximeter.[3] End-tidal CO_2 monitors are rapidly gaining entry into the monitoring armamentarium of many doctors using general anesthesia or IV deep sedation, and somewhat more gradually for IV conscious sedation. Use of the pulse meter and ECG is less essential during parenteral sedation procedures than are techniques for monitoring the respiratory system. The ECG, though desirable, may be considered as an optional monitor for IV conscious sedation.

The most important monitor employed during IV conscious sedation is that of the central nervous system through direct verbal contact with and response from the patient. Patients should be able to respond appropriately to verbal or physical stimulation throughout parenteral conscious sedation procedures.

BASIC INTRAVENOUS TECHNIQUES

The first group of sedation techniques include those that form the backbone of IV conscious sedation. With these techniques availabile the trained doctor will be able to meet the needs of a dental or surgical procedure of any duration and achieve satisfactory sedation in virtually all patients requiring the IV route.

The *Jorgensen technique* is arguably the original IV conscious sedation technique.[4] Despite attempts at improving it, the original Jorgensen technique is still taught today, providing excellent sedation with few reports of any significant complications. The primary indication for the Jorgensen technique is procedures requiring 2 or more hours to complete.

Intravenous conscious sedation using a *benzodiazepine* has become the most popular technique in dentistry.[5] Intravenous benzodiazepine sedation meets the needs of contemporary dental practice, that is, sedation of approximately 1-hour duration. In the few short years since its introduction (1986) midazolam has challenged diazepam for supremacy in the area of 1-hour IV conscious sedation.

With the availability of these two techniques virtually all patients requiring IV sedation will be treated successfully. However, with the major effect of diazepam or midazolam being under 1 hour, and the Jorgensen technique effective for more than 2 hours, a procedure providing effective sedation of from 1 to 2 hours may be needed. This need is effectively met by *promethazine*.

These three basic techniques are described next. The benzodiazepine and Jorgensen techniques will be described in detail. These provide the basic format for the techniques to follow, which will be described in somewhat less detail.

Intravenous benzodiazepine (diazepam or midazolam)
Preliminary appointment

When considering either diazepam or midazolam for use intravenously, specific questions must be asked of the patient concerning any prior experience with the drugs to be used, their response to it, any adverse responses, and any specific contraindications to their use. For diazepam and midazolam these include the following:

> ### CLASSIFICATION OF INTRAVENOUS MEDICATIONS
>
> #### Group A (antianxiety or sedative-hypnotic agents)
> 1. Diazepam
> 2. Midazolam
> 3. Pentobarbital
> 4. Promethazine
>
> #### Group B (opioid-type analgesics)
> 1. Meperidine
> 2. Morphine
> 3. Fentanyl
>   a. Alfenanil
>   b. Sufentanil
> 4. Pentazocine
> 5. Nalbuphine
> 6. Butorphanol
>
> #### Group C (anticholinergics)
> 1. Atropine
> 2. Scopolamine
> 3. Glycopyrrolate

1. Allergy or hypersensitivity to benzodiazepines
2. Glaucoma (untreated)
3. History of phlebitis, thrombophlebitis (contraindication to diazepam)
4. Acute pulmonary insufficiency (contraindication to midazolam)
5. Preexisting respiratory depression

Patients classified as ASA I and II are candidates for IV sedation. Only selected ASA III patients should be considered and then only on a case-by-case basis.

Prior to the day of treatment, the following items concerning the patient's suitability for IV sedation are evaluated by the doctor and staff.

1. Degree of apprehension. Which technique of sedation (oral, IM, inhalation, IV) is most appropriate for this patient? If the IV route is selected, which of the techniques is most appropriate for this patient?

2. Informed consent. If the IV route is selected, informed consent must be provided to the patient, describing the intravenous procedure, its alternatives (e.g., IM, general anesthesia), and the more likely complications associated with its use. The patient is asked to sign the form, which is then added to the patient's dental record.

3. Medical history. The medical history questionnaire, dialogue history, and vital signs are reviewed to determine the presence of contraindications, either relative or absolute, to the use of the drug(s) being considered.

4. Nature and length of dental procedure being contemplated. The degree of trauma associated with the planned procedure must be considered when evaluating a potential sedative technique. In addition, the length of the procedure is also a consideration. Selection of appropriate IV drugs can tailor the length of sedation to almost any duration.

5. Presence of superficial veins. The presence of suitable superficial veins is a primary requisite for elective IV sedative procedures. Lack of suitably visible veins is an acceptable reason for avoiding the IV route and selecting an alternative route of drug administration.

6. Record vital signs. *Baseline vital signs* are obtained at this visit if they have not yet been recorded.

7. Preoperative instructions. Following is an example of preoperative instructions for IV sedation.

1. Arrangements must be made for a responsible adult to drive the patient home after the IV sedation appointment. The patient will be unable to leave the office alone.

COMMENT: When the patient arrives for treatment, the name, address, and telephone number of their escort should immediately be obtained. If treatment is planned to last up to 1 hour, the escort is requested to accompany the patient to the office and remain during the procedure. For procedures lasting more than 2 hours, the escort is still requested to accompany the patient to the office. However, the doctor may elect to permit the escort to leave the office for the duration of the procedure and to return before the procedure is scheduled to end. In either case it is extremely important to have seen or at least spoken to the patient's escort prior to the start of the procedure. It is my policy to cancel the planned procedure whenever a suitable escort is not available at the start of treatment.

When oral sedation is prescribed preoperatively an escort *must* accompany the patient to the office.

2. The patient should have had nothing to eat for approximately 4 hours prior to the procedure.

COMMENT: The attempt here is to provide an empty stomach and gastric fluids with a higher pH in the unlikely event that the patient should become nauseous or vomit during or following the IV procedure. There is less likelihood of aspiration if food is not present in the stomach. Patients may be permitted to ingest clear liquids such as water or apple juice along with any medications they may be required to take (e.g., antihypertensives). If the scheduled appointment is before noon, the patient is told not to eat anything that morning. For afternoon IV sedations, the patient is advised to avoid anything by mouth after 8 A.M. A light, carbohydrate-rich breakfast consisting of dry cereal and juice may be taken prior to 8 A.M. that morning.

3. The patient is advised to wear loose-fitting garments.

COMMENT: This will prevent any possibly excessive respiratory depression caused by mechanical means. The upper garment worn by the patient should be of short-sleeved length or have no sleeves so that access may readily be gained to both arms.

Many doctors employing IV sedation or general anesthesia have the patient change into a surgical shirt (''OR greens''). Loose-fitting and sleeveless, this permits the anesthesia team immediate and unimpeded access to the patient's chest and upper body throughout the procedure.

4. The patient should plan to arrive at the office approximately 15 minutes prior to the scheduled appointment.

5. Should the patient develop a cold, flu, sore throat, or any other illness, the appointment will be cancelled and rescheduled at a time when the patient is more physically fit. The patient should call if any of these symptoms develop.

Recent research has demonstrated that morbidity and mortality following anesthesia in patients with upper respiratory infections (URI) are actually greater in the period of time following the patient's apparent "recovery" from the URI.[6] Most of this morbidity is related to respiratory disease.

6. The medication(s) to be taken prior to arrival in the office for treatment are prescribed and the name of drug, dosage, and instructions are given.

7. The time, date, and place of appointment are given to the patient.

Day of treatment

The day of the scheduled IV sedation and dental treatment arrives, and the patient is in the waiting room. Knowing that the patient is fearful of the upcoming procedures, the doctor will not wish to prolong his wait any longer than necessary, since the patient's anxiety and fears will increase during this time.

An exception to this will be the patient's receiving oral sedation in addition to IV sedation. If the drug is not taken at home the patient should be scheduled to arrive in the office approximately 45 minutes prior to the scheduled start of the IV sedation, the oral drug administered, and the patient asked to remain in the waiting room.

During this time the assistant prepares the IV infusion and drugs for use (Chapter 25). Once all is ready the assistant asks the patient to go to the restroom and void, if necessary, following which the patient is taken to the treatment chair and seated in a semiupright (comfortable) position. The availability of the patient's escort should be determined at this time. *Preoperative* vital signs are monitored and recorded on the anesthesia record sheet for the patient (Fig. 27-1).

Once these procedures are completed, the monitors are placed. The blood pressure cuff is placed on the arm opposite the working side of the doctor and left in place throughout the procedure. The pretracheal stethoscope, ECG electrodes (if used), and pulse oximeter and/or end-tidal CO_2 monitor or pulse monitor are also placed at this time. A nasal cannula or nasal hood is positioned, and a 3- to 6-L/min flow of oxygen is administered throughout the IV procedure. This is standard IV protocol at USC.

Because of an increased incidence of phlebitis when diazepam is administered, it is suggested that when possible, smaller veins such as those on the dorsum of the hand or wrist be avoided when venipuncture is performed.[8] This is not the case with water-soluble midazolam. Venipuncture is completed and the IV infusion established and secured (Chapter 25).

Diazepam

Diazepam may now be administered to the patient. The diazepam has previously been readied for use by the dental assistant. This is now reviewed.

Diazepam is available in a 10-ml vial at a concentration of 5 mg/ml. The assistant takes a sterile, disposable 3- or 5-ml syringe and after wiping the rubber diaphragm of the vial with isopropyl alcohol (and waiting 1 minute for the alcohol to dry) injects 3 ml of air into the vial of diazepam and withdraws an equal volume of the yellowish diazepam solution. The syringe is recapped, labeled "Diazepam 5 mg/ml," and put aside for later use. Syringes containing drugs must always be labeled, even in situations in which only one drug is being used.

Drug administration. The patient is placed into a supine position prior to drug administration. It is good practice to open up the IV infusion so that the rate of flow is rapid during the administration of any drug. This further dilutes the drug, minimizing any local irritation that might develop as the drug comes into contact with the vein wall.

Immediately prior to beginning drug administration the assistant or doctor should make one final check to confirm that the IV infusion is still patent. Squeezing the flash bulb of the tubing (Fig. 27-2) or holding the bag of IV solution below the patient's heart level should disclose blood in the tubing, a sign of a patent IV line (Fig. 27-3).

Diazepam, an oily viscous liquid, has the propensity to cause some patients to complain of a burning sensation when the drug is administered, the sensation lasting until the diazepam is flushed from the injection site. A rapidly running IV drip will minimize this effect. In addition, it is advisable to tell the patient that they may experience a brief period of *warmth* when the drug is injected, and that this is normal and will quickly subside.

A test dose of 0.2 ml (each small delineation on the syringe is 0.2 ml) is administered to determine if any unusual response (hypersensitivity, allergy) is to develop (Fig. 27-4).

After waiting about 15 seconds, the titration of diazepam starts. The recommended injection rate of diazepam is 1 ml per minute; this is equivalent to 5 mg of diazepam per minute.

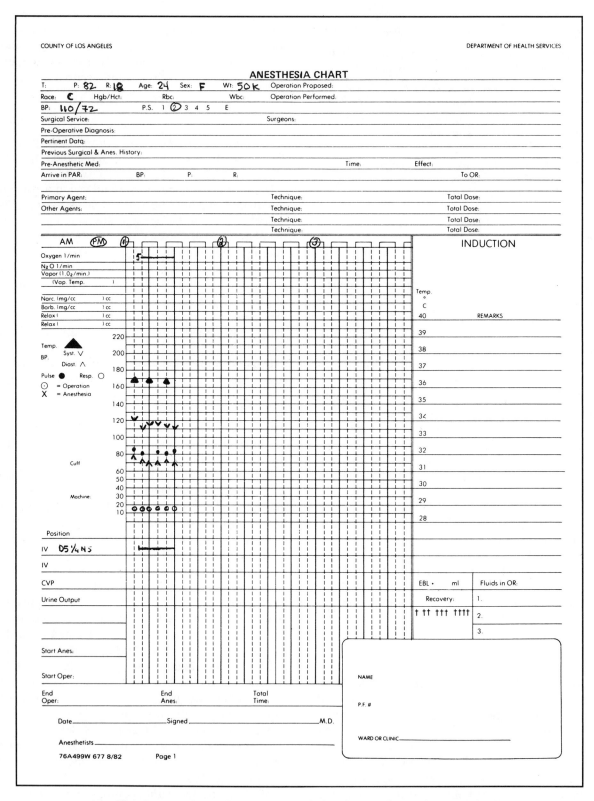

Fig. 27-1. Preoperative vital signs are recorded and entered onto the patient's chart.

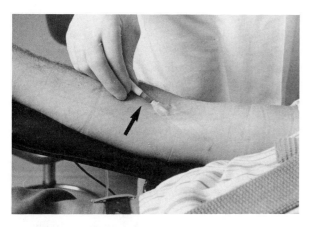

Fig. 27-2. Squeezing and releasing flashbulb should elicit return of blood *(arrow)* as final check of patency of vein.

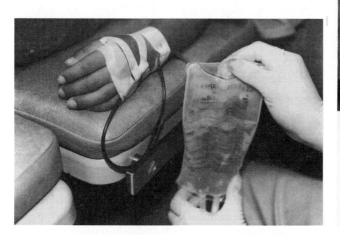

Fig. 27-3. Holding bag of IV solution below level of vein should produce a return of blood into the tubing, a sign of a patent IV.

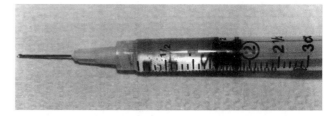

Fig. 27-4. A test dose of 0.2 ml (each small delineation on the syringe is 0.1 ml) is administered to determine if any unusual response (hypersensitivity, allergy) develops.

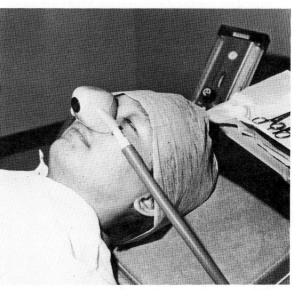

Fig. 27-5. Halfway ptosis of the upper eyelid is often seen when diazepam is employed as an IV sedative. (The patient is receiving 100% O$_2$ via nasal hood.)

Start by administering 0.5 ml slowly and continuously over 30 seconds. Because of the great individual variation in drug response, the doctor must always titrate carefully to each patient's precise level of sedation. Continue to titrate diazepam at a rate of 1 ml per minute until this ideal level of sedation is achieved.

When first learning to use IV sedation, the natural tendency of the doctor will be to cease administration of the diazepam at the very first sign of a change in the patient's level of consciousness. For this reason, based on the uncertainty of the doctor, many patients may, in fact, be inadequately sedated. As clinical experience is gained, the doctor will develop a "feel" for the proper level of sedation.

There are clinical signs and symptoms associated with the desired level of sedation:

The patient will appear to become more relaxed in the dental chair in contrast to his earlier, more tense demeanor. The patient may stretch out, uncross his legs, and relax his grip on the arm of the chair.

The patient's response to questions will be somewhat slower than it was prior to the sedation, and the patient may appear to have some difficulty in putting thoughts together into words.

The patient's eyelids may appear to be drooping. This is *not* to be considered the primary criterion for proper sedation. Halfway ptosis of the upper eyelid, the Verrill sign (Fig. 27-5), usually occurs when the patient is somewhat too heavily sedated.[8,9]

When diazepam is administered at the recommended rate, the typical patient, requiring approximately 10 to 12 mg of diazepam, will be sedated within 2 to 3 minutes of the start of drug administration.

Once the desired level of sedation is reached, the rate of the IV infusion must be slowed. Whenever a drug is not being administered, the infusion rate is adjusted to approximately 1 drop every 5 to 10 seconds. The purpose is to prevent the needle from becoming clotted with blood during the procedure. This slow drip rate is commonly abbreviated as *t.k.o.* (to keep open).

Immediately following completion of the diazepam administration vital signs and the drug dose are recorded on the anesthesia record. Vital signs should be recorded immediately following any subsequent IV drug administration and at 10- to 15-minute intervals throughout the procedure. All drugs administered during the IV sedation procedure, including local anesthetics, must be recorded on the anesthesia record.

Dosage. The average dose of diazepam required to provide clinically adequate IV conscious sedation is between 10 and 12 mg (average of over 2800 cases). The range of these doses is of far greater importance, for it illustrates the tremendous individual variability in response to diazepam (and all drugs). In my experience with diazepam as a sole agent for sedation, clinically adequate sedation has been achieved with as little as 2.5 mg in some patients, whereas others have received in excess of 30 mg and have not even approached the desired level of sedation.

The following is strongly recommended as a means of determining the maximum dose of diazepam for a given patient.

Diazepam is titrated at a rate of 5 mg (1 ml) per minute until ideal sedation is achieved. The average dose of diazepam required to produce this clinical effect is 10 and 12 mg. Once this effect is achieved titration ceases, the IV infusion is slowed to t.k.o., and the operative phase of treatment is started (see later discussion).

However, if a diazepam dose of 20 mg has been administered and the patient does demonstrate some clinical sedation, though not quite at the desired level, additional diazepam may be titrated up to a total of 25 mg. On the other hand, when the patient has received 20 mg of diazepam but exhibits virtually no signs or symptoms of sedation, it is prudent to cease the administration of diazepam. Experience with diazepam has demonstrated that when adequate sedation does not occur by a 20-mg dose, the addition of another 10 or 20 mg probably will not prove beneficial to the patient but may in fact increase the risk of occurrence of several dose-related complications. My recommendation to the neophyte at IV conscious sedation is that when a dose of 20 mg diazepam fails to produce any signs or symptoms of clinical sedation, the administration of diazepam be terminated and the planned dental/surgical procedure attempted without the administration of any additional intravenous drugs.

The doctor experienced in IV sedation and general anesthesia has several options available at this time, but in the hands of the doctor without anesthesiology training the most prudent course of action at this time is to cease IV drug administration and begin the planned procedure. I am continually surprised by the number of patients who, without any signs or symptoms of sedation, do extremely well and who have a significant degree of amnesia at the end of the procedure. Should this attempt to treat fail, the patient should be dismissed (following recovery) and rescheduled for a different IV sedation technique at a later date.

Diazepam

Average sedative dose	10 to 12 mg
Sedative dose range	2.5 to > 30 mg
Maximum dose—no sedation	20 mg
Maximum dose—some sedation	25 mg

Intraoperative period. Local anesthesia is administered to the patient exactly as it would be if the patient were not sedated. This includes the use of topical anesthetic and all of the other steps involved in the atraumatic administration of local anesthetics.[10] The patient may react to any pain associated with the local anesthetic injection, but this usually is nothing more than a slight moan, grimace, or minor movement. Adequate time for the local anesthetic to take effect (3 to 5 minutes) should be allowed before beginning the planned procedure.

During the first 3 to 5 minutes following IV diazepam administration the depth of sedation is greatest. Although overresponse is not common, the patient who has overresponded to diazepam will be somewhat sluggish in response to verbal commands such as "open your mouth." For this reason, the use of a mouth prop should be considered, at least at the beginning of the IV diazepam procedure. Within 5 to 10 minutes the depth of sedation has usually lessened so that the patient's mouth can be voluntarily kept open. A rubber bite block with a piece of string (dental floss) tied around it or a ratchet-type (Molt) mouth prop may be used at this time (Fig. 27-6).

Lack of response to verbal command and more

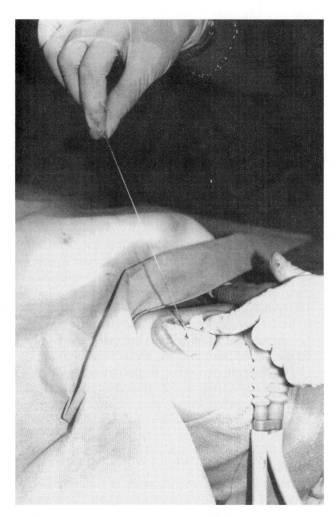

Fig. 27-6. Rubber bite block with string (dental floss) tied to it placed into mouth of sedated patient.

significantly a lack of response to a painful stimulus (i.e., local anesthetic injection) may indicate that the patient is overly sedated. Lack of response is always an indication for the doctor to stop treatment and reevaluate the patient's level of consciousness and airway and ventilatory status.

Following local anesthetic administration, a rubber dam should be applied, if feasible, for the planned procedure. The rubber dam serves two important functions during IV sedation:

It aids in maintaining the mouth in an open position (it may be used in place of the mouth prop).

It prevents extraneous material from falling into the posterior part of the mouth, throat, and pharynx.

Dental treatment begins at this time. Because of the 45-minute duration of sedation provided by IV diazepam, treatment should be planned to fit into this time period.[11] Also, diazepam produces a period of anterograde amnesia in approximately 75% of patients, the amnesic period lasting approximately 10 minutes.[12] It is recommended that potentially painful or traumatic procedures be completed at the start of the treatment in order to take advantage of this amnesic period.

In this manner, as the sedative effect begins to wane (about 30 minutes following drug administration), relatively innocuous procedures will be performed, such as packing alloys, suturing, or adjusting occlusion. In addition, having received local anesthesia earlier, the patient will be pain-free at this time and able to tolerate these procedures without complaint. In most patients actual treatment time, with one initial titrating dose of diazepam, can usually be extended well beyond 1 hour because of the lack of pain and the relative innocuousness of the procedures being carried out at this time.

It is rare for a patient to require a second dose of diazepam if the duration of the planned procedure was appropriate (about 1 hour). As discussed in Chapter 26, diazepam sedation may be divided into three phases—stage one: decreased awareness, good sedation, amnesia; stage two: more aware, good sedation, no amnesia; stage three: alert, aware. With entry into the third phase the patient may opine that he or she feels "normal" once again, and the doctor might be tempted to readminister additional diazepam. However, at this time treatment should be nearing completion, the procedure being performed is usually atraumatic, the patient has effective local anesthesia, and though the patient feels normal, he or she is still anxiety-free if not visibly sedated. Thus it is clear that readministration of diazepam is rarely necessary in the typical 1-hour IV conscious sedation procedure.

Occasionally the readministration of diazepam might become necessary to permit successful completion of the procedure. For example, a patient is scheduled for restorative procedures with IV diazepam. All goes well, but one of the teeth requires endodontic treatment. The patient begins to become increasingly aware of the surroundings approximately 40 minutes into the procedure and has become somewhat apprehensive again. The treating doctor has two options: first, to temporarily fill the canal, dismiss the patient, and reschedule for another IV visit; or second, to retitrate additional diazepam and continue with endodontic care at the same visit.

Should the decision be made to retitrate and continue treatment, the assistant increases the rate of the IV drip and additional diazepam is titrated slowly until the patient becomes sedated once again or until a total dose of 30 mg diazepam is administered. Following retitration, the IV drip rate is again slowed to t.k.o. and treatment continued.

Retitration with diazepam almost always requires a smaller dose than that required initially. For example, if 12 mg were required at first, a dose of 3 or 8 mg might produce the same clinical level of sedation on retitration. For reasons that will be explained in Chapter 28, the total, combined dose of diazepam administered at one appointment should, if possible, be kept under 30 mg.

When diazepam is readministered, the vital signs are recorded on the anesthesia record sheet.

Posttreatment period. Following completion of the planned treatment, the IV infusion may be discontinued if, in the opinion of the doctor, there will be no further need for it. The patient should be responding normally at this time, with no adverse or bizarre signs or symptoms noted (e.g., emergence delirium). The technique for termination of the IV infusion was discussed in Chapter 25. The nasal O_2 can also be terminated at this time.

Recovery criteria. The patient is never discharged alone from the office following IV sedation, regardless of the patient's apparent state of recovery or the degree to which the patient protests. Criteria for discharge from the office will include the vital signs and the reaction of the patient.

Vital signs should be approximately at baseline level (taken at the preliminary visit). If blood pressure appears significantly depressed (more than 30 mm Hg below baseline) and clinical signs and symptoms of sedation are present, the patient should be permitted to recover for a few more minutes while receiving O_2.

The most important criterion for discharge is the patient's response. Under no circumstances should a patient ever be permitted to leave the office feeling poorly or unable to walk without assistance. In some few cases the patient may feel dizzy, mildly nauseous, or weak. This patient should be permitted to rest until he or she feels better (thus the importance of a recovery area in the office supervised by a trained assistant). A sedated patient should never be left unattended in any room for any length of time; the doctor or a trained member of the staff should be physically present at all times.

When it is felt that the patient has recovered sufficiently to be discharged, all monitoring devices are removed and the patient is permitted to stand. A member of the dental team, the doctor or assistant, should position himself or herself in front of the patient so that if the patient's legs are a little weak, that person can support the patient, thus preventing injury and possible litigation.

The position of the chair is adjusted from the semiisupine to a 90-degree position. This should be done slowly, preferably in several steps, allowing the patient's cardiovascular system to readapt to the effect of gravity, thereby preventing postural hypotension, possible dizziness, and syncope.

The patient then sits with his or her legs touching the floor and then stands. If the patient is able to accomplish this without difficulty (following diazepam or midazolam IV conscious sedation there is rarely difficulty in standing after 45 minutes), the patient is requested to take a few steps toward the doctor or assistant. If all is well, the patient is reseated in the dental chair and the escort is called in.

The foremost criterion in permitting patients to be discharged from the office is their ability to take care of themselves should they for any reason be left alone during the remainder of the day. They should be able to walk without assistance. If such is not the case, the patient is allowed additional time to recover.

When diazepam or midazolam is employed for IV sedation, clinical recovery usually appears to be quite complete at 45 to 60 minutes. However, with other drugs (e.g., pentobarbital, promethazine) recovery may not appear nearly as complete.

Once recovery is deemed adequate for discharge, the patient is returned to the dental chair and the escort is called in. In the presence of both persons posttreatment instructions are given verbally and in writing. It is potentially possible, though highly unlikely with diazepam, that the patient may still be amnesic at this time in the procedure; thus the necessity of the companion and written instructions. Instructions given the patient should be recorded on the anesthesia record and/or included in the patient's dental chart.

Usual postsedation instructions are presented in the box. Additional instructions should be included if mandated by the dental treatment. This might include restrictions on diet or the need for ice or heat applications. Once again, these are presented verbally to both the patient and his escort, given to the patient in writing, and recorded on the patient's chart.

POSTSEDATION INSTRUCTIONS

1. Go home and rest for the remainder of the day.
2. Do *not* perform any strenuous activity. You should remain in the company of a responsible adult until you are fully alert.
3. Do *not* attempt to eat a heavy meal immediately. If you are hungry, a light diet (liquids and toast) will be more than adequate.
4. A feeling of nausea may occasionally develop after sedation. The following may help you to feel better:
   a. Lying down for a while
   b. A glass of a cola beverage
5. Do not drive a motor vehicle or perform any hazardous tasks for the remainder of the day.
6. Do not take any alcoholic beverages or any medications for the remainder of the day unless you have contacted me first.
7. The following medication(s) have been ordered for you by the doctor. Take them only as directed below:
8. If you have any unusual problems you may call (office telephone number).

The companion accompanies the patient from the office. A member of the office staff should remain with the patient until the patient is safely in the car with the seat belt secured.

The anesthesia record sheet and the patient's treatment chart are completed, disposable IV equipment (needle, tubing, syringes, and infusion solution) is discarded, and any unused drug is discarded. A note in the chart and anesthesia record sheet is made: "x mg diazepam discarded." Recording of the disposition of all drugs, especially the Schedule II barbiturates and opioid agonists, is a very important part of the IV procedure.

Figure 27-7 illustrates a typical anesthesia record at the conclusion of the IV sedation procedure. The following entry is made in the patient's dental chart when the anesthesia record sheet is included in the chart:

Date. Patient received intravenous conscious sedation. Anesthesia record enclosed. Dental treatment—extraction #27, 30, 31; MOD #15, etc., signature or initals of doctor.

In a situation in which an anesthesia record is not available (every effort should be made to avoid this contingency!) the following chart entry is suggested:

IV started with a 21-gauge indwelling catheter in the left ventral forearm. The patient received 13 mg diazepam in one dose. Duration of IV procedure = 45 minutes, the patient receiving 5 L/min 100% O_2 via nasal hood throughout the procedure. A total of 180 ml of 5% dextrose and water was administered. Monitoring included continuous pulse oximetry and BP q15m. The patient tolerated the procedure well and was discharged from the office in the custody of Mr. John Smith at 12:05 P.M. Postoperative instructions were given verbally and in writing to both the patient and companion.

	Blood pressure	*Heart rate*	*O_2 Sat*
Baseline:	124/68	66	97
Preoperative:	132/74	78	97
Postsedation:	128/70	74	98
Postoperative:	124/72	74	98

Doctor's signature

Though this may appear to be voluminous and perhaps excessive, especially considering the nature of the usual entry in dental records, this type of record keeping is absolutely essential whenever sedative procedures are employed. There should be no doubt at a later date as to exactly what transpired during the sedative procedure.

One more important task remains on the day of the IV sedation: each and every patient who receives IV (or IM) sedation should be contacted by telephone, by the doctor, before he or she leaves the office in the late afternoon if the IV was in the morning, or early that evening if the IV was during the afternoon. This is one of the most important actions a professional can perform for his or her patient. It demonstrates to the patient the doctor's sincerity and concern and is a means of circumventing potential problems (such as developing pain or bleeding) before they become more significant. This conversation is recorded in the patient's chart.

Midazolam

The technique of IV conscious sedation with midazolam is similar to that described for diazepam, with the following exceptions. Midazolam should be administered intravenously in a concentration not to exceed 1 mg/ml. A letter from the drug's manufacturer, Roche Laboratories, recommends use of the 1 mg/ml concentration.[13] When using the 5 mg/ml formulation of midazolam, 1 ml of the drug is placed in a 5-ml syringe and 4 ml of D5 & W or 0.9% sodium chloride is added. This provides a final concentration of 1 mg/ml midazolam.

Because midazolam is water-soluble and phlebitis is rarely noted, the intravenous infusion may be started at any available site, including the dorsum of

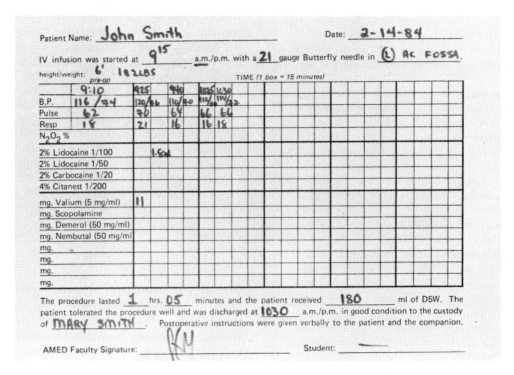

Fig. 27-7. Completed sedation record for an IV diazepam procedure.

the hand and wrist. After increasing the rate of the IV drip, midazolam is administered slowly. The manufacturer recommends a rate of 1 ml every 2 minutes, followed by an additional 2 minutes or more to fully evaluate the sedative effect. The range of midazolam required for "ideal" sedation varies from 1 to 10 mg or more. It is suggested that titration be terminated if sedation is not evident at a dose of 6 to 8 mg. Clinical experience suggests that midazolam is anywhere from two to four times as potent as diazepam.[14] If additional doses of midazolam are required, it is suggested that the total midazolam dose not exceed 10 mg for the entire appointment, if at all possible.

Patients who are receiving benzodiazepines orally for prolonged periods may exhibit a tolerance to the intravenous administration of diazepam or midazolam. Robb et al.[15] reported three cases of patients who required doses of 47 and 50 mg midazolam; 26 mg midazolam; and 30 and 34 mg midazolam for intravenous sedation. Discontinuance of the oral benzodiazepine produces a return to more normal drug response.

The duration of midazolam-induced sedation is slightly shorter than that of diazepam. Clinical experience has demonstrated that recovery, although quite excellent, is not as complete as with diazepam. Patients may exhibit a degree of residual sedation up to 60 minutes following drug administration, though

this is rare. It also appears, subjectively, that the depth of sedation provided by midazolam is not as intense as that noted with diazepam; however, the degree and length of midazolam-induced anterograde amnesia is far greater than that seen with diazepam.

The decision as to which benzodiazepine to employ must take into account several factors, including the following:
1. Possibility of phlebitis (venous inflammation)
2. Requirement for sedation
3. Requirement for amnesia

Posttreatment instructions—verbal and written—must always be given to both the patient and his adult escort. This is especially important with midazolam because of the more likely presence of amnesia persisting into the recovery period. The administration of flumazenil, a benzodiazepine antagonist, may be indicated at this time if continued amnesia is not desirable. Early studies indicated that flumazenil decreased the length of midazolam-induced amnesia.[16] Whether flumazenil should be routinely administered at the termination of midazolam sedation remains to be determined.

The administration of a single titrating dose of either midazolam or diazepam for sedation will provide the doctor with approximately 45 to 60 minutes of sedation. When combined with adequate local anesthesia treatment time easily exceeds 1 hour. There are occasions, however, when treatment requires in excess of 2 hours to complete. For these procedures, use of the Jorgensen technique is indicated.

The Jorgensen technique

The Jorgensen technique is a combination of three drugs administered intravenously that provides for more than 2 hours of conscious sedation. Niels Bjorn Jorgensen first employed this technique, which he called "intravenous premedication," in 1945 at the Loma Linda University School of Medicine.[17] Jorgensen introduced the technique because of his dissatisfaction with the oral and intramuscular routes of sedation. Intravenous drug administration permitted a more precise and reliable level of sedation than was possible by any of the other techniques then available.

This technique has been employed successfully at the Loma Linda University School of Dentistry in excess of 13,000 times since 1965. Originally designed for use during oral surgical procedures, its appropriateness in all branches of dentistry has been reaffirmed many times. The technique became known as the "Loma Linda technique" because of Jorgensen's affiliation with that school, and is now known as the "Jorgensen technique," for the man considered by many to be the father of intravenous sedation in dentistry.

Three drugs are administered in the Jorgensen technique:

1. Pentobarbital, a barbiturate
2. Meperidine, an opioid agonist
3. Scopolamine, an anticholinergic

As will be discussed later in this chapter, polypharmacy, the use of multiple drugs to achieve a therapeutic goal, should be avoided, if possible, for the incidence of drug-drug interactions greatly increases as additional drugs are administered to patients. The Jorgensen technique is a positive example of polypharmacy, but unlike many drug combinations that appear to have no relevance for the drugs being administered, each of the drugs administered in the Jorgensen technique serves an important function.

Everett and Allen[18] discussed the physiological effects of the Jorgensen technique and demonstrated that there is minimal physiologic alteration produced, although three of their subjects did develop nausea. This latter effect was most likely caused by the opioid. In my experience with the Jorgensen technique nausea and vomiting are extremely rare and are rarely significant complications.

Function of the individual drugs

Detailed pharmacology of the drugs used in the Jorgensen technique is found in Chapter 26.

Pentobarbital. Pentobarbital is *the* drug used to produce the desired level of sedation in the Jorgensen technique. Pentobarbital is also the drug that provides the 2- to 4-hour duration of action associated with the Jorgensen technique. Pentobarbital, a generalized CNS depressant, has the disquieting effect of making patients more likely to overreact to stimulation. This is a negative action of the drug and is one reason for inclusion of the opioid in the technique.

Meperidine. Meperidine is a opioid agonist and as such has a number of potentially adverse side effects, including respiratory depression, postural hypotension, nausea, and vomiting. Its functions in the Jorgensen technique are threefold:

1. To provide some additional sedation
2. To provide some analgesia, counterbalancing the negative actions of the barbiturate
3. To provide some euphoria

In the dosage of meperidine used in the Jorgensen technique (not greater than 25 mg) the major effect of meperidine is its analgesic action. Patients who have received pentobarbital alone usually overrespond to painful or traumatic stimulation; however, with the addition of up to 25 mg of meperidine this response is moderated, most patients responding "normally" to stimulation.

Scopolamine. Scopolamine is an anticholinergic with several functions in the Jorgensen technique:

1. Scopolamine provides anterograde amnesia in some patients
2. It inhibits salivary secretions, thus providing a dry operating field
3. It produces a degree of CNS depression, although this is rarely of any significance

Scopolamine may also produce emergence delirium, for which reason it is contraindicated in patients under age 6 years and over age 65 years.

Preliminary appointment

At the visit prior to actual treatment the patient will be evaluated as discussed in the diazepam technique section.

The Jorgensen technique is described to the patient in general terms, mentioning that the drugs are to be administered intravenously and that the patient will feel quite relaxed, perhaps somewhat sleepy. It is important to mention to the patient that he or she will not be unconscious, for this is not general anesthesia, but a safer, equally effective technique called "conscious sedation."

The patient's previous reactions to the drugs involved in the technique must also be determined. Whether the patient has ever received Nembutal, Demerol, or scopolamine is determined, and if so, the patient's reaction is noted. In addition, the patient is questioned about the presence of possible contraindications to the use of one or more of these agents. These include the following.

Contraindications to the Jorgensen technique

1. Allergy or hypersensitivity to any of the three drugs
2. Porphyria (contraindication to barbiturate)
3. Liver disease (contraindication to barbiturate, opioid)
4. Asthma (contraindication to barbiturate, opioid, scopolamine)
5. Respiratory depression (contraindication to barbiturate, opioid)
6. Alcoholism (contraindication to barbiturate, opioid)
7. MAOIs within 14 days (contraindication to opioid)
8. Glaucoma (contraindication to scopolamine)
9. Adhesions between iris and lens (contraindication to scopolamine)
10. Prostate disease (contraindication to scopolamine)
11. Myasthenia gravis (contraindication to scopolamine)
12. Contact lenses (contraindication to scopolamine)

Baseline vital signs are recorded, the presence of superficial veins is determined, preoperative instructions are given to the patient, and the sedation appointment is scheduled.

Day of treatment

On the day of treatment the patient is prepared for the IV procedure as previously described for the benzodiazepines. Because of the inherent length of the Jorgensen technique, the importance of asking the patient to void prior to the start of the procedure is stressed. Venipuncture may be started at any site in which suitable veins are located, there being no prohibitions concerning selection of an IV site with any of the three drugs.

Preparation of drugs. Two 5-ml syringes are required when preparing drugs for use in the Jorgensen technique. The drugs are available as follows:

Pentobarbital: 50 mg/ml in 2-ml ampules and multidose vials
Meperidine: 50 mg/ml in 0.5- and 1-ml ampules
Scopolamine: 0.3 mg in 1.0-ml ampules

Into the first syringe is placed 3 ml (if using the multidose vial) or 4 ml (two 2-ml ampules) of pentobarbital. The syringe is labeled "Pentobarbital 50 mg/ml."

To remove a drug from an ampule the doctor or assistant holds the ampule in the fingers as illustrated in Fig. 27-8. A gauze is used to prevent injury from sharp pieces of glass. Making certain that all of the drug is in the bottom of the ampule, the doctor or assistant cracks the glass at its prescored neck. A microfilter needle (optional) is placed onto the syringe and the drug drawn up into the syringe. The micropore filter is designed to stop any small fragments of glass that may have fallen into the solution from entering the syringe and being injected into the patient. After the syringe is filled with solution, the micropore filter needle is replaced with the original needle. The filter needle can be used in only one direction—either to withdraw solutions into the syringe or to inject them out of the syringe—and it must be replaced with the original needle for the other function.

When a drug is removed from a multidose vial, the rubber stopper is cleansed with an alcohol wipe and permitted to dry. Placing the needle of the syringe into the bottle at an angle to prevent coring (the placing of small pieces of rubber into the solution), a volume of air equal to the volume of solution to be withdrawn is injected into the vial. This makes it much easier for solution to be withdrawn from the vial.

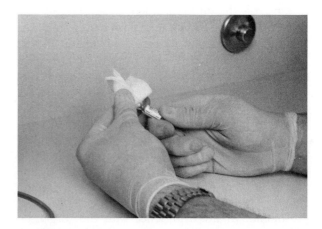

Fig. 27-8. Ampule is held in gauze and cracked at its prescored neck.

In the second syringe will be placed meperidine (25 mg), scopolamine (0.3 mg), and a volume of diluent that may be withdrawn from the IV infusion bag. Assuming in this instance that the meperidine ampule contains 50 mg in 1.0 ml (or 25 mg in 0.5 ml) and the scopolamine contains 0.3 mg in 1.0 ml, the doctor or assistant first inserts the empty syringe into the injection site on the IV infusion bag or the injection site on the IV tubing and withdraws 3.5 ml of solution. Each of the ampules is carefully opened and its contents withdrawn into the syringe. A total of 5 ml of solution should now be in the syringe (3.5 ml of IV solution, 1 ml scopolamine, and 0.5 ml meperidine), containing 25 mg meperidine and 0.3 mg scopolamine. The syringe is labeled "Meperidine 5 mg/ml, scopolamine 0.06 mg/ml."

> ALWAYS READ THE LABEL OF THE DRUG BEING PREPARED FOR USE TO CONFIRM ITS MG/ML FORMULATION

The patient is placed in a semisupine position, monitoring devices attached, preoperative vital signs recorded, and the venipuncture established. There are no prohibitions on venipuncture site for any of the drugs in the Jorgensen technique. Nasal O$_2$ through either a cannula or nasal hood at a rate of 3 to 5 L/min is initiated at this time.

The rate of the IV infusion is increased, and the patency of the IV infusion is rechecked as described for the benzodiazepines. The pentobarbital syringe is placed into the injection site on the IV tubing, and a test dose of 0.2 ml of solution (one small delineation on the syringe) is administered to rule out any allergic reaction or hypersensitivity response. After 30 seconds the doctor or assistant begins the administration of pentobarbital at a rate of 10 mg every 30 seconds (0.2 ml or one small delineation) while continuously conversing with the patient.

The pentobarbital is injected until the patient mentions the presence of the first symptoms of cortical depression. These usually are the following:
- Slight dizziness
- A feeling of being tired
- Decreased apprehension
- Difficulty in focusing on distant objects

Clinical signs that may be noted at this time are the following:
- Relaxation in patients who were initially agitated
- Slight slurring of speech
- Slower response to commands
- Heaviness of the eyelids

It is suggested that a mouth prop be placed in the patient's mouth at this time so that should responses become even more sluggish, the patient will have no difficulty in maintaining an open mouth.

It is important to administer the pentobarbital slowly, for the lag time between injection and the onset of clinical signs and symptoms is somewhat slower than that noted with either diazepam and midazolam, approximately 2 to 4 minutes. In other words, the clinical effect seen at any moment in time was produced by the pentobarbital administered up to 4 minutes earlier.

Jorgensen[19] termed the point of appearance of the first signs of cortical sedation "baseline." The average dose of pentobarbital required to reach baseline is between 125 and 175 mg. The range, however, is quite broad, baseline sedation having been achieved with pentobarbital doses from 30 to 300 mg.

In Jorgensen's[17] original description of the technique he stated that at this point an additional volume of pentobarbital is injected equal to 10% to 15% of the baseline dosage. Thus if 100 mg was required to reach baseline, an additional 10 to 15 mg will be injected and the syringe removed. Having used this technique for 20 years I have found that this additional 10% to 15% need not always be administered, for in many patients additional pentobarbital leads to a greater depth of sedation than is desired. Additional pentobarbital can always be administered if necessary, but once the drug has been injected, there is no way of removing it or of reversing its actions.

Having achieved baseline sedation, the second syringe, containing meperidine and scopolamine, is placed into the injection site. The dose administered is based on the meperidine: it is suggested that it be injected at a rate of 10 mg per minute or, in this instance, 1 ml every 30 seconds.

The maximum dose of meperidine is based on the dose of pentobarbital required to reach baseline sedation. The ratio of pentobarbital to meperidine will be 4:1 mg up to a maximal dose of 25 mg meperidine (Table 27-1). Thus a patient who received 100 mg pentobarbital *may receive up to 25 mg meperidine.* If 60 mg pentobarbital was required, a maximal dose of 15 mg meperidine may be administered. If the patient required 180, 200, or 300 mg pentobarbital to reach baseline, the maximal meperidine dose is still 25 mg. No more than 25 mg meperidine is administered.

As the meperidine-scopolamine combination is administered the patient must be observed carefully for

Table 27-1. Ratio of barbiturate to meperidine in Jorgensen technique

Barbiturate dose (mg) (syringe 1)	Maximal meperidine dose (syringe 2)	
	Milligrams	*Milliliters*
30	7.5	1.5
50	12.5	2.5
60	15	3
80	20	4
100	25	5
200	25	5
300	25	5

signs of increasing sedation. In most instances no noticeable change in depth of sedation will occur, and the maximal calculated dose of meperidine-scopolamine will be administered.

In some instances, however, the patient will be noted to become more deeply sedated as meperidine is administered. Further administration of meperidine-scopolamine should be halted before the patient reaches an overly deep level of sedation. In this situation the maximal calculated dose of meperidine is not administered.

The rate of the IV infusion is now slowed to a rate just fast enough to keep the needle from occluding (t.k.o.). Vital signs are recorded on the anesthesia record sheet following IV drug administration.

The combination of pentobarbital (for its sedation), meperidine (for its analgesia, euphoria, and some additional sedation), and scopolamine (for its amnesic and antisialagogue actions) usually results in a cooperative, relaxed, and sedated patient who willingly accepts 2 or more hours of concentrated restorative or surgical procedures under local anesthesia yet remains conscious and able to assist the doctor when necessary.

Intraoperative period. Local anesthesia is administered and treatment begun. Although virtually all patients will be well sedated and cooperative at this point, it is possible that some few will overreact when treatment is started. This may be an indication for the administration of either additional pentobarbital or of local anesthetic to the patient. If it appears that the patient's movements are related only to painful dental procedures (e.g., excavating cavities, soft tissue surgery) but that they resolve when treating enamel, pain control may be incomplete, requiring the administration of additional local anesthetic. However, if the patient's movements are more generalized—occurring in response to nontraumatic

procedures—the patient is asked how he is feeling. If the patient responds that he is still fearful of the procedure the IV infusion rate is increased and additional pentobarbital titrated until relaxation occurs. Pentobarbital is responsible for the proper level of sedation in the Jorgensen technique. Once an appropriate sedation level is achieved, the pentobarbital syringe is removed and the IV infusion rate is slowed (t.k.o.). No additional meperidine-scopolamine is administered at this time.

In the event that there is a sluggish or absent response, additional drug is not administered. Airway patency is checked immediately. Hypoxia and/or hypercarbia are often noted clinically as restlessness. Ventilation is assessed and controlled if necessary until the patient recovers (sedation lightens) sufficiently to permit resumption of the dental procedure.

The duration of the depth of ideal sedation during the Jorgensen technique is considerably longer than that seen with diazepam or midazolam. Recovery is also somewhat slower—the patient appears sedated even after 3 or 4 hours of treatment.

The following are several points to be aware of during treatment of the sedated patient:

1. *Work efficiently and quietly.* Remember that your patient is awake and able to hear you. Be careful in what you do and say while treating the sedated patient, who may not hear every word that you utter and may misinterpret those they do hear. Be especially careful where you place your hands and instruments. The patient may consider a perfectly innocent gesture as an assault on his or her body (Chapter 18).

2. *When the patient is female (or male if the operator is female), it is important medicolegally for another female to be present in the room with you at all times during the procedure.*

3. *Some patients may complain about the dryness that accompanies the administration of scopolamine.* It may be necessary for the doctor or assistant to moisten the soft tissues of the patient's mouth and throat with small squirts of water from the air-water syringe.

4. *When a scalp vein or straight metal needle is used in the antecubital fossa for the Jorgensen technique, immobilization is required.* Some patients complain that their elbow is sore. They are unable to flex the joint because of the mandatory presence of an elbow immobilizer whenever a nonflexible needle is used for venipuncture. It is therefore suggested that the operator use either an indwelling catheter for venipuncture at any site (including the antecubital fossa) or a scalp vein or straight metal needle in either the

ventral aspect of the forearm or dorsum of the hand where joint immobilization is not necessary.

Posttreatment period. Recovery from the Jorgensen technique is considerably less complete than that seen following either diazepam or midazolam. This is perversely beneficial because the patient is unlikely to want to drive a car or do other potentially hazardous duties after sedation with the Jorgensen technique. The typical patient simply wants to go home and go to bed and sleep. Fitness for discharge will be based on the patient's ability to walk without assistance and on a comparison of the vital signs obtained before, during, and after the procedure, as described in the discussion on benzodiazepine sedation. Record keeping in the patient's chart will include the anesthesia record sheet or a written statement similar to that recommended for the benzodiazepines.

Postoperative instructions are given verbally and in writing to both the patient and his companion. Postoperative analgesics administered during the first 6 to 8 hours should be nonopioid, so as to minimize any additive effects of opioids with those administered intravenously. If pain is expected to be a significant problem postoperatively, administration of a long-acting local anesthetic such as bupivacaine or etidocaine immediately prior to discharge of the patient is suggested.

The patient is escorted out of the office to his vehicle by his escort and a staff member. A telephone call is made later that day to see how the recovery is progressing and to review postoperative instructions.

There is a greater possibility that the patient will not be fully recovered from the effects of the pentobarbital the next day, especially if the sedation procedure occurred during the afternoon. It is preferable therefore for sedation with the Jorgensen technique to be carried out during the morning hours.

Intravenous promethazine

The third of the basic techniques of IV sedation is the administration of promethazine, a phenothiazine derivative with potent sedative and antihistaminic properties. Because promethazine does possess antihistaminic and anticholinergic properties, the addition of an anticholinergic, such as atropine or scopolamine, is usually unnecessary.

The primary indication for promethazine is a dental or surgical procedure expected to require between 1 to 2 hours to complete. Procedures of less than 1 hour are well managed with diazepam or midazolam, whereas with procedures of more than 2

hours the Jorgensen technique is suggested. The following relative and absolute contraindications to promethazine must be sought at the preoperative visit:

1. Allergy or hypersensitivity to promethazine
2. Glaucoma
3. Prostatic hypertrophy
4. Stenosing peptic ulcer
5. Bladder/neck obstruction

If any of these are present, alternative IV techniques should be sought. Diazepam or midazolam is recommended in place of promethazine in most of these patients. The Jorgensen technique is not as suitable, primarily because these same contraindications are present for the anticholinergics used in that technique.

Promethazine is prepared for injection by placing 3 ml of 5% dextrose and water into a 5-ml syringe and then adding 2 ml of promethazine (25 mg/ml). This produces a concentration of 10 mg/ml, the recommended concentration for injection of promethazine. The IV infusion may be established at any convenient site when promethazine is used.

The drug is titrated at a rate of 1 ml per minute to clinical effect. The average dose of promethazine required for sedation is 32.5 mg, the range between 25 and 35 mg. If adequate sedation is not present by 50 mg, drug administration is terminated and the planned treatment begun if possible or the patient rescheduled for another appointment at which time a different intravenous technique will be used.

Although readministration of promethazine is usually not required once the initial titrating dose has been given, readministration may be necessary on occasion. In this situation the suggested absolute maximal dose of promethazine is 75 mg.

Promethazine

Average sedative dose	32.5 mg
Sedative dose range	25 to 35 mg
Maximum dose—no sedation	50 mg
Maximum dose—some sedation	75 mg

Recovery from promethazine sedation is not as clinically complete as that for diazepam or midazolam, the patient still retaining some degree of CNS depression on departing from the office.

Summary

Three techniques that I have classified as basic have been presented. It is my belief that these techniques form the backbone of the doctor's IV sedative armamentarium. When these techniques are used as described, serious complications will not arise. Retrospective studies on the Jorgensen technique and IV diazepam have demonstrated beyond doubt that these procedures are sound, safe, and effective.[20,21]

Availability of these three procedures will enable the doctor to pick an appropriate intravenous technique based on the time allotted for treatment:

Up to 1 hour—diazepam or midazolam
From 1 to 2 hours—promethazine
More than 2 hours—Jorgensen technique

In addition, the following applies to IV drug administration:

- Titrate the drugs slowly.
- Remain within the dosage limits recommended for each technique.
- Failures (the inability to provide adequate sedation within the dosage recommended), though quite rare, will occur. When this happens, no other drug should be administered to the patient (this includes N_2O-O_2). An attempt is made to treat the patient in the best possible manner. If this proves to be futile, the procedure is terminated and rescheduled for another time at which a different technique of sedation will be used. The administration of additional drug or of a different drug to the patient will frequently lead to problems (e.g., unconsciousness, airway obstruction) in the hands of the inexperienced doctor. Finding out the hard way that this is true is not recommended.

MODIFICATION OF BASIC TECHNIQUES

In this section a common modification of a basic technique is described, the addition of an anticholinergic medication to diazepam or midazolam. The Jorgensen technique already includes an anticholinergic, and promethazine possesses anticholinergic properties so that addition of anticholinergics is unnecessary.

Selection of a suitable anticholinergic is based on the needs of the patient and the desired duration of its action. Where a slight degree of sedation and amnesia is desired, scopolamine (0.3 mg) is recommended. Its use is appropriate in a procedure of any duration. If the patient is younger than 6 years or over 65 years of age, scopolamine is not recommended because of the increased incidence of emergence delirium.

Atropine (0.4 mg) is employed where a drying effect is desired without amnesia or additional sedation, and the duration of the procedure is less than 2 hours. Glycopyrrolate (0.2 mg) is recommended

Table 27-2. Indications for anticholinergics

	Salivary secretions	Amnesia	Sedation	Duration (hours)
Atropine	+	−	−	<2
Glycopyrrolate	+	−	−	>2
Scopolamine	+	+	+	<2

for procedures in excess of 2 hours when a drying effect is required.

Table 27-2 summarizes the properties of anticholinergics.

Technique

When anticholinergics, which are aqueous solutions, are administered with diazepam, which is lipid-soluble, they must be administered in a separate syringe. The patient receives diazepam as discussed previously, and the anticholinergic is then administered. Slowly inject the anticholinergic drug over a 1-minute time span.

The use of diazepam and scopolamine (0.3 mg) will provide a greater degree of amnesia in most patients than will either drug alone. Rather than the amnesic period being approximately 10 minutes in duration, it may extend over the entire appointment.

Being water-soluble, midazolam and anticholinergics may be mixed in a single syringe prior to administration and injected together, although in most situations it is more practical to administer the anticholinergic separately, as previously discussed.

One of the disadvantages of employing anticholinergics is that some patients will complain that the drying effect is bothersome, both during the procedure and in some cases following the procedure when they return home. Although drugs are available to reverse anticholinergics (the reversible cholinesterases, neostigmine and physostigmine) their use is not recommended (because of possible undesirable side effects).

ADVANCED TECHNIQUES

In this section techniques will be discussed that include the addition of an opioid to an antianxiety or a sedative hypnotic drug or employ drugs, such as propofol, that require increased care in handling. The box on p. 408 presents a categorization of the drugs discussed in this section.

When used for a well-defined purpose, the combination of a drug from group A (antianxiety/sedative-hypnotic) and one from group B (opioid) is quite rational. As discussed in the preceding section, the addition of an anticholinergic (group C) is suggested whenever a drying effect or amnesia is desirable.

Techniques described in this section should be limited in use to doctors meeting one or both of the following requirements:

1. Doctors who have successfully completed training in general anesthesia techniques and in the management of the airway of an unconscious patient
2. Doctors with extensive experience in the basic techniques of IV sedation

Because these techniques involve administration of two or more CNS depressants, there is an increased risk of development of additive drug effects. Clinically this would produce an increased depth of sedation beyond that which is desirable, and it might require the doctor to terminate dental treatment momentarily and evaluate the patient's status.

When the listed drugs are administered as suggested (dosage, rate of injection, and monitoring), clinical problems are extremely unlikely to develop. Deviation from these guidelines will increase the potential for adverse side effects.

Rationale for advanced techniques

Why discuss the addition of a second drug to the basic intravenous conscious sedation discussed? Two reasons are presented.

First, maximum, safe, and effective doses of each of the basic drugs have been presented. If no clinical effect has developed at that dose, further administration of the same drug is unlikely to produce acceptable sedation unless extremely large doses are given. It was strongly recommended in the discussion of basic techniques that the inexperienced doctor terminate the procedure and attempt a different IV technique at a subsequent appointment.

The doctor who meets one or both of the criteria listed above can, however, administer a second CNS depressant to this patient. Opioids are an excellent choice, with small doses usually providing the additional sedation required for the patient to accept dental treatment and remain comfortable.

Second, a degree of analgesia is provided during painful procedures, or in some cases (barbiturates) the opioid counterbalances the negative effect of a drug on the pain reaction threshold. When used in this regard, a larger dose of opioid is desirable.

The sequence in which the antianxiety or sedative-hypnotic and opioid are administered will depend on the reason for its inclusion in the technique.

Requirement: sedation

In the situation in which the group A drug (diazepam, midazolam, pentobarbital, or promethazine) has been administered to its maximal recommended dose yet the patient remains unsedated, the addition of an opioid will aid in providing the necessary sedation. The opioid is slowly titrated, the doctor and assistant carefully observing the patient for signs of increasing sedation. Titration of the opioid ceases when the desired sedation is reached. The depth of sedation achieved in this manner should be no greater than that observed with the basic techniques.

In this first technique, in which the primary requirement is sedation, the patient will have received a larger dose of the antianxiety drug and a smaller dose of the opioid analgesic, for example, diazepam 20 mg and meperidine 10 mg or promethazine 50 mg and morphine 6 mg.

Requirement: analgesia

When the planned dental procedure involves a potential for pain, such as oral surgery or periodontal surgery, the benefits of an opioid analgesic may be welcomed. The primary technique of pain control during dental treatment will always be local anesthesia. The addition of IV analgesics will help the patient during the procedure should the local anesthetic effect begin to lessen. The nature of the discomfort experienced by the patient will be altered.

When used for this reason the analgesic is administered first, titrated until one of two things occur: (1) clinically adequate sedation develops or (2) the maximal recommended opioid dose is administered. In most situations the slow administration of the opioid does not produce significant sedation so that the maximal recommended dose is usually administered; however, the opioid must always be titrated slowly to prevent a hyperresponding patient from overreacting.

Following opioid administration, if additional sedation is desired, a group A drug may be slowly titrated.

It is obvious that when this technique is employed, the patient will receive a larger dose of the opioid analgesic and a smaller dose of the antianxiety or sedative hypnotic drug, for example, meperidine 50 mg and diazepam 7 mg or pentazocine 30 mg and promethazine 15 mg.

Some patients are quite sensitive to the CNS-depressant actions of opioids and will become adequately sedated at a dose below that of the maximum recommended for that drug. Should this occur, ti-

Table 27-3. Group B drugs: doses and dilutions

	Availability (mg/ml)	Maximal dose (mg)	Dilution for use (mg/ml)
Meperidine	50	50	10
Morphine	10	8	1
Alphaprodine*	40-60	40	10
Fentanyl	0.05	0.08	0.01
Pentazocine	30	30	10
Nalbuphine	10	10	2
Butorphanol	2	2	0.4

*No longer available in the United States.

tration of the opioid is ceased when the desired sedative level is reached, no other group A drug is administered intravenously, and treatment is started.

The maximal doses and the recommended dilutions of group B drugs (opioids) are presented in Table 27-3.

Techniques

Diazepam or midazolam with opioid

When either diazepam or midazolam is the primary drug for sedation, the most appropriate opioids to employ are the shorter-acting ones: meperidine, alphaprodine, fentanyl, and pentazocine. Duration of sedation will usually not be increased; however, it is possible that clinical recovery at 60 minutes will not be as complete as that seen when diazepam or midazolam are administered alone. Administration of longer-acting opioids (morphine) will only delay recovery.

Diazepam or midazolam with opioid plus anticholinergic

Addition of an anticholinergic is based on the criteria previously discussed. The use of glycopyrrolate is not recommended because of its prolonged duration of action compared to diazepam or midazolam.

The anticholinergic may be mixed in the same syringe as the opioid (see the Jorgensen technique for procedure).

Promethazine with opioid

Because the clinical action of promethazine is somewhat longer than that of diazepam or midazolam, longer-acting opioids may be employed if indicated. Nalbuphine, butorphanol, morphine, meperidine, and pentazocine are recommended. Morphine should be used for procedures requiring very close to or more than 2 hours to complete, while

meperidine and pentazocine are for those procedures requiring just slightly over 1 hour.

Promethazine with opioid plus anticholinergic

There is little need for this combination because of the anticholinergic properties of promethazine.

Pentobarbital with opioid

The administration of pentobarbital intravenously as a sole agent for sedation is rarely justified because of the negative action of the drug on the patient's pain reaction threshold. Patients receiving IV barbiturates may overreact to painful stimulation. In addition, many patients become quite talkative and increase their movement in the dental chair following pentobarbital administration.

The administration of an opioid analgesic therefore is almost mandatory whenever pentobarbital is employed unless, of course, the doctor does not wish to increase the sedative level of the patient any further.

Pentobarbital will normally be employed for procedures requiring 2 or more hours to complete. Therefore our choice of opioid is limited to the longer-acting ones:

Meperidine	If duration is just 2 hours
Morphine	2 to 4 hours
Butorphanol	2 to 3 hours
Nalbuphine	2 to 3 hours

Jorgensen technique plus benzodiazepine

As the dental or surgical procedure extends beyond the second hour, some patients may require additional sedation for their treatment to be completed. Because of its long duration of action (2 to 4 hours) the readministration of pentobarbital is not recommended at this time. For this reason, in those few cases in which patients do require additional sedation, a benzodiazepine is administered. Either diazepam (at 5 mg/min) or midazolam (at 1 mg/min) is titrated carefully to clinical effect. This technique provides the additional sedation necessary in the doctor's judgment while not unnecessarily prolonging the duration of the entire sedative procedure.

Opioid with group A drug

In reversing the order of drug administration we seek a greater analgesic effect from our drugs. Anxiety reduction is *not* the primary reason for the IV procedure.

Selection of the opioid and antianxiety or sedative-

Table 27-4. Average drug doses from 1716 cases

Agent(s)		Dose (mg)	
Drug 1	Drug 2	Drug 1	Drug 2
Diazepam	—	12.8	—
Diazepam	Meperidine	19.3	33.0
Meperidine	Diazepam	47.1	8.6
Promethazine	—	41.2	—
Promethazine	Meperidine	48.6	31.1
Meperidine	Promethazine	45.2	21.4

hypnotic should be based on the anticipated duration of the procedure, as discussed.

Anticholinergics (group C) may be added to the opioid syringe if desired. Table 27-4 illustrates the different doses of group A and B drugs required when administered alone or in combination. These results are taken from IV sedation continuing education courses.

When any of these advanced IV techniques are used, the drugs must always be titrated slowly (1 ml per minute), unless otherwise recommended. The patient is observed for signs of increasing sedation so that oversedation does not occur.

Never combine the opioid in the same syringe as the group A antianxiety or sedative-hypnotic. The administrator loses control over drug action when this is done.

Propofol

Propofol has been employed for intravenous sedation in a number of medical specialities, including ophthalmology,[22] radiology,[23] gynecology,[24,25] gastroenterology,[26] neurosurgery,[27] intensive care medicine,[28,29] and pediatric surgery,[30] as well as dentistry.[31-33]

Among its advantages is a very rapid onset of action and an extremely rapid recovery following termination of administration. Following propofol sedation patients are ready for discharge in a considerably shorter period of time than following the IV benzodiazepines, diazepam and midazolam, or barbiturates (methohexital).[34]

Disadvantages of the administration of propofol include the possibility of a burning sensation on intravenous administration and the expense of the drug and infusion pumps. The infusion-pump costs approximately US$3000 (July 1994).

Microcomputer-based syringe pumps have become available, enormously simplifying the delivery of drug infusions on a dose/weight/time basis (e.g.,

microgram/kilogram/minute). Two examples are Medfusion #2010 and the Baxter Auto Syringe #AS20GH-2. The Bard Infusor syringe pump accepts magnetically encoded drug-specific "smart labels" that eliminate any need for the operator to enter the drug concentration manually.[35]

Oei-Lim et al.[33] found that a syringe-infusion pump set at an initial rate of 3 mg/kg/hr induced *conscious sedation* in approximately 11.6 minutes in severely apprehensive or mentally and/or physically handicapped patients. The infusion rate was then adjusted to accommodate for variations in the level of sedation during the dental procedure (average duration of treatment = 55 minutes). The mean infusion rate was 3.6 mg/kg/hr. Sedation was successful in 17/19 patients. Cohen et al.[36] employed an initial bolus of dose of 0.5 mg/kg, followed by an infusion of 4 mg/kg/hr to provide *deep sedation* for ambulatory oral surgery.

Alternatively, propofol may be administered as a bolus by syringe without an infusion pump. Propofol must be administered frequently by this method in order to maintain the patient in a sedated state.

An increasingly common technique of using propofol for conscious sedation is to administer an IV bolus, the dose based on the patient's body weight, and then maintain the level of sedation using the infusion pump.

OTHER TECHNIQUES

Other IV sedation techniques are available. It is my belief, however, that the techniques discussed in this section should *not* be employed unless the doctor has completed a residency program in anesthesiology and is conversant with and able to maintain the airway of the unconscious patient. The depth of sedation is considered deep sedation when compared with the conscious sedation techniques described in the previous sections of this chapter. The point at which deep sedation ends and general anesthesia (the loss of consciousness) starts is a grey area to be avoided by all but the most well-trained individuals. Indeed, many state dental boards and legislative bodies have determined that deep sedation, for all intents and purposes, *is* general anesthesia and must be treated in the same manner.

Diazepam with methohexital (Foreman technique)

The combination of diazepam with methohexital, an ultrashort-acting barbiturate, has been used with success by many persons, foremost among whom is Peter Foreman of New Zealand.[37-40]

After initially titrating diazepam to baseline sedation (see diazepam technique discussion), a dose of 5 to 10 mg of methohexital is employed whenever unpleasant procedures are anticipated. This includes the administration of local anesthetics or surgery on osseous structures. The 5- to 10-mg increments of methohexital provide a deepening of sedation (into deep sedation) that lasts for from 5 to 7 minutes.

Foreman has found this technique to be valuable in dental procedures requiring 30 to 90 minutes for completion. In his experience the usual dose of drugs administered in a procedure lasting more than 1 hour is diazepam 10 to 20 mg and methohexital 50 to 100 mg (in 5- to 10-mg increments). Amnesia is greatly enhanced by addition of the methohexital.

Care must be taken to administer only small increments of methohexital with this technique because larger doses will produce deep sedation bordering on loss of consciousness, with attendant depression of protective reflexes, skeletal muscle relaxation, difficulty in maintaining a patent airway, and possible laryngospasm.

The Berns technique

Joel Berns[41] has developed a technique involving the administration of three drugs, the barbiturate (group A) secobarbital, the opioid (group B) meperidine, and the barbiturate (group A) methohexital.

Secobarbital is administered first, being slowly titrated to baseline sedation (the dose range being from 25 to 75 mg), followed by 25 to 50 mg meperidine. Local anesthesia is administered and the procedure started. Methohexital in increments of 10 to 20 mg is administered just prior to any traumatic procedure, which may include administration of local anesthesia, or extractions.

This technique is similar to the Foreman technique previously described with the barbiturate secobarbital replacing diazepam. The same benefits and potential problems exist in this procedure. An additional consideration is the absence of any pharmacologic antagonist for the barbiturates, while flumazenil is available to reverse any unwanted actions of the benzodiazepines.

The Shane technique

Sylvan Shane,[42,43] from Maryland, developed a technique, first described in 1966, that he calls "intravenous amnesia." The technique consists of two components: (1) a verbal component that precedes drug administration, and (2) a drug component that involves the IV administration of alphaprodine, hydroxyzine, atropine, and methohexital, and local anesthesia for pain control.

The verbal component is extremely important in the Shane technique. Prior to drug administration the patient is told the following:

1. You will be asleep during the procedure.
2. Prior to falling asleep you will feel the calming effects of the medications.
3. "Pentothal" is being administered.
4. No pain will be felt during the procedure.
5. When the procedure is complete, you will express disbelief and insist that you were never asleep. (This must be said to the patient before the patient says it to the dentist.)
6. You will know when the procedure is over, for your lips, tongue, and teeth will feel numb. When you feel the numbness, you will know that "something must have happened," and this numbness confirms the fact that the procedure is over.
7. (The patient is then exposed to the sound of the drill, air blower, and amalgam condenser.) You will hear these sounds, and they also mean that the procedure is over. These instruments are used to polish, carve, and smooth the fillings, and this is done during the hour required for you to awaken sufficiently to get up out of the chair.
8. (Gauze is placed over the patient's eyes [taped in place].) The gauze will be over your eyes when you awaken to keep the polishing dust out of your eyes.
9. (The patient's later response to all of the above is anticipated.) You will swear that you were never asleep, yet the treatment will be completed and you will feel as though only a minute has passed.

The drugs are then administered as listed in Table 27-5.

Table 27-5. Shane technique drug schedule

| Drug | Dose (mg)* | | |
	Age 2 to 6 years	Age 7 to 18 years	Adult
Alphaprodine	6	7-18	18-24
		(Same as age in years)	
Hydroxyzine	25	25-50	50
Atropine	0.3	0.4	0.6

*Normal saline is added to dilute the mixture as needed to a total of 5 ml in the syringe.

Shane recommends combining alphaprodine, hydroxyzine, and atropine in one syringe, the methohexital in a second syringe.

Following the administration of the drugs in the first syringe to clinical effect, 1 to 2 ml (10 to 20 mg) of methohexital is administered. Local anesthesia of the entire oral cavity (as needed) is obtained. On completion of local anesthetic administration the patient is told to close his mouth and nothing is said or done for the next 2 minutes.

The dentist then tells the patient that the treatment is completed, all the fillings are done, and the patient may now go home. Of course, the doctor has not even started treatment yet. Patients normally respond to this by saying, "You're fooling me" or "You're kidding."

The doctor counters this by reminding the patient that his mouth is numb, and that he was told previously that when he awakened, he would be numb. The patient will then lie back in the chair and begin sleeping.

At this point the doctor states, "I am going to be polishing your fillings or trimming your bony spicules from the extraction sites." The actual dental procedure starts.

Shane[44,45] terms the verbal component of the procedure the "therapeutic lie." He has reported on at least 15,000 sedations without fatality.

During the Shane technique the patient is in deep sedation. The doctor employing this technique must be well trained in the management of this level of CNS depression.

Factors that severely limit use of the Shane technique are the recommendation by the manufacturer of hydroxyzine that the drug not be administered intravenously and the removal of alphaprodine from clinical use in the United States.

SUMMARY

A number of techniques of IV conscious sedation have been presented in this chapter. As a rule, there is no necessity for any one doctor to have all of these techniques available for use in his or her dental practice.

The most rational way of employing these techniques is to start out by initially working with the basic techniques. To learn them well will require at least 50 to 100 cases of each technique.

The only means of obtaining the knowledge and training in the safe and effective use of IV conscious

Table 27-6. Summary of intravenous drug doses, duration, amnesia

Drug	Mg/ml used	Average mg	Maximal mg*	Maximal mg†	Duration	Amnesia‡ induced
Group A						
Diazepam	5	10-12	20	30	45 minutes	Yes
Midazolam	2	2.5-7.5	6-8	10	45 minutes	Yes
Pentobarbital	50	125-175	300	500	2-4 hours	Somewhat
Promethazine	10	25-35	50	75	1-2 hours	Somewhat
Group B						
Meperidine	10	37.5	50	50	<1 hour	No
Morphine	1	5-6	8	8	1.5-2.5 hours	No
Alphaprodine§	10	15-20	30	40	30-45 minutes	No
Fentanyl	0.01	0.05-0.06	0.08	0.08	30-45 minutes	No
Pentazocine	10	20	30	30	1 hour	No
Nalbuphine	2	7-8	10	10	1.5-2 hours	No
Butorphanol	0.4	1.5	2	2	1.5-2 hours	No
Group C						
Atropine	0.4	0.4-0.6	0.4 to 0.6	0.4 to 0.6	3-4 hours	No
Scopolamine	0.3	0.3	0.3	0.3	3-4 hours	Yes
Glycopyrrolate	0.1	0.1	0.1	0.2	7 hours	No

*Maximal dose at one titration.
†Maximal total dose at appointment.
‡Amnesic effect when used in maximal dose recommended.
§Not available in the United States.

sedation techniques is through dental school undergraduate, postgraduate, and continuing education courses. The safe administration of IV sedation cannot be learned through the reading of a textbook.

Strict adherence to the recommendations presented for each of the drugs and techniques, without exception, no matter how tempting alterations might appear, is essential. If these simple rules are followed, problems do not often occur. A summary of recommended drugs, dosages, and durations is presented in Table 27-6.

REFERENCES

1. Rosenberg MB, Campbell RL: Guidelines for intraoperative monitoring of dental patients undergoing conscious sedation, deep sedation, and general anesthesia, *Oral Surg* 71(1):2, 1991.
2. University of Southern California School of Dentistry: Guidelines for parenteral sedation, Los Angeles, 1991, University of Southern California.
3. Malamed SF: Survey of doctors using IV sedation, unpublished data, 1993.
4. Jorgensen NB, Hayden J Jr: *Premedication, local and general anesthesia in dentistry.* Philadelphia, 1967, Lea & Febiger.
5. Coughlin MW, Panuska HJ: Direct comparison of midazolam and diazepam for conscious sedation in outpatient oral surgery, *Anesth Prog* 36(4-5):160, 1989.
6. Tait AR, Knight PR: The effects of general anesthesia on upper respiratory tract infection in children, *Anesthesiology* 67:930, 1987.
7. Valium, drug package insert, Roche Laboratories, 1990.
8. O'Neill R, Verrill PJ, Aellig WH et al: Intravenous diazepam in minor oral surgery, *Br Dent J* 128(1):15, 1970.
9. Trieger N: *Pain control.* Chicago, 1974, Quintessence.
10. Malamed SF, Sykes P, Kubota Y et al: Local anesthesia: a review, *J Anesth Pain Contr Dent* 1(1):11, 1992.
11. O'Boyle CA, Barry H, Fox E et al: Controlled comparison of a new sublingual lormetazepam formulation and i.v. diazepam in outpatient minor oral surgery, *Br J Anaesth* 60(4):419, 1988.
12. O'Boyle CA: Benzodiazepine-induced amnesia and anaesthetic practice: a review, *Psychopharmacol Series* 6:146, 1988.
13. Roche Laboratories: Dosing and titration of midazolam (Versed), Letters to doctors, Nutley, NJ, 1987.
14. Nuotto EJ, Kortilla KT, Lichtor JL et al: Sedation and recovery of psychomotor function after intravenous administration of various doses of midazolam and diazepam, *Anesth Analg* 74(2):265, 1992.
15. Robb ND, Hargrave SA: Tolerance to intravenous midazolam as a result of oral benzodiazepine therapy: a potential problem for the provision of conscious sedation in dentistry, *J Anesth Pain Contr Dent* 2(2):94, 1993.
16. The Flumazenil in General Anesthesia in Outpatients Study Group I: Reversal of the central effects of midazolam by intravenous flumazenil after general anesthesia in outpatients: a multicenter double-blind clinical study. *Clin Thera* 14(6):966-977, 1992.
17. Jorgensem NB, Leffingwell FE: Premedication in dentistry, *J South Calif State Dent Assoc* 21:25, 1953.
18. Everett GB, Allen GD: Simultaneous evaluation of cardiorespiratory and analgesic effects of intravenous analgesia using pentobarbital, meperidine, and scopolamine with local analgesia, *JADA* 83:155, 1971.
19. Jorgensen NB, Hayden J Jr: *Sedation, local and general anesthesia in dentistry,* ed 2. Philadelphia, 1972, Lea & Febiger.
20. Shepherd SR, Sims TN, Johnson BW et al: Assessment of stress during periodontal surgery with intravenous sedation and with local anesthesia only, *J Periodontol* 59(3):147, 1988.
21. Daniel SR, Fry HR, Savard EG: Intravenous "conscious" sedation in periodontal surgery: a selective review and report of 1,708 cases, *J West Soc Periodontol/Periodont Abstr* 32(4):133, 1984.
22. Kost M, Emerson D: Propofol-fentanyl versus midazolam-fentanyl: a comparative study of local sedation techniques for cataract surgery, *CRNA* 3(1):7, 1992.
23. Bloomfield EL, Masaryk TJ, Caplin A et al: Intravenous sedation for MR imaging of the brain and spine in children: pentobarbital versus propofol, *Radiology* 186 (1):93, 1993.
24. Sherry E: Admixture of propofol and alfentanil: use for intravenous sedation and analgesia during transvaginal oocyte retrieval, *Anaesthesia* 47(6):477, 1992.
25. Silverman DG: New anesthetic approaches to gynecologic surgery, *Curr Opin Obstet Gynecol* 3(3):375, 1991.
26. Chin NM, Tai HY, Chin MK: Intravenous sedation for upper gastrointestinal endoscopy: midazolam versus propofol, *Singapore Med J* 33(5):478, 1992.
27. Silbergeld DL, Mueller WM, Colley PS et al: Use of propofol (Diprivan) for awake craniotomies: technical note, *Surg Neurol* 38(4):271, 1992.
28. Niccolai I, Barontini L, Paolini P et al: Long-term sedation with propofol in ICU: hemocoagulation problems, *Minerva Anestesiol* 58(6):375, 1992.
29. Ewart MC, Yau KW, Morgan M: 2% propofol for sedation in the intensive care unit: a feasibility study, *Anaesthesia* 47(2):146, 1992.
30. Bifarini G, Spaccatini A, Ciammitti B et al: Sedation with continuously infused propofol in caudal block for elective pediatric surgery, *Minerva Anestesiol* 58(4):181, 1992.
31. Makkes PC, Vermeulen Cranch DM et al: A comparison of the effects of propofol and nitrous oxide on the electroencephalogram in epileptic patients during conscious sedation for dental procedures, *Anesth Analg* 75(5):708, 1992.
32. Rudkin GE, Osborne GA, Curtis NJ: Intra-operative patient-controlled sedation, *Anaesthesia* 46(2):90, 1991.
33. Oei-Lim LB, Vermeulen-Cranch DM, Bouvy-Berends EC: Conscious sedation with propofol in dentistry, *Br Dent J* 170(9):340, 1991.
34. Dembo JB, Kirkwood CA, Marsh RA: A comparison of propofol (Diprivan) and methohexital for outpatient oral surgery. Proceedings of the 40th annual meeting of the American Society of Anesthesiology, Toronto, Ontario, 1993.
35. Doyle DJ: Intravenous infusions in anesthesia. Proceedings of the 40th annual meeting of the American Society of Anesthesiology, Toronto, Ontario, 1993.
36. Cohen M, Eisig S, Kraut RA: Infusion pump for deep conscious sedation with propofol and methohexital. Proceedings of the 40th annual meeting of the American Society of Anesthesiology, Toronto, Ontario, 1993.
37. Foreman PA: Pharmacosedation: intravenous route. In McCarthy EM, editor: *Emergencies in dental practice,* ed 3. Philadelphia, 1979, Saunders.

38. Foreman PA: Control of the anxiety/pain complex in dentistry: intravenous psychosedation with techniques using diazepam, *Oral Surg* 37:337, 1974.

39. Foreman PA: Intravenous diazepam in general dental practice, *NZ Dent J* 65:243, 1969.

40. Foreman PA, Neels R, Willetts PW: Diazepam in dentistry, *Anesth Prog* 15:253, 1968.

41. Berns JM: "Twilight sedation": a substitute for lengthy office intravenous anesthesia, *J Conn Dent Assoc* 37:4, 1963.

42. Shane SM: Intravenous amnesia to obliterate fear, anxiety and pain in ambulatory dental patients, *J Maryland Dent Assoc* 9:94, 1966.

43. Shane SM: Intravenous amnesia for total dentistry in one sitting, *J Oral Surg* 24:27, 1966.

44. Shane SM, Carrel R, Vandenberge J: Intravenous amnesia: an appraisal after seven years and 10,500 administrations, *Anesth Prog* 21:36, 1974.

45. Shane SM: Intravenous amnesia for total dentistry in one sitting: an appraisal after 15,000 administrations. Fifth annual Continuing Education Seminar in Practical Considerations in IV and IM Dental Sedation, Miami Beach, 1979.

CHAPTER 28

Complications

There are a number of complications that can occur when the IV route of drug administration is used. Most, fortunately, are relatively benign and easily managed. Some, however, are more significant and can lead to serious morbidity and to death.

The complications associated with IV drug administration are divided into four groups: those associated with venipuncture, localized complications related to drug administration, general drug-related problems, and specific drug complications. These are outlined below.

Venipuncture complications

Nonrunning IV infusion
Venospasm
Hematoma
Infiltration
Local venous complications
Air embolism
Overhydration

Local complications of drug administration

Extravascular drug administration
Intraarterial drug administration
Local venous complications

General drug-related complications

Nausea and vomiting
Localized allergy
Respiratory depression
Emergence delirium
Laryngospasm

Specific drug complications

Benzodiazepines
   Local venous complications
   Emergence delirium

   Recurrence of amnesia
   Oversedation
Pentobarbital
   Oversedation
   Respiratory depression
Promethazine
   Oversedation
   Extrapyramidal reactions
Opioids
   Nausea and vomiting
   Respiratory depression
   Rigid chest
Scopolamine
   Emergence delirium

VENIPUNCTURE COMPLICATIONS
Nonrunning IV infusion

One of the most common complications of venipuncture and IV sedation is the nonrunning or very slowly running IV infusion. Once a venipuncture has been successfully completed the tourniquet is removed and the IV drip opened. During administration of drugs the drip rate should be increased; at other times the rate should be slowed. The causes of a nonrunning or slowly running IV infusion are listed below.

IV infusion bag too close to the heart level

Gravity forces the solution from the IV bag down into the patient. The greater the difference in height between the bag and the patient's heart, the more rapid will be the flow of solution. A simple experiment will demonstrate this.

The IV bag is held high above the patient's heart level and the rate of flow is checked. With the rate-adjusting knob opened fully the drip should be quite rapid. The bag is gradually lowered toward the level

432

of the patient's heart. The rate of flow of the drip will decrease until, when held at the patient's heart level, the flow ceases entirely. As the bag is lowered below the level of the patient's heart, blood returns into the tubing (Fig. 28-1, *A* and *B*).

This situation might arise when the dental chair is placed low to the floor at the start of a procedure and is elevated at a later time. Lowering the chair or elevating the bag of IV infusion solution will correct the situation.

Bevel of needle against wall of vein

It was recommended that the bevel of the needle be facing upward during venipuncture so as to make entry into the skin as atraumatic as possible. Follow-ing entry into the skin, the needle is advanced into the vein. At this point the tourniquet is removed and the infusion started. If the IV drip rate is rapid un-til the scalp vein or metal needle is taped into posi-tion, and then slows considerably, it is quite possible that in taping the needle into position the bevel was lifted and lies against the wall of the vein. This would prevent or restrict the flow of fluid from the IV drip into the patient.

To determine if this is the cause of the slow or nonrunning drip, the needle is carefully untaped and the wings gently lifted. This will lower the bevel off the wall of the vein. If the drip rate increases then the protective cap from the scalp vein needle (Fig. 28-2), or a 2- × 2-inch gauze square, is carefully

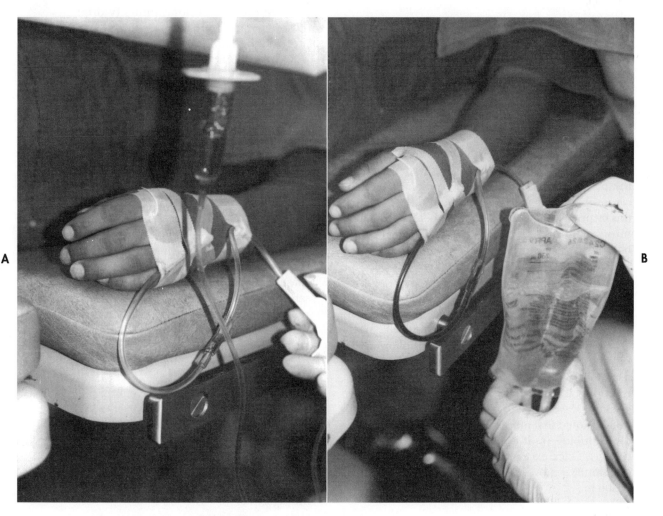

Fig. 28-1. A, Bag of IV solution held above level of patient's heart (vein) allows fluid to run *into* patient. **B,** Lowering bag of IV solution *below* level of patient's heart (vein) allows blood to return into tubing from patient.

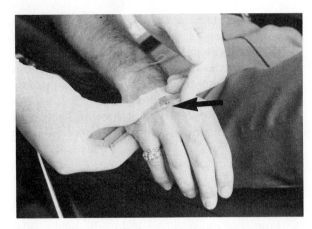

Fig. 28-2. Placing the protective sheath of the needle (or gauze) beneath the wings of the needle *(arrow)* will increase the rate of IV infusion if the bevel is pressing against the vein wall.

placed under the wings of the needle and the needle is retaped.

This is not likely to occur when the indwelling catheter is used for venipuncture because there is no bevel on the catheter. However, when the catheter is positioned in either the dorsum of the hand or the antecubital fossa, it is possible for the end of the catheter tip to lie at a bend in the vein, creating a slow flow of IV solution. Determine this by straightening the patient's wrist or elbow and looking for an increase in the rate of flow of the IV drip. Minimize this by preventing the patient from bending the joint through the use of an elbow immobilizer or wrist board.

Tourniquet left on arm

This is an embarrassing but not uncommon cause of a nonrunning IV drip following successful venipuncture. The tourniquet may have simply been covered by a sleeve that has inched down. Following the return of blood into the IV tubing the doctor or assistant opens up the control knob to start the IV drip. It is noted that the drip is not flowing and that blood does not leave the IV tubing as normally occurs. It is usually noted that more blood appears to be entering the IV tubing (as it is forced from the vein into the tubing). Once excessive blood is noticed in the tubing, simply removing the tourniquet will alleviate the problem.

Infiltration

Following successful entry into the vein the needle becomes dislodged during the securing (taping) of the needle. The doctor and assistant, unaware of this,

open the rate knob but little or no solution flows. If no solution is flowing, check first the three causes of nonrunning IVs discussed. If the drip rate is extremely slow and cannot be increased, look at the site where the needle tip is located beneath the patient's skin. If the needle has left the vein and fluid is still flowing, a small colorless swelling will develop at this site. This is termed an "infiltration."

• • •

In all cases in which an IV drip that was previously running well has either slowed or stopped running entirely, the needle should not be removed from the vein until it has been determined definitely that the needle is no longer within the vein. The following procedure should be followed to determine the cause of the slow or nonrunning IV drip:

1. Open drip rate knob.
2. Elevate bottle. Does flow rate increase?
3. Place bottle below heart level. Does blood return?
4. Check IV site. Is tissue swelling? Does the skin at needle site feel cooler than surrounding tissues? (See Infiltration, p. 436)
5. Elevate wings of needle or straighten patient's arm or wrist, as appropriate. Does flow improve?

Venospasm

Venospasm is a protective mechanism in which the vein wall responds to stimulation from the needle by going into spasm. As the needle approaches the vein, the vein appears to disappear or "collapse." Venospasm is occasionally accompanied by a burning sensation in the immediate area. This burning sensation resolves without treatment. Venospasm may occur before or after entry of the needle into the vein, securing of the needle, and starting of the IV drip.

Prevention

There is no way to prevent venospasm.

Recognition

Venospasm is identified by the disappearance of a vein while attempting venipuncture. A burning sensation may or may not accompany venospasm.

Management

The needle should not be removed from the skin, for the vein has not yet been entered or damaged. The needle is pulled back slightly (1 to 2 mm) and heat applied to the site in an effort to dilate the ves-

sel. When (if) the vein reappears, the venipuncture may be reattempted.

A sensation of burning is associated with several other complications and with one noncomplication. The IV administration of diazepam will occasionally produce a sensation of warmth or burning; however, this sensation will travel up the patient's arm as the drug passes through the veins. Intraarterial injection of a drug produces a burning sensation or pain traveling down the arm toward the fingers. Extravascular injection of a drug produces a burning sensation at the site of injection that remains at the site of administration. The injection of meperidine may cause the release of histamine and a burning or itching sensation along the path of the vein. Venospasm occurs more frequently in apprehensive patients, presumably caused by their higher levels of circulating catecholamines (predisposing to peripheral vasoconstriction).

Hematoma

Hematoma is the most common complication associated with venipuncture. It is the extravasation of blood into the interstitial space surrounding the blood vessel. The presence of blood in this space leads to localized swelling and discoloration.

When venipuncture is successful, the needle itself acts as an obturator, sealing the hole within the vein made during entry of the needle. In some patients, particularly older patients in whom vein walls are less elastic, leakage of blood around the needle may occur during the IV procedure although the needle is still within the vein.

Hematoma may occur at two times during the IV procedure. First, it may develop during the attempt at venipuncture if the vessel is damaged. This is not always preventable. The second cause of hematoma is usually preventable. In this situation the IV procedure has been completed and the needle removed from the vein. Improper application of pressure or inadequate duration of pressure at the venipuncture site can lead to a hematoma.

Recognition

Hematoma is a painless, bluish discoloration under the skin at the site of the needle puncture. It develops during venipuncture attempt or at the conclusion of the IV procedure.

Prevention

It is not always possible to prevent a hematoma during venipuncture, although careful adherence to recommended technique will minimize its occur-

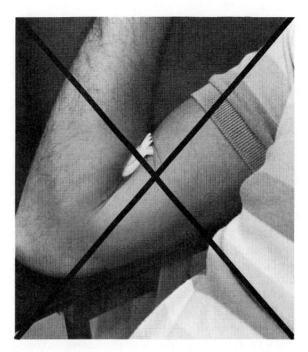

Fig. 28-3. Placing gauze over the injection site and bending the elbow does *not* provide adequate pressure and frequently results in hematoma formation.

rence. Hematoma developing after the procedure can be prevented by the application of firm pressure for a minimum of 5 to 6 minutes. The commonly used technique illustrated in Fig. 28-3 of placing gauze over the venipuncture site in the antecubital fossa and having the patient flex his arm does *not* provide pressure adequate to prevent hematoma.

Management

When *hematoma develops during attempted venipuncture,* the swelling increases rapidly because the tourniquet is still on the patient's arm (increasing blood pressure in the vein). Immediate management consists of the following:

1. Remove the tourniquet to decrease venous blood pressure.
2. Remove the needle from the skin.
3. Apply firm pressure with sterile gauze for 5 to 6 minutes.
4. If the site is tender, ice may be applied in the first few postoperative hours. Ice acts as a vasoconstrictor and as an analgesic.

When *hematoma develops following removal of the IV needle,* immediate management consists solely of direct pressure with gauze and ice. Subsequent management of either form of hematoma can best be described as "tincture of time." It will require approximately 7 to 10 days for the subcutaneous blood to be resorbed by the body. Nothing can be done to speed up this process. Should the patient complain of discomfort or soreness (more likely if the hematoma is located in a joint), he can be advised to use moist heat on the area for 20 minutes every hour. Heat should not be used within the first 4 hours after the onset of the hematoma for it acts as a vasodilator and might induce further bleeding.

Infiltration

Infiltration is similar to a hematoma in that a fluid is being deposited into the tissues surrounding a blood vessel. In fact, a hematoma is actually the infiltration of blood outside of a blood vessel. Extravascular injection of a drug is an infiltration of drug outside of a blood vessel. Infiltration may be defined as a painless, colorless swelling developing at the site of the needle tip when the IV infusion is started.

In this situation we are discussing the deposition of the IV infusion solution into the tissues surrounding the blood vessel. The infiltration discussed here differs from hematoma in that the swelling that develops will not occur until the IV drip is turned on, whereas the hematoma occurs as soon as the vein is punctured.

In the continuous IV infusion technique if infiltration does occur it will only be a solution such as 5% dextrose and water or normal saline, which do not produce any tissue irritation or damage. In contrast, in those IV procedures in which a drug is injected directly into a blood vessel, it is much more likely that the drug will produce tissue damage and/or a delayed onset of sedation if deposited outside the blood vessel.

Prevention

Infiltration can be prevented by careful venipuncture technique and by not starting the IV drip or injecting drugs until it is confirmed that the needle tip lies within the lumen of the vein. Checking for this is quite easy. The flash bulb on the IV tubing may be squeezed and blood will return into the tubing when the pressure is released, or the IV bag may be held below the level of the patient's heart (Fig. 28-4).

Cause

Movement of the metal needle either while it is being secured or through movement of the patient's arm during the sedation procedure may cause the needle to perforate the vein wall and produce an infiltration. The most common causes of a needle's be-

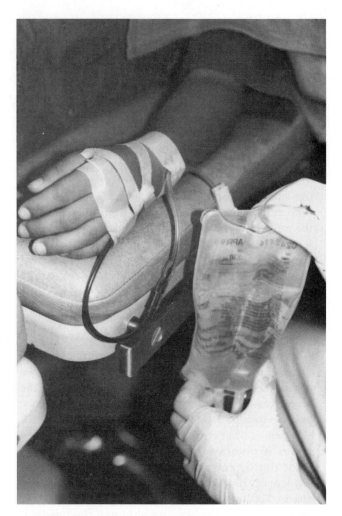

Fig. 28-4. Lowering bag of IV solution *below* level of patient's heart (vein) allows blood to return into tubing from patient.

coming dislodged are (1) attempting to thread (insert) a needle too far into the vein and (2) carelessness during taping of the needle. Infiltration is much less likely to occur when catheters are used for venipuncture.

Recognition

Infiltration is a painless, colorless swelling occurring around the tip of the needle when the IV drip is started. The tissue around the needle tip will be raised and the skin at this site will feel cooler than skin at a distance away from this site. This is because the infusate is at room temperature (72° F), not body temperature.

Management

The IV infusion must be stopped immediately and the needle removed from that site. A 2- × -2-inch gauze is placed at the site and pressure applied for 5 to 6 minutes. Pressure will stop any bleeding as well as spread out any solution within the tissue. This solution will be resorbed into the cardiovascular system. Little or no residual soreness will be noted.

Localized venous complications

Localized venous complications can develop following IV sedation procedures. Many factors are responsible for their development, and indeed there are a number of different clinical expressions that venous complications take. Trauma to the vein wall produced by the needle or cannula is a possible cause of this problem. In the dental outpatient environment the most likely cause of venous complications is chemical irritation of the vein wall produced by the drug being administered, usually diazepam or pentobarbital. Localized venous complications will be discussed further under local complications (see the following section).

Air embolism

Air embolism is a possible, though extremely unlikely, complication of IV sedation. It is best avoided by using a technique that is free of air: eliminating air bubbles from syringes and from the IV tubing prior to the procedure and periodically observing the IV infusion bag to prevent its becoming emptied.

In the highly likely event that one or more small bubbles of air enter into the venous circulation, they will be absorbed quite rapidly by the blood and produce no clinical problem. It is not always possible for all air bubbles to be removed from the IV tubing or syringes, and it is quite probable that they will enter into the venous circulation of the patient. The patient, sighting an air bubble moving slowly down the IV tubing toward his arm, may become quite agitated, thinking that as little as one bubble of air is lethal. Fortunately, this is not so. A rule of thumb in a hospital environment is that a patient can tolerate up to 1 ml/kg of body weight of air in the peripheral venous circulation without adverse effect.[1]

The average IV administration set will hold approximately 13 ml of air.[2] When it is considered that 10 drops of solution (or air) equals 1 ml (adult infusion set), then it can be seen that the chances of introducing large volumes of air into the patient's circulation are quite low. A 50-kg (110-lb) patient can tolerate 50 ml of air. This is equivalent to 750 drops of air from an adult IV administration set.

When managing small children air embolism is a more significant problem, as their bodies cannot tolerate large volumes of air. A 30-lb (13-kg) child is at greater risk of this complication than the larger patient.

Management

Should air embolism occur, management is based on the attempt to prevent this air from entering into the cerebral and pulmonary circulations. This is accomplished by positioning the patient in the dental chair lying on his left side (preventing entry into the pulmonary circulation) and in a head down position (preventing entry into the cerebral circulation).

Overhydration

Overhydration of the patient is not a very common problem during IV sedative procedures in the dental office. The two most likely candidates for overhydration, however, are the patient with congestive heart failure and the child. Signs of overhydration include pulmonary edema, respiratory distress, and an increase in the heart rate and blood pressure. These are also the signs and symptoms occasionally noted in a patient with acute pulmonary edema.

A rule of thumb for replacement of fluid in a patient is that the initial dose of IV solution administered is equal to 1.5 times the number of hours a patient has gone without food times the patient's weight in kilograms.[3] This is the volume of fluid in milliliters required to replace the fluid deficit created by the patient's being **NPO** prior to the procedure. If a patient had taken nothing by mouth for 6 hours prior to coming to the office, the initial volume of milliliters of IV solution administered would be nine times the patient's body weight in kilograms. The maintenance dose of IV solution is 3 ml/kg. The problem of underhydration is not significant in the usual outpatient environment.

When administering IV drugs to pediatric patients, it is recommended that a pediatric infusion set be employed. This set, which permits 60 drops per milliliter instead of the usual 10, allows for a more careful administration of fluids to the younger, smaller patient or to the adult with serious congestive heart failure. In most instances these two classes of patients are not candidates for elective IV sedation procedures in the outpatient setting.

LOCAL COMPLICATIONS OF DRUG ADMINISTRATION
Extravascular drug administration

When a drug is injected into subcutaneous tissues instead of a blood vessel, three problems may develop:

1. Pain
2. Delayed absorption of the drug
3. Tissue damage

Pain associated with extravascular drug administration occurs at the site of the needle tip under the skin and tends to remain localized to that area. This distinguishes extravascular injection from intraarterial and IV injections where a burning sensation will radiate either peripherally or centrally. The patient will complain of discomfort as the drug is being injected in all three situations.

A potentially greater problem is delayed absorption of the drug into the cardiovascular system, especially if larger volumes have been deposited into the tissues. In essence the drug has been administered subcutaneously instead of intravenously. Uptake of the drug is slow with an onset of clinical activity occurring anywhere from about 10 to 30 minutes later.

A third problem that might arise is damage to the tissues into which the drug has been deposited. Some drugs used intravenously are quite irritating to the tissues. This is especially true for diazepam and pentobarbital. The initial reaction in the tissues is for arteriolar and capillary constriction, which decreases the blood supply to the area. If vascular constriction is prolonged or if the chemical is irritating enough, necrosis and sloughing of tissue may occur.

Causes

There are two causes of extravascular drug administration. The first is the needle or cannula slipping out of the vein. This usually leads to an immediate formation of a hematoma that is quickly recognized. No drug is usually injected at this time. The second cause is the needle entering the vein and then being pushed through the other side as the doctor attempts to advance it farther into the vein. Blood will have returned into the tubing as the needle entered the vein originally, thereby giving the impression that the needle is still in the vein. However, with removal of the tourniquet it is unlikely that the blood will leave the tubing, as normally occurs, because the lumen of the needle is no longer in the vein but in subcutaneous tissue. On occasion the blood will reenter the patient and the IV infusion will be running even though the needle tip is no longer in the vein. This will occur when the bag of IV solution is quite high above the patient's heart or if the patient's skin and underlying soft tissues are not "firm," allowing gravity to force the solution into the tissues.

The continuous IV drip technique really minimizes the possibility of extravascular injection of a drug because an infiltration of infusate produces a swelling immediately. Second, prior to administration of any drug it is recommended that the patency of the vein be reconfirmed by squeezing the flash bulb or holding the IV bag below the level of the patient's heart. Despite these precautions, a subtle movement of a patient's wrist or elbow just after this check but just before drug administration can produce this complication if metal needles are used. The administration of a 0.2-ml test dose of a drug is a means of detecting this complication before a larger, potentially more damaging bolus of drug is deposited.

Recognition

As the irritating drug, especially diazepam or pentobarbital, is injected extravascularly, the patient will complain of a more intense pain that occurs at the site of the needle tip and does not migrate up or down the arm. In addition, as a volume of the drug is injected, the tissue at the site of the needle tip will become raised if the solution is being forced into the subcutaneous tissues. If the chemical is irritating, the skin overlying the raised tissue will become ischemic as the blood vessels in the area constrict in response to the irritation. A second possible reaction is for the tissues to become erythematous as a result of inflammation.

Management

The two major problems to be managed are possible delayed absorption of the drug and its effect on the patient and potential damage to the tissues at the site of injection. Management initially consists of removing the needle and the application of pressure at the site of injection to (1) stop the bleeding and (2) disperse the solution deposited under the skin. If less than 1 or 2 ml of drug has been deposited extravascularly, these steps are all that are required for effective management.

In the highly unlikely situation that larger volumes of drug have been deposited extravascularly and the overlying tissue is raised and ischemic, two problems must be addressed: (1) tissue damage and (2) delayed onset sedation. Pressure alone may not be adequate to spread the solution, and drug management may be required. The drug of choice is 1% procaine, a local anesthetic with profound vasodilating properties. Several milliliters of procaine can be infiltrated into the affected tissues, using a single puncture point and a "fan-type" injection. This will increase the rate of drug absorption. A second benefit of the procaine will be to eliminate any discomfort that may be present.

The possible delayed onset of sedation produced by the slow absorption of the drug must be managed symptomatically, with basic life support procedures: maintaining the airway, ventilation, and circulation, implemented, as needed.

In the conscious patient receiving drugs via an IV infusion, it is unlikely that a large volume of drug will be administered extravascularly. If the drug is titrated at the recommended rate of 1 ml per minute, it will become obvious well within a minute that the needle is not in the vein. Further administration of the drug is immediately stopped and the IV patency rechecked.

Intraarterial injection

The most significant of the localized complications of IV sedation is the intraarterial injection of a drug. There are numerous reasons why this serious complication occurs only infrequently. However, when it does occur, immediate and vigorous therapy is indicated in order to prevent tissue damage, gangrene, and possible loss of the limb.[4-8] Drugs injected into an artery produce irritation of the artery wall as the drug is carried peripherally. As the diameter of the artery decreases the drug is increasingly in contact with the artery wall. The immediate response of the artery to this insult is spasm. Arterial spasm, especially if it occurs in one of the larger arteries of the upper limb, as is quite likely in this situation, will compromise the circulation to all, or a large portion, of the tissue distal to the injection site.

Prevention

Prevention is the most important feature in this discussion of intraarterial injections. Fortunately, it is rather difficult to accidentally enter into an artery and even more difficult to accidentally administer a drug into the artery. Many signs and symptoms develop that alert the doctor and assistant to the fact that the needle is not within a vein.

1. The vessel should be palpated prior to venipuncture. *Arteries conduct a pulse that can be palpated **before** the tourniquet is placed on the patient's arm.* Once the tourniquet is in place the artery may not pulsate and the doctor may mistake this vessel for a vein. This is especially likely to happen on the medial aspect of the antecubital fossa where the brachial artery lies somewhat superficial.

2. As the needle approaches the arterial wall the vessel will begin to spasm. Arterial spasm is much more intense than venospasm and is associated with a more intense burning sensation. For this reason alone it is usually very difficult to accidentally (and on many occasions even purposefully) enter into an artery.

3. If the needle enters the artery (or any vessel, for that matter), blood will return into the IV tubing. With the tourniquet in place the return of blood will be similar to that seen in venipuncture; however, the color of the blood is different. Arterial blood is a brighter cherry red, whereas venous blood is a darker maroon color.

4. On removal of the tourniquet a significant difference is noted. Venous blood leaves the IV tubing when the tourniquet is released (lowering the venous blood pressure [to 4 to 6 mm Hg] in the arm) and the IV drip started. Following removal of the tourniquet arterial blood with a much higher blood pressure (e.g., 120/80 mm Hg) will remain in the IV tubing and demonstrate a pulsatile flow with every contraction of the heart.

To this point, nothing damaging has been done to the patient or the artery. If the intraarterial puncture is noted at this time, the needle is carefully removed and firm pressure exerted over the site for at least 10 minutes. If, however, a drug is injected into the artery, problems may develop rapidly.

Recognition

There are a number of signs and symptoms associated with intraarterial injection of a drug:

1. The patient will complain of a severe pain that radiates distally from the site of injection of the drug toward the hand and fingers.

2. The radial pulse should be checked. Absence of the radial pulse indicates that the arterial spasm is quite severe and that immediate management is essential. Presence of the radial pulse, even though it may be quite weak, indicates that at least some arterial blood is entering the hand and fingers. A serious problem may still exist, but it is not as acute.

3. The skin color of the affected hand should be compared with that of the opposite hand. Lack of blood flow into the affected limb will produce a loss of normal skin color. A paler color or a mottled appearance may be noted initially.

4. Both limbs should be felt to determine temperature. The flow of blood to the hand provides

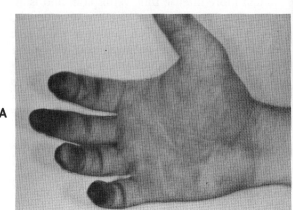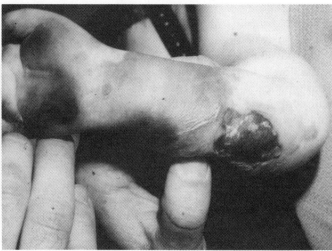

Fig. 28-5. A, Gangrenous fingers secondary to intraarterial drug administration. **B**, Gangrene of forearm, hand, and fingers.

warmth. When blood flow to the limb is compromised, that limb will feel cooler than the opposite limb with normal blood flow.

The major cause of injury from intraarterial injection is chemical endarteritis that results in thrombosis and ischemia. Crystals of the drug precipitate as a result of the change in pH leading to further occlusion of vessels. The result of this ranges from small areas of gangrene to the loss of fingers or a limb (Fig. 28-5).

Management

Management of intraarterial injection is best achieved by the following steps:

1. *Leave the needle in place.* Do not remove the intraarterial needle that has been accidentally placed. It provides an avenue for the administration of the drug used in management of this situation.
2. *Administer procaine.* Slowly inject 1% procaine, to a volume of between 2 and 10 ml, into the artery. Procaine serves four functions at this time:
   a. Anesthetic, to decrease pain
   b. Vasodilator, to break the arterial spasm and initiate return of blood flow
   c. pH about 5, counterbalance for drugs with alkaline pH (pentobarbital)
   d. Diluent, decreasing the concentration of the previously administered IA drug

Procaine frequently breaks the arterial spasm, noted by a return of color and warmth to the limb, as well as a return of a pulse wave equal in strength to that of the opposite limb.

3. *Hospitalize the patient.* All patients having had accidental intraarterial drug administration should be seen in the emergency department of a hospital where a vascular surgeon or anesthesiologist will be consulted. The doctor should accompany the patient to the hospital so that the physicians can be advised of the drug(s) administered intraarterially and the treatment rendered. Additional treatment may also be deemed necessary. Such treatment may consist of a sympathetic nerve block, such as stellate ganglion block or brachial plexus block. Where indicated, general anesthesia or surgical endarterectomy may be required. Heparinization may be employed, if needed, to prevent further thrombosis. If all modalities of treatment fail to return an effective blood flow to the limb, amputation of gangrenous parts may be required. Hyperbaric oxygen is frequently used to force oxygen into the tissues when IA spasm is not readily broken by the above procedures.[9]

The intraarterial injection of a drug is a serious complication that should not occur if basic concepts of venipuncture and IV drug administration recommended in earlier chapters of this section are followed. In the unlikely situation that IA drug administration does occur, management as described above is recommended, followed by accurate record

---

INTRAARTERIAL INJECTION

Prevention

Palpate vessel prior to placing tourniquet
Avoid anatomically risky areas (e.g., median antecubital fossa), if possible

Recognition

Intense pain during venipuncture attempt
Bright cherry red blood
Pulsating flow of blood in IV tubing when tourniquet is removed
Intense pain radiating down arm toward fingers as drug is injected
Loss of color in limb
Loss of warmth in limb
Loss or weakening of radial pulse in limb

---

keeping and contacting the doctor's insurance carrier immediately.

Local venous complications

Following a successful IV sedation procedure, the patient is discharged home. The patient may feel fine through the next day only to find, 2 days after the procedure, that the hand in which the needle and drug were placed is swollen, red, hot, and painful.

The general category of local venous complications is being used here because of the multiple names given to the situation being discussed.

Phlebitis is the inflammation of a vein.

Thrombophlebitis is a condition in which inflammation of the vein wall has preceded the formation of a thrombus (blood clot).

Phlebothrombosis is the presence of a clot within a vein, unassociated with inflammation of the wall of the vein.

Gelfman and Driscoll[10,11] have reported on several prospective and retrospective studies of the problem of local venous complications. Criteria that they established for identification of these entities were:

Thrombophlebitis—pain, induration, and a delay in onset of these symptoms

Phlebothrombosis—a condition of venous thrombosis without inflammation; occurs much more immediately, and pain is not a prominent feature

It appears that the primary problem developing after IV sedation is thrombophlebitis. Clinical features of thrombophlebitis include:

Edema
Inflammation
Tenderness
Delayed onset: 24 to 48 hours, may develop up to a week after venous insult

Causes of thrombophlebitis

Anything that produces either mechanical or chemical irritation of a vein is capable of inducing thrombophlebitis. Among the factors involved in the development of thrombophlebitis are the following:

pH of the infusion liquid
Components of the infusate
pH of the drug(s)
Duration of the IV infusion
Mechanical factors:
    Bevel and dullness of needle
    Technique of venipuncture
    Improper fixation of needle
    Size of needle in relation to vein lumen
    Type of needle (metal vs. plastic catheter)
    Presence of infection or disease
    Age and sex of the patient
    Site of venipuncture

• • •

IV solutions, be they infusions or drugs, that have pH values at either end of the spectrum are associated with a greater incidence of venous complications.

Some of the drugs injected intravenously have vehicles, such as propylene glycol and alcohol, that are irritating to vein walls. Diazepam is an example of a drug containing such a vehicle (propylene glycol). It was mentioned earlier in this section that some patients experience pain on the IV administration of diazepam. Gelfman and Driscoll[11] reported that in patients experiencing such discomfort on injection, the incidence of phlebothrombosis, but not thrombophlebitis, was increased.

The duration of the IV infusion is not as great a concern in outpatient sedation as it is within the hospital, where an IV infusion may be required for days at a time. It is common practice within hospitals for an IV team to change the site of the infusion every few days, thereby minimizing the risk of local venous complications.

Improper technique, use of dull needles (highly unlikely with disposable needles), and improper fixation of the needle are mechanical causes of irritation. A needle that is not well secured will continually irritate the walls of the vein.

Placement of a very large needle within the lumen of a smaller vein will potentially produce greater irritation and an increased risk of thrombophlebitis. As recommended in this section, the 21-gauge needle will not impinge on the walls of any vein within the upper limb.

The site of venipuncture is also a factor. Venipuncture of the femoral or saphenous veins of the leg is associated with a higher incidence of thrombophlebitis and thromboembolism. There are significantly fewer complications with the superficial veins of the arm and the dorsum of the hand. Within the upper limb, there are differences in the incidence of thrombophlebitis. Nordell et al.[12] reported five cases of thrombophlebitis in 52 patients. The following is a summary of the site of venipuncture and incidence of thrombophlebitis:

Site	Number of venipunctures	Number of cases of thrombophlebitis	% of thrombophlebitis
Hand, wrist	26	3	11.5
Forearm	15	2	13.33
Antecubital fossa	11	0	0

Other studies have demonstrated similar statistics. Chambiras found a twofold increase in the incidence of venous complications in the hand when compared to the antecubital fossa.[13]

Prevention

It is not always possible to prevent local venous irritation when one of the factors responsible for its development is mechanical irritation produced by the venipuncture or the needle being used. Fortunately the superficial veins of the upper limb are less likely to suffer serious postinjection complications than are the veins of the leg. Prevention is based on the following:

Use of sharp, sterile needles
Atraumatic, sterile venipuncture technique
Securing the needle firmly in position
Injecting IV drugs slowly into a rapid infusion
Dilution of IV drugs whenever possible
When dilution is not possible (diazepam, propofol), use of larger veins (antecubital fossa and forearm)

Recognition

The patient is usually asymptomatic for 1 or more days after the IV procedure. The inflammatory process requires approximately 24 to 48 hours to fully develop, and at that time the patient usually contacts the office complaining of soreness, (possibly) swelling, redness of the area, and (possibly) warmth.

Management

Management of any localized venous complication requires that the patient return to the office for evaluation. The doctor should examine the patient to determine the nature and the extent of the situation. All findings are recorded in the patient's chart and the patient is examined regularly until the situation resolves. The key to successful management is patient cooperation and satisfaction.

Management of thrombophlebitis includes the following:

1. Activity in the limb must be limited through the use, if possible, of a sling.
2. The affected limb must be elevated whenever possible.
3. Moist heat must be applied for 20 minutes three to four times a day.
4. Should thrombophlebitis occur in a joint (elbow or wrist), immobilization is more difficult but should still be attempted. Constant movement of the affected area leads, in some patients, to increased discomfort. Management of pain consists of the administration of antiinflammatory analgesics (NSAIDs) such as aspirin, every 4 to 6 hours as needed for pain.
5. Anticoagulants and antibiotics are *not* part of the usual therapy and will not be required unless the situation deteriorates. By this time, however, the patient will have been referred to a physician (vascular surgeon) for definitive management.

In the usual course of events, the acute phase, involving tenderness, swelling, and discomfort, resolves within a few days, gradually leading to a chronic phase in which the discomfort is gone but the vein remains hard and knotty. This may occur at the site of the venipuncture or anywhere along the path of this vein and its tributaries. The extent of these lumps and bumps will subside over time. Treatment of choice during this phase is tincture of time.

The patient is seen in the office on a less and less frequent basis as the situation resolves. Records are maintained of the findings at each visit. In most cases full resolution is noted within 3 to 4 weeks, although cases have been reported in which patients have suffered lingering tenderness for over 3 years (wrist vein).

In the unlikely event that fever or malaise develops, consultation with a vascular surgeon (the person most likely to be familiar with the management of this complication) is recommended. In any situation in which a patient is being referred for medical (or dental) consultation it is recommended that the referring doctor speak with the physician (discussing management of the case) before the patient is seen. Another clinical indication for referring of this patient to a physician is patient dissatisfaction. If the patient expresses doubt over the doctor's handling of the problem (after all, this is no longer a dental problem), immediate consultation with an appropriate physician is recommended.

Management of phlebothrombosis, which is a small painless nodule located at the site of venipuncture, is essentially the same as that described for thrombophlebitis:

1. Immobilization of the affected limb
2. Moist heat applied to area
3. Tincture of time

Virtually all cases of local venous complications resolve within a short period of time without residual effects.

GENERAL DRUG-RELATED COMPLICATIONS

In this section systemic reactions brought about through the administration of IV drugs will be discussed.

Nausea and vomiting

The incidence of nausea and vomiting associated with IV conscious sedation is quite low. However, the potential does exist for some of the drugs being administered to produce this problem. Among the drugs recommended for use via the IV route, the opioids are most likely to induce nausea and vomiting. Promethazine and scopolamine, which possess antiemetic properties, are among those drugs least likely to produce nausea and vomiting.

Causes of nausea and vomiting

1. Opioid administration
2. Hypoxia
3. Blood

The potential problem is not in the development of nausea, but in the act of vomiting, especially in the sedated patient. The patient who vomits lying supine in a dental chair facing upward faces the possibility of aspirating vomitus into the trachea and suffocating on the vomitus. The fact that a patient has received a CNS depressant drug only increases this risk because their protective reflexes may be depressed.

As mentioned, it is the general category of opioids in which the incidence of vomiting is greatest. The production of nausea and vomiting related to opioid usage is a dose-related response. The greater the dose of the opioid, the higher the incidence of nausea and vomiting. In the dosages recommended in Chapters 26 and 27, the incidence of vomiting has proved to be virtually zero. When I first began the clinical use of nalbuphine, it was employed in doses greater than those currently recommended. Five of the first 10 patients receiving nalbuphine either became nauseous or vomited later that same day. Decreasing the dosage of the drug has eliminated this as a significant problem.

The incidence of vomiting following opioid administration is increased in ambulatory patients compared with hospitalized, nonambulatory patients.[14] Patients receiving very large doses of opioids during general anesthesia do not have as high an incidence of postoperative vomiting, whereas patients undergoing ambulatory surgery and receiving significantly lower doses of opioids have a greater incidence of vomiting. This increased rate of vomiting is related to the more frequent changes of body position that occur in the ambulatory patient. Unfortunately this is a fact of life with which we must live. Happily, however, when opioid dosages are kept within the limits recommended herein, the incidence of this complication is extremely low.

Management of nausea

Should nausea develop while still in the dental office the patient can be placed back in the dental chair and O_2 administered. This alone usually leads to recovery. Hypoxia is a common cause of nausea. Since recommending that nasal O_2 be administered routinely during IV sedation we have seen a virtual disappearance of nausea in our patient population in the dental office.

If nausea develops after discharge of the patient from the office, postoperative instructions suggest that the patient lie down for awhile and drink a cola beverage if it is available, as this may settle his stomach.

Management of vomiting

Should nausea progress to vomiting when the patient is at home, the most important thing for the patient to remember is that he should not be lying on his back, as the possibility of aspiration of vomitus is greater in this position. This is one of the reasons for strict adherence to the recommendation that the patient be able to manage himself at home before being discharged from the office.

If vomiting should occur during dental treatment (a situation that has only occurred once in over 3000 cases at USC) the airway must immediately be cleared of all dental equipment. Turn the patient's head to the side (away from the operator) so that the vomitus pools on one side of the mouth leaving a patent airway. Suction is then applied so that the remaining vomitus may be removed.

Localized allergy

It is not uncommon for a patient receiving IV drugs to mention that the skin at the site of injection is itching. There may be a localized or diffuse reddening of the tissues. Several possibilities exist as to the cause of this reaction.

The opioid agonist meperidine induces the localized release of histamine. As the drug enters and travels up the vein toward the heart, a red line tracing the course of the vein may be noted (Fig. 28-6). The patient may mention that his arm is itching. *Histamine release is a normal pharmacological property of meperidine and does not represent allergy.* Within 5 to 10 minutes this response will resolve by itself. Treatment is usually not required. If the itching is intense then IV administration of an antihistamine such as diphenhydramine or chlorpheniramine should be considered.

Less frequently it will be observed that the skin around the site of the needle is diffusely erythematous with raised areas noted. The word "blotchy" may appropriately be used to describe its appearance. The site may burn or be quite itchy. The reaction is localized to the immediate area but is not as localized to the path of the blood vessels as is the meperidine-induced histamine reaction. The most frequently observed cause of this type of localized allergic response is the adhesive on the tape used to secure the needle. Many persons are allergic to the adhesives used on tape. The erythematous reaction will appear to be located around the tape. Management of this situation dictates the IV administration of an antihistamine, either diphenhydramine or chlorpheniramine. The use of hypoallergenic tape will prevent recurrence of this reaction.

If the allergic response appears to be more directly related to drug administration, treatment need be more vigorous and more immediate. The chemical mediators of allergy that are released from mast cells into the venous circulation in response to the anti-

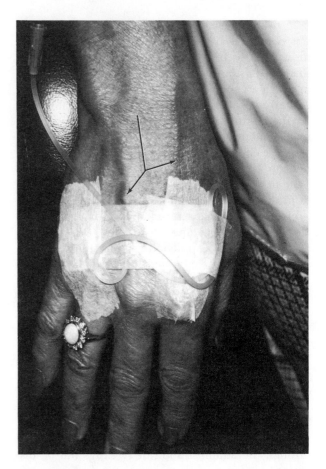

Fig. 28-6. Meperidine-induced localized histamine release along path of vein *(dark lines on wrist)*.

genic challenge will be traveling toward the heart and may soon involve the entire body in the reaction—the skin and respiratory and cardiovascular systems. Management of this potentially life-threatening reaction involves placing a tourniquet high on the patient's arm as soon as the reaction is noted. This will prevent or at least slow the development of a generalized reaction. If the reaction is still limited to the limb, parenteral administration of an antihistamine is recommended; however, once the reaction becomes more generalized, 3 to 5 ml of a 1:10,000 epinephrine solution is administered intravenously, followed by antihistamine administration.

Prevention of allergic reactions is greatly preferred to their management. Prevention is based on a careful pretreatment discussion of the patient's prior allergic history and response to the drugs being administered. The patient should be questioned about any previous reactions to adhesive tape. In addition, the 0.2-ml test dose recommended for all drugs will aid in determining whether or not allergy is present. Although the administration of a dose as small as 0.2 ml of an allergen can, in some cases, induce anaphylactic or anaphylactoid reactions, in most circumstances the observed reaction will be less severe and management can proceed as previously described.

Respiratory depression

Morbidity and mortality from IV sedation has usually been related to the presence of respiratory depression that went undetected and led to respiratory arrest, cardiac dysrhythmias, and cardiac arrest.

All of the sedative drugs discussed in this book are respiratory depressants (though to varying degrees at therapeutic doses). All are capable, in some doses and in some patients, of producing respiratory arrest. Respiratory depression is a more significant problem with certain drugs groups, primarily the opioid agonists and the barbiturates.

Respiratory depression occurring after drug administration is a dose-related response. Smaller doses of the drug produce little or no respiratory depression in the "average (middle of the bell-shaped curve) patient"; however, increasing the dosage of the drug increases its CNS depressant effects and leads ultimately to respiratory depression.

Respiratory depression may occur following extremely low doses of any drug if the patient lies on the hyperresponding slope of the bell-shaped curve. Unfortunately there is little that can be done prior to drug administration to determine this fact. The patient can be questioned as to his usual response to drugs, such as analgesics and tranquilizers (e.g., oral diazepam). A response from a patient who mentions falling asleep after one 2-mg Valium tablet should alert the doctor to the possibility of hyperresponsiveness to benzodiazepines. The 0.2-ml test dose, followed by a wait of 30 seconds before administering any additional drug, is another means of discovering a patient's hypersensitivity to a drug. One other means of accounting for variations in patient response to drugs is titration. Always titrate drugs to clinical effect, if titration is possible. When this is done, oversedation and respiratory depression following IV drug administration should not occur, or will do so only infrequently. The drug doses recommended in Chapters 26 and 27 will provide effective sedation with little or no respiratory depression in the typical patient.

The two drug categories most likely to produce respiratory depression are the opioid analgesics and

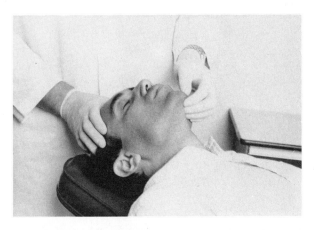

Fig. 28-7. Airway maintenance employing head-tilt, chin-lift.

barbiturates. Opioid-induced respiratory depression is characterized by a decrease in the rate of breathing. The adult respiratory rate, normally between 14 to 18 breaths per minute, may decrease to 5 or 6 deeper breaths per minute. Barbiturate-induced respiratory depression is characterized by a more rapid but shallower respiratory effort than that seen with opioids.

Management of respiratory depression

The initial steps in management of respiratory depression are universal, regardless of the cause of the problem. These are the steps of basic life support.

1. If not already in the supine position, the patient is placed in this position immediately. The patient's feet are elevated slightly (10 to 15 degrees) to aid the return of venous blood to the heart.
2. Probably the most important step in basic life support is maintenance of a patent airway. This is accomplished through head-tilt, chin-lift (Fig. 28-7). Proper performance of this step elevates the tongue from the hypopharynx, providing a patent airway in most circumstances.
3. The doctor or assistant performing the previous step places his or her ear about 1 inch from the patient's mouth and nose, looking at the patient's chest, while listening and feeling for air exiting the patient's mouth and nose and watching the patient's chest for signs of spontaneous ventilatory efforts (Fig. 28-8).
4. In the likely event that the patient is breathing spontaneously but the rate and depth are depressed, the rescuer must assist or control the

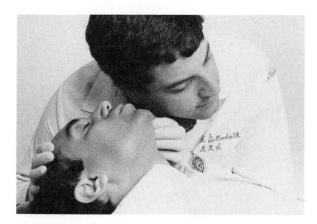

Fig. 28-8. Look, listen, and feel while checking for respiration and airway patency.

patient's breathing. Using a positive pressure O_2 device (Robertshaw or Elder valve) (Fig. 28-9) or a self-inflating bag-valve-mask device (Ambu bag) (Fig. 28-10), the rescuer inflates the patient's lungs every time a spontaneous respiration is attempted. If the patient's respiratory rate is less than 8 per minute, the rescuer will increase the rate of breathing by interposing a controlled ventilation between each of the spontaneous attempts by the patient. The self-inflating bag-valve-mask device is not recommended for use in larger-sized adults unless a reservoir bag is added. It is, however, recommended for use in children.

5. The carotid pulse is checked to determine the functional status of the cardiovascular system. If respiratory depression is recognized early, the carotid pulse will still be strong and regular.
6. If respiratory depression has occurred following opioid administration (either as a sole drug or as one of a combination), an opioid antagonist should be administered to the patient.
Naloxone is currently the drug of choice for reversing opioid-induced respiratory depression. Nalbuphine has been employed with great success; however, more study of this drug is required before it can be recommended for this function.[15] Naloxone should be diluted from its original 0.4 mg/ml concentration by adding 3 ml of diluent (5% dextrose and water, normal saline), producing a 0.1 mg/ml concentration for injection. The patient is continually observed for signs of increased respiration while 0.1 mg (1 ml) is slowly administered every minute. In most cases less than 0.4 mg naloxone

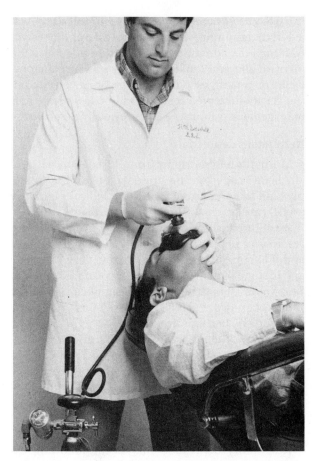

Fig. 28-9. Assisted or controlled ventilation using a positive pressure demand device.

will be required to reverse respiratory depression. In the not too distant past, naloxone was administered in 0.4-mg increments. It was found, however, that larger doses of naloxone also antagonize the analgesic properties of the opioid. If the patient had undergone a painful procedure (e.g., abdominal surgery), the removal of the analgesic actions of the opioid led to an acute onset of pain, which is a significant stimulus to the heart and cardiovascular system. This led to life-threatening emergencies in patients with prior histories of cardiovascular disease.[16] Slow titration of 0.1 mg per minute minimizes this reaction. During the time between the administration of naloxone and its onset of action, the steps of basic life support must be continued.

7. With the return of more rapid and deep respiration the patient begins to look and feel considerably better. He may be unaware of what has

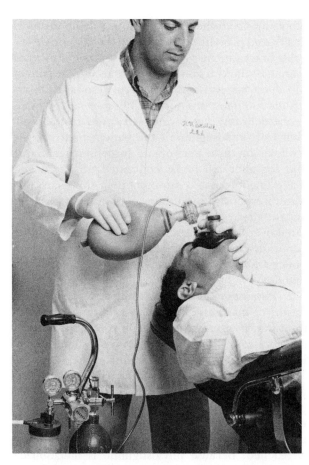

Fig. 28-10. Assisted or controlled ventilation using a self-inflating bag-valve-mask device.

transpired for he has been deeply sedated during this period of time. Dental treatment may be halted, but the patient should not be discharged from the office at this time. Naloxone is a rapid-acting respiratory depressant; however, its duration of action following IV administration is fairly short. It is therefore possible, though unlikely, for respiratory depression to recur approximately 30 minutes after the initial dose of naloxone was given. With the use of the shorter-acting opioids, fentanyl, alfentanil, and sufentanil, this is less likely to occur. When meperidine, pentazocine, morphine, and butorphanol are administered, the likelihood increases. The patient should remain in the office, in a monitored recovery area, for at least 1 hour after the administration of naloxone. Following the initial dose of naloxone and the recovery of the patient, it is recommended by many

persons that 0.4 mg naloxone be administered intramuscularly. The duration of clinical action of IM naloxone is considerably longer than that of IV naloxone, thereby minimizing the risk of recurrence of respiratory depression.

Respiratory depression that is not produced by opioids is not reversible with naloxone administration. The barbiturates are the other drug group most likely to produce respiratory depression. Management of nonopioid-induced respiratory depression is based on the steps of basic life support—airway, breathing, and circulation—until the cerebral blood level of the offending drug has been lowered, through redistribution and metabolism, to the point that breathing is no longer depressed. There are no effective antidotal agents for the barbiturates.

Respiratory depression produced by benzodiazepines is much more uncommon within the dosage ranges presented previously. That respiratory depression can occur with these agents was recently brought to the attention of doctors in the United States by a letter from the manufacturer of midazolam that reemphasized this possibility and recommended appropriate measures to minimize or prevent its development.[17] Management is based upon the basic life support techniques described. The IV administration of the benzodiazepine antagonist flumazenil, in an initial dose of 0.2 mg. (2 ml) with subsequent doses administered every 10 minutes as needed (to a maximum dose of 1.0 mg), will reverse the respiratory depression (and other clinical actions of benzodiazepines) more rapidly.

Emergence delirium

A complication known as emergence delirium has been reported following the administration of many CNS depressants, as well as some adjunctive drugs commonly employed intravenously in sedative procedures. The patient's response is one of transient delirium, hallucination, anxiety, or rage that develops at some time during or immediately after the sedative procedure. Very often the response is associated with recall of an upsetting event in the patient's life. Minichetti and Milles[18] reported a case of a 27-year-old patient receiving 7.5 mg IV diazepam, in addition to meperidine, atropine, N_2O-O_2, and local anesthesia for extraction of several teeth. The patient felt quite comfortable and sedated. Following the administration of an additional 2.5 mg diazepam later in the procedure, the patient became progressively more excited. His eyes closed, he began crying, and he would not respond to verbal commands. Attempts were made to communicate with the patient but he would not respond to questioning. He became hyperexcitable and began thrashing about in the dental chair. Removal of the N_2O and administration of 100% O_2 did not resolve the situation, nor did administration of 0.4 mg naloxone. He continued to hallucinate for about 20 minutes, exhibiting rage and anxiety. He recovered gradually, calmed down, and stopped crying, responding to his name. When questioned later about the reaction he said that he had dreamt about an unpleasant experience he had had in Vietnam.

The drugs most likely to produce emergence delirium are scopolamine, diazepam, and midazolam. Other benzodiazepines, such as lorazepam, have been reported to produce emergence delirium too. Scopolamine, however, is far and away the drug most likely to produce emergence delirium.[19]

The reactions associated with emergence delirium are thought to be manifestations of the central anticholinergic syndrome (CAS).[20,21] CAS includes such paradoxical reactions as acute hyperactivity, anxiety, delirium, hallucinations, and recent memory impairment. In its most severe form CAS produces apnea, medullary paralysis, coma, and death, though these reactions are extremely rare. The dose of scopolamine or benzodiazepine required to produce CAS is extremely small; it is not a dose-related phenomenon. Therefore, the doctor administering IV anticholinergics or benzodiazepines must be aware of the CAS, its prevention, and its management.

Prevention

The incidence of CAS and emergence delirium is considerably lower in patients between the ages of 6 and 65 years. For this reason the use of scopolamine is not recommended in patients under 6 and over 65 years of age. Other anticholinergics, such as atropine and glycopyrrolate, which are less likely to produce CAS are recommended in these patients. Fortunately the indication for IV sedation in these two groups of patients is not great. Slow injection of drugs and use of minimal doses may aid in minimizing these reactions.

Management

Management of the usual form of emergence delirium, in which the patient may exhibit dreaming and appears uncomfortable but does not respond to verbal questioning, takes two forms.

1. Symptomatic management. Monitoring of the patient, assurance of a patent airway and adequate blood supply to the brain (both usually no problem at all), and prevention of injury to the patient are the goals of treatment. Given an appropriate time span (variable) the reaction will terminate and the patient will open his eyes and be able to respond to commands and questions normally. In one case of emergence delirium that I witnessed (prior to the availability of physostigmine), the patient had received scopolamine as a part of the Jorgensen technique and for almost 5 hours continued to dream and make uncoordinated movements in the chair. She was unresponsive to questioning but had a very adequate airway and her vital signs were slightly elevated over baseline. Approximately 5 hours after the administration of the scopolamine, the patient opened her eyes and was able to respond to commands.

2. Physostigmine administration. The second means of managing emergence delirium is the administration of physostigmine, a reversible anticholinesterase. IV administration of physostigmine rapidly reverses emergence delirium and the CAS.

The dose of physostigmine for reversal of emergence delirium is 1.0 mg for the 70-kg adult and 0.5 mg for the child, administered intravenously. One milligram may be administered per minute until the reaction is terminated or a maximum dose of 4 mg is reached. Because physostigmine is metabolized within 30 minutes, the patient must be monitored closely to be certain that signs and symptoms do not recur.

Rapid administration of physostigmine is associated with the possible development of bradycardia, hypersalivation, emesis, and defecation.[22]

Laryngospasm

Laryngospasm is a protective reflex of the body. In the fully conscious (non–CNS-depressed) patient, foreign objects are prevented from entry into the airway (trachea) by the swallowing reflex, the epiglottis, and the cough reflex. As a patient becomes more and more CNS depressed through the administration of drugs, these protective reflexes are progressively depressed to an even greater degree. In conscious sedation, as observed with N_2O-O_2, IV diazepam, midazolam, the Jorgensen technique, and IV promethazine, there is but little impairment of these reflexes. Foreign material such as water and scraps of dental material will be easily removed by the patient as he spits or swallows. Aspiration is not a common occurrence with these techniques of conscious sedation. However, as the level of CNS depression increases through the addition of other drugs or increased doses of the same drugs, the protective reflexes are depressed to a greater degree.[23]

In stage two, ultralight general anesthesia, foreign material present in the area of the larynx will provoke a protective reflex in which the vocal cords adduct in an attempt to seal off the trachea from entry of foreign material. Though this truly is a protective reflex, it is obvious that this reflex will also prevent the passage of air into and out of the trachea and lungs (Fig. 28-11). Laryngospasm will not occur in stage one of anesthesia, which we have called sedation or analgesia, because the other protective reflexes are still intact. It is only when the patient enters stage two that laryngospasm will occur.

Recognition

Recognition of laryngospasm is based on the presence or absence of sounds. A partial laryngospasm is identified by the presence of stridor, an abnormal high-pitched, musical respiratory sound produced as air is forced out through partially adducted vocal folds. A complete laryngospasm is identified by the absence of sound, an ominous "sound" indeed.

The patient will be attempting to breathe against this partially or completely closed airway. Respiratory efforts will be exaggerated, expansion of the chest greater than usual, and accessory muscles of respiration used. Substernal, supraclavicular, and intercostal soft tissue retraction may be observed (Fig. 28-12). This is the drawing in of the soft tissues overlying the spaces between the ribs and sternum as the chest expands and intrathoracic pressure becomes more negative. Soft tissue retraction is a sign of a partially or totally obstructed airway.

Management

1. The first step in managing laryngospasm is the *removal of any offending material from the patient's airway.* A large-diameter suction tip or a tonsil suction is placed into the pharynx to remove any material it finds. This step alone will break the spasm in most cases.
2. *Positive pressure O_2* is administered, either via the self-inflating bag-valve-mask device or positive pressure-demand valve. Very often it is possible to break the spasm by forcing O_2 past the vocal cords. Steps 1 and 2 are highly recommended.
3. Drug administration. The *administration of drugs to terminate laryngospasm is never recommended unless the doctor is well trained in anesthesiology and in management of the apneic patient.* The drug of choice is succinylcholine, a short-acting depolarizing muscle relaxant. Administered in a con-

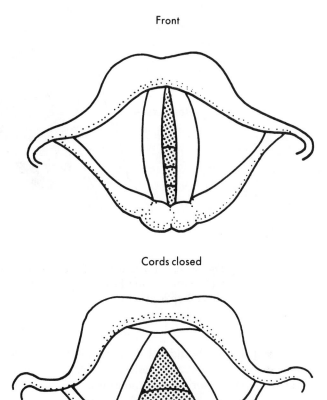

Front

Cords closed

Cords open

Fig. 28-11. View of vocal cords. *Top,* Cords are adducted (closed), thus preventing foreign material and air from entering trachea. *Bottom,* Cords abducted. (From Shibel EM, Moser KM: *Respiratory emergencies.* St Louis, 1977, Mosby.)

centration of 20 mg/ml, an IV dose of 20 to 40 mg is usually adequate to break laryngospasm by paralyzing the muscles of respiration. At this point, however, the patient is no longer breathing and the doctor is responsible for instituting controlled ventilation for the period of 3 to 4 minutes until the typical patient resumes spontaneous ventilation.[24]

4. If no drugs were administered during laryngospasm, the level of CO_2 in the patient's blood would increase, the level of consciousness would decrease, and the laryngospasm would break spontaneously. Though this technique of managing laryngospasm is acceptable, it is not recommended for the untrained doctor.

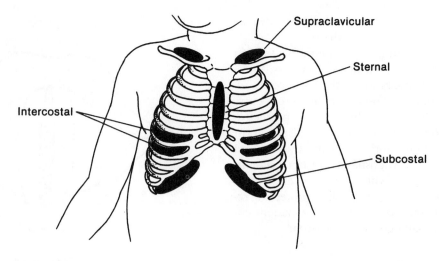

Fig. 28-12. Retractions associated with respiratory distress: intercostal, suprasternal, subcostal, and sternal. (From Eichelberger MR et al: *Brady pediatric emergencies,* Englewood Cliffs, NJ, 1992, Prentice-Hall.)

Laryngospasm should not develop if lighter levels of sedation are maintained and if the airway is kept free of debris, water, blood, and saliva.

SPECIFIC DRUG COMPLICATIONS
Benzodiazepines

The most commonly seen complications associated with diazepam and midazolam administration are the following:
1. Local venous complications (diazepam only)
2. Emergence delirium
3. Recurrences of amnesia (diazepam only)
4. Oversedation

Local venous complications and *emergence delirium* have been discussed previously. The *recurrence of amnesia* following diazepam administration has only occurred twice in my experience over 20 years; however, it was this phenomenon that caused me to decrease the recommended dose of diazepam used for sedation.

Two patients received diazepam, one a dose of 45 mg and the other a dose of 38 mg, and achieved clinically ideal sedation lasting for the usual 45 minutes. Recovery was normal, the patients appearing unsedated after 1 hour. It was later reported that for the first 24 hours after they left the clinic (these cases were done at different times and on different days) their recovery was normal. However, in both cases, approximately 24 hours later the patients experienced a relapse of amnesia. One patient had driven to work, parked his car, and entered his office build-

ing when suddenly he did not remember where he was, how he had gotten there, or what day it was. Within a few minutes the patient's memory returned. No further relapses occurred. The same type of response occurred in the second patient. I am unaware of similar responses developing in patients who have received less than 30 mg of diazepam at a single treatment, thus the recommendation that this dose not be exceeded as a total for one treatment session.

Oversedation is not likely to develop with diazepam or midazolam if the drug is titrated at the recommended rate of 1 ml per minute. However, if a patient becomes oversedated, management is to ensure a patent airway and ventilation. Within a few minutes redistribution of the drug will lead to a lessening of the level of sedation and increased responsiveness. The administration of flumazenil will speed recovery.[25,26]

Pentobarbital

The most common problems associated with pentobarbital administration are *oversedation* and *respiratory depression.* Management of both situations requires implementation, as needed, of basic life support: airway, breathing, and circulation. There are no antidotal drugs that can be administered to reverse barbiturate-induced oversedation or respiratory depression. Unfortunately, because of the prolonged duration of action of pentobarbital, it may take 30 minutes to an hour for the patient to become considerably more responsive.

Promethazine

Promethazine-related complications include *over-sedation* and *extrapyramidal reactions*. Oversedation is managed through basic life support. There is no effective antidote for promethazine-induced oversedation or respiratory depression. Extrapyramidal reactions, though quite rare, do develop following promethazine administration. Four types of reaction are identified: akathisia (motor restlessness), acute dystonias, parkinsonism, and tardive dyskinesias. These are described in Chapter 8. Management requires administration of IV diphenhydramine, 50 mg for the adult and 25 mg for the child.

Opioids

The major side effects of opioid administration are *nausea and vomiting, respiratory depression,* and *rigid chest*. The first two complications are discussed earlier in this chapter.

Rigid chest is an uncommon phenomenon that has been observed primarily following administration of fentanyl but can develop with any opioid.[27-30] It is most commonly seen when N_2O-O_2 has been administered concomitantly.[31] In this situation the skeletal muscles of the thorax appear to be paralyzed and inflation of the chest is impossible. The cause of rigid chest is unknown. The patient will be unable to breath. Efforts to force air into the patient will prove futile as the chest will not expand. The chest has a firm boardlike feel during this reaction. Management of rigid chest involves the following:

1. The airway is supported and an attempt is made to force O_2 into the lungs.
2. IV succinylcholine 20 to 40 mg is administered (only recommended for those trained in anesthesiology).
3. Following the release of the rigid chest (caused by the actions of succinylcholine), the patient will be apneic for approximately 3 to 5 minutes during which time controlled ventilation is absolutely necessary.

Rigid chest has been observed in conjunction with the fentanyl and N_2O combination. Use of this combination is therefore not recommended for routine use in outpatient sedation procedures. The use of combinations of techniques will be discussed in Chapter 29.

Scopolamine

The major problem associated with scopolamine administration is emergence delirium, which was discussed earlier.

Table 28-1. Percentage of doctors who have witnessed IV complications*

	Malamed (n = 114)		Trieger (n = 117)	
	no.	%	no.	%
Hematoma	39	34.2	32	27.0
Infiltration	38	33.3	41	35.0
Pain on injection	29	25.4	50	42.0
Hyperexcitement	29	25.4	11	9.0
Thrombophlebitis	28	24.5	24	20.0
Prolonged sedation	19	16.6	12	10.0
Vomiting	16	14.0	8	6.0
Hypotension	12	10.5	11	9.0
Apnea	1	0.8	0	0.0
Arterial injection	0	0.0	3	2.5

From Malamed SF: *Anesth Prog* 28:158, 1981.
*The statistics illustrate the *number of doctors* who have seen the complication listed, not the *number of times* they have seen it occur. Therefore, a doctor may have seen one case of vomiting in 5000 IV procedures, but since 16 of the 114 reporting doctors reported at least 1 case of vomiting, it is listed as a 14% incidence.

SUMMARY

Complications do occur during IV sedation. Trieger[31] and Malamed[32] conducted independent surveys of doctors having completed their basic IV sedation programs to determine which complications did in fact develop most often. The following chart presents their findings (Table 28-1).

REFERENCES

1. Woodring JH, Fried AM: Nonfatal venous air embolism after contrast-enhanced CT, *Radiology* 167(2):405, 1988.
2. Trieger NT: *Pain control,* ed 2. St Louis, 1994, Mosby.
3. Philip JH: Intravenous access and delivery principles. In Rogers MC, Tinker JH, Covino BG et al, eds: *Principles and practice of anesthesiology.* St Louis, 1993, Mosby, p 1191.
4. Engler HS: Gangrenous extremities resulting from intraarterial injections, *Arch Surg* 94:644, 1967.
5. Albo D Jr: Effect of intra-arterial injection of barbiturates, *Am J Surg* 120:676, 1970.
6. Goldsmith D, Trieger N: Accidental intra-arterial injection: a medical emergency, *Anesth Prog* 22:180, 1975.
7. Lynes RFA, Bisset WIK: Intra-arterial thiopentone: inadvertent injection through a cannula on the back of the hand, *Anaesthesia* 24:257, 1969.
8. Topazian RG: Accidental intra-arterial injection: a hazard of intravenous medication, *JADA* 81:410, 1970.
9. Myers RA, Schnitzer BM: Hyperbaric oxygen use, update 1984, *Postgrad Med* 76(5):83, 1984.
10. Gelfman SS, Dionne RA, Driscoll EJ: Prospective study of venous complications following intravenous diazepam and in dental outpatients, *Anesth Prog* 28:126, 1981.

11. Gelfman SS, Driscoll EJ: Thrombophlebitis following intravenous anesthesia and sedation: an annotated literature review, *Anesth Prog* 24:194, 1977.

12. Nordell K, Mogensen L, Nyquist O et al: Thrombophlebitis following intravenous lidocaine infusion, *Acta Med Scand* 192:263, 1972.

13. Chambiras PG: Sedation in dentistry, intravenous diazepam, *Aust Dent J* 17:17, 1972.

14. Watcha MF, White PF: Postoperative nausea and vomiting: its etiology, treatment, and prevention, *Anesthesiology* 77(1):162, 1992.

15. Blaise GA, Nugent M, McMichan JC et al: Side effects of nalbuphine while reversing opioid-induced respiratory depression: report of four cases, *Canad J Anaesth* 37(7):794, 1990.

16. Pallasch TJ, Gill CJ: Naloxone-associated morbidity and mortality, *Oral Surg* 52:602, 1981.

17. Dosing and titration of midazolam (Versed), Letter to doctors, Roche Laboratories, December 1987.

18. Minichette J, Milles M: Hallucination and delirium reaction to intravenous diazepam administration: case report, *Anesth Prog* 29:144, 1982.

19. Olympio MA: Postanesthetic emergence delirium: historical perspective, *J Clin Anesth* 3(1):60, 1991.

20. Schneck HJ, Rupreht J: Central anticholinergic syndrome (CAS) in anesthesia and intensive care, *Acta Anaesth Belg* 40(3):219, 1989.

21. Rupreht J: The central muscarinic transmission during anaesthesia and recovery—the central anticholinergic syndrome, *Anaesth Reanim* 16(4):250, 1991.

22. Physostigmine, drug package insert, Forest Pharmaceuticals, 1993.

23. Odom JL: Airway emergencies in the post anesthesia care unit, *Nurs Clin North Am* 28(3):483, 1993.

24. Roy WL, Lerman J: Laryngospasm in paediatric anaesthesia, *Can J Anaesth* 35(1):93, 1988.

25. Longmire AW, Seger DL: Topics in clinical pharmacology: flumazenil, a benzodiazepine antagonist, *Am J Med Sci* 306(1):49, 1993.

26. Kulka PJ, Lauven PM: Benzodiazepine antagonists: an update of their role in the emergency care of overdose patients, *Drug Safety* 7(5):381, 1992.

27. Klausner JM, Caspi J, Lelcuk S et al: Delayed muscular rigidity and respiratory depression following fentanyl anesthesia, *Arch Surg* 123(1):66, 1988.

28. Vacanti CA, Silbert BS, Vacanti FX: The effects of thiopental on fentanyl-induced muscle rigidity in a human model, *J Clin Anesth* 3(5):395, 1991.

29. Ackerman WE, Phero JC, Theodore GT: Ineffective ventilation during conscious sedation due to chest wall rigidity after intravenous midazolam and fentanyl, *Anesth Prog* 37(1):46, 1990.

30. Sokoll MD, Hoyt JL, Gergis SD: Studies in muscle rigidity, nitrous oxide, and narcotic analgesic agents, *Anesth Analg* 51:16, 1972.

31. Trieger NT: Teaching intravenous sedation: follow-up of 200 dentists, *Anesth Prog* 25:154, 1978.

32. Malamed SF: Continuing education in intravenous sedation, Part 2: complications and non-use, *Anesth Prog* 28:158, 1981.

CHAPTER *29*

Practical considerations

The following are frequently asked questions that relate to IV sedation.

Who can start the IV and administer IV drugs?

Many doctors wish to delegate the duties of venipuncture and drug administration to auxiliary personnel (i.e., dental assistant, registered dental assistant, dental hygienist, registered nurse). Although the Dental Practice Act in each state must be consulted for specific regulations, it is the law in most states that only the doctor (DDS or equivalent, MD, or certified registered nurse anesthetist [CRNA]) may start a venipuncture and administer intravenous drugs. In some states registered nurses (RN) may also perform venipuncture. As was mentioned in Chapter 25, the auxiliary may perform virtually all of the duties relating to the IV sedation procedure except for the act of venipuncture and the administration of drugs.

What if the patient doesn't respond to the maximal dose of the drug?

The manner in which patients respond to drugs differs greatly, as evidenced by the bell-shaped curve. The fact that titration is possible for virtually all intravenously administered drugs (lorazepam being a notable exception) permits us to determine exactly where the patient fits into this curve. Some patients are hyporesponders. For these patients the clinically observed effect of a given drug at its maximal recommended dose is less than ideal or, in fact, may be nonexistent. The most reasonable approach to take, when the maximal dose of a drug has produced inadequate sedation, is to cease further administration of the drug and attempt the planned dental treatment. As mentioned earlier, I have been pleasantly surprised on numerous occasions with the ease with which treatment proceeds on an apparently nonse-

dated patient. If sedation is truly inadequate to permit the dental care to continue at this time, then the patient should be allowed to recover (despite the apparent lack of symptoms), discharged, and rescheduled at a later date for a different drug technique. For patients in whom diazepam has failed to produce adequate sedation, midazolam or the Jorgensen technique has almost always been successful at subsequent visits and vice versa.

Doses of drugs beyond those recommended should not be administered unless training in anesthesiology has been completed. In many cases, persons with this training will not administer additional drugs because the administration of other drugs can only prolong and complicate recovery in the ambulatory outpatient setting.

The drug doses and techniques recommended in this section have withstood the test of time. When used as recommended the success rate of IV sedation approaches 100%. Occasional failures will occur and must be accepted by the doctor. Inability to accept failure requires the doctor to inject larger and larger doses of more and more drugs, a situation fraught with disaster.

Who should escort the patient from the dental office?

On occasion, usually once in a doctor's career, a patient's escort (ride home) will disappear or never show up. If the IV sedation procedure has not yet begun, I strongly urge that the procedure be cancelled unless another suitable escort can be arranged *before the start of the procedure*. It is tempting and natural for the doctor to want go ahead with the IV procedure because of the time which has been allotted in the day's schedule. The doctor must resist such temptation.

Patients receiving diazepam or midazolam will appear quite recovered 1 hour after drug administration. In the absence of an escort, the patient may insist that he is well enough to leave the office unescorted. *This must never be permitted to happen.* Explain to the patient that although he feels recovered he is not. The feeling is similar to that occurring when one has had some alcohol and feels normal but cannot function at a normal capacity.

Alternative patient escorts that may occur to the patient or to you are a taxicab, a bus or train, walking home, or being accompanied by a member of the office staff. None of these alternatives are acceptable. The only person who should be permitted to escort the patient home is a relative or close friend of the patient, a person who can remain with the patient until he has recovered. The dangers involved in these other alternatives are unacceptable. It is good practice for a member of the office staff to contact the patient the day before the scheduled IV procedure to review preoperative instructions, stressing the need for an escort.

What do you recommend when I first introduce IV sedation into my office?

First, members of the office staff, especially chairside assistants, should also attend the IV sedation course, so that they can learn the techniques firsthand. Very often remarks in a lecture can be misconstrued with a very important concept improperly understood. Having several office personnel attending the course will decrease the chance of this occurring.

Second, the introduction of IV sedation into a dental office will disrupt the normal flow of the office, at least temporarily. It is a new technique and must be used many times before it becomes a regular part of the practice routine. Anticipate the extra time required during the first 50 or so cases. This can best be accomplished by scheduling IV cases immediately before lunch time or as the last appointment of the day, so that if they should become delayed the doctor will not have to worry about a reception room filled with waiting patients. As the technique becomes more accepted by the office staff, IV patients can be scheduled earlier in the day when most apprehensive patients are more ideally treated.

I have more trouble with venipuncture than anything else. How can I become more proficient?

The hardest part of learning to do IV sedation is to become proficient in venipuncture. Administering drugs intravenously is easy (if basic rules are followed). However, without a needle placed within a vein, drug administration is impossible.

Practice makes perfect (almost). Unfortunately, most doctors don't wish to practice venipuncture on their patients. There are several possible sources where one may practice the technique of venipuncture. A local hospital or blood bank may welcome volunteers to help draw blood. Volunteering 1 hour a week will greatly improve venipuncture technique.

What about the use of combinations of techniques?

Unless the doctor is experienced in general anesthesia or has extensive experience with IV conscious sedation, the use of some combinations of techniques is contraindicated. These include the combination of IM and IV sedation (absolute contraindication) and the combination of inhalation and IV sedation (relative contraindication).

When N_2O-O_2 is added to IV sedation, the degree of patient monitoring must increase significantly, as the patient may drift in and out of deeper levels of sedation as the stimulation of the treatment changes. Without the training suggested I do not believe that this combination of techniques should be employed.

There are but few indications for the use of IM and IV sedation together. One is the use of an IM injection for the induction of sedation in a disruptive child or handicapped patient, after which an IV line is established and used for the administration of any additional drugs (see Chapters 36 [pedo] and 39 [handicapped]).

Oral sedation can be used effectively with IV sedation providing that the levels of sedation achieved with the oral drugs remain light (see Chapter 8). Oral drugs are administered the night before the appointment and/or immediately (60 minutes) before treatment in order to take the edge off the last few minutes. Oral drugs should not be used for deep sedation. When the IV line is established, as long as the IV drug is titrated, there should be no problem associated with this combination of techniques. Failure to titrate (i.e., administration of a fixed dose of drug) increases the risk of oversedation and respiratory depression or arrest.

Do I have to titrate IV drugs?

Only if you do not want problems. Fixed drug combinations are frequently mentioned in legal depositions where morbidity or mortality has occurred. A statement frequently heard is, "But I gave this same dose of drugs to 10,000 other patients without ever seeing a problem." Unfortunately for patient number 10,001, he was on the hyperresponding side of the bell-shaped curve, and this "usual" dose was an overdose for this patient. Titration is a safety feature that must always be used.

Is intravenous sedation safe?

A very interesting and provocative question. Newspapers publish lurid accounts of deaths occurring in dental offices.[1-3] Frequently these patients have received IV drugs; whether they received IV sedation or general anesthesia is not often stated. If we were to listen to only the newspaper account, we would have to say that intravenously administered drugs are dangerous. The fact of the matter is quite the opposite. When IV sedation is employed *as taught,* it is the safest of all techniques of parenteral drug administration with the exception of inhalation sedation with N_2O-O_2. The degree of control maintained by the administrator over intravenously administered drugs is second only to that available with inhalation sedation.

If the techniques described in this book are followed, and if the doctor does not experiment with increased dosages or administer drugs with which he or she is unfamiliar or unprepared to use, then serious problems will not occur. In a review of deaths in dental offices related to anesthesia (a general term implying the use of drugs of any type), The Dentists Insurance Company of California (TDIC) stated that three factors were present in most instances where death or serious morbidity occurred[4]:

1. Inadequate preoperative evaluation of the patient
2. Lack of knowledge of the pharmacology of the drugs being employed
3. Inadequate monitoring during the procedure

Education of the doctor and staff can eliminate these sources of problems. Though no long-term studies have been published as to morbidity and mortality associated with IV sedation, several papers have been published from which numbers can be extrapolated. Though scientifically not valid, these numbers do illustrate the safety of the basic techniques discussed in this section. Over 3000 IV diazepam, midazolam, and Jorgensen techniques have been completed without any significant complication during the 17 years of the Basic Intravenous Sedation Course at the USC School of Dentistry. In a survey of 188 doctors having completed this course, it was found that they had completed more than 53,664 cases in private practice without any serious complications.[5] After 6 years of presenting a similar course at the University of Oregon, Foreman and Jastak[6] reported that no complications of a serious nature had been encountered during any of their courses. Extrapolating from data presented by Foreman and Jastak, IV sedation has been successfully employed more than 37,960 times by doctors completing their course.

In a 1975 study published in *The Journal of the American Dental Association,* Jastak and Paravecchio[7] analyzed 1331 cases of sedation and reported that "the safety of IV sedation was also good although not quite as complication free as N_2O-O_2. However, as with N_2O-O_2 sedation, there were no incidents of hypoxia, aspiration, laryngospasm, or other serious sequelae." In their conclusion they stated, "The safety and efficacy of intravenous, oral, combination, and especially inhalation sedation given by individuals not formally trained in general anesthesia appears to have been confirmed."

At the Loma Linda School of Dentisty, where IV sedation in dentistry got its start, more than 15,000 Jorgensen techniques have been successfully performed since 1965 without any serious complications.[8]

REFERENCES

1. Maxwell E: Third patient of dentist being probed dies, *Los Angeles Times* 102, February 20, 1983, p 1.
2. Newcomer K: Dentist waited outside while patient died, Denver, *Rocky Mountain News,* August 4, 1992.
3. Marks P: Boy lapses into coma after dental surgery, *New York Times* 142, May 14, 1993, p B5(L).
4. DeJulien LF: Causes of severe morbidity/mortality cases, *CDAJ* 11(2):45, 1983.
5. Malamed SF: Continuing education in intravenous sedation: part 2, complications and non-use, *Anesth Prog* 28:158, 1981.
6. Foreman PA, Donaldson D, Jastak JT et al: Continuing education in intravenous sedation, *Anesth Prog* 29:163, 1982.
7. Jastak JT, Paravecchio R: An analysis of 1331 sedations using inhalation, intravenous, or other techniques, *JADA* 91:1242, 1975.
8. Anderson D: Personal communication, May 1988.

CHAPTER *30*

Guidelines for teaching

Education and experience are the critical elements that make IV sedation safe. New drugs become available almost every year, and it is only through continuing education that it is possible for the doctor to evaluate these drugs properly, many of which are initially marketed as panaceas.

In 1977 the American Dental Association (ADA), American Dental Society of Anesthesiology (ADSA), and the American Association of Dental Schools (AADS) convened a conference at which *Guidelines for Teaching the Comprehensive Control of Pain and Anxiety in Dentistry,* Part III, were developed for a continuing education program.[1,2] These guidelines have undergone periodic revision, most recently in July 1993.[3] Sections of Part III of the guidelines ("Teaching the Comprehensive Control of Pain and Anxiety in a Continuing Education Program") relating to inhalation sedation were presented in Chapter 20. Material pertaining to continuing education in intravenous (IV) sedation is presented here.

In the section on *objectives* of an intensive course in conscious sedation techniques it is stated:

Upon completion of a course in parenteral techniques of conscious sedation, the dentist should be able to:

a. Describe and demonstrate the technique of venipuncture or any other parenteral technique chosen for the patient.

b. Discuss the pharmacology of the drug(s) selected for administration.

c. Discuss the precautions, contraindications, and adverse reactions associated with the drug(s) selected.

d. Administer the selected drug(s) parenterally to dental patients in a clinical setting in a safe and effective manner.

e. List the complications associated with parenteral techniques of sedation.

f. Discuss the prevention, recognition, and management of these complications.

g. Describe a protocol for management of emergencies in the dental office.

h. List the emergency drugs and equipment required for management of life-threatening situations.

i. Discuss the use of these emergency drugs and equipment in specific life-threatening situations.

j. Discuss principles of advanced cardiac life support (ACLS). Certification in ACLS should be encouraged.

k. Demonstrate the ability to manage life-threatening emergency situations, including cardiopulmonary resuscitation.

The following information related to IV sedation programs was presented later in the document in a discussion of *course content:*

Additional course content for parenteral conscious sedation programs should include:

a. Venipuncture: anatomy, armamentarium, and technique.

b. Sterile techniques in intravenous therapy.

c. Prevention, recognition, and management of local complications of venipuncture.

d. Description and rationale for the technique to be employed.

e. Prevention, recognition, and management of systemic complications of intravenous sedation, with particular attention to airway maintenance and support of the respiratory and cardiovascular systems.

f. Abuse potential of parenteral agents.

The *Guidelines* also address the length of the training programs in parenteral conscious sedation:

Parenteral conscious sedation instruction: A minimum of 60 hours of instruction, plus management of at least 20 pa-

456

tients per participant is required to achieve competency in parenteral conscious sedation techniques. Clinical experience in managing a compromised airway is critical to the prevention of life-threatening emergencies. Participants should be provided supervised opportunities for clinical experience to demonstrate competence in management of the airway. Typically, clinical experience will be provided in managing healthy adult patients. Additional supervised experience is necessary to prepare participants to manage children and medically compromised adults. The faculty should schedule participants to return for additional experience if competency has not been achieved in the time allotted.

In recent years several specialty groups within dentistry have developed guidelines for their members that propose standards for the use of sedation. These groups include oral and maxillofacial surgery,[4,5] pediatric dentistry,[6,7] and periodontology.[8]

Until the early 1980s I presented a continuing education program in basic IV sedation that was 5 days in length (35 hours). The success of this course was apparent, as over 75% of doctors participating in the program still employed IV sedation in their practices 1 year after the program.[9,10] In a survey of these doctors it was determined that in no instance did any doctor encounter a serious emergency situation related to the administration of IV medications.[9]

However, because of a number of well-publicized unfortunate occurrences (usually involving doctors who had received little or, more commonly, no formal training in parenteral sedation or general anesthesia), it became more and more obvious that the length and depth of training in these valuable techniques had to be increased so as to enhance patient safety. As of June 24, 1992, 45 states had adopted legislation or regulations that govern the administration of parenteral sedation.[11] In addition, at least three provinces in Canada has enacted similar regulations (Canadian Dental Association, personal communication, 1993).

In some extreme instances a doctor must complete a 1-year residency in anesthesiology to be eligible to administer IV sedation. Other states and provinces have established less restrictive requirements based on the educational and clinical background of the doctor.

The 1- to 2-day short course in IV sedation is a thing of the past. They served only to scare the doctor away from this technique or to create a potentially very dangerous person—*a doctor who thought he knew how to properly administer IV drugs*. Training programs, at all levels of education—doctoral (dental school),

postdoctoral (residency programs), and continuing education—have been expanded to meet the growing needs of the dental profession and the dental patient.[3]

Training in IV sedation, at all three levels, at the University of Southern California School of Dentistry has been expanded to a program involving a minimum of 174 hours. The program includes four modules that must be completed sequentially:

Module 1 consists of four prerequisite courses that must be completed prior to acceptance into module 2. These are courses in physical evaluation (7 hours), emergency medicine (7 hours), monitoring and the use of emergency equipment (7 hours), and basic life support (provider level—C; 7 hours).

Module 2 is a 35-hour program in basic IV sedation at which time venipuncture and basic techniques of IV conscious sedation are presented. Clinical patient management is included in this module.

Module 3 (IV sedation study club) provides additional experience with clinical management of patients receiving IV drugs in a supervised clinical environment. At the conclusion of modules 2 and 3 it is expected that the doctor will have completed a minimum of 20 cases of IV sedation under direct supervision.

Module 4 permits the doctor to receive clinical experience in airway management of the unconscious patient (80 hours). Doctors use the operating room or outpatient general anesthesia facilities in order to gain hands-on experience in these invaluable and lifesaving procedures.

Following completion of the four modules it is anticipated that the doctor will begin to use IV sedation in the practice of dentistry. A voluntary "certification" program has been established, which a doctor may take advantage of at this time. To receive certification in IV sedation from the University of Southern California School of Dentistry, the doctor must document 50 cases of IV sedation (including those performed under supervision), successfully complete both a written and oral examination in subjects relating to anesthesia (e.g., physical evaluation, emergency medicine, monitoring, pharmacology, technique), and successfully undergo an in-office evaluation in which both the doctor and staff will be observed in their management of IV sedation and of staged emergency situations. It has been our experience that doctors successfully completing this intensive course of study are well trained in all aspects of the safe and effective administration of drugs via the IV and IM routes and have no difficulty in receiving certification from the state or province in which they practice dentistry.

REFERENCES

1. American Dental Association, Council on Dental Education: Guidelines for teaching the comprehensive control of pain and anxiety in dentistry, *J Dent Educ* 36:62, 1972.
2. American Dental Society of Anesthesiology: Guidelines for the teaching of pain and anxiety control and management of related complications in a continuing education program, part III, *Anesth Prog* 26:51, 1979.
3. American Dental Association, Council on Dental Education: Guidelines for teaching the comprehensive control of pain and anxiety in dentistry. Chicago, 1993, The Association.
4. American Association of Oral and Maxillofacial Surgeons, Committee on Anesthesia: *Office anesthesia evaluation manual,* ed 4. Rosemont, Ill, 1991, The Association.
5. American Association of Oral and Maxillofacial Surgeons: Parameters of care for oral and maxillofacial surgery: a guide for practice, monitoring and evaluation (AAOMS parameters of care—92), *J Oral Maxillofac Surg* 50(7) (suppl 2):1, 1992.
6. Committee on Drugs: Guidelines for monitoring and management of pediatric patients during and after sedation for diagnostic and therapeutic procedures, *Pediatrics* 89(6):1110, 1992.
7. American Academy of Pediatric Dentistry: Guidelines for the elective use of conscious sedation, deep sedation, and general anesthesia in pediatric patients. In *1992-1993 reference manual.* Chicago, 1993, The Academy.
8. American Academy of Periodontology, Research, Science, and Therapy Committee: *Guidelines for the use of conscious sedation in periodontics.* Chicago, 1992, The Academy.
9. Malamed SF: Continuing education in intravenous sedation: part 2, complications and non-use, *Anesth Prog* 28:158, 1981.
10. Malamed SF: Continuing education in intravenous sedation: survey of 188 dentists, *Anesth Prog* 28:33, 1981.
11. American Dental Association, Department of State Government Affairs, Chicago, 1992, The Association.

SECTION SIX

General anesthesia

31 BACKGROUND

32 ARMAMENTARIUM, DRUGS, AND TECHNIQUES

*General anesthesia has been an integral part of dental practice ever since 1844 when Horace Wells first used nitrous oxide (N_2O) to induce the loss of consciousness. General anesthesia was for many years an integral part of the pain control armamentarium of dentists, primarily because other techniques of pain control were less well developed. With the introduction of local anesthetics in the 1870s and their steady improvement in the 1900s, with the introduction of procaine and later of the amides in the 1940s, the need for general anesthesia as a primary means of achieving pain control during dental treatment has diminished. A second need for general anesthesia was in the management of dental fears and anxieties. For well over 100 years general anesthesia was **the** primary technique used for this purpose. With the introduction of newer drugs capable of relieving anxiety without inducing the loss of consciousness, our ability to manage dental fears through conscious sedation techniques has increased dramatically, further diminishing the role of general anesthesia in the practice of dentistry.*

In spite of the decreasing reliance being placed on general anesthesia in dentistry today, several significant indications for its use remain. These will be discussed in Chapter 31. The dental profession has been a leader in the development of general anesthesia from the early days of Horace Wells and William Morton to the more recent advances in the field of outpatient general anesthesia.

I have taken the liberty of categorizing general anesthesia in the following three groups:

1. Outpatient general anesthesia using IV barbiturates (ultralight general anesthesia)
2. Outpatient general anesthesia using conventional general anesthetic agents
3. Inpatient general anesthesia

As will be made clear later in this section, the techniques of general anesthesia are not amenable to teaching in a short course. Extensive training must be obtained by the doctor who contemplates using any technique of general anesthesia. The ability to render patients unconscious, safely maintain them in that state during dental treatment, and then return them to a normal state of functioning requires at least 2 years of full-time training in an anesthesiology residency or its equivalent during an oral and maxillofacial surgery residency program. In

459

addition to the 2 years of training, it is becoming increasingly commonplace for individual state boards of dental examiners to require the doctor to obtain a special license or permit before being allowed to use general anesthesia. As of June 1992, 47 states required such licensure.[1]

Many excellent textbooks are available on the subject of general anesthesia, and these books should be consulted by the doctor who is interested in this technique. In the two chapters comprising this section the indications for general anesthesia in dentistry as well as some of the drugs and techniques used will be presented. General anesthesia does indeed form a very valuable technique for the spectrum of pain and anxiety control in both dentistry and medicine.

REFERENCE

1. American Dental Association, Department of State Government Affairs: Chicago, 1992.

CHAPTER *31*

Background

General anesthesia has been defined as a reversible state of unconsciousness produced by anesthetic agents with loss of the sensation of pain over the entire body.[1] Pallasch[2] described general anesthesia as "hypnosis (sleep or loss of consciousness) accompanied by the loss of protective laryngeal reflexes (cough). Ideally, general anesthesia represents the simultaneous presence of analgesia (loss of pain), amnesia (loss of memory) and hypnosis along with reflex inhibition and loss of skeletal muscle tone which allows for safe surgical procedures." When the central nervous system (CNS) is depressed to the extent that consciousness is lost, changes occur in the physiology of the patient that are life threatening in the absence of a "guardian" trained in the management of the unconscious patient. These changes include partial or complete airway obstruction, hypoxia, hypercapnia, loss of the ability to clear the tracheobronchial tree, respiratory depression, blood gas and pH changes, cardiovascular depression, and depressed or absent protective reflexes.

Since the introduction of techniques of conscious and deep sedation in clinical practice, the need for general anesthesia has diminished. Sedative techniques possess a number of advantages, not the least of which is the retention of consciousness as well as maintenance of the airway and protective reflexes. One of the inherent dangers of general anesthesia is that these three factors are lost, making it the obligation of the anesthesiologist to provide a patent airway and to protect the patient during the period of unconsciousness.

Several types of general anesthesia are recognized. The most frequent use of general anesthesia in dentistry is within the specialty of oral and maxillofacial surgery. The oral surgeon has been responsible for the development of outpatient or ambulatory general anesthesia using either IV barbiturates (ultra-light general anesthesia—where the patient is maintained in Guedel stage II of anesthesia) or conventional general anesthetic agents (the patient maintained in Guedel stage III of anesthesia). As hospital costs continue to rise, outpatient general anesthesia has gained popularity within the medical profession. The dentist anesthesiologist, a dentist trained in general anesthesia (minimum of 2 years), has made outpatient general anesthesia available to patients requiring nonoral surgical dental care, such as periodontics, endodontics, implants, and restorative procedures.

A third form of general anesthesia available to the dental patient is traditional inpatient general anesthesia. Whether the anesthesiologist is a dentist or a physician, the patient is admitted to the hospital and brought to the operating room, where anesthesia is induced and the dental procedure is performed. The dentist doing the dentistry need not be trained in general anesthesia for this type of anesthesia to be used because the anesthesiologist is responsible for inducing and maintaining the appropriate depth of anesthesia. Each of these types of general anesthesia will be described in Chapter 32.

ADVANTAGES OF GENERAL ANESTHESIA

1. *Patient cooperation is not absolutely essential for the success of general anesthesia.* One of the disadvantages of all sedative techniques is that a degree of patient cooperation is required in order for the administered drugs to produce the desired clinical effect (the inhalation route), to administer the drugs (intravenous—IV), or to proceed with dental treatment. In cases where the loss of consciousness is the goal (general anesthesia), patient cooperation, though desirable, is not absolutely essential. The patient may, if necessary, be premedicated with intramuscular (IM) drugs and anesthesia induced with inha-

461

lation anesthetics. Once the patient is unconscious, an IV infusion is established and the anesthetic procedure continued in the usual manner.

2. *The patient is unconscious.* The loss of consciousness will be considered both as an advantage and as a disadvantage (see later). The fearful patient, the patient with a management problem, and the mentally or physically disabled patient can receive *quality* dental care in a well-controlled environment, be it a dental office or the operating room of a hospital or of an outpatient surgical facility (e.g., Surgi-center). Dental care may be impossible to undertake or the quality of the care significantly compromised with this patient still conscious.

3. *The patient does not respond to pain.* Although many general anesthetics possess either no or only slight analgesic properties, the level of depression of the patient's CNS occurring in general anesthesia will prevent any response by the patient to the nociceptive stimuli that reach the brain. There will be some variation in this response depending on the level of CNS depression. Local anesthetics may not be administered during some surgical procedures, including dental treatment; however, local anesthetics are frequently administered during general anesthesia in order to prevent any painful stimuli from reaching the brain. In this manner the concentrations or volumes of general anesthetic agents required to maintain a smooth, even level of general anesthesia will be decreased.

During ultralight general anesthesia using IV barbiturates such as methohexital or thiopental, the utilization of local anesthesia is more critical to success. In this procedure the level of unconsciousness (e.g., the depth of CNS depression) is kept as minimal as possible in order to hasten the patient's postoperative recovery. However, when this happens, the patient may respond to noxious stimulation during the dental or surgical procedure.

To prevent this response two things may be done: The level of anesthesia may be deepened, or local anesthesia may be administered. Deepening of the level of general anesthesia through administration of additional drugs prolongs the recovery period, which in outpatient settings is undesirable. Through the administration of local anesthesia, response to painful procedures is prevented both during the operative procedure and, equally important, in the postoperative period.

4. *Amnesia is present.* With loss of consciousness amnesia is present. For many extremely fearful patients, a lack of recall of events occurring during treatment represents *the* major indication for the use of general anesthesia or other techniques that provide amnesia. In cases where amnesia is the primary requirement in a procedure general anesthesia can usually be avoided. The use of IV conscious sedation with diazepam, midazolam, or scopolamine is recommended in place of general anesthesia.

5. *General anesthesia may be the only technique that will prove successful for certain patients,* such as the precooperative child, extremely fearful adult, and patients with either physical or mental disabilities such as multiple sclerosis, cerebral palsy, Down's syndrome, or autism.

6. *The onset of action of general anesthesia is usually quite rapid.* Drugs are administered by the IV or inhalation routes, the two techniques with the most rapid onset of action. In most situations unconsciousness can be induced within approximately 1 minute.

7. *Titration is usually possible,* the patient receiving the smallest volume of drug required to produce the desired effect.

DISADVANTAGES OF GENERAL ANESTHESIA

1. *The patient is unconscious.* Previously discussed as an advantage of general anesthesia, the loss of consciousness must also be considered a disadvantage because of the many changes in the patient's physiology occurring with the loss of consciousness. These changes are deleterious to the well-being of the patient. As Trieger has stated, "Such care requires extensive education and training on the part of the doctor. The management of an individual who has lost his protective reflexes depends upon his anesthetist's ability to ensure his safety and survival."[3]

2. *Protective reflexes are depressed.* The loss of consciousness is accompanied by a progressive depression of the CNS and of the protective reflexes of the patient. Because the dentist is operating in the oral cavity, the potential for debris, water, saliva, or blood entering into the airway and producing an obstruction or laryngospasm is greater in dental cases than with most other surgical procedures. One of the most important tasks of the anesthesiologist is to ensure the integrity of the patient's airway.

3. *Vital signs are depressed.* With the administration of general anesthesia it is normal to see a depression of functioning of the cardiovascular and respiratory systems. The administration of ambulatory general anesthesia for elective dental procedures to high-risk, medically compromised patients (ASA IV and

sometimes ASA III) is contraindicated, in part because of this property of general anesthetic drugs.

4. *Advanced training is required.* In no other technique discussed in this book is the requirement for postgraduate training as important (or as difficult to obtain) as it is for general anesthesia. The doctor (physician or dentist) who wishes to administer general anesthesia must have completed a minimum of 2 years of full-time training in anesthesiology.[4] All staff members participating in the administration of general anesthesia must also have received thorough training, although it need not be as extensive as that of the doctor. Lack of proper training or education on the part of personnel represents an absolute contraindication to the administration of general anesthesia.

5. *An "anesthesia team" is required.* For the administration of a general anesthetic in a dental office there should be a team consisting minimally of the anesthesiologist, an anesthesia assistant, and a circulating nurse. The doctor administering the general anesthetic should not be responsible for performing the dental therapy. Division of labor by one person in anesthesiology can only lead to an increased risk of serious complications. Lack of enough, or inadequate training of, personnel represents an absolute contraindication to the administration of general anesthesia.

6. *Special equipment is required wherever general anesthesia is administered.* Monitoring of the unconscious anesthetized patient is of greater importance than it is for those who are sedated, because in the absence of the ability to communicate with the patient (CNS depression), the only means of determining a patient's status is the level of functioning of various other systems of their body, such as the cardiovascular and respiratory systems.

In addition to monitoring equipment, additional equipment is required for the administration of general anesthesia. Such equipment includes a laryngoscope, endotracheal tubes, and oropharyngeal or nasopharyngeal airways. The absence of adequate equipment either for monitoring or for the administration of general anesthesia represents an absolute contraindication to the use of this technique.

7. *A recovery area must be available for the patient.* Following general anesthesia of any duration or depth, an area must be available for the patient to remain in until she or he has recovered sufficiently to be discharged. Such an area must have equipment, including oxygen and a suction apparatus, and must be monitored on a continual basis while the patient is present. Lack of adequate recovery facilities represents an absolute contraindication to the administration of general anesthesia.

8. *Intraoperative complications are more common during general anesthesia than during sedative procedures.* The patient's physiology has been altered by the administration of CNS–depressant drugs to a greater degree during general anesthesia than during sedation. Problems relating to the cardiovascular and respiratory systems, such as hypotension, tachycardia, bradycardia, dysrhythmias, and respiratory depression are much more frequently encountered in general anesthesia.

9. *Postanesthetic complications are more common during general anesthesia than during sedative procedures.* Postanesthetic problems can include any of those mentioned in the preceding paragraph.

10. *The patient receiving general anesthesia must receive nothing by mouth for 6 hours prior to the procedure.* This is usually easily provided for when the patient is hospitalized but is less of a certainty in the outpatient environment. The presence of food or liquid in the stomach can lead to the extremely dangerous occurrence of vomiting during anesthetic induction or regurgitation during the procedure, with the possibility of airway obstruction or tracheal burning or infection of the lung. Such a risk is negligible during sedative procedures.

11. *Patients receiving general anesthesia must be evaluated more extensively preoperatively than patients receiving conscious sedation.* Laboratory tests are required routinely before general anesthesia is administered. Urinalysis, complete blood count (CBC), and hematocrit and/or hemoglobin determinations are normally obtained. In patients over the age of 35 years, a chest x-ray and electrocardiogram (ECG) are usually required. Such extensive evaluation is not required (nor is it needed) for patients receiving conscious sedation.

CONTRAINDICATIONS

The following are contraindications to the administration of general anesthesia either in a hospital environment or in an outpatient facility such as a dental office or day-surgery center for elective dental care:

1. Lack of adequate training by the doctor
2. Lack of adequately trained personnel
3. Lack of adequate equipment

4. Lack of adequate facilities
5. ASA IV and certain ASA III medically compromised patients

The first four contraindications have been mentioned in the preceding paragraphs on the disadvantages of general anesthesia; however, they are of such great importance that they must be mentioned again. Under absolutely no circumstances should general anesthesia be administered in the absence of any one of these four vital ingredients. Specifics of each of these items will be discussed later in this chapter and in Chapter 32.

Under the fifth contraindication (ASA IV and certain ASA III medically compromised patients) there will be some variance between the outpatient and inpatient forms of general anesthesia. Outpatient general anesthesia, regardless of the type, is generally contraindicated in all but ASA I, ASA II, and some ASA III patients. Other ASA III and all ASA IV patients should be hospitalized with their dental care performed in the more controlled environment of the operating room.

The severely medically compromised patient will benefit from a more thorough preoperative evaluation when hospitalized prior to the start of treatment and from the more immediate availability of medical consultation and emergency care should the occasion(s) arise. Most medically compromised patients are readily identified through the routine medical history and physical examination performed in the dental office. Other patients who may not be candidates for outpatient general anesthesia include:

1. Patients with a history of poliomyelitis in which the chest muscles have been involved
2. Patients with a history of myasthenia gravis
3. Patients with significantly decreased cardiac and/or pulmonary reserve
4. Obese patients, especially those with short, thick necks, which will provide difficulty with airway maintenance

INDICATIONS

1. *Extreme anxiety and fear.* The techniques of sedation that have been discussed will prove to be effective in approximately 97% of apprehensive adult dental patients. In these patients there is little indication for general anesthesia. However, general anesthesia is the only technique available for dental treatment for the remaining 3%. The nature of the general anesthesia to be administered will vary according to the nature of the planned dental treatment—ultralight general anesthesia using IV barbi-

turates for surgical procedures of short duration, or outpatient general anesthesia using conventional general anesthetic agents for longer procedures involving other types of dental treatment. In some cases it may be prudent to hospitalize the patient and utilize the services of the anesthesiologist and operating room in managing this patient.

2. *Adults or children who are mentally and/or physically disabled, senile, or disoriented.* The use of conscious sedation techniques in these patients may be ineffective, thus providing an indication for the administration of general anesthesia. These patients commonly require many forms of dental care such as periodontics, endodontics, oral surgery, and restorative procedures—procedures that generally are long. It is suggested, therefore, that when conscious sedation techniques are unavailable or have proved to be ineffective, these patients be admitted to a hospital or an outpatient surgical facility where they may undergo a more in-depth preoperative evaluation in addition to receiving the usual high standard of care during and after the anesthetic procedure. Many of these dental procedures can be completed on an outpatient basis, but the availability of inpatient facilities is recommended in case the patient should require an extended period of recovery. Management of these patients is discussed in Chapter 39.

3. *Age—infants and children.* The techniques of sedation that have been discussed may be of little use in the very young patient, primarily because of the patient's inability to cooperate. Oral, inhalation, and IV sedation may not be effective in managing these patients, whereas intramuscularly administered drugs are somewhat more effective. In Chapter 36 the use of IM/IV midazolam is presented. This technique has been quite successful in managing this patient population.

When the patient is very young, general anesthesia will be of benefit to both the patient and the dental staff. The trauma involved in dental care is minimized with a properly performed general anesthetic. Dental care may be carried out in a more calm and controlled environment with the patient's safety being ensured by the anesthesiologist.

Smith et al.[5] have estimated that between 2% and 5% of pediatric dental patients will require general anesthesia in order for their dental treatment to be completed successfully. Trapp[6] lists the two indications for pediatric general anesthesia as (1) the healthy patient who is unable to cooperate for office procedures after the standard management armamentarium has been exhausted, and (2) the patient who is medically compromised (e.g., cerebral palsy, severe mental retardation) and unable to tolerate routine dental procedures.

4. *Short, traumatic procedures.* Procedures of short duration (less than 30 minutes) but that are of a traumatic nature, such as the removal of four impacted third molars, may be an indication for the administration of ultralight general anesthesia utilizing IV barbiturates or propofol.

5. *Prolonged, traumatic procedures.* Whereas many adult dental patients can tolerate procedures requiring 1 or 2 hours to complete, some patients may be unable to tolerate these same, or much longer, procedures. Although there are alternatives to the use of general anesthesia in this situation (such as multiple shorter appointments), general anesthesia may be a viable option. Procedures of 4 hours or longer may be performed under general anesthesia in an outpatient setting.

Within the area of general anesthesia the following are indications for the administration of outpatient, versus inpatient, general anesthesia:

1. *Economics.* The use of outpatient general anesthesia has grown in the United States since the 1980s for several reasons. One of these is the decreased cost of outpatient procedures compared to identical inpatient procedures. Schmidt has stated that the cost of outpatient procedures is between 30% and 70% less than identical inpatient procedures.[7]

2. *Psychological benefits.* The major psychological benefit derived from outpatient general anesthesia is in the area of pediatrics, in which the trauma associated with separation of the child from his parents, as well as the strange environment of the hospital, may be minimized.

3. *Reduced exposure to nosocomial infections.* Steward has stated that outpatient general anesthesia in pediatrics results in a decreased incidence of infection because the patient has a reduced exposure to health professionals, hospital wards, and their associated pathogens.[8]

4. *Parental preference.* In surveys of the parents of pediatric patients, the overwhelming majority have indicated their preference for outpatient general anesthetic procedures over inpatient procedures.[7]

TYPES OF GENERAL ANESTHESIA

The following variations of general anesthesia are used in dentistry:

1. Outpatient general anesthesia
   a. Intravenous barbiturates or propofol (less than 30 minutes)
   b. Conventional operating room–type general anesthesia (more than 30 minutes and less than 4 hours)
2. Inpatient general anesthesia

The administration of IV barbiturates to induce and to maintain unconsciousness has become an accepted and relatively common technique of general anesthesia. This form of general anesthesia is used primarily in oral and maxillofacial surgery for relatively short procedures (usually less than 30 minutes), such as the removal of impacted third molars.[9] It is also known as *ultralight general anesthesia,* and the most frequently administered drugs are methohexital (Brevital, Brietal), thiopental (Pentothal), and thiamylal (Surital). Methohexital is by far the most commonly used IV barbiturate in this technique of general anesthesia. Propofol, a new rapid-acting short-duration nonbarbiturate, has become a popular alternative to methohexital, thiopental, thiamylal. Patient recovery is rapid and more complete than with barbiturates.

Patients receiving ultralight general anesthesia may in addition receive other drugs, including nitrous oxide-oxygen (N_2O-O_2), a benzodiazepine, opioids, and local anesthetics that assist in maintenance of a smooth level of general anesthesia. The benzodiazepine and N_2O-O_2 act to prolong the duration of the anesthesia and to potentiate the effect of the IV barbiturate, permitting a smaller dose to be used, thus shortening the patient's recovery period. In addition, the administration of O_2 minimizes the risk of hypoxia. Recent studies utilizing pulse oximeters and end-tidal CO_2 monitors have demonstrated that some degree of hypoxia and hypercarbia is not uncommon during this form of general anesthesia unless supplemental O_2 is provided.[10] Local anesthesia is important, because by preventing noxious stimuli from reaching the brain, the dosage of barbiturate (and other CNS-depressant drugs) may be minimized, once again shortening recovery and discharge of the patient. Postoperative pain control is also aided by the administration of local anesthetics, especially the longer-acting drugs, such as bupivacaine and etidocaine in addition to either oral or parenteral nonsteroidal antiinflammatory drugs (NSAIDs).[11] The typical patient will remain pain free (from the local anesthetic) for from 6 to 12 hours after completion of the surgical procedure. The requirement for administration of postoperative opioid analgesics is therefore minimized.

Lytle and Driscoll et al.[12,13] have reported on mortality rates from outpatient general anesthesia with

IV barbiturates. The rates presented in these studies are approximately one death in 400,000 general anesthetic administrations, a figure that compares quite favorably with figures reported from hospital centers (see later). A more recent study provided similar statistics from Great Britain—a mortality rate of 1:338,536 for outpatient general anesthesia.[14]

The statistics from Great Britain appear to be more reliable than the others primarily because the numbers in the first two studies were extrapolations of data provided voluntarily by dentists, whereas the British numbers were based on reports from the Office of Population Censuses and Surveys, which is responsible for recording basic population data, including deaths, for England and Wales. Regardless of the source of information, it appears that outpatient general anesthesia in ASA I, II, and selected ASA III patients administered by persons with adequate training, possesses a remarkable safety record.

Conventional operating room–type general anesthesia

The second variety of outpatient general anesthesia is utilized for procedures ranging from 30 minutes to 4 hours or longer (Fig. 31-1). The patient will undergo the same general anesthetic preparation and procedure as will the inpatient. Facilities for anesthetic administration may vary from the dental office to an outpatient day-surgery facility to a hospital operating room.

Because of the length of the dental or surgical procedure to be completed, this form of general anesthesia is usually limited to the ASA I, II, and selected ASA III patients. ASA IV patients requiring general

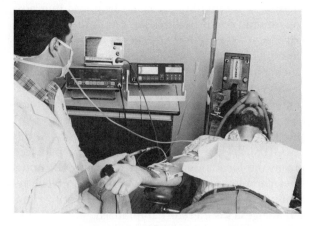

Fig. 31-1. Ultralight general anesthesia employing an IV barbiturate, initial titration.

anesthesia for their dental care will be hospitalized prior to the procedure and remain hospitalized after the procedure.

The person administering the anesthetic to the patient must have completed training in anesthesiology (a minimum of 2 full years). This person may be a physician anesthesiologist, a dentist anesthesiologist, or a Certified Registered Nurse Anesthetist (CRNA). A dentist will be responsible for the dental care. In no circumstance should the same person administer the general anesthetic and perform the dental treatment.

Residency programs in anesthesiology for dentists are available, although they are limited in number. Educational aspects of anesthesiology training are discussed in the following paragraph. The drugs and techniques used in general anesthesia will be discussed below and in Chapter 32.

The mortality rate associated with operating room–type general anesthesia in ASA I and II outpatients, administered by qualified persons, is equal to that for hospital inpatients.[7] Coplans and Curson[14] reported a mortality rate of 1:593,000 for hospital outpatient general anesthesia in which the general anesthetic was judged to be solely responsible for the death of an ASA I patient, and 1:148,000 in which the anesthetic as well as underlying disease (ASA II, III, and IV patients) were implicated. The incidence of hospital admissions as a complication of outpatient general anesthesia is less than 5%.[8,15] This complications rate is associated directly with the duration of the general anesthetic.[16,17] Because of the relationship between duration of anesthesia and the incidence of complications, it is recommended that the duration of an outpatient general anesthetic not exceed 4 hours.[8]

Inpatient general anesthesia

The third form of general anesthesia is inpatient general anesthesia. The patient is admitted to the hospital prior to the planned procedure, undergoes a workup to determine the potential risk of the surgery and anesthesia, undergoes the procedure, and then remains in the hospital at least 1 day postoperatively to recover and for her or his physical condition to stabilize.

In this situation the dentist need not be trained in anesthesiology. The Department of Anesthesiology is responsible for the administration of the anesthetic for the planned procedure. The dentist should be contacted by the anesthesiologist prior to the scheduled procedure to determine if there are any special requirements. In many cases in which prolonged dental treatment is planned, the doctor will request that the patient be intubated through the nose (nasoendotracheal) rather than through the mouth (oroendotracheal), so that there is less danger of the dental procedure interfering with the patient's airway, and vice versa.

Although it may appear at first glance that dental treatment is often a very "minor" procedure to be done under general anesthesia, especially compared with cardiac surgery, neurosurgery, or other forms of surgery, the truth is that the administration of general anesthesia for dental procedures is actually more difficult in many ways. This is because the oral cavity is always being used by the dental surgeon; as a result the potential for airway complications is increased. Many hospitals maintain a dentist anesthesiologist or a physician anesthesiologist who will administer anesthesia for all dental cases requiring general anesthesia. Familiarity with the peculiar requirements of this combination of surgery and anesthesia increases patient safety.

Patients of any ASA classification may be admitted to the hospital for general anesthesia as inpatients; however, it seems prudent to limit this form of general anesthesia to ASA IV and selected ASA III patients and to any other patient for whom outpatient procedures are contraindicated or are not available.

Mortality rates for hospital inpatient anesthesia are somewhat higher than those for outpatient procedures primarily because of the difference in patient risk factor. Most ASA I and II patients are treated as outpatients when anesthesia is administered, whereas ASA III and IV patients are usually hospitalized. In the United States the anesthesia mortality rate in large teaching institutions is 1:1500, whereas in smaller nonteaching hospitals it is 1:9000. The surgical procedure most similar to a simple dental procedure is the removal of tonsils and adenoids (T and A). The mortality rate for this procedure in hospitals in the United States is approximately 1:40,000. The recent British study reported a 1:63,000 general anesthesia mortality rate for hospital inpatients in cases in which the general anesthetic was solely responsible for the death of a healthy, ASA I patient, and 1:26,000 in cases in which the underlying disease as well as the general anesthetic were judged to be responsible.[14]

EDUCATION IN GENERAL ANESTHESIA

In no other area of patient management is thorough educational and clinical experience as important as in the administration of general anesthesia. It is not possible to teach this important technique in short courses, as is possible with some of the other techniques of sedation. Education in general anesthesia requires not less than 2 years of full-time training of the dentist in an accredited anesthesiology residency or its equivalent during oral and maxillofacial surgery residencies.[4]

Although there are a few residency programs designed specifically for dentists (Ohio State, Loma Linda, Medical College of Virginia), there are several that have had a long history of dental residents and that tailor their training program to meet the specific requirements of the dental anesthesiology resident. A list of programs available as of 1993 is presented at the end of this chapter.

Guidelines Relative to the Establishment of a Dental Residency in Anesthesiology*

In 1979 the American Dental Society of Anesthesiology (ADSA) established and approved the following guidelines[18]:

1. Trainee title: Dental Resident in Anesthesiology
2. Suggested qualifications of resident: Although this is not mandatory, it would be desirable for the resident to have satisfactorily completed a minimum of 1 year of previous hospital training, such as a general practice residency or an equivalent program in which training in hospital procedures and inpatient management is emphasized.
3. The training program must be full-time and be a minimum of 1 year's duration.
4. Didactic and clinical program must be structured and resident schedule of duties clearly delineated.
5. The program should be a joint cooperative effort between the department of anesthesiology and the department of dentistry. Accordingly, support and cooperation of the director of anesthesiology is essential in order to establish and conduct a meaningful joint training program.
6. Instruction of both a didactic basic science as well as a clinical nature must be incorporated into the residency program. This instruction must be given in a seminar or conference format or may include formal courses.

---

*More recent guidelines require a minimum of 2 calendar years.

7. The dental resident shall serve on an equal basis with the medical residents in anesthesiology. The programs shall include participation in all the usual duties of anesthesiology residents, including preanesthetic patient evaluation, administration of anesthesia in the operating room on a daily scheduled basis, postanesthetic care and management, and emergency call.

8. The resident's training must include significant experience in anesthetic management for ambulatory outpatient procedures, as well as the use of inhalation and IV sedation techniques. An optimum learning experience for these procedures would be provided in a hospital dental clinic that is properly equipped and staffed for the administration of general anesthesia for ambulatory patients.

9. Individuals responsible for training the resident(s) must include a qualified medical anesthesiologist and at least one qualified dentist who is a fellow in general anesthesia of the ADSA. In addition, the dental director of the program must hold fellowship status in the ADSA.

10. Clinical training should include training in a broad spectrum of pain-control techniques suitable for ambulatory patients. In addition, a clear understanding of pain and pain mechanisms should be developed.

11. The program must conform to that outlined in Part Two (Teaching of Pain Control and Management of Related Complications at the Advanced Education Level) of the *Guidelines for Teaching the Comprehensive Control of Pain and Anxiety in Dentistry* as approved by the ADA Council on Dental Education and the Commission on Accreditation and endorsed by the ASA Committee on Manpower.[4]

12. Dental residents should be encouraged to take the annual In-Service Training Examination in Anesthesiology.

13. The Fellowship Committee of the ADSA will act in an advisory capacity with regard to these guidelines.

The availability of accredited training programs in general anesthesia for dentists has become increasingly important, because almost all states in the United States have adopted regulations that act to restrict the use of this technique to qualified dentists. At the time of publication of the second edition of this textbook in July 1987, 37 states required special licensing for doctors using general anesthesia. As of June 1993 this number had increased to 47.[19]

Although general anesthesia regulations vary, many states have proposed regulations limiting the administration of general anesthesia to doctors who meet one or both of the following criteria: (1) a licensed dentist who has completed a residency program in anesthesiology of not less than 2 calendar years that is approved by the Board of Directors of the American Dental Society of Anesthesiology for eligibility for the Fellowship in General Anesthesia, or has a Fellowship in General Anesthesia, or (2) a licensed dentist who has completed a graduate program in oral and maxillofacial surgery that has been approved by the Commission on Accreditation of the ADA.

The Fellowship in General Anesthesia of the American Dental Society of Anesthesiology is available to dentists and physicians who have completed at least 1 full year of anesthesiology residency in an accredited program or its equivalent in an approved oral and maxillofacial surgery residency program. At this time it appears that the Fellowship has become an important means of defining adequacy of training in general anesthesia in dentistry. In addition, the American Society of Dentist Anesthesiologists (ASDA), an organization composed of dentists who have completed 2 years of training in anesthesiology, has recently been developed.

General anesthesia must never be taken lightly. The doctor who is considering the use of this valuable, but potentially dangerous, technique should explore the means of achieving at least 2 full years of residency training in general anesthesia.

ACCREDITED ANESTHESIOLOGY RESIDENCIES IN WHICH DENTISTS CAN ENROLL

The following is a listing of programs that provide 2 years of training in anesthesiology for qualified dentists. This list was provided by the ADSA and is dated June 1993.[20] It is suggested that persons interested in pursuing training in anesthesiology write directly to the chief of the dentistry department at the hospital of their choice.

California

Loma Linda University
Dr. Russell Seheult, Director
Loma Linda University
School of Dentistry
Loma Linda, CA 92350
  2-year residency program

Florida

University of Miami Affiliated Hospitals
N. W. Craythorne, M.D., Director
University of Miami
School of Medicine R-370
P.O. Box 016370
Miami, FL 33101
   2 years unless stated otherwise

Illinois

Illinois Masonic Medical Center
Harold J. Heyman, M.D.
Director, Anesthesiology Residency Program
Illinois Masonic Medical Center
836 Wellington Avenue
Chicago, IL 60657
   6-month to 1-year residency program

University of Illinois Hospital
Alon P. Winnie, M.D., Director
University of Illinois Hospital
840 S. Wood Street
Chicago, IL 60657
   2 years unless stated otherwise

Massachusetts

Boston City Hospital
Dr. Crocker, Director
Boston City Hospital
818 Harrison Avenue
Boston, MA 02118
   2 years unless stated otherwise

New York

Albert Einstein College of Medicine
Dental Coordinator
Albert Einstein College of Medicine
111 E. 210th Street
Bronx, NY 10467
   2 years unless stated otherwise

Brookdale Hospital Medical Center
Adel R. Abadir, M.D., Director
Brookdale Hospital Medical Center
Department of Anesthesiology
Linden Boulevard at Brookdale Plaza
Brooklyn, NY 11212
   2-year residency program

Long Island Jewish—Hillside Medical Center Program
Sylvan N. Surks, M.D., Director
Department of Anesthesiology
270-05 76th Avenue

Hyde Park, NY 11042
   2 years unless stated otherwise

Maimonides Medical Center Training Program
Philip H. Sechzer, M.D., Director
Maimonides Medical Center
4802 10th Avenue
Brooklyn, NY 11219
   1-year residency program

Montefiore Hospital and Medical Center
Deryck Duncalf, M.D., Director
Montefiore Hospital and Medical Center
111 E. 210th Street
Bronx, NY 10467
   2 years unless stated otherwise

Mount Sinai School of Medicine Affiliated Hospital
Dr. Joel Kaplan, M.D., Director
Mount Sinai Hospital
One Gustave Levy Place
New York, NY 10029
   2 years unless stated otherwise

New York University Medical Center
Dean of the Dental School
New York University
Department of Anesthesiology
550 First Avenue
New York, NY 10016
   2 years unless stated otherwise

SUNY at Stony Brook Affiliated Hospitals
Paul J. Poppers, M.D., Director
University Hospital
Department of Anesthesiology
Level 4-Room 560
Stony Brook, NY 11794
    No stipend. Must have your own malpractice insurance.

Ohio

Cleveland Metropolitan General/Highland View Hospitals
Lee S. Shepard, M.D., Director
Cleveland Metro General/Highland View Hospital
3395 Scranton Road
Cleveland, OH 11794
   2-year residency program

Ohio State University
Joel M. Weaver, D.D.S.
Ohio State University
College of Dentistry
305 W. 12th Avenue

Columbus, OH 43210
2-year residency program

Pennsylvania

Conemaugh Valley Memorial Hospital
John C. Swik, M.D., Director
Conemaugh Valley Memorial Hospital
Division of Anesthesiology
1086 Franklin Street
Johnstown, PA 15905

Medical College of Pennsylvania
Athole G. McNeil Jacobi, M.D.
Medical College of Pennsylvania
1601 Walnut Street
Philadelphia, PA 19102

Utah

University of Utah Affiliated Hospitals
K. C. Wong, M.D., Director
University of Utah Medical Center
50 N. Medical Drive
Salt Lake City, UT 84132

Virginia

Medical College of Virginia
Dr. Robert Campbell, D.D.S., Director
Box 638
Medical College of Virginia
Richmond, VA 23298
2-year residency program
The reader is directed to the ADSA for updated program lists:

Mr. Peter C. Goulding, Executive Director
American Dental Society of Anesthesiology
211 East Chicago Avenue, Suite 948
Chicago, IL 60611
Phone: (312) 664-8270

REFERENCES

1. Snow JC: Intravenous anesthesia. In *Manual of anesthesia.* Boston, 1977, Little, Brown, p 109.
2. Pallasch TJ: *Pharmacology for dental students and practitioners.* Philadelphia, 1980, Lea & Febiger.
3. Trieger NT: *Pain control,* ed 2. St Louis, 1994, Mosby.
4. American Dental Association, Council on Dental Education: *Guidelines for teaching the comprehensive control of pain and anxiety in dentistry,* Chicago, 1993, The Association.
5. Smith F, Deputy BS, Berry FA Jr: Outpatient anesthesia for children undergoing extensive dental treatment, *J Dent Child* 45:38, 1978.
6. Trapp LD: Sedation of children for dental treatment, *Pediatr Dent* 4(1):164, 1982.
7. Schmidt K, editor: Outpatient anesthesia, *Int Anesthesiol Clin* 14:1, 1976.
8. Steward D: Outpatient pediatric anesthesia, *Anesthesiology* 43: 268, 1975.
9. Rosenberg M, Weaver J: General anesthesia, *Anesth Prog* 38(4-5):172, 1991.
10. Jastak JT, Peskin RM: Major morbidity or mortality from office anesthetic procedures: a closed-claim analysis of 13 cases, *Anesth Prog* 38(2):39, 1991.
11. Acute Pain Management Guidelines Panel: *Acute pain management: operative or medical procedures and trauma, Clinical practice guideline,* AHCPR Pub No 92-0032. Rockville, Md, 1992, Agency for Health Care Policy and Research, Public Health Service, US Department of Health and Human Services, pp 25-26.
12. Lytle JJ: Anesthesia morbidity and mortality survey of the Southern California Society of Oral Surgeons, *J Oral Surg* 32: 739, 1974.
13. Driscoll EJ, Herbert CL, Batting CG: Research in anesthesia for ambulatory patients: practical considerations, *Trans Congr Int Assoc Oral Surg,* 1970, p 538.
14. Coplans MP, Curson I: Deaths associated with dentistry, *Br Dent J* 153:357, 1982.
15. Smith F, Deputy BS, Berry FA Jr: Outpatient anesthesia for children undergoing extensive dental treatment, *J Dent Child* 45:38, 1978.
16. Fahy A, Marshall M: Postanaesthetic morbidity in outpatients, *Br J Anaesth* 41:433, 1969.
17. Steward D: Experiences with an outpatient anesthesia service for children, *Anesth Analg* 52:877, 1973.
18. American Dental Society of Anesthesiology: Guidelines relative to the establishment of a dental residency in anesthesiology, *Anesth Prog* 26:177, 1979.
19. American Dental Association, Department of State Government Affairs, Chicago, 1992, The Association.
20. American Dental Society of Anesthesiology: *Accredited dental anesthesiology residencies.* 1993, Chicago, The Society.

CHAPTER 32

Armamentarium, drugs, and techniques

This chapter presents an overview of the equipment, drugs, and techniques that are vitally important to the success of general anesthesia. Many of the drugs discussed have been reviewed in depth elsewhere in this book and will receive only the briefest of notice here. Other drugs will be mentioned for the first time; however, their pharmacology will also be briefly reviewed, for it is not the purpose of this chapter to provide the reader with a feeling that he or she is able to use safely these drugs after having read about them. As discussed in Chapter 31, this section is meant as an introduction to the vast subject of general anesthesia, not as a complete text in that area.

Following a review of the armamentarium and drugs, each of the major techniques of general anesthesia—outpatient general anesthesia with IV barbiturates, operating room–type outpatient general anesthesia, and inpatient general anesthesia—will be discussed.

ARMAMENTARIUM

The equipment required for the administration of general anesthesia may differ according to the type of anesthesia being delivered. In general, the equipment for intravenous (IV) barbiturate general anesthesia will vary somewhat from that required for other types of anesthesia.

The armamentarium for general anesthesia may be divided into the following five groups:

Anesthesia machine
Intravenous equipment
Ancillary anesthesia equipment
Monitoring equipment
Emergency equipment and drugs

Anesthesia machine

The anesthesia machine is able to deliver oxygen (O_2) and inhalation anesthetics to the patient. The inhalation sedation unit used in dental practice is a modification of the anesthesia machine used in the operating room. The primary difference between the two is the number of inhalation anesthetics the operating room unit is capable of delivering. As seen in Fig. 32-1, the anesthesia machine can deliver seven gases: nitrous oxide (N_2O), oxygen, halothane, methoxyflurane, enflurane, isoflurane, and fluroxene. Flowmeters, as well as devices called *vaporizers* that contain the various volatile anesthetics and permit their concentrations to be controlled, are integral parts of the unit.

The anesthesia machine is capable of operating with O_2 and N_2O supplied from either a central cylinder system or portable cylinders mounted on the sides of the unit. In the operating room, many of the fail-safe devices used in dental inhalation units are not present. However, most anesthesia machines have O_2 monitors that sound an alarm if the unit fails to provide a preset minimum percentage of O_2 (i.e., 25%).

During IV barbiturate general anesthesia an inhalation sedation unit, as discussed in Chapter 15, will be used to supplement the patient's ventilation with O_2 and perhaps N_2O. In the other forms of anesthesia a unit similar to that shown in Fig. 32-1 will be used.

The modern anesthesia machine also contains a number of important devices for monitoring patients receiving these agents. Attached to the anesthesia machine shown in Fig. 32-1 are several monitors, including a blood pressure monitor, electrocardio-

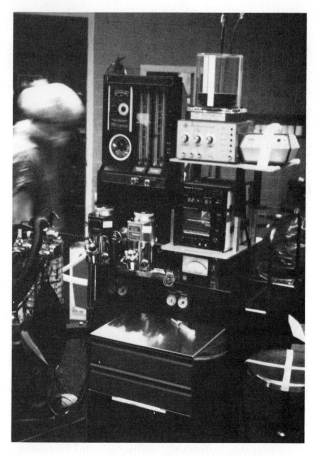

Fig. 32-1. General anesthesia machine can deliver a variety of anesthetic gases and contains multiple monitoring devices.

gram (ECG), pulse oximeter, end-tidal carbon dioxide (CO_2) monitor, electroencephologram (EEG), and a temperature monitor. Attached to the right side of the unit is a ventilator, a device used to control or assist the ventilation of a patient during anesthesia.

Intravenous equipment

A supply of equipment for venipuncture and IV drug administration is required during general anesthesia. A *continuous IV infusion* is recommended for all general anesthetic procedures. Winged needles are rarely used during general anesthesia, except perhaps for the shortest of procedures. Even then, however, *indwelling catheters* are recommended. The gauge of the venipuncture needle or indwelling catheter should not be smaller than 21 (for short procedures), with the 18-gauge needle being most commonly used for routine general anesthetic

procedures and 16-gauge needles used whenever a transfusion of blood may be required. An assortment of needles should be available.

Tubing and bags of IV solution are also required. During short procedures a 250-ml bag may be adequate; however, a 1000-ml size is usually recommended for all procedures lasting over 30 minutes because of the possibility of the patient becoming hypovolemic as a result of a combination of having been NPO (kept without food) prior to surgery, blood loss during surgery, and evaporation of fluids during surgery (especially where the abdominal or thoracic cavities are exposed).

A variety of *disposable syringes* and *needles* should also be available as well as various *tapes* (e.g., paper, hypoallergenic).

Ancillary anesthesia equipment

The following items must also be available whenever general anesthesia is to be administered:

Full-face masks in child and adult sizes and appropriate connectors

Laryngoscope complete with adequate selection of blades and spare batteries and bulb

Adequate selection of endotracheal tubes and appropriate connectors

Adequate selection of oropharyngeal and nasopharyngeal airways

Tonsillar suction tips

Magill intubation forceps

Child- and adult-size sphygmomanometers and stethoscopes

Face Masks

Face masks (Fig. 32-2) are rubber or silicone masks that cover both the mouth and nose of the patient. Face masks are used to deliver O_2, N_2O-O_2, and/or other inhalation anesthetics before, during, and after the anesthetic procedure. Because of the variations in the size and shape of faces, several different sizes of full-face masks should always be available.

Face masks are frequently made of black rubber, which prevents the mouth and nose of the patient from being visualized. Preferred is a clear plastic or rubber face mask that allows the patient's mouth and nose to be seen so that foreign material (e.g., vomitus, blood) may be observed and removed.

Metal connectors that attach the face mask to the tubing of the anesthesia machine are required. These connectors come in a variety of sizes and shapes.

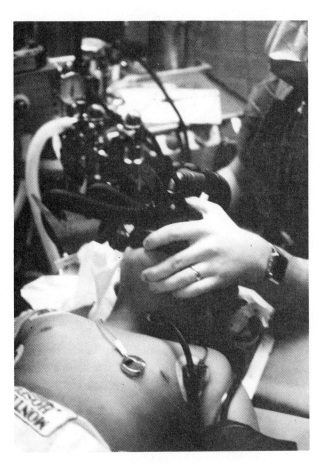

Fig. 32-2. Full-face mask covers both the mouth and nose of the patient. Note precordial stethoscope.

Laryngoscopes

The laryngoscope (Fig. 32-3) is a device designed to assist in the visualization of the trachea during intubation. It consists of two parts: a handle and battery holder, and a blade. The handle is usually made of metal (although some are made of plastic) and contains batteries that are used to operate the light bulb found in the blade.

The blade of the laryngoscope is also usually made of metal, although plastic is also used today. The laryngoscope blade is designed to be placed into the patient's mouth to aid in visualization of the larynx. A small light bulb that illuminates the laryngeal area is attached to the blade. There are two basic types of laryngoscope blade: the curved (Macintosh) and the straight (Miller) blade. Each of these blades is available in a variety of sizes. The technique for using these blades differs.

The curved blade is the more commonly used. The tip of the curved blade is inserted into the vallecula,

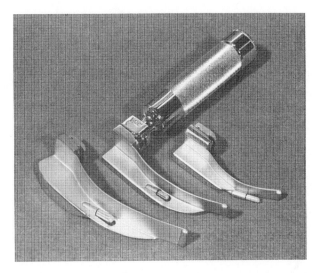

Fig. 32-3. Laryngoscope handle and several sizes of curved blades.

the cul-de-sac between the base of the tongue and the epiglottis (Fig. 32-4). The handle of the laryngoscope is then lifted straight up, a movement that exposes the vocal cords. When the straight blade is used, its tip is placed underneath the laryngeal surface of the epiglottis (Fig. 32-5), and the larynx is exposed by an upward and forward lift of the blade.

Most laryngoscopes and blades are designed to be held in the operator's left hand, with the endotracheal tube held in the right. Special laryngoscope blades are available for left-handed operators.

Endotracheal tubes and connectors

Endotracheal tubes and connectors (Fig. 32-6) are rubber tubes designed to be placed from the mouth (oroendotracheal) or nose (nasoendotracheal) into the patient's trachea. Reusable and disposable endotracheal tubes are available, with disposables being more popular today. Because the diameter of the laryngeal opening and of the trachea varies from patient to patient, endotracheal tubes are manufactured in a variety of diameters. Endotracheal tubes are commonly referred to by their size; for example, a No. 38 tube has an external diameter of 38 mm. For adult patients a No. 36 tube is usually appropriate for a male and a No. 34 tube for a female. Smaller- and larger-size tubes are available to accommodate the child or larger patient.

Endotracheal tubes have an inflatable cuff (Fig. 32-6) located near its distal end. When intubating a patient, the endotracheal tube is inserted into the

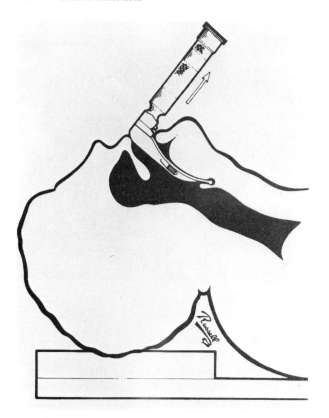

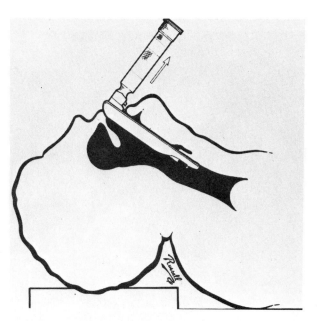

Fig. 32-5. Straight laryngoscope blade is placed beneath epiglottis and lifted, thereby exposing larynx. (From *Advanced cardiac life support manual,* (©) Reproduced with permission. American Heart Association.)

Fig. 32-4. Curved blade is placed between the base of the tongue and the epiglottis. Laryngoscope is then lifted, elevating tongue and exposing larynx. (From *Advanced cardiac life support manual.* (©) Reproduced with permission. American Heart Association.)

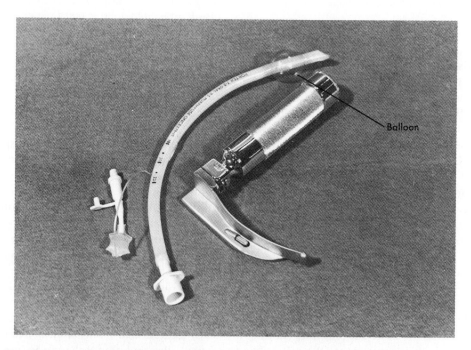

Fig. 32-6. Laryngoscope and endotracheal tube. Distal end of tube has inflatable cuff *(arrow)* designed to provide an airtight seal, preventing entry of substances into the trachea.

trachea so that the cuff just disappears beyond the level of the larynx. Air is then injected into a tube that connects with the cuff and inflates it. Enough air is injected into the cuff to seal the trachea off from the pharynx, thereby preventing foreign material, such as blood, saliva, or vomitus, from entering the trachea and bronchi.

Connectors for endotracheal tubes are the same as those used for full-face masks. They are used to connect the endotracheal tube to the anesthesia machine.

Oropharyngeal and nasopharyngeal airways

Oropharyngeal (Fig. 32-7) and nasopharyngeal airways (Fig. 32-8) are used to assist in maintaining a patent airway during and after the anesthetic procedure. Oropharyngeal airways are plastic, rubber, or metallic devices designed to fit between the base of the tongue and the posterior pharyngeal wall (Fig. 32-9). The nasopharyngeal airway (also known as a nasal trumpet) is a thin, flexible rubber tube designed to be inserted through the nares and to rest between the base of the tongue and posterior pharynx (Fig. 32-10). The purpose of both of these devices is to displace the tongue from the pharynx and thereby permit the patient to exchange air either around or through the airway. The nasopharyngeal airway is better tolerated by the patient, thereby minimizing the occurrence of gagging and vomiting. Nasal airways should be lubricated prior to their insertion in order to speed their placement.

Tonsillar suction tips

The immediate availability of suction devices is absolutely essential before general anesthesia is started. Excessive salivation, bleeding in the mouth or pharynx, or vomiting can produce airway obstruction, laryngospasm, or possible infection of the trachea or bronchi. Tonsillar suction tips are recommended because they can be inserted blindly into the posterior pharynx of the patient without risk of producing bleeding. The end of the tonsillar suction tip is rounded, making this device preferable to others that have sharper tips. Several tonsillar suction tips should be available in the event that one becomes clogged.

Magill intubation forceps

A Magill intubation forceps (Fig. 32-11) is designed to assist in placing the endotracheal tube. It is most frequently used during nasoendotracheal intubation and is therefore a very important item in the armamentarium for general anesthesia for dental procedures.

Sphygmomanometers and stethoscopes

Sphygmomanometers and stethoscopes must also be available during general anesthetic procedures. They will be used for the monitoring of vital signs, specifically blood pressure, heart rate and rhythm, heart sounds, and breath sounds. Appropriate-size sphygmomanometers must be available if accurate blood pressure values are desired.

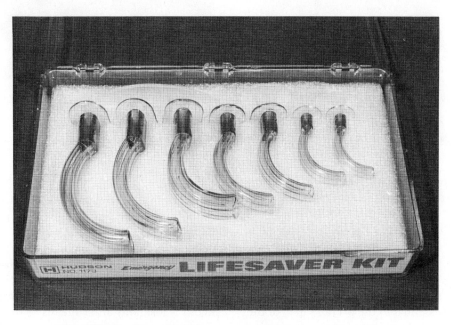

Fig. 32-7. Oropharyngeal airways are available in a variety of sizes.

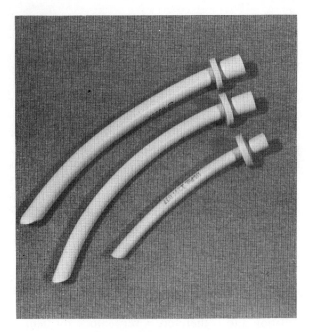

Fig. 32-8. Nasopharyngeal airways.

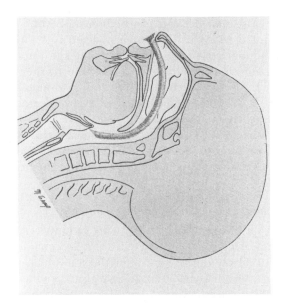

Fig. 32-10. Nasopharyngeal airway is designed to rest between the base of the tongue and pharyngeal wall, thus permitting air to pass between the lungs and the nose. (From Bennett CR: *Monheim's general anesthesia in dental practice,* ed 4. St Louis, 1974, Mosby.)

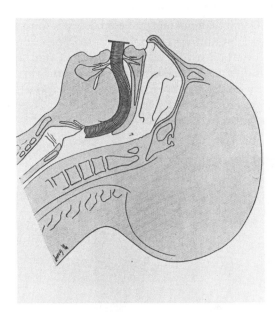

Fig. 32-9. Oropharyngeal airway is designed to lift the tongue off the posterior wall of the pharynx. (From Bennett CR: *Monheim's general anesthesia in dental practice,* ed 4. St Louis, 1974, Mosby.)

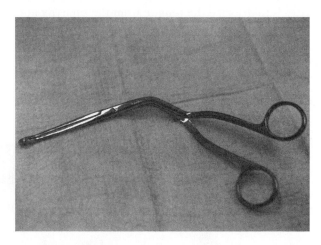

Fig. 32-11. Magill intubation forceps are designed to assist in passage of an endotracheal tube, especially during nasal intubation.

Monitoring equipment

Monitoring of the patient during sedation or general anesthesia is essential to the overall safety of the procedure. During sedative procedures monitoring of the central nervous system (CNS) via direct communication with the patient is of primary importance. Because the patient is able to respond appropriately to verbal command, other, more complex, monitoring devices need not be used routinely.[1] However, once a patient is unconscious (increased CNS depression) their ability to respond to command is lost, and other means of determining their status during anesthesia must be used. For this rea-

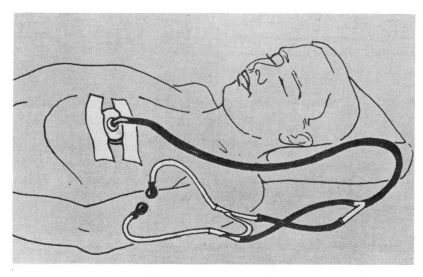

Fig. 32-12. Precordial stethoscope.

son the level of monitoring during general anesthesia is increased over that required for sedative procedures. A monitor is a device that reminds and warns. The department of anesthesiology at the Harvard University School of Medicine recently designed monitoring guidelines for use during general anesthesia.[2] The recommendations in these guidelines have been well received and widely implemented. The following are some of the methods and devices used to monitor patients during general anesthesia:

1. The stethoscope is used with auscultation to monitor the heart rate, heart rhythm, and/or breath sounds. Taped to the chest in the precordial region, the *precordial stethoscope* (Fig. 32-12) provides continuous monitoring of heart sounds, but when placed on the neck directly over the trachea, the *pretracheal stethoscope* permits monitoring of respiration. The pretracheal stethoscope is recommended for use during IV sedation procedures as well as during all forms of general anesthesia. An alternative to the precordial stethoscope during general anesthesia is the *esophageal stethoscope* (Fig. 32-13), a rubber tube inserted into the patient's esophagus after intubation. This device provides continuous monitoring similar to that provided by the precordial stethoscope but is more effective because of its closer proximity to the heart and lungs. Breath and heart sounds can usually be heard more distinctly. Esophageal stethoscopes are not used during sedation procedures and brief outpatient general anesthetics.

2. The *pulse oximeter* (Fig. 32-14) provides a non-invasive means of monitoring the degree of oxygen saturation of hemoglobin in peripheral blood vessels. Pulse oximeters provide continuous monitoring of oxygenation and of the heart rate, permitting a more rapid detection of potential airway problems (there is a time lag of about 20 seconds). The use of pulse oximetry is considered to be a standard of care during general anesthesia.

3. *End-tidal CO$_2$ (ETCO$_2$) monitors* are a recent addition to the monitoring armamentarium during general anesthesia. They help to evaluate the effectiveness of ventilation (Fig. 32-15). Because the ETCO$_2$ monitor evaluates every breath, airway problems may be detected almost instantaneously (a lag time of several seconds exists), permitting their correction before they become significant.

4. The *sphygmomanometer,* or *blood pressure cuff,* is used to monitor blood pressure by indirect determination. During general anesthesia blood pressure, heart rate and rhythm, and respiratory rate are monitored continuously and recorded every 5 minutes. If events warrant, more frequent determinations are obtained.

5. The *ECG* provides a means of monitoring the electrical activity and rhythm of the heart. The ECG permits continuous observation of the rate and rhythm of the heart during general anesthesia. Use of the ECG is considered a standard of care during all forms of general anesthesia.

6. *Continuous temperature monitoring* by rectal or esophageal probe has become increasingly common since the 1980s with the recognition of malignant hyperthermia. Although not done with all patients undergoing general anesthesia, temperature monitoring is considered a standard of care in children,

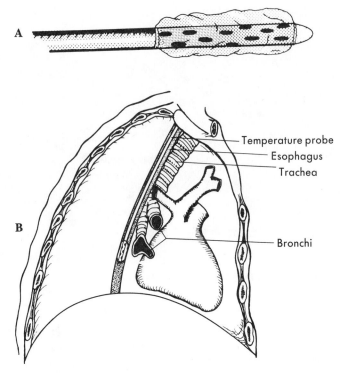

Fig. 32-13. Esophageal stethoscope aids in monitoring both heart and lung sounds. **A,** Distal end of esophageal stethoscope has multiple perforations that aid in picking up sounds in thorax. **B,** Esophageal stethoscope is inserted into esophagus to the level of the heart, thereby maximizing sound amplification. (From Gravenstein JS, Paulus DA: *Monitoring practice in clinical anesthesia,* Philadelphia, 1982, Lippincott.)

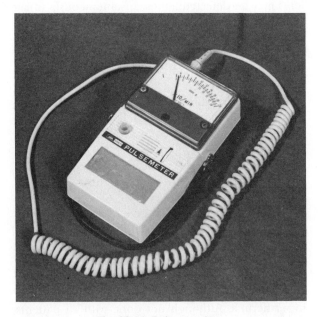

Fig. 32-14. Pulse monitor.

young adults, patients with fever, and patients undergoing procedures involving induced hypothermia.[2]

7. The *EEG* reveals the electrical activity of the brain. Although not used routinely, it can easily be obtained through the use of scalp electrodes. The level of cortical depression associated with anesthesia or the effects of adverse conditions such as hypoxia or hypercapnia may be evaluated.[3]

8. Although not used routinely, direct measurement of arterial blood pressure is frequently of value in the critically ill patient and during cardiopulmonary bypass, major traumatic surgery, and hypotensive or hypothermic anesthesia. Its major advantage over indirect blood pressure methods is that it provides accurate values of intraarterial or intracardiac blood pressure on a continuous basis.

9. Collection and measurement of urinary output are easily obtained in the anesthetized patient whose bladder has been catheterized. Urinary output is a

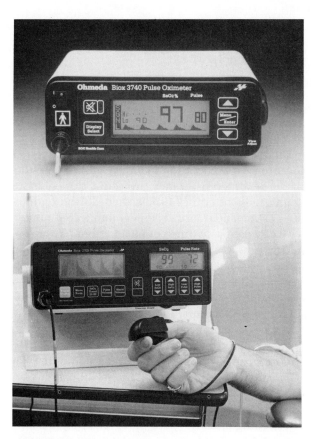

Fig. 32-15. Oximeter *(top)* provides continuous monitoring of arterial O$_2$ saturation by a fingerprobe *(bottom)*. (Courtesy Ohmeda, Littleton, Colo.)

simple method of determining the degree of hydration of the body. During general anesthesia the patient should produce urine at a rate approaching the normal of 40 to 60 ml/hour. Volumes below this may signify dehydration and indicate the need for additional fluid replacement. For routine general anesthetic procedures the monitoring of urinary output is not required.

10. *Central venous pressure (CVP)* measures the pressure exerted by blood returning to the right side of the heart and the ability of the right heart to manage it effectively. Monitoring CVP enables the doctor to distinguish between hemorrhage and congestive heart failure. With extensive blood loss the CVP will fall, whereas in congestive heart failure or overhydration the CVP is elevated.

An invasive procedure, CVP monitoring is recommended in older patients, in patients in whom considerable blood or fluid loss is expected, during major traumatic surgery, in cases in which multiple transfusions are given, and during open heart sur-

gery, among other indications. For the typical ASA I or II ambulatory dental patient undergoing general anesthesia, routine use of CVP is not necessary.

Emergency equipment and drugs

Complications occur during the administration of general anesthesia. Among the more frequently observed complications are hypotension and cardiac dysrhythmias. Monitoring of the anesthetized patient enables the entire anesthesia team to be aware of the presence of these and other potentially lethal problems and to initiate appropriate corrective treatment. The anesthesiologist will have available a supply of emergency drugs and equipment for use in these circumstances. The emergency drugs required by the Board of Dental Examiners in the state of California for doctors using general anesthesia will be listed here.[4] A more thorough discussion of emergency drugs recommended for outpatient facilities will be presented in Chapter 34.

Equipment	*Drugs (by category)*
Portable apparatus for intermittent positive-pressure breathing (IPPB)	Vasopressor(s)
	Corticosteroid(s)
	Bronchodilator(s)
	Succinylcholine
Bag-valve-mask, face masks, connectors	Sodium bicarbonate
	Intravenous replacement fluid
Portable, battery-powered light source	Opioid antagonist(s)
	Antihistamine(s)
Apparatus for emergency tracheotomy or cricothyrotomy	Anticholinergic(s)
	Antidysrhythmic(s)
	Antihypertensive(s)
Electrocardiogram monitor and defibrillator	Drug for arterial dilation

Several of the drugs recommended for the emergency tray are also commonly used during the routine administration of general anesthesia. These include succinylcholine, IV replacement fluid, and opioid antagonists.

DRUGS

An array of drugs may be used during the administration of general anesthesia. Many of these drugs have been discussed in other sections of this book and are listed here with minimal discussion. Other drugs make their first appearance at this time; however, they too will only receive a brief review as it is not the goal of this textbook to provide the reader with an in-depth knowledge of general anesthesia.

The more commonly used drugs in general anesthesia may be divided into the following categories:

Intravenous induction agents
Opioids (agonists and agonist/antagonists)
Neuroleptic agents
Dissociative agents
Muscle relaxants
Inhalation anesthetics

Intravenous induction agents

In the adult patient receiving general anesthesia it is the desire of the anesthesiologist to achieve stage III anesthesia as rapidly as possible. To do so, IV agents are usually preferred to inhalation anesthetics for they are more rapid acting and do not possess the unpleasant odors of some of the gases (i.e., halothane).

Barbiturates

The *barbiturates* remain the most commonly used IV induction agents with methohexital, thiopental, and thiamylal the most frequently administered. Other drugs used intravenously for induction of anesthesia include diazepam, midazolam, lorazepam, etomidate, ketamine, and propofol.

Methohexital is a rapid-onset, short-acting barbiturate. It is most often used as the sole agent to provide general anesthesia for short procedures (less than 30 minutes).[5] Methohexital is less frequently used as an induction agent for general anesthesia. The dosage of methohexital for induction of general anesthesia is 1 mg/kg. It is 2.5 times as potent as the thiobarbiturates (thiopental and thiamylal) and has a more rapid recovery.[6] Proprietary names of methohexital are Brevital (United States) and Brietal (Great Britain). The uses of methohexital in anesthesia are for short-duration outpatient procedures, electroconvulsive therapy,[7] and minor gynecologic or orthopedic procedures.

Thiopental (Pentothal) and *thiamylal* (Surital) are called thiobarbiturates because they possess a sulfa molecule. Pharmacologically they are quite similar. Following IV administration the onset of action of these drugs is rapid (within 30 to 40 seconds) and of short duration. Duration of action of thiopental and thiamylal is, however, longer than that of methohexital.[8]

The induction of general anesthesia with a thiobarbiturate is usually produced by the slow IV injection of 150 to 300 mg over a 15- to 30-second interval. Thiopental and thiamylal are used as 2.5% solutions. After induction of general anesthesia, other longer-acting anesthetics are administered for the maintenance of anesthesia.

Absolute contraindications to the administration of barbiturates include status asthmaticus and latent or manifest porphyria.

Benzodiazepines

Several benzodiazepines are also used as induction agents for general anesthesia. These include diazepam, midazolam, and lorazepam.

Diazepam and midazolam are benzodiazepines that are used on occasion to induce general anesthesia.[9] The benzodiazepines provide a slower, more gradual loss of consciousness than do the barbiturates. The patient initially enters into a comfortable level of sedation, at which point additional diazepam, midazolam, or other IV (e.g., opioids) or inhalation agents (e.g., halothane) may be administered to produce the desired level of unconsciousness. Diazepam and midazolam are also used during short IV barbiturate general anesthetic procedures in order to potentiate the actions of the barbiturate as well as to "smooth out" the anesthesia.

Lorazepam (Ativan) is a benzodiazepine that was *not* recommended earlier for use in outpatients because of its long duration of action and the inability of the administrator to titrate the drug to clinical effect owing to its very slow onset of action. Because the need for rapid and "complete" recovery in inpatient procedures is not as urgent, lorazepam may be used like diazepam or midazolam in these patients.

Other agents

Etomidate (Amidate) was introduced in the United States in 1983 as a nonbarbiturate IV induction agent. Administered in a dose of 0.3 to 0.4 mg/kg, etomidate demonstrates a rapid onset of action combined with less respiratory depression than is seen with the barbiturates.[10] Cardiovascular stability is another positive feature of etomidate. Etomidate is highly lipid soluble, has a half-life of 60 minutes, and is short acting. Recovery of cognitive and psychomotor function is intermediate between thiopental[11] and methohexital.[12] Negative factors associated with etomidate include a burning sensation as the drug is injected in some patients, the occurrence of myoclonic jerks, the inhibition of steroid synthesis, and the occurrence of excitatory effects in approximately 30% of patients receiving it. Etomidate is used for IV induction in children where hemodynamic stability is desirable (hypovolemia) and the hypertension and tachycardia caused by ketamine are unacceptable.

Ketamine, used as either an IV or IM induction agent, primarily in children, is discussed more fully in Chapter 26. Ketamine is most suitable in children who are hemodynamically unstable or hypovolemic.[13] In addition, ketamine is used in asthmatic children because of its bronchodilating properties.[14] When administered by any route, ketamine should be preceded or accompanied by the administration of atropine or glycopyrrolate to attenuate the increase in airway secretions associated with its administration.[10] In addition, benzodiazepine administration is recommended to lessen the dysphoric emergence from anesthesia that may be associated with ketamine.[15]

Propofol (diisopropylphenol) is a nonbarbiturate IV anesthetic agent that is employed in situations in which rapid-onset and short-duration general anesthesia is desired.[16] Propofol is most often compared to methohexital.[17] Pecaro et al. demonstrated that in usual dosages propofol has insignificant cardiovascular and respiratory effects.[18] Moreover, it lacks excitatory or emetic actions. The primary side effect noted with propofol administration was pain on injection (37.5% on dorsum of hand).[19]

The anesthesia induction dose of propofol is 2.5 mg/kg, which makes the drug equipotent with 4 mg/kg of thiopental.[20] McCulloch et al.[19] suggested an induction dose of 2.25 mg/kg in "younger patients" and a dose of 1.5 mg/kg in "older patients." Pharmacokinetically, the terminal half-life of propofol is 286 minutes plus or minus 36 minutes, with clearance in 1803 minutes plus or minus 125 minutes.[21]

Cundy et al.,[22] comparing propofol with methohexital, found that propofol provided a statistically significant superior quality of anesthesia. No difference was noted in recovery time, and postoperatively methohexital patients were significantly more drowsy. Coughing and laryngospasm did not occur with propofol (0/30) as they did with methohexital (5/30). The proprietary name of propofol is Diprivan.

Opioids

The term *opioid* is used in a broad sense to include both the opioid agonists and opioid agonist/antagonists. The pharmacology of these drugs was discussed in some detail in Chapter 26.

Opioids are frequently used for the maintenance of general anesthesia in a technique involving the administration of an opioid, N_2O-O_2, and a muscle relaxant. Anesthesia is induced with one of the short-acting IV agents previously discussed and is maintained with periodic doses of an appropriate opioid. Nitrous oxide-oxygen is administered to minimize the dosage of opioid required. The most commonly used opioids in general anesthesia are morphine, meperidine, fentanyl, and its analogs sufentanil and alfentanil.

Morphine is the standard opioid analgesic drug to which all others are compared. Morphine has strong analgesic and sedative properties. It is used primarily for longer-duration procedures. Morphine is usually injected as a 1-mg/ml solution.

Meperidine (Demerol) is probably the most frequently used opioid analgesic in anesthesia. It is usually used in a concentration of 10 mg/ml. Meperidine is intermediate in duration of action between morphine and fentanyl.

Fentanyl (Sublimaze) is used either as a component of Innovar (droperidol with fentanyl) to provide neuroleptanesthesia or alone during shorter surgical procedures. It is used alone in a concentration of 0.01 mg/ml.

Alfentanil (Alfenta) and *sufentanil* (Sufenta) are rapid-onset, short-duration analogs of fentanyl that have been recently introduced and have gained some popularity.[23,24]

Opioid agonist/antagonists such as *nalbuphine* and *butorphanol* are also used during general anesthesia. Their primary benefit appears to be the ceiling effect on respiratory depression that is noted with their administration.[25] This contrasts to the dose-related respiratory depression observed with opioid agonists.

The opioid antagonist *naloxone* is commonly used when opioids have been administered. At the termination of the anesthetic procedure the anesthesiologist attempts to awaken the patient. If opioids have been used during surgery, the patient's rate of breathing may be quite slow at this time. Titration of naloxone may be necessary to reverse this opioid-induced respiratory depression. Careful monitoring of the patient following reversal with naloxone is required because several of the opioids have a longer duration of action than does naloxone and a return of respiratory depression at a later time is possible. To minimize this potential risk, the administration of an intramuscular (IM) dose of naloxone should be considered following its IV administration.[26] The slower onset and longer duration of the IM dose of naloxone will minimize the risk of a recurrence of significant respiratory depression.

The opioid analgesics are very important anesthetic agents. Their use in a typical anesthetic procedure will be described.

Neuroleptanesthesia

Neuroleptanesthesia and neuroleptanalgesia were discussed in Chapter 26. The neuroleptic state is produced when a neuroleptic drug (another name for a tranquilizer) and a opioid analgesic are administered together to produce a state characterized by the following[27]:

Sleepiness without total unconsciousness
Psychological indifference to the environment
No voluntary movements
Analgesia
Satisfactory amnesia

In clinical practice neuroleptanesthesia is produced through the administration of the following:

Neuroleptic drug
Opioid
Nitrous oxide-oxygen
Muscle relaxant

Innovar, a premixed combination of droperidol (Inapsine)—2.5 mg/ml—and fentanyl (Sublimaze)—0.05 mg/ml—is the drug most frequently used to induce a neuroleptic state. The pharmacologic properties of droperidol and of fentanyl are discussed in Chapter 26. A brief review follows.

Droperidol, a tranquilizer, produces clinical actions within 5 to 10 minutes after IV administration. Long acting, its actions may be observed for 6 to 12 hours following a single injection. Additional properties of droperidol include its antiemetic and its slight α-adrenergic receptor-blocking effects. Disadvantages of droperidol include its long duration of action (a disadvantage in outpatient procedures); its peripheral vasodilating effects, which may produce hypotension; the fact that there is no pharmacologic antagonist for droperidol; and the fact that large doses produce muscle movements similar to extrapyramidal effects—dystonia, akathisia, and oculogyric crisis (see Chapter 8).

Fentanyl, a powerful opioid analgesic, acts rapidly after IV administration, with a duration of action of between 30 and 60 minutes. The analgesic potency of 0.1 mg fentanyl is equal to that of 10 mg morphine. Fentanyl does not release histamine (unlike meperidine, which does), can be reversed by opioid antagonists, produces euphoria, and has negligible effects on the cardiovascular system. Negative features of fentanyl include the fact that it is an emetic and that it produces respiratory depression, miosis, possibly bradycardia and bronchoconstriction, and, with large doses, possibly muscular rigidity (see Chapters 26 and 28).

Neuroleptanesthesia produced by droperidol, fentanyl, N$_2$O-O$_2$, and a muscle relaxant has become a very popular anesthetic technique, especially in the more severely medically compromised patient (ASA III, IV). Snow lists the following advantages of neuroleptanesthesia[28]:

No secretions
No venous or tissue irritation
Stable cardiovascular system
No sensitization of myocardial conduction system to actions of catecholamines
No toxic effects on liver or kidney function
Reduced cerebrospinal fluid (CSF) pressure and intraocular pressure
Nonemetic
Nonexplosive
Prompt recovery
Long periods of analgesia and amnesia induced
In recovery room, longer tolerance of endotracheal tube

The following are disadvantages of neuroleptanesthesia[28]:

Respiratory depression and apnea can be caused by fentanyl and muscle relaxants
Assisted or controlled ventilation is required
Action of muscle relaxants must be reversed

Dissociative anesthesia

Dissociative anesthesia and analgesia, as produced by ketamine, were described in Chapter 26. In the dissociative state patients appear to be awake—their eyes are open and they are capable of involuntary muscular movement, but they are unaware of, or dissociated from, the environment. After IV administration ketamine produces analgesia and unconsciousness within 30 seconds. The usual general anesthesia induction dose of ketamine is 1 to 2 mg/kg, injected at a rate of 0.5 mg/kg per minute.[29]

Ketamine is used as an induction agent for general anesthesia and as the sole agent for short diagnostic and surgical procedures that do not require skeletal muscle relaxation. Ketamine is used frequently in children. It is used especially in surgical procedures in which control of the airway is difficult to maintain, especially for correction of scars and burns of the face and neck—procedures that make intubation and extension of the neck very difficult, if not impossible. The administration of dissociative anesthesia is contraindicated in intraocular surgery and in patients with a history of increased CSF pressure, cerebrovascular accident (CVA), psychiatric problems, and high blood pressure.

Ketamine is nonirritating to blood vessels and tissues. It produces profound analgesia, muscle tone is preserved, and the laryngeal and pharyngeal reflexes are not depressed; therefore, a patent airway can usually be maintained without the need for intubation.

Disadvantages of ketamine include increases in heart rate, blood pressure, and intraocular pressure; in addition, diplopia, eye movements, and nystagmus can occur during anesthesia—thus the recommendation that ketamine not be used in intraocular procedures. There is no antagonist for ketamine. Probably the most serious disadvantage of ketamine is its ability to produce a confused state, associated with unpleasant dreams and frightening or upsetting hallucinations, which occur most commonly in adults during the recovery period.[30,31] These appear much less frequently in children.

Muscle relaxants

Muscle relaxant drugs are also known as neuromuscular blocking agents. These drugs interfere with the transmission of impulses from motor nerves to muscle at the skeletal neuromuscular junction. Prior to the introduction of muscle relaxants into anesthesia, skeletal muscle relaxation was obtained during surgery by inducing deeper levels of anesthesia. Along with muscle relaxation, a greatly increased incidence of complications, morbidity, and mortality was seen. With the introduction of muscle relaxants, deep anesthesia can now be avoided, and the concept and technique of balanced anesthesia have developed. Muscle relaxants are the most commonly used adjuvants in anesthesia practice.

During short-duration outpatient general anesthesia (e.g., with methohexital), there is little or no indication for the administration of muscle relaxants. When longer-duration outpatient procedures are performed, the patient may need to be intubated, a procedure that usually requires the use of the short-acting muscle relaxant *succinylcholine*. Patients undergoing inpatient dental procedures performed under general anesthesia will receive succinylcholine for intubation and may, if necessary, receive other longer-acting muscle relaxants.

There are four mechanisms in which the physiology of neuromuscular transmission may be interfered with to interrupt nerve impulses arriving at the end plate:

1. In *deficiency block* the synthesis and/or transmission of acetylcholine is interfered with. Examples of drugs that act in this manner include local anesthetics; neomycin, kanamycin, and streptomycin; *Clostridium botulinum* toxin; calcium deficiency; and magnesium excess.

2. *Nondepolarizing block* is also known as a competitive block. The drug attaches to cholinergic receptors, preventing acetylcholine from attaching to the receptor, a form of competitive inhibition. Most commonly used muscle relaxants act in this manner. Examples of nondepolarizing muscle relaxants include d-tubocurarine (Curare), pancuronium metocurine, vecuronium atricurium, and gallamine. The actions of nondepolarizing muscle relaxants may be reversed by increasing the concentration of acetylcholine, which is accomplished clinically by administering anticholinesterases such as neostigmine. Nondepolarizing muscle relaxants do not produce fasciculations (skeletal muscle contractions) when administered intravenously.

3. In *depolarizing block* (also known as phase I block) the drug acts in a manner similar to acetylcholine but for a prolonged time. The drug acts to produce muscle contractions, called fasciculations (the equivalent of acetylcholine action), followed by prolonged muscle flaccidity. Two drugs that produce this effect are succinylcholine and decamethonium.

4. *Dual block* is also called *desensitization block*. In dual block the membrane is depolarized (phase I) and is then slowly repolarized. The drug enters into the fiber and acts as a nondepolarizing agent (phase II), even though the membrane potential is restored.

All neuromuscular blockers impair respiration and can produce apnea; therefore, these drugs must never be administered by persons untrained in endotracheal intubation and in the administration of artificial ventilation. Nondepolarizing muscle relaxants are used more frequently during surgery than depolarizing agents because their duration is somewhat longer (20 to 45 minutes). Depolarizing agents are used for endotracheal intubation, laryngoscopy, bronchoscopy, esophagoscopy, and other short procedures.

Patients with myasthenia gravis should receive nondepolarizing muscle relaxants with great caution as they are extremely sensitive to the actions of these drugs. Such patients usually require as little as one tenth the usual dose for clinical effect.

Tubocurarine (Tubarine) remains a commonly used nondepolarizing muscle relaxant in anesthesia. After IV administration the drug produces its actions within 3 minutes and has a duration of 30 to 40 minutes. The average initial dose in adults is 15 to 20 mg. Supplemental doses may be required for prolonged surgical procedures. Muscle fasciculation and postoperative muscle pain do not develop with tubocurarine. Administration of tubocurarine is contraindicated in patients with myasthenia gravis, renal disease, and bronchial asthma (because it releases histamine).

Pancuronium (Pavulon) was introduced in the United States in the early 1970s and has become a very popular nondepolarizing muscle relaxant. It is approximately five times as potent as tubocurarine and has an onset of action within 3 minutes and a duration of action of 30 to 40 minutes.

Pancuronium does not produce muscle fasciculations nor does it produce postanesthetic muscle pain. Unlike tubocurarine, pancuronium does not release histamine. The initial IV dose range is 0.04 to 0.01 mg/kg, with supplemental doses required for prolonged procedures. Small doses of pancuronium in patients with myasthenia gravis will produce profound effects.

Recent additions to the nondepolarizing group of muscle relaxants include *metocurine, vecuronium,* and *atracurium.* The major advantage of these drugs is an elimination half-life shorter than the 2 hours possessed by pancuronium and d-tubocurarine. Vecuronium has an elimination half-life of 70 minutes, atracurium about 20 minutes.

Gallamine (Flaxedil) is another synthetic nondepolarizing muscle relaxant; it is one sixth as potent as tubocurarine. Gallamine does not release histamine and produces no fasciculations and no muscle pain. The range of initial dose is 80 to 120 mg, with a duration of action of 20 to 40 minutes. Supplemental doses of 20 to 40 mg are given as required. Because gallamine is excreted entirely unchanged from the kidney, it is contraindicated in patients with kidney failure.

Succinylcholine (Anectine) is a synthetic, short-acting depolarizing muscle relaxant. After an IV dose of 60 to 80 mg (for a 70-kg patient), relaxation develops within 1 minute. Recovery of muscle tone is rapid and complete within 5 to 15 minutes. For children the usual dose for intubation is 20 mg. Succinylcholine is used routinely for skeletal muscle relaxation prior to tracheal intubation. It may also be used by continuous IV drip for relaxation during abdominal operations. Succinylcholine is used during electroconvulsive therapy (ECT) and as an emergency drug during the treatment of laryngospasm (Chapter

28). Succinylcholine is contraindicated for use in patients with penetrating injuries of the eye and patients with myotonia.

Strong skeletal muscle contractions (fasciculations) follow the administration of succinylcholine. Patients receiving this drug may complain of severe muscle pain for several days after its administration. Fasciculations develop first in the eyebrow and eyelids, then in the shoulder girdle and abdominal muscles, and finally in the muscles of the hands and feet. The severity of fasciculations may be diminished by slow administration of the drug or by the prior administration of tubocurarine (3 to 6 mg) or pancuronium (0.5 to 1 mg).

Succinylcholine may produce hyperkalemia (succinylcholine-induced hyperkalemia), which in certain patients may lead to cardiovascular collapse or cardiac arrest. At-risk patients include those with:

Severe burns
Massive trauma
Tetanus
Spinal cord injury
Brain injury
Uremia with increased serum potassium

Succinylcholine has been implicated as a trigger agent in malignant hyperthermia (MH). In MH-susceptible patients succinylcholine administration is followed by exaggerated fasciculations, rigidity, and difficulty in intubation. Body temperature then increases at an alarming rate. Succinylcholine must not be administered to patients with a MH history.

Metabolized in the serum by plasma pseudocholinesterase, succinylcholine is usually rapidly inactivated (muscle tonus returns to normal within 5 to 15 minutes). However, 1 in 3000 persons has atypical pseudocholinesterase and will exhibit a prolonged response to succinylcholine.[32] The presence of atypical pseudocholinesterase should be suspected in any patient in whom spontaneous respiration has not returned within 15 minutes following the administration of succinylcholine. Management of prolonged apnea requires continued controlled ventilation until spontaneous ventilation returns or until fresh-frozen plasma or blood is administered to restore the pseudocholinesterase level of the plasma.

Decamethonium (Syncurine) is another depolarizing muscle relaxant with actions similar to those of succinylcholine but longer acting. Fasciculations may occur but are usually not as exaggerated as those of succinylcholine. The IV dose of decamethonium is 3 mg (equal to 15 mg of tubocurarine) with a duration of about 20 minutes. It undergoes excretion in the urine unchanged, which explains its longer duration of action.

Muscle relaxants are important adjuvants to general anesthesia. Their presence has permitted abdominal operations to be completed with much more ease and comfort for the patient, surgeon, and anesthesiologist alike. Their use, especially that of the longer-acting nondepolarizing muscle relaxants, is not recommended in outpatient procedures. Succinylcholine is used in outpatient procedures for intubation and in the emergency management of laryngospasm.

Inhalation anesthetics

Inhalation anesthetics are the most frequently used means of producing general anesthesia. They are popular because of their controllability, which is based on the fact that their uptake and elimination are largely affected by pulmonary ventilation. The advantages of inhalation anesthetics were reviewed in Chapters 13 and 14.

The "ideal" inhalation anesthetic has not been found; however, volatile agents that approach the ideal are currently available. The following characteristics are desirable in an inhalation anesthetic:

1. The inhalation anesthetic should be either a gas or a liquid. If it is a gas, it should be easily liquified at moderate pressures.
2. The blood/gas solubility coefficient (ratio) should be low (in the range of 0.3 to 2) so that a high partial pressure is obtained quickly in the alveoli. This will provide a rapid induction of anesthetic effect and an equally rapid elimination of the agent.
3. The oil/water solubility should also be low so

that the drug is not stored in fat, thus avoiding prolonged recovery.

4. The inhalation anesthetic should be neither flammable nor explosive.
5. The inhalation anesthetic should be stable—not decomposing on exposure to moisture, light, or air. It should not corrode or react with rubber, plastic, metal, or CO_2 absorbers.
6. The inhalation anesthetic should have a pleasant odor, be nonirritating, and have minimal postanesthetic sequelae.
7. The inhalation anesthetic should be nontoxic to the organs and nonallergenic.
8. The inhalation anesthetic should be potent enough so that it provides good analgesia and anesthesia and so that at least 50% O_2 may be administered with it.
9. The inhalation anesthetic should be completely inert, being excreted entirely unchanged through the lungs.

The physical and chemical characteristics of major inhalation anesthetics currently used in general anesthesia are presented in Table 32-1. More commonly used inhalation anesthetics include N_2O, halothane, enflurane, isoflurane, desflurane, and sevoflurane. Other inhalation anesthetics, such as cyclopropane, chloroform, diethyl ether, divinyl ether, ethyl vinyl ether, fluroxene, methoxyflurane, and trichloroethylene are no longer used in general anesthesia. These inhalation anesthetics and the reasons for their discontinuance are listed in the following paragraphs.

Cyclopropane provides rapid-induction anesthesia, is nonirritating, and is indicated for poor-risk patients. However, cyclopropane produces broncho-

Table 32-1. Characteristics of inhalation anesthetics

Agent	Partition coefficient at 37°C		Minimum anesthetic concentration (MAC)‡ (percent)	Inspired concentrations (percentage)	
	Fat/blood*	Blood/gas†		Induction	Maintenance
N_2O	2.3	0.47	105.0	75	50-70
Halothane	60	2.3	0.75	1-4	0.5-2.0
Enflurane	36	1.8	1.58	2-5	1.5-3.0
Isoflurane	45	1.4	1.28	1-4	0.8-2.0
Desflurane	27	0.42	4.6-6.0	—	—
Sevoflurane	48	0.59	1.71	—	—

*Fat/blood partition coefficient—lower value, decreased lipid storage, and more rapid recovery.

†Blood/gas partition coefficient—lower value, rapid onset, and rapid recovery.

‡Minimum anesthetic concentration—gas concentration in alveoli, which when in equilibrium with CNS, causes 50% of individuals to move in response to painful cutaneous stimulation (in O_2).

constriction, sensitizes the myocardium to catecholamines (increasing the risk of dysrhythmias), produces vomiting, and is extremely explosive.

Chloroform produces rapid induction, is nonirritating, provides good muscle relaxation, and is nonexplosive and nonflammable. Its major disadvantages are that it produces hepatotoxicity and that it is a myocardial depressant.

Diethyl ether is a bronchodilator, does not depress circulation, is a good muscle relaxant, and is relatively nontoxic and safe. Disadvantages include a relatively slow onset and recovery, irritation produced from its disagreeable odor, which may induce secretion of mucus in the upper airway, its tendency to induce vomiting, and the fact that it is explosive and flammable.

Divinyl ether (Vinethene) provides rapid induction and recovery and is a respiratory stimulant. It is, however, an irritant to the upper airway and larynx, cannot be administered safely for longer than approximately 15 minutes (it is hepatotoxic if administered for longer than 60 minutes), and it is flammable and explosive.

Ethyl vinyl ether (Vinamar) is clinically similar to divinyl ether (see preceding paragraph). It, too, is flammable and explosive.

Trichloroethylene (Trilene) is nonirritating, provides analgesia, maintains a stable blood pressure, and is nonflammable and nonexplosive. Unfortunately, it is a myocardial depressant, sensitizes the myocardium to catecholamines, produces dysrhythmias and tachypnea, is an emetic, and cannot be used with CO_2-absorption systems because it reacts with soda lime or barium hydroxide to form toxic substances such as phosgene (a respiratory tract irritant) and dichloroacetylene (explosive and neurotoxic to cranial nerves V and VII).

Among the inhalation anesthetics that are in use today, N_2O is by far the most common. In fact, N_2O is administered during almost every general anesthetic. The pharmacology of this very important inhalation sedative and general anesthetic was presented in Chapter 14. The primary function of N_2O administration during general anesthesia is to potentiate the actions of other, more potent drugs (IV or inhalation) being administered to produce a controlled state of unconsciousnes.. Its administration (along with O_2) permits a smaller dose or lesser concentration of the primary drug to be administered to produce the desired level of general anesthesia. For example, halothane administered with O_2 alone may require a 4% concentration to produce surgical-

depth anesthesia; however, with the administration of 60% N_2O, halothane effectively provides the same depth of anesthesia at only a 1% concentration. With IV drug administration the same is true.

Halothane was introduced into anesthesia practice in 1956 and had profound effects on the practice of anesthesia and surgery in that it was not flammable. This permitted the use of electrocautery by the surgeon and the introduction of extensive electronic monitoring by the anesthesiologist. Unlike ether, which preceded halothane, it permitted a rapid induction and emergence from anesthesia, also allowing for rapid changes of anesthetic depth during surgery. With the introduction of newer inhalation anesthetics, halothane is used less frequently in adults. Its popularity in pediatric anesthesia remains.

Disadvantages of halothane include myocardial depression, production of cardiac dysrhythmias (at higher concentrations), sensitization of the myocardium to the actions of catecholamines, acting as a potent uterine relaxant and possibly producing shivering or tremor during recovery in patients whose body temperature is low. Probably the most serious disadvantage of halothane is its possible hepatotoxicity. Reports also indicate that halothane may produce postanesthetic jaundice or disturbed liver function and even necrosis. The National Halothane Study concluded that if indeed halothane-induced hepatic necrosis occurs, it is rare.[33]

Although most inhaled halothane is removed through the lungs, metabolites are slowly removed from the body over 2 to 3 weeks. Halothane is administered for outpatient anesthesia and on some occasions is used in lower concentrations to provide sedation.

Methoxyflurane (Penthrane) was synthesized in 1958 and introduced into clinical anesthesiology in 1960. Because of methoxyflurane's high blood/gas solubility coefficient (13), the induction of anesthesia is slow, as is emergence from unconsciousness. The fact that methoxyflurane is also quite soluble in rubber tubing only adds to the slow onset and emergence. High-lipid solubility further delays recovery from methoxyflurane anesthesia.

Methoxyflurane has a high oil/gas solubility coefficient and is the most potent as well as least soluble inhalation anesthetic. Its MAC is 0.16%, with anesthesia induced at concentrations of 2 to 3% and maintained at concentrations of 0.25% to 1%.

Methoxyflurane provides a good margin of safety, is an excellent muscle relaxant, does not sensitize the myocardium to catecholamines, and is nonflammable and nonexplosive. Its major disadvantage is its slow onset of action and the equally prolonged recovery period. In addition, methoxyflurane is nephrotoxic, an action caused by free fluoride ions produced during the metabolic breakdown of the drug. Methoxyflurane is infrequently used for outpatient procedures because of slow recovery from its clinical effects.

Enflurane (Ethrane) was synthesized in 1963 and has clinical and pharmacologic properties similar to those of halothane. Enflurane, however, has the advantage of being compatible with epinephrine—up to 10 ml of a 1:100,000 concentration, with a decreased risk of dysrhythmias developing.[34]

Advantages of enflurane include the fact that it has a pleasant odor; there is rapid induction and recovery; it is nonirritating (produces no secretions); it is a bronchodilator and a good muscle relaxant; it keeps the cardiovascular system fairly stable (dysrhythmias are uncommon); it is not an emetic; it is nonexplosive and nonflammable; and it is compatible with epinephrine. The MAC for enflurane is 1.68%, and anesthesia is induced at concentrations of 2 to 5% and maintained at concentrations of 1.5 to 3%.

Disadvantages of enflurane include myocardial depression; progressive hypotension develops with increase in anesthetic depth; shivering may develop on emergence; there is a possibility of liver damage; it should be avoided in patients with severely compromised renal function; and it produces CNS irritation at higher concentrations, especially if the patient is hypocarbic. Clinically, muscular twitching is noted in the jaw, neck, or extremities, and increased spike activity is noted on the EEG. Enflurane undergoes metabolism only to the extent of 2.5%, the remainder being excreted unchanged through the lungs.

Isoflurane (Forane), synthesized in 1970, is a chemical isomer of enflurane. No abnormal motor activity, such as muscle twitching or convulsions, is noted with isoflurane.

Advantages of isoflurane include that it has a pleasant odor; a rapid induction and recovery; it is nonirritating (produces no secretions); it is a bronchodilator; it provides excellent muscle relaxation; it keeps the cardiac rhythm stable; it is compatible with epinephrine; it is not an emetic; and it is nonexplosive and nonflammable. The MAC for isoflurane is 1.2%; anesthesia is induced at concentrations of 1% to 4% and maintained at concentrations of 0.8% to 2%.

Disadvantages of isoflurane include myocardial depression; blood pressure is depressed as the level of anesthesia is increased; shivering develops postanesthetically; the possibility exists for hepatotoxicity; and it is probably not advised to administer isoflurane to patients with severely compromised renal function.

Sevoflurane and *desflurane* are relatively new inhalation anesthetics. The low solubility of these agents is desirable, producing a rapid onset of anesthesia and equally rapid recovery, but they do so only at the expense of a decreased potency. Desflurane, an investigational drug, does not undergo biotransformation in the body. A principle disadvantage is airway irritation during inhalation induction. Its principle advantage seems to be rapid patient emergence from anesthesia.[35] This may be a valuable property in busy surgical suites where a rapid turnover of patients is required and in surgical outpatients who would especially benefit from the rapid recovery of mental facilities.[36] Sevoflurane is currently in clinical use in Japan and in clinical trials in the United States. Like desflurane, it is noted for its low solubility and rapid induction of, and emergence from, anesthesia.

TECHNIQUES
Inpatient general anesthesia

General anesthesia as administered to the hospitalized patient represents the fundamental technique from which the other forms of general anesthesia have developed. As a rule this form of anesthesia is utilized in dentistry for the medically compromised patient and for patients undergoing extensive and possibly traumatic dental procedures.

The patient is usually admitted to the hospital 1 day prior to the scheduled procedure so that an extensive preoperative evaluation can be completed. A physical examination and laboratory tests such as hematocrit, hemoglobin, complete blood count (CBC, differential), and urinalysis form the minimal evaluation. In adult patients scheduled for general anesthesia a chest x-ray film and ECG are required in most hospitals.

The evening prior to the surgical procedure the anesthesiologist will make a preanesthetic visit, the purpose of which is to evaluate the patient as to any special anesthetic risks (e.g., potential airway maintenance problems); to review the physical examination of the patient and results of the laboratory tests; to discuss the upcoming anesthetic procedure with the patient so as to allay any apprehensions, and to determine if the patient has any special requests as to the type of anesthesia. The anesthesiologist will write preanesthetic orders for the patient. Typical orders include the patient fasting prior to surgery ("npo after midnight") and preoperative medications to be administered intramuscularly either 1 hour prior to the scheduled procedure or "on call to the operating room" if the procedure is scheduled for later in the day. The most frequently prescribed combination of preoperative drugs include an antianxiety drug such as diazepam or midazolam or a barbiturate such as pentobarbital; an opioid (meperidine); and an anticholinergic (scopolamine or atropine). If it is deemed necessary, the patient will also receive a sedative such as flurazepam or secobarbital orally prior to bedtime so as to ensure a good night's sleep prior to surgery.

Prior to the arrival of the patient, the anesthesiologist will have prepared all of the necessary drugs and equipment. On arrival in the operating room the patient will be properly identified by the nursing staff and placed onto the operating room table. Physiologic monitors, such as a blood pressure cuff, a precordial stethoscope, ECG leads, and pulse oximeter are attached.

An IV infusion is established, usually on the arm opposite the blood pressure cuff. An indwelling catheter, not smaller than 18 gauge, is inserted and secured. In procedures in which blood transfusion is considered likely, a 16-gauge indwelling catheter will be used for the IV infusion. A 1000-ml bag of either 5% dextrose and water or lactated Ringer's solution is used for maintenance of the infusion. Vital signs are monitored and recorded on the anesthesia record (Fig. 32-16).

On arrival of the surgical team the induction of anesthesia commences. The patient may be administered (IV) a small dose of benzodiazepine to produce a greater degree of sedation while awaiting the surgical team. A topical anesthetic, frequently cocaine, will be applied to each of the patient's nostrils with a cotton applicator stick to produce both analgesia and hemostasis during nasal intubation. A full-face mask is placed on the patient with a flow of approximately 5 to 7 L/min of 100% O_2.

Thiopental or thiamylal is titrated until the patient loses consciousness (usually 200 to 250 mg). The anesthesiologist will then "bag" the patient (breathe for the patient) to confirm that a patent airway is present prior to administration of a muscle relaxant. Once a patent airway is ensured, a dose of succinylcholine, a depolarizing muscle relaxant, is administered. Fasciculations occur, and then the patient

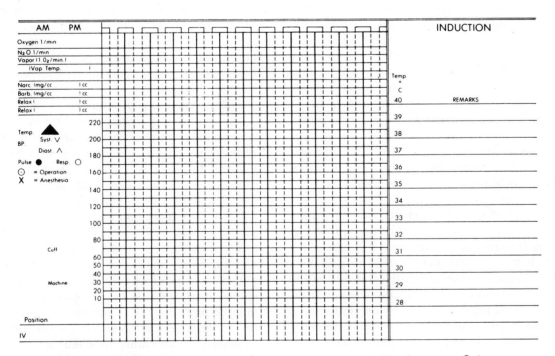

Fig. 32-16. Anesthesia record. ∨, Systolic blood pressure; ∧, diastolic blood pressure; ●, heart rate; ▲, temperature; ○, respiration.

ceases breathing. To prevent or minimize fasciculations, a small dose (1 to 2 ml) of a nondepolarizing muscle relaxant may be administered prior to the succinylcholine.

Once fasciculations occur and the patient becomes apneic, the lubricated nasotracheal tube is placed into a nostril and gently advanced into the nasopharynx (Fig. 32-17). The anesthesiologist visualizes the larynx and the tip of the tube using the laryngoscope. With a Magill intubation forceps the endotracheal tube is gently advanced and placed into the trachea. Once inserted the endotracheal tube is attached to the anesthesia machine, and the patient is ventilated. The drugs to be used for maintenance of anesthesia are administered—for example, a 1.5% to 2% concentration of halothane or a dose of an IV drug such as meperidine. The gas flow on the anesthesia machine is adjusted to 3 L/min of N_2O and 2 L/min of O_2. The endotracheal tube is secured, its

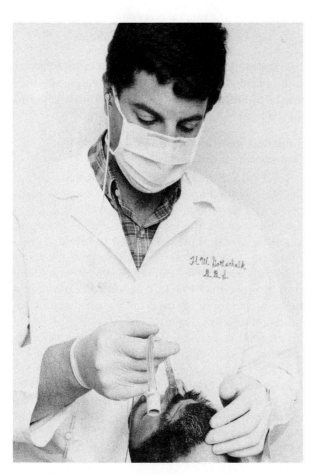

Fig. 32-17. Nasoendotracheal tube is passed through nostril and into nasopharynx. Magill intubation forceps assists in its passage into trachea.

cuff inflated, and the chest auscultated to determine if breath sounds are equal on the right and left sides (the endotracheal tube may have been overinserted with its tip lying in the right mainstem bronchus). A nasogastric tube is frequently inserted through the other nostril to remove any air and gastric secretions that develop during the procedure.

The anesthetized patient is draped and prepared for surgery (Fig. 32-18). During this time the anesthesiologist administers additional doses of the maintenance drug(s) and continues to monitor the patient's vital signs. For most dental procedures local anesthetics will be administered to assist in pain control and hemostasis. When possible, epinephrine will be included in the local anesthetic solution. The response of the patient to stimulation as well as his or her vital signs determines the need for additional anesthetic drugs. With inhalation anesthetics the concentration of the drug will be gradually decreased to as low a level as possible (without adverse patient response). Minimal doses of injectable anesthetic drugs will be administered periodically as determined by the patient's response to surgical stimulation and their vital signs.

During full-mouth reconstructive dental procedures, implants, or extensive surgery, there may be a need for muscular relaxation so that the doctor can more readily gain access to the oral cavity. In most instances the degree of muscle relaxation provided by the primary anesthetic drug, especially inhalation anesthetics, is sufficient. Occasionally, however, it becomes necessary to provide additional muscle relaxation through administration of a neuromuscular blocking agent such as pancuronium or tubocurarine.

As the surgical procedure terminates, the administration of inhalation anesthetics will be stopped and the patient permitted to breathe either 100% O_2 or a combination of N_2O-O_2 and then 100% O_2. The use of inhalation anesthetics usually provides a more rapid emergence from general anesthesia. In cases in which IV opioids, benzodiazepines, and muscle relaxants were used to provide anesthesia, it may be necessary to administer additional drugs to reverse their actions. Naloxone titrated intravenously is used to reverse opioid-induced respiratory depression, and flumazenil for residual benzodiazepine actions, whereas an anticholinesterase such as neostigmine (Prostigmin) is administered to reverse any residual muscle relaxation. Atropine will usually be administered with the neostigmine to prevent bradycardia.

After reversal of the opioid and muscle relaxant or

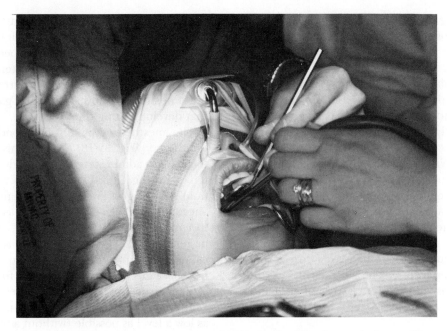

Fig. 32-18. Anesthetized patient is draped and prepared for the surgical procedure.

termination of the flow of inhalation anesthetic, the patient will usually rapidly emerge from anesthesia. When the patient's respiratory movements are deemed adequate, the patient is extubated. Immediately prior to extubation the anesthesiologist must carefully suction the pharynx to remove any salivary secretions, fluids, or debris that may have collected in this region. The cuff of the endotracheal tube is deflated and the tube removed. The face mask is placed on the patient, and 100% O_2 is administered.

The patient is transferred to a recovery room where a trained staff of nurses and anesthesiologists look after him or her in the immediate period following recovery from anesthesia and surgery. The patient in the recovery area will receive O_2 by nasal cannula and have his or her blood pressure, pulse, respirations, and ECG monitored until the vital signs are stable and he or she is alert and awake.

Once the patient has recovered adequately from the effects of anesthesia, he or she will be discharged from the recovery room and readmitted to the surgical ward. The patient will remain in this ward until the surgeon permits him or her to be discharged from the hospital. In many inpatient dental cases the patient remains hospitalized overnight and is discharged the day after surgery. In cases of ASA III and some ASA II patients, stabilization of the medical condition may require more prolonged hospitaliza-

tion. For the ASA I or II patient who is to be admitted to the hospital for extensive dental treatment under general anesthesia, a minimum stay of two nights and approximately 3 days will be the norm.

Outpatient general anesthesia
Conventional general anesthetics

A second technique of general anesthesia is hospital-type general anesthesia on an outpatient basis. The actual anesthetic technique is quite similar to that described for the inpatient stay, with an important exception that the drugs used to produce anesthesia will be shorter acting, so as to permit a more rapid and complete recovery upon completion of the surgical procedure. For this reason inhalation anesthetics are more often used for maintenance of anesthesia than are IV agents.

The patient, an ASA I or II (with the extremely rare exception an ASA III), undergoes a physical examination, including basic laboratory tests, not more than 48 hours prior to the scheduled procedure. The patient will have received explicit, written preoperative instructions that include being NPO for at least 6 to 8 hours prior to treatment.

On the morning of treatment the following must be in order:

1. The patient has been NPO for at least 6 to 8 hours.

2. Results of the basic laboratory tests have been received, examined, and are within normal limits.
3. The patient's medical records are complete, including the medical history and physical examination.
4. The informed consent form has been signed and witnessed.

Immediately prior to the start of the procedure the patient will be asked to void and to remove contact lenses and removable dental prostheses, if present.

Intramuscular premedication is not desirable prior to outpatient general anesthesia because most drugs used for this purpose serve to prolong the recovery period. An anticholinergic such as atropine is recommended for IM or IV administration immediately prior to the induction of general anesthesia.

The patient is placed in either the dental chair or the operating table on which the procedure is to be performed. The anesthesiologist places monitoring devices—an ECG, precordial stethoscope, blood pressure cuff, and pulse oximeter and then starts an IV infusion with an 18-gauge indwelling catheter, using an infusate of either 5% dextrose and water or lactated Ringer's solution (1000 ml). The nasal mucosa is then sprayed with 4% cocaine or 0.5% phenylephrine.

Anesthesia is induced by using a short-acting barbiturate, usually methohexital, or with an inhalation anesthetic. In the small child it may be difficult to start an IV infusion with the patient conscious; as a result induction with inhalation anesthetics is more common in children.

Prior to inserting the nasotracheal tube 1 mg of pancuronium (to prevent fasciculations) and an appropriate dose of succinylcholine are administered. The technique for intubation is similar to that described on p. 473.

Once general anesthesia is induced and the patient prepared for the surgical procedure, anesthesia is maintained with a combination of N_2O, O_2, and halothane or enflurane. Muscle relaxation is rarely required when this procedure is used. The patient's ventilation will be spontaneous but requires assistance from the anesthesiologist. On rare occasions ventilation may be controlled.

Immediately prior to the start of the dental or surgical procedure, the operating dentist places a gauze pack or curtain across the posterior part of the pharynx. This will serve as a screen to collect any debris produced during the dental procedure. A rubber dam is another means of preventing the accumulation of debris in the pharynx.

The administration of local anesthesia is desirable because it decreases the requirement for additional CNS-depressant administration, thereby hastening recovery and discharge of the patient.

At the termination of the procedure the patient receives 100% O_2, and when his or her protective reflexes are intact he or she is extubated and taken to a recovery area that is supplied with a bed, O_2 suction, monitoring equipment, and emergency equipment and drugs and that is staffed by a trained nurse or anesthesia assistant. A minimum of 1 hour of recovery time is recommended and longer if the doctor considers it necessary. On occasion it may be necessary to admit a patient to the hospital overnight to permit more complete recovery when it appears that recovery is slow or incomplete. The possibility of hospitalization should have been discussed with the patient prior to the planned procedure and arrangements made with a nearby hospital for possible patient admittance. In cases in which recovery is adequate, the patient may be discharged from the facility if accompanied by a responsible adult guardian. It is recommended that the patient be contacted later that same day to determine how his or her recovery is progressing.

Intravenous barbiturate general anesthesia

Shorter procedures, usually requiring less than 30 minutes, may be facilitated with the administration of short-acting IV barbiturates or nonbarbiturates, such as propofol. Although several barbiturates are available, thiopental and methohexital have become the mainstays of ambulatory anesthesia practice in the United States and the United Kingdom.

The patient receiving IV general anesthesia in an ambulatory care facility such as a dental office will be an ASA I, II, or, rarely, an ASA III patient. Preoperative assessment will include laboratory tests (CBC, hemoglobin and/or hematocrit, and urinalysis). Patients over the age of approximately 35 years will also receive a chest x-ray film and ECG. Preoperative instructions (Table 32-2) and preoperative preparation are similar to those discussed on p. 488. Monitors include a precordial stethoscope, ECG, blood pressure cuff, and pulse oximeter.

An IV line is established using a scalp vein needle (21 gauge) or catheter (21 gauge) and a 250-ml bag of suitable infusate. A small test dose of 1 or 2 ml of methohexital (1%) or thiopental (2.5%) or propofol

Table 32-2. Preanesthetic instructions

1. If the patient is an adult, he should have nothing to eat or drink after midnight of the night prior to surgery.
2. If the patient is an infant, he should have no solid food or milk for 6 hours prior to surgery. Clear fluids may be given up to 4 hours before anesthesia.
3. It must be emphasized to parents to keep a careful watch on children so that early morning snacks are not eaten.
4. No makeup is to be worn, or at least it must be kept to a minimum.
5. Children must be accompanied by parents or a legal guardian.
6. Adults must be accompanied by another adult and must not drive a motor vehicle for 24 hours after completion of anesthesia.
7. If there is any change in general health before the date of surgery, the patient is advised to contact the doctor or ambulatory care facility in which the procedure is to be performed.

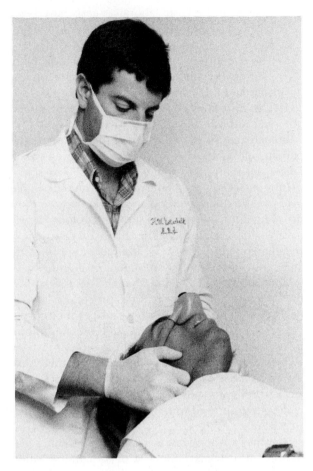

Fig. 32-19. Patent airway is maintained during procedure by an anesthesiologist, nurse anesthetist, or anesthesia assistant.

is administered, and a bite block placed between the patient's teeth to prevent their closing after the loss of consciousness. The IV anesthetic is then titrated slowly until the patient loses consciousness. The loss of the eyelid reflex is a common, though not always reliable, indicator of a light level of unconsciousness. The loss of consciousness commonly occurs approximately 30 to 40 seconds after the titration of the drugs. If a pulse oximeter or ECG is being used, a significant increase in the heart rate will be noted as methohexital begins to exert its effect.

As the patient loses consciousness, the airway must be maintained. This is accomplished by a "head-holder" or "chinner"—an anesthesiologist, dentist, nurse anesthetist, or anesthesia assistant who is responsible for maintenance of a patent airway during the dental procedure (Fig. 32-19). The administration of additional methohexital or thiopental may be necessary during the procedure. The response of the patient to surgical stimulation will serve as a gauge to the need for additional drug administration.

Throughout the procedure a nasal hood is maintained in place, delivering either 100% O_2 or a combination of N_2O-O_2. The latter is used during longer procedures as a means of "smoothing out the anesthetic" and minimizing the dose of barbiturate required. The administration of small IV doses of a benzodiazepine to smooth out the anesthetic, in addition to the O_2 or N_2O-O_2, has become increasingly popular. The administration of diazepam or mida-

zolam does not increase the recovery time from this technique.

The administration of propofol, a short-acting drug, via infusion pump enables the anesthesiologist to maintain a constant level of CNS depression throughout the procedure. Recovery of consciousness is rapid and more complete than with barbiturates following cessation of the infusion.

The back of the oral cavity is screened off with a gauze curtain (a 4- × 8-inch gauze). The surgical assistant is responsible for the maintenance of a dry and relatively clean surgical field and for changing the gauze as often as is required.

Local anesthesia is recommended as a means of blocking painful stimulation, thereby decreasing the total dose of the IV anesthetic required to achieve clinically adequate anesthesia. The continued presence of local anesthesia in the immediate postoperative period enables the patient to recover from the general anesthetic without any discomfort.

After termination of the procedure the patient usually recovers consciousness quite rapidly, not from rapid metabolism of the intravenously administered drugs but, rather, from their redistribution to other organs and storage sites within the body. Be that as it may, the patient appears to recover quite rapidly and is then transferred (most frequently by walking with assistance) to the fully equipped and staffed recovery area, where he or she remains until recovery is deemed adequate to permit discharge home, accompanied by a responsible adult. Contact with the patient later that day or evening is recommended.

SUMMARY

The use of general anesthesia in dentistry dates to the origins of anesthesia itself. Dentists were intimately involved in the discovery of this valuable technique of pain and anxiety control and in many of its subsequent advances. Indeed, dentistry has been in the forefront in the recent evolution of outpatient general anesthesia.

General anesthesia is a technique that requires significantly greater training on the part of the doctor and staff in order for it to be used safely. Under no circumstances should a person without a minimum of 2 years full-time training in anesthesiology or its equivalent in an oral and maxillofacial surgery training program ever consider the administration of general anesthesia.

The indications for general anesthesia in dentistry have diminished over the years as techniques of conscious sedation have evolved. Yet, many indications for its use remain. The selection of the most appropriate type of general anesthesia for use in a given patient must be made after a thorough evaluation of the patient's physical condition, the planned dental treatment, the training and background of the doctor and staff, and the preparedness of the facility.

REFERENCES

1. Rosenberg MB, Campbell RL: Guidelines for intraoperative monitoring of dental patients undergoing conscious sedation, deep sedation, and general anesthesia, *Oral Surg* 71(1):2, 1991.
2. Eichhorn JH, Cooper JB, Cullen DJ et al: Anesthesia practice standards at Harvard: a review, *J Clin Anesth* 1(1):55, 1988.
3. Griffiths MJ, Preece AW, Green JL: Monitoring sedation levels by EEG spectral analysis, *Anesth Prog* 38(6):227, 1991.
4. Board of Dental Examiners: *General anesthesia statute.* Extract from business and professions code, Chapter 4—Dentistry, Article 2.7—Use of general anesthesia, Sacramento, Calif, 1993, The Board.
5. Zink BJ, Darfler K, Salluzzo RF et al: The efficacy and safety of methohexital in the emergency department, *Ann Emerg Med* 20(12):1293, 1991.
6. Gilman AG, Rall TW, Nies AS et al: *Goodman and Gilman's pharmacological basis of therapeutics,* ed 8. New York, 1990, McGraw-Hill, p. 1690.
7. Gaines GY III, Rees DI: Anesthetic considerations for electroconvulsive therapy, *South Med J* 85(5):469, 1992.
8. Van Hemelrijck J, Gonzales JM, White PF: Pharmacology of intravenous anesthetic agents. In Rogers MC, Tinker JH, Covino BG, eds: *Principles and practice of anesthesiology.* St Louis, 1993, Mosby, pp. 1143-1144.
9. Eldor J: High-dose flunitrazepam anesthesia, *Medical Hypotheses* 38(4):352, 1992.
10. Wetzel RC, Maxwell LG: Anesthesia for children. In Rogers MC, Tinker JH, Covino BG, eds: *Principles and practice of anesthesiology.* St Louis, 1993, Mosby, p. 2173.
11. Horrigan RW, Moyers JR, Johnson BH et al: Etomidate vs thiopental with and without fentanyl, a comparative study of awakening in man, *Anesthesiology* 52:362, 1980.
12. Miller BM, Hendry JGB, Lees NW: Etomidate and methohexital, a comparative clinical study in outpatient anesthesia, *Anaesthesia* 33:450, 1978.
13. Waxman K, Shoemaker WC, Lipmann M: Cardiovascular effects of anesthetic induction with ketamine, *Anesth Analg* 59:355, 1980.
14. Tobias JD, Martin LD, Wetzel RC: Ketamine by continuous infusion for sedation in the pediatric intensive care unit, *Crit Care Med* 18:819, 1990.
15. Reich DL, Silvay G: Ketamine: an update on the first twenty-five years of clinical experience, *Can J Anaesth* 36(2):186, 1989.
16. Weightman WM, Zacharias M: Comparison of propofol and thiopentone anaesthesia (with special reference to recovery characteristics), *Anaesth Intensive Care* 15:389, 1987.
17. Rutter DV, Morgan M, Lumley J et al: ICI 35868 (Diprivan): a new intravenous induction agent, *Anaesthesia* 35:1188, 1980.
18. Pecaro BC, Houting T: Diprivan (ICI 35868, 2, 6, di-isopropylphenol), a new intravenous anesthetic, *Oral Surg* 60:586, 1985.
19. McCulloch MJ, Lees NW: Assessment and modification of pain on induction with propofol (Diprivan), *Anaesthesia* 40:1117, 1985.
20. Grounds RM, Twigley AJ, Carli F et al: The haemodynamics of intravenous induction. Comparison of the effects of thiopentone and propofol, *Anaesthesia* 40:735, 1985.
21. Kay NH, Uppington J, Sear JW et al: Use of an emulsion of ICI 35868 (propofol) for the induction and maintenance of anaesthesia, *Br J Anaesthesiol* 57:736, 1985.
22. Cundy JM, Arunasalam K: Use of an emulsion formulation of propofol (Diprivan) in intravenous anaesthesia for termination of pregnancy. A comparison with methohexitone. *Postgrad Med J* 61(suppl 3):129, 1985.
23. Wedell D, Hersh EV: A review of the opioid analgesics fentanyl, alfentanil, and sufentanil, *Compendium* 12(3):184, 1991.
24. Clotz MA, Nahata MC: Clinical uses of fentanyl, sufentanil, and alfentanil, *Clin Pharm* 18(8):581, 1991.
25. Lefevre B, Freysz M, Lepine J et al: Comparison of nalbuphine and fentanyl as intravenous analgesics for medically compromised patients undergoing oral surgery, *Anesth Prog* 39(1-2):13, 1993.

26. Elleby DH, Greenberg PM, Barry LD: Postoperative narcotic and nonnarcotic analgesics, *Clin Podiatr Med Surg* 9(2):365, 1992.

27. Bremang JA: Neuroleptic analgesia in ambulatory (nasal) endoscopies, *J Otolaryngol* 20(6):435, 1991.

28. Snow JC: Intravenous anesthesia. In *Manual of anesthesia*. Boston, 1977, Little, Brown, p. 109.

29. Waxman K, Shoemaker WC, Lipmann M: Cardiovascular effects of anesthetic induction with ketamine, *Anesth Analg* 59:355, 1980.

30. Roelofse JA, Vander Bilj P: Adverse reactions to midazolam and ketamine premedication in children, *Anesth Prog* 38(2):73, 1991.

31. Klausen NO, Wilberg-Jorgensen F, Chraemmer-Jorgensen B: Psychotomimetic reactions after low-dose ketamine infusion. Comparison with neuroleptanaesthesia, *Br J Anaesth* 55(4):297, 1983.

32. Schweinefus R, Schick L: Succinylcholine: ''good guy, bad guy,'' *J Post Anesth Nurs* 6(6):410, 1991.

33. Bunker JP and the National Research Council, Subcommittee on the national halothane study: *The national halothane study: a study of the possible association between halothane anesthesia and postoperative hepatic necrosis: report.* Bethesda, Md, National Institute of General Medical Science, 1969.

34. Ogawa A, Oi K: Use of N_2O/O_2 enflurane anesthesia for dental treatment of the handicapped, *J Oral Maxillofac Surg* 49(4):343, 1991.

35. Smiley RM, Ornstein E, Matteo RS et al: Desflurane and isoflurane in surgical patients: comparison of emergence time, *Anesthesiology* 74:425, 1991.

36. Fletcher JE, Sebel PS, Murphy MR et al: Psychomotor performance after desflurane anesthesia: a comparison with isoflurane, *Anesth Analg* 73:260, 1991.

SECTION SEVEN

Emergency preparation and management

Whenever drugs are administered or prescribed, adverse reactions are possible. Fortunately, with the vast majority of drugs currently used in the management of pain and anxiety, the incidence of adverse drug reactions (ADRs) is quite low. Indeed, those drugs that, although therapeutically useful, have a greater incidence of ADRs are very rapidly replaced in the physician's and dentist's armamentarium by newer, equally useful drugs possessing a lesser risk of ADRs.

Indiscriminate utilization of drugs is one of the major causes of the increase in the number of serious incidents of drug-related, life-threatening emergencies that are reported in the medical and dental literature.[1,2] It is hoped that whenever a drug is administered or prescribed, a rational purpose exists for its administration. Most drug-related emergency situations are classified as one aspect of iatrogenic disease, a category that encompasses a spectrum of adverse effects produced unintentionally by health professionals during patient management.

The frequency of occurrence of ADRs as reported in the medical and dental literature has ranged from 3% to 20% of all hospital admissions.[1-4] Of patients hospitalized for other reasons, 5% to 40% will experience an ADR during their hospitalization. Furthermore, another 10% to 18% of those patients hospitalized because of an ADR will have yet another ADR while in the hospital, which results in the length of their hospitalization being prolonged.[4]

Because the overwhelming majority of drugs discussed in this text are CNS depressants administered to patients for the purpose of managing their treatment-related fears and anxieties, it is quite likely that ADRs will be noted at some time. For this reason the doctor and the entire office staff must be able to recognize and be prepared to manage these situations rapidly and effectively.

This section is divided into three chapters. The first two chapters discuss the subject of preparation—of the office, of office personnel, and the requirement for emergency drugs and equipment—and the third chapter reviews the management of systemic emergencies that might develop during sedative procedures. Localized complications have been reviewed with each of the major techniques of sedation (see Chapter 11 for intramuscular sedation, Chapter 17 for inhalation sedation, and Chapter 28 for intravenous sedation). The need for emergency preparedness exists in a dental or medical practice regardless of whether or not sedative techniques are employed. Indeed, as discussed in Chapter 5, the medically compromised patient who is fearful or experiences pain during treatment is more likely to suffer an acute exacerbation of a medical problem in this stressful situation than is a more relaxed, pain-free patient with the same medical problem. In one report 77% of systemic emergencies associated with dental care occurred either during or immediately following the administration of local anesthetic (54.9%) or during the ensuing dental treatment (22.9%), arguably the most psychologically and physiologically stressful portions of the entire dental experience.[5] The types of dental treatment most frequently being attempted at the time the systemic emergency occurred were tooth extraction and pulpal extirpation—procedures in which complete pain control may prove elusive.[5]

OCCURRENCE OF SYSTEMIC COMPLICATIONS

Just before treatment	1.5%
During/after local anesthesia	54.9%
During treatment*	22.9%
After treatment	15.2%
After leaving office	5.5%

*See next box for specific treatment during emergency.

TYPE OF DENTAL TREATMENT DURING OCCURRENCE OF SYSTEMIC COMPLICATION

Tooth extraction	38.9%
Pulpal extirpation	26.9%
Unknown	12.3%
Other treatment	9.0%
Preparation	7.3%
Filling	2.3%
Incision	1.7%
Apicoectomy	0.7%
Removal of fillings	0.7%
Alveolar plastics	0.3%

Basic preparation of the dental/medical office and office staff will be the same whether or not sedative procedures are used. There will, however, be some drugs and items of emergency equipment that the doctor using sedation techniques will have available that are unnecessary in the offices of doctors not using sedation. Emergency equipment will be reviewed along with the components of the basic emergency kit.

Most, but not all, drug-related emergencies can be prevented. The doctor administering or prescribing drugs for a patient must always keep the following three principles of toxicology in mind[6]:

1. No drug ever exerts a single action.
2. No clinically useful drug is entirely devoid of toxicity.
3. Potential toxicity of a drug rests in the hands of the user.

Ideally the right drug in the right dose will be administered by the right route to the right patient at the right time for the right reason and will not produce any unwanted effects. Unfortunately, this clinical situation rarely, if ever, occurs because no drug is so specific that it produces only the desired effects in all patients. It must also be remembered that ADRs may occur when the wrong drug is administered to the wrong patient in the wrong dose by the wrong route at the wrong time and for the wrong reason. The most important safety factors in drug administration are the knowledge and ability of the person administering the drug. Before administering any drug, the doctor should be fully prepared to manage any ADR that might develop.

REFERENCES

1. Naranjo CA, Shear NH, Lanctot KL: Advances in the diagnosis of adverse drug reactions, *J Clin Pharmacol* 32(10):897, 1992.
2. Waller PC: Measuring the frequency of adverse drug reactions, *Br J Clinic Pharmacol* 33(3):249, 1992.
3. Einarson TR: Drug-related hospital admissions, *Ann Pharmacother* 27(7-8):832, 1993.
4. Bates DW, Leape LL, Petrycki S: Incidence and preventability of adverse drug events in hospitalized adults, *J Gen Intern Med* 8(6):289, 1993.
5. Matsuura H: Analysis of systemic complications and death during dental treatment in Japan, *Anesth Prog* 36:219, 1990.
6. Pallasch TJ: *Pharmacology for dental students and practitioners*. Philadelphia, 1980, Lea & Febiger.

CHAPTER *33*

Preparation for emergencies

Although the prevention of life-threatening emergencies is our primary goal, there still exist occasions on which potentially catastrophic situations will develop in spite of the doctor's best efforts. Through proper patient evaluation prior to the start of any treatment, appropriate treatment modification if necessary, selection of appropriate techniques and drugs for pain and anxiety control, adherence to proper techniques of drug administration and adequate monitoring throughout the procedure, it is unlikely that emergency situations will arise. However, in the event that an emergency does occur, it becomes extremely important for the office to be properly prepared and for all office personnel to be trained to recognize and manage such situations in a prompt and effective manner.

Table 33-1 summarizes the suggested preparation of the medical/dental office and office staff for emergency situations.

OFFICE

With all office personnel trained in the recognition and management of life-threatening situations, it is possible for each of them to maintain the life of a victim alone or as a member of a trained emergency team. Although management of most emergencies is possible with but a single rescuer, the concerted efforts of several trained persons is usually more efficient. Because most dental and medical offices have a number of staff persons present during working hours, the development of a team approach to emergency management is possible.

OFFICE PERSONNEL

An important factor in preparation of the medical/dental office for management of emergency situations will be the training of *all* office personnel, including nonchairside personnel, in the recognition and management of emergency situations. Training should include an annual refresher course in all aspects of emergency medicine—a course reviewing situations such as seizures, chest pain, unconsciousness, altered consciousness, drug-related emergencies, and respiratory difficulty, not simply basic life support (BLS). Such continuing education programs are available and a list is published biannually by the American Dental Association.[1] In the dental office in which sedation techniques are used, refresher courses in these techniques, including their complications, are also recommended.

Basic life support

Of significantly greater importance than the overall emergency review program is the requirement for the clinical ability to perform BLS, more commonly known as CPR (cardiopulmonary resuscitation). It is my opinion that no other preparatory step is as important as this one, since training in BLS enables the rescuer to recognize an acute life-threatening situation and to know what to do. The steps of BLS require no additional equipment; the mouth, hands, and knowledge of the rescuer are quite adequate in most cases to maintain life. When involved with drug-related emergencies, BLS most often proves to be the first and, quite often, most important step in management.

The doctor should mandate that all office personnel remain proficient in BLS techniques after having received their initial course. As CPR chairman for one of the divisions of the Greater Los Angeles Affiliate of the American Heart Association, I saw dramatic examples of the rapid decline in CPR skills following an initial BLS training program. Within 6 months of completing a Provider-level training program, the average person loses approximately 60% of his ability to perform adequate BLS.[2] Maintaining

Table 33-1. Summary of preparation

Office

Team approach to emergency management
Drugs and equipment checked regularly
Emergency telephone numbers available
    Paramedics
    Oral and maxillofacial surgeon
    Emergency ambulance service
    Hospital with 24-hour, fully staffed emergency room
    Physician
Emergency practice drills

Office personnel

Semiannual certification as BLS provider
Annual review program in emergency medicine

proficiency is important because even when BLS is performed perfectly the delivery of oxygenated blood to the victim's brain is only 25% to 33% of normal.[3] Faulty technique leads to a diminished cerebral blood flow and a decreased likelihood of survival for the victim.

If the doctor, assistant, or hygienist was working in an office with only one other person present and was the victim of cardiac arrest, this second person would be the only one available to provide BLS. *Making certain that all personnel are proficient in BLS thus becomes the single most important step in assuring that medical emergencies are managed efficiently and effectively.*

Advanced cardiac life support

Advanced cardiac life support (ACLS) involves the use of adjunctive equipment and drugs to further stabilize and manage the victim of a cardiac arrest or other serious cardiac rhythm disturbance. The ACLS course includes training and evaluation in technique of venipuncture and endotracheal intubation, interpretation of ECG rhythms, and management of cardiac dysrhythmias through drug therapy and defibrillation.

Doctors using IV conscious sedation should consider becoming trained in ACLS. With the availability of the IV route of drug administration the doctor with ACLS training will be better able to treat such situations. It is my belief that doctors employing deep sedation or general anesthesia should be certified in advanced cardiac life support. Provider-level programs in ACLS are available in most vicinities to eligible persons only. These include the physician, nurse, pharmacist, and dentist who have previously

been certified in BLS. In some jurisdictions paramedical personnel are ACLS-trained. ACLS programs are usually presented within a hospital under the auspices of the American Heart Association (AHA). Contact your local AHA affiliate for more information about these courses.

Team approach to emergency management

An office emergency team consists of two or three members, each of whom has a well-defined role in the management of an emergency situation. The doctor leads the team and is responsible for directing the activities of its other members (unless it is the doctor who is the victim of the emergency). In most situations the doctor will be responsible for performing the steps of BLS (airway maintenance and breathing) and will administer emergency drugs to the victim if indicated.

The second team member will be responsible for emergency drugs and equipment. This person is assigned to check the emergency kit and equipment on a regular basis to make certain that they will be available when needed (see Chapter 34). When an emergency does occur, this team member gathers the emergency kit and equipment and immediately brings it to the site of the emergency. Should emergency drug administration be required, this team member prepares the drugs for administration by the doctor. Other possible roles for this team member include administration of BLS, monitoring of vital signs, and summoning medical assistance. In BLS this team member will be an integral part of the emergency management and will ventilate the victim and/or perform external chest compression.

A third team member may be utilized when available. This member reports immediately to the site of the emergency and remains available as a circulating member, assisting as required. Roles for this member include monitoring vital signs, summoning medical assistance, administering BLS, and recordkeeping. During CPR this member will be available to relieve the first or second member.

Where the dental office is located in a large, multioffice building, a team member is directed to be certain an elevator is readily available for the emergency team and to direct the team to the correct office.

It is important that all office personnel be capable of participating in the emergency team. In addition, all team members should be able to carry out any of the functions of the entire team. Practice thus becomes vitally important.

EMERGENCY PRACTICE DRILLS

If life-threatening situations occurred regularly in medical and dental offices, there would be little need for emergency practice sessions. Team members would receive their training under actual emergency conditions. Fortunately, life-threatening situations do not occur with any degree of frequency. Because of this, team members quickly become rusty from the lack of opportunity to use their newly acquired knowledge and skill. Annual refresher courses in emergency medicine are invaluable in maintaining the level of overall knowledge of the emergency team members.

Of greater importance, however, is the team's ability to perform well in the office setting. In-office emergency drills are one means of maintaining an efficient emergency team in the absence of true emergency situations. On an irregular basis the doctor may stage a simulated life-threatening emergency. All team members should be able to respond exactly as they must under emergency conditions. Many doctors have even purchased mannequins for practicing BLS and hold frequent practice sessions for their staff.

Oral and maxillofacial surgeons have used a system of in-office evaluation for general anesthetic technique and emergency preparedness. A group of examiners (other doctors) assesses the preparedness of the oral surgery office under evaluation by staging mock emergencies (e.g., laryngospasm, cardiac arrest, bronchospasm) and viewing the office staff's response.[4] Created by the Southern California Society of Oral and Maxillofacial Surgeons, the in-office evaluation has become a requirement for membership in the American Association of Oral and Maxillofacial Surgeons. Similar programs have been instituted by dental boards of many of the 48 states that require a dentist to obtain a permit in order to utilize general anesthesia or parenteral sedation.[5] A voluntary program in office emergency preparedness, part of an IV conscious sedation certification program, has been in existence for 10 years at the University of Southern California School of Dentistry.[6]

OUTSIDE MEDICAL ASSISTANCE

Although most emergency situations are transient in nature and readily managed by the emergency team, there may be occasion to seek outside medical assistance. In situations involving ADRs following the administration of CNS depressants, follow-up evaluation by well-trained individuals is frequently rec-ommended. For these reasons, telephone numbers of emergency services personnel should be readily available and conspicuously posted by each telephone in the office (Fig. 33-1). With the availability of programmable telephones it is strongly suggested that these telephone numbers be included:

Local emergency medical services (EMS) (i.e., 9-1-1)

A *well-trained* dental or medical colleague

Emergency ambulance service with BLS- or BLS/ACLS-trained personnel

An AHA-certified hospital emergency department

Many communities have instituted the universal emergency telephone number 9-1-1 to expedite activation of their EMS. This number immediately connects the caller to the rescue service (usually fire, police, and medical). When emergency medical care is required in the dental office, the community EMS is usually the preferred source of immediate assistance. However, since not all areas have instituted the 9-1-1 system, appropriate telephone numbers must be available.

A *well-trained* dental or medical colleague can also serve as a source of emergency medical care. It is important, however, to discuss this arrangement prior to its actual need. The doctor seeking assistance must be absolutely certain that the person called is, in fact, well versed in emergency medicine and is likely to be available during office hours.[7] In offices in which more than one well-trained doctor is usually present, such a system is easily adopted. It has been my experience that the individuals with the best training in emergency medicine are emergency room physicians, anesthesiologists, surgeons (physi-

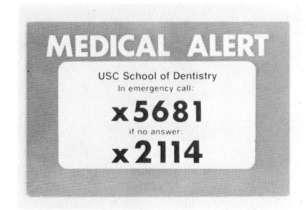

Fig. 33-1. Emergency telephone numbers should be posted clearly at every telephone.

cians), and oral and maxillofacial surgeons (dentists). Unfortunately for the doctor working in a private dental practice, the first two groups are normally hospital-based and are not readily available to the non-hospital-based dental practitioner. A surgeon (MD) or an oral and maxillofacial surgeon may be more readily available in the non-hospital setting. Prior arrangement with these persons will avoid potential misunderstandings and increase their effectiveness in emergency situations.

Most emergency ambulance services require their personnel to be trained as emergency medical technicians (EMT). This may serve as an alternate source of assistance should other rescuers be unavailable.

The location of the hospital closest to your office that has a 24-hour emergency department staffed with fully trained emergency personnel should be determined in the event that a victim requires transport to the facility for evaluation or management. The American Heart Association evaluates and certifies those emergency departments that meet their rigid criteria.

SUMMARY

Adequate training of all members of the office staff is absolutely essential if potentially life-threatening situations are to be adequately managed. Prepara-

tion of the staff must occur before emergencies occur. The recommended steps in preparing both the office staff and the office for such situations have been discussed. In the following chapters the components of the emergency drug kit and emergency equipment will be reviewed as well as the management of specific emergency situations related to drug administration.

REFERENCES

1. Council on Dental Education: Continuing education course list for January-June, 1994, Chicago, ADA.
2. Bossaert LL, Putzeys T, Monsieurs KG et al: Knowledge, skills and counselling behavior of Belgian general practitioners on CPR-related issues, *Resuscitation* 24(1):49, 1992.
3. Paradis NA, Martin GB, Goetting MG et al: Simultaneous aortic, jugular bulb, and right atrial pressures during cardiopulmonary resuscitation in humans: insight into mechanisms, *Circulation* 80:361, 1989.
4. American Association of Oral and Maxillofacial Surgeons, Committee on Anesthesia, *Office anesthesia evaluation manual*, ed 4. Rosemont, Ill, The Association, 1991.
5. Department of State Government Affairs, American Dental Association, 1992.
6. Malamed SF: Evolution of an undergraduate program in pain and anxiety control: a 15-year history, *J Dent Educ* 53(5/6):277, 1989.
7. Peter R: Sudden unconsciousness during local anesthetic, *Anesth Pain Control Dent* 2(3), 140, 1993.

CHAPTER 34

Emergency equipment

Emergency drugs and equipment must be available in every medical and dental office whether or not sedation and/or general anesthesia techniques are employed. Although most emergency situations do not require drug administration, emergency drug administration may prove to be lifesaving on occasion. In the acute systemic allergic response—anaphylaxis, for example—the administration of epinephrine is essential. In most other emergencies, however, drug administration is afforded a secondary role in overall management. In situations in which ADRs develop after the administration of drugs used for sedation and pain control it may be possible, in some cases, to significantly improve the clinical picture through the administration of an antidotal drug.

The emergency drug kit will be discussed at several different levels of complexity. The entry level represents the basic emergency kit, which I believe should be available in all dental and medical offices regardless of whether or not sedative techniques are used. The second group of drugs will be recommended for doctors who have received more advanced training in the care and handling of medical emergencies. Following this, drugs recommended for possible administration in ACLS are discussed, with drugs required for the management of ADRs associated with parenteral drug administration concluding our discussion.[1]

The emergency kit need not and indeed should not be overly complex. As Pallasch[2] has stated, "Complexity in a time of adversity breeds chaos."

The American Dental Association does not recommend any proprietary emergency kit, since "emergency kits should be individualized to meet the special needs and capabilities of each clinician. Practitioners are encouraged to assemble their own individual kit that will be safe and effective in their hands or to purchase a kit that contains drugs that they are fully trained to administer."[3]

The emergency drug kit maintained by the doctor employing parenteral sedation or general anesthesia will, of necessity, include drugs that are not recommended for inclusion in emergency kits of doctors who are not well trained in anesthesia (used in its broadest sense). No currently available proprietary emergency kit meets these requirements. The Council on Dental Therapeutics of the American Dental Association, many state dental boards, and speciality organizations have developed and published either recommendations or requirements for the inclusion of specific emergency drugs and equipment for offices in which either parenteral sedation and/or general anesthesia are administered (Tables 34-1 and 34-2).[4-6]

A plastic container for fishing tackle can be used to store these drugs (Fig. 34-1). A more inclusive emergency kit might be developed from a mobile tool chest (Fig. 34-2). Labels are applied to each container with both the generic and proprietary names of the drug and its dosage, for example, diazepam (Valium), 5 mg/ml. The emergency kit must be maintained in an area where it may be easily located. All emergency drugs and equipment should be checked on a weekly basis and reordered prior to their expiration date; O_2 should be checked daily.

The following are guidelines for the development of an office emergency kit. Categories of drugs will be listed with a suggestion for specific drug(s) within each grouping. Space precludes lengthy descriptions of the rationale for selecting each drug. Readers desiring more in-depth information are referred to Chapter 3 of Malamed's *Medical Emergencies in the Dental Office* (1993).

Table 34-1. Emergency drugs required by California State Board of Dental Examiners for Conscious Sedation Permit and General Anesthesia

1. Vasopressor
2. Corticosteroid
3. Bronchodilator
4. Appropriate drug antagonists
5. Antihistaminic
6. Anticholinergic
7. Coronary artery vasodilator
8. Anticonvulsants
9. Oxygen
10. 50% dextrose or other antihypoglycemic
11. Muscle relaxant*
12. Intravenous medication for treatment of cardiopulmonary arrest*
13. Antiarrhythmic*
14. Antihypertensive*

*Use for general anesthesia only.

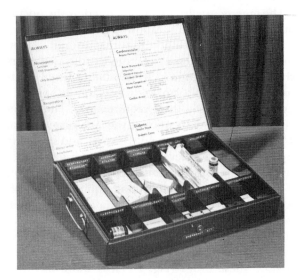

Fig. 34-1. Emergency kit.

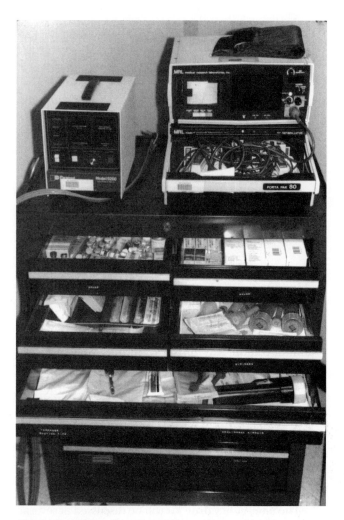

Fig. 34-2. Fully equipped, mobile emergency kit. (Courtesy Department of Oral and Maxillofacial Surgery, University of Southern California, School of Dentistry.)

All of the drug categories presented next should be considered for inclusion in the emergency kit; however, the doctor should select only those drugs with which he or she is familiar. The doctor must carefully evaluate everything that goes into the emergency kit. All drugs come with a drug package insert. This insert should be saved and read and important information concerning the drug noted, such as usual dose, contraindications, adverse reactions, and expiration date. Two categories of drugs, injectables and noninjectables, will be included in the emergency kit. Emergency equipment will be discussed later. The types of drugs and equipment included in the emergency kit must be appropriate for the level of training of the office personnel who will be called upon to use the kit. Table 34-4 lists drugs that should be included in a basic emergency kit.

LEVEL ONE: BASIC EMERGENCY KIT (Table 34-3)
Injectable drugs

The following two categories are considered to be primary critical drugs and should be included in *all* emergency kits:

1. Epinephrine (for management of acute allergic reactions)
2. Histamine blocker (antihistamine)

Epinephrine (Adrenalin) is the drug of choice in management of the acute allergic reaction involving the respiratory or cardiovascular system. In addition, epinephrine administration is indicated in broncho-

Table 34-2. Suggested emergency equipment and drugs

Suggested equipment

A. Source of oxygen and equipment to deliver positive-pressure ventilation
B. Respiratory support equipment
   1. Oral airways/nasal airways
   2. Endotracheal tubes with stylets
   3. Laryngoscope and suitable blades (plus extra bulbs and batteries)
   4. McGill forceps or other suitable instruments
   5. Coniotomy set with connector
C. Stethoscope
D. Blood pressure cuff
E. DC defibrillator
F. ECG or electrocardioscope with leads and electropaste
G. Equipment to establish intravenous infusion
   1. Needles, syringes, intravenous sets, and connectors
   2. Intravenous cutdown set
   3. Tourniquets for venipuncture
   4. Adhesive tape
H. Pulse oximeter

Suggested drugs

The following are examples of drugs that will be helpful in the treatment of anesthetic emergencies. The list should not be considered mandatory or all-inclusive.

A. Intravenous fluids
   1. Water for injection and/or mixing or dilution of drugs
   2. Intravenous fluids
B. Cardiotonic drugs
   1. Verapamil
   2. Digoxin
   3. Coronary dilators
      a. Amyl nitrite (ampules or pearls)
      b. Nitroglycerin (Nitrostat)
C. Vasopressors
   1. Dopamine hydrochloride (Intropin)
   2. Epinephrine 1:1000 or 1:10,000
   3. Dobutamine
   4. Isoproterenol (Isuprel)
   5. Phenylephrine (Neo-Synephrine)
D. Antiarrhythmic agents
   1. Atropine sulfate
   2. Lidocaine 2%
   3. Propranolol (Inderal)
   4. Procainamide
   5. Verapamil
   6. Vertillium or Bretylium
E. Antihypertensive agents (Immediate)
   1. Diazoxide (Hyperstat)
   2. Chlorpromazine (Thorazine)
   3. Nitroprusside
   4. Nitroglycerin
F. Diuretics
   1. Furosemide (Lasix)
G. Antiemetics (Droperidol, Compazine)
H. Narcotic antagonist
   1. Naloxone (Narcan)
I. Anticholinergic antagonist
   1. Physostigmine salicylate (Antilirium)
J. Accessory drugs
   1. Dextrose 50%
   2. Hydrocortisone sodium succinate (Solu-Cortef)
   3. Dexamethasone (Decadron)
   4. Aminophylline
   5. Atropine sulfate
   6. Glycopyrrolate (Robinul)
   7. Diazepam (Valium)
   8. Methohexital 1% (Brevital)
   9. Sodium thiopental 2.5% (Pentothal)
   10. Diphenhydramine (Benadryl)
   11. Isuprel (Medihaler)
   12. Midazolam (Versed)
   13. Succinylcholine (Anectine)
   14. Morphine sulphate

Adapted from: *Office Anesthesia Evaluation Manual*, ed 4. Rosemont IL, 1991, American Association of Oral and Maxillofacial Surgeons.

Table 34-3. Level one: basic emergency kit

Category	Drug Generic name	Proprietary name	Dosage (mg/ml)	Quantity
Injectable drugs				
Allergy	Epinephrine	Adrenalin	1	1 preloaded syringe; 2-3 1-ml ampules
Antihistamine	Diphenhydramine	Benadryl	50	2-3 ampules
Noninjectable drugs				
O₂	O₂		Minimum—1	E cylinder
Vasodilator	Nitroglycerin	Nitrolingual spray	0.4	1 spray container

spasm (asthma) and cardiac arrest. Suggested for the emergency kit are one preloaded syringe (1:1000) (Fig. 34-3) and three to four ampules of 1:1000 epinephrine. For doctors comfortable with venipuncture and intravenous drug administration epinephrine is available as a 1:10,000 dilution (1 mg in 10 ml).

There are several *histamine blockers* available for parenteral administration. Those most frequently used in emergency situations are diphenhydramine (Benadryl) and chlorpheniramine (Chlor-Trime-

ton). Indications for the administration of a histamine blocker include management of delayed allergic response, definitive management of acute allergy, and as a local anesthetic when a history of allergy is present. Suggested for the emergency kit are several 1-ml ampules of either 10 mg/ml of chlorpheniramine or 50 mg/ml of diphenhydramine.

Noninjectable drugs

Two noninjectable drugs, O_2 and a vasodilator, are recommended as essential for all emergency kits. *Oxygen* is probably the most important drug included in the emergency kit. Although available in a variety of cylinder sizes (Chapter 15), it is the E cylinder that is most highly recommended for emergency use. Therapeutic indications for the administration of O_2 include any situation in which respiratory distress is evident. The minimal suggested amount for the emergency kit is one E cylinder (an apparatus for O_2 delivery must also be available and is discussed later).

Vasodilators will be administered in the immediate management of chest pain. The drug of choice is nitroglycerin in a translingual spray. Suggested for the emergency kit is one bottle of Nitrolingual Spray (0.4 mg/spray).

LEVEL TWO: ADVANCED EMERGENCY KIT *(Table 34-4)*
Injectable drugs

Five injectable drugs—an anticonvulsant, analgesic, vasopressor, corticosteroid, and antihypogly-

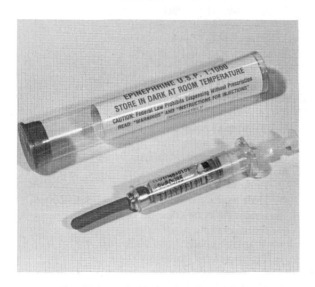

Fig. 34-3. Preloaded epinephrine syringe.

Table 34-4. Level two: advanced emergency kit

| | Drug | | | |
Category	Generic name	Proprietary name	Dosage (mg/ml)	Quantity
Injectable drugs				
Anticonvulsant	Diazepam	Valium	5	1 10-ml vial
Analgesic	Morphine sulfate (N_2O-O_2 may be substituted)		10	2-3 ampules
Vasopressor	Methoxamine	Vasoxyl	20	2-3 1-ml ampules
Corticosteroid	Hydrocortisone sodium succinate	Solu-Cortef	50	1 2-ml vial
Antihypoglycemic	50% dextrose		500	1 50-ml vial
Noninjectable drugs				
Respiratory stimulant	Aromatic ammonia		0.3 mg	6-12 vaporoles
Antihypoglycemic	Carbohydrate		1 dose of any form	
Bronchodilator	Albuterol	Ventolin	1-2 doses/hour	1 inhaler

cemic—are recommended for inclusion in the emergency kit of doctors who have received advanced training in emergency medicine and/or anesthesia. Such persons include oral and maxillofacial surgeons; dentist anesthesiologists; pedodontic, periodontic, endodontic, and other dental specialists who have completed a hospital training program; and general practitioners who have completed a general practice residency.

The *anticonvulsant* of choice is a benzodiazepine, either diazepam or midazolam. It must be administered intravenously in order to terminate a tonic/clonic seizure, whether in a patient with a history of prior seizure disorders or in management of local anesthetic overdose. Other therapeutic indications for the emergency administration of a benzodiazepine include termination of febrile convulsions, hyperventilation (for sedation), and thyroid storm (for sedation). Suggested for the emergency kit is either 5 mg/ml of diazepam or midazolam 1 mg/ml in a 10-ml multidose vial.

An *analgesic* drug will be valuable during situations in which acute pain or anxiety are present. Management of pain during acute myocardial infarction represents a common indication for administration of analgesics. Other therapeutic indications include intense, prolonged pain or anxiety and as a sedative in the management of CHF. Opioid analgesics are the drugs of choice, with morphine sulfate most highly recommended. In recent years, however, the use of N_2O-O_2 in management of pain during myocardial infarction has increased in popularity.[7] N_2O-O_2 is administered in a concentration of 35% N_2O and 65% O_2. If nitrous oxide is not available, then morphine sulfate, 10 mg/ml (two to three 1-ml ampules) is recommended.

Vasopressors are administered in the management of hypotension. One vasopressor, epinephrine, has already been included in the basic emergency kit; however, its administration in most cases of mild hypotension is not recommended. A vasopressor with less profound actions is usually desirable. Within this category many drugs are available; methoxamine is selected because of its ability to increase blood pressure with little secondary effect on the workload of the myocardium. Indications for vasopressor administration include management of hypotension as seen in syncopal reactions, drug-overdose reactions, postseizure states, acute adrenal insufficiency, and allergy. Recommended for the emergency kit is 10 mg/ml of methoxamine (two to three 1-ml ampules).

Corticosteroids are administered in the management of the acute allergic reaction, but only after epinephrine and the histamine blockers have proved effective. Another indication for their administration is management of acute adrenal insufficiency. Recommended for the emergency kit is 50 mg/ml of hydrocortisone sodium succinate (one 2-ml vial).

Antihypoglycemics are administered parenterally in the definitive management of hypoglycemia and in the differential diagnosis of unexplained unconsciousness or seizures of unknown origin. The recommended agent, 50% dextrose solution, must be administered intravenously. Recommended for the emergency kit is one vial (50 ml) of 50% dextrose. An alternative is glucagon, available as 1 mg/ml in a 2-ml ampule. Glucagon may be administered either intravenously or IM.

Noninjectable drugs

Three noninjectable drugs—a respiratory stimulant, an antihypoglycemic (oral), and a bronchodilator—are recommended for the emergency kit of persons with some advanced training in emergency medicine. *Aromatic ammonia* is the recommended respiratory stimulant for the emergency kit. Its use is not limited to persons with advanced training in emergency medicine. It is included as a secondary emergency drug because I consider it to be an important, but not an essential, drug. Available in a silver-gray vaporole, it is crushed between the rescuer's fingers and placed beneath the nose of the victim. Indications for use of aromatic ammonia include respiratory depression not induced by opioid analgesics and vasodepressor syncope. Recommended for the emergency kit is one box of vaporoles of aromatic ammonia.

COMMENT: Aromatic ammonia will be one of the most frequently used drugs in the emergency kit. It is suggested that one or two vaporoles be placed close to every treatment area so that required time will not be spent waiting for the emergency kit to arrive. Several vaporoles should remain in the emergency kit for use in other areas of the office.

Hypoglycemia is not an uncommon occurrence. Most hypoglycemic patients, whether diabetic or not, remain conscious but behave oddly. Treatment of such situations involves administration of an *antihypoglycemic* either intravenously, IM, or orally (see previous discussion). There are several commercially produced oral antihypoglycemia products available, such as Glucola, Gluco-Stat, and Insta-glucose. In addition to these, nondietetic soft drinks, fruit juices, and simple sugar are available. Suggested for the emergency kit of the conscious hypoglycemic is some form of oral glucose. A tube of decorative cake icing is suggested for use in the hypoglycemic who loses consciousness and where parenteral drug therapy is unavailable.

Bronchodilators will be required in the definitive management of bronchospasm. Epinephrine, probably the most highly recommended bronchodilator, has been included in the emergency kit as an injectable drug. Other drugs, equally effective as bronchodilators (beta-$_2$ actions) but with fewer cardiovascular (beta-$_1$) side effects are available and can be administered directly into the bronchi by aerosol inhalation (as can epinephrine). Recommended for use in the medical or dental office is albuterol, a drug with excellent beta-$_2$ effects but minimal beta-$_1$ actions. Therapeutic indications for administration of bronchodilators include respiratory distress as seen in asthma and allergic reactions with a significant respiratory component. Suggested for the emergency kit is one albuterol inhaler.

LEVEL THREE: ADVANCED CARDIAC LIFE SUPPORT (Table 34-5)

The following drugs are classified as essential drugs in emergency cardiac care by the American Heart Asociation.[8] Their use is restricted to persons trained in advanced cardiac life support. These drugs should be included in the emergency kit, or in a separate kit, in those offices in which the doctor has been certified in ACLS. Essential drugs for ACLS include the following, some of which have been discussed previously: O$_2$, epinephrine, atropine, lidocaine, and morphine.

Atropine sulfate is used in the management of severe sinus bradycardia when accompanied by symptomatic hypotension or hypotension that might impair coronary artery blood flow. *Lidocaine* is recommended for management of ventricular premature beats as well as ventricular tachycardia and ventricular fibrillation that is refractory to defibrillation. Sodium bicarbonate and calcium chloride were removed in 1986 from the list of essential ACLS drugs.[9]

LEVEL FOUR: ANTIDOTAL DRUGS (Table 34-6)

Antidotal drugs reverse some, or all, of the actions of other drugs that have been previously administered. These drugs should be available in the emergency drug kit where any technique of parenteral sedation is employed in patient management (IM, submucosal, IV, or general anesthesia). The pharmacology of these drugs has been presented in Chapter 26. In this section only a brief description of each drug will be presented. These drugs include opioid antagonists, a benzodiazepine antagonist, a drug for reversal of emergence delirium, and a vasodilator.

Opioid antagonists reverse the actions of opioid agonists (i.e., meperidine, morphine, fentanyl). In clinical practice opioid antagonists are administered primarily to reverse respiratory depression produced by opioids. Naloxone (Narcan) is available in a 0.4 mg/ml dosage form (for adults). It is administered at a rate of 0.1 mg every 2 to 3 minutes to the adult up to 2.0 mg, with the patient's response being monitored constantly. In children an initial IV dose of 0.01 mg/kg is suggested.[10] It is important to remember that in addition to reversing the respiratory-depressant actions of the opioid analgesic, naloxone also reverses its analgesic effects. Therefore patients who receive opioid analgesics for anesthesia and undergo their surgical procedure without the benefit of local anesthesia and then receive naloxone may experi-

Table 34-5. Level three: ACLS injectable drugs

Generic name	Dosage	Quantity
Epinephrine	0.1 mg/ml	2 syringes
Atropine	0.5 mg/ml	1 syringe plus 2-3 ampules
Lidocaine (Xylocaine)	20 mg/ml	1 ampule
Morphine	10 mg/ml	2-3 ampules

Table 34-6. Level four: Antidotal drugs

Category	Drug		Dosage (mg/ml)	Quantity
	Generic name	Proprietary name		
Narcotic antagonist	Naloxone	Narcan	0.4	2-3 1-ml ampules
Agent for reversal of emergence delirium	Physostigmine	Antilirium	1.0	2-3 2-ml ampules
Vasodilator	Procaine	Novocain	10.0	2-3 2-ml ampules
Benzodiazepine antagonist	Flumazenil	Romazicon	0.1	2 5-ml bottles

ence severe postsurgical pain.[11] Nalbuphine, an opioid agonist/antagonist, has also been shown to be effective in reversing opioid-induced respiratory depression. A major advantage of nalbuphine over naloxone is that the analgesic properties of the opioid remain.[12]

Recommended for the emergency kit is 0.4 mg/ml of naloxone (two to three 1-ml ampules) for use in adults. Naloxone is also available as a 0.02 mg/ml concentration for pediatric use.

The *benzodiazepine antagonist* flumazenil (Romazicon) specifically counteracts the clinical actions of diazepam and midazolam (as well as other benzodiazepines). Recovery from sedation is hastened and the length of amnesia is decreased when flumazenil is administered.[13] Recommended for intravenous use only, the initial dose of flumazenil is 0.2 mg administered IV over 15 seconds. After waiting an additional 45 seconds, a further dose of 0.2 mg can be administered and repeated at 60-second intervals where necessary to a maximal dose of 1.0 mg. Most patients respond to 0.6 to 1.0 mg.[14] Suggested for the drug emergency kit is one 10-ml multidose vial of 0.1 mg/ml flumazenil.

Emergence delirium (central anticholinergic syndrome) is an uncommon ADR developing after administration of anticholinergics (primarily scopolamine) or the benzodiazepines. Emergence delirium may be terminated through the administration of *physostigmine* (Antilirium). Dosage is 0.5 to 1.0 mg IM or IV. No more than 1 mg should be administered per minute. Additional doses may be administered every 10 to 30 minutes if the desired patient response is not obtained. Recommended for the emergency kit is 1.0 mg/ml of physostigmine (two to three 2-ml ampules).

A *vasodilator* is recommended for the emergency kit in the event that an extravascular injection of an irritating drug (e.g., diazepam, pentobarbital) occurs or in the more unlikely event of an intraarterial injection of a drug. Procaine (Novocain) is the drug of choice because of its potent vasodilating properties and its anesthetic actions.

Recommended for the emergency kit is two to three 2-ml ampules of 1% procaine.

EMERGENCY EQUIPMENT

Emergency equipment has a very definite place in the management of life-threatening situations. As with drugs, however, it is important for the doctor to know his or her limitations when it comes to using this equipment. Improper use of emergency equip-ment may further increase the danger to the patient. There are two categories of emergency equipment: primary or basic equipment, which I believe should be available in every medical and dental office, and secondary or advanced equipment, for those persons who have received training and are experienced in its use.

Merely having items of emergency equipment available does not in and of itself make the office better equipped or the staff any more prepared to manage medical emergencies. Personnel expected to use emergency equipment must be well trained in emergency management and in the proper use of these items. Unfortunately, many of the emergency items commonly found in dental and medical offices can prove to be useless or, more significantly, hazardous if used improperly or on the wrong patient. Training in the proper use of some of these items, such as the laryngoscope and oropharyngeal airway, can best be obtained only by caring for patients under general anesthesia, a situation usually not readily available. Many of the items of emergency equipment listed in this section are therefore recommended for use only by trained personnel. All of the secondary equipment falls into this category; unfortunately, several items listed as primary are also included (e.g., O_2 delivery system). Although all dentists and physicians should be trained in the use of O_2 delivery systems, courses in which these techniques are taught to clinical proficiency are particularly difficult to locate.

Primary (basic) emergency equipment

The basic level of emergency equipment includes the following items:

1. O_2 delivery system
2. Suction and suction tips
3. Syringes for drug administration
4. Tourniquets
5. Magill intubation forceps

An O_2 delivery system adaptable to an E cylinder of O_2 must permit the delivery of positive-pressure O_2. Examples of this type of device include the positive-pressure/demand valve and the reservoir bag on all inhalation sedation units. The Robertshaw Valve and the Elder Valve (Fig. 34-4) are examples of such devices. When properly placed on the victim's face these devices provide O_2 on demand when the patient takes a spontaneous ventilation. Negative pressure created beneath the mask triggers the device to provide O_2 under positive pressure. In this regard the positive-pressure/demand valve operates

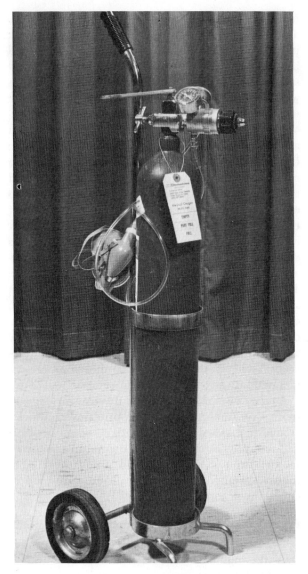

Fig. 34-4. O_2 delivery system consisting of an E cylinder and a full-face mask.

positive-pressure/demand valve ceases to function once the O_2 cylinder is depleted.

A portable, self-inflating, bag-valve-mask device is a self-contained unit that is easily transported to any site within the dental or medical office (Fig. 34-5). It does not require a compressed gas cylinder of O_2 in order to operate and therefore has a wider area of potential use than the positive-pressure device. As with the positive-pressure device, the rescuer must be able to maintain a patent airway and an airtight seal of the mask on the patient's face with only one hand, the other being used to squeeze the bellows bag and inflate the victim's lungs. This device is known by a variety of proprietary names, including the Ambu-Bag and the Pulmonary Manual Resuscitator (PMR).

The self-inflating bag-valve-mask device may be used to deliver 21% O_2 (ambient or atmospheric air), or, by attaching an O_2 delivery tube to the end of the bellows bag, enriched O_2 (greater than 21% but less than 100% O_2) may be supplied to the patient.

The self-inflating bag-valve-mask device is recommended for use in pediatric and smaller adult patients (because of their smaller lung capacity); however, the same device is not recommended for use in the average- to large-sized adult. Tests have demonstrated that even in the hands of well-trained ventilators these devices do not deliver an adequate volume of air to a large adult victim's lungs.[15] Addition of a reservoir bag that provides additional volume can make this device adequate for use in the large adult.

Face masks must be available if either the positive-pressure mask or BVM is to be used. The face mask should be constructed of a clear plastic or of rubber,

like a scuba mask and is readily usable by almost all rescuers. It is in the use of this device for controlled ventilation (positive-pressure ventilation) that difficulties arise. In order to properly ventilate an apneic patient using the positive-pressure mask, the rescuer *must* be able to maintain a patent airway and an airtight seal with the mask on the patient's face with but one hand. Their other hand is used to activate the valve that supplies O_2 to the patient. The positive-pressure/demand valve is one means of providing the victim with 100% O_2. In order for this device to be used, a source of 100% O_2 must be available. The

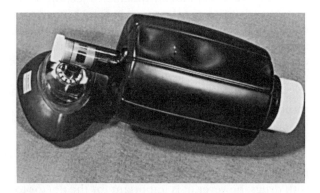

Fig. 34-5. Portable, self-inflating bag-valve-mask device delivers atmospheric or O_2-enriched air to patient.

which permits the efficient delivery of O_2 or air to the patient while permitting the rescuer to visually inspect the mouth for the presence of foreign matter (e.g., vomitus, blood). A variety of sizes of face mask should be available. Suggested for the emergency kit is one portable O_2 cylinder (E cylinder) with a positive-pressure/demand valve and/or one portable self-inflating, bag-valve-mask device.

COMMENT: Advanced training is required for the safe and effective use of these devices.

It is essential that an effective suction system and a number of suction tips be available in the office. The disposable saliva ejector is entirely inadequate in situations in which anything other than tiny objects must be evacuated from the mouth of a patient. Suction tips should be of large diameter and rounded so that there is little hazard of inducing bleeding should it become necessary to suction the hypopharynx. Plastic evacuators and tonsil suction tips are quite adequate for this purpose. The minimal suggested number for the emergency kit is two plastic evacuators or tonsil suction tips.

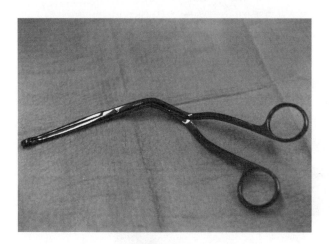

Fig. 34-6. Magill intubation forceps.

Plastic disposable syringes with an 18- to 21-gauge needle are required for drug administration. Many syringe sizes are available, but a 2-ml syringe is quite adequate. Suggested for the emergency kit are two to three 2-ml disposable syringes with an 18- to 21-gauge needle.

A tourniquet is required if IV drug administration is contemplated. In addition, three tourniquets will be needed for management of acute pulmonary edema. A sphygmomanometer (blood pressure cuff) may be used as a tourniquet by inflating the cuff to a reading that falls between the diastolic and systolic measurements. Suggested for the emergency kit are two to three tourniquets and a sphygmomanometer.

A Magill intubation forceps aids in the recovery of small objects that have fallen into the distal part of the oral cavity or pharynx (Fig. 34-6). Cotten pliers and hemostats may be employed but are considerably more difficult to use and are less efficient than the Magill intubation forceps.

Table 34-7 summarizes the basic equipment for the emergency kit.

Secondary (advanced) emergency equipment

Several other items of equipment are available for use in emergency situations. Advanced training is required for the safe and effective use of these devices. It is recommended, therefore, that the following equipment *not* be used unless adequate training and experience has been obtained:

Scalpel or cricothyrotomy needle
Artificial airways
Airway adjuncts

As a final step in the management of an obstructed airway, it may be necessary to perform a cricothyrotomy. Although this procedure is highly unlikely to ever be required, there are occasions in which the recommended procedures involving abdominal or chest thrusts may prove to be ineffective in opening

Table 34-7. Primary (basic) emergency equipment

Device	Description	Quantity
O_2 delivery system*	Demand valve or self-inflating bag-valve-mask *and* clear full face masks	1 of either plus various face masks
Suction plus suction tips	Large diameter, round-ended suction tips or tonsil suction tips	2 or more
Syringes	Disposable syringes for drug administration	2-3 2-ml syringes with 18- to 21-gauge needle
Tourniquets	Rubber tourniquet, latex tubing, or sphygmomanometer	Minimum, 1

*Advanced training is required for safe and effective use of this device. *All* dental and medical personnel should be trained in its use.

an airway that has become obstructed by a foreign object.[16] One clinical situation in which the latter procedures will prove fruitless is laryngeal edema, a form of allergic response in which the soft tissues of the larynx swell, thereby restricting the flow of air into and out of the trachea. The usual airway maneuvers fail to provide a patent airway because a foreign object is not present. Cricothyrotomy is necessary to provide O_2 to the victim. It is recommended that in the office of a doctor who is trained in the technique the emergency kit should contain a *scalpel* or a *cricothyrotomy needle* (Fig. 34-7). The latter need only be a 13-gauge ½-inch-length needle. Technique of cricothyrotomy will be reviewed in Chapter 35. Suggested for the emergency kit is one scalpel with disposable blade and/or one 13-gauge ½-inch cricothyrotomy needle.

Plastic or rubber *oropharyngeal* and *nasopharyngeal airways* are used to assist in maintenance of a patent airway. These devices are used almost routinely during and after general anesthesia to assist in airway maintenance in the unconscious or semiconscious patient. The oropharyngeal airway is designed to lie between the base of the tongue and the posterior wall of the pharynx, lifting the tongue off of the pharyngeal wall and thus aiding in airway maintenance. Use of the oropharyngeal airway (Fig. 34-8) must be

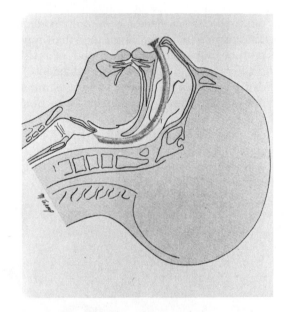

Fig. 34-9. Nasopharyngeal airway.

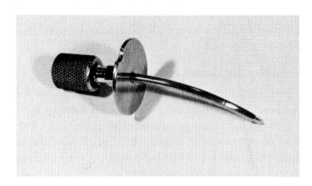

Fig. 34-7. Cricothyrotomy needle.

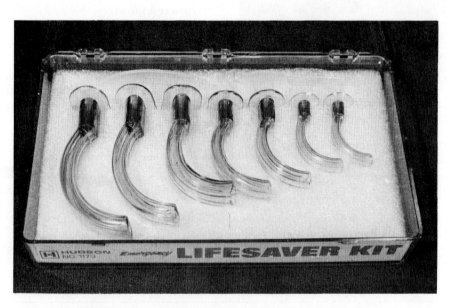

Fig. 34-8. Oropharyngeal airways are available in a variety of sizes.

restricted to persons trained in its insertion since improper placement will force the base of the tongue farther back into the pharynx, thereby increasing the degree of obstruction. If it is placed into the pharynx of a patient who is not deeply unconscious, the patient will react to the presence of the airway by gagging (not too bad), vomiting or regurgitating (worse), or having a laryngospasm (worse yet). Placing an orophryngeal airway in a still reactive patient is the equivalent of placing your finger deep down in your throat. In properly placing the oropharyngeal airway, the tip of the tongue of the patient is grabbed with a piece of gauze and pulled anteriorly while the airway is being inserted.

Nasopharyngeal airways are better tolerated by most patients. It is lubricated (KY jelly or Xylocaine viscous) prior to insertion into one nostril (usually the right) and then gently advanced into position (Fig. 34-9). Because it lies in the nasopharynx, not the oropharynx, gagging, vomiting, regurgitation, and laryngospasm are rarely a problem even in the conscious patient.

Use of these devices is recommended only in situations where manual methods of airway maintenance have been ineffective. Training and experience in the use of oral and nasal airways is mandatory if they are to be used effectively and safely. Suggested for the emergency kit is a set of adult- and child-sized airways (either oropharyngeal or nasopharyngeal).

The final category of equipment is airway adjuncts and consists of a number of devices that are used to assist in airway maintenance. Included for possible consideration are the S tube airway, the esophageal obturator airway, the laryngoscope, and the endotracheal tube. As with other devices in this category, training and experience in the use of each item are absolutely essential.

The S tube airway is a modification of the oropharyngeal airway that permits the rescuer to maintain a patent airway and deliver exhaled air ventilation without physically contacting the victim's mouth. Problems encountered with improper patient evaluation or insertion include further obstruction of the airway, gagging, regurgitation, or vomiting, and laryngospasm. Of greater importance is the fact that this device severely limits the rescuer's ability to perform one-person BLS: to ventilate the victim with the S tube the rescuer must be at the head of the victim, not astride his or her head. The S tube airway is *not* recommended for inclusion in the emergency kit.

The *esophageal obturator airway* (EOA) (Fig. 34-10) is a rubber tube similar in appearance to the endotracheal tube except that its distal end is sealed and there are many small holes placed along the length of the tube. The EOA is designed to be placed blindly into the airway without the benefit of a laryngoscope. As noted in the following paragraph, when placed

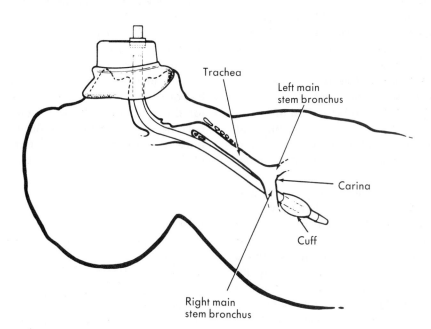

Fig. 34-10. Esophageal obturator airway in position. (From *Advanced cardiac life support manual*. Reproduced with permission. American Heart Association.)

Table 34-8. Secondary (advanced) emergency equipment

Device	Description	Quantity
Scalpel or cricothyrotomy needle*	Scalpel with straight blade or 13-gauge ½-inch needle	1
Artificial airways*	Oropharyngeal and/or nasopharyngeal airways	1 small (child) 1 medium (small adult) 1 large (large adult)
Airway adjuncts*	S tube airway	*Not recommended*
	Esophageal obturator airway	*Not recommended*
	Laryngoscope and endotracheal tubes	1 laryngoscope plus various sizes of blades and tubes

*Advanced training is required for safe and effective use of this device. This *should not be included in the emergency kit* if the person using the emergency kit is not trained to use this device properly.

blindly into the airway an endotracheal tube will frequently pass into the esophagus, thereby preventing air from entering the patient's lungs. The EOA uses this "problem" with the endotracheal tube to advantage. After lubrication the EOA is passed blindly into the patient's esophagus and a cuff is inflated. The proximal end of the EOA is attached to a positive-pressure device and air forced through the tube. This air escapes from the holes along the side of the EOA and is forced into the trachea. Although this device is still used by some paramedical personnel in the field, its use has diminished as several problems have been noted over the years: first, approximately 10% of EOAs enter into the trachea instead of the esophagus, thereby preventing delivery of O_2 to the patient's lungs, unless the rescuer quickly discovers the error (the abdomen will inflate with each ventilation, the chest does not). Second, a significant percentage of persons with EOAs inserted regurgitate or vomit when the device is removed from their airway. The esophageal obturator airway, although a potentially valuable airway adjunct, should be limited in its use to persons who have received extensive training and experience with it under careful supervision. It is not recommended for the emergency kit in most dental offices.

Endotracheal intubation using a *laryngoscope* and *endotracheal tube* provides the ultimate in airway maintenance. The use of endotracheal intubation must be strictly limited to persons who are well trained in this technique. Quite realistically this limits its usefulness to anesthesiologists, nurse anesthetists, trained paramedical personnel, and those few dentists and physicians who have received training in anesthesiology. The most common mistakes noted during intubation are accidental intubation of the esophagus and taking too long to intubate (it should take no longer than 15 seconds to intubate a patient).

Table 34-8 summarizes the secondary or advanced emergency equipment.

SUMMARY

The selection of emergency drugs and equipment for the dental or medical office must be based on the training and background of the doctor who is responsible for its use. Because of the diversity in emergency preparedness training among both dentists and physicians, no stereotyped emergency kit is appropriate for all practitioners. I have attempted to describe several levels of drugs and equipment that I believe would be appropriate at different levels of expertise in emergency medicine. In addition, many states and provinces have established credentialing bodies that regulate the use of parenteral sedation and general anesthesia. Specific mandatory drug lists are included in many of these regulations. Regardless of the nature of drugs and equipment selected for the emergency kit, it is vital for the doctor to become familiar with the indications, contraindications, dosages, and method of administration of each of these drugs and be able to correctly operate any available equipment.

REFERENCES

1. Malamed SF: Managing medical emergencies, *JADA* 124:40, 1993.
2. Pallasch TJ: This emergency kit belongs in your office, *Dent Management* 16:43, 1976.
3. Council on Dental Therapeutics: Emergency kits, *JADA* 87:909, 1973.
4. American Dental Association Council on Dental Education: Guidelines for teaching the comprehensive control of pain

and anxiety in dentistry. Part II, Chicago 1992, The Association.

5. California State Board of Dental Examiners: Conscious sedation and general anesthesia regulations. Extract from California Code of Regulations. Title 16, Chapter 10, Article 5—General anesthesia and Conscious Sedation, 1993.

6. American Association of Oral and Maxillofacial Surgeons, Committee on Anesthesia: *Office anesthesia evaluation manual,* ed 4, Rosemont, Ill, 1991, The Association.

7. O'Leary U, Puglia C, Friehling TD et al: Nitrous oxide anesthesia in patients with ischemic chest discomfort: effect on beta-endorphins, *J Clin Pharmacol* 27(12):957, 1987.

8. Emergency Cardiac Care Committee and Subcommittees, American Heart Association: Guidelines for cardiopulmonary resuscitation and emergency cardiac care. III, adult advanced cardiac life support, *JAMA* 268:2199, 1992.

9. American Heart Association and the National Academy of Sciences, National Research Council: Standards for cardiopulmonary resuscitation (CPR) and emergency cardiac care (ECC), *JAMA* 255:2905, 1986.

10. Naloxone, drug package insert, Du Pont Multi-Source Products, 1993.

11. Pallasch TJ, Gill CJ: Naloxone-associated morbidity and mortality, *Oral Surg* 52:602, 1981.

12. Hu C, Flecknell PA, Liles JH: Fentanyl and medetomidine anaesthesia in the rat and its reversal using atipamazole and either nalbuphine or butorphanol, *Lab Anim* 26(1):15, 1992.

13. Longmire AW, Seger DL: Topics in clinical pharmacology: flumazenil, a benzodiazepene antagonist, *Am J Med Sci* 306(1): 49, 1993.

14. Romazicon, drug package insert, Roche Laboratories, April 1993.

15. Carden E, Hughes T: An evaluation of manually operated self-inflating resuscitation bags, *Anesth Analg* 54:133, 1975.

16. Heimlich HJ: A life-saving maneuver to prevent food choking, *JAMA* 234:398, 1975.

CHAPTER 35

Management of emergencies

Despite efforts at prevention, complications and ADRs still arise during and following the administration of drugs for the management of pain or anxiety. In the office that has prepared for these situations *prior* to their occurrence there is greater likelihood of a successful outcome than in the unprepared or ill-prepared office. Many states, provinces, and speciality groups require that the dental office team be capable of correctly identifying and managing specific ADRs associated with parenteral sedation and general anesthesia.[1,2] These emergencies are reviewed in this chapter.

Pallasch[3] has proposed a classification of ADRs.

Toxicity due to direct extension of pharmacologic effects

1. Side effects
2. Abnormal dosage (overdosage)
3. Local toxic effects

Toxicity due to altered recipient

1. Presence of pathology
2. Emotional disturbances
3. Genetic aberrations (idiosyncrasy)
4. Teratogenicity
5. Drug-drug interactions

Toxicity due to drug allergy

According to Pallasch's system there are three major methods by which drugs may produce adverse reactions:

1. A direct extension of the pharmacological actions of the drug
2. A deleterious effect on a chemically, genetically, metabolically, or morphologically altered recipient
3. Initiation of an immune (allergic) response

Most drug reactions are not life-threatening. There are, however, potential responses that are life-threatening, requiring immediate and effective management if the patient is to fully recover. These include the overdose reaction and the allergic response. A third, the idiosyncratic reaction, is also reviewed.

Overdose reaction refers to those symptoms manifested as a result of an absolute or relative overadministration of a drug that produces elevated blood or plasma levels of that drug in specific organs of the body. For CNS-depressant drugs an overdose occurs when the blood level of the drug becomes overly high in the cerebral circulation.[4] Clinical manifestations of overdose are related to a direct extension of the normal pharmacological actions of the agent. For example, in therapeutic doses barbiturates produce a mild depression of the central nervous system, resulting in sedation or hypnosis (desirable effects). Barbiturate overdosage produces a more profound depression of the central nervous system with respiratory or cardiovascular depression and a potential loss of consciousness.

Allergy is defined as a hypersensitive state acquired through exposure to a particular allergen, reexposure to which brings about a heightened capacity to react.[5] Clinically there are a variety of manifestations through which allergy expresses itself. These include drug fever, angioedema, urticaria, dermatitis, depression of blood-forming organs, photosensitivity, and anaphylaxis. Certain drugs are more likely to elicit allergic reactions than others, and allergic reaction is possible with any substance.

In contrast to overdose, in which clinical manifestations are related directly to the pharmacological properties of the causative agent, the clinical response observed in the allergic reaction is mediated by the exaggerated response of the immune system of the body. The level of this response determines the severity of the allergic reaction. Allergic responses to a barbiturate, a local anesthetic, and an antibiotic are produced by the same mechanism and may appear clinically similar. All require the same basic management, whereas overdose reactions to these three agents are quite dissimilar clinically and require entirely different management.

Idiosyncrasy or idiosyncratic reactions are defined as those ADRs that cannot be explained by any known pharmacological or biochemical mechanism. Another definition is that an idiosyncratic reaction is any ADR that is neither an overdose nor an allergic reaction. An example of an idiosyncratic reaction is CNS stimulation (excitation, agitation) produced following the administration of a known CNS depressant such as a barbiturate.

Idiosyncratic reactions span an extremely wide range of clinical manifestations. For example, depression following administration of a stimulant, stimulation following administration of a depressant, and hyperpyrexia following administration of a muscle relaxant are all idiosyncratic reactions. It is virtually impossible to predict in advance the person in whom such reactions will develop or indeed the nature of the resulting idiosyncratic reaction.

Because of the unpredictability of the nature and occurrence of idiosyncratic reactions, their management is of necessity symptomatic. Of primary importance in the management of idiosyncrasy is basic life support: maintenance of the airway, ensuring adequate ventilation and circulation. If seizures develop, management is based on airway maintenance and prevention of injury during the seizure.

It is thought today that virtually all instances of idiosyncrasy have an underlying genetic mechanism.[6] These genetic aberrations remain undetected until the individual receives a specific drug, such as succinylcholine, which then produces its bizarre (nonpharmacological) clinical expression.

Two major forms of ADRs, overdose and allergy, will be reviewed; in addition, other emergency situations will also be discussed. Successful demonstration of the management of these situations is frequently a requirement of parenteral sedation and general anesthesia permits. These complications are listed in the adjacent box.

OVERDOSE

Whenever CNS-depressant drugs are administered to a patient, the possibility always exists that an exaggerated level of CNS depression might develop. This might be noted clinically as a slightly overse-

---

EMERGENCY SITUATIONS IDENTIFIED FOR PARENTERAL SEDATION AND GENERAL ANESTHESIA[1,2]

1. Airway obstruction, p. 541
2. Laryngospasm, p. 543
3. Bronchospasm, p. 529
4. Emesis and aspiration of foreign material under anesthesia, p. 543
5. Angina pectoris, p. 540
6. Myocardial infarction, p. 541
7. Cardiopulmonary resuscitation, p. 539
   a. Bradycardia
   b. Ventricular tachycardia
   c. Ventricular fibrillation
   d. Asystole
   e. Electromechanical dissociation (EMD)
8. Hypotension, p. 533
9. Hypertensive crisis, p. 537
10. Acute allergic reaction, p. 526
11. Convulsions, p. 546
12. Hypoglycemia, p. 547
13. Syncope, p. 548
14. Hyperventilation, p. 544
15. Respiratory depression, p. 545

---

dated patient, or it might result in an unconscious patient who has ceased breathing.

The group of drugs most likely to produce an overdose is the barbiturates. This group represented the first major breakthrough in the pharmacological management of anxiety, and because of this, adverse reactions, such as allergy, addiction, and overdose, were tolerated. With the introduction of newer antianxiety drugs (e.g., benzodiazepines) that do not possess the same potential for abuse and overdose, the clinical use of barbiturates has declined. However, the barbiturates still remain a useful group in the dentist's and physician's armamentarium for the management of treatment-related anxiety.

Although the barbiturates present the greatest potential for adverse reaction, the opioid analgesics are involved with the greatest number of clinically significant episodes of overdose and respiratory depression. This is simply because opioids are used to a much greater degree than the barbiturates. As has been discussed previously (Chapters 8, 11, and 36), the use of opioids is popular in pediatric sedation. Opioids are often employed intravenously, in conjunction with antianxiety drugs, to aid in sedation and pain control in the adult patient. Goodson and

Moore[7] reported on 14 cases in pediatric dentistry in which the administration of opioids (and other drugs) led to seven deaths and three cases of brain damage. Several opioids were implicated in these reactions: alphaprodine (7), meperidine (6), and pentazocine (1).

Predisposing factors and prevention

Since the barbiturates and opioids are commonly used for the management of pretreatment fear and anxiety, they are most often administered orally or intramuscularly. The clinical efficacy of a drug depends, in large part, on its absorption into the cardiovascular system and subsequent blood levels of the drug in various organs of the body. Only the inhalation and intravenous routes of drug administration allow for titration. With oral and intramuscular drug administration absorption is erratic, as demonstrated by the wide range of variability in clinical effectiveness. The normal distribution curve becomes important when drugs are used via those routes in which titration is not possible. "Average" drug doses are based on this curve; therefore secobarbital, 100 mg orally, provides a desired effect (mild sedation) in the majority of patients receiving it. For some patients (about 15% of the population), however, the 100-mg dose is ineffective, these persons requiring a larger dose to attain the same clinical level of sedation. These persons are not at risk for potential overdose given the average dose, since a lack of adequate sedation is the clinical result.

The potential danger in the use of drugs lies with patients for whom an average 100-mg dose of secobarbital is too great. These are persons who are quite sensitive (not allergic) to this drug and require smaller than usual doses to obtain clinically effective sedation. It is normally not possible to predict in advance the 15% of the population that will react in this manner. Only a previous history of an ADR can provide a clue to this occurrence. The medical history questionnaire should be carefully examined in relation to all drug reactions. When a history of drug sensitivity is obtained, great care must be exercised when barbiturates and opioid analgesics are to be used. Lower-than-average doses should be administered or different drug categories substituted. Nonbarbiturate sedative-hypnotic drugs, such as the benzodiazepines and the opioid agonist/antagonists, may be used in place of these drugs.

Although the clinical nature of the overdose cannot always be predicted in advance, there is another way in which these drugs can produce this reaction, a way that is preventable. It relates entirely to the goal being sought by the doctor when these drugs are administered. Some clinicians use barbiturates or opioids to achieve deep levels of sedation on apprehensive patients. When used in this manner via the oral or IM routes of drug administration, the potential for overdose is increased. Most doctors who administer barbiturates in their practices have encountered patients who became uncooperative (less inhibited) after receiving these drugs. The planned procedure could not be completed because of the difficulty in managing a patient who was slightly overdosed on barbiturates. Larger doses of the barbiturate given to an anxious patient in an attempt to produce deeper levels of sedation may produce greater degrees of CNS depression with possible loss of consciousness and respiratory depression.

Administering any CNS depressant in order to obtain deeper levels of sedation via routes of administration in which titration is not possible is foolhardy and an invitation to overdose. It should not be condoned. Only those techniques permitting titration should be employed to achieve deeper levels of sedation, and then only where the doctor and entire team are thoroughly familiar with both the technique and the drugs to be administered and are able to manage all possible complications associated with the procedure.

The inhalation and IV routes are the only ones that permit titration. A factor to be remembered regarding inhalation and IV sedation is that absorption of the drug(s) into the systemic circulation occurs rapidly so that drug responses (both therapeutic and adverse) develop quite suddenly. Titration remains the greatest safety feature these techniques possess and should always be employed whenever possible.

Table 35-1 summarizes the recommendations made throughout this book for the various routes of drug administration.

Clinical manifestations
Barbiturate and nonbarbiturate sedative hypnotics

Barbiturates produce depression of a number of physiological properties including nerve tissue, respiration, and skeletal, smooth, and cardiac muscle. The mechanism of action (sedation and hypnosis) is depression at the level of the hypothalamus and the ascending reticular activating system (RAS), which produces a decrease in the transmission of impulses to the cerebral cortex. Further increases in barbiturate blood level produce depression at other levels of the central nervous system, such as profound cortical depression, depression of motor function, and

Table 35-1. Summary of routes of drug administration

Route of administration	Control		Recommended safe sedative levels
	Titrate	Rapid reversal	
Oral	No	No	Light only
Rectal	No	No	Light only
IM	No	No	Adults: light, moderate
			Children: light, moderate, deep
IV	Yes	No (most drugs); yes (opioids, benzodiazepines)	Adults and children*: light, moderate, deep
Inhalation	Yes	Yes	Any sedation level

Modified from Malamed SF: *Handbook of medical emergencies in the dental office,* ed 4. St Louis, 1993, Mosby.
*There is usually little need for IV sedation in normal healthy children. Most children who will permit a venipuncture will also permit a local anesthetic to be administered intraorally. IV sedation is of great benefit in managing disabled children and adults.

finally depression of the medulla. This is represented diagrammatically as follows:

Sedation (calming) → Hypnosis (sleep) → General anesthesia (unconsciousness with progressive respiratory and cardiovascular depression) → Respiratory arrest

Sedation and deep sedation. At low (therapeutic) blood levels the patient appears calm and cooperative (sedated). As the barbiturate level in the blood increases, the patient falls into what initially is a rousable sleep (hypnosis). The doctor will notice the patient's inability to keep his mouth open despite constant reminders to do so. In addition, patients at this level of barbiturate-induced CNS depression have a tendency to overrespond to stimulation, especially that of a noxious nature. The unsedated adult patient may grimace in response to pain; the oversedated adult given barbiturates has an exaggerated response, perhaps yelling or jumping. This reflects the loss of self-control over emotion that is associated with the CNS-depressant action of the barbiturate.

Hypnosis. With continued elevation of the barbiturate level in the blood, hypnosis (sleep) ensues, with a minor degree of respiratory depression (decreased depth and increased rate of ventilation). At this level there is usually no adverse action on the cardiovascular system, only a slight decrease in blood pressure and heart rate similar to that occurring in normal sleep. Dental treatment cannot be continued at this level of CNS depression since the patient is unable to cooperate with the doctor by keeping his mouth open and may well require assistance in maintaining airway patency (head tilt). The patient still responds to noxious stimulation but in a sluggish manner.

General anesthesia. With further increases in the barbiturate blood level the degree of CNS depression broadens so that the patient is now unconscious (incapable of response to sensory stimulation, loss of protective reflexes with attendant inability to maintain an airway). Respiratory efforts are still present; however, with further increase in barbiturate blood levels, medullary depression occurs and is clinically evident as respiratory and cardiovascular depression. Respiratory depression is seen as shallow breathing movements at a slow or rapid rate. Ventilatory excursions of the chest do not indicate that air is entering or leaving the lungs but only that the patient is attempting to bring air into the lungs. Cardiovascular depression is evident as a continued decrease in blood pressure (caused by medullary depression and direct depression of the myocardium and vascular smooth muscle) and an increased heart rate. The patient develops a shocklike appearance, with a weak and rapid pulse, and cold, moist skin.

Respiratory arrest. As the barbiturate blood level continues to increase or if the patient does not receive adequate therapy in the previous stage, respiratory arrest will occur. Respiratory arrest may readily be managed with artificial ventilation. If ventilation is not adequately provided, cardiac arrest will ensue.

• • •

Other nonbarbiturate sedative-hypnotic drugs (i.e., benzodiazepines) also possess the potential to produce overdose, though this is not as likely to occur as with the barbiturates. The potential for overdose varies greatly from drug to drug, but to some degree all sedative hypnotic drugs have this potential.

Opioid agonists

Meperidine, morphine, fentanyl, alfentanil, and sufentanil are the most frequently used parenteral opioids, with meperidine and fentanyl the most popular.

Meperidine, like most opioid agonists, exerts its chief pharmacological actions on the central nervous system. Therapeutic doses of meperidine produce analgesia, sedation, euphoria, and a degree of respiratory depression. Of principle concern, of course, is the respiratory depressant effect of the opioid agonists. They are direct depressants of the medullary respiratory center. In human subjects respiratory depression from opioid agonists is evident even at doses that do not disturb the level of consciousness. The degree of respiratory depression produced by opioids is dose dependent: the greater the dose of the drug, the more significant the level of respiratory depression. The opioid agonist/antagonists nalbuphine and butorphanol offer the combination of analgesia and sedation with minimal respiratory depression.

Death from opioid overdose almost always results from respiratory arrest. All phases of respiration are depressed—rate, minute volume, and tidal volume. The respiratory rate may fall below 10 per minute. Rates of 5 to 6 per minute are not uncommon. The cause of the decreased respiratory activity is a reduction in responsiveness of the medullary respiratory centers to increases in carbon dioxide tension (PCO_2) and also a depression of the pontine and medullary centers that are responsible for respiratory rhythm.

The cardiovascular effects of meperidine are not clinically significant when the drug is administered within its usual therapeutic dose range. Following IV administration of meperidine, however, there is normally an increase in the heart rate produced by the atropine-like vagolytic properties of meperidine. At overdose levels the blood pressure remains quite stable until late in the course of the reaction, when it falls, primarily as a result of hypoxia. The administration of O_2 at this time will produce an increase in blood pressure despite continued medullary depression. Overly high blood levels of opioid agonists can lead to the loss of consciousness.

Overdose reactions to both the sedative-hypnotics and opioid agonists are produced by a progressive depression of the central nervous system that is manifested by alterations in the level of consciousness and as respiratory depression that ultimately results in respiratory arrest. The loss of consciousness produced by barbiturates or opioid agonists is not always the result of unintentional overdose—these drugs are very commonly administered as the primary agents in general anesthesia (Chapter 32). However, where sedation is the goal, the loss of consciousness and respiratory depression must be considered to be complications of drug administration.

The duration and the degree of this clinical reaction will vary according to the route of administration, the dose administered, and the patient's individual sensitivity to the drug. In most situations oral and rectal administration result in less CNS depression but with a longer duration; IM and submucosal administration result in a more profound level of depression of relatively long duration, whereas IV administration produces the most profound level of depression of a shorter duration than that seen with the other techniques. The onset of respiratory depression following IV administration may be quite rapid while that following oral or rectal administration is considerably slower. Onset is intermediate in IM and subcutaneous administration.

Management
Sedative-hypnotic drugs

Management of an overdose to sedative-hypnotic drug administration is concerned with correction of the clinical effects of CNS depression. Of primary importance is the management of respiratory depression through the administration of BLS. Unfortunately, there is no pharmacologic antagonist able to reverse the CNS-depressant properties of the barbiturate sedative-hypnotic drugs. Flumazenil effectively reverses benzodiazepine-induced overdose.

Step one. The patient is placed supine with the feet elevated slightly (Fig. 35-1). The goal in this situation, regardless of the patient's level of consciousness (or unconsciousness), is to ensure adequate cerebral blood flow.

Step two. A patent airway must be ensured and the adequacy of breathing checked. Head-tilt/chin-lift is used at this time (Fig. 35-2). The presence or adequacy of the patient's spontaneous ventilatory efforts is next assessed by the rescuer, who places his or her ear 1 inch from the patient's mouth and nose and listens and feels for exhaled air while watching the patient's chest to see if he is attempting to breathe spontaneously.

Maintenance of a patent airway is the most important step in management of the patient. The next step, adequate oxygenation, is contingent on successful maintenance of a patent airway.

Step three. The patient may exhibit many different degrees of depressed or compromised breathing. The patient may be conscious but overly sedated—responsive, but sluggishly, to painful stimulation. In this situation the patient is usually able to maintain

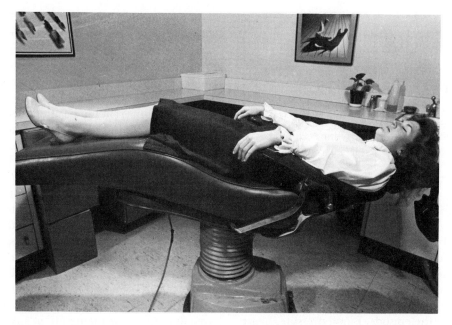

Fig. 35-1. Unconscious patient is placed in supine position with feet elevated slightly.

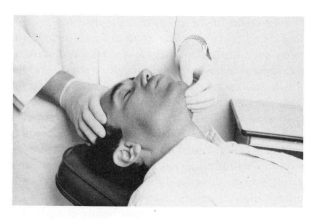

Fig. 35-2. Head-tilt/chin-lift technique of airway maintenance.

his own airway and to breathe spontaneously and rather effectively. The rescuer need only monitor the patient and, if desired, administer O₂ via a demand valve.

The patient may also be more deeply sedated and barely responsive to stimulation, with the airway partially or totally obstructed (Table 35-2 and the box on the next page). In this situation airway maintenance is necessary in addition to assisted ventilation. With patency of the airway ensured the patient should receive O₂ via a full face mask. If spontaneous breathing is present but shallow, then assisted positive-pressure ventilation is required. This is accomplished with the full face mask sealed on the patient's face and O₂ forced into the lungs at the start of each respiration. When the positive-pressure mask is used, this is accomplished by depressing the button on top of the mask until the chest rises and then releasing the button. With a self-inflating bag-valve-mask (BVM) device the bellows bag is squeezed at the onset of each inhalation. Head-tilt must be maintained at all times. Remember that the BVM device is not recommended for use in larger adults.

Should respiratory arrest occur, controlled artificial ventilation must be started immediately. The recommended rate for the adult is one breath every 5 seconds (12 per minute), and one breath every 3 seconds for the child aged 1 year through 8 years and for the infant under 1 year of age (20 per minute).

Table 35-2. Causes of airway obstruction

Sound heard	Probable cause	Degree of obstruction
Snoring	Hypopharyngeal obstruction by the tongue	Partial
Gurgling	Foreign material in airway	Partial
Wheezing	Bronchospasm (asthma)	Partial
Crowing	Laryngospasm (partial)	Partial
None	Any of above to a greater degree	Total

From Malamed SF: *Handbook of medical emergencies in the dental office,* ed 4. St Louis, 1993, Mosby.

SIGNS AND SYMPTOMS OF POOR AIR EXCHANGE

Weak, ineffective cough
High-pitched "crowing" sound on inhalation
Increased respiratory difficulty
Ashen grey color of skin
Possible cyanosis of mucous membranes and nail beds

From Malamed SF: *Medical emergencies in the dental office*, ed 4. St Louis, 1993, Mosby.

Successful ventilation is noted by elevation of the patient's chest. Overinflation is to be avoided because this leads to abdominal distention and increases the risk of regurgitation and/or impaired ventilation.

Step four. The patient's vital signs must be monitored throughout the episode. Blood pressure, heart rate and rhythm, and respiratory rate are recorded every 5 minutes and a written record maintained. A second member of the emergency team is responsible for this task. If the blood level of the sedative-hypnotic drug increases significantly, blood pressure will progressively decrease while the heart rate increases. Should blood pressure and a palpable pulse be absent, external chest compression must be instituted immediately.

In most cases of barbiturate or other sedative-hypnotic overdose the patient is maintained in this manner until the blood level of the drug is decreased and the patient demonstrates clinical recovery. In most cases this apparent recovery is the result of a redistribution of the drug, not its biotransformation. Regardless, the patient appears more conscious (more alert and responsive), breathing improves (becomes deeper), and if depressed, the blood pressure returns to approximately baseline levels. The length of time this process will require depends on the drug administered and its route of administration.

Step five. In some cases it may be prudent to summon medical assistance. The need for this will, of course, vary with the training of the doctor and staff, the nature of the incident, and the availability of medical assistance. This step must be considered when judged necessary by the doctor.

Step six. If an IV infusion had not previously been established (oral, IM administration), it is prudent to establish one at this time, if possible. Although there are no effective antidotal drugs for barbiturate sedative-hypnotic overdose, benzodiazepine overdose

and hypotension may be treated effectively through intravenously administered drugs or fluids. As blood pressure falls veins will become progressively more difficult to locate and cannulate. Establishing an IV line at the earliest possible time may prove invaluable later.

Venipuncture should be attempted only if the doctor is trained in this technique, has available the necessary equipment, and the patient is receiving adequate care (BLS) from other personnel. *A patent airway is more important than a patent vein.*

Step seven. Definitive management of this situation is based primarily on the maintenance of an adequate airway and ventilation until the patient recovers. Where a benzodiazepine is responsible for the overdose, flumazenil may be administered in a dose of 0.2 mg (2 ml) IV over 15 seconds with additional doses of 0.2 mg administered at 60-second intervals if the desired level of response is not observed. A maximum dose of 1.0 mg (10 ml) is recommended.[8]

Signs and symptoms of hypotension are sought. (Management of hypotension is reviewed later in this chapter.)

Step eight. In the event that the overdose is profound and requires the assistance of outside medical personnel, the patient may require transportation to a hospital for observation and full recovery. Should this be necessary, the doctor should always accompany the patient to the hospital.

In most cases, however, the overdose is less severe, with diminished responsiveness and slight respiratory depression noted clinically. Management consists of positioning, airway maintenance, and assisted ventilation until recovery with antagonist drug administration, if appropriate. The patient should be observed for not less than 1 hour before considering discharge. Prior to discharge (in the custody of a responsible adult) the patient must be capable of standing and walking without assistance. Under no circumstances must the patient be discharged alone or if he is not adequately recovered. The same criteria used for patient discharge following IM and IV sedation are recommended here.

The following list of actions pertains to the management of overdose to sedative-hypnotic drugs.

1. Position the patient—supine.
2. Maintain patent airway and check effectiveness of breathing.
3. Start artificial ventilation and administer O_2 as needed.
4. Monitor and record vital signs.
5. Summon medical assistance, if necessary.

6. Start IV infusion, if available and practical.
7. Start definitive management (as required): flumazenil 0.2 mg IV q60 seconds for benzodiazepine); methoxamine 20 mg IM or IV for prolonged hypotension.
8. Permit recovery for at least 1 hour.
9. Discharge patient home (with responsible adult) or to hospital (doctor accompanies), as indicated.

Opioid analgesics

Oversedation and respiratory depression are the primary clinical manifestations of opioid overdose. Cardiovascular depression does not usually develop until quite late in the overdose reaction. Management of the patient who has received an absolute or relative overdose of an opioid is similar to that described for sedative-hypnotic drugs with one major addition: specific antagonist drugs are available that rapidly reverse the clinical effects of the opioids. Steps in management of an opioid overdose follow.

Step one. The patient is placed in the supine position with feet elevated slightly.

Step two. The presence of a patent airway is ensured, and breathing is monitored.

Step three. O_2 or artificial ventilation is administered if necessary. The administration of O_2 is especially important in the early management of opioid overdose. Minimal cardiovascular depression is normally observed and in most cases it occurs as a result of hypoxia secondary to respiratory depression. The administration of O_2 to a patient with a patent airway prevents or reverses any cardiovascular depression that is evident.

Step four. Vital signs are monitored every 5 minutes and entered on the record sheet. Should pulse and blood pressure ever be absent, cardiopulmonary resuscitation is initiated immediately.

Step five. Definitive management is available in cases in which an opioid has been administered to the patient. Even in situations in which what is normally considered to be a small dose of the opioid has been administered, an opioid antagonist should be administered when overdose is evident.

Nothing is administered to the patient until a patent airway and adequate ventilation have been ensured and vital signs are monitored. At this point an opioid antagonist is administered. The agent of choice, naloxone (Chapters 26 and 34), is administered intravenously, if possible, to take advantage of the more rapid onset of clinical activity with this route. If the IV route is unavailable, IM administration will suffice. The onset of action is slower, but the drug will prove effective if the respiratory depression is opioid induced. Regardless of the route of administration of naloxone, the doctor must continue to provide BLS as indicated during the period from naloxone administration until patient recovery, as determined by increased patient responsiveness and more adequate and rapid ventilatory efforts. Following IV administration, naloxone will demonstrate its actions within 1 to 2 minutes, within 10 minutes following IM administration.

Naloxone is available in a 1-ml ampule with 0.4 mg of the drug. The drug is loaded into a plastic disposable syringe, and if the IV route is available, 3 ml of diluent (any IV fluid) is added to the syringe, producing a final concentration of 0.1 mg naloxone per ml. The drug is then administered to the patient at a rate of 0.1 mg (1 ml) per minute until the patient's ventilatory rate increases. If administered IM, an undiluted dose of 0.4 mg is administered into a suitable muscle mass, preferably the mid-deltoid region of the upper arm.

Naloxone is also available in a pediatric concentration of 0.02 mg/ml. The initial dose is 0.01 mg/kg of body weight IV. Subsequent doses of 0.01 mg/kg may be administered if the desired response is not noted.[9]

A potential problem with naloxone is that its duration of clinical activity may be shorter than that of the opioid it is being used to reverse. This is especially true in cases in which morphine is being used, less likely with meperidine, and less likely still with fentanyl and its analogues. Should this occur, the doctor and staff would notice an initial improvement of the patient's clinical appearance as naloxone begins to act, only to see a recurrence of CNS depression develop approximately 30 or more minutes later. Because the opioid producing the overdose is continually undergoing redistribution and biotransformation during this time, in the event that such a recurrence does occur it would quite likely be of a much milder nature than the initial response. It may be prudent, in cases in which longer-acting opioids have been administered intramuscularly or submucosally, to follow the original IV dose of naloxone with an IM dose (0.4 mg [adult]). In this manner, as the clinical effect of the original naloxone dose diminishes, the naloxone from the IM dose will reach a peak blood level, preventing a relapse reaction.

The administration of naloxone in cases of opioid overdose is a very important step in overall patient management (see following discussion).

Step six. The patient is observed in the period following naloxone administration and apparent clinical recovery. The patient may be transported to a recovery area but must remain there under constant supervision for at least 1 hour. On the other hand, if recovery is deemed to be complete and if the doctor so desires, the planned treatment may continue. Vital signs should be recorded every 5 minutes, O₂ and suction must be available, and trained personnel must be present.

Step seven. The need for medical assistance is at the doctor's discretion.

Step eight. The discharge of the patient may require the transport of the patient to a hospital facility for observation or follow-up treatment. Regardless of the indication for hospitalization, the doctor responsible for treating this patient should accompany the patient to the hospital or physician's office.

In most cases this will prove unnecessary. Following a period of recovery in the dental or medical office, the patient can be dismissed in the custody of a responsible adult companion using the same criteria established for IV and IM sedation. The patient must be able to stand and walk without aid from another person.

The following is a summary of the management of the opioid-induced overdose:

1. Position the patient—supine, feet elevated.
2. Ensure patent airway, check for breathing.
3. Start artificial ventilation; administer O₂ as indicated.
4. Monitor and record vital signs, q5m.
5. Start definitive management: naloxone 0.4 mg IM or IV (titrate 0.1 mg/ml).
6. Observe patient recovery for at least 1 hour.
7. Summon medical personnel, if indicated.
8. Discharge patient with responsible adult.

Summary

The previous discussion dealt with overdose reactions of varying severity that occur following the administration of a single drug. Although this is not uncommon, especially following intramuscular or submucosal administration, most reported overdose reactions involve administration of more than one drug. In many of these cases drugs such as an antianxiety drug (category A, Chapter 26) are combined with an opioid analgesic (category B) to provide sedation and some analgesia. To these may be added a local anesthetic for the control of operative pain, and nitrous oxide and oxygen inhalation sedation.

It has been stressed several times in this book that when CNS-depressant drugs are being used together, the dosages of both agents must be reduced from their usual dosage to prevent an exaggerated, undesirable clinical response. As demonstrated in Table 35-3, in most of the cases reported by Goodson and Moore reduced drug dosages were not employed.[7]

Another factor must be considered, one that, as a rule, is not given much thought when sedative techniques are used. That is the fact that local anesthetics are CNS depressants and can produce additive actions when administered in conjunction with the drugs commonly employed for sedation. The maximal dosage of local anesthetic to be administered to any patient, but especially to a child or lighter-weight adult, should be based on the patient's body weight in kilograms or pounds. When no other CNS depressant is to be administered this maximal dose could be reached without adverse reaction (if the patient is an ASA I and lies within the normal response range on the bell-shaped curve). Maximal doses of the most commonly used local anesthetics are presented in Table 35-4. When used in conjunction with other CNS depressants, the dosage of the local anesthetic should be minimized.

It was mentioned earlier that a goal of sedation is to produce a cooperative patient who still maintains protective reflexes. Whenever possible, this goal should be achieved using the simplest technique available as well as the fewest number of drugs possible. Polypharmacy, the combination of several drugs, may be necessary in some patients to achieve the desired clinical effects of sedation and analgesia. However, if this same level can be produced with one drug, the combination of drugs ought not be employed. Drug combinations increase the opportunity for ADRs as well as making it less obvious which drug has produced the problem, thereby making management of the situation more complicated.

Within the individual techniques of sedation the recommendation was made that single-drug regimens were preferred to combinations of drugs. Rational drug combinations were presented for use where they were specifically indicated. With IV drug administration the problem of severe ADRs should not occur if the technique of titration is adhered to at all times. With intramuscular and oral drug administration, however, where titration is not available, the doctor must adjust drug dosages prior to their administration. Serious ADRs are more likely to occur when titration is unavailable.

Consideration must also be given to the use of mul-

Table 35-3. Dose administered relative to recommended maximum dose

Case	Narcotic analgesics (percentage)*	Antiemetic sedatives (percentage)*	Local anesthetics (percentage)*	N₂O-O₂	Result
1	216	36	172	−	Fatality
2	173	145	237	−	Fatality
3	336	0	342	−	Fatality
4	127	27	267	+	Fatality
5	309	372	230	+	Brain damage
6	436	?	?	−	Fatality
7	100	136	107	−	Fatality
8	167	300	219	+	Brain damage
9	66	0	60	−	Recovery
10	66	92	?	+	Recovery
11	183	0	?	−	Recovery
12	200	558	0	−	Recovery
13	250	136	127	−	Brain damage
14	50	0	370	+	Fatality

From Goodson JM, Moore PA: *JADA* 107:239, 1983. Copyright by the American Dental Association. Reprinted by permission.
*Expressed as percentage of maximal recommended dose for that patient.

Table 35-4. Maximal recommended local anesthetic doses

Drug	Dose Mg/kg	Dose Mg/lb	Absolute maximal dose
Lidocaine	4.4	2.0	300
Mepivacaine	4.4	2.0	300
Prilocaine	6.0	2.7	400
Bupivacaine	2.0	0.9	90

tiple techniques of sedation in a patient. It will not be uncommon for a patient who presents a management problem to receive an oral antianxiety drug prior to arrival in the office, followed by either IM, submucosal, IV, and/or inhalation sedation in addition to local anesthesia during treatment. Wherever oral sedation with CNS depressants has been used, the dosages of all other CNS depressants should be decreased. This is critical when the IM or submucosal routes are used, since titration is unavailable. With inhalation and IV sedation, careful titration of drugs to the patient who has been orally sedated will usually produce the desired sedation level with a lower dose of the IV or inhalation drug being used.

How then may overdose reactions best be prevented? Goodson and Moore made the following recommendations concerning the use of sedative techniques in which opioids are being administered.[7]

1. Be prepared for emergencies.

Continuous monitoring of the cardiovascular and respiratory systems should be employed. An emergency kit containing drugs such as epinephrine, O₂, and naloxone should be readily available, in addition to equipment and trained personnel. In their article Goodson and Moore state that "because multiple sedative drug techniques can easily induce unconsciousness, respiratory arrest and convulsions, practitioners should be prepared and trained to recognize and control these occurrences."

2. Individualize drug dosage.

When drugs are used in combination, the dosage of each drug must be carefully selected. The toxic effects of drug combinations appear to be additive. Drug selection must be based on the patient's general health history. The presence of systemic disease usually indicates the need for a reduction of dosage.

Since most sedative drugs are available in quite concentrated form, and since children will require very small dosages, extreme care must be taken when these drugs are being prepared for administration.

Fixed-dose administration of drugs based on a range of ages (e.g., 4 to 6 years: 50 mg) should not be employed. Preferred are dosages based on body weight or surface area of the patient or titration if possible.

Should the selected drug dosage prove to be inadequate, it is prudent to consider a change in the technique of sedation or in the drugs being used (at a subsequent appointment), rather than increasing the drug dosage to a higher and potentially more dangerous level.

3. Recognize and expect adverse drug effects.

When combinations of CNS-depressant drugs have been administered, the potential for excessive CNS and respiratory depression is increased and they should be expected.

• • •

The Dentists Insurance Company (TDIC) in a retrospective study of deaths and morbidity in dental practice over a 3-year period concluded that in those incidents related to the administration of drugs there were three common factors in most of the events[10]:

1. Improper preoperative evaluation of the patient
2. Lack of knowledge of drug pharmacology by the doctor
3. Lack of adequate monitoring during procedure

These three factors greatly increased the risk of serious ADRs developing, with a negative outcome.

Overdose reactions to the administration of CNS-depressant drugs may not always be preventable; however, with care on the part of the doctor the incidence of these events should be extremely low, and a successful outcome should occur every time. With techniques such as IV and inhalation sedation, in which titration is possible, overdosage should develop rarely, if at all. With oral, IM, and SM drug administration, where the doctor has no control over drug effect because of the inability to titrate, greater care must be expended in preoperative evaluation of the patient, determination of the appropriate drug dosage, and monitoring throughout the procedure so that excessive CNS or respiratory depression may be detected and treated immediately. When the oral, SM, and IM routes of administration are employed, the onset of adverse reactions may be delayed. The adverse reaction may not develop until after the rubber dam is in place and the dental procedure has started. Monitoring during the procedure therefore becomes critically important to patient safety.

ALLERGY

Allergy is defined as a hypersensitive state acquired through exposure to a particular allergen, reexposure to which produces a heightened capacity to react. Allergic reactions cover a broad range of clinical manifestations, from mild, delayed-onset reactions occurring as long as 48 hours after exposure to immediate and life-threatening reactions developing within seconds of exposure. Although all allergic phenomena are important and require thorough evaluation by the doctor, only one form, the type I, or immediate, reaction will be discussed at this time, for it may present the doctor with a life-threatening emergency situation. A classification of allergy types is presented in Table 35-5.

Allergic reactions are mediated through immunologic mechanisms that are similar regardless of the specific antigen responsible for precipitating the response. Therefore an allergic reaction to the venom of a stinging insect may be identical to that seen following aspirin or penicillin administration in a previously sensitized individual. Allergic reactions must be differentiated from the overdose, or toxic, reaction previously discussed, which is the result of a direct extension of the normal pharmacological properties of the drug administered. Overdose reactions are much more frequently encountered than are allergic drug reactions. Of all ADRs, 85% result from the pharmacologic actions of drugs; 15% are immunologic reactions.[11] To the nonmedical individual, however, any adverse drug response is frequently labeled "allergic."

Allergy is a frightening word to those health professionals responsible for primary care of patients. Though none of the drugs commonly employed for the management of pain and anxiety has a significantly high rate of allergenicity, allergic phenomena may occur with any of these agents. The only drugs mentioned in this book that to my knowledge have never been shown to have produced allergy are N_2O and O_2. Although the concept of prevention has been stressed repeatedly throughout this book, in no other situation is this concept of greater importance than in allergy. Although allergy is not the most common ADR, it is frequently involved with the more serious of these reactions.

Of the many antianxiety drugs employed, the barbiturates probably possess the greatest potential for sensitization of patients. Although not nearly as common as allergy to penicillin or aspirin, barbiturate allergy usually manifests itself in the form of skin lesions such as hives and urticaria or less frequently in the form of blood dyscrasias such as agranulocytosis or thrombocytopenia. Allergy to barbiturates occurs much more frequently in persons with a history of asthma, urticaria, and angioedema.[12] A documented history of allergy to any of the barbiturates represents

Table 35-5. Classification of allergic diseases (after Gell and Coombs)

Type	Mechanism	Principal antibody or cell	Time of reactions	Clinical examples
I	Anaphylactic (immediate, homocytotropic, antigen-induced, antibody-mediated)	IgE	Second to minutes	Anaphylaxis (drugs, insect venom, antisera)
				Atopic bronchial asthma
				Allergic rhinitis
				Urticaria
				Angioedema
				Hay fever
II	Cytotoxic (antimembrane)	IgG	—	Transfursion reactions
		IgM (activated complement)		Goodpasture's syndrome
				Autoimmune hemolysis
				Hemolytic anemia
				Certain drug reactions
				Membranous glomerulonephrosis
III	Immune complex (serum sickness-like)	IgG (form complexes with complement)	6 to 8 hours	Serum sickness
				Lupus nephritis
				Occupational allergic alveolitis
				Acute viral hepatitis
IV	Cell-mediated (delayed) or tuberculin-type response	—	48 hours	Allergic contact dermatitis
				Infectious granulomas (tuberculosis, mycoses)
				Tissue graft rejection
				Chronic hepatitis

Reproduced, with permission, from Krupp MA, Chatton MJ: *Current medical diagnosis & treatment,* copyright Lange Medical Publications, 1984.

an absolute contraindication to use of any of these related drugs.

Among the opioids, meperidine is capable of releasing histamine locally. When meperidine is administered intravenously, this localized histamine release develops along the path of the vein through which the drug travels. This reaction is not allergy and requires no therapeutic management. The reaction resolves after the drug leaves the area of its administration. Use of meperidine is relatively contraindicated in asthmatics because of potential bronchospasm induced by histamine release.

Atropine, an anticholinergic, may produce flushing of a patient's face, neck, and upper chest following IV administration. This phenomenon is called *atropine flush,* and though not common, does occur, is not allergic in nature, and requires no therapeutic intervention since spontaneous resolution occurs within a brief time. This response is most often seen following overdose of atropine. However, in certain sensitive individuals (those who are hyperresponders on the bell-shaped curve), the usual therapeutic dose may provoke this response.

Prevention of allergy

Whenever any drug or combination of drugs is being considered for administration to a patient, the doctor should question the patient about any prior exposure to that drug or members of the same drug family. In addition, the patient's medical history questionnaire must be evaluated. All questionnaires include questions concerning current drug use and prior ADRs. These two steps will, in most cases, enable the doctor to determine in advance the possibility of an adverse drug response. Should a positive history be elicited, questioning is undertaken to determine the nature of the previous reactions. Though the questioning may vary, basic questions to be asked include the following:

1. What drug was used?
2. What happened? The patient describes the sequence of events that ensued.
3. What treatment was required? Was epinephrine or an antihistamine administered? O_2 or aromatic ammonia?
4. Were the services of a physician or paramedical personnel required? Were you hospitalized?
5. What is the name and address of the doctor (physician or dentist) who treated you at that time?

Knowledge of the signs and symptoms of the "reaction" and the method of treating it can go far in aiding the doctor in diagnosing the alleged "allergy."

The need for hospitalization or assistance of another health professional usually indicates a more serious ADR. If possible, it may be prudent to speak directly to the doctor involved with the patient at that time.

Following a thorough dialogue history and a review of the medical history questionnaire, it is usually possible to form a general opinion about the reaction. If the doctor is convinced that an allergic response did occur, then other drugs structurally dissimilar to the offending drug should be selected for administration. In most cases, however, it will become obvious that the "allergy" was in fact a side effect of the drug (e.g., nausea from codeine) or that the response was anxiety induced. If doubt remains as to the precise nature of the problem, the patient should be managed, at that time, with drugs unrelated to the one(s) in question, followed by consultation with an allergist so that more definitive testing may be started.

Clinical manifestations

Most allergic drug reactions are immediate, in particular the type I, or anaphylactic, reaction. The term *immediate,* relating to allergic phenomena, indicates that the onset of clinical signs and symptoms developed within 60 minutes of exposure to the allergen.

A number of organs and tissues are affected during immediate allergic reactions, particularly the skin, respiratory system, cardiovascular system, and gastrointestinal tract. Generalized, or systemic, anaphylaxis by definition affects all the systems mentioned. If hypotension is also a clinical component of the response, the term *anaphylactic shock* is correctly employed.

Immediate allergic reactions also manifest through any number of combinations involving these organs. Reactions involving one system are referred to as "localized anaphylaxis"—for example, asthmatic attack, in which the respiratory system is the target, and urticaria, in which the skin is the target organ.

Onset

The time elapsing between exposure of the patient to the antigen and the development of clinical signs and symptoms is of great importance. In general, *the more rapidly signs and symptoms evolve following exposure, the more intense the ultimate response.* Conversely, the greater the length of time between exposure and onset, the less intense the reaction. However, cases of anaphylaxis have been reported to arise many hours following exposure. Of importance, too, is the rate of progression of the signs and symptoms once they appear. If they appear and increase in severity rapidly, the reaction is more likely to become life-threatening than one that progresses slowly or not at all.

Skin reaction

Allergic skin reactions are the most common sensitization reaction to drug administration. Many types of allergic skin reaction may occur, the two most important types being localized anaphylaxis and drug eruption. Drug eruption constitutes the most common group of skin manifestations of drug allergy. Included in this category are urticaria, erythema (reddening), and angioedema (localized swelling).

Urticaria is associated with wheals (smooth, slightly elevated patches of skin) and frequently with intense itching (pruritis). Angioedema is a process in which localized swelling occurs in response to an allergen. Several forms of angioedema exist, but clinically they appear to be similar. The skin is usually of normal color (unless accompanied by urticaria or erythema) and temperature, and pain and itching are uncommon. The areas most frequently involved include the hands, face, feet, and genitalia. Of special concern is the potential involvement of the lips, tongue, pharynx, and larynx, leading to obstruction of the airway (laryngeal edema).

Allergic skin reactions, if the sole manifestation of allergy, are usually not considered to be life-threatening. Yet a skin reaction that develops rapidly following drug administration may be the first indication of the generalized reaction to follow.

The adhesive tape employed during IV sedation is a not uncommon cause of dermatologic reactions, the adhesive being the allergen. The usual response to this tape is erythema and urticaria developing around the site where the tape has been placed. In adhesive-allergic individuals, hypoallergenic tapes are recommended for use.

Respiratory reactions

Clinical signs and symptoms of allergy may be related entirely to the respiratory tract, or signs and symptoms of respiratory tract involvement may occur along with other systemic responses. In a slowly developing generalized allergic reaction, respiratory tract involvement usually follows the skin response but precedes cardiovascular signs and symptoms. Bronchospasm is the classic respiratory manifestation of allergy. It represents the clinical result of constriction of bronchial smooth muscle. Signs and symptoms include respiratory distress, dyspnea, wheezing, flushing, possible cyanosis, perspiration, tachycardia, greatly increased anxiety, and the use of accessory muscles of respiration.

A second respiratory manifestation of acute allergy may be the extension of angioedema to the larynx, which produces a swelling of the vocal apparatus with subsequent obstruction of the airway. Clinical manifestations include little or no air exchange from the lungs (chest is not moving, little or no air is felt), wheezing, indicating partial airway obstruction, or no sound, indicating total obstruction. The occur-

rence of significant angioedema represents one of the most ominous of clinical signs. Acute airway obstruction leads rapidly to death of the patient unless immediately corrected.

Generalized anaphylaxis

Generalized anaphylaxis is the most dramatic and acutely life-threatening allergic reaction and may cause clinical death within a few minutes. It may develop following the administration of an antigen via any route but is most likely to occur following parenteral administration. The time from antigenic challenge to the onset of reaction is quite variable, but typically the reaction develops rapidly, reaching a maximum within 5 to 30 minutes. Delayed responses of an hour or more have also been reported. It is believed that this is the result of the rate at which the antigen enters into the circulatory system.

Signs and symptoms of generalized anaphylaxis are highly variable. Four major clinical syndromes are recognized: skin reactions, smooth muscle spasm (gastrointestinal and genitourinary tracts and respiratory smooth muscle), respiratory distress, and cardiovascular collapse. In typical generalized anaphylaxis the symptoms progressively move through these four areas; however, in cases of fatal anaphylaxis, respiratory and cardiovascular disturbances predominate and are evident early in the reaction.

In the typical generalized anaphylactic reaction the patient may begin to complain of feeling sick and develop intense itching, flushing, and giant hives over the face and upper chest. Nausea, possibly followed by vomiting, may also occur. These early symptoms are primarily related to the skin. Other responses noted early in the reaction include conjunctivitis, vasomotor rhinitis (increased mucous secretion in nose), and pilomotor erection (the feeling of hair standing on end).

Associated with the development of skin symptoms are various gastrointestinal and genitourinary disturbances related to spasm of smooth muscle. Severe abdominal cramps, nausea and vomiting, diarrhea, and fecal and urinary incontinence may occur.

Respiratory symptoms normally follow. However, in rapidly developing reactions all symptoms may occur within a short time with considerable overlap, and in particularly severe reactions respiratory and cardiovascular symptoms may be the only signs present.

Respiratory symptoms begin with a feeling of substernal tightness or pain in the chest. A cough may develop in addition to wheezing and dyspnea. If the respiratory disturbances are severe, cyanosis may ensue, noted initially in mucous membranes and nail beds. Laryngeal edema may also develop, producing acute airway obstruction.

Signs and symptoms of cardiovascular disturbance appear next and include pallor, lightheadedness, palpitation, tachycardia, hypotension, and cardiac dysrhythmias followed by loss of consciousness and cardiac arrest. With loss of consciousness the anaphylactic reaction may more properly be called "anaphylactic shock."

The duration of the reaction or any part of it may vary from minutes to a day or more. With prompt and appropriate therapy the entire reaction may be terminated rapidly; however, the two most serious sequelae, hypotension and laryngeal edema, may persist for hours to days in spite of vigorous therapy. Death may occur at any time, the usual cause being upper airway obstruction produced by laryngeal edema.

Management
Skin reactions

Skin reactions may range from localized angioedema to diffuse erythema, urticaria, and pruritis. Management of these reactions is based on the speed at which they appear following antigenic challenge (drug administration).

Delayed skin reactions

Skin reactions that appear more than 60 minutes after antigenic exposure and do not progress are not considered to be life-threatening. These include a mild skin reaction following IM or submucosal injection or localized reaction to adhesive tape.

When this occurs during parenteral sedation, the first step in management is the IM or IV administration of a histamine blocker (antihistamine) such as diphenhydramine 50 mg or chlorpheniramine 10 mg. The patient is then given a prescription for antihistamine to be taken orally for approximately 3 to 5 days.

Medical consultation should follow with the patient's physician or an allergist to determine the nature of the allergy(ies).

If the skin reaction is mild but the patient has left the office before noticing it, the patient should be requested to return to the office, where the same therapy as described would be employed. Should the reaction be noted at a time when the patient is unable to return to the office for evaluation, the patient is advised to see a physician at a local hospital emergency room. The treating dentist should arrange to meet the patient at the hospital, if possible.

Histamine-blocking agents inhibit the actions of histamine by occupying receptor sites on the effector cell (competitive antagonism), thereby preventing the agonist molecules (histamine) from occupying these same sites. The protective responses from histamine blockers include control of edema formation and itch. Other allergic responses such as hypotension and bronchoconstriction are influenced little if at all by histamine blockers. Histamine blockers are only of value in mild allergic responses in which only small quantities of histamine have been released or to prevent reactions in allergic individuals.

Immediate skin reactions

Allergic skin reactions developing within 60 minutes should be managed more vigorously. Other allergic symptoms of a relatively mild nature included in this section are conjunctivitis, rhinitis, urticaria, pruritis, and erythema.

Epinephrine is administered intravenously, intramuscularly, or subcutaneously in an adult dose of 0.3 mg. A histamine blocker (diphenhydramine or chlorpheniramine) is then administered. Medical consultation is requested.

In most cases in which a patient has required the administration of epinephrine it is my belief that the patient should be fully evaluated prior to discharge from the office or hospital. In most cases the patient should be observed for not less than 1 hour, and in the absence of a return of signs and symptoms may be discharged home in the company of a responsible adult. If the reaction is more severe, medical consultation prior to discharge is indicated.

Respiratory reactions

Bronchospasm. Treatment is terminated and the patient placed in a comfortable (usually semierect) position. O_2 is administered via a full-face mask (demand valve) or nasal inhaler.

A bronchodilator, such as epinephrine or albuterol, is administered either via aerosol administration or via injection (epinephrine 0.3 mg). The potent bronchodilating actions of epinephrine usually terminate bronchospasm within 1 to 2 minutes. Albuterol aerosol will act just as rapidly and should be used in the absence of epinephrine or in the presence of bronchospasm and a history of cardiovascular disease. Aminophylline can also be used in the treatment of bronchospasm. Aminophylline is administered *slowly* intravenously at a rate of 50 mg per minute until the desired response is obtained. Hypotension and reflex tachycardia may be noted with aminophylline administration.

Following administration of the bronchodilator, the patient should be observed for possible recurrence of symptoms for approximately 1 hour. The administration of a histamine blocker and a suitable steroid such as dexamethasone, 20 mg, intramuscularly or intravenously, will decrease the risk of a recurrence.[2]

Laryngeal edema. The second and probably more life-threatening respiratory manifestation of allergy is the development of laryngeal edema. It may be diagnosed when little or no air movement can be heard or felt through the mouth and nose despite spontaneous respiratory efforts. A partially obstructed airway in the presence of spontaneous respiratory efforts produces a characteristically high-pitched crowing sound, whereas total obstruction is accompanied by an ominous silence. The patient soon loses consciousness from a lack of oxygen.

The patient must immediately be placed into the supine position with the legs elevated slightly to improve venous return to the heart. Epinephrine is administered (0.3 mg intravenously, intramuscularly, or submucosally) and a patent airway is provided. Epinephrine administration for a partially obstructed airway may halt or even reverse laryngeal edema. Medical assistance should be obtained as soon as possible.

A totally obstructed airway may not be improved (or improved rapidly enough) by epinephrine administration. In this case it is necessary to create an emergency airway to save the patient's life. Time is of the essence, and it is not possible to delay action until the arrival of medical assistance. A cricothyrotomy is the procedure of choice for establishment of an airway in this situation (Fig. 35-3).[13]

The patient's neck is hyperextended to permit identification of the thyroid and cricoid cartilages and the cricothyroid membrane. A roll of towels may be placed beneath the patient's neck to aid in hyperextension. The thyroid cartilage is held steady between the thumb and second finger while the index finger identifies the cricothyroid membrane.

A vertical skin incision is made in the midline over the thyroid and cricoid cartilages. Vessels are retracted from the midline with the thumb and index finger of the opposite hand. As the wound is opened by finger dissection the cricothyroid membrane becomes readily apparent. A horizontal incision is

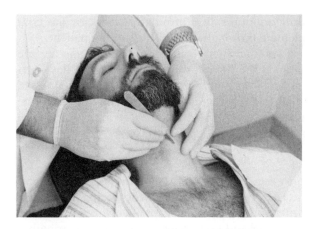

Fig. 35-3. Cricothyrotomy technique. With fingers placed on thyroid and cricoid cartilages, a vertical skin incision is made, followed by a horizontal incision into the trachea. (From Malamed SF: *Handbook of medical emergencies,* ed 3. St Louis, 1987, Mosby.)

made into the cricothyroid membrane as close as possible to the cricoid cartilage to minimize bleeding.

Enlarge the cricothyroid space by inserting the handle of the scalpel into the horizontal incision and rotating it 90 degrees to open the airway. If available, a cricothyroid or tracheotomy tube can be inserted temporarily. Properly performed, a cricothyrotomy can be accomplished in 15 to 30 seconds.

Anesthesia is not necessary as the patient is unconscious and unable to react to the stimulation of the scalpel. It is not unusual for the patient to cough once the trachea is entered.

Once an airway is obtained, O_2 must be administered, artificial ventilation employed if needed, and vital signs monitored. A histamine blocker and corticosteroid should be administered intravenously or intramuscularly. These drugs can halt the progress of the reaction or even reverse it. The patient will require hospitalization following transfer from the office to the hospital by paramedical personnel.

Generalized anaphylaxis

In generalized anaphylaxis a wide range of clinical manifestations may appear; however, the cardiovascular system is involved in virtually all reactions. In a rapidly progressing anaphylactic reaction cardiovascular collapse may develop within minutes of the onset of symptoms. Immediate and vigorous management of the situation is imperative if a successful result is to be achieved. It is highly unlikely that this situation will develop following parenteral or enteral drug administration provided the doctor has completed a thorough drug history on the patient.

Two other life-threatening situations may also develop at the time of drug administration that might on occasion mimic anaphylaxis: vasodepressor syncope (fainting) and an overdose reaction. In immediate management there must be an attempt to diagnose the actual causative event.

Signs of allergy present

In the event that signs and symptoms such as urticaria, erythema, pruritus, or wheezing are evident prior to the patient's collapse, a diagnosis of allergy is obvious and management proceeds accordingly.

The patient should be placed into the supine position with his feet elevated slightly, and BLS should be instituted as soon as possible. Emergency personnel are summoned immediately (i.e., 9-1-1).

The emergency drug kit is brought to the site of the emergency and the preloaded syringe of epinephrine readied for use. An adult dose of 0.3-mg (0.3 ml of a 1:1000 solution) epinephrine is administered intramuscularly or subcutaneously as quickly as possible. If administered intravenously, a 1:10,000 epinephrine solution is used, and 3 ml is administered over 30 seconds.

Epinephrine administration usually produces clinical improvement in generalized anaphylaxis. Respiratory and cardiovascular signs and symptoms should begin to resolve. Should the clinical picture fail to improve or continue to deteriorate within 3 to 5 minutes of the first IV epinephrine dose or 5 to 10 minutes of the IM or subcutaneous dose, a second 0.3-mg dose is administered. Subsequent doses of 0.3 mg may be administered as needed, always keeping in mind the potential risk of epinephrine administration (excessive cardiovascular stimulation).

BLS will be provided for the patient throughout the period until epinephrine exerts its clinical actions or medical assistance becomes available. During this time vital signs are monitored continuously and recorded. O_2 may be administered to the patient. CPR must be initiated immediately should cardiac arrest occur.

During the acute, life-threatening phase of the obvious anaphylactic reaction, management consists of the administration of O_2 and epinephrine, with continual monitoring of vital signs. Until improvement in the patient's status is observed, no additional drug therapy is warranted.

Once clinical improvement is noted (increased blood pressure, decreased bronchospasm), addi-

tional therapy may be instituted. This includes the administration of a histamine blocker and a corticosteroid either intramuscularly or intravenously. Their function is to minimize the risk of recurrence of signs and symptoms and to obviate the need to continue the administration of epinephrine. They are not administered during the acute phase of the reaction because they are too slow in onset of action and they do not do enough immediate good to justify their early administration. Epinephrine and O_2 are the only drugs administered during the acute phase of the anaphylactic reaction.

No signs of allergy

A second clinical picture of the acute allergic reaction might well be one in which a patient receiving an IM or IV injection loses consciousness immediately following drug administration and no clinical signs or symptoms of allergy were or are obvious.

The unconscious patient is placed in the supine position with the feet elevated, and BLS is initiated. A victim of vasodepressor syncope rapidly recovers consciousness (within 10 seconds) once properly positioned with a patent airway. The patient who does not recover at this point should continue to receive BLS.

The patient's vital signs must be monitored continuously during the episode, with CPR instituted immediately if indicated. Medical assistance is summoned when the patient has failed to recover spontaneously within 10 seconds after instituting BLS. In the absence of definitive signs and symptoms of an allergic reaction, the administration of epinephrine and other drugs is not indicated. A number of other situations might be the cause of the loss of consciousness, for example, CVA, overdose reaction, hypoglycemia, acute adrenal insufficiency, or convulsive episodes. The most prudent course of action in the absence of definitive evidence of allergy is to continue the administration of BLS until medical assistance becomes available.

O_2 may be administered to the patient at any time during management.

Laryngeal edema is yet another possible development during the generalized anaphylactic reaction. Should ventilation become difficult in spite of adequate head-tilt and a clear pharynx (obtained by suctioning), it may become necessary to perform a cricothyrotomy to obtain an airway. Laryngeal edema is a manifestation of allergy. Once a patent airway has been assured (cricothyrotomy), epinephrine (0.3 mg) may be administered, followed by a histamine blocker and corticosteroid as outlined previously. Once stabilized, the patient must be transferred to a hospital for definitive management and observation.

Overdose and allergy represent the most serious of the complications associated with the administration of anesthesia and sedation. There are other complications that also produce life-threatening situations. These include hypotension, cardiac dysrhythmias, respiratory depression, and laryngospasm. The latter two have been reviewed previously in the discussion of complications of IV sedation (Chapter 28).

HYPOTENSION

A slight decrease in a patient's blood pressure during general anesthesia or conscious sedation is not unusual. Such decreases in blood pressure are usually minimal, especially during conscious sedation. More significant reductions in arterial blood pressure are clinically important because of the necessity to maintain adequate tissue perfusion. A systolic blood pressure of 80 mm Hg in an ASA I adult might not require treatment, whereas the same blood pressure in an elderly hypertensive patient might constitute a life-threatening situation. The need to treat hypotension is based on the ability of the circulation to adequately perfuse the tissues. Clinical signs and symptoms associated with hypotension and inadequate tissue perfusion are found in Table 35-6 and include the presence of chest pain, dyspnea, or a systolic blood pressure (adult) below 90 mm Hg.[14]

In the child, hypotension is considered to be present where the systolic blood pressure is less than 70 mm Hg plus 2 times the age in years. Thus, the lowest acceptable blood pressure in a 4-year-old child would be 78 mm Hg $(70 + [2 \times 4])$.[15]

Table 35-6. Signs and symptoms associated with significant hypotension

Chest pain
Dyspnea
Hypotension (systolic bp <90 mm Hg)
Congestive heart failure
Ischemia
Infarction
Restlessness
Anxiety
Disorientation
Pallor
Cold, clammy skin
Dilated pupils
Prolonged capillary refill time

Always consider the difficulty in assessing blood pressure accurately in the smaller child patient. Use of a blood pressure cuff that is too small (narrow) for the arm produces artificially elevated readings, while use of too large a cuff (e.g., an adult cuff on a small child) produces artificially decreased readings. The reader is referred to Chapter 5 for a description of the proper technique of recording blood pressure.

In the conscious patient who develops hypotension, cerebral ischemia occurs secondarily and is associated with restlessness, anxiety, and disorientation. Circulatory inadequacy is suggested by pallor, cold clammy skin, and dilated pupils. The rate of capillary refill can be used as a gauge of peripheral perfusion. In hypotensive states capillary refill time is prolonged.

During sedative procedures hypotension can be diagnosed in one or more of several ways:

1. Monitoring of blood pressure throughout procedure.
2. Observing and communicating with patient.
3. Observation of the operative field: during surgical procedures in which bleeding is normal, the doctor and assistant will notice that the surgical field is considerably drier than usual. This should lead to an immediate checking of the patient's blood pressure.

If a blood pressure cuff is not immediately available, a quick estimate of the systolic blood pressure may be obtained by palpating peripheral pulses at the radial, brachial, and/or carotid arteries.

Pulse present	Systolic pressure is at least
Radial artery	80 mm Hg
Brachial artery	70 mm Hg
Carotid artery	60 mm Hg

For example, if a carotid pulse is palpated but the brachial is absent the systolic blood pressure is greater than 60 mm Hg but lower than 70 mm Hg.

Causes of hypotension

Possible causes of hypotension include the following:

Excessive premedication
The action of therapeutic drugs taken prior to the sedative/anesthetic procedure by the patient for preexisting disease
Overdose of sedatives/anesthetics
Reflex (light anesthesia, pain)
Vascular absorption of local anesthetics
Hemorrhage
Positional changes of patient

Hypoxia and hypercarbia
Abnormalities of circulatory system
Adrenocortical insufficiency
Metabolic derangement (i.e., diabetic coma)

Excessive premedication or the administration of a relative overdose to a "sensitive" patient can provoke hypotension. Following oral administration, this is unlikely to occur; however, following the administration of an IM drug, especially an opioid agonist, hypotension has been documented. Opioids produce this effect through their depressant actions on the vasomotor center, reducing muscle tone, decreasing ventilation, and dilating peripheral blood vessels.

The influence of *therapeutic drugs* required by the patient for a preexisting disorder might result in hypotension. Drugs such as corticosteroids, antihypertensives, and tranquilizers such as chlorpromazine may produce hypotension.

Overdose of sedatives/anesthetics is unlikely to develop when these drugs are administered carefully via techniques in which titration is available and is used. These techniques are the inhalation and IV routes of administration. When these drugs are administered intramuscularly or submucosally, however, there is a greater likelihood of overdose and hypotension because of the lack of control over the ultimate drug effect. In addition, the opioids are the drugs most often administered in these techniques, drugs that are more likely to produce hypotension if administered to excess. Conversely, *anesthesia that is too light or the presence of pain* are capable of inducing hypotension reflexly.

Vascular absorption of local anesthetics is another potential cause of hypotension. Many causes of local anesthetic overdose and hypotension are possible, including overadministration (relative or absolute), intravascular administration, rapid absorption, slow elimination, or slow biotransformation. The primary means of preventing hypotension and overdose from local anesthetics are aspiration prior to every injection and slow administration of the smallest volume of solution that will provide adequate pain control. The reader is recommended to other texts for a more in-depth description of local anesthetic overdose.[16]

Hemorrhage is unlikely to be severe enough during a dental procedure to produce a drop in blood pressure; however, this is not an uncommon cause of hypotension within the hospital during major surgical procedures.

Change in position of the patient is more likely to produce postural or orthostatic hypotension, partic-

Table 35-7. Drugs producing orthostatic hypotension

Category	Generic name	Proprietary name
Antihypertensives	Guanethidine	Ismelin
Phenothiazines	Chlorpromazine	Thorazine
	Thioridazine	Mellaril
Tricyclic antidepressants	Doxepin	Sinequan
	Amitriptyline	Elavil
	Imipramine	Tofranil
		Presamine
Opioids	Meperidine	Demerol
	Morphine	Morphine
Antiparkinson drugs	Levodopa (L-dopa)	Dopar
		Larodopa

From Malamed SF: *Medical emergencies in the dental office*, ed 4, St Louis, 1993, Mosby.

ularly in elderly patients, patients receiving certain drugs (Table 35-7), and those who have received CNS-depressant drugs, particularly opioids.

Positional changes of the dental chair or the patient standing up from the chair should be accomplished gradually to permit the cardiovascular system to adapt to the increased effect of gravity as the patient becomes more upright. It has been mentioned throughout this book that the recommended position of the patient during procedures in which CNS depressants have been administered is supine with legs elevated slightly or a semisupine position. The upright (erect) position should be avoided during treatment unless absolutely essential.

Hypoxia and hypercarbia are additional possible causes of hypotension. Adequate management of the patient's airway during deep sedation or general anesthesia is of critical importance.

Cardiovascular abnormalities are another possible cause of hypotension during sedative or anesthetic procedures. The occurrence of myocardial ischemia or infarction during a procedure may result in a profound drop in systemic blood pressure. In the conscious, albeit sedated, patient other clinical signs and symptoms would usually be available (pain radiating in a classic pattern, nausea, dusky appearance, cyanosis of mucous membranes) that would aid in diagnosis; however, in the unconscious patient such a diagnosis would be more difficult to establish. Other cardiovascular causes of hypotension, all of which are extremely unlikely to develop in the outpatient setting on ASA I or II patients, include embolism to the brain (CVA) or lungs (pulmonary infarction), hypovolemia caused by the patient's poor physical condition prior to the start of the procedure (unlikely to be observed in the outpatient setting), heart failure, and anaphylactic shock.

Adrenocortical insufficiency may produce hypotension and shock. When a patient has received exogenous corticosteroid therapy in the recent past (the rule of twos, Chapter 5), prophylactic corticosteroid administration prior to the start of any traumatic procedure is strongly recommended.

Metabolic derangements such as diabetic coma (hyperglycemia and ketoacidosis) or insulin shock (hypoglycemia) are other possible causes of hypotension that should be considered when the reason for a hypotensive episode is being sought. A history of diabetes mellitus in such a patient would provide a definite indication that this is a likely cause of the hypotension. Hypoglycemia is a much more likely cause than hyperglycemia in the patient who is able to stand and walk.

Management of hypotension

Treatment of hypotension is directed to its etiology. However, there are certain basic steps that must be carried out when hypotension occurs.

Step one. The procedure is terminated and the patient placed into the supine position with his feet elevated to increase blood flow to the brain and aid in return of venous blood from the legs. BLS procedures (airway, breathing, circulation) are initiated as needed. The patient will likely be attempting to breathe spontaneously, although the airway may or may not be patent. The pulse will be weak and probably rapid (tachycardia frequently accompanies hypotension). Blood pressure will be decreased from the patient's baseline values. O_2 may be administered to the patient at any time during management.

Step two. If an inhalation anesthetic such as N_2O (or any other gaseous agent) is being administered, its concentration is decreased. This step alone will usually lead to an increase in blood pressure. Although the patient is receiving a concentration of the agent that is within normal limits, a relative overdose of the drug may be administered if the patient is unusually sensitive to its actions.

If barbiturates have been administered intramuscularly or intravenously, general supportive measures (BLS) must be continued until the patient improves because no effective antagonistic drug for the barbiturates exists.

If opioids or a benzodiazepine have been administered, the appropriate antagonist (naloxone or flumazenil) may be administered intravenously or in-

tramuscularly. Though the primary effect of naloxone is to improve respiratory depression induced by the opioids, a slight elevation in blood pressure may also be observed because the analgesia from the opioid also decreases and the patient begins to respond to painful stimuli if local anesthesia is absent.

Step three. When hypotension develops during an IV sedation procedure or if an IV infusion can be started, a relatively effective and safe means of managing hypotension is available, especially in the ASA I or II patient. The rapid IV infusion of solution (5% dextrose and water, physiologic saline, or lactated Ringer's solution) will provide extra fluid volume in the cardiovascular system and an increase in blood pressure. The 250-ml bag of solution should be opened and permitted to flow rapidly until it is observed that the blood pressure has increased. Mild decreases in systemic blood pressure may usually be reversed in this simple manner.

The administration of vasopressors is reserved for hypotension that is more severe and persists following these preceding measures. A number of vasopressors are available. It is recommended in Chapter

---

ACTIONS OF ALPHA AND BETA RECEPTORS

Alpha receptors

Peripheral vasoconstriction: skin, mucosa, intestine, kidney
Mydriasis
Myometrial contraction

Beta receptors

Beta receptors are subdivided into two groups: beta-1 and beta-2 receptors. Stimulation of these receptors produces the following reactions.

Beta-1 receptors

Bronchodilation
Tachycardia
Palpitation
Hypertension
Insomnia
Tremor
Increased cardiac contractility

Beta-2 receptors

Bronchodilation
Vasodilation

Table 35-8. Vasopressors: summary of actions on receptors

Agent	Alpha	Beta 1	Beta 2	Usual dose IV	Usual dose IM
Epinephrine (most potent agent to alpha receptor)	+	+	+	0.1 mg	0.2-0.3 mg
Norepinephrine bitartrate	+	+	+	Used as continuous IV drip; not recommended IM	
Isoproterenol	–	+	+	0.025 µg/kg/min IV drip; not recommended IM	
Phenylephrine	+	–	–	0.25-0.5 mg	2-3 mg
Mephenteramine	+	+	+	5-15 mg	10-30 mg
Ephedrine	+	+	+	10-25 mg followed by IM dose	25-50 mg
Metaraminol	+	+	–	0.5-2 mg	2-5 mg
Methoxamine	+	–	–	2-5 mg	5-10 mg
Dopamine	–	+	–	Via continuous IV infusion (200 mg in 250 or 500 ml 5% dextrose and water)	
Propranolol		+	+	0.5 to 1 mg up to maximum of 2 mg IV	

34 that methoxamine or mephenteramine be available in the emergency drug kit. *Methoxamine* exerts its effect by stimulating alpha receptors, producing constriction in vascular smooth muscle in the skin, mucosa, kidney, and splanchnic region. Methoxamine has little or no direct effect on beta receptors that increase the workload of the heart (box on previous page). A reflex bradycardia may be associated with methoxamine administration. *Mephenteramine* increases blood pressure by enhancing cardiac contraction but does not increase peripheral resistance. Mephenteramine is usually safe and effective for the management of unexplained hypotension during local or general anesthesia and sedation. In the absence of greater knowledge of the status of the patient's cardiovascular system and heart, the administration of other drugs (Table 35-8) with beta actions or mixed alpha and beta actions is not recommended.

Most vasopressors stimulate both alpha and beta receptors, but the degree of stimulation by each drug varies. Table 35-8 summarizes the clinical action of the more commonly used vasopressors, and the accompanying box lists the actions of the various receptors. Other vasopressors may be employed in place of methoxamine, provided the doctor is conversant with the pharmacology, indications, contraindications, precautions, adverse reactions, and recommended dosage of the drug. Methoxamine, in a dose of 5 to 10 mg intramuscularly or 2 to 5 mg intravenously, or mephenteramine, 15 to 30 mg, are

recommended. An IM dose is suggested; the IV route is reserved for emergency situations in which a more immediate response is required. The onset of activity is 15 minutes after IM administration and 2 to 3 minutes after IV administration. Duration of action is approximately 30 minutes to 1 hour (IV).

The following actions relate to the management of hypotension occurring during anesthesia or sedation:

1. Terminate the procedure and position the patient supine with feet elevated.
2. Initiate BLS as indicated (airway, breathing, circulation).
3. Administer O_2.
4. Monitor vital signs.
5. Observe for signs and symptoms of cause of hypotension.
6. Definitive therapy:
   - Decrease concentration of inhalation anesthetics
   - Reverse opioid actions with naloxone
   - Reverse benzodiazepine actions with flumazenil
   - If patient has diabetes, consider hypoglycemia and manage appropriately
   - Monitor and look for signs and symptoms of cardiovascular system involvement (angina, myocardial infarction)
   - Determine any history of recent corticosteroid therapy: IV administration of corticosteroids (see later discussion)

7. If IV route is available, administer IV infusate rapidly (up to 500 ml in ASA I, 250 ml in ASA II).
8. If IV route is not available or if hypotension is refractory to preceding steps, administer IM or IV vasopressor.
9. Summon medical assistance if deemed appropriate.

Hypotension in patients receiving corticosteroid therapy

Patients receiving corticosteroids or having recently completed a long course of steroid therapy are more likely to encounter hypotensive episodes during surgery and anesthesia. This is related to their inability to release adequate levels of steroids in response to surgical stress producing acute adrenal insufficiency. Preoperative administration of steroids (in consultation with the patient's physician) can minimize this risk. Where hypotensive episodes develop during treatment, large intravenous doses of corticosteroids and vasopressors are usually required to prevent morbidity or death.

Hypotension in patients receiving beta-blockers

Patients who are beta-blocked do not experience an elevation in their heart rate with simple exercise. Management of hypotension in the beta-blocked patient consists of[2]:

1. *Isoproterenol* (Isuprel), administered slowly intravenously at a rate of 0.2 mg at 1-minute intervals. Dose is determined by the patient's response. In the presence of total beta-blockade, a large dose of isoproterenol may be required.
2. Where the hypotensive episode continues despite isoproterenol administration, intravenous *glucagon* is administered.
3. *Atropine* (0.5 to 1.0 mg) is administered intravenously wherever severe bradycardia is present.

HYPERTENSION

Hypertension, or elevated blood pressure, may be noted during surgical and dental procedures when the level of pain control is inadequate. Transient elevations in blood pressure may be prevented through the administration (or readministration) of local anesthesia. Transient minor elevations in blood pressure (hypertensive urgencies) are usually well tolerated and of little danger to the patient. Sustained and/or significant elevations in blood pressure (hypertensive emergencies or crises) must be treated aggressively.

Guidelines for the evaluation of blood pressure in both adult and pediatric patients were presented in Chapter 5.

Causes of episodes of high blood pressure during dental treatment, surgery and anesthesia (sedation, general anesthesia) include the following[2]:

1. Light anesthesia or sedation
2. Pain
3. Hypercarbia
4. Hypoxia
5. Emergence delirium
6. Fluid overload (overhydration)
7. Hyperthermia

The most common causes of hypertension during dental procedures, surgery and anesthesia are light anesthesia or sedation and the presence of pain. Management is directed at providing adequate sedation, anesthesia, and pain control. Blood pressure usually decreases as the quality of anesthesia improves.

Hypercarbia and hypoxia are the next most frequent causes of elevated blood pressure. Catecholamine release is increased with both hypercarbia and hypoxia. Airway management and ventilation will reverse this cause of elevations in blood pressure.

Postoperatively, pain, hypercarbia, and emergence delirium are common causes of elevated blood pressure. Strict management of the airway and the administration of oxygen preclude hypoxia and hypercarbia. The administration of physostigmine will terminate episodes of emergence delirium, while the use of local anesthesia or the administration of opioids or NSAIDs will help to manage posttreatment pain.

Fluid overload is not a frequent cause of high blood pressure in the dental outpatient, especially when the 250-ml bag of IV infusate is administered. ASA III and IV patients with congestive heart failure may be at risk for acute pulmonary edema when larger volumes of intravenous fluids are received.

Hyperthermia is associated with increased metabolic rates, increased heart rate, and increased blood pressure. A patient's temperature should be recorded prior to conscious sedation whenever there is an indication that infection may be present or the patient appears warm or flushed. Temperature should be recorded preoperatively and intraoperatively when general anesthesia is administered.

Management of a hypertensive crisis

A hypertensive crisis is said to exist when the systolic blood pressure is 250 mm Hg or greater and/

or the diastolic pressure is 130 mm Hg or more.[17] Hypertensive crisis usually occurs in patients with a history of chronic, stable hypertension. The goal in management is to avoid rapid changes in blood pressure without compromising cerebral perfusion.[18] To this end, antihypertensive therapy is not recommended in any patient unless there is severe hypertension (>200/130).[19] Hypertensive crisis must be distinguished from a modest and transient elevation in blood pressure from causes previously listed. Deepening of the anesthesia or eliminating pain through the readministration of local anesthetics will bring with it a return of the elevated blood pressure towards baseline values. However, when elevated, blood pressure does not return to acceptable levels within a few minutes of onset, or if it continues to increase, the possibility of a hypertensive crisis must be considered and steps initiated to manage it.

Among the possible acute causes of the hypertensive crisis are cardiovascular complications, such as myocardial infarction and dissecting aortic aneurysm, while other potential causes include recreational drugs (e.g., cocaine), patients receiving monoamine oxidase inhibitors, pheochromocytoma, and thyroid crisis.[18] It is important when evaluating the hypertensive crisis to distinguish whether the cause is cardiac or noncardiac.[2]

When significant elevation is noted in the patient's blood pressure, proceed as follows:

Step 1. Terminate dental treatment.
Step 2. Position the patient in an erect position (45 degrees upright or more).
Step 3. Monitor blood pressure and heart rate/ rhythm every 5 minutes.
Step 4. Administer oxygen.
Step 5. Activate EMS.
Step 6. Establish an IV infusion, if not already present.

Where the cause of the hypertensive crisis is cardiac, such as congestive heart failure, proceed as follows:

Step 7. Titrate nitroprusside (Nipride) at an infusion rate of 5 µg/kg/min until the blood pressure is lowered to a desired point. The average therapeutic range is between 0.5 and 10 µg/kg/min.

Where ischemic heart disease (MI) or CHF are present, proceed as follows:

Step 7. IV nitroglycerin, a drug similar to nitroprusside, is administered as a 50-µg bolus followed by an infusion of 10 to 20 µg/min. The infusion may be increased 5 to 10 µg per minute until the desired blood pressure response is noted.[2,18]

When a noncardiac cause of the hypertensive crisis is present (e.g., anxiety, allergy, CVA), proceed as follows:

Step 7. Administer diazoxide (Hyperstat) IV in doses of 1 to 3 mg/kg up to 150 mg. This dose may be repeated every 5 to 10 minutes up to 600 mg.
Step 8. In those situations in which anxiety is a major component of the hypertensive crisis, midazolam or diazepam may be of some utility in managing the hypertension.

Table 35-9 summarizes the drugs employed in management of the hypertensive crisis.

There may arise situations in which an IV infusion cannot be started and/or the appropriate parenteral antihypertensive drugs are not available for administration. In such instances the following regimen is suggested:

Step 1. Terminate dental treatment.
Step 2. Position the patient in an erect position (45 degrees upright or more).
Step 3. Monitor blood pressure and heart rate/ rhythm every 5 minutes.

Table 35-9. Parenteral drugs used in treatment of hypertensive crisis

Drug	Administration	Onset	Duration	Dosage	Side Effects
Sodium nitroprusside	IV fusion	Immediate	2-3 min	0.5-10 µg/kg/min	Hypotension, nausea, vomiting, apprehension
Diazoxide	IV bolus	q5-10 min, up to 600 mg	1-5 min	6-12 hr 50-100 mg	Hypotension, tachycardia, nausea, vomiting, fluid retention; exacerbate myocardiac ischemia, heart failure, or aortic dissection
Nitroglycerin	IV infusion	1-2 min	3-5 min	5-100 µg/min	Headache, nausea, vomiting

Step 4. Administer oxygen.

Step 5. Activate EMS.

Step 6. Administer sublingual nitroglycerin tablets (2 tablets of 0.3 mg) or 2 sprays of nitrolingual spray onto the mucous membrane of the tongue. This dose may be repeated every 5 to 10 minutes if necessary.

Step 7. Upon arrival of emergency medical assistance, an intravenous infusion will be established and appropriate drugs administered. The patient will usually require a period of hospitalization to ensure stabilization of the blood pressure.

CARDIAC DYSRHYTHMIAS

A dysrhythmia is any deviation from the normal sinus rhythm. It was reported as the most common intraoperative complication occurring in 112,721 patients studied.[20] The incidence of perioperative dysrhythmias under general anesthesia has been reported by different sources to be from 4% to 60%.[21,22] Driscoll has reported the incidence of dysrhythmias during extraction of erupted bicuspids in patients receiving local anesthesia and sedation to be 24.19%.[23]

Fortunately, the majority of dysrhythmias encountered during sedative and general anesthetic procedures will rarely require treatment. Indeed, if bradycardia (<60 beats per minute) and tachycardia (>100 beats per minute) are discounted, the incidence of dysrhythmias requiring drug therapy is exceedingly low. However, the presence of a cardiac dysrhythmia can be a warning that some physiological or pharmacological problem exists that does require immediate management. DeRango[24] makes some generalizations about the incidence of cardiac dysrhythmias:

1. The majority of anesthetized patients who are continuously monitored (ECG) will demonstrate some dysrhythmia during the anesthetic period.
2. The incidence of dysrhythmias is higher in patients with a history of heart disease than in those without such a history.
3. The incidence of dysrhythmias is higher in patients whose trachea is intubated.
4. The incidence of dysrhythmias is more frequent in patients undergoing surgery lasting more than 3 hours than in patients undergoing shorter procedures.
5. Patients receiving digitalis preoperatively have a higher incidence of dysrhythmias than patients not receiving digitalis.

From a review of the preceding information it appears that the incidence of cardiac dysrhythmias during outpatient procedures in ASA I or II patients should be considerably lower than that for in-hospital procedures. The very nature of the patient (healthier) and of the procedure (shorter duration, trachea rarely intubated) being performed are reasons for a decreased incidence of serious dysrhythmias during outpatient procedures.

Precipitating factors

Dysrhythmias may be produced in patients receiving anesthesia and sedation by the following means:

1. Anesthetic agents
2. Carbon dioxide
3. Stimulation under light planes of anesthesia
4. Vagal responses
5. Intubation
6. Anoxia
7. Duration of the procedure

Anesthetic agents may provoke dysrhythmias. Among commonly used inhalation anesthetics halothane is associated with a greater incidence of dysrhythmias than enflurane, isoflurane, desflurane, and sevoflurane.

Carbon dioxide retention (hypercarbia) is a frequent cause of dysrhythmias during anesthesia and sedation. The mechanism of dysrhythmia generation is the release of catecholamines by the increasing CO_2 tension in the blood. Many anesthetic drugs sensitize the myocardium to the effects of these catecholamines, and dysrhythmias are the result.

Stimulation of the patient during a procedure while the patient is under general anesthesia or sedation is a common cause of dysrhythmias. Stimulation (i.e., pain) leads to vagal and sympathetic responses that are ultimately responsible for most dysrhythmias. Management consists of either deepening the level of general anesthesia or sedation (to decrease patient response to stimulation) or to provide more adequate pain control (local anesthesia).

Vagal responses produce a slowing of the sinus rate, which can lead to dysrhythmias such as sinus bradycardia, sinus arrest, junctional rhythms, and most frequently PVCs. Vagal responses are much more likely to develop during general anesthesia than in sedative procedures. Most often these responses occur in response to non-dental surgical stimulation such as traction on intraabdominal structures, traction on extraocular muscles, pressure on the globe, and carotid sinus stimulation.

Tracheal intubation is probably responsible for the greatest incidence of dysrhythmias during general anesthesia, especially when the patient is in a light plane of anesthesia. Most often the dysrhythmias seen are tachydysrhythmias associated with elevations in blood pressure. These dysrhythmias are normally transient and require no drug therapy. Management consists of adequate ventilation and a deepening of the level of anesthesia.

Anoxia, or *severe hypoxia,* during general anesthesia or sedation is another cause of dysrhythmias. Anoxia is associated with the development of hypercarbia (see previous discussion). Management consists of adequate ventilation.

The *duration of surgery* or of the procedure is related to the incidence of dysrhythmias. The incidence of dysrhythmias in procedures under 3 hours is considerably lower than in those requiring more than 3 hours to complete. The body's ability to handle stress is compromised as the procedure lengthens. Increased levels of catecholamines appear in the blood, and dysrhythmias are the result.

Dysrhythmias are significant because they may indicate dysfunction of the myocardial conduction system, which if the dysrhythmia is severe, may lead to cerebral, myocardial, or renal ischemia; CHF and pulmonary edema; myocardial infarction; or ventricular fibrillation (cardiac arrest).

Again, the overwhelming majority of dysrhythmias occurring during general anesthesia and especially during sedative procedures are transient in nature and relatively benign and require no formal drug management. Management usually consists of assuring adequate ventilation, increasing or decreasing (as appropriate) the level of anesthesia or sedation, and providing adequate pain control.

Continuous ECG monitoring of the patient receiving general anesthesia is required; however, the routine use of the ECG during sedative procedures is not necessary, though if available it should be employed in patients with a history of cardiovascular disease.

Dysrhythmias may be discovered through the use of a pulse oximeter or other pulse monitoring device, or more simply by keeping a finger on the patient's pulse. Common dysrhythmias are discussed in Chapter 5. The reader is referred to that chapter for a review of this subject and to advanced cardiac life support textbooks for in-depth discussion of the significance and management of cardiac dysrhythmias.[2,25]

Angina pectoris

Stable angina pectoris is defined as a characteristic thoracic pain, usually substernal; precipitated chiefly by exercise, emotion, or a heavy meal; relieved by vasodilator drugs and a few minutes rest; and a result of a mild inadequacy of the coronary circulation.[5] Several anginal syndromes are identified, including stable angina (ASA III), vasoplastic angina (coronary artery spasm, atypical angina, variant angina, Prinzmetal's angina; ASA III) and unstable angina (preinfarction or crescendo angina, intermediate coronary syndrome and impending MI; ASA IV). Drugs used for the management of acute anginal episodes include nitroglycerin (sublingual tablets, translingual spray, or transdermal patch), for the management of stable and vasospastic angina. Calcium channel blockers (nifedipine, diltiazem, and verapamil) are effective in managing the vasospastic component of angina.

Signs and symptoms

The "pain" of angina is rarely described as such by the patient. More frequently an acute anginal episode is described as a "tightness," "constricting feeling," or a "heavy weight" on the chest. The patient will usually stop whatever he/she is doing and seek relief by sitting upright and administering nitroglycerin. A typical anginal episode lasts but minutes with drug therapy but may persist for up to an hour. Chest pain of long duration, however, is more likely to lead to a presumptive diagnosis of myocardial infarction than angina. Additional signs and symptoms associated with angina include palpitation, faintness, dizziness, dyspnea, and "indigestion."

It is important to note that *the pain of angina is quickly relieved by nitroglycerin administration and that it does not return.*

Management

Step 1. Terminate dental care.
Step 2. Position patient comfortably.
Step 3. Administer oxygen.
Step 4. Administer nitroglycerin.

If a history of angina exists, the patient should be allowed to take his usual dose of sublingual or translingual nitroglycerin. This dose may be repeated in 2 to 5 minutes if the episode persists.

In the absence of a history of angina a dose of two translingual sprays is administered. It is also recommended that in the absence of any history of angina, emergency medical assistance be procured as soon as is possible.

If the episode terminates, proceed as follows:
Step 5. Seek to determine the cause of the episode and modify treatment to preclude further acute episodes of angina during dental treat-

ment. Dental care may continue if both the doctor and patient agree to proceed.

When the episode continues, proceed as follows:

Step 5. If the initial dose of nitroglycerin does not end the episode, two additional doses may be administered. If the patient's nitroglycerin tablets were used initially it is recommended that nitroglycerin spray be used for the subsequent doses.

Step 6. Monitors should be attached, if not already in use. This includes blood pressure, pulse oximetry, and ECG (if available)

Step 7. Summon EMS when chest pain persists following a third dose of nitroglycerin OR sooner if the anginal patient desires it (anginal patients usually know if their episode is anginal or not).

Myocardial infarction

Prolonged ischemia of the myocardium produced by partial or complete occlusion of blood flow through one or more coronary arteries leads to necrosis of heart muscle. Severe chest pain and dysrhythmias are commonly present during myocardial infarction. Cessation of effective cardiac function may occur, producing cardiac arrest and necessitating the immediate institution of basic life support.

Signs and symptoms

Myocardial infarction frequently mimics angina at its onset. One striking difference (in the nondental setting) is that 55% of patients are *at rest* when myocardial infarction occurs whereas angina is associated with an increase in myocardial activity.

Patients experience a more severe and more prolonged pain that, though it may seem anginal at onset, progressively increases in severity. The patient is quite apprehensive and may exhibit weakness, dia-

phoresis, hypotension, and dysrhythmias. Dysrhythmias develop in 95% of myocardial infarcts and increase the rate of morbidity and mortality associated with MI.[27] Hypotension is noted in 80% of patients with myocardial infarction.[28]

Management

Management of myocardial infarction progresses from that described for angina.

Step 1. Terminate all dental care.

Step 2. Position patient comfortably.

Step 3. Administer O_2.

Step 4. Administer nitroglycerin (as described; see angina).

Step 5. Activate EMS when pain does not subside following 3 doses of nitroglycerin or if pain subsides and returns.

Step 6. Monitor patient. Blood pressure, heart rate and rhythm, pulse, oximetry and ECG.

Step 7. Establish an IV infusion.

Step 8. Manage pain with IV morphine 2 to 5 mg every 15 minutes. A 35% nitrous oxide/65% oxygen concentration is an acceptable alternative.

Step 9. Attempt to remain calm during this period. Seek to alleviate the patient's apprehensions.

Step 10. Prepare to administer basic life support should cardiac arrest occur.

Airway obstruction

The most common cause of airway obstruction during sedation or general anesthesia is the posterior displacement of the tongue into the pharynx as muscle tonus is lost as a result of CNS depression produced by the administered drugs. A second possible cause of airway obstruction is a foreign object, such

Table 35-10. Breathing sounds and their management

Sound	Probable Cause	Management
Quiet whooshing	Normal, unobstructed airway	None required
None/no respiratory efforts	Apnea	Controlled ventilation
None/exaggerated respiratory efforts	Complete obstruction	1. Head-tilt/chin-lift 2. Anterior displacement of tongue with hemostat or gauze 3. Pharyngeal suctioning 4. Abdominal thrusts 5. Cricothyrotomy
Snoring	Soft tissue (tongue) displaced in pharynx	1. Head-tilt/chin-lift 2. Anterior displacement of tongue with hemostat or gauze
Gurgling	Fluid in airway	Pharyngeal suction
Wheezing	Bronchospasm	Administer bronchodilator

as a crown or tooth that becomes displaced, although these commonly do not produce total obstruction, but rather a partial airway obstruction. Fluids: blood, saliva, water, and vomitus can also be responsible for airway obstruction.

Airways may become partially or completely obstructed. Distinctive sounds are associated with airway obstruction produced by various causes. These sounds must be detected, diagnosed, and treated as expeditiously as possible. Use of the pretracheal stethoscope during parenteral sedation and general anesthesia allows for instantaneous detection of airway problems.

Normal, unobstructed air flow through the mouth and nose has a very distinct low whooshing sound. Movement of the chest during respiration is minimal and looks "smooth." No soft tissue retraction is present. A *complete obstruction* of the airway is associated with the absence of sound. If the patient is attempting spontaneous ventilation, the observed respiratory movements will appear exaggerated with evident supraclavicular and intercostal soft tissue retraction. The use of abdominal muscles during respiration will also be evident. *Partial airway obstruction resulting from the tongue* being displaced posteriorly is associated with a snoring sound that frequently can be heard by all persons in the treatment room. The presence of *fluid in the airway* is detected by a gurgling sound. One other sound that is heard is that of wheezing, the product of a partial obstruction of the lower airway due to *bronchospasm*. Mild bronchospasm is associated with loud wheezing, while in more severe bronchospasm, in which little air is being exchanged, wheezing may be absent. Table 35-10 summarizes the sounds associated with breathing and their management.

Management of airway obstruction
Complete obstruction associated with exaggerated respiratory efforts

Proceed with each of the following steps until a patent airway is obtained, as will be noted by the return of sounds associated with spontaneous breathing.

Step 1. Head-tilt/chin-lift. If obstruction is still present, proceed to next step.

Step 2. Physically displace the tongue anteriorly by grabbing it with a hemostat or gauze sponge.

Step 3. Using a tonsillar suction tip, suction the posterior pharynx to remove any fluids that may be present.

Step 4. Abdominal thrusts (Heimlich maneuver) until a patent airway is obtained, as determined by the passage of air through the mouth and nose and the return of "sound."

Step 5. Activate EMS.

Step 6. Cricothyrotomy: When each of the preceding steps has failed to reestablish a patent airway, it may be necessary to perform a cricothyrotomy. Cricothyrotomy should be carried out only when the doctor is well trained in the procedure. Cricothyrotomy technique is described in other texts.[16]

Complete obstruction associated with apnea

In fact, when apnea occurs it will not usually be immediately known if a total airway obstruction is present. Following unsuccessful attempts at controlled ventilation it will become evident that something other than the tongue is responsible for the airway problem.

Step 1. Once apea is detected efforts at controlled ventilation are initiated (+ pressure O_2; bag/valve/mask) employing head-tilt/chin-lift. If the chest does not rise with each attempted breath, proceed to step 2.

Step 2. Physically displace the tongue anteriorly by grabbing it with a hemostat or gauze sponge. Attempt to ventilate. If unsuccessful, proceed to step 3.

Step 3. Using a tonsillar suction tip, suction the posterior pharynx to remove any fluids that may be present.

Step 4. Abdominal thrusts (Heimlich maneuver) are administered until a patent airway is obtained, as determined by the passage of air through the mouth and nose and the return of "sound." Following the abdominal thrust a "finger sweep" is used to remove the dislodged object. Suction may also be used.

Step 5. Activate EMS.

Step 6. Cricothyrotomy: When each of the preceding steps has failed to reestablish a patent airway, it may be necessary to perform a cricothyrotomy. Cricothyrotomy should be carried out only when the doctor is well trained in the procedure. Cricothyrotomy technique is described in other texts.[29]

Following each step in this sequence, efforts at controlled ventilation should be attempted.

Partial airway obstruction associated with "snoring"

Step 1. Perform head-tilt/chin-lift.

Step 2. Physically displace the tongue anteriorly by grabbing it with a hemostat or gauze sponge.

Partial airway obstruction associated with "gurgling"

Step 1. Perform head-tilt/chin-lift.

Step 2. Using a tonsillar suction tip, suction the posterior pharynx until all fluids are removed.

Partial airway obstruction associated with "wheezing"

The management of wheezing was discussed previously in the section on respiratory allergic reactions.

Laryngospasm

Laryngospasm is a protective reflex that is designed to maintain the integrity of the airway by preventing foreign matter from entering into the larynx, trachea, and lungs. Laryngospasm is considered to be a complication associated with deep sedation and ultralight general anesthesia, not an emergency.[2]

Laryngospasm is extraordinarily uncommon during conscious sedation. In conscious sedation the patient retains his protective airway reflexes: coughing, gagging, or swallowing foreign matter to prevent its entry into the airway. Laryngospasm is also not seen during stage 3 of anesthesia (see Chapter 3). The degree of CNS depression present at this time is such that these reflexes are lost. Material entering into the airway will not provoke a response from the patient. Ensuring the integrity of the airway is a prime obligation of the anesthesiologist during general anesthesia.

Laryngospasm may be partial or complete. Partial laryngospasm is associated with a high-pitched crowing sound and increased difficulty in ventilation, whereas a complete laryngospasm is associated with the absence of sound in the presence of exaggerated respiratory efforts and soft tissue retraction in the supraclavicular and intercostal regions.

Management of laryngospasm

Upon recognition of laryngospasm:

Step 1. Administer 100% O_2 via nasal hood. In most instances the patient will already be receiving N_2O-O_2 during his treatment. Simply terminate the flow of N_2O and increase the O_2 flow to about 5 to 8 lpm.

Step 2. Quickly remove all materials from the patient's mouth. If bleeding is present the area should be packed with surgical gauze to prevent bleeding into the pharynx at this time.

Step 3. Physically displace the tongue anteriorly by grabbing it with a hemostat or gauze sponge.

Step 4. Using a tonsillar suction tip, completely and rapidly suction the oral cavity and posterior pharynx to remove any foreign matter.

Step 5. Keeping your ear close to the patient's mouth and nose, push on the patient's chest. If a rush of air is heard and felt the spasm has been broken and the airway is patent. If no air is heard or felt, proceed to step 6.

Step 6. Positive-pressure O_2 is administered in an effort to mechanically break the spasm by physically forcing oxygen through the vocal cords. The absolute importance of effective suctioning prior to this step is evident as foreign material may be forced into the trachea by the positive-pressure oxygen flow.

Step 7. Succinylcholine. If the preceding steps are unsuccessful, succinylcholine administration is required. Succinylcholine should be administered only by doctors who have received prior training in its administration and in the management of the patient *after* succinylcholine administration. An initial succinylcholine dose of 10 mg IV is recommended for the partial or incomplete laryngospasm, with a dose of 20 to 40 mg recommended for complete spasm or spasm that continues after the initial 10-mg dose is administered.

Step 8. Following succinylcholine administration apnea may be present for a period of up to 4 minutes. Controlled ventilation is mandatory until the return of spontaneous respiratory efforts. Succinylcholine administration, especially in larger doses, produces hyperkalemia which, in turn, can provoke cardiac dysrhythmias (bradycardia, asystole). Monitoring of the blood pressure, heart rate, and rhythm should be continued throughout the recovery period.

Emesis and aspiration of foreign material under anesthesia

Emesis (vomiting) and the possible aspiration of this material into the airway is one of the most frightening of potential emergencies arising during general anesthesia or deep sedation. Fortunately it is also one of the least likely situations to develop when proper patient management techniques are followed. Where protective airway reflexes remain intact (conscious sedation), aspiration of vomitus is unlikely to occur.

Vomiting itself is rarely a significant problem. The act of vomiting requires the forceful contraction of many muscle groups, including the diaphragm, resulting in a projectile elimination of the vomitus from the patient's GI tract and mouth. Aspiration of vomitus, though a possibility, is unlikely. During deep sedation and general anesthesia, where protective airway reflexes and muscle tonus are depressed or absent, vomiting does not occur. Regurgitation, the passive reflux of stomach contents into the esophagus and pharynx can occur and represents a significant danger. Regurgitation is passive (no muscular contraction), and quiet. In nondental situations (podiatry or orthopedic surgery as examples) regurgitation may go unnoticed unless someone is monitoring the airway constantly. A pretracheal stethoscope will enable the gurgling sound of vomitus to be detected almost immediately after it occurs. In dental situations vomitus may be observed in the posterior of the mouth or pharynx.

Stomach contents are extremely acidic. Morbidity and death are more likely to occur the lower the pH of the aspirated materials.[30]

When vomitus is aspirated into the trachea, the potential for disaster exists. The makeup of the material aspirated will have a profound effect on the resulting clinical situation. The aspiration of solid material may produce acute airway obstruction progressing to death unless managed immediately and aggressively.

When liquid is aspirated, the usual airway response is bronchospasm. Rales, dyspnea, tachycardia, partial airway obstruction, and cyanosis develop within seconds, followed shortly thereafter by hypotension.[2]

Management of aspiration of foreign material

Step 1. Immediately place the patient into the Trendelenberg position with a head-down tilt of at least 15 degrees. To assist gravity in directing the vomitus into the pharynx (not into the lungs) turn the patient onto his right side.

Step 2. Activate EMS as soon as possible after diagnosing aspiration.

Step 3. Suction the pharynx, removing any vomitus that may be present.

Step 4. Intubation should be accomplished, if possible. The patient is turned onto his back for intubation.

Step 5. Administer oxygen, if not already administered.

Step 6. Tracheal lavage should be performed if the patient has been intubated. Following slight elevation of the patient's head, a bolus of 10 to 20 ml of either normal saline or sodium bicarbonate is administered into the endotracheal tube. Larger volumes of solution are contraindicated as this might propel the aspirated material further into the trachea and lungs. Immediately following lavage, suction and oxygenation are necessary. This procedure can be repeated several times.

Step 7. Administer IV steroids. To minimize the development of inflammation, edema and aspiration pneumonitis steroids should be administered. There is some controversy associated with steroid administration due to its ability to depress the immune response of these patients who may develop aspiration pneumonitis.

Hyperventilation

Hyperventilation is usually an anxiety-induced response to the threat of dental treatment. Losing control of breathing, the patient breathes more rapidly (tachypnea) and deeply (hyperpnea) than usual. Carbon dioxide is eliminated in excess, producing hypocapnea, which is associated with signs and symptoms including a feeling of coldness and tingling which lead to parasthesia of the fingers, toes, and circumoral region. The patient may become lightheaded or experience a feeling of a tightness in the chest (mimicking the discomfort of angina pectoris). This adds to the anxieties over dentistry and the inability to control breathing. Continued hyperventilation can lead to a spasmodic contraction of the hands and feet termed carpopedal tetany and eventually to seizures and the loss of consciousness. Though hyperventilation may occur in any patient, it appears that patients between their late teens and late thirties are more likely to hyperventilate.

Management of hyperventilation

Step 1. Terminate dental care.

Step 2. Position patient comfortably.

Step 3. Attempt to "talk patient down." If necessary, proceed to step 4.

Step 4. Elevate CO_2 levels by having patient rebreathe his exhaled air. The preferred method of doing this is to have the patient cup his hands in front of his mouth and nose and simply rebreathe. This has two benefits. First, the warm, moist exhaled air will warm the patients cold hands—a psychological boost to the frightened patient, and second, the CO_2 level of the patient's blood will increase relieving the signs and symptoms noted. The technique of rebreathing exhaled air from a paper bag is no longer recommended.

Step 5. If hyperventilation continues, an IV infusion should be started and either diazepam or midazolam titrated very slowly until the patient relaxes and his breathing becomes normal.

Step 6. Activate EMS in the highly unlikely event that the hyperventilation episode continues or if carpopedal tetany or seizures occur.

Respiratory depression

Respiratory depression may develop secondary to the administration of CNS-depressant drugs. It is most likely to be observed during deep sedation and general anesthesia and where certain drug groups, such as the barbiturates and opioids, are employed. Respiratory depression is less likely to occur during oral or inhalation sedation and when benzodiazepines are used during parenteral sedation techniques.

Respiratory depression may be observed as either a decreased rate of respiration (to apnea) and/or decreased ventilatory effort. Monitoring during parenteral sedation and general anesthesia is based primarily on ensuring adequacy of the airway and ventilation. The pretracheal stethoscope is the most significant monitor in this regard, permitting the evaluation of each and every breath taken by the patient. Respiratory problems may be detected virtually instantaneously with the pretracheal stethoscope. Use of the pretracheal stethoscope is suggested for all parenteral sedation and general anesthesia cases. Pulse oximetry permits evaluation of the degree of oxygenation of the blood. Though effective, there is a 10- to 20-second time lag between respiratory changes and notification on the oximeter screen. In addition, blood levels of CO_2 are not evaluated by the pulse oximeter. Use of the pulse oximeter is recommended for all parenteral sedation, deep sedation, and general anesthesia cases. The capnograph permits virtually instantaneous evaluation of the effectiveness of ventilation through monitoring of the end tidal CO_2 for each breath. Airway obstruction as well as diminished ventilatory effort may be detected immediately, permitting corrective actions to be instituted rapidly. Use of the capnograph is currently recommended for operating room general anesthesia.

When respiratory depression is the result of drug administration, it is possible to administer reversal agents in some cases. Naloxone is available when opioids have been administered, while benzodiazepines may be reversed with flumazenil. No specific antagonists exist for either barbiturates or propofol. Propofol, a rapid-acting and short-acting, drug will rarely produce respiratory depression persisting more than a few seconds.

Respiratory depression rarely represents a major problem where the doctor has received appropriate training in the administration of anesthetic drugs. Outside medical assistance is not usually necessary, for the period of respiratory depression is usually transitory, with no adverse effects to the patient occurring.

Management of respiratory depression

Step 1. Immediately terminate the dental procedure and place the patient in the supine position.

Step 2. Provide airway maintenance and evaluate respiratory effectiveness (i.e., look, listen, feel). In most instances assisted ventilation will be required to increase the patient's inspired air volume. In some few instances where apnea is present controlled ventilation is necessary.

Step 3. Administer oxygen.

Step 4. Monitor patient with pulse oximeter, blood pressure, heart rate, and rhythm.

Step 5. Start intravenous infusion, if not already present.

Step 6. Though their administration is not usually necessary, consider antidotal drug administration:

When *opioids* have been administered, slowly titrate *naloxone* at 0.1 mg per minute until improved ventilation is noted. In children a dose of 0.005 mg per minute is administered until improved ventilation is observed.[31]

Following *benzodiazepine* administration *flumazenil* should be considered at an IV dose of 0.2 mg per minute until respiratory efforts improve. A usual adult dose of flumazenil is 0.5 mg.[32]

When *barbiturates* have been administered, no effective antagonist exists. Continued assisted or controlled ventilation is necessary until spontaneous breathing returns.

No effective antagonist exists for *propofol,* but prolonged respiratory depression is unlikely to be observed with this drug due to its extremely short duration of action.

Step 7. Following return of ventilatory adequacy after a brief period of respiratory depression it may be possible to continue with the dental treatment. Where the period of respiratory depression was significant in depth or duration the doctor may elect to terminate the dental procedure. At the end of the planned dental treatment or following termination of the treatment consider the IM administration of an antidotal drug. In situations in which IM opioids or benzodiazepines have been administered, or where long-acting drugs such as morphine and lorazepam have been administered IV, the potential for a rebound depression exists (though this is highly unlikely to occur). IV antagonists have a rapid onset of clinical action, but their duration following IV administration may be shorter than that of the offending drug. An IM dose of either flumazenil or naloxone should be considered in these situations.

Step 8. Discharge of the patient from the office should be in the custody of a responsible adult companion and only when the treating doctor feels that the patient's recovery (from his sedation or general anesthesia) is adequate to permit his safe dismissal from the office. Outside medical assistance is rarely required in respiratory depression.

Convulsions

Convulsions (or seizures) are not uncommon during dental treatment. Epileptics are the most likely persons to have seizures in the dental environment, as stressful situations may provoke seizures even in well-controlled epileptics. Over 90% of epileptics have generalized tonic-clonic seizures, also known as grand mal seizures.[33] Local anesthetic overdose is another possible cause of seizures in the dental environment. The inadvertent intravascular (IV or IA) administration of local anesthetics will produce a seizure within seconds of injection. The administration of too large a total dose will bring on seizure activity more gradually, the patient developing progressively severe signs and symptoms until frank tonic-clonic convulsions occur. Hyperventilation may be associated with seizures if the episode is permitted to continue for a long duration. Seizures will also be associated with extreme hypoxia or anoxia and hypercarbia secondary to airway management problems or apnea.

Seizures are usually readily managed with injury, morbidity or mortality being infrequent results. The primary goals in seizure management are the prevention of injury to the patient during the seizure and ensuring the adequacy of ventilation. Ventilatory adequacy is of particular importance during the local anesthetic-induced seizure as pH changes alter the seizure threshold of the local anesthetic.[34] Acidosis, the result of hypoxia, hypercarbia, and lactic acid production during the seizure, lowers the seizure threshold for the local anesthetic, thereby prolonging the seizure and increasing the risk of serious postictal damage or death. Adequate ventilation will eliminate/prevent CO_2 retention and minimize the duration of the seizure.

The administration of anticonvulsants is rarely necessary during seizures as most seizures are self-limiting, rarely lasting more than 2 to 5 minutes (grand mal epilepsy). However, EMS assistance will be recommended early in our management for two reasons: first, to aid in the definitive management of the patient following the seizure, and second, to administer IV anticonvulsants if the seizure is still present on the patient's arrival.

Management of seizures

Step 1. Terminate dental care and place patient into a supine position in the dental chair.

Step 2. Protect the patient during the clonic phase of the seizure (generalized muscle contractions). *Gently* hold the patient's arms and legs. Movement of the limbs should be permitted but within limits so as to prevent injury. Do not totally restrict movement as this may cause injury to the patient. DO NOT ATTEMPT TO PLACE ANY OBJECT INTO THE MOUTH OF A CONVULSING VICTIM as this will usually injure (fracture, avulse) the teeth and injure the soft tissues.

Step 3. Activate EMS.

Step 4. Ensure airway patency and administer oxygen to minimize hypoxia and hypercarbia.
The *epileptic generalized tonic-clonic convulsion* will cease spontaneously within 2 to 5 minutes. In some few cases a seizure may con-

tinue beyond 5 minutes or a seizure may stop and recur before the patient recovers consciousness. These are the two definitions of status epilepticus, a situation representing an acutely life-threatening emergency.[35] Seizures secondary to *local anesthetic overdose* will continue until the cerebral blood level of the local anesthetic falls below the seizure threshold for that drug. With adequate airway maintenance and oxygenation local anesthetic-induced seizures do not persist for more than 5 minutes. Though extremely rare, seizures occurring during *hyperventilation* will persist until the CO_2 level of the blood is elevated to close to normal levels. Seizures secondary to *severe airway obstruction* or *anoxia* are associated with extreme morbidity or death. Airway patency and oxygenation must be ensured.

Step 5. If the seizure persists, attempt to start an intravenous infusion. A catheter is recommended as its flexibility will minimize the risk of its being accidentally dislodged by the patient.

Step 6. Consider the administration of intravenous anticonvulsants where the seizure is prolonged. To be effective anticonvulsants must be administered intravenously. Diazepam or midazolam should be titrated slowly, diazepam at a rate of 5 mg/min, midazolam at 1 mg/min, until seizure activity ceases. Anticonvulsant administration should be considered only where the doctor is well trained in management of the unconscious, apneic patient, for this is entirely possible in the postseizure state when anticonvulsants have been administered. Intravenous barbiturates may also be administered (thiopental, methohexital, pentobarbital), but the incidence of postseizure apnea is increased.

Step 7. Postseizure management. The *epileptic patient,* who has not received anticonvulsants, will usually be sleeping deeply and perhaps snoring in the immediate postseizure stage. Snoring is an indication of a partial airway obstruction produced by the tongue. Management requires head-tilt/chin-lift and the administration of oxygen. The epileptic patient will also be mentally disoriented. The treating doctor should talk to the patient telling him where he is, what has happened, and that everything is all right. Complete recovery from a generalized tonic-clonic seizure requires

several hours. EMS personnel will evaluate the patient to determine whether he requires a period of hospitalization or if he may be discharged from the office in the custody of an adult companion.

Patients who have had a local anesthetic-induced seizure will normally be hospitalized for an indefinite period in order to fully evaluate their neurological status. Hospitalization will usually be suggested following hyperventilation-induced seizures, but the period of observation is usually minimal.

Seizures secondary to severe anoxia will require hospitalization and intensive care for an undetermined period of time. Patients who have received anticonvulsant drugs to terminate their seizures will usually be hospitalized.

Hypoglycemia

Hypoglycemia, or low blood sugar, is a not uncommon occurrence in the type I, insulin-dependent diabetic (IDDM). The type II, non–insulin-dependent diabetic (NIDDM) is much less likely to become hypoglycemic. Recent changes in the recommendations for management of type I diabetes suggest the more frequent administration of insulin (perhaps 3 to 5 times per day) as a means of preventing the onset of the chronic complications associated with diabetes. However, increased insulin administration will bring with it an estimated threefold increase in the incidence of acute hypoglycemia.[36]

Inadequate cerebral blood levels of sugar lead to diminished CNS functioning. Clinical signs and symptoms associated with mild hypoglycemia include mental confusion, mild muscle tremor, diaphoresis, a feeling of coldness, and tachycardia. This is a likely scenario in a dental practice when the type I diabetic does not eat prior to the scheduled appointment. A telephone call the day prior to the scheduled dental appointment reminding the patient to eat will minimize this occurrence. Where parenteral sedation or general anesthesia is scheduled, a period of fast is necessary. The patient's insulin requirement will be decreased and should be so adjusted either by the patient or after consultation with the physician. The use of 5% dextrose and water as the infusate is not contraindicated in the type I diabetic. The patient appears in the office slightly hypoglycemic following their fast. D5W will provide a needed elevation in the blood sugar level.

When blood sugar levels fall too far consciousness

is lost and seizures may be noted, though the latter should be unlikely in the dental situation. Mild hypoglycemia is easily treated with a rapid return to normal CNS functioning. The need for EMS and hospitalization is minimal. When hypoglycemia produces unconsciousness and/or seizures, EMS assistance is desirable and a period of hospitalization is the norm.

Management of hypoglycemia

Step 1. As soon as signs and symptoms of hypoglycemia are noted, cease dental treatment and place the patient into a comfortable position.

Step 2. Determine if the patient has taken an insulin dose or if he has eaten food recently.

Step 3. If hypoglycemia is considered a possibility, do not hesitate to administer sugar to the patient orally. Most type I diabetics prefer orange juice, feeling that they recover faster than with other liquids (soft drinks). Permit the patient to drink 8 to 12 ounces of orange juice in 4-ounce increments over about 10 minutes. Return to normal CNS status is rapid. Some diabetics prefer candy bars. The planned dental care may continue if the doctor and patient agree.

Step 4. If the episode continues or if the patient loses consciousness, summon EMS immediately.

Step 5. In the presence of unconsciousness the patient must be placed into the supine position and basic life support administered as needed. In most instances airway maintenance is all that is required.

Step 6. Establish an IV infusion, if not already present.

Step 7. Administer antihypoglycemic. A dose of 50 ml of 50% dextrose is administered intravenously. The return of consciousness is usually quite rapid. The pediatric dose is 50 ml of a 25% dextrose solution. Where an IV cannot be started or when 50% (or 25%) dextrose is unavailable, glucagon may be administered IM or IV. The dose of glucagon is 0.5 to 1.0 mg administered subcutaneously, IM or IV. Consciousness usually returns within 15 minutes with the dose repeated every 15 minutes if necessary. When the patient does not respond to glucagon, intravenous glucose must be administered.[37]

Step 8. Once consciousness returns, the patient should be monitored until the arrival of EMS personnel. A period of hospitalization is usually necessary when unconsciousness occurs.

Syncope

Syncope, a transient loss of consciousness, is not uncommon in the practice of dentistry. In a recent survey of emergencies in dental practice, 50% of 30,000 emergencies were listed as syncope.[38] Produced by a sudden drop in blood pressure which decreases oxygen delivery to the CNS, other names for syncope are "vasodepressor syncope," "vasovagal syncope," "common faint," and "psychogenic syncope."

In stressful situations as might develop in the dental office, such as a sudden unexpected pain, or the sight of blood or dental instruments such as needles or the drill, blood is directed into skeletal muscle in the arms and legs to prepare the body for the "fight or flight response." In the absence of movement venous return to the heart and blood flow to the brain are decreased. Signs and symptoms of a slight decrease in cerebral blood flow are a feeling of warmth, the loss of color (pale or ashen gray skin tone), diaphoresis, complaints of feeling "bad" or "faint," and nausea, along with the development of a tachycardia. The tachycardia enables the body to compensate for the decrease in cardiac output and to maintain a minimally adequate blood flow to the brain, which maintains consciousness. In the absence of definitive treatment of this patient decompensation occurs, consisting of a significant bradycardia (heart rate ± 30 beats per minute with significant periods of asystole frequently observed), which severely decreases cerebral blood flow and induces the loss of consciousness.[39] Placement of the patient in the supine position with his legs elevated increases venous return while airway maintenance ensures the delivery of oxygen to the blood. Recovery of consciousness is normally quite rapid, within 10 to 15 seconds. EMS is rarely necessary, nor is hospitalization. Indeed, where consciousness was never lost, the planned dental procedure may continue; however, when consciousness was lost for any period of time, it is prudent to postpone treatment until a later time. Modification of future dental care should be considered so as to avoid recurrence of this episode.

Syncope is unlikely to occur in the sedated patient. More likely is the scenario of the fearful patient, unmedicated, collapsing in the reception area or in the dental chair upon seeing the needle of the local anesthetic syringe. Pretreatment diagnosis of the patient's dental fears and modifications in dental care should prevent syncope from occurring. Most incidents of fainting occur with the patient seated in an upright position. With most dental patients now placed in a reclined position (or supine) in the dental chair, the loss of consciousness from syncope is becoming less common.

Management of syncope

Step 1. On recognizing any signs and symptoms of presyncope, terminate dental care and place the patient into the supine position with the feet elevated.

Step 2. Remove any dental equipment from the patient's field of vision.

Step 3. Administer oxygen.

Step 4. Administer ammonia. Ammonia inhalants should be kept in every treatment room as well as being included in the emergency kit. Crushed between the rescuer's fingers, the inhalant is held under the patient's nose. Inhalation of ammonia, a noxious odor, provokes muscular movement of the arms and legs, thereby increasing the return of venous blood to the heart and increasing cardiac output and blood flow to the brain.

Step 5. The episode will rapidly resolve, the patient feeling considerably better once positioned and breathing oxygen. If both the doctor and the patient agree, the planned dental procedure may proceed. Consider modification of dental care to diminish any anxiety that may be present.

Step 6. Should unconsciousness occur, place the patient into the supine position with their feet elevated, and if not already done, employ head-tilt/chin-lift and evaluate the airway. The patient will usually be breathing spontaneously, and the heart rate will be slow ($\pm$ 30 beats per minute).

Step 7. Consciousness should return within 10 to 15 seconds. The postsyncopal period is marked by the patient feeling poorly. The patient is nauseous (and will probably vomit), feels achy all over, and will require approximately 24 hours to fully return to a normal state of function. Oxygen should be administered to the patient via nasal cannula or nasal hood during the recovery period. Vital signs should be monitored and recorded.

Step 8. If consciousness does not return within 10 to 15 seconds, activate EMS. There are many other potential causes for unconsciousness. These will not respond to the treatment described. Whenever unconsciousness persists for longer than 10 seconds, it is recommended that emergency assistance be sought immediately.

Step 9. Discharge of the patient from the office should only be considered after a lengthy period of recovery (approximately 1 hour) during which time the patient remains under direct observation. Patients who have lost consciousness should not be permitted to leave the office alone nor to drive their car or any other vehicle (bicycle, skate board, etc.). The patient should be discharged in the company of a responsible adult companion. There is rarely a need for EMS assistance or for hospitalization in the common episode of faint.

SUMMARY

Emergency situations can and do arise in the dental and medical office. In this chapter several potential emergency situations that are associated with the administration of drugs for anesthesia, sedation, or pain control have been reviewed. The best treatment for these emergencies is their prevention. Adequate preoperative patient evaluation, adherence to proper technique, intraoperative monitoring, and postoperative management will prevent virtually all of these complications.

Other medical emergencies that occur during medical and dental treatment were described. Patients who are at risk (ASA II, III, and IV) are unable to tolerate the normal stresses associated with operative or surgical procedures and are more likely to develop acute medical problems related to their underlying disease. The appropriate use of sedation and pain control in these patients will greatly decrease their risk during treatment.

REFERENCES

1. California State Board of Dental Examiners: Conscious sedation evaluation protocol, Sacramento, 1993.
2. American Association of Oral & Maxillofacial Surgeons: *Office anesthesia evaluation manual*, ed 4. Rosemont, Ill, 1991, The Association
3. Pallasch TJ: *Pharmacology for dental students and practitioners.* Philadelphia, 1980, Lea & Febiger.
4. Dupont RL, Saylor KE: Depressant substances in adolescent medicine, *Pediatr Rev* 13:(10):381, 1992.
5. *Mosby's medical, nursing, and allied health dictionary*, ed 3. St Louis, 1990, Mosby.
6. Boobis AR: Molecular basis for differences in susceptibility to toxicants: introduction, *Toxicol Let* 64–65:109, 1992.
7. Goodson JM, Moore PA: Life-threatening reactions after pedodontic sedation: an assessment of narcotic, local anesthetic, and antiemetic drug interaction, *JADA* 107:239, 1983.
8. Flumazenil, drug package insert, Roche Laboratories, 1993.
9. Naloxone, drug package insert, DuPont Multi-Source Products, 1993.

10. deJulien LF: Causes of severe morbidity/mortality cases, *J Cal Dent Assoc* 11:45, 1983.
11. Bates DW, Leape LLI, Petrycki S: Incidence and preventability of adverse drug events in hospitalized patients, *J Gen Intern Med* 8(6):289, 1993.
12. Dolovich J et al: Anaphylaxis due to thiopental sodium anesthesia, *Can Med Assoc J* 123:292, 1980.
13. Milner SM, Bennett JD: Emergency cricothyrotomy, *J Laryngol Otology* 105(11):883, 1991.
14. American Heart Association: *Textbook of advanced cardiac life support,* Dallas, Tex, 1987, American Heart Association.
15. Emergency Cardiac Care Committee and Subcommittees, American Heart Association: Guidelines for cardiopulmonary resuscitation and emergency cardiac care, *JAMA* 268:2251, 1992.
16. Malamed SF: *Medical emergencies in the dental office,* ed 4. St Louis, 1993, Mosby.
17. Hulyalkar AR, Miller ED Jr: Evaluation of the hypertensive patient. In Rogers MC Tinker JH, Covino BC et al, eds: *Principles and practice of anesthesiology.* St Louis, 1993, Mosby.
18. Calhoun SC, Oparil S: Treatment of hypertensive crisis, *N Engl J Med* 323:1177, 1990.
19. Opie LH: Treatment of severe hypertension. In Kaplan NM, Brenner BM, Laragh JH, eds: *New therapeutic strategies in hypertension.* New York, 1989, Raven Press.
20. Cohen MM, Duncan PG, Pope WDB, et al: A survey of 112,000 anaesthetics at one teaching hospital (1975–1983, *Can J Anaesth* 33:22, 1986.
21. Atlee JL: *Perioperative cardiac dysrhythmias: mechanisms, recognition, management,* ed 2. Chicago, 1989, Year Book Medical.
22. Wingard DW: What is a normal heart rate prior to surgery? *Anesthesiology* 63:130, 1985.
23. Driscoll EJ, Smilack ZH, Lightbody PM et al: Sedation with intravenous diazepam, *J Oral Surg* 30:332, 1972.
24. DeRango FJ: Management of common medical problems. In Lichtiger M, Moya F, eds: *Introduction to the practice of anesthesia,* ed 2. Hagerstown, Md, 1978, Harper & Row.
25. Emergency Cardiac Care Committee and Subcommittees, American Heart Association: Guidelines for cardiopulmonary resuscitation and emergency cardiac care, III. Adult advanced cardiac life support, *JAMA* 268:2215, 1992.
26. Reference deleted in proofs.
27. Ferraris VA et al: Predictors of postoperative ventricular dysrhythmias: a multivariate study, *J Cardiovasc Surg* 32(1):12, 1991.
28. Liau CS, Hahn LC, Tjung JJ et al: The clinical characteristics of acute myocardial infarction in aged patients, *J Formosan Med Assoc* 90(2):122, 1991.
29. Reference deleted in proofs.
30. Hollingsworth HM, Irwin RS: Acute respiratory failure in pregnancy, *Clin Chest Med* 13(4):723, 1992.
31. Barsan WG, Tomassoni AJ, Seger D et al: Safety assessment of high-dose narcotic analgesia for emergency department procedures, *Ann Emerg Med* 22(9):1444, 1993.
32. Kulka PJ, Lauven PM: Benzodiazepine antagonists: an update of their role in the emergency care of overdose patients, *Drug Safety* 7(5):381, 1992.
33. Earnest MP: Seizures, *Neurol Clin* 11(3):563, 1993.
34. Covino BG: Toxicity of local anesthetic agents, *Acta Anaesthesiol Belg* 39(suppl 2):159, 1988.
35. Treatment of convulsive status epilepticus: recommendations of the epilepsy foundation of America's working group on status epilepticus, *JAMA* 270(7):854, 1993.
36. The diabetes control and complications trial research group: The effect of intensive treatment of diabetes on the development and progression of long-term complications in insulin-dependent diabetes mellitus. *N Engl J Med* 329(14):977, 1993.
37. Glucagon, drug package insert, Eli Lilly, 1989.
38. Malamed SF: Managing medical emergencies, *JADA* 124(8): 40, 1993.
39. van Lieshout JJ et al: The vasovagal response, *Clin Sci* 81(5): 575, 1991.

SECTION EIGHT

Special considerations

In this concluding section, several groups of patients for whom the management of pain and anxiety will require greater attention from the doctor and staff are discussed. For these patients, the overall risks of unwanted drug effects, acute medical problems, and unsuccessful results are greater than in other groups of patients. For these patients too, the rewards for successful treatment (in terms of personal satisfaction and accomplishment) are also infinitely greater.

The pediatric patient represents a group in which the various techniques of sedation and general anesthesia are frequently required. Yet pediatric patients cannot be treated as though they were simply small adults. Drug dosages must usually be altered to meet children's specific needs. Unfortunately, a disproportionate number of the serious problems that have occurred with the use of sedative techniques in dental and medical outpatient practices over the past few years have occurred in the pediatric patient.[1] In this chapter, drugs and techniques that have proved successful in the pediatric patient are reviewed.

The geriatric patient also presents a greater risk of adverse drug response when CNS depressants (and other drugs) are administered. Although the requirement for sedation is not usually as great in this rapidly growing group as in younger groups, there are some specific modifications in therapy that are appropriate when managing the geriatric patient.

In Chapters 38 and 39 the medically and physically compromised patient will be reviewed. Growing numbers of these patients are seeking treatment at dental and medical offices. The nature of the patient's underlying medical problem(s) will have a significant impact on the administration of drugs for the management of pain and anxiety. In some cases the patient may prove to be unable to communicate or to cooperate with the doctor, making monitoring during the procedure somewhat more difficult but ever more important. Most of the patients discussed in Chapter 39 can be successfully treated on an outpatient basis if specific treatment modifications are employed.

551

In prior chapters of this book specific contraindications to the administration of drugs were listed as the pharmacology of the drug was discussed. In this section the disease process will be introduced and the various techniques of sedation and specific drugs will be reviewed as to their appropriateness for these patients.

REFERENCE

1. Goodson JM, Moore PA: Life-threatening reactions after pedodontic sedation: an assessment of opioid, local anesthetic, and antiemetic drug interaction, *JADA* 107:239, 1983.

CHAPTER *36*

The pediatric patient

As important as patient management is in the realm of adult dentistry, it is in pediatric dentistry that proper patient management assumes the utmost importance. The young child, approaching a visit to the dentist for the first time, is influenced by a number of sources, some positive and others potentially negative, that will affect his or her attitude and behavior during treatment. Some factors are controllable by the doctor and staff, but others are outside of their control. Proper patient management, especially in the younger, more impressionable patient, will go far toward producing a patient with positive attitudes toward future dental and medical care; conversely, too many unfavorable influences will cause the patient to look upon the prospect of future dental and medical care with increasing fear and trepidation.

In this chapter some of the basic concepts involved in the management of the pediatric patient are discussed briefly. For a more in-depth discussion of this subject, the reader is referred to the following textbooks:

McDonald RE, Avery DR: *Dentistry for the child and adolescent,* ed 6. St Louis, 1994, Mosby.

Pinkham JR: *Pediatric dentistry: infancy through adolescence.* Philadelphia, 1988, Saunders.

Wei SH: *Pediatric dentistry: total child patient care.* Philadelphia, 1988, Lea & Febiger.

FACTORS INFLUENCING PATIENT RESPONSE

A number of factors will interact to determine whether the pediatric patient will face the scheduled visit to the dentist or physician with eager anticipation or with fearful dread. These include the influence of the parent, of the child's peers, of the doctor, and of the office staff. Another factor is the child's prior experience with health professionals.

Parental attitudes in general, and toward dentistry in particular, have a profound influence on a child's behavior. Factors thought to be of importance include the age of the parents and their level of maturity. Positive dental attitudes in parents will create an environment for the child that is conducive to the acceptance of ideal dentistry. It is frequently heard that the greatest difficulty in patient management occurs when a child is accompanied to the dental office by the grandparent. The grandparents often represent the ultimate authority in the family and will do things as they see fit to do them, not as the doctor may desire. This may be a significant factor when decisions are made as to the site and route of administration of sedative drugs.

The parents' prior experience with medical and dental health professionals will greatly influence their child's attitudes. Although few, if any, parents will intentionally tell their children of prior traumatic experiences they have had, such attitudes and feelings will be transferred to the child via nonverbal communication. Children may overhear their parents discussing their experiences or may see their parent suffering either before or after a dental appointment. Children are surprisingly astute observers and will pick up the many clues that parents drop relating to their attitudes toward health care.

Parents may make statements to their children that influence the children's behavior or put the children on guard, expecting that something unpleasant might be in the offing. Simply telling a child, "If you behave yourself at the dentist I will buy you a treat

I would like to thank Drs. Ronald Johnson and Hugh Kopel of the Department of Pediatric Dentistry at the University of Southern California for the assistance offered me in preparation of this chapter. The protocols for use of oral and IM medications were originally prepared by Drs. Johnson and Kopel for use in pediatric dentistry at U.S.C.

later'' may tell the child to anticipate something unpleasant.

The *influence of other children,* either siblings or acquaintances, must never be discounted. Such influence may be either positive or negative. In a family in which several children have undergone dental treatment without difficulty, younger children receive positive reinforcement prior to their visit. However, if prior appointments have been traumatic, such influence may be negative. The same is true for the friends of the child. In my experience, I have found that young friends tend to accentuate the more negative aspects of dentistry and medicine.

Yet another factor influencing the child's behavior during treatment is *their* prior experience with other health professions. Traumatic experiences provoke negative behavior in the patient, and positive experiences lead to a better-behaved child.

Some children are fearful at their first visit to the dental office. The collective influence of the parents, siblings, and friends have produced this unwarranted apprehension. Although the goals of the doctor and staff will be somewhat more difficult to accomplish, the attitude of the office staff can dramatically change this child's feelings toward dentistry.

The factors that have been discussed above are truly out of the control of the doctor. Fortunately, the doctor is able to control several other factors. These include the attitudes of the doctor and staff, as well as the environment (the office) in which the patient will be treated.

The *doctor* sets the behavior standard in the office. Kimmelman[1] has stated that firmness with kindness and a soft, clear voice are an asset in dealing with children. The dress of the doctor is important: White uniforms may provoke negative feelings in younger patients, and colorful uniforms or the absence of uniforms may evoke a more positive response. With universal precautions (gloves, glasses, and masks being mandatory), explanations and role playing with the child to make them comfortable with our safety garb is suggested.

The same guidelines are important for members of the *office staff.* In the management of the pediatric patient, the auxiliary may have significantly greater contact with the patient than does the doctor; therefore, the attitude and attire of the staff are at least equally, if not more, important as that of the doctor.

The time of day at which the appointment is scheduled may have bearing on a child's behavior, especially the younger child. Interference with a child's sleep or eating habits should be avoided, if possible.

The young child accustomed to a midday nap may be irritable if he is in the dental chair instead of his bed at that time. It has been demonstrated that younger patients are most easily managed early in the day. This is also true for the apprehensive patient and the premedicated patient (Chapter 5). The basic concepts presented in the stress-reduction protocols are of great importance in managing the pediatric patient. The length of the appointment should not exceed the child's attention span. Younger patients will be less able to tolerate longer appointments than will older more mature children. Most children are able to tolerate 45-minute appointments with little difficulty.[2]

The *office environment* is another factor that influences the patient's behavior. An office in which many children are treated should offer an environment that is appealing to children. Although most pediatric medical and dental offices are designed with this in mind, even in the office of the busy generalist a separate area of the reception area might be set aside for younger patients. The very fact that this area requires the patient to leave the parent will be more conducive to the separation from the parent that occurs at the time of dental treatment. The color of the office, sound-proofing, and odors are important factors to consider when designing the pediatric office or reception room. Many pediatricians and pediatric dentists offer their patients a gift as they leave the office. These gifts are used as a display of friendship, not as a reward for good behavior.

BEHAVIORAL EVALUATION OF THE PEDIATRIC PATIENT

Granted that there are innumerable factors that interact to influence a child's behavior in the dental office, the doctor must still be able to evaluate this patient's ability to cope with the planned treatment. A number of systems have been developed to aid in classification of a child's behavior and the potential for successful dental treatment. Two of the more commonly used systems are the Frankl Behavioral Rating Scale [3] and the system devised by Wright.[4]

In the Frankl system the observer (doctor) places the child's behavior into one of four categories:

1. Definitely positive behavior
2. Positive behavior
3. Negative behavior
4. Definitely negative behavior

Johnson has stated that the Frankl scale appears to be closely related to the attitude of the parent toward dentistry.[5]

Wright's classification presents three major groups: (1) cooperative, (2) lacking cooperative ability, and (3) potentially uncooperative behavior, with multiple subgroups. Wright has stated that most doctors, either consciously or subconsciously, categorize the behavior of children into one of these groups. These classifications permit the doctor more readily to determine the appropriate means of overcoming the management problems presented by the patient[4]:

1. Cooperative: Most children (can be treated by a tell-show-do approach)
2. Lacking cooperative ability
   a. Very young children with whom communication cannot be established nor comprehension expected
   b. Children with specific debilitating or handicapping conditions
3. Potentially uncooperative behavior
   a. Uncontrolled behavior: Tantrums with flailing of arms and legs, suggestive of acute anxiety and fear (usually seen in young children 3 to 6 years of age on the occasion of the first dental visit)
   b. Defiant behavior: May use passive resistance (most often seen in older children approaching adolescence)
   c. Timid behavior
      I. May hid behind the parent, but usually little resistance to separation
      II. Stalls or hesitates when given directions
      III. Often withholds tears
      IV. Highly anxious
      V. Does not always hear or comprehend instructions
   d. Tense cooperative behavior
      I. Accepts treatment as it is provided
      II. Voice may have a tremor when speaking
      III. Body may tremble
      IV. Most often perspires noticeably on the palm of the hand or brow
      V. Controls emotions
   e. Whining behavior
      I. Allows dentist to proceed, but whines throughout
      II. Frequently complains of pain
      III. Emits sounds constantly

Successful treatment of the patient who lacks the ability to cooperate usually requires the use of one of the techniques of sedation. Should these techniques fail to prove adequate, general anesthesia may be required.

The potentially uncooperative patient may or may not require the use of sedation for successful treatment. The attitudes and technical abilities of the doctor and office staff will be the deciding factors with these patients.

DETERMINING THE NEED FOR SEDATION

The determination to use a technique of sedation should be made only after consideration of several factors:

1. Assessment of dental need
2. Patient cooperation
3. Parental cooperation and involvement
4. Economic considerations
5. Alternative treatment plans
6. Preoperative health evaluation
7. Preoperative behavioral assessment
8. Training and experience of doctor and staff

If only minimal treatment (e.g., one filling) is necessary, the need for sedation is negligible. This is especially true for the parenteral techniques (intramuscular [IM], subcutaneous [SC], submucosal [SM], intravenous [IV]) where prolonged durations of drug effects are involved. Inhalation sedation may be the most appropriate technique for this patient. If full-mouth treatment is necessary (e.g., nursing bottle syndrome), the use of deep IV sedation or general anesthesia might be considered.

Patient cooperation is obviously a deciding factor in opting to use a sedative technique. It is the opinion of most pediatric dentists that at least one and preferably two attempts at treatment should be made prior to considering sedation or general anesthesia for a patient. With experience, it may become quite obvious to the doctor that a patient will require the use of sedation or general anesthesia prior to the initiation of any treatment. Patients who are screaming as they walk through the parking lot to the dental office are more likely to be candidates for sedation. On the other hand, the patient who sits in the dental chair and cries throughout the treatment may be manageable without the use of adjunctive drug therapy. Crying, in the absence of overt disruptive behavior, may not be an indication for the administration of sedative drugs.

Parental attitudes must be taken into account when considering the use of sedation. Unfortunately, the use of sedation in dentistry has periodically received negative publicity, a factor that has conditioned some parents against the use of these techniques in their children. The desires of the parent should always be considered when formulating the patient's treatment plan; however, the doctor must always make the final decision. Several deaths have occurred in pediatric patients, in part because of the doctor's desires to accommodate the parent's wishes that all the dental treatment be completed at one visit. The parent's ability to follow directions must be determined if the doctor is considering the administration of oral drugs to the patient at home prior to their appointment. If doubt exists, the child should be scheduled early, and the drug administered by the doctor in the office.[6]

Economic considerations are also of importance in determining the nature of the sedative procedure to be employed. One reason for the increased use of outpatient sedation in dentistry and medicine has been the high cost (in both financial and emotional terms) of hospitalization. Outpatient procedures are usually a fraction of the cost of the same procedure performed in a hospital. In situations in which the economic status of the family is such that they are unable to afford even the minimal fee for sedation, it might be prudent to not charge the patient for the service. The cooperation of the patient and family is readily obtained and treatment becomes less traumatic for the entire staff and the patient.

Alternative modes of treatment should be considered. Which technique of sedation is most likely to be effective in this patient? Many doctors develop the disturbing practice of using the same technique (and in some cases the same drugs and dosages) on all patients. Consideration in selection of the technique and drugs involves multiple factors, including the degree of cooperation of the patient and the patient's medical history (allergies, illnesses). There is no one technique of sedation that will be effective in all patients. Indeed, in pediatric dentistry the failure rate for sedation is considerably greater than that seen in the adult patient. Trapp has stated that a failure rate of 20% to 40% is not unusual unless the doctor is administering general anesthesia.[7] Recent experience with pediatric sedation has demonstrated a 20% to 40% failure rate with oral sedation, but a 5% failure rate with IM/IV sedation. The greater the number of techniques available to the doctor, the greater the likelihood of a successful outcome.

The preoperative physical evaluation of the child will aid in determining the technique of choice for the patient. Among the items to be determined are the presence of allergies, medications being taken by the patient, and any prior hospitalizations. Behavioral evaluation will also aid in a determination of the requirement for sedation or general anesthesia. In addition, training and experience of the doctor

and staff will be important in determining the appropriate sedative technique. Only those techniques with which the doctor and the staff are well acquainted should be considered for use. The requirements for adequate training in each of the commonly used techniques are discussed earlier in this text.

GOALS AND TECHNIQUES

All of the techniques of sedation discussed in this book are available for use in the pediatric patient. In addition, drug administration by the SM route is occasionally used in pediatric dentistry. Each of these techniques will be reviewed with an eye toward their applicability in the pediatric patient.

Kopel[8] has stated that sedative premedication in the pediatric patient should be used to "train" or "retrain" the patient in an understanding of dental procedures and their importance. He continues by listing the following goals of pediatric premedication.

1. To make the child cooperative and comfortable
2. To decrease anxiety for the patient
3. To decrease strain, apprehension, and excessive fatigue for the doctor and staff
4. To minimize the need for hospitalization and its attendant problems.

Listed are the techniques of patient management involving drug administration that are available in pediatric dentistry. These techniques are presented in the order of their desirability, from most to least desirable (according to this author):

1. Inhalation sedation with nitrous oxide-oxygen (N_2O-O_2)
2. Oral sedation
3. Oral and inhalation sedation
4. Intravenous sedation with or without inhalation sedation
5. Intramuscular and IV sedation with or without inhalation sedation
6. Intramuscular, SM, or SC injection with or without inhalation sedation
7. Use of any of the above with body and oral restraints
8. General anesthesia in the hospital

The goal in using sedation in the pediatric patient is the same as with the adult: to use the most controllable and least profound technique that is capable of providing the desired goal.

Once a technique of sedation has been selected for the pediatric patient, the next task is the determination of the appropriate dosage of the drug(s). Physiological functions in children may vary considerably from those same functions in the older patient. The metabolic rate is increased in the younger patient. Conversely, enzyme systems responsible for the biotransformation of specific drugs may not yet be fully functional in certain younger patients. This factor and others lead to the increased possibility of higher blood levels developing when pediatric drug dosages are simply calculated from the adult dosage forms commonly supplied with drugs. Many cases of morbidity and mortality have been reported in instances in which drug doses within acceptable adult limits were administered to children.

There is no simple answer to the question of proper drug dosage. Many factors act to complicate drug selection and drug action in children. Additionally, the desired level of drug action varies considerably from patient to patient and from doctor to doctor. The most reliable factor in predicting adequate drug effect is a patient's previous clinical experience with the drug in question. Once a drug has been administered to a patient, subsequent dosages can be modified according to this initial response. This is termed *titration by appointment*.[5] Although previous clinical experience can provide guidelines leading to safer and more effective drug administration, it is still necessary to determine a safe and effective drug dose for a first appointment.

Many drug package inserts provide prescribing information concerning pediatric dosages. However, many of the drugs introduced for pain and anxiety control in recent years have not undergone adequate clinical trial in children to permit recommendations concerning pediatric dosage. Conversely, many of these drugs provide only adult dosage forms or indicate that "information [in children] is inadequate to establish dosage." Wilson[9] in a review of the 1963 *Physicians' Desk Reference* found that 62% of listed drugs were not indicated for pediatric use, whereas an additional 16% were without recommendation for pediatric dosage. This number has steadily increased in recent years.

In those instances in which pediatric dosages were indicated, the doses were those used in normal, nonstressful situations. Administration of this dosage form, although adequate to help a child to fall asleep at home, might prove to be entirely inadequate for sedation in a stressful environment, such as the dental office. Most package inserts and pharmacology textbooks indicate the usual, nondental dosage of a drug. Pediatric dentistry texts should be consulted for appropriate dental treatment doses of these drugs.

Various factors govern the determination of drug dosages for children. These are generalizations, with exceptions to be anticipated:

1. Age of the child. In general the older the child the larger the dosage required to achieve the desired clinical action.
2. Weight of the child. This is very often used as the major factor in determining pediatric drug dosages, especially for parenterally administered drugs. In pediatric drug administration, more and more drugs are being prescribed in terms of body surface area, a factor thought to be a more reliable guide to drug dose than body weight.
3. Mental attitude of the child. The greater the degree of anxiety and fear, the larger the dose of drug(s) required.
4. Level of sedation desired. The individual doctor will seek to achieve ideal sedation in a given patient. However, the definition of ideal sedation will vary considerably. To some doctors, ideal sedation will exist only if a patient makes no movement or sound during treatment; others will consider sedation ideal if the planned treatment can be completed in a more relaxed atmosphere (for the staff and patient) in spite of occasional movement and verbalization from the patient. Light levels of conscious sedation may prove appropriate for the mildly apprehensive older child, whereas deep sedation may be required for the precooperative younger patient.
5. Physical activity of the child. The hyperactive, overly responsive child will commonly require increased drug dosages.
6. Contents of the stomach. Following oral administration the presence of food in the stomach will greatly influence the rate of drug absorption into the blood.
7. Time of day. Larger doses of drugs are required for sedation early in the day when the patient is fresh and alert; lower doses are in order later in the day when the patient is more fatigued.
8. Ability to titrate. Whenever possible titration of drugs should be employed. The ability to titrate eliminates any guessing from the calculation of the appropriate drug dosage for a patient. The two techniques of drug administration that permit titration, IV and inhalation sedation, are increasingly popular in pediatric dentistry. Oral, IM, SM, and SC administration do not permit titration.

Formulas, such as Young's rule and Clark's rule, have been suggested as aids in determining pediatric drug dosages as a fraction of the adult dose. The success of such rules is haphazard at best and cannot be recommended.

Young's rule

$$\frac{\text{Age of patient}}{\text{Age} + 12} = \text{Fraction of adult dose for children}$$

Clark's rule

$$\frac{\text{Weight in pounds}}{150} \text{ or } \frac{\text{Weight in kilograms}}{70}$$
$$= \text{Fraction of adult dose for children}$$

Although age and weight are frequently employed in determining pediatric drug dosage, they present certain problems. Because there is significant variation in size among children of the same age, this factor (age) ought not to be of primary consideration. Body weight is more frequently employed in pediatric dose determination; however, the dose of many drugs is not always a simple linear function of body weight and to calculate dosages as mg/lb or mg/kg leads to inaccuracies. Surface area, rather than body weight, has been shown to be a more accurate method of determining drug dosage for a patient. Unfortunately, manufacturers of virtually all drugs marketed today still present dosage recommendations in other units, that is mg/kg.

MONITORING

Monitoring of the sedated patient is discussed in Chapter 6. As important as monitoring is for all sedated patients, in the pediatric patient monitoring is possibly of even greater importance. Because of the relative lack of communication available between the doctor and the very young, precooperative or the handicapped patient, one of the most important means of communication—verbal—is often not present. In addition, because of the inability to titrate drugs administered orally, intramuscularly, or sub-

Table 36-1. Recommended monitoring for pediatric patients

Monitor	Local anesthesia			Oral			IM/SM			Inhalation			IV			General anesthesia					
																Outpatient			Inpatient		
	Pr	In	Po	Pr	In	Po	Pr	In	Po	Pr	In	Po	Pr	In	Po	Pr	In	Po	Pr	In	Po
Heart rate	**	0	*	**	**	**	**	**	**	**	**	**	**	**	**	**	**	**	**	**	**
					Cont.			Cont.			Cont.			Cont.			Cont.			Cont.	
Blood pressure	**	*	*	**	**	**	**	**	**	**	**	**	**	**	**	**	**	**	**	**	**
					q 15 m			q 15 m			q 15 m			q 5 m			q 5 m			q 5 m	
ECG	0	0	0	0	0	0	*	*	0	0	0	0	*	*	*	**	**	**	**	**	**
Respiration	**	0	0	**	**	**	**	**	**	**	**	**	**	**	**	**	**	**	**	**	**
	V			V	PT		V	PT	V	V	V/PT	V	V	PT	V	V	PT	V	V	PT/E	V
Oximetry	0	0	0	0	0	0	0	*	*	0	0	0	0	**	**	*	**	**	*	**	**
Temperature	*	0	0	*	0	0	*	*	*	*	0	0	*	*	*	**	**	**	**	**	**

Legends: 0, not essential; *, optional; **, recommended; *Pr,* preoperative; *In,* intraoperative; *Po,* postoperative; *Cont.,* continuous; *V,* visual; *PT,* pretracheal stethoscope; *E,* esophageal stethoscope; *q_m,* every_minutes.

Heart rate: Heart rate may be monitored by palpation in both the pre- and postoperative periods; however, it is suggested that during intraoperative monitoring an electrical monitor providing a continuous reading be used. Devices such as the pulse meter, pulse oximeter, and ECG provide continuous heart rate monitoring.

Blood pressure (BP): When blood pressure monitoring is recommended, I suggest that the BP cuff be kept on the patient's arm throughout the entire procedure.

ECG: By its very design the ECG provides continuous monitoring of the electrical activity of the heart as well as the heart rate.

Respiration: Visual implies a causal monitoring of the movements of the patient's chest for 30 to 60 seconds to obtain a respiratory rate. PT is the pretracheal stethoscope, providing continuous monitoring of respiratory sounds (and perhaps heart sounds as well). E is the esophageal stethoscope, a device inserted into the esophagus during general anesthesia that provides excellent sound quality for both heart and lung sounds.

Oximetry: By its nature oximetry provides continuous monitoring of arterial oxygen saturation.

Temperature: Preoperative temperature monitoring may be done manually, but when intraoperative monitoring of body temperature is recommended, continuous monitoring is more readily accomplished with a rectal or esophageal probe.

mucosally, the possibility of a relative overdose developing is somewhat enhanced. Constant monitoring of the patient is essential.

Baseline vital signs (blood pressure, heart rate and rhythm, respiratory rate) should be recorded prior to treatment if the patient is cooperative. Very often in the younger, precooperative patient this is not possible. Until the child has been sedated it may be physically impossible to monitor the vital signs; however, while the child is screaming, yelling, and moving around, monitoring is actually being done by simply watching the child's reactions. As soon as the child becomes quiet, more objective monitoring must be initiated. Vital signs should be recorded and a pretracheal stethoscope placed in position and respirations monitored throughout the procedure.

The pretracheal stethoscope is probably the most valuable piece of monitoring equipment available (and the least expensive). With it the doctor is able to monitor continuously both breath sounds and, in many cases, heart sounds. The value of the pretracheal stethoscope cannot be overestimated.

Monitoring of breath sounds in the pediatric patient is of great value because the vast majority of complications seen in sedation of younger patients are associated with respiratory depression or airway management problems. Decreased or altered breath sounds or a slowed rate of breathing should be a warning to the doctor to evaluate the patient's airway and respiratory status. Most cardiac problems in pediatric patients develop secondary to respiratory distress.

Recommended monitoring for pediatric sedation includes:
1. Preoperative vital signs (if possible)
2. Vital signs periodically during treatment (recorded every 15 minutes)
   a. Heart rate and rhythm—monitored continuously
   b. Blood pressure—monitored every 5 minutes
3. Pretracheal stethoscope
4. Pulse oximetry

Optional monitoring for the pediatric patient includes:
1. End-tidal carbon-dioxide (CO_2) ($ETCO_2$) monitoring
2. Electrocardiograph (ECG)

Supplemental O_2 or N_2O-O_2 administration via nasal hood or cannula is recommended for all pediatric sedation cases in which the patient tolerates it. Table 36-1 summarizes pediatric monitoring recommendations.

PHYSICAL RESTRAINT

On occasion it may become necessary to employ physical restraint in order to treat the patient properly. Bed sheets may be easily employed, tied around the patient and then secured with wide adhesive tape. Velcro strips and ties are also available. Parental informed consent must be obtained prior to the use of any form of physical restraint in the pediatric patient. Use without prior consent has led to charges of assault and battery being filed against the doctor.[10]

Two devices are available and popular in pediatric dentistry. The Pedi-Wrap (Clark Associates, Inc., Worcester, Mass.) (Fig. 36-1) is similar to the bed sheet but employs Velcro strips to secure the material. It is made of a netlike material that enables the patient to remain somewhat cooler while being restrained. Because the Pedi-Wrap is somewhat like a blanket, some children will quiet down once secured in it. The Papoose Board (Fig. 36-2) (Olympic Medical Corporation, Seattle, Wash.) is quite effective in restraining the head, torso, and upper limbs.

These devices should not be wrapped too tightly, for the patient may become more agitated, but of greater importance, an overly tight wrap across the patient's chest may restrict respiratory movements that have already been somewhat compromised through the administration of central nervous system (CNS) depressants. The lower (abdominal and leg) restraints may be tightened if necessary.

The use of restraints also makes it more difficult for the doctor and assistant to monitor respiratory movements. The pretracheal stethoscope becomes even more important at these times.

MOUTH-STABILIZING DEVICES

Despite the fact that the patient has been restrained, it may still be difficult, if not impossible, for the doctor to examine and treat the patient safely and adequately. Several devices are used as aids to stabilize the mouth during treatment. Rubber bite blocks are available in a variety of sizes; when inserted between the teeth of the patient on the side opposite treatment, the patient may bite down onto the block but is unable to close the jaws. A long piece of dental floss should always be tied around the bite block and left outside the patient's mouth to aid in its retrieval, if necessary (Fig. 36-3). A ratchet-type mouth prop (Molt prop) is also available. An advantage to the Molt prop is that the patient need open but a few millimeters for the device to be slipped between their teeth. Once in the mouth, the device can be opened

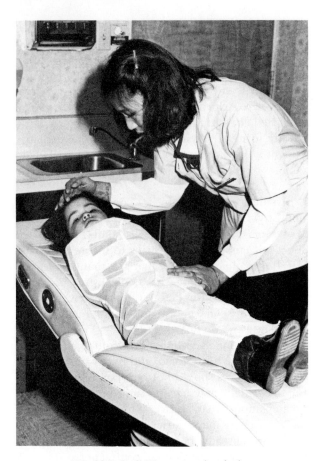

Fig. 36-1. Pedi-Wrap restraint device.

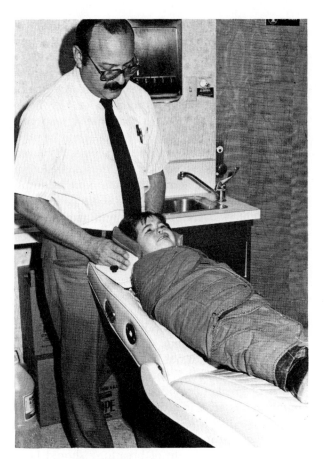

Fig. 36-2. Papoose board restraint device.

to the desired level. When either device is used, the assistant should remain in contact with them to stabilize and prevent their accidentally being dislodged.

DRUGS

Prior to discussing specific routes of drug administration and their use in pediatric dentistry, the drugs that are in most common use in pediatric sedation will be listed (Table 36-2). These statistics are the results of a survey of 409 pedodontists.[11,12] Although this survey is 20 years old, the currently popular pediatric sedatives remain the same with only a few exceptions. Two routes of drug administration predominate, with more than 60% of the respondents indicating that they employ the oral route and approximately 43% employing inhalation sedation. It also becomes evident that although a wide variety of drugs are available for the management of anxiety, pediatric dentists and general practitioners who manage large numbers of children rely on a rather

limited number of well-established drugs. Even more pronounced is the choice of drugs for combination therapy via the oral route, in which promethazine and meperidine stand virtually alone.

General rules for preoperative medication

The usual preoperative and postoperative instructions given to the parent or guardian of children receiving medications for the control of their dental fears are listed in the box.

In addition to these instructions, Album also lists these general rules regarding the administration of sedatives to pediatric patients[13]:

1. There must be strict supervision of the patient while in the office.
2. Adequate time must be provided for the drug(s) to act.
3. A quiet environment is necessary.
4. Vital reflexes must not be impaired.
5. Drugs must not be administered during acute or chronic illness.

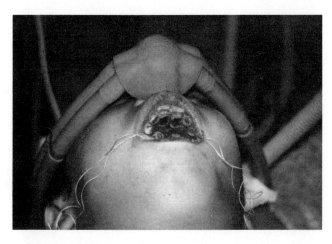

Fig. 36-3. Strings of dental floss tied to two bite blocks placed into mouth of sedated patient permits their easy retrieval.

Table 36-2. Commonly used drugs in pediatric dentistry

Proprietary name	Approximate percentage of pedodontists prescribing
Agents used alone*	
Atarax	27
Chloral hydrate	24
Vistaril	23
Phenergan	16
Demerol	12
Valium	10
Seconal	8
Nisentil	7
Phenobarbital	5
Agents used in combination†	
Demerol	35
Phenergan	35
Atarax	19
Chloral hydrate	18
Vistaril	17
Nisentil	13
Thorazine	6
Seconal	5
Nembutal	5

Modified from Malamed SF. In Braham RL, Morris ME: *Textbook of pediatric denistry.* © 1980, The Williams & Wilkins Co., Baltimore.
*Less than 5% prescribing: Nembutal, Librium, Thorazine, Equanil, Miltown, Pentothal, Sparine, Trilafon.
†Less than 5% prescribing: Equanil, Miltown, Valium, Sparine, Pentothal, Trilafon, Librium.

6. Parents must be informed of postoperative care.
7. Doctor must be familiar with side effects of medications.
8. Resuscitative equipment must be readily available.

Oral sedation

Oral sedation is a valuable technique in pediatric dentistry. One of its major advantages is the fact that there is no need for the use of a needle (IM, SM, SC, IV) or of a nasal hood (inhalation) to produce a clinical effect. Where appropriate, the parent or guardian of the patient may administer the drug at home prior to departing for the office. This practice is, however, somewhat controversial because there are numerous cases on record in which a parent has inadvertently oversedated the child, thinking perhaps that if 1 teaspoon of the drug is good, 2 or 3 teaspoons (or tablespoons) must be better.[6] A way of

---

PEDIATRIC SEDATION:
PREOPERATIVE INSTRUCTIONS

It is necessary to use sedative drugs to obtain dental care for your child. Please be aware of the following:
1. It is most important that you tell the doctor of any drug reactions, medical history, or illness and hospitalization your child has had.
2. The child must be accompanied by a parent or guardian for all appointments.
3. The first appointment will be necessary for adjustment of the proper drug dosage; therefore, little dental work may be accomplished.
4. The child may remain sleepy for a time. Do not be alarmed, as the drugs are "wearing off." Your child may be irritable as this occurs.
5. Do not allow the child to bite his lip, tongue, or cheek, if a local anesthetic has been used.
6. After dental care, your child should be under adult supervision and not be allowed to play near streets, stairways, and other areas where he may be injured by falling.
7. Cold drinks, such as ginger ale or colas, will help reduce any nausea and help to stimulate the patient to be more alert.
8. Should any unusual situation arise, please call the doctor, and notify him as soon as possible.

Modified from Kopel H: Lecture notes, AMED 750, August 1983.

avoiding this potentially dangerous situation is to prescribe only one dose of the drug. In addition, very explicit verbal as well as written instructions should be given to the person who will administer the drug to the patient.

If the doctor does not feel that the parent or guardian is reliable, the patient should be scheduled approximately 1 hour prior to the start of treatment and the oral drugs should be administered by the parent in the presence of a member of the office staff. Another consideration, when the drug has been administered in the office, is monitoring of the patient. If the office is busy, it must still be a staff member's responsibility periodically to check on the child (who is in the waiting room with his parent or guardian). In addition, a busy office environment is not conducive to adequate sedation. A more quiet, relaxed environment is desirable during this waiting period. A quiet room, in which the patient and parent may stay, is often employed for the administration of oral drugs and during the period of onset of drug action.

Younger children may not tolerate tablets and capsules well, the parent having to fight for the child to take the drug. Obviously, if the goal being sought is relaxation of the patient, this type of action is not recommended. Many of the drugs that are administered orally to children are available as an elixir or syrup, which may prove more palatable to the patient. In those cases in which the child refuses to accept the liquid medication on a spoon, the drug may be administered through an irrigation syringe, the drug squirted into the buccal vestibule of the patient, not down their throat.

Drugs that have an unpleasant taste or odor may occasionally be mixed with other foods. Orange juice is frequently used; however, the addition of drugs may alter its taste. For smaller children, drugs may be mixed with applesauce, jellies, baby foods, or yogurt, although these may have an adverse effect on drug absorption from the gastrointestinal (GI) tract. Recently midazolam for oral administration has been made into gelatin cubes,[14] and fentanyl has been added to a lollipop.[15]

The drugs most frequently administered orally in pediatric dentistry are chloral hydrate, hydroxyzine, diazepam, the combination of chloral hydrate and promethazine, and meperidine in combination with chloral hydrate, hydroxyzine, diazepam, or promethazine. Recently, midazolam has been used via the oral route in children with good success.[14,16] The pharmacology of these drugs was reviewed

in Chapter 8. Pediatric use of these agents is discussed now.

Chloral hydrate

Chloral hydrate is most effective for the very young patient and the mentally or physically handicapped patient. Available orally as capsules, elixir, and rectal suppositories, it is most effective in the management of mild to moderate anxiety. The usual oral dosage form of the elixir is 500 mg/5 ml (1 teaspoon).

Initial dosage. Chloral hydrate is administered 30 to 45 minutes prior to the planned appointment. The patient should have had nothing to eat or drink for 2 hours.

Age (years)	Weight (kg)	Dose (to nearest ½ tsp)			
		40 mg/kg	50 mg/kg	60 mg/kg	70 mg/kg
2-3	12-14	500	500-750	500-750	750-1000
3-4	14-16	500	750	750-1000	1000-1250
4-5	16-18	750	750-1000	1000-1250	1250-1500
5-6	18-21	750	1000-1250	1000-1250	1500
6-8	21-25	750-1000	1000-1250	1250-1500	1500-1750
8-10	25-30	1000-1250	1250-1500	1250-1500	1750-2000

The dosage of chloral hydrate may range from 500 to 2000 mg, with the usual range between 750 and 1500 mg. The elixir forms of chloral hydrate usually contain syrups of orange or citric acid to mask its bitter taste. Because of its disagreeable taste and GI-upsetting tendencies, chloral hydrate should be diluted still further with water, orange juice, or soda before being given to the child. Chloral hydrate must never be diluted in or added to alcohol. The duration of action of chloral hydrate is not more than 1 hour.

Comment: In the case of the very young child, it is suggested that a restraint such as a papoose board or a Pedi-Wrap be used during treatment.

Inhalation sedation with N_2O-O_2 may also be used as an alternative to increasing dosages of the oral drug if moderate to no success has been achieved with the original dosage. It is my feeling, however, that when the first dose of a premedicating drug fails to provide the desired effect, additional doses should not be administered nor should different drugs be given to the patient at that appointment. Rather, it is more prudent to discharge the patient and reschedule treatment for another day, reevaluating the choice of drugs and their dosage. The concept of "titration by appointment" suggests that a different dosage schedule be considered for subsequent appointments based on the response of the patient to the initial dose.

For maximum benefit to be obtained from the use of chloral hydrate, the scheduled appointment should not be longer than 1 hour. The parents of the patient should be advised of the possibility of a postoperative period of irritability or excitation as the effects of chloral hydrate wear off. Chloral hydrate, when administered as a solo agent, has proved to be one of the most effective and relatively safe drugs for pediatric sedation.

Hydroxyzine

Hydroxyzine hydrochloride (Atarax—Roerig) and hydroxyzine pamoate (Vistaril—Pfizer) are indicated for administration in patients who are over the age of 3 years, including adolescents. It is most effective in the management of very apprehensive, excited, agitated, and emotionally disturbed children. Additional indications for use of hydroxyzine include hyperactivity, autism, and severe behavioral problems.

Hydroxyzine hydrochloride is available as a syrup in 10 mg/5 cc (1 teaspoon). Hydroxyzine pamoate is available as an oral suspension as 25 mg/5 ml.

Dosage. For the nervous apprehensive child, 50 mg should be administered 2 hours prior to the appointment followed by the same dosage 1 hour before the appointment. In the hyperkinetic, agitated, or behavioral problem patient, 25 mg is administered three times the day prior to treatment, and then 50 mg is administered 2 hours and then again 1 hour prior to treatment. In the less apprehensive patient, one dose of 50 to 75 mg hydroxyzine may be administered 1 hour prior to treatment. Another method of administering hydroxyzine is to give divided doses of the agent; for example, the patient receives 25 mg 1 hour before bed the evening prior to treatment, 25 mg on the morning of treatment, and another 25 mg 1 hour prior to the scheduled appointment (for an appointment between 11 A.M. and 1 P.M.). Hydroxyzine will produce clinical actions within 30 to 60 minutes, with a maximal clinical duration of effective sedation between 1 and 2 hours.

Comment: Hydroxyzine is an excellent drug to give for the introduction of N_2O-O_2 to the apprehensive patient. The banana-flavored pamoate form of hydroxyzine, Vistaril, is more pleasant tasting to most patients than is the hydrochloride (vanilla flavored). Because of the relatively wide margin of safety observed with hydroxyzine, it may be used effectively with N_2O-O_2 and opioid analgesics, provided that reduced dosages of these drugs are used and that careful monitoring of the patient is maintained.

Promethazine

Promethazine (Phenergan) is most often used in combination with other drugs for preoperative sedation (chloral hydrate, hydroxyzine, meperidine, alphaprodine). As a sole agent for sedation, promethazine is most often used to manage a child with lesser degrees of anxiety. By itself it is not suitable for management of extreme apprehension or a disruptive, unmanageable child. Promethazine is available for oral administration as a tablet and a syrup.

Initial dosage. The oral dosage of promethazine is based on 1 mg/kg.

Age (years)	Weight (kgs)	Dose (mg)
2-3	12-14	12.5
3-4	14-16	12.5
4-5	16-18	25
5-6	18-20	25
6-8	20-25	25
8-10	25-30	37.5
10-12	30-36	37.5
12-14	36-45	50

Diazepam

Diazepam (Valium) is administered orally to the hyperactive, highly anxious, and excitable child over the age of 4 years. It is effective in cerebral palsy patients, especially those with athetoid cerebral palsy and in the mentally retarded patient. Diazepam is available in tablet form and as a suspension in 5 mg/5 ml.

Initial dosage. The initial dose of diazepam is 0.2 to 0.5 mg/kg. For the average child between the ages of 4 and 6 years, 2 to 5 mg is administered three times before treatment with the last dose administered 1 hour prior to treatment. In children above 6 years of age, 5 to 10 mg diazepam is administered three times before the appointment with the last dose 1 hour prior to treatment. The actions of diazepam are noted within 1 hour and continue for approximately 2 more hours.

Oral combinations
Chloral hydrate plus promethazine

Chloral hydrate is frequently combined with promethazine for administration to the patient younger than 3 years with rampant caries who is too young for the tell-show-do technique to be effective. Other indications for this combination are the mentally retarded or physically handicapped patient in younger age groups.

Initial dosage. The dose for the 2- to 3-year-old patient is 1000 mg (2 teaspoons) chloral hydrate combined with 25 mg (1 teaspoon) promethazine. The dose for the 3- to 6-year-old patient is up to 1500 mg (3 teaspoons) chloral hydrate combined with 25 mg (1 teaspoon) promethazine. This combination is mixed together and then added to a fruit drink or soft drink and administered 30 to 45 minutes prior to the appointment. The patient should take nothing by mouth for 2 hours prior to its administration. Clinical effectiveness will be noted within 45 minutes; maximal clinical benefit occurs at 1 hour.

Comment: The availability of a restraint, such as the Pedi-Wrap or papoose board, is recommended when managing the very young, apprehensive patient. For greatest benefit to be obtained from this combination of drugs the maximal length of the appointment ought not to exceed 1 hour. The parents or guardian of the patient must be advised of the possibility of postoperative irritability or excitement as the drug effects wear off.

Promethazine plus meperidine

Meperidine (Demerol) and promethazine (Phenergan) are available as a premixed combination for both oral and parenteral administration. The combination is called Mepergan (Wyeth) and the oral form contains 25 mg promethazine and 50 mg meperidine. The combination is a rational one in that the opioid provides for a sedative and analgesic effect while promethazine potentiates the opioid effect and adds an antiemetic action (to counter any possible nausea produced by meperidine). Indications for the administration of this combination are:

1. Recalcitrant, defiant, and uncooperative behavior in children over 6 years of age who may require extensive treatment in a prolonged appointment
2. Severe mental retardation in children

Initial dosage. For the child weighing approximately 25 lbs (10 kg), the initial dose is 25 mg meperidine plus 12.5 mg promethazine. For the child weighing approximately 35 lbs (15 kg), the initial dose is 25 mg meperidine plus 25 mg promethazine. For the child weighing approximately 50 lbs (22 kg), the initial dose is 50 mg meperidine plus 25 mg promethazine. For ease of administration the contents of the capsule may be added to a flavored vehicle (liquid or food).

Comment: Opioid administration is associated with respiratory depression. The doctor should be experienced in the use of opioids, be able to recognize respiratory depression (monitoring the patient throughout the procedure), and have naloxone

readily available whenever this combination is employed.

Because it is difficult to calculate the proper dosage in children when one employs a premixed combination (Mepergan), it is recommended that the doctor make the combination by simply mixing the two ingredients together in the appropriate dosages.

Parenteral sedation

Parenteral sedation techniques in pediatric dentistry include the IM, subcutaneous IV, inhalation, and SM routes of drug administration. In this first section only IM, SC, and SM drug administration will be discussed. Use of IM with IV and/or inhalation routes will be discussed later in this chapter.

The IM, SC, and SM routes of drug administration are of greater importance in pediatric dentistry than for adult patients, primarily because of the decreased need for patient cooperation in these techniques. In order to administer a drug via these routes the patient merely need be restrained for a moment during the injection. As is discussed in Chapters 4 and 11, there are significant drawbacks to these techniques, the most significant of which is the lack of control over the ultimate drug action maintained by the doctor. Titration is not possible via these routes of drug administration; therefore, the risk of oversedation is increased. As the most commonly used drugs in these techniques have traditionally been the opioids, respiratory depression is an ever-present danger. The introduction of IM midazolam has decreased this risk.

Of the three routes of administration, IM, SC, and SM, the slowest onset of action will occur following SC administration (poorest blood supply); IM administration will produce a more rapid onset of action, and SM administration produces the most rapid onset. Trapp and others have demonstrated that SM administration into the oral buccal mucosa produces blood levels at a rate exceeded only by direct IV administration (Fig. 36-4).[17,18] Although this rapid onset of action might be looked on favorably, the fact that opioids (e.g., alphaprodine, meperidine) are administered via this route also means that the adverse effects of these drugs, such as respiratory depression, will also develop rapidly. The doctor employing the SM route of drug administration must be ever vigilant in monitoring these patients.

Monitoring of the patient receiving deep sedation via the IM, SC, or SM routes is essential. The pretracheal stethoscope is an essential piece of equipment.

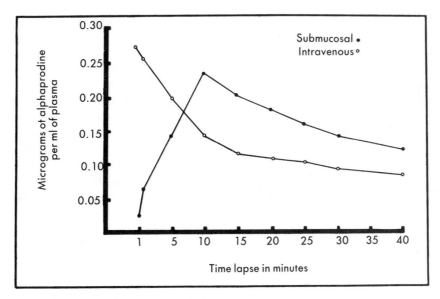

Fig. 36-4. Mean plasma levels of alphaprodine following IV and submucosal administration. (From Caudill WA et al: *Pediatr Dent* 4[special issue 1]:168, 1982.)

As these parenteral techniques are usually reserved for more difficult management problems, the use of physical restraint is required more often than not. The possibility of further respiratory embarrassment exists. Supplemental O_2 should always be administered throughout the procedure whenever IM, SC, or SM drugs are administered.

Alphaprodine

Alphaprodine (Nisentil—Roche) was the drug most commonly administered via SM injection. Alphaprodine was voluntarily withdrawn from the U.S. market by its manufacturer following a number of adverse incidents.[19-23] It is still available and used in many countries, thus its inclusion in this chapter. Indications for its administration include:

1. Children under 3 years of age in good physical condition with rampant or nursing bottle caries
2. Younger retarded children without respiratory or cardiovascular problems

Alphaprodine is available for parenteral administration in 1-ml ampules containing 40 mg/ml and 10-ml vials containing 60 mg/ml.

Comment: There is a significant difference in dose between the 1-ml and 10-ml dose forms of alphaprodine (40 mg versus 60 mg). The potential for inadvertently administering a larger than desired dose therefore exists, especially if a doctor accustomed to using a 1-ml ampule switches to the 10-ml dosage form. The label of the bottle or vial from which a drug is being taken must *always* be checked to verify the concentration of the solution.

Initial dosage. Dosage forms of alphaprodine are administered on the basis of the patient's body weight. In recent years, because of a disproportionately high number of cases of morbidity and mortality, the dose of alphaprodine recommended by its manufacturer, Roche Laboratories, has been decreased to 0.3 to 0.6 mg/kg. This equates to 0.136 to 0.27 mg/lb.

Submucosal injections of alphaprodine are administered into the maxillary buccal vestibule on the side opposite that on which local anesthetic is administered. A 1-ml tuberculin syringe with a 3/8-inch 30-gauge needle (Fig. 36-5) is employed to administer the drug.

The patient to receive SC alphaprodine will usually be premedicated with oral promethazine. The patient is given 1 teaspoon (5 ml) or 25 mg promethazine 1 hour prior to the injection of the alphaprodine. The child is then placed in a restraint (Pedi-Wrap or papoose board), and topical anesthetic is applied in the buccal vestibule at the site where alphaprodine is to be injected (opposite to the side on which local anesthetic is to be injected). Then alphaprodine is administered. It is recommended that the dose of alphaprodine at the initial appointment be calculated at 0.3 mg/kg of body weight ("titration by appointment").

At least 10 minutes should elapse prior to attempt-

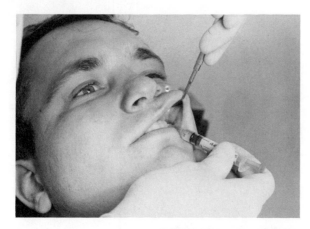

Fig. 36-5. Alphaprodine is administered via a tuberculin syringe into the maxillary buccal fold.

ing treatment. Should the effect of the drugs be inadequate at 10 minutes, additional alphaprodine must not be administered. Two viable options exist at this point: (1) the procedure may be cancelled and rescheduled, or (2) low concentrations of N_2O-O_2 may be administered with the patient carefully titrated and monitored throughout the procedure. This second option is recommended exclusively for those doctors trained in general anesthesia.

The duration of clinical action of alphaprodine is between 45 and 90 minutes. Naloxone should always be available whenever opioids are administered. The usual pediatric dose of naloxone is 0.01 mg/kg. A subsequent dose of 0.1 mg/kg may be administered if the response to the initial dose is inadequate.[24] Routine naloxone reversal of alphaprodine prior to patient discharge is not recommended.

Meperidine plus promethazine

The combination of meperidine and promethazine, known as Mepergan, was discussed previously in the section on oral combinations. It is an effective combination for patients with severe management problems or severe mental retardation. The primary difference between this technique and alphaprodine plus promethazine is the increase in duration of clinical action provided by meperidine. A second difference is that this combination is injected intramuscularly, not submucosally. This combination is especially recommended when procedures requiring 2 hours or more are planned.

Mepergan (Wyeth) is available in 10-ml vials and in 2-ml preloaded syringes. Each milliliter contains 25 mg meperidine and 25 mg promethazine.

Initial dosage. The IM dose of this combination is based on 0.5 mg/lb or 1 mg/kg of body weight.

Lytic cocktail

The combination of meperidine (Demerol), promethazine (Phenergan), and chlorpromazine (Thorazine) is termed the *lytic cocktail*, or *DPT*.[25] This combination has been employed for many years in both pediatric dentistry and medicine. Its popularity in dentistry is waning because of erratic patient responses; however, the lytic cocktail is still quite popular in pediatric medicine. Recently published *Clinical Practice Guidelines for Acute Pain Management in Infants, Children, and Adolescents* raises serious doubt as to the rationale for continued use of this technique.[26] The following is excepted from the *Guidelines:*

Exercise caution when using the mixture of meperidine (Demerol), promethazine (Phenergan), and chlorpromazine (Thorazine), also known as DPT. DPT—given intramuscularly—has been used for painful procedures. The efficacy of this mixture is poor when compared with alternative approaches, and it has been associated with a high frequency of adverse effects.[27] It is not recommended for general use and should be used only in exceptional circumstances.

The drugs are combined in one syringe and are administered intramuscularly. The patient remains with his or her parent for a few minutes until he or she is quiet and is then placed in the dental chair in a restraint. Monitoring devices are applied, supplemental oxygen and local anesthetic are administered, and the procedure is started.

Extrapyramidal reactions, especially tardive dyskinesia, are not uncommon side effects of the phenothiazines (promethazine and chlorpromazine). Should these develop, management requires the administration of diphenhydramine (see Chapter 8).

Midazolam

The water-soluble benzodiazepine midazolam has received considerable attention as an IM drug for pediatric sedation and has become the IM drug of choice in many institutions.[28] Midazolam has been employed successfully intramuscularly as a sole agent for pediatric sedation, and it has been used in conjunction with IV midazolam. This technique is discussed in the section on pediatric IV sedation. The IM dose of midazolam that has been most successfully employed is 0.15 to 0.2 mg/kg.[29,30] Midazolam produces a clinical effect within 10 minutes of its injection, so the patient may usually be placed in the

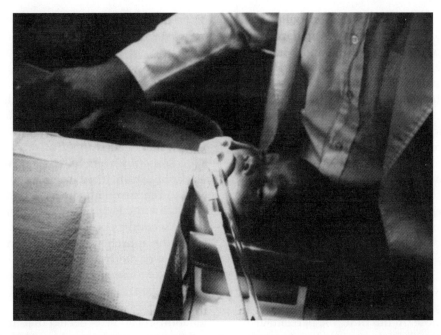

Fig. 36-6. In a crying or screaming patient the nasal hood may be held over the patient's mouth, thereby increasing N_2O delivery.

dental chair with minimal difficulty. When used in conjunction with IV sedation, the duration of dental treatment is indefinite. As with all parenteral sedation techniques, monitoring is essential to patient safety.

Ketamine

Ketamine, a dissociative anesthetic most commonly employed as a general anesthetic, has been used with success in pediatric dentistry in subanesthetic doses.[31] When administered IM, a dose of 2 to 4 mg/kg is administered with an expected onset of dissociation within about 10 minutes. The patient can usually be discharged from the office within 90 minutes after the end of the procedure. It must be stated once again that ketamine should never be administered by anyone who has not been thoroughly trained in general anesthesia and in the management of the unconscious airway.

Inhalation sedation

Inhalation sedation with N_2O-O_2 remains the most nearly ideal technique of sedation in pediatric dentistry. The advantages and indications for the administration of inhalation sedation in children are the same as for the adult patient. The major difficulties encountered with this technique in children are twofold: first, the lack of potency of N_2O-O_2 may render

the technique ineffective in the management of the more apprehensive patient, and second, some children will object to the placement of the nasal hood. In most cases, this second objection can be overcome by altering the usual technique of administration of N_2O-O_2 (Chapter 16) to meet more realistically the requirements of the pediatric patient.

Dosage. The primary advantage of inhalation sedation is the ease with which it may be titrated. Concentrations of N_2O required to provide clinically adequate sedation in the child who readily accepts the nasal hood are virtually identical to those seen in adults. The overwhelming majority of children receiving N_2O-O_2 are adequately sedated at concentrations between 30% and 40% N_2O. Some patients may require less than 30% and some few more than 40% N_2O.

Screaming and crying patients will breathe through their mouth to a much greater degree than is usual and therefore do not receive as great a volume of N_2O being delivered through the nasal hood. A means of overcoming this problem is demonstrated in Fig. 36-6. The doctor removes the nasal hood from the patient's nose and holds it over the mouth so that as the child inhales he or she will receive greater volumes of N_2O. As illustrated in the figure, the patient is rather young (age 4) and has been placed in a restraint. The nasal hood is held over the patient's mouth until he quiets down, at which time it is once again placed on the patient's nose and treatment continued. This process may need to be repeated throughout the dental treatment in some patients.

The patient who will not permit the nasal hood to be placed on the nose poses a greater problem. The following technique will, however, provide the doctor with an increased chance of success. With the child restrained, the nasal hood is placed as close to the child's face as is practical. The concentration of N_2O is maximal (70%), with a high-flow rate (10 to 15 L/min). The patient may be attempting to move his face away from the nasal hood and be crying or screaming; however, he will be receiving a high concentration of N_2O (not 70% because of air dilution) at this time. The nasal hood should be maintained close to, but not on, the face for a few moments until the child quiets. The nasal hood should then be placed onto the nose. At this time, the percentage of N_2O must be lowered to approximately 25% to 30% and then titrated to an appropriate level for the patient.

One of the more unpleasant problems when using N_2O-O_2 in pediatric patients is vomiting. Although not frequent, the incidence of vomiting in pediatric patients is significantly greater than that seen in adults. Two reasons for this are (1) the lack of ability of the doctor to judge the level of the patient's sedation, which may lead to oversedation, and (2) children's greater tendency to mouth-breathe. Mouth breathing decreases the volume of N_2O being inhaled and lessens the level of sedation. When the patient returns to nose breathing, the sedation level deepens. Constant fluctuation in N_2O concentration is one cause of vomiting. Two techniques are available that decrease mouth breathing. First, simplest and most effective is the use of the rubber dam. I strongly recommend its application whenever inhalation sedation (or for that matter any sedative technique) is used. It prevents mouth breathing almost entirely. Another method, used in the absence of a rubber dam, is to tell the mouth-breathing patient that you are placing some "special water" into his mouth and that he cannot swallow it. A small volume of water from the air-water syringe should be placed into the patient's mouth. To keep the water in his mouth, the patient will have to raise his tongue to the roof of his mouth, thereby eliminating mouth breathing.

Several methods of determining a younger patient's level of sedation are available. The first may be used with a patient who is somewhat cooperative and is able and willing to communicate with the doctor. The child will probably be unable to understand the terms usually used to describe the sensations associated with N_2O for the adult patient. The doctor will have to come to the level of the child's understanding. Playing a game with the child is an effective means of determining the level of sedation. The child pretends he is an astronaut and the nasal hood is his space mask. As he inhales through this space mask, the astronaut will begin to float in space. Questioning the astronaut about his feelings can help to determine the level of sedation (that is, floating).

The second technique will be used in situations in which the apprehensive child is less communicative. Titration of the N_2O-O_2 continues at the usual rate, the doctor observing the degree of tension in the patient's body. Watching and touching the patient's hands provides an excellent gauge as to the level of sedation. It can be expected that the patient's hands will become more relaxed as sedation increases. The eyelids of the patient will begin to close, and the patient may yawn occasionally. When the doctor feels that the patient is adequately sedated, treatment is attempted. Changes in N_2O-O_2 concentrations will be based on the patient's response or lack of response to this treatment.

Nitrous oxide-oxygen with other techniques

Nitrous oxide-oxygen is frequently added to other techniques of sedation in order to increase their effectiveness. As discussed in Chapter 29, I believe that there is potential risk involved in this procedure if used by the inexperienced doctor who is not trained in recognizing and managing the airway of the unconscious patient. Where adequate operating room and outpatient sedation experience and training have been received (e.g., pediatric dentistry residency, general practice residency, anesthesiology residency), the combinations of oral plus inhalation sedation; IM or SM plus inhalation sedation; or IM and IV plus inhalation sedation, may be employed safely. Adequate monitoring of the patient, especially of the respiratory system, is essential. Nitrous oxide-oxygen must always be titrated; fixed concentrations should not be administered to all patients because not all patients react in the same manner.

Intravenous sedation

Traditionally, the IV route has seldom been employed in the management of pediatric dental or medical patients. Although this technique of drug administration is the most reliable and, when used as described, the safest, its use is seldom taught in pediatric dentistry training programs.

Because of the problems that have been associated with the administration of IM/SC/SM opioids in past years, alternative agents and techniques have been vigorously sought. With the introduction of midazolam into clinical use a new group of drugs, the benzodiazepines, is now being used for IM/SC/SM sedation in pediatrics.

When administered via these routes, these drugs have a fixed, somewhat short duration of clinical action (<1 hour). It was our thought to combine the administration of IM midazolam (for initial patient management) with IV midazolam or other IV drugs (for continued patient management) in pediatric dental patients.

The technique for IV sedation is briefly described. Following a pretreatment visit at which the patient is thoroughly evaluated (medically, dentally, psychologically) for suitability for sedation and after presedation instructions have been given to the parent or guardian, the patient is brought to the dental office.

Pretreatment instructions include the necessity of being NPO for a minimum of 4 to 6 hours prior to treatment, though smaller children require shorter NPO periods to prevent dehydration.

In a quiet room, with the lights turned down, the IM dose of midazolam (0.15 to 2 mg/kg) is administered to the patient (lateral aspect of thigh), while he or she is being held in the parent's arms. A pulse oximeter probe is immediately placed on the patient's toe or finger, and the patient is left with the parent for approximately 10 minutes. The patient is monitored continuously (via pulse oximetry) during this induction period.

At 10 minutes the patient is placed into the dental chair, enveloped in a physical restraint, and inhalation sedation is added (30% to 50% N_2O). The patient is usually somewhat cooperative, but perhaps not relaxed enough to permit the dental treatment to commence. A venipuncture is performed in every patient, a continuous IV infusion (D_5W with pediatric infusion set) is established and monitors placed. These include the pretracheal stethoscope, ECG, and vital signs monitor in addition to the already placed pulse oximeter. Guidelines for parenteral sedation at the University of Southern California School of Dentistry (see appendix) require the use of two continuous monitors at all times during pediatric parenteral sedation.

If possible, dental treatment is started at this time.

However, in many situations the patient is not yet fully cooperative. Small incremental doses (0.5 to 1 mg) of midazolam are added until the desired level of sedation is reached through titration. At this point, local anesthesia is administered and dental treatment can be started.

If at a later time additional sedation is desired, 0.5- to 1-mg doses of midazolam may be administered intravenously. On some occasions, other IV drugs may be given. When longer procedures are contemplated or when x ray films are necessary, we will follow the IM midazolam with small IV doses (12.5 to 25 mg) of pentobarbital. However, the barbiturate is only administered during the early phase of treatment so as to minimize the recovery time of the patient. There is no pharmacologic antagonist for barbiturates.

Meperidine is occasionally administered to these patients to aid in sedation and when a degree of analgesia is desirable at the conclusion of the dental procedure. Doses of 5 to 10 mg are administered IV as needed.

Propofol has been used during pediatric parenteral sedation when a rapid onset of short-duration sedation is required. In this manner propofol is being used as methohexital was during surgical procedures. Immediately (20 to 30 seconds) prior to the administration of a palatal local anesthetic, a dose of 5 to 10 mg of propofol is injected as a bolus. In addition, propofol is being administered toward the end of the procedure when the patient begins to get too light and movements interfere with the completion of the treatment. Increments of 10 mg of propofol enable the procedure to be completed successfully without prolonging the recovery period.

At the completion of treatment the patient receives 100% O_2, the lights in the room are turned on, and the dental chair positioned so as to make the patient somewhat uncomfortable. Our goal at this time is to arouse the patient and hasten his or her recovery and discharge. Monitoring is continued throughout the recovery period. When recovery is deemed adequate, the patient is dismissed in the custody of a parent or guardian. A telephone call to the family that evening to inquire as to the patient's status is recommended.

This technique should only be employed by persons well versed in deep sedation, general anesthesia, and airway management. When deep sedation is employed, a second individual should be solely responsible for the sedation while another does the required dentistry. Using this technique of IM/IV and inhalation sedation, we have been able to manage

Table 36-3. Parenteral sedation discharge criteria

The following should be completed when considering the discharge of a patient following parenteral sedation. The patient postsedation score must be approximately equal their baseline (presedation) score.

Patient's name: ssn: Date:

Physical Signs	*(Pretreatment)*	*Baseline/Discharge Comments*

A. MOVEMENT
  2—able to walk (where appropriate)
  1—able to move extremities
  0—unable to move any extremity		

B. RESPIRATIONS
  2—able to breathe deeply & cough
  1—limited respiratory effort
  0—no spontaneous respiratory effort		

C. CIRCULATION
  2—systolic BP +/−20% baseline level
  1—systolic BP +/−40% baseline level
  0—systolic BP >+/−40% baseline
    level		

D. CONSCIOUSNESS
  2—full alertness seen in ability to
    answer questions appropriately
  1—aroused when called by name
  0—unresponsive to verbal stimulation		

E. COLOR
  2—normal skin color and appearance
  1—any alteration in skin color
  0—frank cyanosis or extreme pale		

TOTAL SCORE: Dr's signature:		

From *Guidelines for the use of parenteral sedation.* Los Angeles, 1991, The University of Southern California School of Dentistry.

the dental needs of patients ranging from 18 months to 10 years of age.

DISCHARGE FROM THE OFFICE

Pediatric patients who have been sedated may not be discharged from the office until the doctor is convinced that they have recovered adequately. The following are subjective discharge criteria for the pediatric patient:

1. The patient must be able to stand up and respond to questioning and stimulation. If the child is unable to walk alone or must be carried, he or she should not be released from the office.

2. In any situation in which the parent or guardian insists on taking the child before the doctor considers the patient adequately recovered, this must be immediately noted in the patient's chart, and it must be countersigned by a second person who is present at the time. It is the doctor who must be the final judge of the patient's ability to be discharged safely from the office. Until such time, the patient should remain in the recovery area of the office. Table 36-3 presents a list of objective criteria for discharge of the postsedation patient.

RECORDKEEPING

As with the adult patient, sedation records must be maintained for the pediatric patient. An example of one such form was presented in Chapter 27. Two other forms are shown in Fig. 36-7.

GENERAL ANESTHESIA

Approximately 2% to 5% of pediatric patients will require general anesthesia for their dental care to be

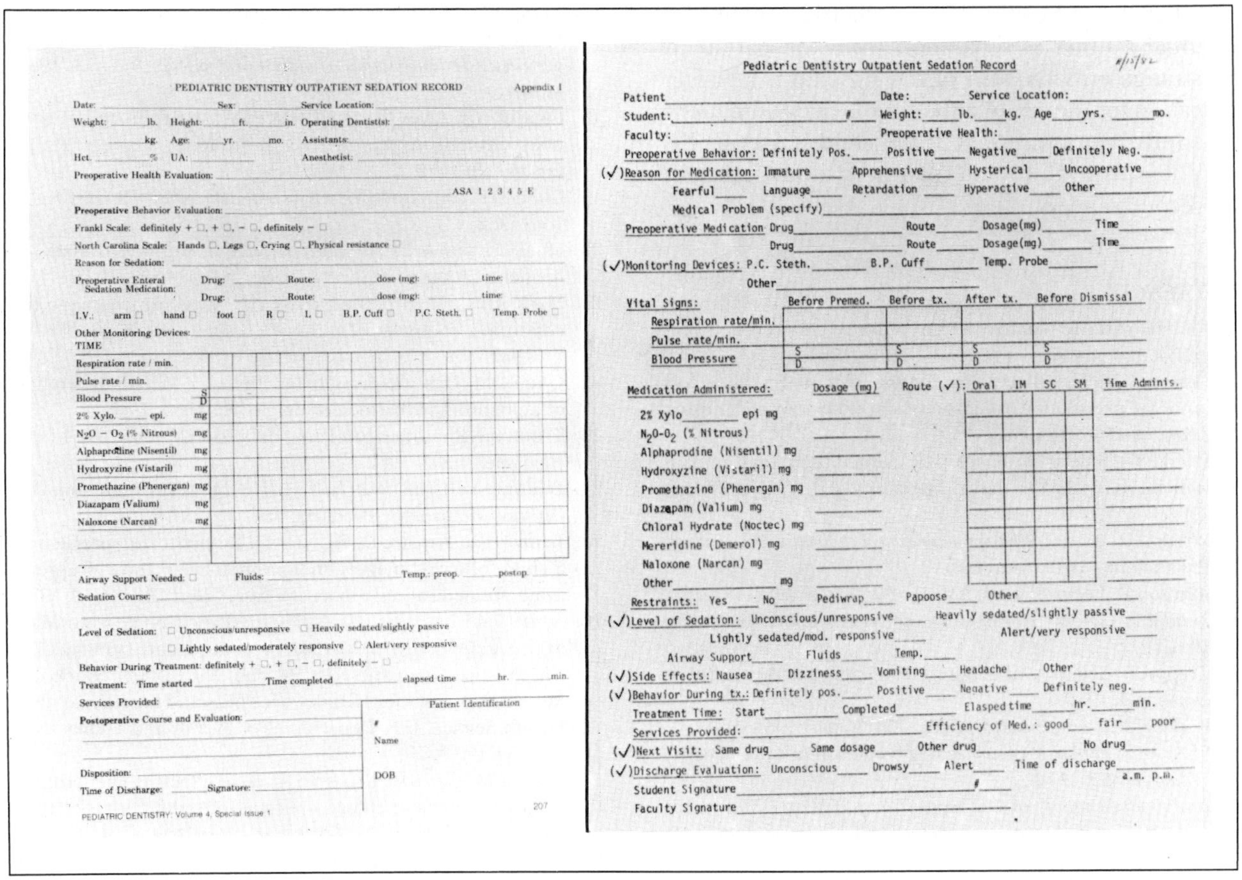

PEDIATRIC DENTISTRY OUTPATIENT SEDATION RECORD — Appendix I

Date: ____ Sex: ____ Service Location: ____
Weight: ____ lb. Height: ____ ft. ____ in. Operating Dentist(s): ____
____ kg. Age: ____ yr. ____ mo. Assistants: ____
Hct. ____ % UA: ____ Anesthetist: ____
Preoperative Health Evaluation: ____
ASA 1 2 3 4 5 E
Preoperative Behavior Evaluation: ____
Frankl Scale: definitely + ☐, + ☐, − ☐, definitely − ☐
North Carolina Scale: Hands ☐, Legs ☐, Crying ☐, Physical resistance ☐
Reason for Sedation: ____
Preoperative Enteral Sedation Medication: Drug: ____ Route: ____ dose (mg): ____ time: ____
Drug: ____ Route: ____ dose (mg): ____ time: ____
I.V.: arm ☐ hand ☐ foot ☐ R ☐ L ☐ B.P. Cuff ☐ P.C. Steth. ☐ Temp. Probe ☐
Other Monitoring Devices: ____
TIME
Respiration rate / min.
Pulse rate / min.
Blood Pressure S/D
2% Xylo. ____ epi. mg
$N_2O - O_2$ (% Nitrous) mg
Alphaprodine (Nisentil) mg
Hydroxyzine (Vistaril) mg
Promethazine (Phenergan) mg
Diazapam (Valium) mg
Naloxone (Narcan) mg
Airway Support Needed: ☐ Fluids: ____ Temp.: preop. ____ postop. ____
Sedation Course: ____
Level of Sedation: ☐ Unconscious/unresponsive ☐ Heavily sedated/slightly passive ☐ Lightly sedated/moderately responsive ☐ Alert/very responsive
Behavior During Treatment: definitely + ☐, + ☐, − ☐, definitely − ☐
Treatment: Time started ____ Time completed ____ elapsed time ____ hr. ____ min.
Services Provided: ____
Postoperative Course and Evaluation: ____
Disposition: ____
Time of Discharge: ____ Signature: ____
Patient Identification
#
Name
DOB
PEDIATRIC DENTISTRY: Volume 4, Special Issue 1 — 207

Pediatric Dentistry Outpatient Sedation Record

Patient ____ Date: ____ Service Location: ____
Student: ____ # ____ Weight: ____ lb. ____ kg. Age ____ yrs. ____ mo.
Faculty: ____ Preoperative Health: ____
Preoperative Behavior: Definitely Pos. ____ Positive ____ Negative ____ Definitely Neg. ____
(✓)Reason for Medication: Immature ____ Apprehensive ____ Hysterical ____ Uncooperative ____
Fearful ____ Language ____ Retardation ____ Hyperactive ____ Other ____
Medical Problem (specify) ____
Preoperative Medication Drug ____ Route ____ Dosage(mg) ____ Time ____
Drug ____ Route ____ Dosage(mg) ____ Time ____
(✓)Monitoring Devices: P.C. Steth. ____ B.P. Cuff ____ Temp. Probe ____
Other ____
Vital Signs: Before Premed. | Before tx. | After tx. | Before Dismissal
Respiration rate/min.
Pulse rate/min.
Blood Pressure S/D
Medication Administered: Dosage (mg) Route (✓): Oral IM SC SM Time Adminis.
2% Xylo ____ epi mg
N_2O-O_2 (% Nitrous)
Alphaprodine (Nisentil) mg
Hydroxyzine (Vistaril) mg
Promethazine (Phenergan) mg
Diazepam (Valium) mg
Chloral Hydrate (Noctec) mg
Mereridine (Demerol) mg
Naloxone (Narcan) mg
Other ____ mg
Restraints: Yes ____ No ____ Pediwrap ____ Papoose ____ Other ____
(✓)Level of Sedation: Unconscious/unresponsive ____ Heavily sedated/slightly passive ____
Lightly sedated/mod. responsive ____ Alert/very responsive ____
Airway Support ____ Fluids ____ Temp. ____
(✓)Side Effects: Nausea ____ Dizziness ____ Vomiting ____ Headache ____ Other ____
(✓)Behavior During tx.: Definitely pos. ____ Positive ____ Negative ____ Definitely neg. ____
Treatment Time: Start ____ Completed ____ Elasped time ____ hr. ____ min.
Services Provided: ____ Efficiency of Med.: good ____ fair ____ poor ____
(✓)Next Visit: Same drug ____ Same dosage ____ Other drug ____ No drug ____
(✓)Discharge Evaluation: Unconscious ____ Drowsy ____ Alert ____ Time of discharge ____ a.m. p.m.
Student Signature ____ # ____
Faculty Signature ____

Fig. 36-7. Two pediatric sedation records. (**A,** from Troutman KC: *Pediatr Dent* 4[special issue 1]:207, 1982.)

successfully completed. Dummett[32] lists the following indications for the administration of general anesthesia to the pediatric patient:

1. Extensive dental needs in uncooperative children who resist all means of conventional management procedures, including premedication and restraints
2. Extensive dental needs in the young, immature, and precommunicative child whose behavior deters dental treatment
3. Multiple pulpally involved teeth in a child with cardiac disease where immediate treatment is indicated for the sake of the child's health
4. Extensive dental needs in the severely physically and sensorially handicapped (e.g., deafness and blindness) where communication cannot be achieved
5. Extensive dental needs in children with blood dyscrasias who may need transfusions
6. Extensive dental needs in children with mental retardation whose behavior deters dental treatment and impairs dentist–patient communication
7. Extensive dental needs in children who are allergic to local anesthetics

As mentioned, before a decision is reached to employ general anesthesia in order to complete treatment, at least two attempts should be made to treat the patient in the office using sedation techniques. Sedation combined with local anesthesia is a highly effective means of managing most patients. When attempts using these procedures have been unsuccessful and signs of progressive improvement in behavior and cooperation have not been demonstrated, general anesthesia should be considered.

Pediatric general anesthesia may be administered in one of three settings: in the dental office, in the hospital or outpatient surgical center as a day admission, or on an inpatient basis in the hospital. When considering the healthy ASA I pediatric patient, the potential trauma of separation from the parent in the strange environment of the hospital is a strong indication for the use of either in-office or outpatient day-admission procedures. If the child is ASA II, III, or IV, hospitalization and treatment as an inpatient are recommended.

REFERENCES

1. Kimmelman BB: Management of sensitive children in a general dental practice, *J Dent Child* 31:146, 1964.
2. Lenchner V: The effect of appointment length on the behavior of the pedodontic patient and his attitude toward dentistry, *J Dent Child* 33:61, 1966.
3. Frankl SN, Shiere FR, Fogelo HR: Should the parent remain with the child in the dental operatory? *J Dent Child* 29:150, 1962.
4. Wright GZ, editor: *Behavior management in dentistry for children.* Philadelphia, 1975, Saunders.
5. Johnson R: Lecture notes, AMED 750, August 1983.
6. Zendell E: Chloral hydrate overdose: a case report, *Anesth Prog* 19:6, 1972.
7. Trapp LD: Sedation of children for dental treatment, *Pediatr Dent* 4:164, 1982.
8. Kopel HM: Lecture notes, AMED 750, August 1983.
9. Wilson JT: Pediatric pharmacology: who will test the drugs? *J Pediatr* 80:855, 1972.
10. American Academy of Pediatrics Committee on Child Abuse and Neglect: Behavior management of pediatric dental patients, *Pediatrics* 90(4):651, 1992.
11. Wright GZ, McAuley DJ: Current premedicating trends in pedodontics, *J Dent Child* 40:185, 1973.
12. Malamed SF: Pharmacology and therapeutics of anxiety and pain control. In Braham RL, Morris ME, eds: *Textbook of pediatric dentistry.* Baltimore, 1980, Williams & Wilkins.
13. Album MM: Meperidine and promethazine hydrochloride for handicapped patients, *J Dent Res* 40:1036, 1961.
14. Rosen DA, Rosen KR: A palatable gelatin vehicle for midazolam and ketamine, *Anesthesiology* 75(5):914, 1991 (letter).
15. Harrison P: Lollipop successful in providing analgesia to children before painful procedures, *Canad Med Assoc J* 145(5):521, 1991.
16. Vetter TR: A comparison of midazolam, diazepam, and placebo as oral anesthetic premedicants in younger children, *J Clin Anesth* 5(1):58, 1993.
17. Trapp LD: Pharmacologic management of pain and anxiety. In Stewart RE, Barber TK, Troutman KC et al, eds: *Pediatric dentistry: scientific foundation and clinical practice.* St Louis, 1981, Mosby.
18. Caudill WA, Alvin JD, Nazif MM et al: Absorption rates of alphaprodine from the buccal and intravenous routes, *Pediatr Dent* 4:168, 1982.
19. Chen DT: Alphaprodine HCI: characteristics, *Pediatr Dent* 4:158, 1982.
20. Hine CH, Pasi A: Fatality after use of alphaprodine in analgesia for dental surgery: report of a case, *JADA* 84:858, 1972.
21. Mack RB: Alphaprodine-hydroxyzine sedation technique for children: a conservative approach, *Pediatr Dent* 4(special issue 1), 1982.
22. Okuji DM: Hypoxic encephalopathy after the administration of alphaprodine hydrochloride, *JADA* 103:50, 1981.
23. Troutman K, moderator: Panel discussion, *Pediatr Dent* 4 (special issue 1):207, 1982.
24. DuPont: *Naloxone. Drug Package Insert.* 1990, Wilmington, DE, DuPont Multisource Products.
25. Benusis KP, Kapaun D, Furnam LJ: Respiratory depression in a child following meperidine, promethazine and chlorpromazine premedication: report of a case, *J Dent Child* 46:50, 1979.
26. Acute Pain Management Guideline Panel: Acute Pain Management: Operative or Medical Procedures and Trauma. Clinical Practice Guideline, AHCPR Pub. No. 92-0032, Rockville, Md, 1992, Agency for Health Care Policy and Research, Public Health Service, U.S. Department of Health and Human Services, p. 45.
27. Nahata M, Clotz M, Krogg E: Adverse effects of meperidine, promethazine, and chlorpromazine for sedation in pediatric patients, *Clin Pediatr* 24:558, 1985.
28. Silvasi DL, Rosen DA, Rosen KR: Continuous intravenous midazolam infusion for sedation in the pediatric intensive care unit, *Anesth Analg* 67(3):286, 1988.
29. Thiessen O, Boileau S, Wahl D et al: Sedation with intranasal midazolam for endoscopy of the upper digestive tract, *Ann Fr Anesth Reanim* 10(5):450, 1991.
30. Malamed SF, Quinn CL, Hatch HG: Pediatric sedation with intramuscular and intravenous midazolam, *Anesth Prog* 36(4-5):155, 1989.
31. Rosen DA, Rosen KR, Elkins TE et al: Outpatient sedation: an essential addition to gynecologic care for persons with mental retardation, *Am J Obstet Gynecol* 164(3):825, 1991.
32. Dummett CO Jr: Guidelines for hospital admission and discharge of pedodontic patients for restorative dentistry under general anesthesia. New Orleans, 1976, Department of Pedodontics, Louisiana State University School of Dentistry.

CHAPTER 37

The geriatric patient

Christine L. Quinn

Classically, age 65 is the beginning of the geriatric period. This arbitrary age cutoff is believed to have originated from two different sources, the first of which is imperial Germany. The Bismarck government decided that they had only enough money to provide benefits for those 65 years of age and older. The second source is a group of English physicians who decided to care exclusively for the elderly. They decided, based on population alone, that they would only have time for those over 65 years of age.[1]

It is important to remember, though, that no matter what age is chosen as the beginning of the geriatric phase, everyone ages in two ways: chronologically and biologically.[1] This makes elderly individuals a physiologically diverse group because there is no correlation of biological age with chronological age because of the effects of concomitant diseases.

The geriatric patient presents possibly an increased risk during dental and medical procedures. By the year 2000 it is estimated that 15% of the U.S. population will be over the age of 65.[2] In some areas of the country the percentage of geriatric individuals exceeds 66%. The number of geriatric persons will continue to rise over the years as the birth rate declines and the life expectancy continues to increase. In 1987 12.3% of the total population was 65 years of age or older. The people comprising the age group of 85 years or older is the population showing the greatest increase in numbers.[3]

The aging process involves both physiological and pathological changes that may alter patients' ability to respond to stress as well as their response to drug administration. Geriatric patients have a decreased functional reserve—their organs function at or near capacity during ordinary activities. When subjected to stress, this inadequacy contributes to an overall difficulty in handling a situation or illness. Many physiological and pathological changes are encountered in the geriatric patient (Table 37-1). Decrease in tissue elasticity is a major physiological change that has significant effect on organs throughout the body. For example, in patients 75 years of age, cerebral blood flow is 80% of what it was in patients at 30 years of age. Cardiac output has declined to 65%, renal blood flow has decreased to 45% of its volume, and hepatic blood flow has also decreased.[4] The decrease in renal perfusion has potentially significant bearing on the actions of certain drugs, primarily those in which urinary excretion is a principal means of removing the drug and its metabolites from the body. This decrease is probably the most responsible for increased plasma drug concentrations. Drugs such as penicillin, tetracycline, and digoxin exhibit greatly increased β–half-lives in geriatric patients.

Decreased tissue elasticity also affects the lungs; pulmonary compliance decreases with aging and may progress to senile emphysema. Other pulmonary factors that tend to diminish respiratory function include chronic exposure to smoke, dust, and pollutants. These factors may produce respiratory disorders. Pulmonary function is considerably diminished compared to that in the younger individual (Table 37-2).

Cardiovascular and respiratory function may be impaired in the normal, healthy geriatric patient. Because of the probable decrease in physiological functioning, the geriatric patient is considered an ASA II patient or greater if disease is present.

Quite often the geriatric patient has multiple chronic disease processes, each of which requires one or more medications. In the geriatric population 85% suffer from at least one chronic condition, and

Table 37-1. Physiologic and pathologic changes in geriatric patients

Central nervous system (CNS)

Decreased number of brain cells
Cerebral arteriosclerosis
    Cerebrovascular accident
    Decreased memory
    Emotional changes
Parkinsonism

Cardiovascular system

Coronary artery disease
    Angina pectoris
    Myocardial infarction
    Dysrhythmias
    Decreased contractility
High blood pressure
    Renovascular disease
    Cerebrovascular disease
    Cardiac disease

Respiratory system

Senile emphysema
Arthritic changes in thorax
Pulmonary problems related to pollutants
Interstitial fibrosis

Genitourinary system

Decreased renal blood flow
Decreased number of functioning glomeruli
Decreased tubular reabsorption
Benign prostatic hypertrophy

Endocrine system

Decreased response to stress
Maturity–onset diabetes mellitus

Modified from Lichtiger M, Moya F: Physiologic and pathologic considerations in the geriatric patient, *Curr Rev Nurse Anesth* 1(1): 1, 1978.

Table 37-2. Pulmonary changes in geriatric patients

Function	Percentage of control at age 30 years
Total lung capacity	100
Vital capacity	58
O₂ uptake during exercise	50
Maximum breathing capacity	55

From data in Lichtiger M, Moya F: Physiologic and pathologic considerations in the geriatric patient, *Curr Rev Nurse Anesth* 1(1):1, 1978.

42% may be limited in activity because of chronic conditions.[5] Some of the more commonly seen diseases are arthritis, hypertension, atherosclerotic heart disease, angina pectoris, emphysema, glaucoma, and prostatitis. The leading cause of death in geriatric individuals continues to be heart disease.

Because of the probability of disease and the requirement for chronic use of medications in the geriatric patient, it becomes extremely important that the doctor receive an accurate and thorough medical history questionnaire from the patient. In 1980 Brady and Martinoff[6] evaluated the validity of patient-completed health history questionnaires and came to the conclusion that dentists should not assume that patients are reliable historians of their own health history. It would be prudent to obtain a physician consult on any patient that you may have questions about. Special emphasis should be placed on the use of any prescription or over-the-counter medications. Adverse drug reactions are more likely to develop in patients over the age of 65 years than in younger patients.[7] Halpern found that 18% of his total patient population were taking medication on a regular basis. The incidence increased with age: at age 60 years or older, 41% of patients were regularly taking medications.[8]

COMMON HEALTH PROBLEMS

Some of the more commonly seen ailments and diseases of the geriatric population are discussed briefly in the following paragraphs, along with possible implications for dental treatment.

Arthritis

The arthritic patient may exhibit difficulty with positioning in the dental chair. Modification of positioning may be necessary for successful and comfortable treatment. Drug management of arthritis commonly includes administration of salicylates (aspirin) and nonsteroidal antiinflammatory drugs (NSAIDs) such as ibuprofen and naproxen. Some increased bleeding may be noted in patients taking NSAIDs.

High blood pressure

Patients with high blood pressure will be receiving antihypertensive medications to lower blood pressure. A desirable level for blood pressure is below 140/90 without the patient experiencing unwanted symptomatology. Side effects may be seen with all antihypertensive medications. Postural hypotension is the most commonly seen side effect, and the antihypertensive agents may accentuate this same effect produced by some of the CNS depressants used for sedation. Careful change of patient position and slow titration of sedative medications will help to minimize the significance of this side effect.

Atherosclerosis

Atherosclerotic heart disease (ASHD) will be present in differing degrees in all patients over the age of 65 years. Possible signs and symptoms of ASHD include elevated blood pressure, irregularities in cardiac rhythm, undue fatigue, and "discomfort" in the chest upon exertion. The administration of sedative medications may be indicated in these patients as a method of minimizing the development of potentially serious complications.

Angina pectoris is a common clinical manifestation of ASHD. Angina may also be seen in the postmyocardial infarction patient. This patient may be at greater risk of a medical emergency during treatment. Inhalation sedation with nitrous oxide-oxygen (N_2O-O_2) is an excellent sedative technique for this patient. Drug therapy for angina pectoris includes the administration of nitrates, which act as vasodilators. Postural hypotension may develop when these agents are administered in the management of an acute episode. Proper positioning will minimize the development of postural hypotension.

Emphysema

Emphysema is one form of chronic obstructive pulmonary disease (COPD) that may be seen in the geriatric population. Chronic exposure to pollutants (e.g., cigarette smoke, air pollution) is the most common cause of emphysema. Because the patient's respiratory reserves are quite diminished, stress-reduction protocol becomes important in patient management. There is no specific drug therapy available for emphysema.

Glaucoma

In glaucoma there is an abnormal accumulation of aqueous humor within the eye that leads to an increase in intraocular pressure. Patients suffering from narrow-angle glaucoma may be treated with pilocarpine eye drops. The action of this medication is to constrict the pupils so that the aqueous humor may drain; however, when an anticholinergic medication such as atropine is administered, the iris folds back into the angle of the anterior chamber and blocks the outflow of the aqueous humor. This effect usually requires larger than therapeutic doses of atropine (more than 1 mg). Atropine in the usual therapeutic dose (0.4 mg) is not absolutely contraindicated in these patients. Timolol, a β-adrenergic blocking agent, is now being used as an antiglaucoma agent. It may be administered alone or in combination with other intraocular pressure-lowering agents.

MANAGEMENT OF PAIN AND ANXIETY

The need for adequate pain control during treatment is as compelling in the geriatric patient as in any other patient group. There are no specific contraindications in the geriatric patient to the administration of any local anesthetic or the utilization of any anesthetic technique in particular. Local anesthetic drug dosages should be kept as low as possible in this age group because of the unknown degree of hepatic and renal dysfunction that may be present. The elimination half-life of the local anesthetic may be considerably prolonged, and plasma levels may remain elevated for extended periods. Block injections are preferred to infiltration because a smaller volume is used to achieve a wider area of anesthesia. The use of vasoconstrictors is not contraindicated in the normotensive or the controlled hypertensive individual. Caution should be exercised in using vasoconstrictors in the geriatric patient with untreated systolic hypertension. The benefits should be weighed against the risks of increased blood pressure, increased heart rate, and possible arrhythmias.[9]

The geriatric patient may also be dental phobic. Central nervous system–depressant drugs may be indicated in these cases. As stated, the geriatric patient is twice as likely to develop adverse drug reactions (ADRs) as is the younger adult patient. The older patient appears to "hyperrespond" to the usual doses of many medications. Extreme care must be exhibited whenever CNS depressants are administered.

Age exerts pharmacokinetic and pharmacodynamic changes in the elderly individual. These changes can help to account for the overreaction to drugs. As a simple review: pharmacokinetic variables determine the relationship between the dose of the drug administered and the concentration delivered to the site of action. Pharmacodynamics determine the relationship between the concentration of the drug at the site of action and the intensity of the effect produced; that is, pharmacokinetics are what the drug does to the body.[10,11] Table 37-3 illustrates this relationship.

The following are some specific reasons for the exaggerated effect of drugs in the elderly[12]:

1. The presence of pathology, such as hepatic dysfunction or decrease in hepatic blood flow, will produce increased plasma levels of drugs and therefore exaggerated clinical actions as well as prolonged duration of action.

2. Drug-drug interactions between the medications that the geriatric patient may be taking on a chronic basis can also potentiate or augment the actions of drugs administered for dental treatment.

3. Renal changes, such as decreased renal perfusion, will also lead to increased plasma levels of the drugs and their associated actions.

4. Changes in intestinal absorption affect the rate and degree to which an orally administered drug will be absorbed.

5. There is a decrease in drug binding due to a decrease in albumin production; therefore, a greater percentage of the drug is available to produce its actions. For example, diazepam is approximately 98.5% bound (1.5% free and available to exert its effect) in younger individuals. In older patients it is only 97% bound. This leaves twice as much diazepam available (3 versus 1.5%) to produce its clinical actions. Given the same drug dosage, the patient with diminished drug binding will exhibit more profound clinical actions.

6. There is a decrease in the number of receptors present in a given tissue, but the receptors apparently function normally. Because of this decrease, lower blood level of the drug may be required to achieve a given response.

7. Lean body mass declines with increasing age. Total body fat increases, which will have the effect of increasing the elimination half-life of a lipid-soluble drug. For example, the elimination half-life of diazepam in a 20-year-old is 20 hours, but it is 90 hours for an 80-year-old individual.[13]

Oral sedation is indicated in geriatric patients. Because orally administered drugs cannot be precisely titrated, it is recommended that smaller dosages be used on the initial visit and titrated by appointment as is necessary. Diazepam and other benzodiazepines are popular premedicants for the geriatric patient. It may be prudent to select a benzodiazepine, such as lorazepam, oxazepam, or trizolam, that is not metabolized into active metabolites. Small dosages usually provide good sedation. As with other patients, barbiturates are not a first-choice drug because of their long duration of action and generalized CNS-depressant effect. They may occasionally produce delirium in the geriatric patient. The use of barbiturates should be avoided if possible. Antihistaminic agents can be used for premedication but should be avoided in the patient with COPD because of their drying actions on the bronchial mucosa.

Intramuscular (IM) sedation is not generally recommended because of the inability to titrate the medication. This technique is usually used on uncooperative patients. When required, midazolam is the medication typically used. Supplemental oxygen administration is recommended whenever IM drugs are administered.

Inhalation sedation is probably the most highly recommended technique of sedation for the geriatric patient. It offers the advantage of providing a light sedative technique with the benefits of supplemental oxygenation.

Table 37-3. Relationship between pharmacokinetic and pharmacodynamic factors

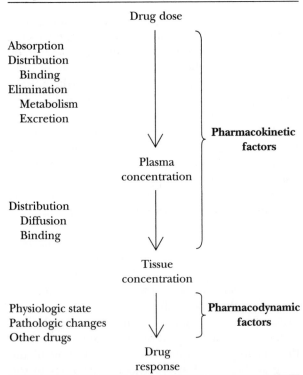

From Craig DB, McLeskey CH, Mitenko PA et al: Geriatric anaesthesia, *Can J Anaesth* 34(2):156, 1987.

Intravenous (IV) sedation is recommended for those patients with intense anxiety. Veins of the older patient may be more difficult to enter because of a loss of elasticity and are very fragile. Titration is the ultimate safeguard in IV sedation. Titration should occur even more slowly in the geriatric individual because of the pharmacokinetic and pharmacodynamic changes that occur. The patient should be maintained at as light a sedative level as possible. Supplemental oxygen administration is recommended for all IV sedation procedures.

Outpatient general anesthesia is not usually recommended for dental treatment of the geriatric individual. Decisions on whether an individual can safely undergo outpatient general anesthesia are based on the overall health of the patient and the absence of significant systemic disease.

REFERENCES

1. Gambert SR: Aging—an overview, *Spec Care Dent* 3:147, 1983.
2. Chow G: Oral surgical consideration of the aged, *Spec Care Dent* 7:17, 1983.
3. US Department of Commerce, Bureau of Census: State population and household estimates with age, sex and components of change: 1981–1987. In *Current population reports, population estimates and projections,* series P-25, number 1024, Washington, DC, 1988, US Government Printing Office. p 5.
4. Stoelting RK, Dierdorf SF, McCammon RL, editors: Geriatric patients. In *Anesthesia and co-existing diseases,* ed 2. New York, 1988, Churchill Livingstone.
5. Kane R et al: *Geriatrics in the U.S.: manpower projections and training considerations,* Santa Monica, Calif, 1980, Rand Publication Series, Rand Corp.
6. Brady WF, Martinoff JT: Validity of health history data collected from dental patients and patient perception of health status, *JADA* 101(4):642, 1980.
7. Vestal R, Cusack B: Drug therapy in the elderly. In *Clinical geriatric dentistry: biomedical and psychosocial aspects,* Chicago, American Dental Association, 1985.
8. Halpern IL: Patient's medical status: a factor in dental treatment, *Oral Surg Oral Med Oral Pathol* 39:216, 1975.
9. Malamed SF: Anxiety and pain control in the older patient, *Spec Care Dent* 7(1):22, 1987.
10. McLeskey C: New views of uptake and distribution of inhalation and intravenous agents in the aging patient, Atlanta, Ga, 1987, ASA 1987 Annual Meeting.
11. Neidle EA: The geriatric dental patient: some pharmacological implications, *Spec Care Dent* 7:12, 1987.
12. Greenblatt DJ, Sellers EM, Shader RI: Drug disposition in old age, *N Engl J Med* 306:(18):1081, 1982.
13. Klotz U et al: The effects of age and liver disease on the disposition and elimination of diazepam in adult man, *J Clin Invest* 55:347, 1975.

BIBLIOGRAPHY

Miller RD: Anesthesia for the elderly. In Miller RD, ed: *Anesthesia,* ed 2. New York, 1986, Churchill Livingstone.

Neidle EA, Picozzi A: Geriatric pharmacology. In Neidle EA, Yagiela JA, eds: *Pharmacology and therapeutics for dentistry,* ed 3. St Louis, 1989, Mosby.

Stoelting RK, Dierdorf SF, McCammon RL, eds: Geriatric patients. In *Anesthesia and co-existing diseases,* ed 3. New York, 1993, Churchill Livingstone.

Stoelting RK, Miller RD: Elderly patients. In *Basics of anesthesia,* ed 2. New York, 1994, Churchill Livingstone.

CHAPTER 38

The medically compromised patient

In our earlier discussion of the management of stress related to medical and dental treatment, it was brought out that there are many patients who are unable to tolerate the usual degree of stress related to dental therapy or, in fact, to everyday existence. These persons usually have an underlying medical problem that limits their ability to manage stress in a normal manner. When faced with increased stress, the probability of this patient undergoing an acute exacerbation of the disease process greatly increases. Examples of this might include the patient with a history of coronary artery disease suffering from chest pain, the epileptic having a tonic-clonic seizure, or an asthmatic having an acute episode of bronchospasm during periods of increased stress such as during dental treatment.

Because of advances in medicine and pharmacotherapeutics, many more of these patients have become increasingly functional to the degree that their existence is no longer limited to their home. They may now be gainfully employed and partially or fully ambulatory and seek out dental and medical care as would any other patient. These persons, however, represent a greater degree of risk during stressful times. How then may these patients be better managed? Reduction of stress associated with treatment will be a primary goal in the management of these patients. Knowledge of the underlying disease process is also essential. In this chapter various disease entities that are seen more commonly in the ambulatory setting will be reviewed. A brief description of the disease process will be presented, followed by a listing of those factors that tend to exacerbate it and a review of the methods available to successfully minimize perioperative stress in this patient.

CARDIOVASCULAR DISEASE

Cardiovascular disease ranks as the number one cause of death in the United States, United Kingdom, and other industrialized nations. It is estimated that the number of persons in the United States with signs and symptoms of cardiovascular disease exceeds 64.9 million. In 1985 991,332 persons died from cardiovascular disease in the United States. Cancer, the second leading cause, was responsible for 457,700 deaths.

Significant advances have occurred in the surgical and pharmacological management of many cardiovascular disorders. Patients who once suffered from extremely severe anginal pains caused by coronary artery disease are today asymptomatic as a result of coronary artery bypass and graft procedures. Newer drugs such as the beta-adrenergic blockers (e.g., propranolol) and calcium channel blockers (e.g., verapamil, nifedipine) have enabled patients to lead more normal lives in spite of the continued presence of a serious underlying cardiovascular disorder.

In view of the fact that more than 10% of the American population has signs and symptoms of clinically significant cardiovascular disease, it stands to reason that the dentist will be managing the oral health needs of many cardiovascular risk patients. Although there are many causes for the various cardiovascular diseases, there is one factor that, when present, is responsible for dramatically increasing the risk of an acute exacerbation. This factor is a myocardial O_2 requirement that exceeds the supply capability of the coronary arteries. When such oxygen deprivation occurs, the patient responds with an acute exacerbation of the underlying problem. For example, chest pain and/or dysrhythmias may develop in the patient with angina, and dyspnea will occur in the patient with CHF.

Patients at cardiovascular risk can usually receive dental care. Modifications in planned dental care are based on the severity (ASA II, III, or IV) of the disease process as determined by the evaluation of the patient (see Chapter 5). Sedation and pain control are of much greater importance in these patients than in the ASA I patient. Specific details that relate to the management of patients at cardiovascular risk are discussed in the following section.

Angina pectoris

Angina is usually a result of arteriosclerotic heart disease but may occasionally occur in the absence of significant disease by coronary artery spasm, severe aortic stenosis, or aortic insufficiency. The basic mechanism producing angina is a discrepancy between the myocardial O_2 demands and the amount of O_2 delivered through the coronary arteries. The pain produced is described as a squeezing or pressure-like pain, retrosternal or slightly to the left of the sternum, that appears suddenly during exertion, may radiate in a set pattern (Fig. 38-1), and subsides with rest or the administration of nitrates. Patients with angina may be taking long-acting nitrates in order to prevent the occurrence of acute episodes. These drugs include isosorbide dinitrate (Isordil, Sorbitrate), pentaerythritol tetranitrate (Peritrate), and erythrityl tetranitrate (Cardilate). In 1981 nitroglycerin ointment became available. It comes in a fixed dose on an adhesive pad that is worn on the patient's chest, providing continuous nitroglycerin therapy. A spray form of nitroglycerin (Nitrolingual Spray [Rhone-Poulenc Rorer]) as well as the traditional sublingual nitroglycerin tablets are available for management of acute episodes of anginal pain.

The patient with stable angina represents an ASA III risk. Persons with infrequent episodes that are easily managed might be classified as an ASA II, and persons who have daily episodes or episodes that appear to be increasing in frequency or severity (unstable angina) are in the ASA IV category.

Factors that produce an acute exacerbation in the anginal patient are as follows:

Physical activity
Hot, humid environment
Cold weather
Large meals
Emotional stress (argument, anxiety, sexual excitement)

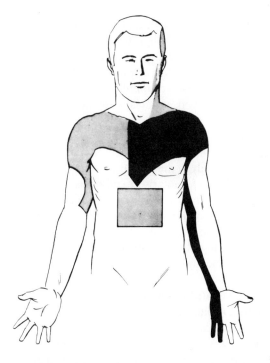

■ Substernal pain projected to left shoulder and arm (ulanar nerve distribution)

▒ Less frequent referred sites including right shoulder and arm, left jaw, neck, and epigastrium

Fig. 38-1. Radiation patterns of chest pain. (From Jastak JT, Cowan FF Jr: *Dent Clin North Am* 17:363, 1973.

Caffeine ingestion
Fever, anemia, thyrotoxicosis
Cigarette smoking
Smoke from other persons' cigarettes
Smog
High altitudes

As with all patients, many anginal patients will exhibit heightened anxiety prior to dental or surgical treatment. Sedation is especially indicated in these patients because of the negative effects of anxiety on the cardiovascular system. Increased blood levels of catecholamines (epinephrine and norepinephrine) produce an increase in the rate of the heart as well as an increase in the strength of each contraction. The net result of these is an increase in the O_2 demand of the myocardium. In the presence of coronary artery disease this demand may not be met and an acute anginal episode results. Dysrhythmias may also develop at this time. Minimizing stress as well as maximizing oxygenation of the patient are the desired goals in prevention of anginal episodes.

Oral sedation is indicated. Light levels of sedation prevent possible clinically significant respiratory depression, which could induce myocardial ischemia. Although not essential, the continuous delivery of O_2 through a nasal cannula or nasal hood during treatment is recommended, especially in the ASA III or IV anginal patient.

IM sedation is not indicated. The use of IM sedation in adult patients is rarely indicated, the IM route being used primarily in the pediatric or handicapped patient. Should occasion arise to administer IM sedative drugs to an anginal patient (as when all other techniques have proved inadequate or unavailable), the level of sedation should be kept light to moderate. O_2 should be delivered through a nasal cannula or nasal hood throughout the procedure and recovery period.

Inhalation sedation is highly recommended. N_2O-O_2 inhalation sedation is the preferred technique of sedation for the anginal patient. Since anginal episodes are provoked by an unmet myocardial O_2 requirement, the administration of N_2O-O_2 will serve the following purposes: (1) sedation of the patient, (2) increase in the pain reaction threshold, and (3) increased oxygenation of the patient's body, including the myocardium. Not only will N_2O-O_2 minimize any increase in myocardial activity as a result of its sedative and analgesic properties, the patient will usually be receiving more than 50%, or at the least approximately 25%, O_2. This represents a 25% to 50% increase in O_2 available to the cells of the patient's body. N_2O-O_2 is the most nearly ideal sedative technique for the anginal patient.

IV sedation is recommended for the more fearful anginal patient. Levels of sedation should be kept light (e.g., diazepam or midazolam) to minimize respiratory depression, hypoxia, and myocardial ischemia. In addition, the patient should receive O_2 by nasal cannula or nasal hood throughout the procedure.

General anesthesia is not recommended for all anginal patients. Outpatient general anesthesia in the patient with angina is generally not indicated because of the increased risk of hypoxia during anesthesia as well as the stress of general anesthesia and the surgical procedure. Anginal patients requiring general anesthesia usually require hospitalization and treatment as described for inpatient procedures.

Unstable angina

Unstable angina is also known as intermediate coronary syndrome, preinfarction angina, premature or impending myocardial infarction, or coronary insufficiency. It is a syndrome intermediate between angina pectoris and acute myocardial infarction.

Since the mortality rate from acute myocardial infarction is greatest within the first few hours, recognition of a syndrome that has an increased likelihood of impending myocardial infarction requires immediate hospitalization and monitoring of the patient in an intensive care unit to prevent sudden dysrhythmias and death.

Unstable angina is recognized by the appearance of pain that is different in character, duration, radiation, and severity from the typical stable anginal episode or pain that, over a period of hours or days, demonstrates progressive ease of induction (decreased exercise tolerance) or that develops at rest or during the night.

Patients with unstable angina who do not develop signs and symptoms of acute myocardial infarction are considered to be in precarious balance between coronary artery supply and myocardial demand and should be treated as though they they had suffered a myocardial infarction.

Patients with unstable angina are ASA IV risks and are not candidates for elective dental or surgical care. Immediate medical consultation is recommended. In the event that emergency care is required, hospitalization of the patient should receive serious consideration. O_2, delivered by nasal cannula or nasal hood, is recommended throughout the procedure, and N_2O-O_2 inhalation sedation is the only sedative technique to be considered for this patient. Medical consultation is definitely indicated before any treatment on this very high-risk individual is contemplated.

Oral sedation is indicated if absolutely necessary. Light levels of CNS depression only should be sought. The administration of O_2 to this patient throughout the procedure is recommended.

IM sedation is not recommended in unstable angina because of the possibility of hypotension, which would further compromise coronary blood flow, and respiratory depression.

Inhalation sedation is recommended in unstable angina because of the increased O_2 delivery to the patient throughout the procedure.

IV sedation is not recommended in unstable angina unless the situation absolutely demands it. The possibilities of hypotension and respiratory depression, although minimal, could further aggravate the precarious balance between coronary O_2 supply and demand. Lighter levels of sedation, such as that achieved with benzodiazepines, plus supplemental O_2 would best serve this patient.

Myocardial infarction

Myocardial infarction is defined as a clinical syndrome resulting from a deficient coronary arterial blood supply to a region of myocardium. It results in cellular death and necrosis. Synonyms for myocardial infarction include *coronary occlusion, coronary thrombosis,* and *heart attack.*

More than 1,500,000 Americans suffer acute myocardial infarction annually. In 1985 ischemic heart disease and acute myocardial infarction (MI) were responsible for 801,700 deaths in the United States.[1] It is the leading cause of death in the United States and is responsible for 35% of deaths occurring in men between the ages of 35 and 50 years.

Patients who are status post-MI (patients who have suffered an acute myocardial infarction and survived) represent a definite risk during dental and surgical treatment. Immediately after the myocardial infarction the incidence of reinfarction is quite high (36% reinfarction rate on surgical patients within 3 months of first myocardial infarction).[2,3] With the passage of time and the formation of a myocardial scar, the incidence of reinfarction declines. The incidence falls to 16% at 5 months for post-MI patients undergoing surgical procedures and to 5% at 6 months after infarction. The reinfarction rate then levels off at 5% and remains at that point indefinitely. By comparison, the infarction rate during surgical procedures for a patient who has not had a myocardial infarction is less than 0.1%.

Status post-MI patients may be receiving a number of drugs to manage post-myocardial infarction complications such as CHF, angina, and dysrhythmias. Drug categories include anticoagulants, antidysrhythmics, digitalis, vasodilators such as nitroglycerin, and medications for high blood pressure.

The status post-MI[1] patient is considered an ASA III patient if more than 6 months have passed since the initial myocardial infarction and no further cardiovascular complications have developed. In the event that cardiovascular complications have developed following the myocardial infarction, medical consultation should be obtained. This patient will be classified as either an ASA III or IV risk depending on the severity of the prior myocardial infarction and the degree of cardiovascular dysfunction still present. In the 6 months following the myocardial infarction the patient is an ASA IV risk and should have elective treatment deferred until a full 6 months after the infarction. In the event that emergency care is required, hospitalization should be seriously considered.

An acute myocardial infarction may be precipitated when the patient undergoes unusual stress, whether physical (pain) or emotional (anxiety). Unfortunately, however, the patient need not be undergoing any physical activity at the time of onset of the myocardial infarction. Alpert and Braunwald[4] reported that 51% of patients were at rest and 8% were asleep when the signs and symptoms of myocardial infarction initially developed. Of the patients 18% were performing moderate or usual exertion, whereas only 13% were physically exerting themselves. It therefore appears to be more a matter of (bad) timing than a result of dental treatment when an acute myocardial infarction develops in the dental office. Stress, however, will increase the risk to the status post-myocardial infarction patient and must be considered.

Sedation in the status post-MI patient is extremely valuable since these patients are usually intolerant of stress. Increased myocardial O_2 demand that is not met can lead to serious complications, including anginal pain, increased severity of CHF, serious dysrhythmias, and reinfarction.

Oral sedation is recommended for light levels of sedation (see Chapter 8). More profound sedation increases the risk of hypotension and respiratory depression with hypoxia. In the event that this does occur, airway maintenance and the administration of supplemental O_2 are essential. IM sedation is not recommended unless other techniques are unavailable or ineffective. Only light-to-moderate sedation is indicated, and the administration of O_2 by nasal cannula or nasal hood is recommended.

Inhalation sedation is highly recommended. N_2O-O_2 inhalation sedation provides the myocardium with excess O_2 throughout the procedure. N_2O-O_2 has been used by paramedical and medical personnel in the management of the patient during the acute myocardial infarction and has proved valuable in decreasing or eliminating the pain of myocardial infarction.[5]

IV sedation is recommended in cases in which inhalation sedation has proved ineffective. Lighter levels of sedation only are recommended in the ASA III patient with supplemental O_2 administered. Hospitalization should be considered for the ASA III patient and is highly recommended for the ASA IV patient for whom only emergency care is recommended and then only in a controlled environment.

Both outpatient and inpatient general anesthesia for elective dental or medical procedures are relatively contraindicated in the status post-MI patient. The risk of reinfarction in this patient during general anesthesia is such that other techniques should be attempted before considering the use of general anesthesia.

High blood pressure

Elevations in blood pressure are not uncommon within the dental office, since the stress associated with treatment leads to increased catecholamine release and subsequent elevations in the rate of the heart and blood pressure. In Chapter 5 the ASA classifications for blood pressure were presented. The two categories that must be reviewed are the ASA III and IV patients. ASA III patients have a blood pressure reading of 160 to 199 mm Hg (ASA IIIa 160-179 mm Hg, IIIb 180-199 mm Hg) systolic, and/or 95 to 115 mm Hg (IIIa 95-104 mm Hg, IIIb 105-115 mm Hg), diastolic. Patients in this classification may receive dental care; however, steps should be taken to prevent any further increase in blood pressure. Two of the most important steps are the management of pain through the effective use of local anesthesia (vasopressors are not contraindicated) and the management of fear and anxiety. The ASA IV patient has a systolic blood pressure above 200 mm Hg and/or a diastolic blood pressure in excess of 115 mm Hg. Elective dental care should be postponed until the blood pressure is better controlled. Emergency procedures may be performed; however, sedation and effective pain control are mandatory to prevent any further elevation in blood pressure. Hospitalization of the ASA IV patient who requires emergency dental care should receive serious consideration.

Further elevation of the hypertensive patient's blood pressure may lead to a number of acute cardiovascular crises, including CVA (stroke), acute myocardial infarction, acute renal failure, and acute heart failure (pulmonary edema).

Most patients with high blood pressure are receiving antihypertensive drugs to lower their blood pressure. Many drugs, each of which has its own side effects, are used in the management of high blood pressure. The doctor must be aware of these side effects and possible drug-drug interactions and take steps to minimize their occurrence or at least be able to manage them successfully. Table 38-1 lists the major categories of antihypertensive drugs and their more common side effects.

The primary side effects of antihypertensive drugs of concern during ambulatory patient care are orthostatic hypotension, CNS-depression, and sedation. Prevention of serious orthostatic hypotension requires that alterations in chair position be made gradually, permitting the patient to adapt to the increasing effect of gravity as he or she rises. Many CNS-depressant drugs, especially the opioids, can enhance this effect of the antihypertensive drugs. The use of sedatives in patients who are somewhat depressed or sedated from their high blood pressure drugs must be handled with extreme care in order to prevent excessive sedation from developing. Techniques in which titration is possible are, as always, preferred.

Elevations in a patient's blood pressure can be expected during dental procedures, especially those that are potentially traumatic. The stress-reduction protocols are especially valuable in these patients. Adequate pain control through the use of local anesthetics with vasopressors (if indicated) and anxiety reduction will enable these patients to receive dental care with a minimum of risk.

In the patient with elevated blood pressure, additional stress will further elevate blood pressure. Increased blood pressure can lead to acute medical crises. The use of sedative techniques will minimize or eliminate any further blood pressure elevations and thereby decrease patient risk during treatment.

Oral sedation is recommended.

IM sedation is recommended. Opioid analgesics can enhance orthostatic hypotension produced by some antihypertensive drugs.

Inhalation sedation is recommended. Inhalation sedation may be used in patients who have blood pressure readings slightly above the ASA IV level (i.e., 206/112 mm Hg). N_2O-O_2 is titrated to the point at which the patient is comfortably relaxed. The patient's blood pressure is rechecked at this time. If it has decreased below the ASA IV level, the scheduled treatment may proceed; however, in cases in which the blood pressure remains elevated (above 200/115 mm Hg), treatment should be cancelled, and the patient oxygenated and dismissed.

IV sedation is recommended. Opioid analgesics can enhance orthostatic hypotension produced by some antihypertensive drugs.

General anesthesia is indicated in patients with minimal increases in blood pressure (ASA II or IIIa) for traumatic procedures in which sedative techniques are not indicated or have proved ineffective.

Table 38-1. Side effects and drug interactions of antihypertensive medications

Drug	Major side effects	Drug interations
ACE-inhibitors	Hypotension	
	Reversible renal insufficiency	
	Reversible hyperkalemia	
Clonidine	Drowsiness	
	Orthostatic hypotension	
	Xerostomia	
Guanethidine	Orthostatic hypotension	Alcohol increases orthostatic hypotension
Hydralazine	Tachycardia	
	Palpitation	
	Increased angina	
	Increased CHF	
Loop diuretics	Hypokalemia	
α-Methyldopa	Orthostatic hypotension	
	Drowsiness	
	Depression	
	Xerostomia	
Potassium-sparing diuretics	Hyperkalemia	
	Nausea (triamterene)	
Prazosin	Orthostatic hypotension with syncope	
	Dizziness	
	Weakness	
	Blurred vision	
	Nausea	
	Headache	
	Palpitation	
Propranolol	Bradycardia	Epinephrine may induce bradycardia
	CHF	
	Increased asthma	
	Weakness	
	Depression	
Reserpine	Drowsiness	Hypotension with general anesthesia
	Sedation	
	Weakness	
	Depression	
	Bradycardia	
Thiazide diuretics	GI upset	
	Weakness	
	Hypokalemia	
	Hyperglycemia	

The ASA II patient may be managed as an outpatient, whereas it has been suggested that ASA III and IV patients might be better managed as inpatients.

Dysrhythmias

Rhythm disturbances of the myocardium are not uncommon. Fortunately most dysrhythmias are of a relatively benign nature, in that the myocardium is still able to function effectively as a pump. However, there are some dysrhythmias that are potentially more dangerous, requiring treatment or immediate referral to a physician for management.

Patients with dysrhythmias of significance will be taking antidysrhythmic drugs. These include propranolol, procainamide, quinidine, and disopyramide.

In the absence of the ECG and training in its interpretation, the dentist is frequently unable to determine the nature of the dysrhythmia that is detected. Termination of dental treatment, the administration of O_2, and the consideration for immediate medical consultation are indicated in such cases.

Dysrhythmias may develop in the heart with organic disease, for example, in the status postmyocardial infarction patient, as well as in the "normal, healthy" heart. Stress, the ingestion of certain substances, or the administration of certain drugs can precipitate or exacerbate cardiac dysrhythmias. Caffeine and nicotine are examples of two substances that may precipitate dysrhythmias, whereas several of the inhalation anesthetics, including halothane, sensitize the myocardium to catecholamines. Stress releases large volumes of the catecholamines, epinephrine and norepinephrine, into the blood, increasing myocardial workload as well as inducing dysrhythmias.

The use of sedation is indicated for patients with most rhythm disturbances. Although all techniques may be used, it is important that hypoxia and hypotension be avoided because of their dysrhythmogenic characteristics.

Oral sedation is recommended.

IM sedation is recommended in cases in which other sedative procedures have proved ineffective. The use of supplemental O_2 delivered by nasal cannula or nasal hood is recommended.

Inhalation sedation is recommended. Use of N_2O-O_2 increases oxygenation, thereby eliminating one possible cause of dysrhythmias.

IV sedation is recommended. O_2 supplementation is warranted to minimize hypoxia.

In patients in whom the dysrhythmia is well controlled through the use of medications and no other cardiovascular disease is evident, IV outpatient general anesthesia might be considered, although this patient should be considered a candidate for hospitalization. ECG monitoring throughout the procedure is recommended, as well as supplemental nasal O_2. The administration of inhalation anesthetics such as halothane, which sensitize the myocardium to catecholamines, is contraindicated. A commonly used general anesthesia technique for patients with dysrhythmias is N_2O-O_2 and intravenous opioids.

Local anesthesia is recommended for intraoperative pain management. The use of vasopressor-containing solutions is not contraindicated in most ASA II, and III patients. Epinephrine-impregnated gingival retraction cord should not be used in these patients.

Table 38-2 lists contraindications (absolute and relative) to the inclusion of vasopressors in local anesthetic solutions.

Congestive heart failure

Heart failure is a pathophysiological state in which an abnormality in cardiac function is responsible for failure of the heart to pump blood in a volume adequate to meet the requirements of the metabolizing tissues. Left heart failure is associated with signs and symptoms related to pulmonary vascular congestion; right heart failure commonly exhibits signs and symptoms of systemic venous and capillary engorgement. Left and right heart failure may develop independently or they may coexist. The term *congestive heart failure* (CHF) refers to the combination of left and right heart failure in which there is evidence of both pulmonary and systemic congestion.

Pulmonary edema is usually an acute condition marked by excess serous fluid in the alveolar spaces or interstitial tissues of the lungs accompanied by extreme difficulty in breathing.

Heart failure may be produced by a number of etiological factors, including coronary artery disease;

Table 38-2. Contraindications to use of vasoconstrictors

Absolute contraindications

1. Unstable angina pectoris (preinfarction angina, crescendo angina)
2. Recent myocardial infarction (<6 months)
3. Recent coronary artery bypass surgery (<6 months)
4. Refractory dysrhythmias
5. Untreated or uncontrolled severe hypertension (>200 and/or >115)
6. Untreated or uncontrolled severe congestive heart failure
7. Uncontrolled hyperthyroidism
8. Uncontrolled diabetes
9. Sulfite sensitivity
10. Pheochromocytoma

Relative contraindications

1. Patients taking tricyclic antidepressants
2. Patients taking phenothiazine compounds
3. Patients taking monoamine oxidase inhibitors (MAO-Is)
4. Patients taking nonselective beta-blockers
5. Cocaine abuser

Modified from Perusse R, Goulet JP, Turcotte JY: Contraindications to vasoconstrictors in dentistry, *Oral Surg* 74:679, 1992.

myocarditis; hypertension; aortic or pulmonary valve stenosis; hypertrophic cardiomyopathy; aortic, mitral, or tricuspid valve insufficiency; thyrotoxicosis; anemia; pregnancy; and congenital left-to-right shunts. Heart failure is a common sequela of myocardial infarction.

The annual rate of development of heart failure is 2.3 per 1000 in males and 1.4 per 1000 in females (Framingham study).[6] The incidence rises considerably after the age of 50 years. High blood pressure is a common precursor with over 75% of patients with CHF having a history of preexisting high blood pressure.

Patients with heart failure frequently take medications to control their high blood pressure and digitalis preparations. Digitalis increases cardiac output, decreases right atrial pressure, decreases venous pressure, and increases the excretion of sodium and water.

There is considerable variation in the degree of severity of heart failure. A commonly used method of classification of CHF is called the "functional reserve category." Four classes are recognized, based on a patient's ability to climb a normal flight of stairs (Fig. 38-2). The functional reserve classification is defined as follows:

1. Patient is able to climb a normal flight of stairs without pausing and can continue walking without resting.
2. Patient is able to climb a normal flight of stairs without pausing but must stop at top of the stairs to catch his breath.
3. Patient is able to climb a normal flight of stairs but must pause before reaching the top of the stairs to catch his breath.
4. Patient is unable to climb a normal flight of stairs.

These numbers can be considered the ASA physical status classification for CHF.

Hypoxia or stress can increase the degree of heart failure by increasing the workload of the myocardium and by increasing its requirement for oxygen. Use of the stress-reduction protocol is of considerable importance in management of CHF patients. Scheduled appointments early in the morning when the patient is well rested, limiting the length of the appointment so as not to exceed the limit of the patient's tolerance, and monitoring vital signs preoperatively are recommended. Should the weather be extremely warm or humid or if the patient appears somewhat fatigued prior to the start of treatment, it is prudent to postpone the planned treatment to another day. Intraoperatively, the need for effective pain and anxiety control is quite important since increased stress produces an increased myocardial workload and an increase in the degree of heart failure.

Positioning of patients with CHF may require modification from that recommended for the sedated patient. Although the supine or semisupine position is strongly recommended for patients during sedative procedures, the patient with CHF may demonstrate orthopnea, which may preclude the use of this position. Should this occur, the patient should be positioned in the most recumbent position in which he can still breathe comfortably.

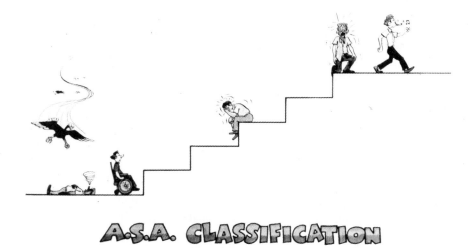

Fig. 38-2. ASA classification for CHF. (Courtesy Dr. Lawrence Day.)

Local anesthetics containing vasopressors are indicated for pain control in the patient with CHF. The recommended concentration of epinephrine is 1:100,000 or 1:200,000.

There are no contraindications to the use of any of the techniques of sedation in the patient with CHF. It is important to remember that the primary problem in this patient is the failure of the heart to deliver an adequate volume of blood and O_2 to the tissues of the body. Because all of the drugs used in sedative techniques are CNS, respiratory, and potential cardiovascular depressants, it is essential that any additional hypoxia be prevented from developing during the procedure. The ASA II patient is an excellent candidate for sedation with any technique, whereas the ASA III patient should be restricted to lighter levels of sedation by oral or inhalation sedation.

Oral sedation is quite appropriate for the patient with CHF (ASA II or III) for preoperative anxiety control. Light levels of sedation only should be sought, such as that obtained with the benzodiazepines.

IM sedation should be reserved for the patient in whom other more controllable techniques have proved ineffective. Light to moderate levels of sedation should be sought with O_2 supplementation throughout the procedure in the ASA II patient only. Drugs such as opioids and barbiturates, which are potent respiratory depressants, should be used with considerable care, if at all.

N_2O-O_2 inhalation sedation is an appropriate technique for the ASA II or III CHF patient because it provides sedation and analgesia as well as additional O_2 for the patient.

Light to moderate levels of IV sedation are recommended for the ASA II patient with CHF. Supplemental O_2 is recommended for all IV sedative procedures. The use of IV sedation is not recommended for use in the ASA III CHF patient unless it is considered essential by the doctor, in which case only lighter levels of sedation are recommended (with O_2 supplementation).

Outpatient general anesthesia is not recommended for the ASA II, III, or IV patient with CHF. In-hospital general anesthesia should be considered in cases in which other sedative techniques have proved inadequate in patient management.

Congenital heart disease

The incidence of congenital heart disease is 9:1000 live births. Some of these defects develop as a result of genetic abnormalities; however, most congenital heart lesions occur in the absence of any detectable chromosomal abnormality. Although there are a tremendous number of congenital lesions, those listed in Table 38-3 account for more than 80% of those seen in children with congenital heart disease. Ventricular septal defects account for approximately one-third of all lesions, and atrial septal defects and patent ductus arteriosus account for 10% each; other relatively common defects include pulmonary stenosis and coarctation of the aorta. Others, although less common, are tetralogy of Fallot, aortic stenosis, and transposition of the great arteries.

Because of the great variation noted in the clinical signs and symptoms and relevance toward dental care of the congenital heart lesions, a thorough medical history, dialogue history, and clinical evaluation are absolutely essential. Once a history of congenital heart disease is obtained, medical consultation with the patient's (child or adult) physician is recommended.

Primary concerns associated with dental management of this patient include the exacerbation of heart failure and cardiac dysrhythmias caused by the stresses involved with dental therapy, and the possibility of infection leading to bacterial endocarditis. Consulting recent AHA, AMA, and ADA guidelines for prophylaxis and possible medical consultation with the patient's physician will provide a determi-

Table 38-3. Congenital heart lesions

Acynotic heart lesions with left-to-right shunts
Ostium secundum atrial septal defect
Anomalous pulmonary venous return
Endocardial cushion defects
Ostium primum atrial septal defect
Atrioventricular canal
Ventricular septal defects
Patent ductus arteriosus
Aorticopulmonary window and truncus arteriosus

Acyanotic heart disease with obstructive lesions
Coarctation of the aorta
Aortic stenosis
Pulmonary stenosis

Cyanotic heart lesions
Tricuspid artresia
Pulmonary artresia
Tetralogy of Fallot
Ebstein's anomaly of the tricuspid valve
Transposition of the great arteries

nation as to the requirement for prophylactic antibiotics.[7] In many patients with surgically repaired defects, the need for antibiotic coverage during dental care exists for life.

As specifically relates to the management of pain and anxiety in patients with congenital heart disease, pain control through the use of local anesthetics is a vitally important means of minimizing stress. The administration of local anesthetics containing vasopressors is not contraindicated in these patients.

Sedative techniques will be indicated as a method of minimizing intraoperative stress in this patient. The primary goal during sedation will be to provide adequate sedation without producing hypoxia. The myocardium of patients with congenital heart disease is less able to tolerate hypoxic episodes than healthy heart muscle.

Oral sedation is indicated for light levels of sedation. Deep sedation administered by the oral route is not indicated.

IM sedation should be reserved as a last-choice technique in cases where other sedative procedures have proved ineffective. Light-to-moderate levels of sedation only are recommended by the IM route along with supplemental O_2 throughout the procedure.

Inhalation sedation is an excellent sedation technique for these patients primarily because additional levels of O_2 are supplied throughout the procedure.

IV sedation is also recommended, provided the level of sedation remains light to moderate. Deep sedation is not recommended because of the increased likelihood of hypoxia and a depression of respiratory and cardiovascular function. Supplemental O_2 should be administered when IV sedation is used.

Outpatient general anesthesia is not recommended in patients with congenital heart lesions, whether repaired or not. General anesthesia should be reserved for those patients in whom sedative procedures have been ineffective. The patient will be admitted to the hospital prior to the procedure to receive a more in-depth medical evaluation due to the nature of his underlying disease.

Valvular heart disease

Valvular heart disease is a common sequela of rheumatic fever. The incidence of valvular heart disease from rheumatic fever has been diminishing in the past two decades; however, congenital valvular lesions are being diagnosed with increasing regularity. It is estimated that more than 18,000 cardiac valvular replacements are performed annually in the United States.[8]

Most patients who have received valvular replacements have had their life expectancy prolonged. Along with this benefit, however, is the ever-present prospect of bacterial endocarditis. The reader is referred to the guidelines for prophylaxis, which present detailed antibiotic regimens for these patients.[7] The patient's physician should be consulted prior to dental treatment.

The primary concern during the dental management of the patient with valvular heart disease will be the prevention of bacterial endocarditis. In addition, stress must be minimized through the use of effective local anesthesia and the administration of sedative drugs, as indicated. Hypoxia should be avoided.

The administration of local anesthetics with vasopressors is indicated, if needed, in patients with valvular replacement.

Oral sedation is indicated for the management of lesser degrees of preoperative anxiety. Light levels of sedation only are recommended.

IM sedation is recommended in cases in which other sedative modalities have proved ineffective. Intraoperative O_2 administration is recommended for the light-to-moderate sedation recommended by the IM route.

Inhalation sedation with N_2O-O_2 is highly recommended for anxiety control in patients with valvular prostheses.

IV sedation is also recommended, with light-to-moderate levels only suggested. Intraoperative O_2 administration is suggested.

Outpatient general anesthesia is not recommended for the patient with a valvular prosthesis. Hospitalization and thorough work-up are strongly suggested.

RENAL DISEASE

Glomerulonephritis, pyelonephritis, nephrotic syndrome, chronic renal insufficiency, and chronic renal failure are among the more common disorders of renal function that are encountered. Renal dialysis and transplantation are used in the management of chronic renal failure. In 1984 it was estimated that more than 55,000 persons were undergoing dialysis for end-stage renal disease.[9] Approximately 4000 patients undergo renal transplantation annually in the United States.

Most patients with renal failure may be safely managed in the outpatient setting and represent ASA II,

III, or IV risks. Specific questioning and examination will determine the degree of risk of the patient.

All patients with altered renal function—especially those undergoing dialysis, in the days just prior to their dialysis appointments—must be managed carefully since their blood chemistries may be in disarray. It is recommended that dental appointments be scheduled on the day following dialysis so that the patient's metabolic status is optimal and the effects of systemic anticoagulation are minimal.

Prophylactic antibiotics may be required prior to dental care in the patient with renal disease, especially the renal transplant patient. Consultation with the patient's physician is strongly recommended to determine an appropriate regimen.

Many patients with chronic renal disease, especially patients having undergone renal transplantation, receive long-term corticosteroid therapy. Such therapy diminishes the patient's capacity to respond appropriately to increased stress. The administration of additional corticosteroid may be necessary prior to particularly traumatic (emotionally or physically) procedures. Medical consultation is recommended.

Patients undergoing renal dialysis as well as renal transplant patients are considered to be high risks for contracting hepatitis B and should be evaluated prior to the start of dental care. Patients who are surface-antigen negative and surface-antibody positive may be treated in the usual manner, whereas those who are surface-antigen positive should be treated using current recommendations to minimize transmission of hepatitis B. There is also an increased risk of HIV and AIDS infection. This increased risk should be considered prior to the use of parenteral techniques of sedation.

Most drugs are excreted through the kidneys, a percentage of the drug unchanged along with its major metabolites. Drugs such as cocaine and gallamine, which are excreted entirely unchanged in the urine, should not be administered to patients undergoing renal dialysis. Blood levels of these drugs would be overly high, leading to a greater risk of overdose or toxic reaction. Approximately 10% to 15% of most amide local anesthetics are excreted unchanged in the urine, whereas virtually no ester local anesthetic is found unchanged in the urine, having undergone metabolism in the blood. Among drugs used for sedation, there is little problem in that only very small amounts of unchanged drug are found in the urine. Benzodiazepines and the opioids may be administered in the usual manner in both the patient with renal insufficiency and the functionally anephric patient. Aspirin is a drug that must have its dosage regimen changed from the usual every 3 to 5 hours to every 4 to 6 hours in renal insufficiency and to every 8 to 12 hours in the anephric patient.

Amide local anesthetics may be administered normally and there are no contraindications to the inclusion of vasopressors.

Oral sedation is indicated for light-to-moderate levels of sedation.

IM sedation is indicated for light-to-moderate levels of sedation. The increased risk of hepatitis B or AIDS in the dialysis patient must be considered prior to IM sedation.

Inhalation sedation is indicated.

IV sedation is indicated. The increased risk of hepatitis B or AIDS in the dialysis patient must be considered prior to IV sedation.

General anesthesia on an outpatient basis is not recommended in the patient with chronic renal disease. Because of the potential presence of metabolic disorders, the patient should be hospitalized and thoroughly evaluated prior to general anesthesia.

RESPIRATORY DISEASE

The patient with respiratory disease must be evaluated carefully prior to dental treatment and especially prior to the administration of any drug, such as a CNS depressant, that may further inhibit the patient's respiratory efforts. Many patients with chronic respiratory disorders have respiratory centers that are less sensitive to the normal stimulus for breathing: increased arterial CO_2 tension. Instead, these patients develop decreased arterial O_2 tension as their respiratory stimulus. Such patients may be described as hypercarbic (increased CO_2 tension) and hypoxic (decreased O_2 tension).

It is likely that many of these patients will be able to tolerate the stresses associated with their dental care with little or no modification necessary in their treatment. However, the addition of stress can greatly increase the risk of a serious exacerbation of their disease process. Sedative drugs, which possess varying degrees of potential for respiratory depression, must be used with great care in order to minimize any further reduction in the patient's respiratory drive.

Evaluation of the patient with chronic respiratory disease will primarily revolve around his ability to exchange O_2 and CO_2 effectively. Inability to do so will be demonstrated by the presence of clinical signs and symptoms. The most frequently observed respiratory disorders include asthma, COPD, bronchiectasis, and pneumonia.

Asthma

Asthma is a clinical state of hyperreactivity of the tracheobronchial tree, characterized by recurrent paroxysms of dyspnea and wheezing, which are the result of bronchospasm, bronchial wall edema, and hypersecretion by mucous glands. Several forms of asthma—extrinsic asthma, also known as allergic asthma; intrinsic asthma (nonallergic asthma); drug-induced asthma; exercise-induced asthma; and occupational asthma—are recognized.

It is estimated that asthma affects 6 to 8 million persons in the United States.[10] The typical asthmatic patient is asymptomatic between acute episodes but has varying degrees of respiratory distress during the acute asthmatic attack. Although the degree of respiratory distress is usually moderate, many persons die each year in the United States from asthma-related disorders.[11] The goal in the dental management of the asthmatic patient is to prevent the acute exacerbation.

The acute asthmatic episode may be triggered by any of the following items, probably the most significant of which in the dental management of this patient is increased stress:

Psychic stress
Antigen-antibody reaction (allergy)
Bronchial infection
Dust, fumes
Climate (smog, cold)
Drugs

Determination of the type of asthma present and its degree of severity are of primary importance to the doctor prior to the start of treatment. The typical asthmatic will be classified as ASA II, with an ASA III patient being defined as a patient with a frequency of more than one acute episode per week or with episodes at any frequency that are difficult to manage without medical attention.

Because the asthmatic patient appears asymptomatic between episodes, the doctor must be quite thorough in the dialogue history and physical examination of this patient. The doctor should determine which drug(s) the patient uses for management of acute episodes and request that the medication(s) be brought to all appointments. The acute asthmatic attack is in great part an episode of bronchial smooth muscle spasm (bronchospasm). To this is added the secretion of copious volumes of mucous and of bronchial wall edema. The drugs used to manage the asthmatic episode are termed bronchodilators, the more common being listed in Table 38-4.

The use of sedation in the asthmatic patient may be quite important in the prevention of acute episodes in situations in which stress or anxiety play a role. However, some of the drugs that are commonly used in the management of stress have the potential to provoke an acute episode of bronchospasm. Two examples of these are the barbiturates and opioids (especially meperidine), which are histamine-releasing drugs. These drugs should not be administered to the asthmatic patient.

Oral sedation is recommended for light-to-moderate levels of sedation. If possible, barbiturates and opioids should be avoided because of the potential for acute exacerbation. Chloral hydrate and hydroxyzine are frequently used effectively in the management of the asthmatic child.

IM sedation is recommended in the pediatric patient for whom other techniques are ineffective. Opioids and barbiturates, two commonly used drug groups, are relatively contraindicated in the asthmatic and should be avoided if possible. Nasal O_2 throughout the procedure is recommended. Inhalation sedation with N_2O-O_2 is the most recommended sedative technique for both pediatric and adult asthmatic patients. Although N_2O does not possess bronchodilating properties similar to halothane,

Table 38-4. Common medications used in long-term management of asthma

Drug group	Examples (generic names)
Sympathomimetic amines	Epinephrine
	Isoproterenol
	Metaproterenol
	Ephedrine
	Pseudoephedrine
	Terbutaline
Xanthine derivatives	Aminophylline
	Theophylline
	Oxtriphylline
	Dyphylline
Corticosteroids	Hydrocortisone
	Prednisone
	Beclomethasone
Sodium cromoglycate	Cromolyn sodium
Steroids	Azmacort

its sedative properties and the additional O_2 administered along with it effectively prevent acute asthmatic episodes from developing. The occasional misguided medical consultation recommends against use of N_2O-O_2 because some individuals believe that this technique may provoke bronchospasm. Inhalation agents that irritate the respiratory mucosa are, in fact, capable of provoking the acute attack; however, N_2O is not an irritating vapor and may be administered without increased risk (in fact, with decreased risk).

IV conscious sedation is recommended with the addition of O_2 by nasal administration. Opioids and barbiturates are contraindicated (the Jorgensen technique) in these patients.

Outpatient general anesthesia should be avoided in these patients because of the increased risk of bronchospasm during general anesthesia. Dental and medical care for the asthmatic patient requiring general anesthesia should be completed in the more controlled setting of the operating room of a hospital or day-surgery center.

Chronic obstructive pulmonary disease

Chronic obstructive pulmonary disease (COPD) is the most common cause of death and disability resulting from lung disease in the United States. There are two primary disease entities that comprise COPD—emphysema and chronic bronchitis. Unlike the patient with asthma who is essentially asymptomatic in periods between acute episodes, the COPD patient will appear more debilitated and chronically ill and represents a greater risk during treatment. The typical COPD patient is classified as an ASA III.

Emphysema

Emphysema represents a disease entity in which the interalveolar septa (including blood vessels) are destroyed, producing a coalescence of air spaces to form abnormally large cystic or bullous areas in the lungs that do not function in gas exchange. The primary symptom presented in emphysema is a variable degree of dyspnea on exertion. The chest is often enlarged in a hyperinflated (barrel-chest) position. A chronic cough with sputum production may be present, although this is not characteristic of the disease.

There is no effective treatment for emphysema. Medical management is symptomatic, attempting to improve the patient's quality and length of life. Patients are cautioned to avoid all toxic inhalants such as cigarette smoke and toxic fumes. Minor pulmo-

nary infection may readily produce respiratory failure in these patients; therefore, extraordinary care is maintained and vigorous treatment instituted at the first signs of infectious respiratory processes. Supplemental O_2 administered by low-flow nasal cannula (2 to 3 L/min) at home using portable O_2 devices is frequently required for these patients.

Chronic bronchitis

Chronic bronchitis is probably the most common debilitating disease in the United States. A strong relationship exists between chronic bronchitis and inhalation of irritating substances, most frequently cigarette smoke and various pollutants. Pathological findings in chronic bronchitis include hyperplasia and hypertrophy of the submucosal bronchial mucous glands, hyperplasia of bronchiolar goblet cells, squamous metaplasia of bronchial mucosal cells, chronic and acute inflammatory infiltrates in the bronchial submucosa, profuse inflammatory exudates in the lumens of bronchi and bronchioles, and denudation of bronchial mucosa. Primary clinical symptomatology includes chronic cough and sputum production. Chronic bronchitis is most often seen in smokers over the age of 35 years. For a diagnosis of chronic bronchitis to be established, a productive cough must have been present for a minimum of 3 months in the year in at least 2 consecutive years. As the disease progresses it is marked by recurrent episodes of acute respiratory failure resulting from infectious exacerbations of the bronchi. These episodes are marked by increased cough, change in sputum from clear to purulent, fever, dyspnea, and varying degrees of respiratory distress, managed with antibiotics, bronchodilators, and respiratory therapy.

Medical management of chronic bronchitis includes cessation of cigarette smoking and exposure to toxic inhalants and the prevention or vigorous management of any respiratory infections. Bronchodilators are also useful in the chronic management of these patients. Other measures included in management of some of these patients are home O_2 administration by nasal cannula and treatment of right heart failure (with diuretics), which occasionally develops in chronic bronchitis.

The progress and prognosis of chronic bronchitis is quite variable; however, in general there is a progressive deterioration of pulmonary function with increasing frequency of episodes of respiratory failure until death. The life expectancy in the typical patient once severe symptoms develop is rarely more than 5 to 10 years.

The typical patient with chronic bronchitis represents an ASA III risk; those with more mild symptomatology are ASA II and those who require supplemental O_2 at all times, have severe orthopnea, and a severe, productive cough are classified ASA IV. ASA IV patients should have their dental care postponed until a time when their health improves. If dental care is urgent, hospitalization is recommended.

Dental management of COPD patients may require altering the position of the patient from the recommended supine position because of the presence of orthopnea. The COPD patient should be positioned in the most recumbent position in which he is still able to breathe comfortably. Supplemental O_2 at low flows (2 to 3 L/min) may be administered by nasal cannula or nasal hood throughout the dental appointment, whether or not a sedative procedure is used.

Local anesthesia is indicated for the COPD patient. Vasopressors are not contraindicated.

Oral sedation may be indicated, but only for light levels of sedation. Opioids and barbiturates specifically are not recommended because of their greater propensity to depress respiration. Anticholinergics (atropine, scopolamine, and glycopyrrolate) and antihistamines (hydroxyzine) are contraindicated because they increase the viscosity of secretions in the respiratory tract.

IM sedation is rarely considered in the COPD patient, primarily because these disease processes are almost always seen in older adults. Because of the ability of many intramuscularly administered drugs to produce respiratory depression, this technique of drug administration is not recommended. If IM sedation is used, opioids and barbiturates are contraindicated, anticholinergics and antihistamines should not be used, and O_2 must be administered in a 2- to 3-L/min flow throughout the procedure. The benzodiazepine midazolam is the preferred IM sedative agent.

Inhalation sedation may be the only sedative technique that can be used in the COPD patient with an expectation of success that does not significantly increase the patient's risk of acute respiratory failure. Theoretically it is possible for the higher levels of O_2 administered with N_2O-O_2 to remove the stimulus for breathing in this patient (decreased arterial O_2 tension). In clinical practice, however, this situation is unlikely to develop and N_2O-O_2 remains the sedative technique of choice in COPD.

IV sedation is not recommended as a primary technique in COPD because of the increased sensitivity of these patients to hypoxia and respiratory depression. Opioids, barbiturates, antihistamines, and anticholinergics are contraindicated. Should IV sedation be necessary, light levels of sedation only, with agents that do not produce significant respiratory depression (benzodiazepines, propofol), and the administration of 2- to 3-L/min nasal O_2 throughout the procedure are recommended.

Outpatient general anesthesia is contraindicated in COPD. General anesthetic procedures should be relegated to inpatient procedures within the operating room, where thorough preoperative evaluation is obtainable and the patient can be observed both during and after the procedure prior to discharge.

NEUROLOGICAL DISORDERS

Neurological disorders, especially seizure disorders, CVA, and myasthenia gravis, are of concern to the practicing dentist and physician. The patient who has a disorder of the central nervous system must be evaluated carefully, especially when the use of the CNS-depressant drugs is contemplated.

Seizure disorders

Seizure disorders are characterized by abrupt transient symptoms of a motor, sensory, psychic, or autonomic nature, often associated with changes in consciousness. These changes are secondary to sudden transient changes in brain function associated with excessive rapid electrical discharges in the gray matter.

The outline in the box on p. 592 lists various types of seizure activity. The incidence of epilepsy (recurrent seizure activity) among the general population in North America is 0.5% to 1.0%.[12] It is estimated that more than 10 million persons have suffered at least one convulsion and more than 2 million have suffered two or more episodes. It is also estimated that more than 200,000 Americans have seizures more than once a month despite medical treatment.

Seizures encountered most frequently and those possessing the greatest potential for morbidity and mortality are those in group II: generalized seizures or seizures without local onset. Within this group are the tonic-clonic convulsive episode, represented clinically as grand mal or major epilepsy, and petit mal or minor epilepsy (also termed an "absence attack").

Among epileptics 70% have only one type of seizure, the remainder having two or more types. Gen-

---

INTERNATIONAL CLASSIFICATION OF EPILEPTIC SEIZURES

I. Partial seizures (seizures beginning locally)
   A. Partial seizures with elementary symptoms (generally without impairment of consciousness)
      1. With motor symptoms (includes Jacksonian seizures)
      2. With special sensory or somatosensory symptoms
      3. With autonomic symptoms
      4. Compound forms
   B. Partial seizures with complex symptoms (generally with impairment of consciousness), temporal lobe, or psychomotor seizures
      1. With impairment of consciousness only
      2. With cognitive symptoms
      3. With affective symptoms
      4. With "psychosensory" symptoms
      5. With "psychomotor" symptoms
      6. Compound forms
   C. Partial seizures secondarily generalized
II. Generalized seizures (bilaterally symmetric and without local onset)
      1. Absences (petit mal)
      2. Bilateral massive epileptic myoclonus
      3. Infantile spasms
      4. Clonic seizures
      5. Tonic seizures
      6. Tonic-clonic seizures (grand mal)
      7. Atonic seizures
      8. Akinetic seizures
III. Unilateral seizures (or predominantly)
IV. Unclassified seizures (due to incomplete data)

From Gastaut H: Clinical and electroencephalographical classification of epileptic seizures. *Epilepsia* 11:102, 1970. Reprinted with permission of Raven Press, Publishers, New York.

---

eralized tonic-clonic seizures are present in 90% of all epileptics (60% only grand mal; 30% grand mal plus others). Petit mal seizures are seen in 25% of epileptics (4% alone; 21% with other types). Petit mal is seen most often in children under 16 years of age. Psychomotor seizures are seen in approximately 18% of epileptics (6% alone; 12% mixed) and are minor seizures in which the victim loses contact with the environment for 1 or 2 minutes.

Epileptics are managed with anticonvulsant drugs, the goal being to prevent the occurrence of seizure activity by depressing the neuronal focus in the brain. Table 38-5 lists commonly used anticonvulsants. Primary dental treatment concerns with these patients are the prevention of seizure activity and the management of the patient should a seizure develop. Factors acting to exacerbate seizures include psychological stress and fatigue. In the presence of apprehension over the planned procedure, sedative techniques should be considered. The use of alcohol is absolutely contraindicated in epileptic patients, since it may precipitate seizure activity. No patient with a history of epilepsy should be treated if it is obvious that alcohol has recently been ingested, and alcohol should not be used as a sedative in epileptics. Most well-controlled epileptics (seizures developing rarely, less than one a month) are considered ASA II risks, with those having seizures more frequently considered ASA III. The degree of control over seizure activity is the primary factor in determining the risk involved in management of this patient.

Local anesthesia is indicated in the epileptic patient. Although the intravenous administration or the administration of overly large doses of local anesthetics may provoke seizure activity (generalized tonic-clonic), it is unlikely that careful administration, following aspiration and slow injection of minimal volumes of the local anesthetic, will produce a problem. Vasopressors may be included in the local anesthetic if required for adequate duration or hemostasis.

The use of sedative techniques in the epileptic is indicated, for they serve to decrease the patient's fears of dentistry. It is important, however, that cerebral hypoxia be avoided, because in the absence of adequate O_2 a seizure may be provoked. Adequate oxygenation is therefore quite important for the epileptic patient.

Oral sedation is indicated for the preoperative management of anxiety. When used to produce light levels of CNS depression only, supplemental O_2 is not required.

IM sedation is indicated in cases in which other techniques of sedation have proved ineffective. Supplemental O_2 is strongly recommended throughout the sedative treatment.

Inhalation sedation is an excellent technique for use in the epileptic patient. Occasional reports indicate that N_2O is capable of inducing seizure activity (it is allegedly epileptogenic) in seizure-prone patients.[13] Clinical experience with N_2O-O_2 over more than 100 years has conclusively proved its safety in the seizure-prone patient.[14,15]

Table 38-5. Drugs used in long-term management of epilepsy

Generic name	Proprietary name	Type of seizure	Side effects
Acetazolamide	Diamox	Grand mal, petit mal	Drowsiness, paresthesia
Carbamazepine	Tegretol	Psychomotor, grand mal	Diplopia, transient blurred vision, drowsiness, ataxia, bone marrow depression
Clonazepam	Clonopin	Petit mal, atypical petit mal, myoclonic, akinetic	Drowsiness, ataxia, agitation
Ethosuximide	Zarontin	Petit mal	Drowsiness, nausea, vomiting
Methsuximide	Celontin	Petit mal, psychomotor	Ataxia, drowsiness
Mephenytoin	Mesantoin	Grand mal, some cases of psychomotor; effective when petit mal and grand mal coexist	Nervousness, ataxia, nystagmus, pancytopenia, exofoliative dermatitis
Phenacemide	Phenurone	Psychomotor	Hepatitis, benign proteinuria, dermatitis, headache, and personality changes
Phenobarbital	—	One of the safest drugs for all seizures; may aggravate psychomotor seizures	Drowsiness, dermatitis
Phenytoin sodium	Dilantin	Safest drug for grand mal and some cases of psychomotor epilepsy; may accentuate petit mal	Gingival hypertrophy, rash, nervousness, ataxia, drowsiness, nystagmus
Primidone	Mysoline	Grand mal, especially in conjunction with other drugs	Drowsiness, ataxia
Valproic acid	Depakene	Petit mal, atypical petit mal, myoclonic, akinetic	Nausea and vomiting, drowsiness; interferes with platelets (similar to aspirin) and therefore may increase bleeding

IV sedation is also recommended in the fearful epileptic patient. Techniques that include the administration of benzodiazepines or barbiturates are favored since these drugs have anticonvulsant properties. The administration of supplemental O_2 throughout the procedure to minimize the possibility of hypoxia is strongly recommended. IV drugs such as ketamine, which provokes high-frequency EEG activity, are not recommended in epileptic patients.

General anesthesia in the epileptic patient should be limited to in-hospital procedures.

Cerebrovascular accident

Cerebrovascular accident (CVA) is a focal neurological disorder caused by the destruction of brain substance as a result of intracerebral hemorrhage, thrombosis, embolism, or vascular insufficiency. Synonyms for CVA include *stroke* and *cerebral apoplexy*.

CVAs are not uncommon in the adult population, although their occurrence in persons under the age of 40 years is quite rare. In the United States approx-imately 400,000 new acute CVAs are reported annually.[1] Although mortality rates from various types of CVA differ markedly, the overall rate is relatively high. More than 200,000 deaths are reported annually from CVA, making it the third leading cause of death in the United States (behind cardiovascular disease and cancer). The frequency with which CVA develops is emphasized by the fact that approximately 25% of routine autopsies (death from all causes) demonstrate evidence of prior CVA. CVAs are the most common form of brain disease. The average age of persons at the time of their first CVA is approximately 64 years. Fortunately, recent evidence demonstrates that the incidence of CVA is declining. For every 100 first episodes of CVA that occurred in a unit of adult population between 1945 and 1949, only 55 first episodes of CVA occurred between 1970 and 1974.[16] This decline is noted in both sexes and all age groups but is most notable in the elderly.

A number of factors that increase the risk of CVA have been identified. These include high blood pressure, diabetes mellitus, cardiac enlargement, hypercholesterolemia, the use of oral contraceptives, and cigarette smoking. Consistently elevated blood pressure has been demonstrated to be a major risk factor in development of both hemorrhagic and atherosclerotic forms of CVA. Evidence from the Framingham study has led to the belief that high blood pressure may well be the major risk factor in the development of acute hemorrhagic CVA.[17] It is estimated that the risk of developing an acute CVA increases by 30% for every 10-mm Hg elevation in systolic blood pressure above 160 mm Hg.

The status post-CVA patient represents a significant risk within the dental or medical office during treatment. Survivors of CVAs have a very good chance of recovering some degree of function. Gresham (1975) showed that 84% of CVA survivors were living at home, 80% were capable of independent mobility, and 69% had total independence in the normal activities of daily living, yet only 10% exhibited no functional deficit.[17] With independent mobility the status post-CVA patient expects to receive dental and surgical care; however, it must be kept in mind that the recurrence rate of CVAs is high and that pain and anxiety only add to the risk presented by these patients.

Patients who are status post-CVA will be receiving some or all of the following drugs: anticoagulants, antihypertensives, and aspirin. Anticoagulants are used in the status post-CVA patient primarily to minimize the risk of recurrence. Antihypertensive drugs are important in status post-CVA patients in whom high blood pressure is present. This includes approximately two-thirds of all CVA patients. The treating doctor must be aware of the many side effects of the antihypertensive drugs (Table 38-1). Low-dose aspirin therapy (300 mg four times a day) has been demonstrated to decrease the risk of CVA in men with transient cerebral ischemia (TCI).[18]

The typical status post-CVA patient represents an ASA II or III patient—ASA II if the patient has had a CVA more than 6 months prior and has no evidence of residual neurological deficit, ASA III if the patient has had a CVA more than 6 months earlier but has some degree of neurological deficit. The status post-CVA patient is classified as ASA IV if the CVA occurred less than 6 months earlier or if significant residual deficit remains.

Stress must be minimized in the status post-CVA patient. The stress-reduction protocol, especially shorter appointments, effective pain control, and the management of apprehension, is of great importance in these patients.

All CNS depressants are relatively contraindicated in the status post-CVA patient. Any of these drugs may produce hypoxia, which may provoke increased confusion, aphasia, and other potentially serious complications, such as seizures. It has been my experience that lighter levels of sedation, as produced with inhalation sedation, are quite safe and highly effective in reducing stress in the status post-CVA patient. However, sedative techniques should be reserved for the status post-CVA patient in whom their use is truly justified.

Local anesthetics with vasopressors are not contraindicated in the status post-CVA patient provided that negative aspiration precedes the slow administration of the drug and that blood pressure is not overly elevated.

Oral sedation will be quite valuable in the status post-CVA patient demonstrating a greater degree of preoperative anxiety. Only light levels of sedation are recommended, using drugs such as the benzodiazepines and hydroxyzine. Medical consultation with the patient's physician is recommended prior to the administration of these drugs.

IM sedation is contraindicated in the status post-CVA patient because of the lack of control maintained over the actions of the drugs and the increased potential for hypoxia.

Inhalation sedation remains the most highly recommended sedative technique for use in the status post-CVA patient. Medical consultation prior to its administration is recommended since some physicians may object to the use of this technique because of the fact that higher concentrations of O_2 may produce constriction of cerebral arteries, thus producing diminished cerebral blood flow with possible hypoxia. However, when sedation is required in the status post-CVA patient, inhalation sedation with N_2O-O_2 remains the preferred technique.

IV sedation should be reserved for only the most apprehensive status post-CVA patients and then only after medical consultation. Once again an increased possibility of hypoxia after IV drug administration mitigates against use of this technique. When considered essential to the success of therapy, lighter levels of sedation, as obtained with the benzodiazepines, are recommended. Supplemental oxygenation is strongly recommended. General anesthesia in the status post-CVA patient should be reserved for the hospital operating room environment, with the patient being admitted for a complete workup prior to the procedure and permitted to remain in the hospital until recovery is complete.

Myasthenia gravis

Myasthenia gravis is a neuromuscular disorder characterized by a marked weakness and easy fatigability of muscles. Although almost any muscle within the body may be affected, those muscles innervated by the bulbar nuclei (facial, oculomotor, laryngeal, pharyngeal, and respiratory muscles) are most often involved. The cause of myasthenia gravis is unknown, although investigators believe that it is a result of an autoimmune response.[19] Muscle fatigability is worsened by exertion and improved by rest.

Myasthenia gravis occurs in 1:20,000 persons and is more common in females (3:2), appearing most often between the ages of 20 and 30 years.

Clinical signs and symptoms include pronounced fatigability of muscles with subsequent weakness and paralysis. Weakness of extraocular muscles results in diplopia and strabismus. Ptosis of the eyelids is most pronounced later in the day. Difficulty with speech and swallowing may develop after prolonged use of these functions. The patient may have difficulty in use of the tongue, as well as a high-pitched nasal voice. The so-called myasthenic smile, a snarling, nasal smile, may be evident. Fluctuations in the severity of the disease (exacerbations and remissions) are common and unpredictable. Weakness is intensified by infection and certain drugs, such as increased dosages of anticholinesterases (e.g., physostigmine, neostigmine, edrophonium), aminoglycoside antibiotics (e.g., neomycin), and membrane stabilizers (e.g., procainamide and phenytoin).

Patients with myasthenia gravis are managed with anticholinesterases (see following box). In cases in which anticholinesterase drug management is ineffective, surgical removal of the thymus (thymectomy) or corticosteroid therapy is recommended. Side effects of anticholinesterase therapy include abdominal cramps, nausea, and vomiting. The addition of atropine or atropine-like drugs to the treatment regimen may alleviate or prevent side effects. In recent years plasmaphoresis has been demonstrated to have a beneficial effect in the control of acute exacerbations of myasthenia gravis.[20]

The prognosis for myasthenia gravis is that approximately 75% of myasthenic patients improve after thymectomy and many go into remission. Myas-

---

> ### DRUGS USED IN MYASTHENIA GRAVIS
>
> Pyridostigmine bromide (Mestinon)—especially effective in treatment of bulbar muscle weakness
> Neostigmine bromide
> Ambenonium chloride (Mytelase)—longer acting than neostigmine, with fewer side effects
> Edrophonium bromide (Tensilon)
> Ephedrine sulfate—administered with each dose of neostigmine; appears to enhance effectiveness of neostigmine

---

thenic crisis may occur, with sudden death from respiratory failure. Overtreatment with neostigmine or other anticholinesterases may produce extreme muscular weakness that may simulate myasthenic crisis.

Physostigmine (Antilirium) is administered in the management of emergence dilirium occurring from the administration of scopolamine or benzodiazepines. Exacerbation of myasthenia gravis occurs with infection and stress. A myasthenic crisis may be induced by a dental abscess or heightened anxiety about dental or surgical care. The myasthenic patient with a history of repeat crises should receive such therapy within the confines of a hospital or other facility where acute airway management, including intubation, is readily available.

The administration of drugs with muscle-relaxant properties should be reserved for those situations in which they are essential. Few such occasions will arise in the typical outpatient dental or surgical setting.

Local anesthetics are the preferred drugs for the management of pain in the myasthenic patient. Indeed, even in the hospitalized myasthenic the use of regional nerve block anesthesia is preferred to general anesthesia. Vasopressors are not contraindicated.

Sedative techniques may be used, but care must be taken to avoid the administration of skeletal muscle relaxants such as diazepam and midazolam. Medical consultation is definitely indicated prior to the start of treatment in the myasthenic patient.

Oral, IM, inhalation, and IV techniques may be used on an outpatient basis if it is determined that they are absolutely necessary after medical consultation. Agents that produce muscle relaxation, especially nondepolarizing muscle relaxants such as tubocurarine, are contraindicated in the myasthenic patient.

LIVER DISEASE

Liver disease is of great importance because the liver is responsible, in large part, for the biotransformation of most drugs. Hepatic dysfunction may be responsible for prolonged and exaggerated effects of many drugs utilized for pain and anxiety control. A thorough history must be elicited when liver disease is suspected.

Probably the most easily recognized sign of possible liver disease is the presence of jaundice, a yellowish appearance of the skin and sclera. Jaundice is evidence of the accumulation of bilirubin in body tissues. Another less common and less obvious sign of liver dysfunction is fetor hepaticus, a sweet, musty odor on the breath of the patient. Liver diseases of significance include viral hepatitis (type A, type B, and non-A non-B), chronic hepatitis, alcoholic hepatitis, fatty liver, nodular cirrhosis, and biliary cirrhosis.

It is extremely unlikely that the doctor will be called upon to treat the patient with active acute hepatitis. In the event that such an occasion develops, the primary concern on the part of the doctor and staff will be to prevent cross-contamination. Precautions will include masking and gloving as well as sterilization of all equipment. Vaccination of the doctor and staff with the hepatitis B vaccine is recommended. The degree of liver dysfunction evident in the patient during the acute phase of hepatitis should be known prior to treatment. Most local anesthetics (especially the commonly used amides) and CNS depressants are biotransformed in the liver. These drugs should be administered only if absolutely essential and then only in the smallest effective dose. Medical consultation prior to treatment is suggested. During the acute phase of hepatitis the patient may be quite debilitated and unable to tolerate additional stress. Treatment of an emergency nature only is recommended at this time.

Chronic hepatitis is defined as a chronic inflammatory reaction of the liver that persists for more than 6 months. Although different forms of this disease are seen, the doctor must make a determination of the state of liver dysfunction in the patient prior to the administration of drugs. Chronic active hepatitis is characterized by progression to cirrhosis, although milder cases may resolve spontaneously. When deterioration of the patient's condition is ev-

ident, approximately 66% of patients die within 5 years of the onset of symptoms.

Alcoholic hepatitis is the most common form of chronic hepatitis. A history of heavy drinking over many years is always found. Parenchymal necrosis of the liver occurs as a result of alcohol abuse. Alcoholic hepatitis is the precursor of alcoholic cirrhosis. Alcoholic hepatitis may be reversible, depending on the degree of liver damage. In those cases in which the prothrombin time has been prolonged (to the degree at which liver biopsy cannot be performed), the mortality rate is 42%.

Drug-induced liver disease may result from toxic responses to the administration of various therapeutic agents. Drug-induced liver disease can mimic viral hepatitis or biliary tract obstruction. Examples of drug-induced liver disease follow:

Viral hepatitis–like reactions
   Halothane
   Methoxyflurane
Cholestatic reactions—inflammation of portal areas, with features of allergy (eosinophilia)
   Chlorpromazine
   Prochlorperazine
   Promazine
   Chronic active hepatitis
   Chlorpromazine

The most common cause of nodular cirrhosis is the chronic abuse of alcohol. This disease involves hepatocellular injury, which leads to both fibrosis and nodular degeneration throughout the liver. Cirrhosis is a serious and irreversible disease that when advanced has a very poor prognosis. The response of the patient to most CNS-depressant drugs may be exaggerated and prolonged.

Primary biliary cirrhosis is a chronic liver disease manifested by cholestasis. Insidious in onset, it is seen most frequently in women between the ages of 40 and 60 years. Its primary symptom is pruritus, with jaundice developing within 2 years of its onset. Secondary biliary cirrhosis follows chronic obstruction to bile flow, which is usually produced by a calculus, neoplasm, stricture, or biliary atresia.

The major concerns facing the doctor when asked to manage a patient with liver disease include the possibly debilitated condition of the patient, the degree of hepatic dysfunction, and the possibility of cross-contamination of the office staff. ASA classifications for patients with liver disease will range from class II to class IV, based on signs and symptoms and the results of medical consultation.

In cases in which debilitation is obvious, elective dental care should be deferred until such time as the patient is better able to withstand the stresses involved in the treatment. Emergency care should be considered only after consultation with the patient's physician and managed in the least traumatic manner. Definitive care may be instituted after the patient's return to a better state of health.

The administration of drugs to the patient with serious liver damage increases the risk of development of ADRs because of the fact that the drug will undergo biotransformation into inactive metabolites at a considerably slower rate than usual. For example, the β-half-life of lidocaine in the healthy patient is 90 minutes, whereas with cirrhosis lidocaine's half-life may approach 450 minutes.[21] Elevated blood levels of the drug develop, resulting in a prolonged duration of clinical action of CNS-depressant drugs as well as a greater risk of side effects and overdose reactions. Most drugs used for the management of pain and anxiety undergo a significant percentage of their biotransformation in the liver. Dosages of these drugs must be determined after carefully considering the effects of diminished liver function. In general, drug dosages should be decreased to approximately 50% of the usual dose in that patient. It is even more prudent to avoid the administration of such drugs where possible. The problem of cross-contamination has been previously discussed.

Local anesthesia is recommended in these patients. Vasopressors are not contraindicated. Since the half-life of amide local anesthetics may be considerably prolonged when significant liver disease is present, minimal volumes of amide local anesthetics should be administered. Nerve blocks are recommended over large areas of infiltration, except in those patients in whom prothrombin times have been increased because of the extent of liver damage. In these patients infiltration, or nerve blocks which have a minimal risk of hemorrhage, are recommended.

Oral sedation is recommended as an excellent means of providing light levels of sedation. Drugs such as the benzodiazepines can be used with little increased risk in the patient with hepatic dysfunction.

IM sedation should be avoided wherever possible in the patient with hepatic dysfunction since the actions of the drug(s) will be prolonged and exaggerated. Opioids, a group of drugs commonly used in IM sedation, demonstrate an exaggerated clinical action in the presence of liver dysfunction and should be avoided.

Inhalation sedation with N_2O-O_2 is, without doubt, the safest and most effective sedative technique in the patient with hepatic dysfunction. Neither of these gases undergoes biotransformation in the liver, and neither demonstrates exaggerated clinical actions in the presence of liver disease. IV sedation is also relatively contraindicated in the presence of severe liver disease. Barbiturates and opioids may exhibit exaggerated and prolonged responses in these patients. The use of benzodiazepines is preferred in cases in which IV sedation is considered necessary.

Outpatient general anesthesia is also contraindicated in the presence of severe liver dysfunction. The patient for whom general anesthesia is contemplated should be hospitalized for a thorough preoperative evaluation, his condition stabilized, and the procedure completed in the operating room under careful monitoring.

ENDOCRINE DISORDERS

Several potentially important disease entities are related to dysfunction of the endocrine glands, including the thyroid, adrenal, pituitary, and parathyroid glands. Especially important to the practicing dentist and physician will be disorders of the thyroid and adrenal glands, specifically hyperthyroidism, hypothyroidism, hyperadrenocorticism (Cushing's syndrome), and hypoadrenocorticism (Addison's disease).

Thyroid gland dysfunction

Located in the neck on either side of the trachea, the thyroid gland produces and secretes hormones that perform an important function in regulating the level of biochemical activity in most tissues of the body. Proper functioning of the thyroid gland is essential for normal growth and development.

Dysfunction of the thyroid gland is a relatively common medical disorder. If diabetes mellitus is excluded, thyroid dysfunction accounts for 80% of all endocrine disorders. Dysfunction of the thyroid gland may occur through overproduction (hyperthyroidism) or underproduction (hypothyroidism) of thyroid hormone. In both instances clinical manifestations cover a broad spectrum ranging from subclinical dysfunction to acute life-threatening situations. Fortunately, however, most patients with thyroid dysfunction have milder forms of the disease.

Hyperthyroidism

Hyperthyroidism is also known by several other names, including thyrotoxicosis, toxic goiter (diffuse or nodular), Basedow's disease, Graves' disease, Parry's disease, and Plummer's disease. It may be defined as a state of heightened thyroid gland activity associated with the production of excessive quantities of the thyroid hormones thyroxine (T4) and triiodothyronine (T3). Because the thyroid hormones affect the cellular metabolism of virtually all organ systems, the signs and symptoms of hyperthyroidism may be noted in any part of the body. Untreated hyperthyroidism may lead to thyroid storm or crisis, which manifests itself in part as severe hypermetabolism.

The incidence of thyroid gland hyperfunction is 3 per 10,000 adults per year and is seen in females in a 5:1 ratio over males. Its peak incidence occurs between the ages of 20 and 40 years. Although its etiology is unknown, hyperthyroidism is more common in areas of iodine deficiency and has been demonstrated to have familial tendencies. It may manifest itself initially during periods of emotional and physical stress.

Patients with hyperfunction of the thyroid gland undergo treatment aimed at halting the excessive secretion of thyroid hormone. Management may involve surgical removal of all or part of the thyroid gland, long-term drug therapy with antithyroid drugs to achieve remission of the disease, or radioactive iodine therapy, rather than surgical excision. Frequently prescribed antithyroid drugs include thiouracil, propylthiouracil, methimazole (Tapazole), iothiouracil, and iodine.

Common signs and symptoms of hyperthyroidism are presented in Table 38-6. Mild degrees of thyroid hyperfunction may pass for acute anxiety, with little increase in clinical risk to the patient. It must be noted that several cardiovascular disorders, primarily angina pectoris, are exaggerated in hyperthyroidism. Severe hyperfunction is an indication for immediate medical consultation. Dental treatment should not begin until the underlying metabolic disturbance has been corrected.

Additional considerations in hyperthyroid patients include contraindications to the administration of several drugs:

1. Atropine and other anticholinergics—because of their vagolytic properties, which produce an increase in heart rate. This may be a factor in precipitating thyroid crisis.
2. Vasopressors—drugs such as epinephrine,

Table 38-6. Clinical manifestations of hyperthyroidism

Symptoms	Signs
Nervousness	Tachycardia
Increased sweating	Goiter
Hypersensitivity to heat	Skin changes
Palpitation	Tremor
Fatigue	Bruit over thyroid
Weight loss	Eye signs
Tachycardia	Atrial fibrillation
Dyspnea	
Weakness	
Increased appetite	
Eye complaints	

From Williams RH: *Textbook of endocrinology*, ed 6. Philadelphia, 1981, Saunders.

which act as cardiovascular stimulants and in the presence of a cardiovascular system already stimulated by the hyperthyroid state may precipitate cardiac dysrhythmias or thyroid storm. Local anesthetics with vasopressors may be used since they possess minimal epinephrine concentrations (1:100,000 and 1:200,000). Of greater risk, however, is the use of racemic epinephrine for gingival retraction. This substance is likely to precipitate unwanted side effects.

Patients who are mildly hyperthyroid might easily be mistaken for apprehensive patients. The use of conscious sedation is not contraindicated. Since the cause of the apparent nervousness is not truly dental in origin, but hormonal, the effectiveness of sedative drugs may be less than ideal.

Hypothyroidism

Hypothyroidism is a clinical state in which the tissues of the body receive an inadequate supply of thyroid hormones. The clinical picture of hypothyroidism relates to the patient's age at the time of onset and to the degree and duration of the hormonal deficiency. Cretinism is a clinical syndrome encountered in infants and children, resulting from deficiency of thyroid hormone during fetal and early life. Severe hypothyroidism developing in an adult is termed *myxedema*. Myxedema refers to the appearance of mucinous infiltrates beneath the skin. Severe, unmanaged hypothyroidism may ultimately lead to the loss of consciousness, a state termed *myxedema coma*.

Hypothyroidism in the adult usually develops as a result of idiopathic atrophy of the thyroid gland, a

Table 38-7. Clinical manifestations of hypothyroidism

Symptoms	
Weakness	Thick tongue
Dry skin	Edema of face
Coarse skin	Coarseness of hair
Lethargy	Pallor of skin
Slow speech	Memory impairment
Edema of eyelids	Constipation
Sensation of cold	Gain in weight
Decreased sweating	Loss of hair
Cold skin	Pallor of lips

From Williams RH: *Textbook of endocrinology*, ed 6. Philadelphia, 1981, Saunders.

process currently thought to occur through an autoimmune mechanism. Other causes of hypothyroidism include total thyroidectomy, ablation following radioactive iodine therapy (both procedures are frequently used in the management of hyperthyroidism), and chronic thyroiditis. Hypofunction of the thyroid gland is seen much more commonly in females, with a peak incidence about the time of menopause.

Patients with thyroid hypofunction receive thyroid extract or a synthetic preparation. The most frequently used drug and the one considered to be the drug of choice is levothyroxine sodium (Synthroid). Other drugs used in the management of hypothyroidism include liotrix (Euthyroid, Thyrolar) and dextrothyroxine (Choloxin).

Signs and symptoms of hypothyroidism are listed in Table 38-7. Patients who are clinically hypothyroid may represent an increased risk during medical and dental treatment involving the administration of CNS depressants. The hypothyroid patient is unusually sensitive to sedatives, opioids, tranquilizers, and other CNS depressants, including local anesthetics. Normal therapeutic doses of these agents may result in overdose reactions in the hypothyroid patient.

Prior to the start of treatment on the hypothyroid patient the following are recommended:
1. Medical consultation with the patient's physician
2. Use of CNS depressants with extreme caution
3. Seeking the presence of cardiovascular disease

NOTE: in the clinically hypothyroid patient there is an increased incidence of cardiovascular disease, especially in cases that have persisted for many years.

The patient who is hypothyroid or hyperthyroid, is receiving treatment, and is asymptomatic represents an ASA II risk, whereas the patient with clinical signs and symptoms is considered ASA III. The following are recommendations for the use of pain- and anxiety-control techniques for both hypothyroid and hyperthyroid individuals.

Local anesthesia is recommended in both conditions. The use of vasopressors is not contraindicated in the hyperthyroid individual; however, minimal volumes of the least concentrated solution should be employed. In the clinically hypothyroid patient the volume of local anesthetic should be minimized in order to prevent blood levels from becoming elevated. Overdose thresholds for local anesthetics in the hypothyroid patient may be decreased.

Oral sedation is recommended for both patients. The use of CNS depressants is relatively contraindicated in the clinically hypothyroid patient. In cases in which oral sedation is necessary, the barbiturates and opioids should NOT be used; instead, the benzodiazepines and nonbarbiturate sedative/hypnotics are preferred.

IM sedation is recommended for use only in cases in which other techniques have proved inadequate. The use of opioids and barbiturates is not recommended in the hypothyroid individual.

Inhalation sedation is highly recommended because of the degree of control maintained over the drugs action. In the hypothyroid patient, lower than usual concentrations of N_2O often prove adequate, whereas the hyperthyroid individual may require greater than usual concentrations or the technique may prove to be unsuccessful.

IV sedation should be used with extreme care in the hypothyroid patient, since the actions of most commonly used drugs will be exaggerated. This is especially true for the opioids and barbiturates, but is also true to a lesser degree with benzodiazepines. Careful, slow titration minimizes any adverse response. The hyperthyroid patient may prove difficult to sedate adequately within the dosage limits presented earlier (Chapter 27). Failure of the technique to provide adequate sedation is preferred to the administration of dosages in excess of those recommended.

Outpatient general anesthesia is contraindicated in the clinically hyperthyroid or hypothyroid patient. Hospitalization prior to the procedure, complete medical evaluation, and stabilization of the disease process should be considered prior to the administration of any general anesthetic in these patients.

Patients with thyroid gland dysfunction, whether hyperfunction or hypofunction, who are receiving or have received treatment, have normal levels of circulating thyroid hormones, and are asymptomatic, are considered to be euthyroid (ASA II). Euthyroid patients may receive dental and medical treatment in the usual manner.

Adrenal disorders

The adrenal gland is a combination of two glands, the cortex and the medulla, which are fused together yet remain distinct and identifiable. The adrenal cortex produces and secretes over 30 steroid hormones. Cortisol, one of the glucocorticoids, is considered to be the most important product of the adrenal cortex. It permits the body to adapt to stress and is therefore extremely vital to continued survival.

Adrenal hypersecretion of cortisol leads to increased fat deposition in certain areas—the face (Fig. 38-3, *A*) and a "buffalo hump" (Fig. 38-3, *B*) on the back—increases in blood pressure, and alterations in blood cell distribution (eosinopenia and lymphopenia). Clinically cortisol hypersecretion is referred to as Cushing's syndrome and is usually readily corrected through surgical removal of a part or all of the adrenal gland. Renal and adrenal surgery are important factors in the development of primary adrenal cortical insufficiency.

The Cushing's syndrome patient is a class II risk. The doctor should evaluate the patient carefully for high blood pressure, signs and symptoms of heart failure, diabetes mellitus, and possible emotional disorders (depression). The use of local anesthetics and other CNS depressants for sedation is not contraindicated in these patients. Medical consultation is recommended prior to beginning therapy.

Inadequate production and secretion of cortisol, on the other hand, may lead to the relatively rapid

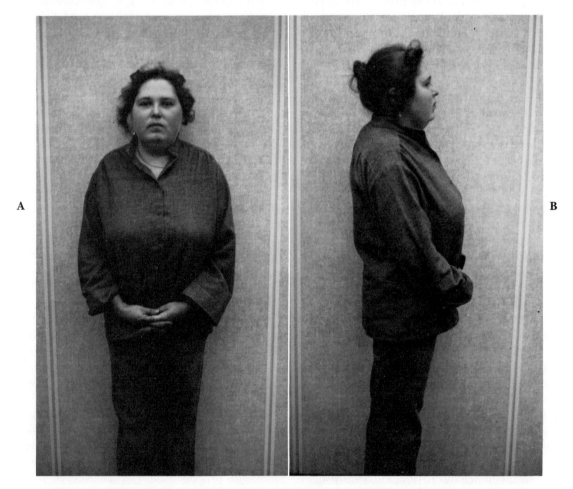

Fig. 38-3. Hypersecretion of the adrenal cortex, or chronic administration of corticosteroids leads to an increased fat deposition in the face (**A**) and back (**B**).

development of signs and symptoms. Primary adrenocortical insufficiency is termed Addison's disease, an insidious and usually progressive disease. The incidence of Addison's disease is estimated at 0.3 to 1.0 per 100,000 persons, occurring equally in both sexes and in all age groups. Although all corticosteroids may be deficient in this disease state, it is important to note that the administration of physiological doses of cortisol will correct most of the pathophysiological effects. Clinical manifestations of adrenal insufficiency do not develop until at least 90% of the adrenal cortex has been destroyed.

A second form of adrenocortical hypofunction may be produced through the administration of exogenous glucocorticosteroids to a patient with normal adrenal cortices. In the development of acute adrenal crisis, secondary adrenal insufficiency is a much greater potential threat than Addison's disease. Glucocorticosteroid drugs are widely prescribed in pharmacological doses for the symptomatic relief of a wide variety of disorders. When utilized in this way, glucocorticosteroid administration produces disuse atrophy of the adrenal cortex, decreasing the ability of the adrenal cortex to produce the levels of corticosteroid necessary to cope with stressful situations, which in turn leads to the development of signs and symptoms of acute adrenal insufficiency.

Patients with Addison's disease require corticosteroid administration in replacement (physiological) doses for life. However, patients receiving glucocorticosteroids for symptomatic treatment of their disorders commonly receive larger (pharmacologic or therapeutic) doses. These large doses may produce suppression of the normal adrenal cortex if continued for any length of time.

The "Rule of Two's" is valuable in determining risk in patients who are currently taking or have recently taken glucocorticosteroids.[22] It states that adrenocortical suppression should be suspected if a patient has received glucocorticosteroid therapy:

1. In a dose of 20 mg or more of cortisone or its equivalent daily
2. By the oral or parenteral route for a continuous period of 2 weeks or longer
3. Within 2 years of dental therapy

Following long-term exogenous corticosteroid therapy the adrenal cortex may require up to 9 months for a full recovery to normal function. Others have estimated that normal function may not return for as long as 2 years following long-term corticosteroid use.[23]

Since patients in these two categories are unable to adapt to stress in the usual manner, dental treatment must be modified to meet their needs. The stress-reduction protocol is extremely important in the overall management of these persons. In addition, both groups of patients require increased doses of their glucocorticosteroid drugs during and after the treatment period. Fig. 38-4 is an example of a corticosteroid coverage protocol. Since stress represents a significant factor in increasing the risk involved in treatment of these patients, the requirement for adequate pain and anxiety control is critical.

Local anesthetics, with and without vasopressors, are indicated for use in these patients.

All techniques of sedation are indicated. There are no contraindications to any technique or to specific drugs discussed previously.

Outpatient general anesthesia is contraindicated because of the increased stress associated with its administration, even in the best of situations. The patient with adrenal insufficiency, either primary or secondary, should be hospitalized for any general anesthetic procedure.

METABOLIC AND GENETIC DISORDERS

A number of disorders of metabolism and genetics are of potential importance in the management of pain and anxiety. The following disorders—diabetes mellitus, porphyria, malignant hyperthermia, and atypical plasma colinesterase—are discussed in the following paragraphs.

Diabetes mellitus

Diabetes mellitus is a chronic systemic disease characterized by disorders in the production or utilization of insulin, in the metabolism of carbohydrate, fats, and protein, and in the structure and function of blood vessels. Diabetes is characterized by an inappropriately elevated level of glucose in the blood, termed *hyperglycemia*.

Diabetes mellitus is present in 1% to 2% of the population of the United States. This represents approximately 2 to 4 million persons and includes only diagnosed diabetic persons. Another 1% to 2% of the population is believed to have undiagnosed or subclinical diabetes. Although diabetes is considered a disease of the elderly (its incidence peaks in the fifth and sixth decades), it also occurs in young adults and children.

Two acute complications may develop in the diabetic: hyperglycemia (leading to diabetic coma) and, more importantly and commonly, hypoglycemia

---

Card for Patient on Corticosteroid Therapy

Mr.
Mrs.
Miss _ _ _ _ _ _ _ _ _ is being treated for _ _ _ (disorder) _

with _ (corticosteroid) _ in a dose of _ _ _ (dose) _ _ _. In the

event of "stress", the steroid dosage should be increased thus:

    1. Mild "Stress" (eg, common cold, single dental extraction,

mild trauma): use double doses daily.

    2. Moderate "Stress" (eg, flu, surgery under local anesthesia,

several dental extractions): use hydrocortisone, 100 mg, or

prednisolone, 20 mg, or dexamethasone, 4 mg daily.

    3. Severe "Stress" (eg, general surgery, pneumonia or other

systemic infections, high fever, severe trauma): use hydro-

cortisone, 200 mg, or prednisolone, 40 mg, or dexamethasone

8 mg daily.

    When vomiting or diarrhea precludes absorption of oral doses,

give dexamethasone 1 to 4 mg intramuscularly every 6 hours.

             (Signed) _____ M.D.

             (Address) _____

Fig. 38-4. Sample corticosteroid coverage protocol for patient receiving corticosteroid therapy. (From Streeten DHP: *JAMA* 232:944, 1975. Copyright 1975, American Medical Association.)

(leading to insulin shock). Whereas these complications must be looked for and managed if they develop, it is other, more chronic complications that are responsible for the majority of deaths occurring in diabetic persons. Table 38-8 lists the chronic complications associated with diabetes mellitus. Three major categories of chronic complications are large blood vessel disease, small blood vessel disease (termed *microangiopathy*), and increased susceptibility to infection. The doctor treating the diabetic patient should carefully evaluate the patient for clinical signs and symptoms of cardiovascular disease, which is the most common cause of death in the diabetic patient.[24]

Knowledge on the part of the doctor of the type of diabetes—type I or insulin-dependent (IDDM) or type 2, non–insulin-dependent (NIDDM)—and the degree of control the patient maintains over his dis-

ease will enable the doctor to establish a risk factor for this patient. In general, the well-controlled type II diabetic who demonstrates no associated disease is classified as an ASA II risk; type I diabetics (patients with no beta-cell activity) are ASA III or IV risks depending on the severity of the disease and their level of control.

It is important for the doctor to speak with the diabetic patient prior to treatment to discuss the possible effect of the dental care on the patient's eating habits. The diabetic must attempt to maintain a normal eating pattern so that he does not become hypoglycemic after insulin administration. With recent changes in recommendations for management of type I diabetes (increased frequency of insulin administration) it is expected that the incidence of hypoglycemic episodes will triple.[25] Alterations in insulin dosages may be required in some situations in

Table 38-8. Chronic complications of diabetes mellitus

Affected part or condition	Complication
Vascular system	Atherosclerosis
	Large blood vessel disease
	Microangiopathy
Kidneys	Diabetic glomerulonephritis
	Arteriolar nephrosclerosis
	Pyelonephritis
Nervous system	Motor, sensory, and autonomic neuropathy
Eyes	Retinopathy
	Cataract formation
	Glaucoma
	Extraocular muscle palsies
Skin	Xanthoma diabeticorum
	Necrobiosis lipoidica diabeticorum
	Pruritus
	Furunculosis
	Mycosis
Mouth	Gingivitis
	Greater incidence of dental caries and periodontal disease
	Alveolar bone loss
Pregnancy	Greater incidence of large babies, stillbirths, miscarriages, neonatal deaths, and congenital defects

From Malamed SF: *Handbook of medical emergencies in the dental office,* ed 3. St Louis, 1987, Mosby.

which alterations in the patient's eating habits are unavoidable. Medical consultation may be indicated prior to adjustment of insulin dosage.

In the management of pain and anxiety, the diabetic does not present any unusual problems. Most techniques of pain and anxiety control are recommended for use in the diabetic patient. Treatment modification will be required in the ASA III and IV diabetic according to the severity of the associated medical complications. The following relates to the diabetic patient who is classified as an ASA II risk.

Local anesthesia is recommended for use in the diabetic patient, with no restrictions regarding either the choice of local anesthetic or the vasopressor.

Oral sedation is recommended for use in the diabetic patient with no restrictions.

IM sedation is recommended for the diabetic patient in cases in which other techniques of sedation have proved ineffective. There are no specific contraindications to the administration of IM drugs.

Inhalation sedation is recommended for use in the diabetic, with no restrictions.

IV sedation is recommended in the diabetic patient, with no restrictions. The use of a 5% dextrose in water infusion will not produce any significant alteration in the patient's blood sugar level, especially when one considers that the patient receiving IV sedation will be NPO for at least 4 to 5 hours prior to the procedure and will be slightly hypoglycemic.

Outpatient general anesthesia is usually contraindicated in the type I diabetic. The type II, non–insulin-dependent diabetic is a good risk for outpatient general anesthesia. Most insulin-dependent diabetics requiring general anesthesia should be hospitalized so that their diabetic condition can be stabilized and monitored closely both during and after the procedure.

Porphyria

Porphyrins are cyclic compounds that are the precursors of heme and other important enzymes and pigments. Heme is the complex of iron and porphyrin that unites with the protein globin to form hemoglobin. The porphyrias are disorders of porphyrin metabolism in which a marked increase in the production and excretion of porphyrins and their precursors is noted. Porphyria may be either hereditary or acquired. Porphyrias are classified in two main categories, hepatic porphyrins and erythropoietic porphyrins, depending on whether the excessive porphyrin production occurs within the liver or in the bone marrow.

It is important to be aware of the presence of latent or manifest porphyria because of the potential for some drugs to provoke episodes of acute intermittent porphyria. This rare disorder is exacerbated by the administration of barbiturates, sulfonamides, and griseofulvin, which cause a marked increase in porphyrin synthesis. Clinically this is associated with acute episodes of abdominal pain, paresthesia, neuritic pain, convulsions, muscle paralysis, psychiatric disturbances, and the passage of a reddish urine. Death results from respiratory paralysis in up to 25% of patients with acute episodes. Such paralysis may not develop for several days after drug administration.

Patients who have porphyria are classified as either ASA II or ASA III patients, depending on the severity of the disorder and the incidence of acute exacerbations.

Local anesthetics with and without vasopressors are recommended in the patient with porphyria. Oral sedation is recommended; however, barbiturates are absolutely contraindicated. IM sedation is recommended; however, administration of any barbiturate is absolutely contraindicated. Inhalation sedation is recommended in the patient with porphyria. IV sedation is recommended; however, the administration of barbiturates is absolutely contraindicated.

Outpatient general anesthesia is contraindicated in the patient with porphyria. The patient with porphyria who requires a general anesthetic should be hospitalized prior to administration of the general anesthetic. Barbiturates are absolutely contraindicated in the patient with porphyria.

Malignant hyperthermia

Malignant hyperthermia (malignant hyperpyrexia) is a pharmacogenetic disorder in which a genetic variant in the patient alters his response to certain drugs. The problem is, however, that prior to exposure to specific drugs it may be impossible to recognize an MH-susceptible patient. The genetic defect manifests itself as a flaw in the control of calcium levels in skeletal muscle when the normal intracellular environment is altered by certain drugs.[26] The concentration of calcium in the sarcoplasm is abnormally high. The list of drugs implicated as triggering malignant hyperthermia is large and includes many of the most commonly used general anesthetics:

Halothane
Enflurane
Methoxyflurane
Succinylcholine
Dextrotubocurarine
Gallamine
Ether
Cyclopropane

Acute clinical manifestations of malignant hyperthermia include the following: *Muscle rigidity,* which occurs in 80% of cases, may appear immediately after the administration of succinylcholine, a muscle relaxant. Masseteric rigidity is a common first sign. Rigidity may develop up to 2 hours after the beginning of a procedure when inhalation anesthetics are used. *Tachycardia* is almost universally present in malignant hyperthermia. *Tachypnea* develops simultaneously with the tachycardia; however, in cases in which mus-

cle relaxants have been administered, this symptom may be masked. *Fever* is the primary feature of malignant hyperthermia. It is the rate of rise, not the absolute temperature, that is of importance in MH. In general anesthetic procedures the use of a temperature probe is universally recommended. An elevation of temperature of more than 0.5°C should be suspect. Fever is usually a late sign, being noted after tachypnea and tachycardia. Other clinical signs include *dysrhythmias, cyanosis, dark venous blood* in the surgical field, *red urine,* and *hot skin.*

The mortality rate of patients with malignant hyperthermia was 63% to 73% prior to the introduction of dantrolene sodium, an intravenous agent used to terminate episodes.[27] Dantrolene sodium inhibits the release of calcium from intracellular organelles such as mitochondria and the sarcoplasmic reticulum. Since its introduction the mortality rate from malignant hyperthermia has decreased. Dantrolene sodium is also available in an oral form that has enabled susceptible patients to receive prophylaxis prior to their exposure to drugs that might induce malignant hyperthermia.

The incidence of malignant hyperthermia is approximately 1:15,000 in children and 1:50,000 in adults.[28] The majority of cases occur in children, adolescents, and young adults. Males develop malignant hyperthermia more frequently than do females. Malignant hyperthermia is encountered with much greater frequency in certain areas of North America where families with the genetic trait have settled. Three areas of concentration include Toronto, Canada, and Wisconsin and Nebraska in the United States.

Patients with documented malignant hyperthermia or those who are possibly susceptible are classified as ASA III risks. Definite treatment modification is in order to minimize risk for these patients during therapy. Medical consultation is recommended, discussing the proposed treatment, including drugs.

Local anesthetics of the amide group—lidocaine, mepivacaine, prilocaine, etidocaine, bupivacaine, and articaine—were considered to be contraindicated in MH patients. It was felt that these drugs were capable of triggering the MH response. Research has demonstrated conclusively that the *amide local anesthetics are not contrainidicated* in the MH-susceptible patient.[29-31] Neither is there any contraindication to the administration of the ester local anesthetics. The inclusion of vasopressors in the anesthetic solution is not contraindicated.

Oral sedation is recommended. Barbiturates,

opioids, and benzodiazepines may be administered with no increased risk in MH patients.

IM sedation may be administered, although I would probably have serious second thoughts about the administration of any parenteral sedation technique on an outpatient basis to a child with a history of malignant hyperpyrexia. Hospitalization would appear to be a more prudent approach to this patient's management.

Inhalation sedation with N_2O-O_2 is recommended in the MH patient. Following consultation the use of inhalation sedation on an outpatient basis might prove to be most favored.

IV sedation is recommended; however, as with IM sedation, I personally believe that it is more prudent to consider hospitalization of the MH-susceptible patient requiring parenteral sedation, unless the patient is well controlled through the administration of dantrolene sodium.

Outpatient general anesthesia is contraindicated in the patient with malignant hyperthermia. Hospital-based care is recommended for the patient with malignant hyperthermia who requires general anesthesia. Because of the risk involved in general anesthesia for this patient, the benefits to be gained by using general anesthesia should be carefully weighed against its risk before it is used.

Atypical plasma cholinesterase

Atypical plasma cholinesterase is another pharmacogenetic disorder. Two commonly used drugs—succinylcholine, a short-acting, depolarizing muscle relaxant used during intubation in general anesthesia, and the ester local anesthetics, such as procaine, chloroprocaine, and propoxycaine—are metabolized by the enzyme plasma cholinesterase. One in 2820 persons has an atypical form of this enzyme, called atypical plasma cholinesterase.[31] Patients with atypical plasma cholinesterase are unable to metabolize these drugs at a normal rate and are therefore more likely to exhibit clinical signs and symptoms of (1) prolonged clinical activity and/or (2) drug overdose. When succinylcholine is administered, the clinical duration of muscular relaxation in these patients is considerably prolonged beyond the usual 5 minutes. In cases in which an ester local anesthetic has been administered, elevated blood levels, which increase the risk of drug overdose developing, are noted. Clinical duration of action (pain control) is not prolonged when local anesthetics are administered to these patients. Patients with atypical plasma cholinesterase are considered ASA II risks.

Amide local anesthetics are recommended in these patients. Vasopressors are not contraindicated. Ester local anesthetics should be avoided in patients with atypical plasma cholinesterase; however, if they must be administered, the smallest effective volume is recommended.

Oral sedation, IM sedation, and inhalation sedation are recommended without specific contraindications. IV sedation is recommended with the warning that succinylcholine not be administered to these patients.

Outpatient general anesthesia may be administered if succinylcholine is not administered to this patient. It is prudent, however, to consider hospitalization of this patient if general anesthesia is required.

DISORDERS OF THE BLOOD

Several disorders of potential significance to the administration of drugs—anemia, sickle cell anemia, polycythemia vera, and hemophilia—are included in this category.

Anemia

Anemia is a condition in which an insufficient number of red blood cells produces a decrease in the total O_2-carrying capacity of the blood. Causes of anemia include hemorrhage (either external or internal), diminished manufacture of erythrocytes in the body, and a shortened life span of red blood cells. McCarthy has listed the following three categories of anemia[33]:

1. Reduction below the normal number of erythrocytes—megaloblastic anemia, pernicious anemia, folic acid deficiency, aplastic anemia
2. Reduction in the quantity of hemoglobin—iron deficiency anemia, sickle cell anemia
3. Reduction in the volume of packed red cells—bleeding or destruction (hemolytic anemia)

Signs and symptoms of anemia include ease of fatigability, dyspnea, pallor, palpitation, angina pectoris, and tachycardia. With a normal adult hemoglobin level of 12 to 18 g/100 ml of blood, levels below 9 g/100 ml are considered to be indicative of anemia. The ASA risk categories for anemic individuals vary according to the severity of clinical signs and symptoms; however, in general, the anemic patient with a hemoglobin level above 9 g/100 ml will be classified as ASA II, whereas the patient with a hemoglobin level below 9 g/100 ml is classified as ASA III.

Stress reduction is required for the anemic patient. The primary modification will be the recommendation that the patient receive O_2 via nasal cannula throughout his treatment.

Local anesthetics are indicated with or without vasopressors. Prilocaine and articaine are relatively contraindicated in anemic individuals, especially those with methemoglobinemia.[34] Large volumes of these local anesthetics can produce cyanosis (managed with the administration of IV methylene blue).[35] Other amide and ester local anesthetics do not produce elevations in methemoglobin.

Oral sedation is recommended with no specific contraindications.

IM sedation is recommended. Supplemental O_2 administered by nasal cannula throughout the procedure is suggested.

Inhalation sedation is recommended. The supplemental O_2 administered along with the N_2O is quite beneficial to the patient.

IV sedation is indicated. Supplemental O_2 administered by nasal cannula is suggested.

Outpatient general anesthesia is relatively contraindicated in anemic patients because of the decreased O_2-carrying capacity of the blood. In cases in which the anemia is mild and the patient asymptomatic, outpatient general anesthesia may be contemplated. In most cases, however, the patient should be hospitalized for the general anesthetic procedure.

Sickle cell anemia

Sickle cell anemia is a hereditary disorder essentially confined to blacks. Abnormal hemoglobin is transmitted as a dominant trait. Heterozygous carriers have mixtures of normal and sickle hemoglobin in all of their red blood cells. Sickling of erythrocytes occurs at a low O_2 tension, especially when the pH of blood is also low (acidosis). The S (sickle) hemoglobin (HbS), which is present in this disease, is less soluble in its deoxygenated (reduced) form, leading to an increase in the viscosity of whole blood. Increased viscosity results in stasis and obstruction of blood flow through capillaries, venules, and terminal arterioles, which results in pain and swelling in the involved organs.[36]

It is estimated that 50,000 Americans, primarily blacks, have sickle cell disease, in which HbSS is present in all red blood cells. This is approximately 1:600 blacks. Sickle cell trait, which another 2 million black Americans may carry, rarely causes signs and symptoms since their red blood cells contain both sickle and normal hemoglobin, HgAS.

The patient with sickle cell disease represents an increased risk during treatment, particularly treatment that involves the administration of drugs with the potential to produce respiratory depression. A sickle cell crisis might be precipitated by CNS-depressant drugs as well as infection and extreme cold. When a sickle cell crisis occurs, the organs most often involved are the brain, kidneys, spleen, liver, and bones. The patient with sickle cell trait, although unlikely to develop crisis, may, in circumstances of extreme stress, such as physical exertion and general anesthesia, suffer a sickle cell crisis.

Most patients with sickle cell disease represent an ASA III risk during therapy. Those with sickle cell trait may be categorized as ASA II patients. Treatment modifications involve the provision for adequate oxygenation at all times in these patients, the prevention of acidosis, and the management of stress.

Local anesthetics are recommended either with or without vasopressors. No specific contraindications exist to any drug.

Oral sedation is recommended for light levels of preoperative anxiety control. Should moderate levels of sedation be sought by this route, the administration of supplemental O_2 by nasal cannula is recommended.

IM sedation is recommended in cases in which other techniques of sedation have been ineffective. O_2 administered by nasal cannula throughout the procedure is recommended.

Inhalation sedation with N_2O-O_2 is ideally suited for the patient with a history of sickle cell disease. Increased levels of O_2 are provided the patient throughout the procedure.

IV sedation is recommended with no specific contraindications to any drugs. Supplemental O_2 administered by nasal cannula is recommended.

Outpatient general anesthesia is not recommended since the potential risk of hypoxia may be increased. Hospitalization of the patient is strongly recommended for the administration of general anesthesia.

Polycythemia vera

Polycythemia vera is an overproduction of one or more types of blood cells, such as RBCs, WBCs, or platelets. Symptomatology is produced by an increased viscosity of blood and hypermetabolism. Although polycythemia vera may develop at any age, it is commonly observed after the age of 50 years. It is more common in males and is seen more often in Jews from Eastern Europe. Polycythemia vera is rarely encountered in blacks and Latin Americans.[37]

Clinical signs and symptoms include headache, inability to concentrate, hearing loss, itching, pain in fingers and toes, a decreased feeling of well-being, and a loss of energy.

Complications of polycythemia vera include hemorrhage (GI bleeding) and thrombosis, especially in uncontrolled polycythemia vera. Excessive bleeding is common during surgery. Management of polycythemia vera consists of administration of radiophosphorus and phlebotomy. Survival averages 13 years in properly treated patients. Acute leukemia causes the death of 5% of patients.

The typical patient with polycythemia vera represents an ASA II risk during treatment. Excessive bleeding is likely to occur during dental and surgical treatment. The use of supplemental O_2 is recommended during all treatment in these patients.

Local anesthesia is recommended with no specific contraindications to any local anesthetic drug or vasopressor. Nerve block anesthesia, especially those techniques in which a high percentage of positive aspiration is likely to occur, such as inferior alveolar nerve block, should be avoided because of the potential risk of excessive bleeding. Alternative techniques such as the Gow-Gates mandibular block, periodontal ligament injection, or infiltration are preferred in these patients.

Oral sedation is recommended without specific contraindications.

Parenteral sedation techniques are relatively contraindicated due to the increased risk of excessive bleeding and venous thrombosis. IM sedation should be reserved for those patients in whom it is absolutely necessary and in whom the benefits of its use outweigh the potential risks. Supplemental O_2 is recommended.

Inhalation sedation is highly recommended.

IV sedation is relatively contraindicated because of the potential for increased bleeding and venous thrombosis. Risks should be carefully weighed against benefits when IV sedation is being considered. Supplemental O_2 is recommended.

Outpatient general anesthesia is relatively contraindicated in the patient with polycythemia vera. Hospitalization and treatment as an in-patient should be given careful consideration.

Hemophilia

Hemophilia is an inherited disorder of coagulation characterized by a lifelong history of abnormal bleeding. Hemophilia A and hemophilia B are the most common of the inherited bleeding disorders.

Hemophilia A is classic hemophilia resulting from a deficiency of antihemophilic factor (AHF) activity. Because of its absence from plasma, thromboplastin formation is affected. Christmas disease—hemophilia B—is a deficiency in plasma thromboplastin component (factor IX).

Patients with hemophilia rarely have massive hemorrhages. Bleeding is usually a prolonged oozing that develops after minor surgery or trauma. Of special concern during dental care is the administration of local anesthesia for pain control (see following discussion). Management of patients with hemophilia consists primarily of the prevention of bleeding and the administration of the appropriate factor (VII or IX) to the patient either prophylactically prior to surgical procedures or when bleeding does occur as following dental extractions.

Aspirin-containing analgesics should be avoided in persons with hemophilia since it prolongs bleeding for 24 to 48 hours. Acetaminophen, nonsteroidal antiinflammatory drugs (NSAIDs), or other non-aspirin-containing analgesics may be used.

Local anesthesia is recommended with no specific contraindications to the administration of any local anesthetic drug with or without a vasopressor. The administration of regional nerve block anesthesia, especially techniques with a greater incidence of positive aspiration (inferior alveolar nerve block, posterior superior alveolar nerve block, and mental nerve block), should be avoided in the hemophiliac. Alternative techniques, such as the Gow-Gates mandibular block, infiltration, and the PDL are recommended.

Oral sedation is recommended with no specific contraindications.

IM sedation is contraindicated because of the increased potential for prolonged bleeding.

Inhalation sedation is recommended with no specific contraindications.

IV sedation is recommended if the patient has received replacement therapy. Outpatient general anesthesia is contraindicated because of the increased risk of prolonged bleeding. In-patient general anesthesia is preferred, with the patient well controlled prior to the procedure. Oral intubation is preferred to nasal intubation because of the lesser chance of bleeding.

REFERENCES

1. American Heart Association: 1993 Heart Facts, Dallas, Tex, 1993, The Association.
2. Tarhan S, Giuliani ER: General anesthesia and myocardial infarction, *Am Heart J* 87:137, 1974.

3. Weinblatt E, Shapiro S, Frank CW et al: Prognosis of men after first myocardial infarction: mortality and first recurrence in relation to selected parameters, *Am J Public Health* 58:1329, 1968.

4. Albert JS, Braunwald E: Pathological and clinical manifestations of acute myocardial infarctions. In Braunwald E, ed: *Heart disease: a textbook of cardiovascular medicine.* Philadelphia, 1980, Saunders.

5. Stern MS et al: Nitrous oxide and oxygen in acute myocardial infarction, *Circulation* 58 (suppl II):171, 1978.

6. Katz AM: Congestive heart failure, *N Engl J Med* 293:1184, 1975.

7. Committee on Rheumatic Fever, Endocarditis, and Kawasaki Disease of the Council on Cardiovascular Disease in the Young of the American Heart Association: Prevention of bacterial endocarditis—recommendations by the American Heart Association, *JAMA* 264:2919, 1990.

8. Atkins CW: Mechanical cardiac valvular prosthesis, *Ann Thorac Surg* 52(1):161, 1991.

9. Port FK: The end-stage renal disease program: trends over the past 18 years, *Am J Kidney Dis* 20(1) suppl 1:37, 1992.

10. Burr ML: Epidemiology of asthma, *Monogr Allergy* 31:80, 1993.

11. Weiss KB, Gergen PJ, Wagener DK: Breathing better or wheezing worse? The changing epidemiology of asthma morbidity and mortality, *Ann Rev Public Health* 14:491, 1993.

12. Hauser WA: Seizure disorders: the changes with age, *Epilepsia* 33(suppl 4):S6, 1992.

13. Krenn J, Porges P, Steinbereithner K: Ein fall von karkosepkramphen unter stickoxydul-halothan-narkose, *Anaesthetist* 16:83, 1976.

14. Melon E, Homs JB: Nitrous oxide in neurosurgery: its safety in the seizure-prone patient, *Agressologie* 32(8–9):429, 1991.

15. Ito BM, Sato S, Kufta CV et al: Effect of isoflurane and enflurane on the electrocorticogram of epileptic patients, *Neurology* 38(6):924, 1988.

16. Manton KG, Corder LS, Stallard E: Estimates of change in chronic disability and institutional incidence and prevalence rates in the U.S. elderly population from the 1982, 1984, and 1989 national long term care survey, *J Gerontol* 48(4):S153, 1993.

17. Gresham GE, Fitzpatrick TE, Wolf PA: Residual durability in survivors of stroke: the Framingham study, *N Engl J Med* 293:954, 1975.

18. Sila CA: Prophylaxis and treatment of stroke: the state of the art in 1993, *Drugs* 45(3):329, 1993.

19. Oosterhuis HJ, Kuks JB: Myasthenia gravis and myasthenic syndromes, *Curr Opin Neurol Neurosurg* 5(5):638, 1992.

20. Genkins G, Sivak M, Tartter PI: Treatment strategies in myasthenia gravis, *Ann NY Acad Sci* 681:603, 1993.

21. Sawyer DR, Ludden TM, Crawford MH: Continuous infusion of lidocaine in patients with cardiac arrhythmias: unpredictability of plasma concentrations, *Arch Intern Med* 141:34, 1981.

22. McCarthy FM: Adrenal insufficiency. In McCarthy FM, ed: *Essentials of safe dentistry for the medically compromised patient.* Philadelphia, 1989, Saunders.

23. Streeten DHP: Corticosteroid therapy. II. Complications and therapeutic indications, *JAMA* 232:1046, 1975.

24. Fuller JH: Mortality trends and causes of death in diabetic patients, *Diabete Metab* 19(1):96, 1993.

25. The Diabetes Control and Complications Trial Research Group: The effect of intensive treatment of diabetes on the development and progression of long-term complications in insulin-dependent diabetes mellitus, *N Engl J Med* 329(14):977, 1993.

26. Strazis KP, Fox AW: Malignant hyperthermia: a review of published cases, *Anesth Analg* 77(2):297, 1993.

27. Moore JL, Rice EL: Malignant hyperthermia, *Am Fam Physician* 45(5):2245, 1992.

28. Saleh KL: Practical points in the management of malignant hyperthermia, *J Post Anesthes Nursing* 7(5):327, 1992.

29. Dershwitz M, Ryan JF, Guralnick W: Safety of amide local anesthetics in patients susceptible to malignant hyperthermia, *JADA* 118(3):276, 1989.

30. Jelic JS, Moore PA: Malignant hyperthermia and amide local anesthetics, *Pennsyl Dent J* 55(4):35, 1988.

31. Minasian A, Yagiela JA: The use of amide local anesthetics in patients susceptible to malignant hyperthermia, *Oral Surg* 66(4):405, 1988.

32. Metrowitz MR, Mauro JV, Aston R et al: Prolonged succinylcholine-induced apnea caused by atypical cholinesterase: report of a case, *J Oral Surg* 38:387, 1980.

33. McCarthy FM: Physical evaluation and treatment modification. In McCarthy FM, ed: *Emergencies in dental practice,* ed 3. Philadelphia, 1979, Saunders.

34. Bellamy MC, Hopkins PM, Halsall PJ et al: A study into the incidence of methaemoglobinaemia after "three-in-one" block with prilocaine, *Anaesthesia* 47(12):1084, 1992.

35. Bhutani A, Bhutani MS, Patel R: Methemoglobinemia in a patient undergoing gastrointestinal endoscopy, *Ann Pharmacother* 26(10):1239, 1992.

36. Sansevere JJ, Milles M: Management of the oral and maxillofacial surgery patient with sickle cell disease and related hemoglobinopathies, *J Oral Maxillofac Surg* 51(8):912, 1993.

37. Murphy S: Polycythemia vera, *Dis Month* 38(3):153, 1992.

CHAPTER 39

The physically compromised patient

Christine L. Quinn

Gross disabilities that involve the neuromuscular and skeletal systems can present the dentist and staff with many difficulties during treatment. The "care of the handicapped patient should not be considered as a negative aspect of dentistry any more than the pathologies and problems which constitute the bulk of dental practice . . . Rather it should be viewed as a challenging area of practice which can provide its own unique rewards."[1]

NEUROMUSCULAR DISORDERS

The neuromuscular disorders encompass many different diseases and all age groups. The disorders to be discussed include muscular dystrophy, cerebral palsy, multiple sclerosis, and Parkinson's disease.

Muscular dystrophy

Muscular dystrophy is characterized by a progressive muscular degeneration without neurologic pathosis. There are elemental types of muscular dystrophy with the most common and severe form being pseudohypertrophic dystrophy (Duchenne muscular dystrophy). The muscular dystrophies are transmitted genetically.

Pseudohypertrophic dystrophy usually develops within the first 3 years of life and leads to a progressive loss of ambulation. The affected skeletal muscles may become large due to fatty infiltration, and the use of a wheelchair by the age of 12 is common. Late in the disease the patient becomes too weak to move or stand without assistance. Patients have compromised pulmonary function due to chronic weakness of inspiratory respiratory muscles and a decreased ability to cough, making pneumonia a common complication. They also may suffer from congestive heart failure due to myocardial muscle involvement. Patients usually die as young adults due to congestive heart failure and pneumonia. There is also an increased incidence of malignant hyperthermia in these patients.

Medical management of patients with muscular dystrophy is based on physical therapy and the prevention of complications. Dental treatment modifications may be required in positioning the patient to accommodate patient comfort.

Local anesthetics, with and without vasoconstrictors, are recommended without any specific contraindications.

Oral sedation is recommended for lighter levels of preoperative anxiety control.

IM and IV sedation are relatively contraindicated because of the possible adverse effects that CNS depressants may have on the already weakened musculature.

General anesthesia is not recommended due to the complicating medical problems that these patients have. It should only be considered after the dentist has attempted to treat the patient with local anesthetics and perhaps light sedation. If the patient does require general anesthesia it should only be done on an inpatient basis due to the risk of malignant hyperthermia, and cardiac and pulmonary compromise.

Cerebral palsy

Cerebral palsy is a term encompassing a group of conditions that result from damage to the motor areas of the brain before, during, or after birth. Other names for this disorder include Little's disease and spastic paralysis. Cerebral palsy incidence is 6 in 1000 births, making it one of the most common developmental disabilities.

Cerebral palsy is usually associated with multiple disabilities since brain damage may affect more than just the motor areas of the brain. Several types of cerebral palsy are recognized and described by the clinical features of the motor dysfunction (Table 39-1). Spasticity is the most prevalent type of cerebral palsy. It is characterized by stiff, awkward, jerky, and uncontrolled voluntary movements. Spasticity is the result of damage to the motor area of the cerebral cortex. Choreoathetosis is the result of damage to the extrapyramidal system. Clinically it manifests as both fast and jerky (choreoid) and slow and writhing (athetoid) involuntary movements, usually of the distal extremities.

Medical management of the patient with cerebral palsy is based on physical, educational, and social rehabilitation. Also included is the prevention of complications, especially those involving the respiratory system, because of the patient's decreased ability to cough. The patient with cerebral palsy may be classified as ASA II, III, or IV according to risk, depending on the severity of the disability and the associated complications.

Thorough preoperative evaluation of the patient is essential to determine the level of respiratory, neurologic, and musculoskeletal involvement. Uncontrolled movements tend to be the major problem in managing these patients. Stress seems to accentuate these movements so stress reduction procedures are beneficial. Patient positioning may require modification, and gentle restraint may be indicated, with the patient's consent. Use of a rubber dam is recommended since it prevents intrusion of the tongue into the operative site.

Local anesthesia is recommended with no specific contraindications to drugs or vasoconstrictors. *Oral sedation* is extremely useful for patients with preoperative anxiety. It may also help in decreasing uncontrolled movements. No specific contraindications to any common oral sedative drug exist. *IM sedation* is useful in those instances in which other techniques have proved ineffective. *Inhalation sedation* is recommended, but it may be difficult to maintain the nasal hood in proper position because of involuntary movements. *IV sedation* is recommended. Basic techniques are usually quite effective since most often the patient only needs to be sedated to eliminate involuntary movements. Outpatient general anesthesia is not contraindicated but is usually reserved as a last attempt at patient management.

Multiple sclerosis

Multiple sclerosis is the most common of the human demyelinating diseases. It is characterized by the onset of progressive diffuse neurologic disturbances, usually in early adult life. These disturbances undergo irregular periods of exacerbation and apparent remission. Although the disease has been known for almost a century, its cause is not yet known.

Table 39-1. Classification of types of cerebral palsy

Type	Incidence (percentage)	Descriptions
Spasticity	40-66	Stiff, awkward, jerky, involuntary movements; results in scissor gait, elbow flexion, and forearm pronation
Choreoathetosis	19-45	Involvement of the extrapyramidal system resulting in slow involuntary, twisting, unpredictable, and purposeless motion; effort to control motions only appears to intensify them; difficulties common in postural maintenance, speech, and swallowing
Ataxia	5-8	Poor motor coordination (poor balance and muscle coordination)
Rigidity	4-5	Associated with severe mental retardation; diminished motion results from brain damage, causing resistance of antagonist muscles and to a lesser degree contracting muscles
Tremor	2-5	Rhythmic, vibrating movements of involuntary nature that are caused by an imbalance of antagonistic muscle groups
Mixed	1	Though most cerebral palsy patients have a combination of the five types listed above, they are usually categorized by the predominant type. The "mixed" category is reserved for patients with severe involvement and multiple handicaps.

The initial attack and subsequent relapses may follow acute infection, trauma, vaccination, pregnancy, and stress. The signs of the disease are generalized CNS involvement, including slurred speech, tremor of intent, nystagmus, incontinence, spastic paralysis, and increased deep tendon reflexes. As the disease progresses euphoria develops. In general, multiple sclerosis is characterized by (1) widespread neurologic lesions that cannot be explained on a single anatomic basis and (2) signs and symptoms that are subject to repeated exacerbation and remission.[2]

There is no specific treatment for multiple sclerosis, although many courses of therapy have been advocated and tried. Adequate sleep at night and rest during the day have been found to make the patient more comfortable. Sudden changes in temperature, especially heat, exacerbates the condition.

The course of multiple sclerosis is variable, with exacerbations and remissions occurring at irregular intervals. The average survival time following the onset of symptoms has been reported to be 27 years. Death is usually caused by some complicating disease, such as kidney or bladder infection.

The patient with multiple sclerosis may be classified as ASA II, III, or IV according to risk depending on the severity of signs and symptoms. *Local anesthesia* may be administered without undue risk to the patient. The patient with paresthesia in the oral cavity should be advised that signs and symptoms of local anesthesia may mimic this but will resolve within a short period of time (depending on the local anesthetic used). All types of sedation may be used for these patients (*oral, IM, inhalation, IV*). Stress reduction procedures should be followed in these individuals due to the negative impact that stress has on the disease. *General anesthesia* is relatively contraindicated in these individuals because the stress of the general anesthesia could cause exacerbation of the disease. There are, though, no interactions between the disease and the general anesthetic agents that are typically used.

Parkinson's disease

Parkinson's disease, also known as parkinsonism or paralysis agitans, is characterized by a triad of symptoms: tremor, rigidity, and hypokinesia. Parkinson's disease was first described in 1817 by James Parkinson. It is a degenerative central nervous system disease in which there is a loss of dopaminergic fibers in the basal ganglia of the brain, resulting in a decrease of dopamine. A decrease in dopamine is thought to result in the unopposed action of cholinergic neurons in the basal ganglia. The treatment of parkinsonism is aimed at improving the dopaminergic-cholinergic imbalance. The actual cause of the disease cannot be determined in most cases. The disease has an insidious onset usually after the age of 40.

Signs and symptoms include a fixed or less mobile than normal facial expression. Body movements become slower, with a gradually increasing rigidity and decreased movement of the arms while walking. Legs may feel heavy and stiff, leading to a slow, shuffling gait. The posture becomes stooped with the arms at the sides, elbows slightly flexed, and the fingers abducted. Patients with parkinsonism will have a resting tremor involving the fingers and wrist in a "pill-rolling" movement. A to-and-fro tremor of the head may also be noticed.

Management of parkinsonism is usually through the use of drug therapy aimed at decreasing the signs and symptoms (Table 39-2). In certain patients, surgical destruction of portions of the globus pallidus or ventrolateral nucleus of the thalamus has proven beneficial. Physical therapy is also a very important measure in the management of these patients. Because the patient's mental faculties are unimpaired in parkinsonism, the patient must receive reassurance and psychological support. These patients may live for many years with this disease. Disability tends to increase as the disease progresses, with the patient becoming increasingly depressed, anxious, and possibly showing signs of dementia.

The patient with parkinsonism can be classified as

Table 39-2. Drugs used in the treatment of Parkinsonism

Generic name	Proprietary name
Anticholinergics	
Procyclidine	Kemadrin
Trihexiphenidyl	Artane
Benztropine	Cogentin
Biperiden	Akineton
Ethopropazine	Parsidol
Diphenhydramine	Benedryl
Dopaminergic agents	
Levodopa	Larodopa, Dopar
Carbidopa/levodopa	Sinemet
Amantadine	Symmetrel
Bromocriptine	Parlodel
Pergolide	Permax
Selegiline	Eldepryl

ASA II, III, or IV according to risk depending on the presence of other age-related medical problems. Most patients are taking levodopa or the combination of levodopa/carbidopa. These patients are at risk for orthostatic hypotension, and appropriate precautions should be instituted. It is also important to stress that the patient take his normal medication prior to treatment. Abrupt withdrawal of levodopa could result in skeletal muscle rigidity.

Local anesthetics are recommended with no specific contraindications.

Oral sedation is recommended. Sedation is probably best achieved with the use of a benzodiazepine.

Inhalation sedation is recommended.

IV sedation is recommended. Phenothiazines and butyrophenones are contraindicated due to their ability to antagonize the effects of dopamine. A concern with IV sedation is the risk of aspiration due to the decreased ability to swallow as the disease progresses.

Outpatient general anesthesia is relatively contraindicated. Patients should be evaluated on a case-by-case basis.

MENTAL RETARDATION

Mental retardation is defined by the American Association of Mental Retardation as follows: significantly subaverage general intellectual functioning existing concurrently with deficits in adaptive behavior, manifested during the developmental period. As Sanger states, "Persons who are mentally retarded are not suffering from mental illness, which often originates after the developmental period, but from maladjustment in intellectual maturation, learning, and social adjustment."[3]

It is estimated that approximately 6 million persons in the United States are mentally retarded, the vast majority being mildly to moderately impaired. The incidence of mental retardation is approximately 3 to 5 per 100 persons.

In the recent past these people were institutionalized, isolated from the community, and ignored. Because of this the dental and medical professions were seldom called on to treat these individuals. Since the early 1970s there has been a movement toward normalization of these individuals. This philosophy believes that the individuals should be maintained as much as possible in their natural homes and communities. This change in management emphasis has made it possible for the dental and medical professionals to treat the oral and other health needs of this population.

Mental retardation may occur as an isolated entity. This is termed *nonsyndromic mental retardation* and accounts for a small percentage of all mental retardation. More often, mental retardation occurs concurrently with other diseases or disorders and is termed *syndromic mental retardation*. There are numerous causes of mental retardation, a few of which are listed in Table 39-3.

Nonsyndromic mental retardation

Patients with nonsyndromic mental retardation have no other developmental abnormalities. They are essentially healthy persons who happen to have a degree of mental retardation. Medical management of these individuals is based on educational and social rehabilitation.

Dental care for these patients is managed in a manner as close to usual as possible. Indeed, for most of these patients there will be absolutely no difficulty in successfully completing the planned dental therapy. Patients with nonsyndromic mental retardation do not represent an increased risk during treatment. They may be categorized as an ASA II risk.

Many persons have preconceived stereotypes of those with mental retardation. Each patient must be treated as an individual. Most dental personnel, when confronted with individuals who are mentally retarded, become overly reserved, withdrawn, and reluctant to express their personal feelings. Dental personnel must learn to act naturally. Positive attitudes from the treating staff will often produce a return of positive feelings from the patient. Mentally retarded patients should be scheduled at times when the doctor and staff are alert, fresh, and not rushed by a busy schedule.

Many mild to moderately retarded persons can be managed with behavior modification techniques. Behavior modification can be a very positive means of producing good patient conduct. The major disadvantages are that it is time consuming and does not work for a small percentage of severely or profoundly mentally retarded persons.[4]

The specific method of behavior management should be determined by the first appointment with the patient. The doctor should gather a complete history and interact with the patient to discover possible management difficulties. If it appears that pharmacological management is necessary, this is a good time to familiarize the patient with specific monitors and instruments that will be used during the sedation and to gather baseline vital statistics. This appointment also permits the doctor to evaluate the patient's

Table 39-3. Etiologic factors in mental retardation

Etiologic factor	Associated disease of condition
Infection	Prenatal
	Rubella
	Syphilis
	Postnatal cerebral infection
	Bacterial
	Viral
Intoxication	Toxemia of pregnancy
	Maternal phenylketonuria
	Postimmunization encephalopathy
Trauma or physical agent	Prenatal injury
	Mechanical injury at birth
	Hypoxia at birth
	Postnatal injury
Disorder of metabolism, growth, or nutrition	Tay-Sachs disease
	Phenylketonuria
	Marfan's syndrome
	Hypothyroidism
	Maple syrup urine disease
New growths	von Recklinghausen's disease
	Intracranial neoplasm
Unknown prenatal influence	Anencephaly
	Congenital hydrocephalus
	Macrocephaly
	Down syndrome
Unknown or uncertain cause with structural reactions manifest	Encephalopathy associated with diffuse sclerosis of brain
	Encephalopathy associated with prematurity
Uncertain cause with functional reaction alone manifest	Cultural-familial origin
	Associated with maternal deprivation
	Associated with emotional disturbance

Modified from Sanger RG, Casamassimo PS: *Dent Clin North Am* 27:363, 1983.

airway (i.e., short neck, mouth breather) and venous access.

The use of *local anesthesia* is not contraindicated. In fact, minimizing pain and discomfort with local anesthesia is paramount to the management of these patients. It is also important to be aware that the patient may not be familiar with the sensation of local anesthesia. Remind the care provider to watch the patient to prevent postoperative trauma to the lips, cheeks, and/or tongue.

Sedation, whether oral, inhalation, or parenteral, is the treatment of choice for those patients that do not respond to behavior modification. The same indications for use of these techniques are valid in the mentally retarded patient as in the nonretarded individual. No specific contraindications exist to the use of any drug or technique. It should be remembered that individual response varies and that it is possible for some patients to experience paradoxical reac-

tions to sedative drugs. The doctor should also be aware that some of these patients are chronically medicated, which could affect their response to certain drugs. General anesthesia is typically considered as the last technique for management in view of the increased risk to the patient. *Outpatient general anesthesia* is not contraindicated for routine procedures.

Syndromic mental retardation

Syndromic mental retardation is found in the majority of individuals with mental retardation. These patients have associated medical disorders of varying severity. The systemic disorders that may occur in these individuals are cardiovascular abnormalities, respiratory disorders, renal disorders, and metabolic and endocrine disturbances.

The most frequently encountered syndrome is trisomy 21 (Down syndrome). Down syndrome occurs in 1:600-700 live births and is more common with advanced maternal age (75% of the cases) and advanced paternal age. Patients with trisomy 21 have a characteristic look: single palmar crease, flat facies, and oblique palpebral fissures. Congenital heart disease is fairly common, occurring in 40% of the individuals. Most of the defects are endocardial cushion defects and ventricular septal defects.[5]

Medical management of syndromic mental retardation involves the same degree of social and educational rehabilitation as with the nonsyndromic patient, as well as specific management aimed at correction of the associated medical disorders. The ASA classification for the syndromic mentally retarded patient depends on the nature and severity of the underlying disorders. Patients could have an ASA classification ranging from II to IV.

Dental management must take into account both the degree of mental retardation and the underlying medical problems. The patient can usually tolerate dental treatment with few modifications. *Sedation* (oral, inhalation, IM, IV) is an option if indicated as long as the associated medical disorders do not preclude its use. The treating dentist needs to be aware of medications the patient may be taking and whether there is a risk of adverse drug interactions with the sedative medications. Patients with underlying congenital cardiovascular disorders will probably require antibiotic prophylaxis prior to dental treatment. *General anesthesia* is a consideration as long as the patient can medically tolerate the procedure.

Autism

Autism was first written about in 1867, but it was not until 1944 when Kanner described a clinical syndrome in 11 children that it was given the name "early infantile autism." Autism was originally considered to be an emotional disorder but is now recognized as a developmental disability. It can include a variety of disabilities that can have a differing range of severity. There are a variety of biological factors that may produce the syndrome. These include genetic factors (Fragile X), rubella virus, cerebral lipidosis, neurofibromatosis, Rett syndrome, and tuberous sclerosis.[6]

The syndrome is characterized by an early onset (prior to the age of 3 to 5 years old), severe abnormalities in communication and socialization, and behaviors, activities, and interests that tend to be restricted, repetitive, and stereotyped. Autistic individuals typically have a language deficiency in which speech may be lacking or echolalic (echoing of words or sentences) and a variety of behaviors that are ritualistic and create isolation. Autistics are known to rock back and forth and be self-abusive. Even so, no two autistics display exactly the same symptoms. A definitive diagnosis for the syndrome is an abnormal response to sensory stimuli. Children with autism often want to smell people and objects. This behavior is not seen in mentally retarded individuals without autistic features.[6]

As the autistic child approaches adulthood, changes in behavior take place. A positive side of these changes is that there is a decrease in activity level, making behavior more manageable, and self-help skills improve. The negative side is that one third of adolescent or young adult autistics develop seizure disorders. This is seen more commonly among the autistics that are mentally retarded. It is estimated that approximately 67% to 88% of autistics are mentally retarded. The practitioner may experience increased difficulties in treating the autistic adult because aggressive and self-abusive behaviors may become more problematic. Oftentimes it is just the fact that adults are larger and stronger that makes them more difficult to manage than children.

Autistic individuals are frequently taking anticonvulsive medication (Table 39-4) and medication to help control behavior. They may be taking a phenothiazine to help decrease agitation, psychotic behavior, and activity. Some individuals are taking regular doses of the beta-blocking agent propranolol to help control rage behaviors.

Autistics are especially susceptible to dental disease because of the tendency toward abnormal eating habits and food preferences, combined with the usual absence of good oral hygiene practice. Rampant dental and periodontal disease can produce sig-

Table 39-4. Anticonvulsant medications

Generic	Proprietary
Primidone	Mysoline
Phenobarbital	Phenobarbital
Phenytoin	Dilantin
Carbamazepine	Tegretol
Ethosuximide	Zarontin
Clonazepam	Klonipine
Diazepam	Valium
Valproic acid	Depakote/Depakene

nificant discomfort and, secondarily, behavioral and nutritional problems.

Dental evaluation and treatment of the autistic patient may prove to be difficult. Management of these individuals depends on the degree of mental retardation present. Directions should be given in a very simple manner. Communication is achieved through touch and tell-show-do modalities. Care should be taken to keep the autistic patient's anxiety and frustration to a minimum, since these are thought to bring about aggressive behaviors.[7]

Mildly retarded autistic adults can be managed with behavior modification and tell-show-do techniques. The more severely retarded the individual, the more difficulty in cooperating with dental treatment. It may be necessary to use a pharmacological approach for the management of the patient.

No specific contraindications exist to the use of any drug or technique for sedation and pain control in the autistic patient. The same indications are valid for the autistic patient as for the nonautistic patient. It should be kept in mind though that the autistic patient may be chronically medicated, which could alter the response to central nervous system depressants.

Dementia and Alzheimer's disease

Dementia is an impairment of all cognitive functions and learned behaviors. It is a nonspecific clinical syndrome that can result from any of the pathologic processes that affect the central nervous system.[8] Dementia is the major psychiatric disorder of the elderly. It is estimated that 15% of elderly persons in the United States exhibit some degree of dementia.[9]

This section will focus on the senile dementia of the Alzheimer's type. This disease was first described in 1907 by Alas Alzheimer. It has historically been divided into two diseases. Onset prior to 65 years of age was labeled Alzheimer's or presenile dementia. Disease onset after 65 years of age was called senile dementia. More recently it is felt that both are probably the same disease and should be called dementia of the Alzheimer's type.[10]

Of the 15% of elderly persons suffering from dementia, 65% reportedly have Alzheimer's disease.[9] As the percentage of elderly increase in the population, more patients who have Alzheimer's disease will be requiring dental care. Therefore it is important that dentists become familiar with this disease.

In Alzheimer's disease there is a progressive loss of neurons from the cerebral cortex. As this occurs, the cerebral hemispheres lose their ability to control behaviors, and commands begin to originate from the more primitive portions of the brain (diencephalic and brainstem reflex levels). This is the reverse of our ontogenic development where learned behavior replaces reflex behavior.

There are two major pathological changes associated with Alzheimer's disease. There is the development of neuritic plaques and neurofibrillary tangles. Gross atrophy of the brain also occurs. These morphologic and microscopic changes also occur in the brain of a normal elderly individual, making it difficult to assess the degree of nerve loss in the cortex. The neural loss that occurs in Alzheimer's is believed to be five times greater than that found in normal aging.[10] The etiology of Alzheimer's is not known but it is associated with a variety of disorders such as head trauma, viral infection, and genetic disorders (Down syndrome and familial Alzheimer's).

Alzheimer's disease has been divided into stages that correspond to an evolution of behavioral signs and symptoms. Although not all patients manifest this classic course of symptoms, the clinical diagnosis of Alzheimer's disease necessitates documentation of a progression of symptoms. The progression is usually insidious but will appear in a stepwise fashion with changes in the severity of symptoms.[8]

In the early stage, sometimes referred to as the forgetfulness phase, there is some memory loss (both recent and remote).[10] It is sometimes difficult to differentiate between benign and malignant forgetfulness. The latter is characterized by an inability to recall both important and unimportant facts. The patient may demonstrate a loss of judgment and spatial or temporal orientation. There may be mood changes and a collapse of social relationships. Patients are usually aware that something is wrong and may become depressed.

The middle or confusional phase is characterized by a definite impairment of cognitive functioning. The patient may be unable to recognize his own face in the mirror.[9] Aberrations in language become more apparent, perseveration will frequently occur, or the patient may become dysphasic. There may be episodes of irritability in which the patient may be overly anxious, uncooperative, and hyperactive.[10]

In the third or terminal phase the patient is severely disoriented, and behavioral problems are quite apparent. At this point individuals are most often placed in long-term care facilities. The individual

Table 39-5. Treatment planning approaches by severity of Alzheimer's disease

Approach	Mild	Moderate	Severe
General considerations	Minimal changes	⟵ Sedation may be necessary; short ⟶ appointments; more frequent recall visits	
Specific considerations		Aggressive prevention, including use of topical ⟵ fluorides, daily oral hygiene care, and oral health ⟶ education of caregivers	
	Design treatment plan anticipating decline	Design treatment plan with minimal changes (reline denture rather than remake, if possible)	Maintenance of dentition
	Restore to function quickly as possible		Emergency care

From Neissen LC: Alzheimer's disease: a guide for dental professionals, *Special Care in Denistry* 6:6-12, Jan-Feb, 1987.

cannot retain a thought long enough to know what to do next. Psychotic symptoms, hallucinations, delusions, and paranoia may appear. There is motor restlessness and neurological abnormalities appear. Eventually the patient will develop seizures. Patients become extremely susceptible to infection at this point because of their debilitated state.[10]

Dental management of the Alzheimer's patient varies with the stage of the disease and the presence of other systemic diseases. The first dental visit for the Alzheimer's patient will probably represent the best cognitive functioning level of the patient. The patient's ability to cooperate during dental treatment depends on the severity of the disease. A person whose disease is in the early stage will probably be more cooperative than someone whose disease has progressed further. The patient with moderate disease may require sedation for dental treatment. Treatment of these patients generally consists of prevention and maintenance (Table 39-5).

Local anesthesia is recommended with no specific contraindications as to drugs or vasoconstrictors, keeping in mind the mental status of the patient and possible underlying systemic disease. Sedation, in general, is not contraindicated. It is important, however, to remember that the patient is elderly and the metabolism of drugs is affected (see geriatric chapter). *Oral sedation* is the least desirable because of its inherent inability to titrate to a desired clinical effect. *Inhalation sedation* is an excellent route of sedation but requires patient cooperation. *Intravenous sedation*

is a good choice for sedation because of the ability to titrate intravenous drugs. These patients may be exquisitely susceptible to the respiratory depressant effects of medications, so the doctor administering the medication needs to be vigilant. *General anesthesia* is not contraindicated as long as the patient does not have coexisting systemic disease that increases the risk of anesthesia.

REFERENCES

1. Kanar HL: Cerebral palsy and other gross motor or skeletal problems. In Wessels KE, ed: *Dentistry and the handicapped patient*, Littleton, Colo, 1978, PSG Publishing.
2. Poser CM: Exacerbations, activity and progression in multiple sclerosis, *Arch Neurol* 37:471, 1980.
3. Sanger RG, Casamassimo PS: The physically and mentally disabled patient, *Dent Clin North Am* 27:363, 1978.
4. Steifel DJ: Dentistry for persons with mental and physical disabilities. In Levine N, ed: *Current treatment in dental practice*. Philadelphia, 1986, Saunders.
5. Stoelting RK, Dierdorf SF, McCammon RL, eds: *Anesthesia and co-existing diseases*, ed 2. New York, 1988, Churchill Livingstone.
6. Gillberg C, Coleman M, eds: *The biology of autistic syndromes*, ed 2. London, 1992, Mac Keith.
7. Lowe O: Assessment of the autistic patient's dental needs and ability to undergo dental exam, *Assoc J Dent Child* 52:29:1985.
8. Kwentus JA, Hart R, Ligon N et al: Alzheimer's disease, *Am J Med* 81:92, 1986.
9. Neissen LC, Jones JA, Zocchi M et al: Dental care for the patient with Alzheimer's disease, *JADA* 110:207, 1985.
10. Shapiro S, Hamby CL, Shapiro D: Alzheimer's disease: an emerging affliction of the aging population, *JADA* 111:287, 1985.

BIBLIOGRAPHY

Felpel LP: Antiparkinson agents. In Neidle EA, YagielaAJA, eds: *Pharmacology and therapeutics for dentistry,* ed 3. St Louis, 1989, Mosby.

Furukawa T, Peter JB: The muscular dystrophies and related disorders, Part I, *JAMA* 239:1537, 1978.

Furukawa T, Peter JB: The muscular dystrophies and related disorders, Part II, *JAMA* 239:1654, 1978.

Grossman HJ: *Manual on terminology and classification of mental retardation.* Washington, DC, 1973, American Association on Mental Deficiency.

Nowak AJ: *Dentistry for the handicapped patient,* St Louis, 1976, Mosby.

Rose LF, Kaye D: *Internal medicine for dentistry,* St Louis, 1983, Mosby.

St. Franks A: Society and the special patient. In Levine N, ed: *Current treatment in dental practice.* Philadelphia, 1986, Saunders.

Stoelting RK, Dierdorf SF, McCammon RL, eds: *Anesthesia and co-existing diseases,* ed 2. New York, 1988, Churchill Livingston.

Troutman K: Behavioral management of the mentally retarded, *Dent Clin North Am* 21:621, 1977.

Wessels KE: *Dentistry and the handicapped patient.* Littleton, Colo, 1978, PSG Publishing.

APPENDIX

Guidelines for the use of parenteral sedation University of Southern California School of Dentistry

INTRODUCTION

This protocol was developed to provide guidelines for the safe and effective use of parenteral (intramuscular—IM and intravenous—IV) sedation procedures in the clinical environment. They are meant to be guidelines, flexible and dictated by the requirements of the specific clinical situation. Additionally these guidelines will require periodic revision as newer developments arise in the area of parenteral sedation.

PRELIMINARY EVALUATION

Candidates for parenteral sedation must be fully evaluated prior to the procedure as to their physical status and need for sedation.

1. An approved medical history must be completed, dated, and contain all indicated signatures.
2. Parenteral sedation is *not* contraindicated for use in the ASA I and II patient.
3. Parenteral sedation may be employed in *selected* ASA III patients following evaluation and consent from the supervising faculty.

Appropriate written informed consent (or special behavior management consent form) must be obtained from the patient, parent, or guardian of the patient prior to the procedure.

The medical history and planned sedation must be reviewed by the responsible faculty person and students.

Pretreatment instructions will be explained and a written form given to the patient, parent, or guardian of the patient. A sample of these instructions is attached as *Addendum A*.

Prior to each treatment appointment, the medical history data base is updated as necessary. Minimum questioning shall be: "Has there been any change in your medical history, health, or medicines since your last appointment?" All responses, positive and negative, will be noted in a dated, signed treatment note.

Minimum preoperative vital signs consisting of blood pressure and heart rate/rhythm must be measured at each treatment appointment and noted in the records.

It is understood that with some patients being discussed in this protocol it may prove to be impossible to obtain preoperative vital signs. In such cases vital signs will be monitored immediately upon induction of sedation.

MONITORING

All patients receiving parenteral sedation will be monitored by direct observation (e.g., skin, mucous membrane color, respiratory movements). In addition, the following continuous monitoring must be employed:

pulse oximetry *and/or* capnography
and
pretracheal stethoscope
and

(Version 1.1-7/28/91)

618

automatic vital signs monitor [every 5 minutes]
—blood pressure
—heart rate
and the following where indicated:
electrocardioscope
capnograph

If an automatic vital signs monitor is not available, manual monitoring is performed every 5 minutes.

The information obtained must be recorded onto a suitable anesthesia/sedation record at appropriate intervals (q5-15 min).

EMERGENCY DRUGS AND EQUIPMENT

In all parenteral sedation procedures emergency equipment and drugs must be available. The following is included (as a minimum):

Emergency Drugs	Equipment
Epinephrine	Positive-pressure 02
Antihistamine (e.g., diphenydramine)	Face masks (pediatric + adult)
Ephedrine	Laryngoscope
Anticonvulsant (e.g., midazolam)	Endotracheal tubes (p + a)
Corticosteroid (e.g., hydrocortisone)	Lubricant jelly
Vasodilator (e.g., nitroglycerin)	Suction tips
Drug for emergence delirium (physostigmine)	Oropharyngeal airways (p + a)*
Narcotic antagonist (e.g., naloxone)	Defibrillator
Hydralazine (Diazoxide)	Blood pressure cuff (p + a + t)*
Bronchodilator (albuterol—as inhaler)	Stethoscope
(Epinephrine, aminophylline, Isuprel—IV drugs)	Nasopharyngeal airways (p + a)*
	Magill forceps

Emergency equipment must be located either in the operatory or adjacent to the treatment area.

Emergency procedure protocols should be available and monitored periodically.

TECHNIQUE
Preliminary appointment

Evaluation of:
1. Need for parenteral sedation
2. Medical history obtained and reviewed
3. Dental treatment plan, if possible
4. Selection of IV/IM procedure
5. Check for presence of superficial veins (if IV)
6. Obtain baseline vital signs, if possible

---

* *p*, pediatric; *a*, adult; *t*, thigh

7. Preoperative instructions to patient, parent/guardian (*addendum A*)
8. Patient education, as possible
9. Informed consent signed
10. Medical consultation, medically compromised patients at least annually; biannually for all other candidates for parenteral sedation or at discretion of supervising faculty

Day of treatment

The treatment team will consist of the following [minimal] personnel:

IV sedation	*Special patient*	*Pediatric patient*
AMED IV student	AMED IV student	AMED IV student
AMED faculty	AMED faculty	AMED faculty
Dental assistant	Dental student	Pediatric dentistry student
Dental student	DMPH faculty	Pediatric dentistry faculty
	Second dental student or dental assistant	Dental assistant

Oral & Maxillofacial Surgery (OMS)

OMS—resident*, **
SCSOMS program certified oral surgery assistant
OMS faculty

Suggested protocol

1. Review informed consent, physical examination, medical history, and NPO status
2. Prepare drugs and equipment
3. Patient to restroom
4. Patient seated in dental chair (if possible)
   a. IM medications may be necessary in certain patients

---

*Where OMS resident *has completed* an anesthesiology rotation, OMS faculty will be physically present in the operating room at the induction of sedation to baseline (acceptable sedation) levels, and again at discharge of the patient from the clinic.

**Where OMS resident has *not* completed an anesthesiology rotation, either the OMS faculty must be physically present in the operating room for the duration (induction to discharge) of the sedation or a second OMS resident, who has completed anesthesiology training, will be present throughout the procedure as the third member of the team, and is responsible solely for the sedation of the patient.

In addition to the faculty supervisor trained in basic life support (BLS), there must be present at least one other member of the team.

5. Monitoring devices applied [see "Monitoring" section]
6. Preoperative vital signs obtained
7. Intravenous infusion started (if appropriate)
8. Supplemental oxygen or nitrous oxide/oxygen administered
9. Drug(s) are administered IM/IV
10. Administer local anesthesia and commence dental treatment when adequate level of sedation is obtained.
11. Vital signs are monitored every five minutes [q 5 m] throughout treatment and into the recovery period.
12. Vital signs are monitored and recorded at the termination of the dental treatment and the patient evaluated for recovery and discharge from the clinic [see "Discharge" section below].
13. Postoperative dentistry and sedation instructions are explained and a written form given to the patient and the patient's parent or guardian. A sample of these instructions is attached as *addendum C.*
14. Patients will be dismissed from the clinic via wheelchair [wherever possible], in the custody of their parent or guardian, accompanied by an IV sedation student doctor and the treating dental student, and secured in their vehicle.
15. A post-treatment telephone call will be made by the treating dental or IV student that evening to ascertain the patient's post-treatment status and documented in the patients chart.

MAXIMUM SEDATION/ANESTHESIA DRUG DOSAGES

The following are maximum intravenous dosages of the medications discussed in this protocol:

Drug	Maximum mg (IV. pedo. SP)	Maximum mg (OMS)
Diazepam	25	25
Midazolam	12.5 IV	12.5 IV
Midazolam	7.5 IM	7.5 IM
Meperidine	50	200*
Pentobarbital	200	200
Propofol	300	300
Nalbuphine	10	10
Butorphanol	2	2
Fentanyl	100 ug	150 ug*

---

*Administration of fentanyl or meperidine in excess of usual recommended doses requires authorization of, and direct presence in treatment room of, OMS faculty.

Recovery

Following completion of the dental care the patient must be permitted to recover from the sedation until such time as he is considered able to be safely dismissed from the clinic (see section on discharge). During the recovery period the patient will either remain in the treatment chair or be removed to a separate recovery area. In both cases there must be at least one person trained in anesthesia and sedation. Positive-pressure oxygen and a suction apparatus must be available in the recovery area.

Discharge

Patients may be dismissed from the USCSD clinic following parenteral sedation when their postsedation discharge criteria are acceptable to the individuals responsible for recovery. These five categories are movement, respirations, circulation, consciousness, and color. *Addendum "B"* describes these criteria more fully. Post-operative dentistry and post-operative parenteral sedation instructions are explained and a written form given to the patient and to the patient's parent, guardian, or adult escort. A sample of the post-operative parenteral sedation instructions is attached as *addendum "C".*

Patients will be dismissed from the clinic via wheelchair (whenever possible), in the custody of their parent, guardian, or adult escort, and accompanied by an IV sedation doctor and the treating dental student. The latter two will remain with the patient until he is safely in his vehicle.

Post-treatment follow-up

A post-treatment telephone call will be made that evening to determine the patient's status. A note of this will be recorded into the patient's progress notes.

This contact is to be made by the dental student or resident of record. An AMED faculty will be available via telephone for consultation in the event of problems.

The student/resident should maintain a copy of the sedation record for evening review. The student resident should have the AMED or OMS faculty telephone number or air page alert. Faculty should be on air page alert for at least 24 hours after the sedation has been terminated.

Patient's name: *ssn:*   *date:*

Physical Signs	(Pretreatment)	Baseline/Discharge Comments
A. MOVEMENT 2—able to walk (where appropriate) 1—able to move extremities 0—unable to move any extremity		
B. RESPIRATIONS 2—able to breathe deeply & cough 1—limited respiratory effort 0—no spontaneous respiratory effort		
C. CIRCULATION 2—systolic BP +/−20% baseline level 1—systolic BP +/−40% baseline level 0—systolic BP >+/−40% baseline level		
D. CONSCIOUSNESS 2—full alertness seen in ability to answer questions appropriately 1—aroused when called by name 0—unresponsive to verbal stimulation		
E. COLOR 2—normal skin color and appearance 1—any alteration in skin color 0—frank cyanosis or extreme pale		
TOTAL SCORE: Dr's signature:		

Addendum A

PRESEDATION INSTRUCTIONS

1. Arrangements must be made for a responsible adult to drive the patient home after IV/IM sedation. The patient will be unable to leave the clinic if unescorted.

2. The *adult* patient should have nothing to eat or drink for eight (8) hours prior to the procedure. *Pediatric* patients should not have anything to eat for eight (8) hours prior to the procedure and no liquids four (4) hours prior for 0 to 3 years of age, six (6) hours prior for 3 to 6 years of age, and eight (8) hours prior for 7 years and over (or un-less specifically advised otherwise by the attending faculty).

3. The patient is advised to wear loose-fitting garments and a shirt/blouse with short sleeves.

4. The patient should plan to arrive in the office approximately 15 minutes prior to the scheduled appointment.

5. Should the patient develop a cold, flu, sore throat, or any other illness, the appointment should be rescheduled to a time when the patient is more physically fit. The patient, parent, or guardian should call the office if any of these symptoms develop.

6. If there are medication(s) to be taken as part of

the sedation treatment, they will be prescribed and the name of the drug, dosage, and instructions will be given to the patient.

7. The patient should continue to take his/her usual medications as prescribed for other conditions only after consultation with the supervising faculty. Such medications should be taken with minimal water if there is a morning or presedation dose.

8. The date, time, and place of appointment are given to the patient.

Addendum B

PARENTERAL SEDATION DISCHARGE CRITERIA

The following should be completed when considering the discharge of a patient following parenteral sedation. The patient postsedation score must approximately equal his baseline (presedation) score.

Addendum C

POSTSEDATION INSTRUCTIONS

1. Go home and rest for the remainder of the day.
2. Do NOT perform any strenuous activity. You should remain in the company of a responsible adult until you are fully alert.
3. Do not attempt to eat a heavy meal immediately. If you are hungry, a light diet (liquids or soft foods) will be more than adequate.
4. A feeling of nausea may occasionally develop after IV or IM sedation. The following may help you to feel better:
   a. Lying down for a while
   b. A glass of a cola beverage (or 7-Up)
   If nausea persists for more than 4 hours for adults or 1 hour for children, call the dentist who provided the sedation.
5. Do not drive a car or perform any hazardous tasks for the remainder of the day.
6. Do not take any alcoholic beverages or any medications for the remainder of the day unless you have contacted me first.
7. The following medication(s) have been ordered for you by the doctor. Take them only as directed.
8. If you have any unusual problems or any questions you may call:
   1. The dentist who provided your sedation.
   2. If you are unable to contact the dentist who provided the sedation, please call one of the following appropriate Emergency Room numbers:

Adults:
Los Angeles County/U.S.C. Medical Center, (213) 226-2622 or 226-7322

Children:
Children's Hospital of Los Angeles: 213/669-2120
or
Long Beach Miller Memorial Medical Center: 213/595-2133

Index

Page numbers in *italics* indicate illustrations. Page numbers followed by t indicate tables.